Patient Assessment in Pharmacy Practice

PATIENT ASSESSMENT IN PHARMACY PRACTICE

RHONDA M. JONES, Pharm.D.
Associate Professor and Coordinator, Professional Experience Program
Department of Pharmacy Practice
School of Pharmacy and Health Professions
Creighton University
Omaha, Nebraska

RAYLENE M. ROSPOND, Pharm.D., BCPS
Associate Dean and Chair
Department of Pharmacy Practice
College of Pharmacy and Health Sciences
Drake University
Des Moines, Iowa

Editor: David Troy
Managing Editor: Matt Hauber
Marketing Manager: Paul Jarecha
Production Editor: Jennifer Ajello
Designer: Armen Kojoyian
Compositor: Graphic World
Printer:Quebecor World

351 West Camden Street
Baltimore, MD 21201

530 Walnut Street
Philadelphia, PA 19106

Printed in the United States of America

Library of Congress Cataloging-in-Publication Data is available
ISBN: 0-683-30256-6

To purchase additional copies of this book, call our customer service department at **(800) 638-3030** or fax orders to **(301) 824-7390.** International customers should call **(301) 714-2324.**

Visit Lippincott Williams & Wilkins on the Internet: http://www.LWW.com. Lippincott Williams & Wilkins customer service representatives are available from 8:30 am to 6:00 pm, EST.

02 03 04 05 06
1 2 3 4 5 6 7 8 9 10

I dedicate this book to my husband, Mike, and to my children, Monica, Emily, and Adam.

Rhonda M. Jones

I dedicate this book to my husband, Scott, and to my children, Joshua, Heather, Bethany, and Ethan.

Raylene M. Rospond

Preface

Patient Assessment in Pharmacy Practice, a textbook for pharmacy students and practitioners, presents a practical approach to assessing the patient's health-related problems. With the implementation of pharmaceutical care, the pharmacist is responsible for not only delivery of the drug product, but also improving the health outcomes of the patient. An integral part of the pharmaceutical care process involves patient assessment skills.

Unfortunately, most currently available health assessment books, which are intended primarily for medical and nursing students, focus on physical examination skills. While this is a very important piece of patient assessment, it is not the focus of pharmacy practice. The focus of pharmacy practice is gathering patient-specific information, evaluating that information, identifying drug-related problems, and formulating and implementing a pharmaceutical care plan. Physical examination data plays a limited role as compared to the information gathered through the health and medication history. That is why we developed this book. It has been written with one main goal in mind—to provide students and practitioners with a practical text that relates patient assessment skills to pharmacy practice.

ORGANIZATIONAL PHILOSOPHY

Patient Assessment in Pharmacy Practice is divided into two parts. The chapters in Part 1 discuss global issues that are related to assessment. In addition, Part 1 contains chapters that discuss health-related problems that span many body systems (e.g., pain and nutrition). Dependent on the subject matter, some of these chapters are organized similarly to chapters in Part 2.

Part 2 is presented through a body-system, head-to-toe approach, which is the most efficient and logical method for assessing a patient and for student learning. Within each chapter, we use a patient symptom approach, since that is the most common way a patient assessment situation will arise for the pharmacist.

CHAPTER STRUCTURE

Each chapter in Part 2 has four major sections: Anatomy and Physiology Overview, Pathology Overview, System Assessment (i.e., subjective information and objective information), and Application to Patient Symptoms (i.e., case studies).

- **Anatomy and Physiology Overview:** This section provides a basic overview—not extensive—so all readers have the same starting point. Preparatory levels may vary for students and practitioners, so we felt that a basic, similar starting point was needed as a foundation for subsequent patient assessment discussion. For more extensive information on anatomy and physiology, the reader is referred to specialty textbooks in these areas.
- **Pathology Overview:** This section discusses the most common disease states a pharmacist will encounter, as well as the most prevalent disease states for that particular body system. This is not meant to be an all-inclusive discussion of these disease states, but rather a basic overview. Since a large part of patient assessment entails correlating signs and symptoms with possible diseases, we felt that a basic foundational discussion was necessary.
- **System Assessment:**
  - **Subjective Information:** The primary skill that a pharmacist utilizes in nearly all practice settings is communication or, more specifically, patient interviewing to obtain the health and medication history (e.g., symptoms and medication utilization). The interviewing technique (? INTERVIEW) that we utilize is a combination of open-ended questions as a starting point and then closed-ended questions to elicit more specific symptom data concerning the particular symptom. The goal is to provide focused direction to elucidate information relative to the specific disease states/symptoms discussed.
  - **Objective Information:** Physical examination and lab/diagnostic tests are discussed as objective information. The physical examination is covered using a step-by-step approach with each technique (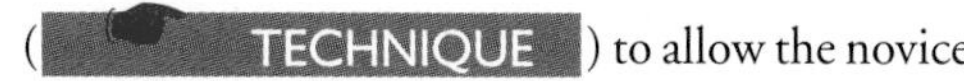) to allow the novice learner to be able to easily follow the appropriate procedures. Normal findings are described with the technique and abnormalities (ABNORMALITIES) and are highlighted as a separate section after each technique. In addition, specific cautions (CAUTION) are highlighted to emphasize particular maneuvers that are sensitive to error or misinterpretation of results
- **Application to Patient Symptoms:** This section is designed as patient cases to illustrate a practice situation in which pharmacists utilize patient assessment skills. We have attempted to vary the practice settings in which these cases occur; however, the majority are in the community environment.

  Each case includes:
  - *Patient-pharmacist* initial interaction.
  - *Interview questions* with patient responses.
  - *Objective assessment information* pertinent to the patient situation.
  - *Discussion* to assist the student in analysis/evaluation of the subjective and objective patient data (i.e., the patient assessment process).
  - *Patient assessment algorithms, or decision trees,* to illustrate the assessment steps that may be used for that particular case. These decision trees provide a logical approach to triaging the patient and determining when a patient may require referral to another health care professional.

- *Pharmaceutical care plan* Documentation is required for all health care professionals. However, pharmacists are relatively new in documenting their patient care interactions. The pharmaceutical care plan provides an example of documentation that should accompany pharmaceutical care activities. We chose the SOAP note approach since it is the most common method of documentation used across all health care professions.
- *Self-assessment and critical thinking questions* to assist the student in learning important information from the chapter. Answers to the self-assessment questions are provided at the end of the book.

PEDAGOGICAL FEATURES

Nearly all chapters include numerous pedagogical features that enhance the book's mission as a practical text that applies patient assessment skills to the pharmacy practice setting.

- **Boxes and Tables:**
  Throughout each chapter, special boxes highlight consistent categories of information from chapter to chapter. These include:
  - Signs and Symptoms: list the most common subjective and objective findings related to the primary disease states discussed in that chapter.
  - Drug-Induced Symptoms: list drugs that may causes signs or symptoms that are discussed in that chapter.
  - Causes of Disease: list common non-drug-related causes of diseases.
  - General boxes: list content material that requires emphasis but does not fit the previous categories.
  - Tables are also utilized throughout the text to highlight important information that may be more challenging for the reader/student to understand in basic text format.
- **Key Terms** (boldface text) for each chapter are listed immediately prior to the Anatomy and Physiology Overview. These terms are defined textually directly following each term as well as in the glossary at the end of the book.

ART

To illustrate the textbook, figures have been chosen that will assist the reader's understanding of the patient assessment process. Specifically, photographs are used in nearly all chapters to illustrate physical examination techniques and abnormal findings. Line drawings are used to illustrate normal anatomy and physiology. In addition, a color-plate insert of abnormal findings is included at the beginning of the book.

SPECIAL INCLUSIONS/EXCLUSIONS

It was a challenge to the authors to decide how to approach the physical examination techniques in this text. As previously stated, this area of pharmacy practice is frequently limited. However, the role of the pharmacist is expanding. Collaborative drug therapy management is on the rise, and thus the role of the pharmacist in pharmaceutical care is growing. In addition, schools and colleges of pharmacy take varied approaches when teaching this material in their curriculum. Therefore, we chose to include physical examination techniques that are commonly used in practice today (e.g., blood pressure measurement), as well as techniques that may be used only in specialty practices today or may provide future practice opportunities (e.g., auscultating breath sounds).

SUMMARY

Patient Assessment in Pharmacy Practice is a textbook that assists the student in applying patient assessment skills to the pharmacy practice setting. It is the result of years of pharmacy practice experience and teaching. Throughout the manuscript preparation and book production, every effort has been made to develop a book that is informative, instructive, and practical. It is our hope that we have accomplished these goals.

Acknowledgments

It is our pleasure to recognize the many wonderful people who helped make this textbook possible. For their encouragement, help, and support, we send our gratitude:

To our friend and colleague, Amy Haddad, RN, PhD, who inspired and encouraged us to write this book. Without her guidance, expertise, and continual encouragement, this book would only be a wish and dream. In addition, many other friends and colleagues were a willing resource of information, constructive comments, and encouragement. We are particularly grateful to Michael Monaghan, Pharm.D., BCPS, and Victoria Roche, PhD, for their support and inspiration.

To all our contributing authors who are listed at the beginning of each chapter we extend our thanks for their professional contribution to the content. To the pharmacy faculty and students who reviewed our draft manuscripts and provided valuable feedback for revision.

To our colleague, Jean DeMartinis, PhD, who provided guidance and expertise with the physical examination photos.

To the tenacious team at Lippincott Williams & Wilkins, who have the skills, expertise, and persistence to mold our manuscript into a professional product. Their patience, assistance, and encouragement made this book possible. Specifically, thank you to David Troy, Acquisitions Editor; Matt Hauber, Senior Managing Editor; and Jenn Ajello, Production Editor. Special thanks also go to Laura Bonnazzoli, the Development Editor throughout this project, and to Donna Balado, former acquisitions editor at LWW who worked with us originally to get the project off the ground.

To our administrative assistants, Margaret Hansen at Creighton University and Mary Jane Murchison at Drake University, who cheerfully assisted us with the editorial process.

To our pharmacy students whose enthusiastic response and energy for learning were an inspiration for this book.

To the many patients with whom we have worked throughout the years—they are the source from which came many of the cases in this book and have always been an inspiration for our passion of pharmacy practice. It is our hope that students will apply the skills and principles of this text to enhance patient care.

Most importantly, we are grateful to our wonderful families. Their love, and steadfast support and encouragement kept us going when discouragement seemed rampant.

Rhonda M. Jones, Pharm.D.
Raylene M. Rospond, Pharm.D.

Contributors

Jeffrey L. Crabtree, MS, OTD, OTR, FAOTA
Associate Professor and Program Director
Occupational Therapy Program
College of Health Sciences
University of Texas at El Paso
El Paso, Texas

Jean E. DeMartinis, PhD, FNPc
Nurse Practitioner, Cardiology
Methodist Health Systems, Physicians Clinic
Omaha, Nebraska

Edward M. DeSimone II, R.Ph., PhD
Professor
Department of Pharmacy Sciences
School of Pharmacy and Health Professions
Creighton University
Omaha, Nebraska

Michele A. Faulkner, Pharm.D.
Assistant Professor
Department of Pharmacy Practice
School of Pharmacy and Health Professions
Creighton University
Omaha, Nebraska

Julie A. Hixson-Wallace, Pharm.D, BCPS
Clinical Associate Professor
Department of Clinical and Administrative Sciences
Mercer University Southern School of Pharmacy
Atlanta, Georgia

Rhonda M. Jones, Pharm.D.
Associate Professor and Coordinator, Professional Experience Program
Department of Pharmacy Practice
School of Pharmacy and Health Professions
Creighton University
Omaha, Nebraska

Wendy Mills, Pharm.D.
Clinical Assistant Professor
Department of Pharmacy Practice
College of Pharmacy
University of Iowa
Iowa City, Iowa

Michael S. Monaghan, Pharm.D., BCPS
Associate Professor and Vice Chair
Department of Pharmacy Practice
School of Pharmacy and Health Professions
Creighton University
Omaha, NE

Paul L. Price, Pharm.D., BCPP
Assistant Professor
Department of Pharmacy Practice
School of Pharmacy and Health Professions
Creighton University
Omaha, Nebraska

Raylene M. Rospond, Pharm.D., BCPS
Associate Dean and Chair
College of Pharmacy and Health Sciences
Drake University
Des Moines, Iowa

Matin A. Royeen, PhD
Dean for Student Services
College of Health Sciences
Roanoke, Virginia

Sarah J. Shoemaker, Pharm.D.
Social and Administrative Pharmacy Graduate Student
College of Pharmacy
University of Minnesota
Minneapolis, MN

Maryann Z. Skrabal, Pharm.D., CDE
Assistant Professor and Coordinator, Professional Experience Program
Department of Pharmacy Practice
School of Pharmacy and Health Professions
Creighton University
Omaha, Nebraska

Karen A. Theesen, Pharm.D. MBA
Board Certified Psychiatric Pharmacist
Senior Regional Medical Scientist
GlaxoSmithKline
Research Triangle Park, North Carolina

Amy Friedman Wilson, Pharm.D.
Assistant Professor
Department of Pharmacy Practice
School of Pharmacy and Health Professions
Creighton University
Omaha, Nebraska

Contents

Part One
Overview of Patient Assessment

Color Plates

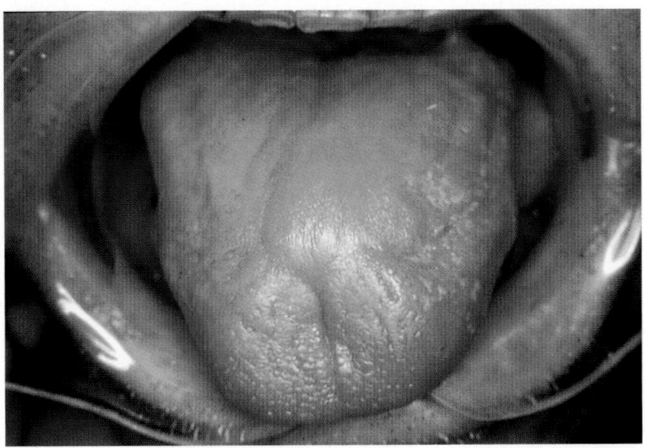

PLATE 1 ■ Atrophic "bald" tongue.

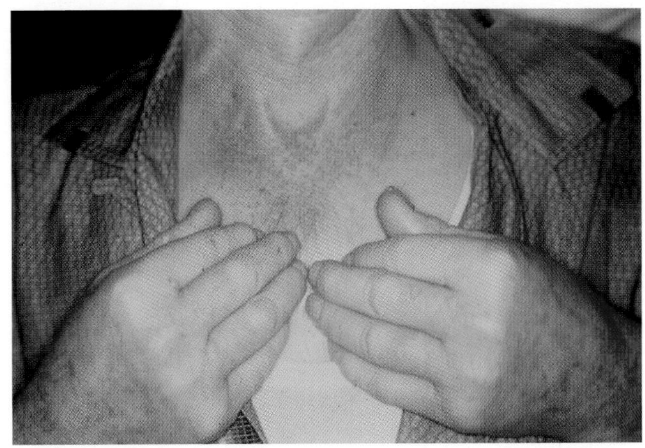

PLATE 2 ■ Pellegra.

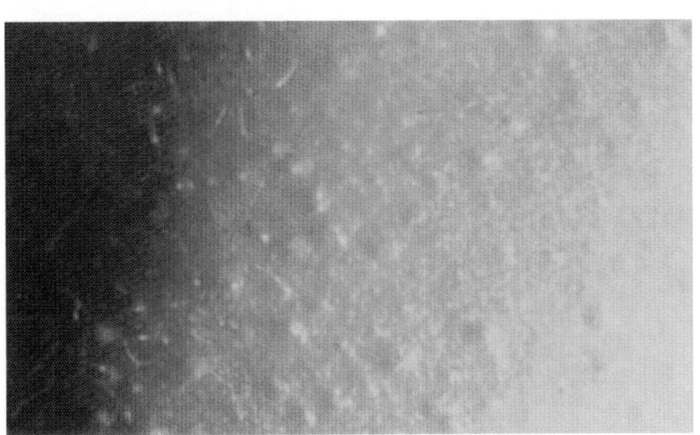

PLATE 3 ■ Follicular hyperkeratosis.

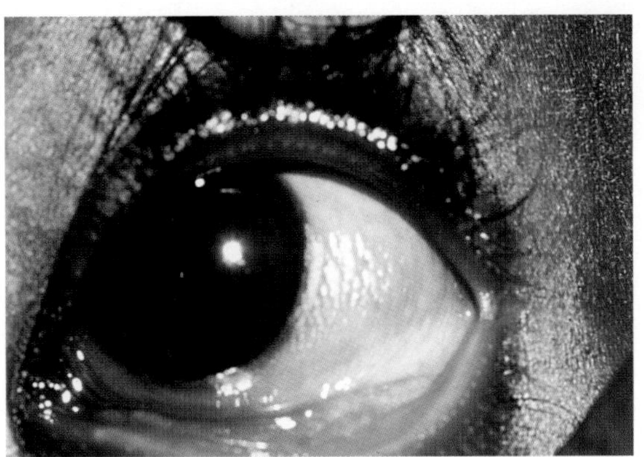

PLATE 4 ■ Bitot's Spots.

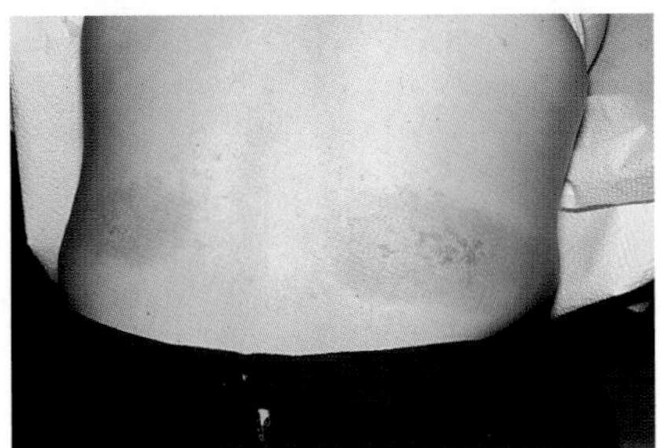

PLATE 5 ■ Contact Dermatitis.

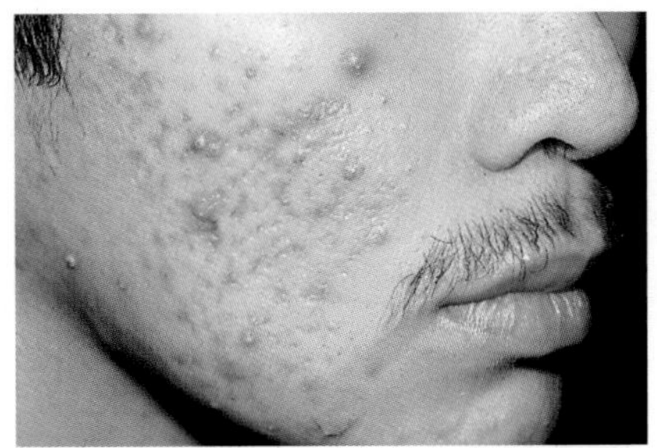

PLATE 6 ■ Acne.

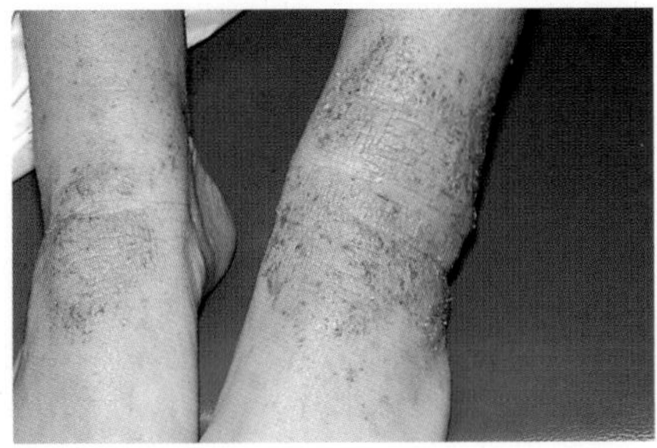

PLATE 7 ■ Atopic Dermatitis. (eczema).

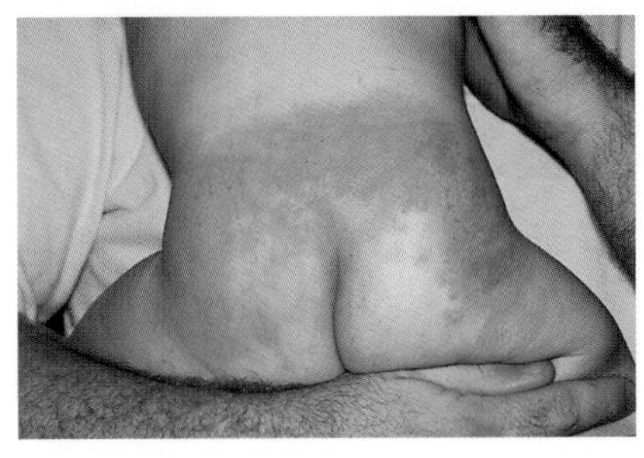

PLATE 8 ■ Diaper Rash.

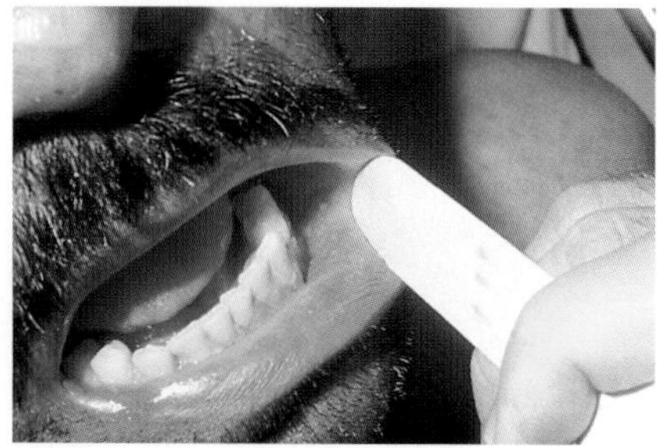

PLATE 9 ■ Koplik's spots with measles.

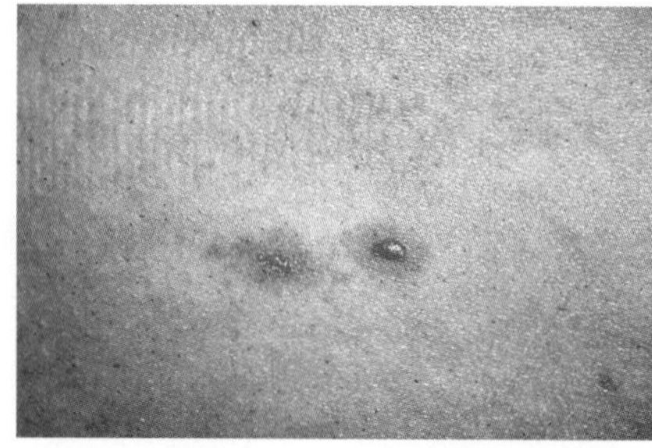

PLATE 10 ■ Varicella (chicken pox).

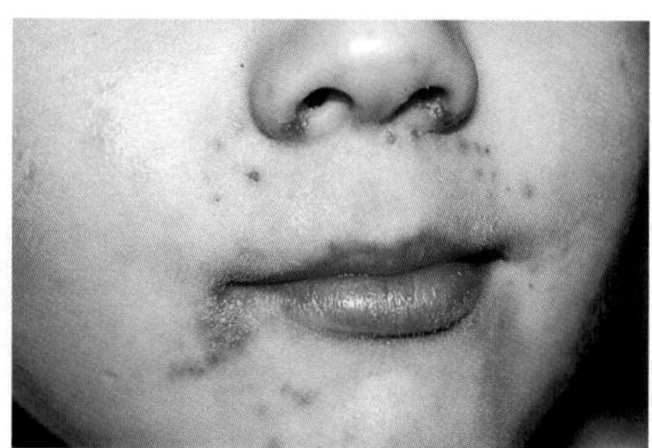

PLATE 11 ■ Impetigo.

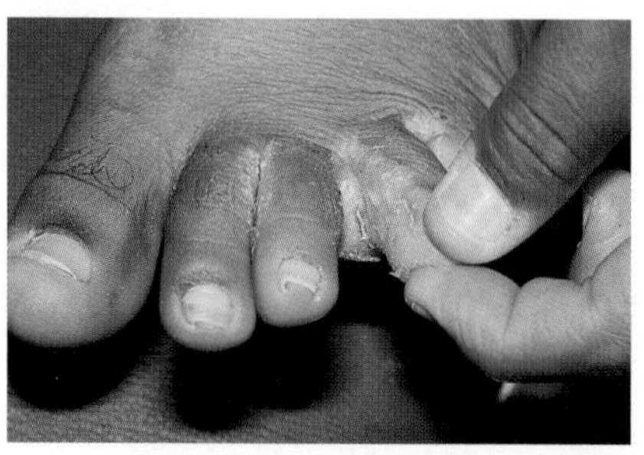

PLATE 12 ■ Tinea pedis (athlete's foot).

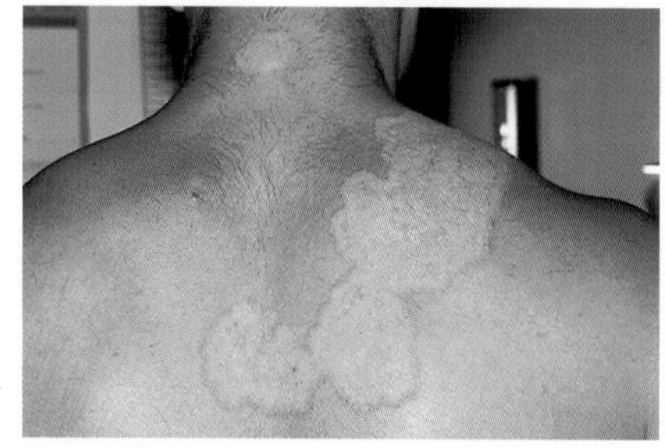

PLATE 13 ■ Tinea corporis (ringworm).

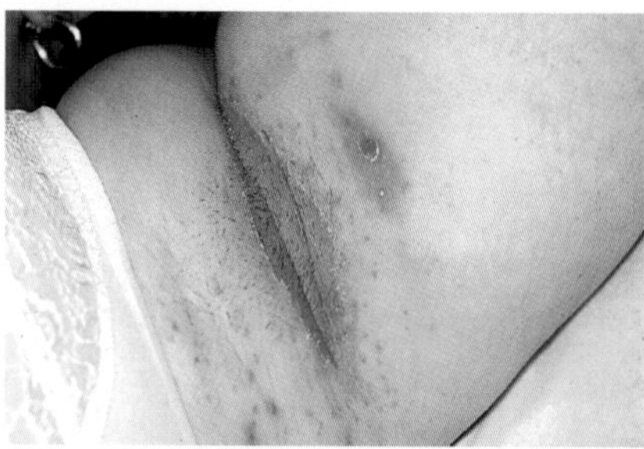

PLATE 14 ■ Candidiasis.

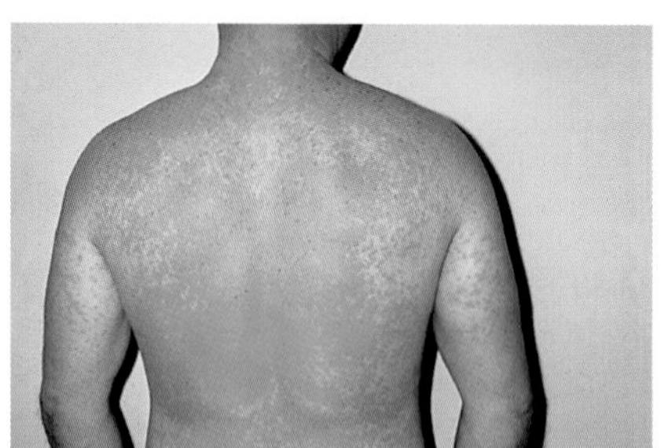

PLATE 15 ■ Drug Reaction.

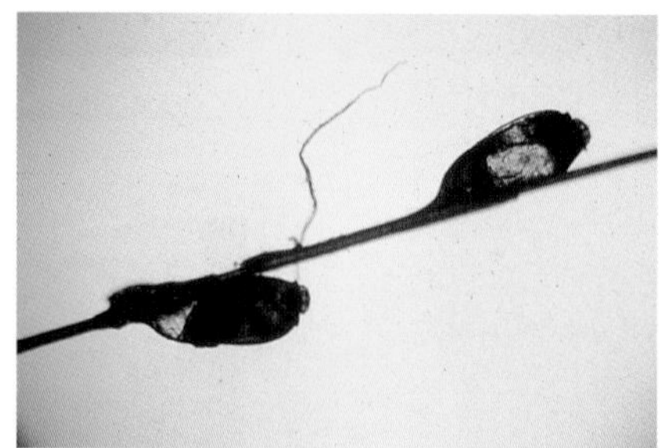

PLATE 16 ■ Pediculosis (lice).

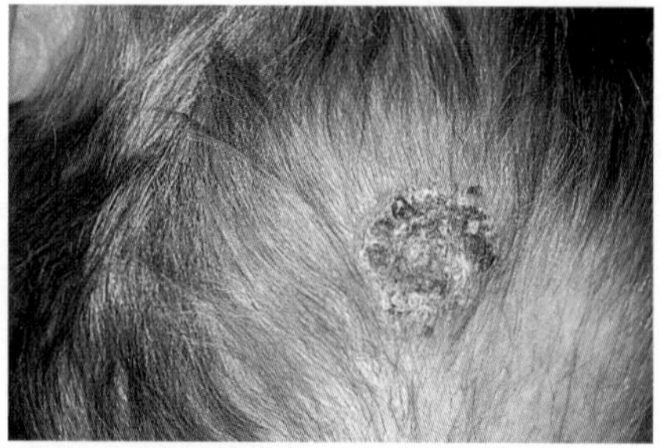

PLATE 17 ■ Basal cell carcinoma.

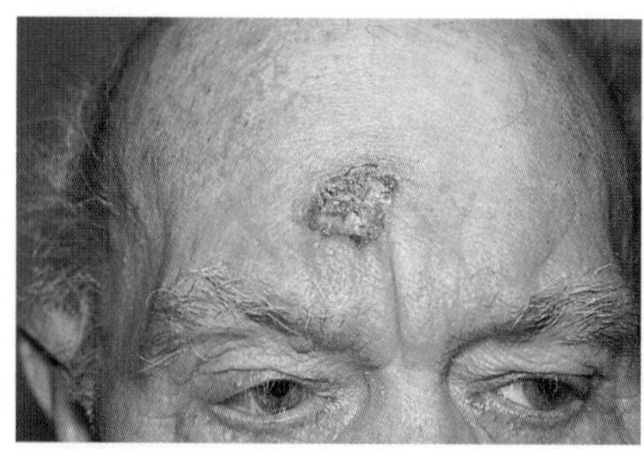

PLATE 18 ■ Squamous cell carcinoma.

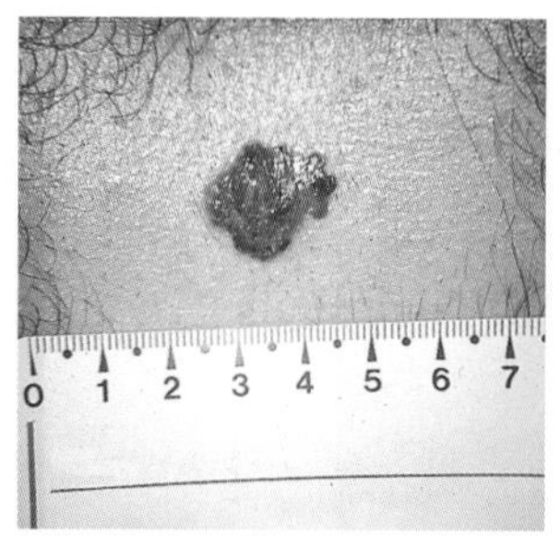

PLATE 19 ■ Melanoma.

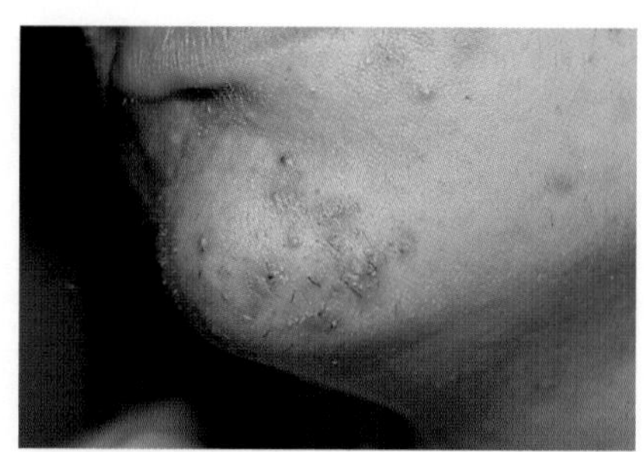

PLATE 20 ■ Folliculitis.

PLATE 21 ■ Onychomycosis.

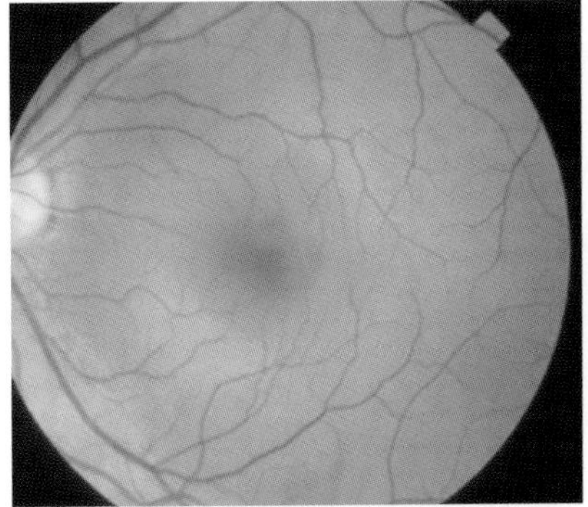

PLATE 22 ■ Fundus of the eye: retina.

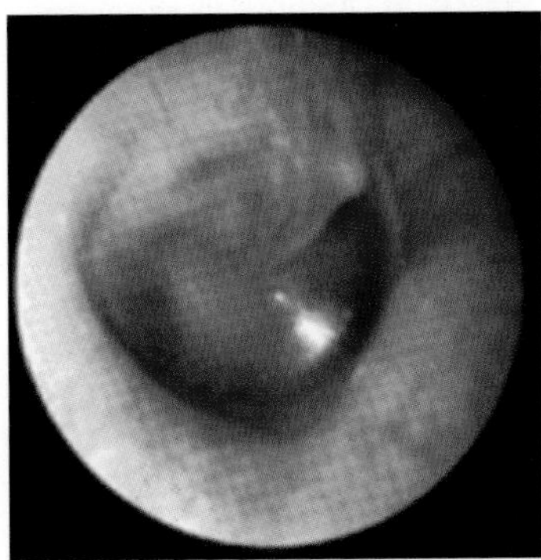

PLATE 23 ■ Otoscopic view of the normal tympanic membrane.

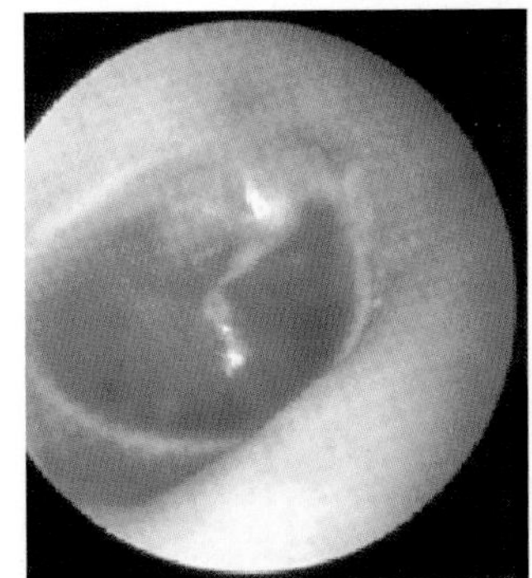

PLATE 24 ■ Acute otitis media.

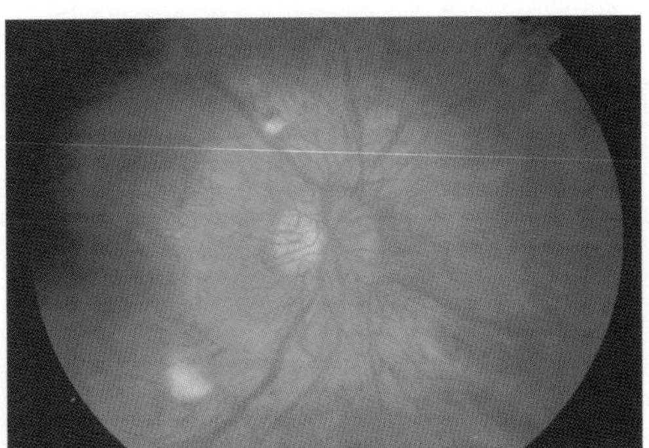

PLATE 25 ■ Diabetic retinopathy.

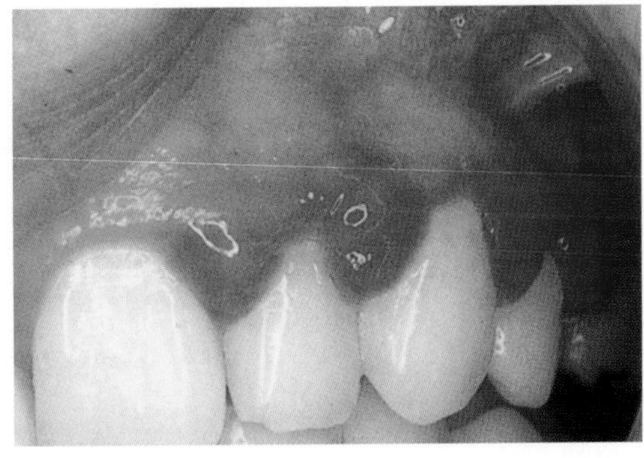

PLATE 26 ■ Gingivitis.

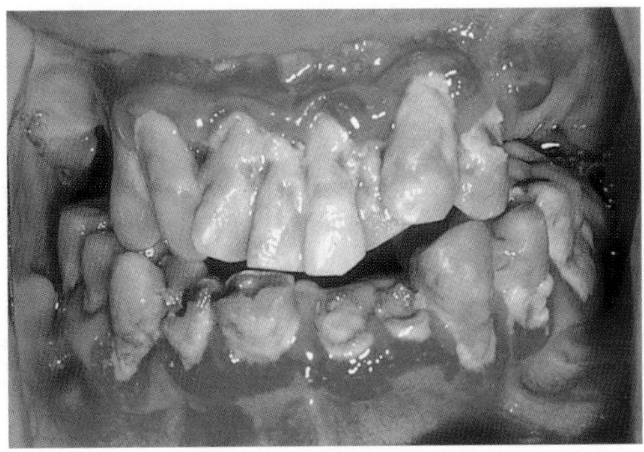

PLATE 27 ■ Periodontitis.

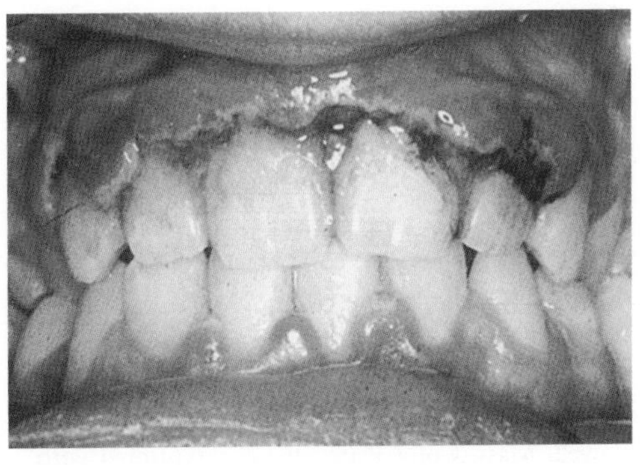

PLATE 28 ■ Acute necrotizing ulcerative gingivitis.

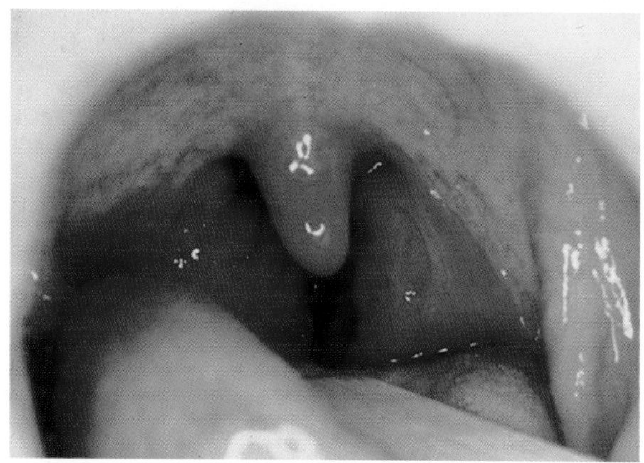

PLATE 29 ■ Severe pharyngitis.

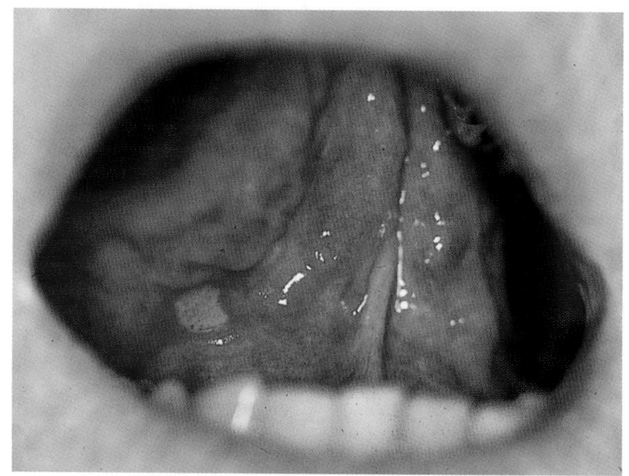

PLATE 30 ■ Apthous ulcer.

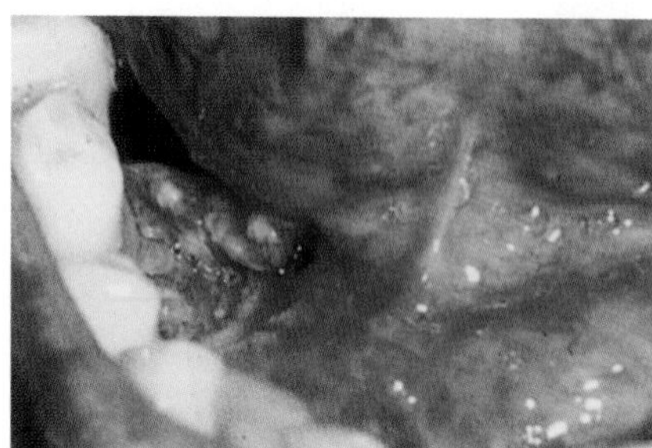

PLATE 31 ■ Carcinoma of the mouth.

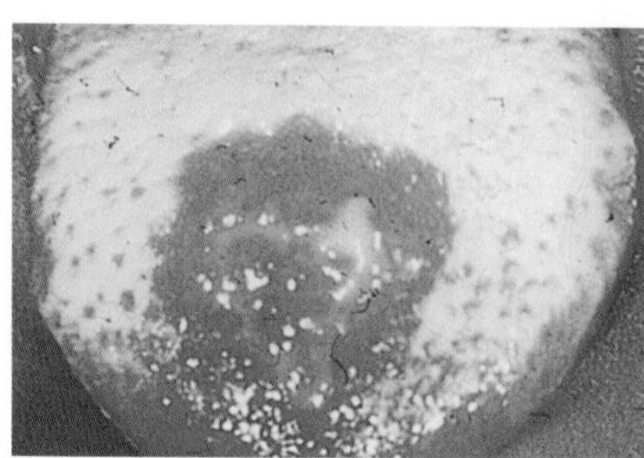

PLATE 32 ■ Candidiasis.

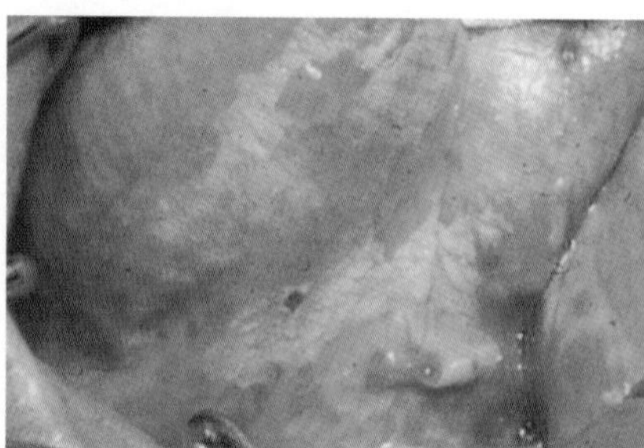

PLATE 33 ■ Leukoplakia.

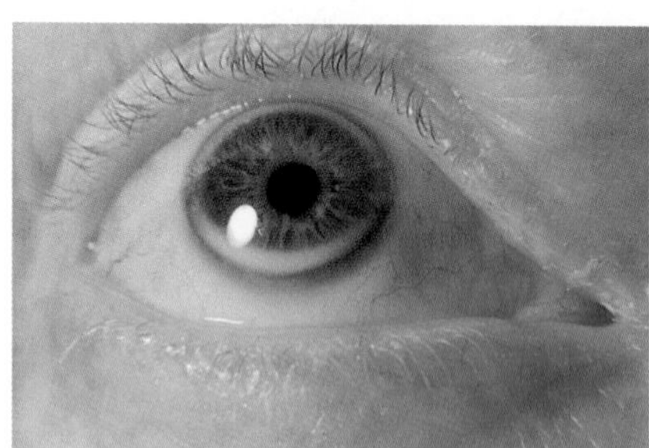

PLATE 34 ■ Corneal arcus.

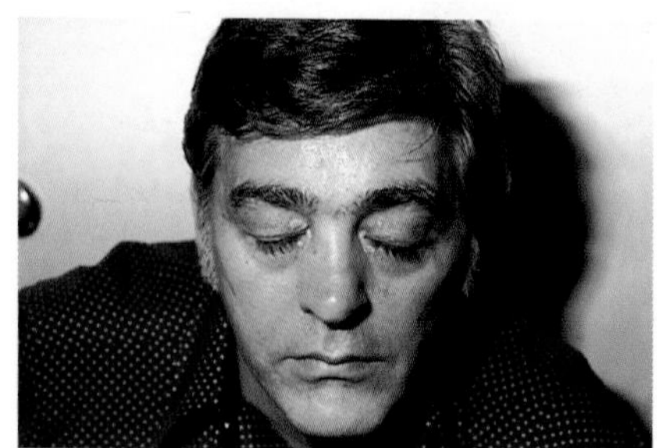

PLATE 35 ■ Xanthelasma.

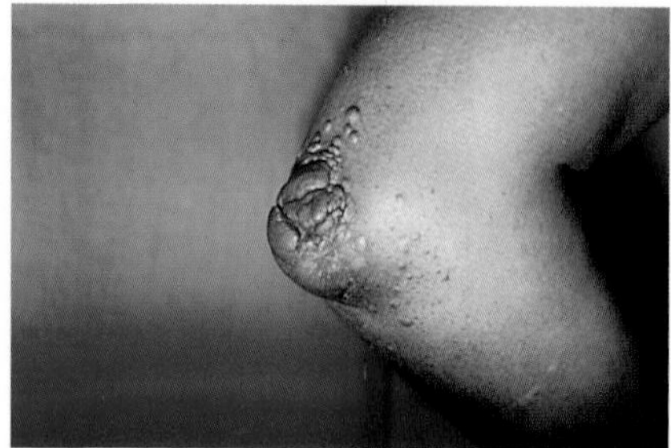

PLATE 36 ■ Xanthomas.

Color Plates 1, 2: Reprinted with permission from Neville BW, et al. Color Atlas of Clinical Pathology. 2nd Ed. Baltimore: Williams & Wilkins, 1999. Color Plate 3: Reprinted with permission from Taylor KB, Anthony LE. Clinical Nutrition. New York, McGraw-Hill, 1983, copyright by Harold H. Sandstead, MD. Color Plate 4: Courtesy of D.E. Silverstone, M.D., New Haven, CT. Color Plates 5-21, 35, 36: Reprinted with permission from Goodheart HP. A Photoguide of Common Skin Disorders: Diagnosis and Management. Philadelphia: Lippincott Williams & Wilkins, 1999. Color Plates 22, 25: National Eye Institute, National Institutes of Health. Color Plates 23, 24: Lowell General Hospital, Lowell, Mass. Color Plates 26, 28: Reprinted with permission from Tyldesley WR. A Colour Atlas of Orofacial Diseases. 2nd Ed. London: Wolfe Medical Publications, 1991. Color Plate 27: Courtesy of Dr. Tom McDavid. Color Plates 29, 30: Reprinted with permission from Bickley LS. Bates Guide to Physical Examination and History Taking. 7th Ed., Philadelphia: Lippincott Williams & Wilkins. Color Plates 31, 33: Reprinted with permission from Robinson HBG, Miller AS: Colby, Kerr, and Robinson's Color Atlas of Oral Pathology. Philadelphia: JB Lippincott, 1990. Color Plate 32: The Wellcome Trust, National Medical Slide Bank, London, UK. Color Plate 34: Reprinted with permission from Tasman, W, et al. The Wills Eye Hospital Atlas of Clinical Ophthalmology. 2nd Ed. Philadelphia: Lippincott Williams & Wilkins, 2001.

PART *One*

OVERVIEW OF PATIENT ASSESSMENT

CHAPTER

1

Patient Assessment and the Pharmaceutical Care Process

Rhonda M. Jones

GLOSSARY TERMS

- Drug therapy problem
- Patient assessment
- Pharmaceutical care

JB is a 74-year-old man who comes to the pharmacy for a refill of his antihypertensive medication, atenolol. As he approaches the pharmacy counter, he loses his balance slightly, but he catches himself on the counter. The pharmacist asks, "Are you okay, Joe?" The patient answers, "Oh, yes, I'm fine. I just stumbled a little. I do that quite often these days. I need a refill of my blood pressure medicine." The pharmacist pulls up Joe's drug therapy profile on the computer screen and asks, "What's the name of the medication?" The patient answers, "I need my atenolol."

In the real-life example of an interaction between a patient and a pharmacist cited above, there exists an opportunity for the pharmacist to gather patient information (both subjective and objective), to assess the data, and possibly, to identify, resolve, and even prevent a drug-related problem (or problems). In other words, the pharmacist has the opportunity to put into practice the philosophy of pharmaceutical care.

Pharmaceutical care is defined by Hepler and Strand as the "responsible provision of drug therapy for the purpose of achieving definite outcomes that improve a patient's quality of life. These outcomes are (1) cure of a disease, (2) elimination or reduction of a patient's symptomatology, (3) arresting or slowing of a disease process, or (4) preventing a disease or symptomatology." The central component of pharmaceutical care is caring about the patient. If the pharmacist cares about the patient, then that pharmacist will incorporate the pharmaceutical care process into his or her practice of pharmacy, regardless of the practice setting (e.g., community, acute care/hospital, ambulatory care, home care, nursing home, etc.).

HISTORY AND EVOLUTION OF PHARMACEUTICAL CARE

During the past 100 years, significant growth and development have occurred in the field of pharmacy. These changes have occurred primarily in four major stages.

During the first stage, from the late 1850s to early 1900s, the classic form of the corner drugstore began to emerge. The major influence during this stage was the entrance of large-scale drug manufacturing. Because drugs began to be manufactured/compounded outside of the actual pharmacy, the work of the pharmacist was simplified into procuring, preparing, evaluating, and selling drug products. The pharmacist was responsible for delivering pure and unadulterated medications and for providing good advice to the customers. In addition, many drugstores were remodeled to move the prescription area to the back of the store, which allowed the front to be opened up for the sale of tobacco, specialty items, and most importantly, soda fountain items. Inclusion of the soda fountain revolutionized the public's view of the "corner drugstore" as an American way of life during the early 1900s. As the pharmacy industry continued to grow, more and more medications were sold as prefabricated drug products rather than as medications that the pharmacist needed to compound. At the same time, the prescription of drugs by physicians was on the rise. Both these factors (i.e., increasing manufacturing and physician prescriptions) began to narrowly constrain the pharmacist's role within the emerging health care system.

During the second stage, from the early 1900s to the mid-1960s, attention focused primarily on educational reform as the method to advance the profession. The leaders in pharmacy education were demanding more rigorous and consistent education for pharmacists, however, many changes were occurring within the practice of pharmacy itself. Several new, very effective medications came on the market during the 1950s, which increased the number of prescriptions being filled by 50%. At the same time, a prescription-only legal status for most drugs was established in 1951. In addition, the American Pharmaceutical Association (APhA) Code of Ethics from 1922 to 1969 prohibited pharmacists from discussing the therapeutic effects or the composition of a prescription with a patient. All these factors greatly influenced the decline of the pharmacist's responsibilities to that of "count, pour, lick, and stick," thus restricting pharmacists to machine-like tasks. In short, pharmacists were considered to be overeducated for a diminishing professional function.

During the third stage, from the late 1960s to 1980s, the pharmacist's role was in transition. The functions of the role expanded rapidly, increasing professional diversity. The pharmacist was beginning to provide new "clinical" services, such as pharmacokinetics, drug information, and drug-use control, primarily in the institutional setting. In 1969, the APhA Code of Ethics was revised to encourage pharmacists to consider the patient's health and safety first as they dispensed medications, fully utilizing all their abilities and training as health care practitioners.

This revision to the APhA Code of Ethics allowed pharmacists to talk with patients about their medications, but the pharmacist's role still focused primarily on drugs and their delivery. An element was still missing: the pharmacist's acceptance of responsibility for the patient's health and welfare, which was greatly needed. Thus, during the 1990s, the fourth stage—the patient care stage—emerged, along with the concept of "pharmaceutical care." During this new era, pharmacists share responsibility for patient health outcomes, which, in turn, improves the patient's quality of life.

PHARMACEUTICAL CARE

The philosophy of pharmaceutical care is centered on four primary elements: (1) a societal need for pharmacists to address drug-related problems, (2) a patient-centered approach to meet this need, (3) a practice based on "caring" about and for patients, and (4) a responsibility for finding and responding to the patient's drug therapy problems. Drug-related problems within society cause a significant amount of morbidity and mortality. It has been estimated that drug-related morbidity in the United States costs several billion dollars annually. Based on the pharmaceutical care philosophy, pharmacists, as well as other health care professionals, are responsible for meeting society's need for appropriate, effective, and safe drug therapy. To do so, pharmacists must focus their practice on the patient as a whole individual, as one who has general health care needs as well as specific drug-related needs. The pharmacist who practices pharmaceutical care will respond to all the patient's health and medication needs while developing and continuing a therapeutic relationship with the patient. This type of relationship requires pharmacists to instill within themselves an ethic of caring about and for the patient, which translates into a demonstration of concern for his or her well-being. Caring behavior primarily involves mutual respect, trust, honesty, integrity, empathy, and sensitivity. In addition to these general characteristics, caring within the pharmaceutical care philosophy requires the pharmacist to put the patient first, to be responsible for ensuring that the patient's medications are as effective and safe as possible, and to ensure that the patient understands how to appropriately take his or her medications.

In addition to these general responsibilities, the pharmacist also has three primary responsibilities within the practice of pharmaceutical care: (1) to ensure that the patient's drug therapy is appropriately indicated, the most effective available, the safest possible, the most convenient to take, and the most economical; (2) to identify, resolve, and prevent any drug therapy problems; and (3) to ensure that the patient's therapeutic goals are met and that optimal health-related outcomes are attained. These responsibilities focus on addressing the patient's drug therapy problems.

A **drug therapy problem** is any undesirable event experienced by the patient that involves drug therapy and that actually (or potentially) interferes with a desired patient outcome. Common drug therapy problems and their causes are listed in Table 1-1, which groups drug therapy problems into seven major categories. For the pharmacist to resolve identified drug therapy problems and to prevent future problems, he or she must understand the causes of these problems. Those listed in Table 1-1 are not all-inclusive, but they do focus on the most common causes of the various drug-related problems.

To fulfill these responsibilities as well as the goals of therapy (i.e., appropriate, effective, safe, convenient, and economical drug therapy), the pharmacist must use a consistent, systematic, and comprehensive process. The pharmaceutical care process, as illustrated in Figure 1-1, starts with initiating a relationship with the patient. This relationship can begin with the patient bringing a new prescription to the pharmacy or asking a question about a nonprescription product. During the next step, the pharmacist gathers all the pertinent information to evaluate the patient's health and drug therapy appropriately. The specific actions involved with this step will vary according to the patient's health problems, drug therapy, and any corresponding drug therapy problems. The information that is obtained may be both subjective (e.g., patient complaints or symptoms) and objective (e.g., medication profile, vital signs, or other physical assessment data). Ways in which this information can be obtained include reviewing the prescription, drug therapy profile, or other pharmacy records; talking with the patient as well as with his or her caregiver, physician, or other health care professional;

TABLE 1-1 ➤ COMMON DRUG THERAPY PROBLEMS AND THEIR CAUSES

DRUG THERAPY PROBLEMS	POSSIBLE CAUSES
Unnecessary drug therapy	No indication Duplicate therapy
Wrong drug	Contraindications present Drug not indicated for condition More effective medication available Drug interaction Indication refractory to drug Inappropriate dosage form
Dose too low	Wrong dose Inappropriate frequency Inappropriate duration Incorrect storage Incorrect administration Drug interaction
Dose too high	Wrong dose Inappropriate frequency Inappropriate duration Incorrect administration Drug interaction
Adverse drug reaction	Undesirable drug side effect Allergic reaction Drug interaction Incorrect administration Dose changed too quickly Unsafe drug for the patient
Noncompliance	Cannot afford drug Does not understand instructions on how to take the drug Cannot swallow/administer the drug Prefers not to take the drug Drug not available
Additional drug therapy	Untreated condition Prophylactic therapy Synergistic therapy

Adapted from Cipolle RJ, Strand LM, Morley PC. Drug therapy problems. In: Pharmaceutical care practice. New York:. McGraw-Hill, 1998: 82–83. Tomochko MA, Strand LM, Morley PC, et al. Q and A from the pharmaceutical care project in Minnesota. Am Pharm 1995; NS35(4): 30–39.

reviewing the patient's medical record, if available; and obtaining physical assessment data (e.g., measuring vital signs).

Once all the pertinent information has been obtained, the pharmacist assesses that information, and looks for drug therapy problems (Table 1-1). The drug therapy problems are then prioritized, along with corresponding goals and goal criteria (i.e., patient outcomes), and they are documented in the pharmaceutical care plan (PCP). Integral to the PCP are the solutions to these problems, which are commonly known as interventions. *Interventions* are the actions that you need to make to resolve identified drug therapy problems or to prevent potential problems in the future. These may include (but are not limited to) educating and counseling the patient about drug therapy or health-related issues, contacting another health care professional to obtain more patient information or to make recommendations about drug therapy, recommending new or alternate (drug and nondrug) therapy, and referring the patient to another health care professional. The choice varies according to the patient's needs and the drug therapy problems that are identified.

Another part of the PCP is the monitoring plan, which outlines factors that will determine attainment of the desired patient outcomes (e.g., blood pressure measurement, laboratory data, or talking with the patient). In selecting the most appropriate intervention and monitoring plan, the pharmacist should also actively consider the patient's needs and desires and incorporate these into development of the plan. Ideally, the patient should be involved throughout the entire pharmaceutical care process.

The final step of the PCP, which is frequently overlooked, is follow-up, which includes implementing the monitoring plan. For example, the pharmacist may contact the patient to evaluate drug therapy compliance or drug side effects. Other follow-up actions may include measuring vital signs or checking other physical or laboratory data. (Note that after the plan has been implemented, the pharmaceutical care process recycles once again. The pharmacist may need to gather more data, assess the patient's progress, and adjust the plan appropriately.)

In summary, the pharmaceutical care process allows the pharmacist to interact with the patient and other health care professionals to develop, implement, and monitor a care plan that will identify, resolve, and prevent drug therapy problems as well as attain specific therapeutic outcomes for the patient.

PHARMACEUTICAL CARE AND PATIENT ASSESSMENT

A key component of the pharmaceutical care process just described is *assessment* of the patient's health and drug-related information. For pharmacists to successfully incorporate pharma-

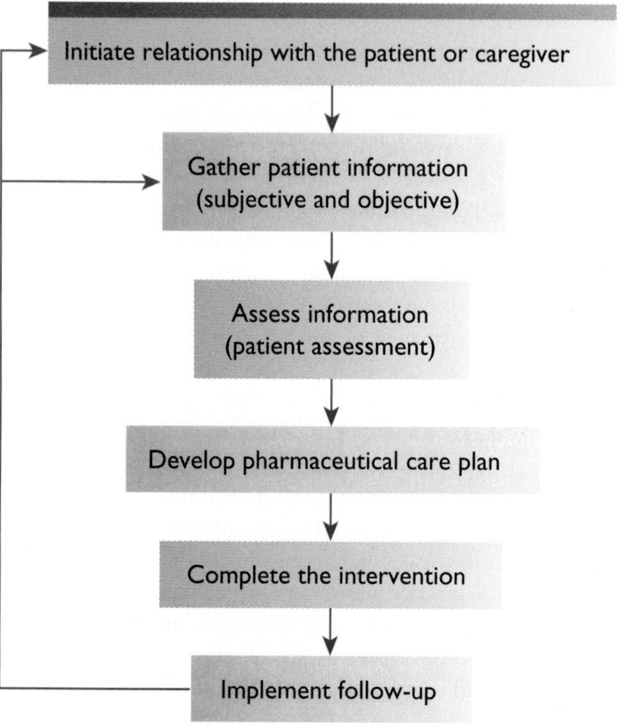

FIGURE 1-1 ■ Pharmaceutical care process.

ceutical care into their practice, they must have knowledge and skills in *patient assessment.* **Patient assessment** is defined as the process through which the pharmacist evaluates patient information (both subjective and objective) that was gathered from the patient and other sources (e.g., drug therapy profile, medical record, etc.) and makes decisions regarding: (1) the health status of the patient; (2) drug therapy needs and problems; (3) interventions that will resolve identified drug problems and prevent future problems; and (4) follow-up to ensure that patient outcomes are being met. The primary purpose of patient assessment is to identify, resolve, and prevent drug therapy problems. Because the responsibilities of pharmaceutical care and patient assessment are so intertwined, a pharmacist cannot adequately provide pharmaceutical care without assessing patients.

For a consistent and comprehensive patient assessment, you should ask yourself a series of questions (Table 1-2) that will guide you through the assessment process. For experienced pharmacists, these questions typically are answered simultaneously while gathering patient information during the health and medication history and physical assessment (for a detailed discussion concerning the health and medication history, see Chapter 3). Physical assessment of the patient is a new and growing skill for pharmacists. Examples of physical assessment techniques that are being applied within pharmacy practice include inspection of skin abnormalities, obtainment of vital signs, peak flow readings, blood glucose levels, and cholesterol values. Whether physical assessment is performed by a pharmacist or another health care professional, pharmacists must have an understanding of the physical assessment process and the corresponding data obtained if they are to provide adequate pharmaceutical care to patients.

TABLE 1-2 ➤ PATIENT ASSESSMENT QUESTIONS

- Are any of the patient's complaints/symptoms or abnormal objective/physical findings due to drug therapy?
  - Consider possible adverse effects of drug therapy.
- What are the other possible causes of the patient's complaints/symptoms or abnormal objective/physical findings?
  - Consider other medical conditions.
- Are each of the medications appropriately indicated?
  - Appropriate medical condition for each drug?
- Are each of the medications the most efficacious and the safest possible?
  - For the medical condition?
  - For the patient? (Consider age, gender, renal and liver function, other medical conditions, and adverse effects.)
- Is the dose the most effective and the safest possible?
  - Correct dose? (Consider age, renal and liver function, weight, and other medical conditions.)
- Is the patient experiencing any adverse effects from the drug therapy?
  - If yes, can any of the adverse effects be resolved?
- Are there any drug interactions that will impair efficacy or safety?
  - Consider prescription and nonprescription drugs.
  - Are there any drug–food or drug–laboratory test interactions?
- Is the patient able to follow the drug regimen?
  - Does the patient understand how to appropriately take the medications?
  - Can the patient afford the drug therapy?
- Does the patient need additional drug therapy for an untreated indication? Synergism with current therapy? Prophylaxis?

Based on information in Tomechko MA, Strand LM, Morley PC, et al. Q and A from the pharmaceutical care project in Minnesota. Am Pharm 1995;NS35(4):30–39.

DOCUMENTATION

Documenting a patient care encounter is a critical step in the pharmaceutical care process, because it creates a valuable communication tool for future encounters with that patient and with other health care professionals. Other reasons why documentation is so valuable to the pharmaceutical care process are listed in Table 1-3. Currently, several different methods are used to document patient care and PCPs, and various printed forms and computer software are available to assist the pharmacist with this process. Good documentation is more than just filling out a form, however; it should facilitate good patient care. Characteristics of useful patient records include:

- Information that is neat, organized, and able to be found quickly.
- Information that is easily understandable, so that any health care professional can determine what the problems were, what actions were taken, and what follow-up is needed.
- Accurate subjective and objective information.
- An assessment of the patient information, focusing on drug therapy problems.
- A plan to resolve any problems that were identified.
- A plan for future follow-up to ensure that any problems are resolved and that patient outcomes are met.

SOAP Note

The most common—and universally recognized—format for documenting patient information in the health care system is the SOAP note, which is an acronym that stands for *S*ubjective, *O*bjective, *A*ssessment, and *P*lan. Each term reflects a section of the note that contains a specific type of information.

TABLE 1-3 ➤ VALUE OF DOCUMENTATION

- Provides a permanent record of patient information.
- Provides a permanent record and evidence of pharmaceutical care activities by the pharmacist.
- Communicates essential information to other pharmacists and health care professionals.
- Serves as a legal record of patient care that was provided.
- Provides back-up for billing purposes.

Based on information in Rovers JP, et al. Documentation. In: A practical guide to pharmaceutical care. Washington DC: American Pharmaceutical Association, 1998: 103–118.

The subjective section includes information that is given by the patient, family members, significant others, or caregivers. The type of information in this section includes:

- Complaints/symptoms from the patient in his or her own words (chief complaint).
- Recent history that pertains to those symptoms (history of present illness).
- Past medical history.
- Medication history, including compliance and adverse effects.
- Allergies.
- Social and/or family history.
- Review of systems.

The objective section includes data that are obtained from the patient and that can be measured objectively. Common information in this section includes:

- Vital signs.
- Physical findings or physical examination (if possible).
- Laboratory test results (if available).
- Serum drug concentrations (if available).
- Various diagnostic test results (if available).
- Computerized medication profile with refill information (if available).

Because other health care professionals also commonly generate certain objective data (e.g., physical examination data generated by physicians or physician assistants, or laboratory test data generated in a clinic or an institutional setting), it is helpful if the date is included with the specific data that are documented.

The assessment section of the SOAP note involves critical thinking and analysis by the pharmacist. The pharmacist analyzes the subjective and objective information and determines the health status of the patient, if the patient is experiencing any drug-related problems, and if the patient's health outcomes are being met. If a problem is identified for the first time, adding a notation of "newly identified" after the problem (e.g., "Hypertension—newly identified.") is helpful. Likewise, for a follow-up assessment or re-evaluation of a problem, adding "resolved," "worsened," or "stable" (e.g., "Gastritis caused by glucophage therapy—resolved.") is also helpful. In addition, the assessment section provides the basis or rationale for the plan section.

The plan section involves actions that were—or need to be—taken to resolve any problems that have been identified. Include sufficient detail, but without being too lengthy, so that future pharmacists or other health care professionals can easily understand what took place during the patient encounter and what follow-up actions are necessary. Thus, a critical component of the plan is follow-up to ensure that problems are actually corrected and that future problems do not develop. The follow-up should include monitoring parameters that need to be assessed as well as the interval for the next assessments (e.g., "Check blood pressure—2 weeks."). It is also helpful to include guidelines concerning what should be done with the data at the time of the follow-up (e.g., "Check blood pressure in 2 weeks. If <140/90 mm Hg and no side effects, continue current medications. If 140–160/90–100 mm Hg, recheck blood pressure in 2 weeks. If >160/100 mm Hg, increase lisinopril to 40 mg QID. If having side effects [cough, light-headedness, dizziness], may need to change to doxazosin, 2 mg QHS."). This information expedites the follow-up process, especially if a different pharmacist sees the patient at this time. A general rule of thumb is that a colleague should be able to read, interpret, and act on the plan if the pharmacist who documented the note is not available.

Problem-Oriented Note

In the problem-oriented note, a patient's active problems are listed, and a SOAP note is written for each problem or closely related group of problems. The problems may be regarding the patient's disease states or may be drug therapy problems. If the patient assessment does not reveal any drug therapy problems, then the note should be so titled (e.g., "No drug therapy problems identified."), and sufficient data that led to this conclusion should be included in the SOAP note. Because both the SOAP note (with all the problems documented in one note) and the problem-oriented note are commonly used, either format is acceptable. The same format, however, should be used consistently from pharmacist-to-pharmacist at a particular practice site. Throughout this book, the SOAP note format is used to document the PCP when illustrating patient case scenarios.

OPPORTUNITIES FOR PATIENT ASSESSMENT

As described previously, patient assessment is an integral part of the pharmaceutical care process, and pharmacists have several opportunities to incorporate patient assessment skills into their practice. The most common settings are directly involved, in some manner, with patient care. These include hospitals, long-term care facilities, ambulatory/outpatient clinics, and community pharmacies. In the hospital setting, pharmacists routinely evaluate patient charts and drug therapy regimens, counsel patients about their medications on discharge from the hospital, and provide specialty clinical services, such as pharmacokinetics, drug and nutrition information, pediatrics, critical care, and cardiology. Long-term care facilities offer unique patient assessment opportunities, because a pharmacist's review and evaluation of each patient's medical record and drug therapy on a monthly basis is mandated by the U.S. federal government. In ambulatory/outpatient clinics, pharmacists counsel and educate the patient about medications as well as evaluate the patient's medical record and drug therapy regimens. Typical areas of focus for patient assessment activities include anticoagulation, diabetes, hypertension, and lipid clinics. Ambulatory clinics are the most common setting in which pharmacists perform physical examination activities with patients (e.g., blood pressure measurement).

Because community pharmacies are typically associated with the drug product rather than with patient care, they are sometimes overlooked as a setting for pharmaceutical care or patient assessment activities; however, the converse is actually true. The community pharmacy provides abundant opportunities for

CASE STUDY

JB is a 74-year-old man who comes to the pharmacy for a refill of his antihypertensive medication, atenolol. As he approaches the pharmacy counter, he loses his balance slightly, but he catches himself on the counter. The pharmacist asks, "Are you okay, Joe?" The patient answers, "Oh, yes, I'm fine. I just stumbled a little. I do that quite often these days. I need a refill of my blood pressure medicine." The pharmacist pulls up Joe's drug therapy profile on the computer screen and asks, "What's the name of the medication?" The patient answers, "I need my atenolol."

ASSESSMENT OF THE PATIENT

Pharmacist: So how long have you been having problems with your balance?
Joe: Oh, it's not a problem. I've just been a little light-headed the past couple of weeks. I guess it's just old age.
Pharmacist: How is your energy level?
Joe: I don't do a whole lot anymore, so I guess I don't need much energy at my age.
Pharmacist: How have you been feeling otherwise? Have you been having any other problems?
Joe: No, otherwise I feel okay.
Pharmacist: I notice in your profile that you just started taking the atenolol 2 weeks ago. How have you been taking it?
Joe: I take it with breakfast and supper. Just like my other blood pressure medicine.
Pharmacist: Actually, you should be taking it just once a day. Why don't you have a seat over here and let me check your blood pressure and heart rate. They could be too low from the atenolol, and that could be causing your light-headedness and low energy.

Joe's heart rate is 48 bpm, and his blood pressure is 114/72 and 112/70 mm Hg.

Pharmacist: Your heart rate and blood pressure are lower than they should be. I think this is probably due to taking the atenolol twice a day rather than once a day, and this is probably causing the light-headedness and decreased energy. I'll go ahead and get the refill for you, but make sure that you take it just once a day.
Joe: Okay. I guess I never paid any attention to it. I just figured it was the same as the other medicine I'm taking. From now on, I'll take it with my breakfast every morning.
Pharmacist: That would be fine. I also want you to come back in a week so that I can recheck your blood pressure and heart rate and see if you're feeling better.
Joe: That sounds like a good idea to me. Thanks for taking the time to check into this.

PHARMACEUTICAL CARE PLAN

Patient Name: JB

Date: 9/8/02

Medical Problems:
Hypertension

Current Medications:
Atenolol, 25 mg, one tablet once daily
Captopril, 12.5 mg, one tablet twice a day

S: Comes in for atenolol refill. C/O occasional light-headedness, decreased energy level, and loss of balance over the past 2 weeks. No other C/O. Currently taking the atenolol twice a day for the past 2 weeks

O: Saw patient lose his balance on way to the pharmacy counter.

Heart rate: 48 bpm

Blood pressure: 114/72, 112/70 mm Hg

A: Bradycardia and hypotension—new onset—probably due to noncompliance with the atenolol.

P:
1. Instructed patient to take the atenolol once a day with breakfast and captopril twice a day as he has been doing.
2. Follow up in 1 week to recheck heart rate and blood pressure. If still low, call the physician and see about possibly D/Cing the atenolol.

Pharmacist: *Rachel Smith, Pharm.D.*

patient assessment. First, the community pharmacist is the most accessible health care professional, and he or she is routinely trusted by society. Second, with the self-care revolution, the number of individuals who are treating themselves using nonprescription products is continually increasing. Third, the number of prescription drugs that are being reclassified as nonprescription drugs is also increasing. Finally, the elderly population (age, >65 years) is escalating at a rapid pace, which is expected to continue for several years. These individuals consume the majority of prescription medications and one-third of nonprescription medications. Because of all these circumstances, the community pharmacist has frequent opportunities to assess patient information on a daily basis.

Example

The case from the beginning of the chapter is reproduced and continued below.

Self-Assessment Questions

1. Briefly describe the concept of pharmaceutical care.
2. What are the pharmacist's primary responsibilities in providing pharmaceutical care to patients?
3. Briefly describe how the concept of patient assessment is intertwined with pharmaceutical care.

Critical Thinking Question

1. In the patient case example discussed in this chapter, the patient's bradycardia and hypotension were probably caused by noncompliance with the atenolol. As a pharmacist who provides pharmaceutical care, what would you do if the patient comes back to the pharmacy a week later, has been taking the atenolol correctly (i.e., once daily), but still has a low heart rate and blood pressure?

Bibliography

American Pharmaceutical Association. APhA principles of practice for pharmaceutical care. Washington, DC: American Pharmaceutical Association, 1996.

American Pharmaceutical Association. Patient assessment and consultation. In: Nonprescription products: patient assessment handbook. Washington, DC: American Pharmaceutical Association, 1997:7–24.

American Pharmaceutical Association. Self-care and nonprescription pharmacotherapy. In: Nonprescription products: patient assessment handbook. Washington, DC: American Pharmaceutical Association, 1997:1–6.

American Society of Health-System Pharmacists. ASHP guidelines on a standardized method for pharmaceutical care. Am J Health-Syst Pharm 1996;53:1713–1716.

Cipolle RJ, Strand LM, Morley PC. A new professional practice. In: Pharmaceutical care practice. New York: McGraw-Hill, 1998:1–36.

Cipolle RJ, Strand LM, Morley PC. Identifying, resolving, and preventing drug therapy problems: the pharmacist's responsibility. In: Pharmaceutical care practice. New York: McGraw-Hill, 1998:73–120.

Cipolle RJ, Strand LM, Morley PC. The patient care process. In: Pharmaceutical care practice. New York: McGraw-Hill, 1998:121–176.

Grainger-Rousseau TJ, Miralles MA, Hepler CD, et al. Therapeutic outcomes monitoring: applications of pharmaceutical care guidelines to community pharmacy. J Am Pharm Assoc 1997;NS37:647–661.

Hepler CD, Strand LM. Opportunities and responsibilities in pharmaceutical care. Am J Hosp Pharm 1990;47:533–543.

Higby GJ. From compounding to caring: an abridged history of American pharmacy. In: Knowlton CH, Penna RP, eds. Pharmaceutical care. New York: Chapman & Hall, 1996;18–45.

Kane MP, Briceland LL, Hamilton RA. Solving drug-related problems. US Pharm 1995;20:55–74.

Rovers JP, Currie JD, Hagel HP, et al. Documentation. In: A practical guide to pharmaceutical care. Washington, DC: American Pharmaceutical Association, 1998:103–118.

Rovers JP, Currie JD, Hagel HP, et al., Identifying drug therapy problems. In: A practical guide to pharmaceutical care. Washington, DC: American Pharmaceutical Association, 1998:15–25.

Rovers JP, Currie JD, Hagel HP, et al. Patient data evaluation. In: A practical guide to pharmaceutical care. Washington, DC: American Pharmaceutical Association, 1998:56–76.

Rovers JP, Currie JD, Hagel HP, et al. The case for pharmaceutical care. In: A practical guide to pharmaceutical care. Washington, DC: American Pharmaceutical Association, 1998:1–14.

Tomechko MA, Strand LM, Morley PC, et al. Q and A from the pharmaceutical care project in Minnesota. Am Pharm 1995;NS35(4):30–39.

CHAPTER 2

Cultural Considerations in Patient Assessment

Rhonda M. Jones, Matin Royeen, and Jeffrey L. Crabtree

GLOSSARY TERMS

- Cultural pluralism
- Culture
- Ethnicity
- Ethnocentrism
- Prejudice
- Race
- Stereotype
- Subculture

For centuries, millions of people, representing hundreds of different cultures and nationalities, have left their countries of birth to make the United States their home. Until recently, many of these immigrants willingly surrendered their individual cultural identity and adopted the European-American culture and the English language as their own, thereby leading to the familiar characterization of the United States as a "melting pot." Today, however, sequestration rather than assimilation may be more accurate when describing the prevalent behavior of various ethnic groups. Recent immigrants now often confine themselves to their own cultural enclaves and interact mainly within their own cultural groups. In light of these changes, the term *cultural pluralism* has been coined. **Cultural pluralism** (or *multiculturalism*) refers to the United States as having tremendous cultural diversity rather than one dominant "American" culture. This diversity requires us, as pharmacists, to become aware of our own culturally determined preferences, values, and behaviors and to appreciate those of other cultures. It also challenges us to examine the issues and problems associated with cultural diversity in our daily practice.

Because cultural belief systems have a significant impact on an individual's health-related behaviors, pharmacists must demonstrate a genuine respect for cultural differences while, at the same time, providing effective pharmaceutical care. As described in Chapter 1, the pharmacist's role is to identify, to resolve, and to prevent medication-related problems, which enhance positive patient outcomes. This specifically involves interviewing patients, taking health and medication histories, obtaining physical assessment data, monitoring and evaluating patient information (both subjective and objective), evaluating patient compliance, and educating as well as counseling patients. In addition, pharmacists frequently interact with colleagues and other health care professionals who represent different sociocultural segments of society. Considering these various aspects, the provision of pharmaceutical care requires a pharmacist to possess effective cross-cultural skills when dealing with patients, colleagues, and other health care professionals. Cross-cultural competency is essential for providing quality care in today's health care environment.

WHAT IS CULTURE?

Culture is a simple word with complex meanings that encompass the entire domain of human activities. Specifically, **culture** is defined as a complex pattern of shared meanings, beliefs, and behaviors that are learned and acquired by a group of people during the course of history. Culture reflects the whole of human behavior, including values, attitudes, and ways of relating to and communicating with each other. It also encompasses an individual's concepts of self, universe, time and space, as well as health, disease, and illness. Because we all have varied aspects to our life, individuals typically belong to more than one cultural group or **subculture,** which refers to separate groups within a larger cultural context. These multiple cultural groups can result from a person's religion, occupation, gender, age, illness, and many other factors. For example, an Irish, Catholic, female patient with cancer will reflect various aspects, in some degree, of all these cultural groups. The term *culture* should not be confused with the term *race,* however. **Race** refers to groupings of people with the same biological and familial heredity. A person's race typically is reflected in physical characteristics, such as skin color, and is continued through generations. Lipson defines **ethnicity** as "a socially, culturally, and politically constructed group of individuals that holds a common set of characteristics not shared by others with whom its members come in contract."

Characteristics of Culture

Culture has four primary characteristics: (1) It is learned from birth through group socialization and language acquisition; (2) it is adapted to specific conditions (i.e., environmental and technical factors); (3) it is dynamic and ever-changing; and (4) it is shared by most, if not all, members of that particular cultural group. Common features of culture include patterns of interaction and communication, social organizations, role expectation, politics, geography, and economics. A person's culture is expressed through shared norms (i.e., cultural boundaries), meanings, and values. In addition, culture helps people to learn and to define their relationship with immediate groups and with members of society in general. Our culture influences the way that we think as well as how we interact and conduct our activities of daily living.

Culture is shaped by a person's nationality, socioeconomic and professional groupings, special needs, and lifestyle preferences. Our attitudes, beliefs, and customs are determined by our cultural heritage, which defines our identity. Sometimes, our culture provides us with unlimited opportunities and personal freedom to exercise our own free will. At other times, it imposes enormous restrictions by preventing us from stepping outside cultural boundaries (i.e., norms).

Ethnocentrism, Prejudice, and Stereotypes

Culture also influences how people view and judge those who seem to be different. Pharmacists reflect society's cultural mix as well as represent their own cultural group as a health care profession. To provide pharmaceutical care appropriately, pharmacists must accept a wide variety of beliefs, practices, and ideas about health and illness that may differ from their own. A major portion of pharmaceutical care relies on communication with patients and other health care professionals, so pharmacists must also recognize and accept variations in communication skills and behaviors that result from differing cultural backgrounds.

Ethnocentrism is the belief in the superiority of one's own group or culture while also expressing disdain and contempt for other groups and cultures. A European-American pharmacist working in a clinic in a Mexican-American border town would be displaying ethnocentrism if he or she arbitrarily dismissed a patient's herbal remedy as being ineffective.

Prejudice is the preconceived judgment or opinion of another person based on direct or indirect experiences. An Anglo-American pharmacist working in a clinic in an inner city environment who recommends oral contraceptives to all African-American females based on the belief that these women have children indiscriminately would be displaying prejudice.

Stereotypes are fixed perceptions or images of a group that reject the existence of individuality within that group. This can occur even with the best of intentions. Table 2-1 outlines generalizations that may apply to various ethnic groups; however, when this type of cultural information is applied indiscriminately, without considering the uniqueness of the individual, stereotyping can occur. Stereotyping is an even greater risk when pharmacists do not recognize their own values and beliefs. A pharmacist who displays ethnocentrism or prejudice, or who stereotypes individuals, will gather data selectively and in accordance with his or her own personal values and judgments. These biases can limit—or even prevent—important patient information from being obtained and, in turn, distort the corresponding assessment of the patient and his or her drug therapy problems.

To apply general cultural information, pharmacists must seek further information to determine whether the cultural generalizations fit the individual. Thus, as you begin to work with various patients, be aware of and sensitive to cultural differences. Box 2-1 identifies ways to develop cultural sensitivity. The first step is to examine your own culturally based values, beliefs, attitudes, and practices—especially concerning health and illness. Also, keep in mind that pharmacists have been socialized into a distinct professional culture, and that this culture (like others) instills its own beliefs and norms regarding health and illness. For the majority of pharmacists, this professional culture includes an acceptance of the biomedical theory of health and illness. (This theory and its alternatives are discussed in more depth in the following section.) In addition, each pharmacist has a culture that is defined by his or her own personal situation.

When a pharmacist interacts with someone from a culture with differing beliefs, conflict can result. Because of this potential conflict, it is helpful to explore your own perception, beliefs, and understanding of health and illness that have developed from your cultural background. Sometimes, this requires significant introspection. To assist with your cultural self-assessment, answer the questions in Box 2-2. After answering these questions, reflect on professional situations in which you have encountered beliefs that differ from your own. Did you accept these differences, or did you discount them in favor of your own? Develop a plan for how you will react in the future.

TABLE 2-1 ➤ CULTURAL CHARACTERISTICS RELATED TO HEALTHCARE

CULTURAL GROUP	HEALTH BELIEFS AND PRACTICES	FAMILY RELATIONSHIPS	COMMUNICATION	HEALTH CARE AND MEDICATION USE
European Americans	Health is a state of well-being, both physically and mentally. Cause of most illnesses explained by germ theory, stress, or improper diet. Frequently seek health care. Utilize self-help products.	Independence and individuality are emphasized. Strong nuclear family rather than extended family.	English is dominant language. Frequent eye contact. Frequent nod of head or "uh-huh" for agreement.	Frequently seek health care. Frequently use prescription, over-the-counter, and herbal products. Increasing use of self-help products.
African Americans	Illness is caused by natural (e.g., cold air, pollution, food) and unnatural (e.g., witchcraft, voodoo) forces.	Strong bonds with extended family. Family helps in time of crisis/illness. Strong sense of peoplehood, even if not related.	English or slang/"Black" English is dominant language. Alert to discrimination. High level of caution and distrust of majority group. Nonverbal behavior is important.	Use home remedies before seeking health care. Frequent use of folk medicine and self-care. Prayer is common means of prevention and treatment.
Arab Americans	Health is a gift from God. Illness is caused by evil eye, bad luck, stress, germs, or an imbalance of hot/dry and cold/wet. Mental illness should be able to be controlled by the patient.	Strong extended family bonds. Women take care of the sick. Family makes health care decisions	Use English or Arabic language. Eye contact considered disrespectful and/or inappropriate between men and women. Touch inappropriate between men and women.	Commonly seek and use health care. May use home/folk remedies (e.g., sweating, herbal teas) and religious rituals.
Chinese Americans	Health maintaining balance between yin and yang in body and environment. Most physical illness caused by imbalance between yin and yang. Harmony important to maintain body, mind, and spirit.	Extended families common; two or three generations often live in same household. Patriarchal society—oldest male makes decisions.	Cantonese and Mandarin most common languages. Eye contact avoided with authority figures as sign of respect. Being on time not valued. Address formally. Keep respectful distance. Silence may be sign of respect.	May use home remedies, herbalists, and acupuncturists in conjunction with Western medicine or before seeking medical help. Diet major source of promoting health.
Japanese Americans	Good health related to taking care of yourself. Balance between self, society, and universe.	Family-oriented cultural group; self subordinate to family. Men usual spokesman, although women can be involved in decision making. Women considered subordinate in more traditional families.	Japanese is the preferred language, but usually able to understand and speak English. Quiet and polite. Little direct eye contact. Touching uncommon. Controlled facial expressions. Promptness important.	Western beliefs in health promotion becoming more accepted. Screening may be inhibited if issues are sensitive. Herbal remedies may be used. Prayer and offerings may be used in conjunction with Western medicine. Western medicine generally accepted.
Vietnamese	Health based on harmony and balance within themselves. Illness related to natural causes, imbalance in yin/yang, punishment for fault or violation of religious taboo.	Highly family oriented, may be extended or nuclear family. Father or eldest son spokesman. Women who are not wage-earners more subordinate in decision making.	Three major languages: Vietnamese, French, and Chinese. Head may be considered sacred and feet profane. Respect shown by avoiding eye contact. More distant personal space. Open expression of emotions is in bad taste.	Treated with herbal medicine, spiritual practices, and acupuncture. Other health practices include cupping, coin rubbing, pinching skin, inhaling aromatic oils, herbal teas, or wearing strings. Believe in both Western medicine and folk medicine. Will seek screening only if emphasized by doctor or nurse.

(Continued)

TABLE 2-1 ➤ *Continued*

CULTURAL GROUP	HEALTH BELIEFS AND PRACTICES	FAMILY RELATIONSHIPS	COMMUNICATION	HEALTH CARE AND MEDICATION USE
Mexican Americans	Health is feeling well and being able to maintain roles. Disease based on imbalance between individual and environment. Do not usually subscribe to maintenance and illness prevention due to present time orientation and belief that future is in God's hands	Mostly nuclear families, with extended family and godparents.	May use English or Spanish. Differences in word usage depending on home region. Direct eye contact frequently avoided with authority figures. Silence may indicate lack of agreement. Touch by strangers generally unappreciated. High degree of modesty. Women may not share information about contraceptive activities. Men disclose feelings less often.	Seek help from *curandero* or *curandera*, who receives power through a calling or dream/vision. Frequently use herbs, rituals, and religious objects.
Puerto Ricans	Health is viewed as the absence of mental, spiritual, or physical discomforts. Being underweight or thin is also seen as unhealthy. Illness might be seen as hereditary, punishment, sin, or the result of evil. Realistic, serene view of life. Some believe destiny or spiritual forces are in control of life situations, health, and even death.	Nuclear and extended family structure. All decisions conceived around family. Women assume active role in caring for the sick.	May use English or Spanish. Express gratitude by providing goods. Speak and give instructions slowly. Relativistic view of time; negotiate for time of appointment.	Multivitamins commonly used. Health screening procedures often avoided, except for children. Home and folk-remedies used before or in combination with Western medicine. Pharmacist has significant role in care-seeking.
Cubans	Traditional Cubans think of someone overweight and rosy-cheeked as being healthy. Modern germ theory well understood, although may believe that extreme nervousness or stress can cause illness.	Family oriented. Extended family important; often three family generations in household. Men expected to make decisions and protect family. Women usually in submissive supportive role.	Use Castilian Spanish, but speak quickly, shorten words, and incorporate English words. Typically outgoing and confronting. Close contact and touching acceptable. Eye contact expected during conversation. Often follow Western business time.	Seek care first from Western medical facilities; prayer and religious assistance used concurrently. Health promotion and illness prevention becoming more accepted. Health screening acceptable to most. Herbal medicine often used. Many food prescriptions used as home remedies.
Native Americans	Health is a state of harmony with nature and universe. Illness is caused by supernatural forces (e.g., witchcraft, evil spirits). Respect for self/body and nature.	Strong extended family bonds. Respect for elderly. Elderly have leadership roles.	Speak English and/or native Indian language. Nonverbal communication important.	Seek help from medicine men. Frequently use herbs and rituals. May wear objects to protect against supernatural forces. Religion and medicine intertwined.

Box 2-1

WAYS TO DEVELOP CULTURAL SENSITIVITY

- Recognize that cultural diversity exists.
- Identify and examine your own cultural beliefs.
- Demonstrate respect for people as unique individuals, with culture as only one factor that contributes to their uniqueness.
- Respect the unfamiliar.
- Recognize that some cultural groups have definitions of health and illness, as well as practices that attempt to promote health and to cure illness, that may differ from your own.
- Be willing to modify health care delivery in keeping with the patient's cultural background.
- Do not expect all members of one cultural group to conduct themselves in exactly the same way.
- Appreciate that each person's cultural values are ingrained and, therefore, difficult to change.

Adapted from Stulc P. In Cookfair JN, ed. Nursing process and practice in the community. St. Louis: Mosby–Year Book, 1990.

Box 2-2

CULTURAL SELF-ASSESSMENT QUESTIONS CONCERNING HEALTH AND ILLNESS

- How do you define *health?*
- How do you define *illness?*
- How do you keep yourself healthy?
- Do you believe in preventative medical practices? If so, which ones (e.g., immunizations, cholesterol monitoring, estrogen replacement therapy)?
- What would you consider as a minor, or nonserious, medical problem? Give examples.
- How do you know when a health problem needs medical attention?
- Do you diagnose your own health problems? Give examples.
- Do you use over-the-counter medications? If so, which ones, and when?
- Do you believe in the use of alternative or complementary medicines? If so, which ones, and when?
- Do you believe that others outside the medical professions have the power to heal?
- Do you consider certain therapies (traditional or nontraditional) to be unacceptable? If so, which, and why?
- Do you make your own health decisions, or do you involve family members in your decision-making process?

Adapted from Spector R. Cultural diversity in health and illness. Stamford, CT: Appleton and Lange, 1996.

CULTURAL VARIABLES THAT AFFECT PATIENT ASSESSMENT

A person's culture is expressed in numerous ways, such as values, beliefs, and customs. For the purposes of this chapter, however, only the variables that most closely affect the process of patient assessment are discussed. When working with patients, cultural differences will undoubtedly exist. You must be sensitive to these differences and be certain that you understand exactly what the patient means—and what the patient thinks *you* mean. This is an underlying necessity during all patient assessments, no matter with which cultural variable you are working. The cultural beliefs and behaviors that affect assessment of the patient as well as development of an appropriate and acceptable pharmaceutical care plan include those involving (1) health beliefs and practices, (2) family relationships, and (3) communication.

Differing Views of Health and Illness

The term *disease* describes an abnormal structure and function of the body that is generally treatable by modern medicine. The term *illness,* however, describes something less objective. Illness is synonymous with changes in social function and a general state of well-being; in other words, it describes how a person might respond to a disease or to changes in his or her function or well-being. Illness may interfere with a person's role in the family and community.

Health care professionals have an exceptional understanding of disease, but the causes of illness are not as well understood. Keep in mind that patients will have various views of health, illness, disease, and cure that are shaped by their particular cultural and/or religious beliefs. One of the fundamental components of illness is what the patient believes causes disease and illness. Disease causation may be viewed in three ways: (1) biomedical, (2) naturalistic, and (3) magico-religious.

Biomedical

The biomedical or scientific theory of disease causation is based on a cause-and-effect relationship: There are specific causes for disease and specific medications to treat the disease and/or its cause. For example, bacteria and viruses are responsible for certain infectious diseases, and antibiotics cure the infection. The biomedical theory of disease is also based on the assumptions that the human body is a mechanically functioning machine, that all life can be reduced into smaller parts, and that all reality can be observed and measured. This approach to health and medical care is commonly embraced by the Western world and is taught in most educational programs for pharmacists and other health care workers.

Naturalistic

Many cultures embrace a more naturalistic or holistic approach to describing the cause of illness. People whose beliefs are congruent with this theory hold that humans are only one part of nature and the general order of the cosmos. The forces of nature—some of which are good and some of which are bad—must be kept in balance or harmony for a person to remain well or healthy. This is exemplified by the *yin/yang theory*, which is the basis for Eastern or Chinese medicine and is commonly embraced by Asian Americans.

The *yin/yang theory* states that all organisms and objects in the universe consist of yin (i.e., cold) and yang (i.e., hot) energies. Yin (or female) energy represents forces, such as darkness, cold, and emptiness, whereas yang (or male) energy represents forces, such as light, warmth, and fullness. Many Asians believe that the balance between yang and yin energies is very important for maintaining good health. Balanced yang and yin assures peaceful interaction of mind and body and, thus, good health. If this balance is disturbed, then illness or disease result.

Yang represents the five visceral organs, or the liver, heart, spleen, lungs, and kidneys. According to this view, an excess of yang can cause "hot" conditions, such as skin rashes, fevers, and constipation. On the other hand, yin represents the gallbladder, stomach, intestine, bladder, and lymph system. An excess of yin can contribute to "cold" conditions, such as diarrhea, headache, and stomach cramps. In addition, foods are classified as hot and cold and are transformed into yin and yang energies as they are metabolized in the body. Yin foods (e.g., fresh vegetables, dairy products, honey) are cold and should be eaten during a hot illness; yang foods (e.g., cheese, eggs, hard liquor) are hot and should be eaten during a cold illness.

Another naturalistic theory is the *hot/cold theory* of health and illness. Similar to the yin/yang theory, the hot/cold theory describes a needed balance between good and bad forces for well-being. The individual as a whole, rather than just a particular disease, is significant. Many Hispanic, African, Asian, and Middle-Eastern Americans embrace this theory and believe that health encompasses a state of total well-being, including physical, psychological, spiritual, and social aspects of the person. In this theory, basic bodily functions are described in terms of temperature, dryness, and moisture, and they are regulated by the four humors of the body (i.e., blood, phlegm, black bile, and yellow bile). Diseases as well as medicines, foods, and beverages are classified as "hot" or "cold" according to their effect on the body, not their physical characteristics. For example, earaches, chest cramps, and gastrointestinal discomfort are believed to be caused by cold entering the body; whereas sore throats and rashes are believed to be caused by the body overheating. According to this theory, treatment of illness includes adding or subtracting cold, heat, dryness, or moisture to restore the balance of the four humors.

Magico-Religious

The third major view of health and illness is the *magico-religious* perspective. This model is based on the belief that supernatural forces, both good and evil, dominate the world. These supernatural forces, which cannot be controlled by people, cause certain types of illness, and the fate of the person depends on the action of these forces. Thus, an illness may occur in a "sinful" person who, without God's protection, becomes vulnerable and falls prey to the demands of evil spirits. Alternatively, a wicked person can cast an evil spell over a good person, thereby causing illness, injury, or bad luck. Because evil spirits are believed to have stronger powers than good spirits, a great deal of energy and time is spent to rid the evil spirits from the body by offering gifts or performing rituals. Some African Americans believe in magical causes of illness, such as voodoo or witchcraft, whereas certain Christian religions (e.g., Catholicism, Mormonism) believe in various faith-healing rituals and practices.

Family Relationships

Despite the high divorce rate in the United States, the family remains the basic social unit for most people. A *family* is defined as a group of individuals living together as one unit. Several variations are common, however, and these include:

- *Nuclear:* husband, wife, and children.
- *Extended:* nuclear family plus blood relatives.
- *Blended:* husband, wife, and children from previous relationships.
- *Single parent:* mother or father and at least one child.
- *Communal:* group of men, women, and children.
- *Cohabitation:* unmarried man and woman sharing a household with children.

Because the family is an integral part of most people's lives, it affects how they view and, ultimately, how they utilize health care services, including pharmacy services. The family serves as the original source of an individual's socialization and acquisition of values and beliefs, which guide the person's attitudes and behaviors throughout life. A hundred years ago, the extended family was a crucial part of traditional American life. Parents, grandparents, and other family members lived together under one roof. In contrast, the contemporary European- American family most commonly consists of a parent(s)-child(ren) unit such as the nuclear or single-parent families. European-American families teach the values of individual freedom and personal independence to children, who are then expected to make their own life decisions in areas such as education and careers. Most children from European-American families are taught to be self-reliant, are encouraged to sleep in their own rooms, and are expected to learn—and to perform—independent self-care skills, such as eating and dressing, at an early age. In addition, these children are expected to leave home on completion of their education.

In contrast, many individuals from other cultural groups not only live with extended families but also base their personal decisions on what is considered to be good for the entire family. In other words, they value the common good of the family. In fact, the common good of the family often is so important that praise of personal accomplishments may cause embarrassment to some members of these cultural groups. These cultural values are also seen during health care decision-making. Whereas European-American culture values individual autonomy in making health decisions, family consensus is prevalent in other cultures. Typically, the individual consults with the extended family before seeking health care. Additionally, it is not unusual in some cultural groups for family members to accompany the sick person to his or her medical appointments and the pharmacy. Consequently, any health care decisions need to be approved by other family members, especially older members of the immediate family.

Because family roles, relationships, and responsibilities vary from culture to culture, pharmacists must be able to identify key decision-makers and caregivers. These may—or may not—be the biological parents, as is typical in European-American culture. Some cultures expect the sick person to be cared for by other family members, whereas European-American culture emphasizes self-reliance and self-care even when a person is sick. Thus, it is important to explore how a particular illness, disease, or medication will affect the patient's ability to do his or her usual activities (e.g., If help is needed, who will help? How will they help the patient?). Because some cultures include family members in making health care decisions, you should also include other family members in the discussions when interviewing a patient or developing pharmaceutical care plans. Such acknowledgement and acceptance of diverse family relationships will strengthen the quality of health care for members of certain cultures.

Communication

Good communication skills are an absolute necessity to practice pharmaceutical care, because the first step in any pharmaceutical care process is gathering and evaluating patient-related information. Communication and culture are closely intertwined, especially in the way that feelings are expressed, both verbally and nonverbally. If you are unaware of cultural differences in communication, you may misinterpret patient information and assess the patient inaccurately.

First, determine how well the patient understands written and spoken English. When the patient does not speak English, a translator or interpreter can be very helpful. Many times, a family member will be expected to serve as an interpreter; however, in some cultures, this may be very challenging and uncomfortable for the family member because of family role conflicts or lack of medical terminology. In addition, the family member may relay messages to both the patient and the pharmacist based on their own perception of the situation—or even withhold important information because it may embarrass the patient or the family member.

Because of these possible problems, use of a professionally trained interpreter is recommended. Tips to assist you when working with an interpreter are listed in Box 2-3. When working with an interpreter, remember to look at and speak directly to the patient, not the interpreter. This is a common error when first working with an interpreter.

Even if you and the patient speak the same language, differences in culturally based values and beliefs can still make communication difficult. Culture-based variations can occur in both verbal (e.g., word meanings, conversational style) as well as nonverbal (e.g., eye contact, personal space, touch, time orientation) communication.

Verbal

The meaning of a given word may differ from group to group, even if it is spoken in English. For example, *bad* may have a negative implication in one culture and a positive meaning in another. Some groups also may have common lay terms for specific types of medical problems. For example, hypertension may be described as "high blood" and anemia as "low blood." Once you have become familiar with the common lay terms utilized by a patient, incorporate these into your speech when interviewing and counseling the patient. These various lay terms will differ between ethnic and cultural groups, so clarify your understanding of the term with the patient. This can be accomplished by asking the patient to describe what they mean by "low blood" or stating your own understanding of "low blood" and then asking the patient if that is correct.

Conversational style also varies from culture to culture, from a direct and to-the-point style to a more indirect style, during which the patient may provide information through an abundant amount of words or, possibly, with stories. A loud voice may mean anger, simple emphasis, or passionate feelings concerning a subject. For example, European Americans tend to talk more directly and loudly, whereas the English speak in more

Box 2-3

TIPS FOR WORKING WITH AN INTERPRETER

- If possible, meet with the interpreter before the session to explain the purpose of the interaction.
- If possible, have the interpreter meet with the patient before the session to learn the patient's attitudes and beliefs about health, illness, and health care.
- Be patient. An interpreted interview may take twice as long as an ordinary interchange.
- Speak in short sentences. Avoid long, involved sentences or discussion involving more than one topic.
- Use simple language. Avoid technical terminology and professional jargon.
- During the interview, look at and speak directly to the patient rather than the interpreter.
- Listen to the patient, and watch for nonverbal communication.
- Encourage translation of the patient's own words rather than paraphrasing in professional jargon.
- Instruct the interpreter not to insert his or her own interpretations or ideas or to omit any information.
- Check the patient's understanding—and the accuracy of the translation—by asking the patient to repeat the information, message, or instructions back to you through the interpreter.

Adapted from Lipson JG. Culturally competent nursing care. In Lipson JG, Dibble SL, Minarik PA, eds. Culture and nursing care: a pocket guide. San Francisco: UCSF Nursing Press, 1996.

accentuated tones and with a softer voice. The use of silence also may have different meanings. In some cultures, it may indicate respect or acknowledgement that the speaker was heard; in others, it may mean "No" or seem rude. European Americans also tend to respond in conversation by nodding their head and/or saying "I see" or "Uh-huh" to indicate understanding, whereas the English tend to blink their eyes to indicate the same. In addition, the speed or ease of the conversation may vary between various cultural groups. Pharmacists should tailor their conversational style to that of the patient, ask questions to clarify their understanding, and observe for consistency in the conversational style of the patient. Inconsistent patterns in conversational style may be a symptom of an underlying pathologic condition. For example, rapid speech accompanied by restlessness may be displayed in patients suffering from anxiety.

Nonverbal

Nonverbal messages are considered to be a very critical and complex part of human communication. Understanding nonverbal communication is very challenging, however, because of the variations with which human beings express themselves. Understanding the features of nonverbal communication can be a useful tool in cross-cultural communication.

Culturally appropriate eye contact will vary from direct to fleeting. In the European-American culture, direct eye contact while you are speaking to a person is considered to be appropriate. In other cultures (e.g., Asian, Arab, Native American), direct eye contact may be a sign of disrespect or aggression, an invasion of someone's privacy, or inappropriate behavior between men and women. Culturally based avoidance of direct eye contact can easily be misinterpreted in the mainstream American culture as a negative personality trait of being "shy" or "quiet." Similarly, use of body language, such as movements of the body, limbs, face, and eyes, are used with considerable variation in communication; some gestures that may be complimentary in one cultural group may be very offensive in others.

The amount of personal space that is comfortable also varies, from very close to distant, based on a person's cultural background. For example, if you are too close to the patient while talking, he or she may perceive you as being aggressive and be very uncomfortable and untrusting. On the other hand, the opposite may also be true: If you back away when the patient approaches, you may be perceived as being rude and distant. Keep in mind that the comfortable amount of personal space varies from patient to patient, and adjust the distance between you and the patient accordingly.

Different cultural groups also have different norms concerning how and when people should touch each other. Some groups use touch to communicate feelings; others view touch as an invasion of privacy. In addition, certain parts of the body are considered to be sacred in some cultural groups (e.g., the head among Asians) and should not be touched. In other groups, touch (e.g., greeting with a hug or an embrace) is appropriate with the same gender but inappropriate with an unrelated person of the opposite gender.

In the European-American culture, being "on time" is important. In addition, life is paced according to the clock, whereas personal or subjective time is less important and is squeezed in as a person's schedule allows. Some other cultures (e.g., Native American), however, value involvement with other people and completion of interpersonal encounters more than being "on time."

The variations described here are only a few examples of how communication, both verbal and nonverbal, can differ between cultural groups. As with all specific examples that describe a particular cultural group in this chapter, these should not be considered as rigid characteristics of all individuals in that group. They are meant to be basic generalizations to provide insight during a particular situation and, thus, to help avoid a misunderstanding. You should recognize, accept, and adapt to differences in verbal and nonverbal communication styles to accurately assess the patient and to maximize the potential for a positive health care experience.

Expression of Symptoms

Another specific area of variation in communication is the manner in which certain symptoms and diseases are expressed, perceived, diagnosed, labeled, and treated. Do not assume that a patient will express symptoms or complaints in a way that has the same meaning as that in the dominant American culture. Symptoms are reported and perceived in a variety of ways. For example, Chinese patients somaticize emotional symptoms and may describe complaints associated with the heart (because it is the center of emotion) rather than tell you they are sad due to the recent death of a family member. To illustrate the cross-cultural variability of a common and universal symptom, this section describes variations in the expression of pain.

Pain is a subjective experience that is influenced by a person's cultural background. The expression, expectation, and treatment of pain are all shaped through a cultural context and personal history. In addition, cross-cultural research has found that pain is a highly individual experience, depending on cultural learning and on the meaning of the situation. For example, Anglo Americans tend to value "silent suffering" as a response to pain, because they have been socialized that "self-control" is better than open expression of feelings. Thus, the coping strategy among Anglo Americans suffering from chronic pain is often "to work and keep busy." Other cultural groups (e.g., Puerto Ricans), however, may openly express pain. In addition, patients will compare and validate the expression of pain with their social environment (i.e., family, friends, coworkers, etc.). Research studying nurses' attitudes toward pain has found that the way in which patients express pain may affect a nurse's assessment of both physical and psychological pain. A female Anglo-American nurse caring for a male Puerto Rican patient may consider the patient to be "faking" when he openly moans and groans as an expression of his pain. In addition, nurses who infer greater patient pain tended to report their own experiences as being more painful.

Because of cultural variation in the expression, meaning, and perception of symptoms, you must fully understand the symptoms or complaints from the patient's perspective rather than from your own—or even from that of the patient's cultural group. This is a critical first step in accurately assessing the patient and in providing pharmaceutical care.

HEALTH-RELATED BELIEFS OF SELECTED GROUPS

The United States has a rich diversity of cultural characteristics among different ethnic groups. This chapter does not include a detailed exploration of all health-related beliefs and characteristics of all cultures, but this section does describe generalizations about the most common cultural groups. It is important to note that not all members of a culture will share all the preferences, values, beliefs, or traits that are described. Each person within the group has his or her own personal traits and characteristics. Thus, you cannot predict a person's character or behavior merely on the basis of common cultural beliefs and practices. In other words, it is inappropriate to stereotype individuals from a particular cultural group. As part of the assessment process, you must acknowledge and recognize the characteristics of the individual with whom you are interacting while also taking into account common cultural behavior. Box 2-4 list questions that are useful in exploring the patient's cultural beliefs about health, illness, and treatment.

Before outlining some cultural generalizations (see Table 2-1), it must be acknowledged that numerous factors affect how closely an individual's culture will mimic the generalizations regarding a specific cultural group. Two of these factors are the *degree of heritage consistency* and *generation.* The degree of heritage consistency refers to how closely an individual relates to his or her original heritage. This factor is closely intertwined with the issue of generation. For example, an individual who immigrated from Cuba to the United States within the last year may closely identify with generalizations about the Cuban culture. In contrast, an individual whose grandparents immigrated to the United States from Cuba may identify more closely with the Anglo-American culture. Then again, that same individual may live in a very cloistered environment in South Florida that closely holds to the culture of their native country; in this case, the generation factor would be overshadowed by the high degree of heritage consistency.

In addition, care must be taken in how broadly cultural generalizations are made. In today's society, many references are made to Hispanics, so a pharmacist may be tempted to apply generalizations regarding Hispanics to all individuals from Spanish-speaking nations. Mexican Americans, Spanish Americans, Central Americans, Cubans, and Puerto Ricans have vastly different cultures, however. This same error can also be made by classifying all individuals from Japan, Vietnam, China, and India as Asian Americans.

Box 2-4

CULTURAL ASSESSMENT QUESTIONS CONCERNING ILLNESS

- What do you think caused your problem?
- When did it start?
- Why do you think it started when it did?
- What does your sickness do to you?
- How does it work?
- How bad is your sickness?
- How long do you think it will last?
- What should be done to get rid of it?
- How have you treated the illness?
- What benefit will you get from the treatment?
- What are the most important problems your sickness has caused for you?
- What worries you and frightens you the most about your sickness?

Adapted from Narayan MC. Cultural assessment in home healthcare. Home Healthcare Nurse 1997;15:663–672.

European Americans

Europeans have been immigrating to the United States for more than 300 years and have diverse origins. The most common countries of origin include Germany, Italy, England, Ireland, Canada, and Russia. Because European (i.e., white) Americans encompass the majority of the U.S. population, it is very difficult to identify all the cultural differences. Thus, some of the basic beliefs regarding health and illness that dominate the American culture are described.

Most European Americans view health as something more than just not being ill; they view health as a state of physical and mental well-being. If an individual is healthy, then he or she can accomplish his or her activities of daily living, will have positive energy to do things, and will be able to enjoy life. Illness is viewed as an absence of well-being or, in other words, the presence of pain, malfunction of body organs, not being able to do what you want, a disorder of the body, or a blessing from God to suffer. Most illnesses are believed to result from infection, stress-related conditions, or improper diet. Although European Americans frequently seek health care and use prescription medications, they also routinely utilize self-help products (e.g., over-the-counter medications, herbal products, vitamins, etc.), because the dominant American culture emphasizes independence and individuality.

African Americans

In many cases, African-American health beliefs stem from traditional cultural beliefs: Illness is a lack of harmony with nature caused by evil spirits. This notion of illness involves a disruption of the unity of mind, body, and soul. In *Cultural Diversity in Health and Illness,* Rachel Spector describes the following beliefs in the African-American culture regarding illness:

- Coldness enters the body and reduces an individual's resistance to illness. During winter, human blood should thicken as a protective mechanism. Consequently, those elderly and young persons with thinner blood become more susceptible to illness and should avoid any conditions that cause chilliness in their systems.
- Dirt or impurities in the body are associated with hot conditions that produce fever, inflammation, measles,

and cancer. Menstruation, digestion, and elimination help to rid the body of these impurities.

- Dietary factors determine health conditions. Improper diet causes fluctuations of high and low blood in the body. Red foods, such as beets, carrots, red wine, and red meats, are considered to be "blood builders" that cause symptoms of dizziness and headaches. Colorless substances, such as vinegar, lemon juice, pickle juice, and garlic, are used to reduce high blood in the body.
- Unnatural illness is caused by unfriendly and hostile forces in the environment. Traditional healers, employing different forms of magic, are used to control these undesirable human conditions.

Many African Americans value general good health, which they define as maintaining rest, exercise, and a good relationship with God and other human beings. African-American spiritual healers focus on achieving physical, social, and spiritual balance in life. Other methods of treatment include the use of herbs, roots, oils, powders, and amulets. The pharmacist should work with the African-American patient and family members to provide a holistic approach to the patient's health needs. Most important, the pharmacist must work hard to win the trust of African-American patients who, for the most part, perceive their interaction with the health care system as a very degrading and humiliating experience. Considering the discrimination and racism that African Americans experience in American society, this view is easily understandable.

Arab Americans

To many Arab (i.e., Middle Eastern) Americans, health is a gift from God and is defined as being able to eat well, meet social obligations, and have strength. Physical illness is thought to result from several different things, such as an evil eye, bad luck, stress in the family, germs, winds, drafts, or an imbalance of hot/dry and cold/moist. Sudden fears, pretending to be ill to manipulate family, or the wrath of God may cause mental illness.

Individuals who are physically sick are treated well and typically are cared for by female family members (e.g., mother, sister, grandmother, sister-in-law, daughter). Physically ill patients expect to be pampered by female family members or health care professionals. Male family members are responsible for logistic arrangements, such as patient transportation, financial needs, and funeral plans, rather than for caring for daily needs. Arab Americans believe that mentally ill patients should be able to control their illness; consequently, individuals suffering from mental illness may not be treated as well. Patients are expected to be passive in any decisions regarding themselves or others. Arab Americans utilize home and folk remedies, such as sweating, religious rituals, herbal teas, chicken soup, and enemas; however, they also commonly respect and seek Western health care services and pharmaceutical medications.

Asian Americans

As previously mentioned, Asian-American cultures vary greatly in their beliefs and values; however, many Asian Americans are influenced by Confucian beliefs, traditional shamans, herbalists, and Chinese traditional medicine. These beliefs include the five elements of wood, fire, earth, metal, and water, which correspond to different hot and cold seasons within the organs of the body. Good health is the proper balance between hot (i.e., yang) and cold (i.e., yin) forces. A hot state may be caused by excessive consumption of hot foods, with symptoms of dry mouth, constipation, and exhaustion. Cold conditions result from drinking milk and eating fruits and vegetables, which can cause respiratory problems, dizziness, and blurred vision. Other Asian Americans view disease as a result of contact with bodily fluids, corpses, or the like.

Common medical problems are treated with acupuncture, coin-rubbing, dietary changes, massage, exercises, steam baths, and setting of bones (to name a few). In addition, those who believe that disease results from contact with bodily fluids or corpses are likely to engage in bathing rituals and to use herbal cathartics.

Hispanic Americans

The U.S. Census Bureau uses the term *Hispanic* or *Latino* to collectively describe individuals of Mexican, Cuban, Central American, Spanish, and Puerto Rican heritage. As previously stated, individuals descended from these nations may have significantly different cultural backgrounds (see Table 2-1).

Many Hispanics believe that illness may be God's punishment for man's transgressions or result from an imbalance in different areas of life, such as self-care, play, and work. Magic or witchcraft, in which an evil spirit invades the person's body, also causes illness. For example, a child can become sick as a result of an evil eye. Natural causes of illness include undigested amounts of food in the abdomen, which causes nausea, vomiting, and fever. Additionally, emotional, mental, and interpersonal problems can trigger illness in this belief system.

For a disease caused by an imbalance in life, treatment may include foods, beverages, and medications. Many Hispanic Americans characterize these diseases as being either hot or cold. They use hot food, such as oils, beef, hard liquor, and chili peppers, to relieve "cold diseases" and cold food, such as fresh vegetables, fruits, and dairy products to relieve "hot diseases." Various items, such as necklaces and medallions, are worn to keep the evil spirits away. In addition to using the Western approach of treatment, many Hispanic Americans use traditional methods of intervention, such as praying, visiting shrines, and making promises to God in return for health.

Native Americans

Traditional health beliefs and practices vary widely among the more than 500 Native American tribes throughout the United States. In general, a Native American's health and wellness is deeply manifested in psychological, physical, and spiritual dimensions of life, all coexisting in harmony with nature. Thus, health is a state of harmony with self, family, friends, and nature. Harming nature is considered to be harming yourself, which results in illness. Respect for both self and nature through proper care and harmony results in good health.

Illness, both physical and emotional, is caused by supernatural forces (e.g., witchcraft), breaking rules, or evil spirits of humans and animals intruding into the body. Some people carry objects to protect themselves against supernatural powers. Others do nothing for protection, however, because they view this form of illness as a punishment for violating tribal rules. Healers among the various Native American tribes, known as medicine men, are believed to have psychic power to diagnose and treat illness. The goal of this healing is the restoration of harmony between the sick individual and nature. According to Spector, some healers are capable of generating positive forces essential for maintaining the group's cultural identity. Others use witchcraft to harm the group's enemies. A third type of healers can only diagnose illness. Treatment of illness includes using herbs and performing feats to recover the lost soul. Faith healing and religion are widely used by medicine men for health recovery. Sweat baths and hot springs are used for cleansing and to provide physical relief against colds, sinus infections, and arthritis and to alleviate psychological stress.

Americans in Poverty

This chapter has focused on how culture, as defined by national heritage, can affect the patient assessment process and the provision of health care. All the cultural variations described thus far may be viewed as barriers that may prohibit or limit our ability to provide adequate pharmacy services. In addition to the barriers of language, family relationships, and differing views on health, disease, and illness previously discussed, many Americans also suffer from the culture of poverty. Poverty or low socioeconomic status presents significant barriers to adequate health care, one of which is accessibility of services.

Socioeconomic Status

Americans in poverty place high priority on meeting the basic needs of daily survival (e.g., food, shelter) rather than on promotion of health and prevention of illness. Although any individual may suffer in poverty, ethnic minorities tend more often to be members of this cultural group. Individuals of low socioeconomic status frequently seek medical assistance only after their health condition interferes with their ability to work.

The "cycle of poverty" contributes to the continued poor health experienced by these disadvantaged individuals. In this cycle, the person lives in an environment that may cause poor physical and intellectual development as well as poor economic productivity and, subsequently, poor nutrition. This leads to an increase in illness and a further decrease in productivity. In turn, all these circumstances lead to higher morbidity and accident rates, which increase health care costs. The resulting high cost of health care then discourages the poor patient from seeking medical assistance, thereby causing more illness and decreased productivity and continuing the cycle of poverty.

Accessibility

In addition to limited financial resources, several factors may cause difficulty in accessing appropriate health care: (1) location of medical facilities, (2) transportation to these facilities, (3) immigration status, and (4) lack of insurance. Many disadvantaged Americans must depend on family or friends for transportation to health care and pharmacy facilities, whether because of geographic distance or because of financial and language barriers that may prevent these individuals from utilizing public transportation. (In other words, they may not be able to communicate with the operator, to read signs and directions, or to afford the fare.) In addition, those suffering in poverty usually do not have insurance and, thus, cannot afford the needed health care and/or medications. Programs designed to aid the underinsured or the uninsured may not be available to individuals with a questionable immigration status. All these factors may cause minorities to underutilize health care and pharmacy opportunities, which contributes to the inequality of medical care among different ethnic groups.

RECOMMENDATIONS TO ENHANCE CULTURAL SENSITIVITY

As modern medicine becomes increasingly concerned with the treatment of disease using the best technology and drugs available, its practitioners—including pharmacists—tend to overlook cultural differences among their patients. Thus, pharmacists often miss opportunities to talk with their patients and to understand their patients' beliefs, concerns, and fears. Pharmacists who truly practice "pharmaceutical care" will learn as much as they can about their patient, including their cultural beliefs, fears, and concerns about health, illness, and health care services. This allows pharmacists to tailor their recommendations to the individual as well as to the medical condition involved. The following recommendations are ways to enhance your cultural sensitivity when interacting with patients of diverse backgrounds:

- Do a cultural self-assessment, and maintain an awareness of your own culturally derived preferences and values.
- Get to know the patient and members of the patient's family. This will increase the level of trust between you, the patient, and the family members.
- Listen actively, and observe the patient's verbal and nonverbal cues to help put multicultural differences into the proper context for effective intervention. Remember, in multicultural situations, you will likely face new and different sets of rules and norms.
- Develop a genuine tolerance, acceptance, and respect for the cultural values of the patient. In other words, do not impose or force your own personal and professional views and beliefs on the patient.
- Acknowledge that you do not know everything, and ask questions about different features of your patient's culture. This is the key that opens the doors of communication for understanding the world of your patient.
- Do not label different customs, norms, and habits as "good" or "bad." A nonjudgmental approach to serving your patients will maximize quality pharmaceutical services.

- Develop courage, patience, and tolerance for the ambiguity created by serving a multicultural population.
- Be empathic, and help the patient to deal with an atmosphere of cultural uncertainty, confusion, and ambiguity.
- Approach every cross-cultural interaction with a willingness to encounter new experiences, and be willing to explore your patient's world.
- Accept that cross-cultural interactions with your patients can be, at times, exhilarating, anxiety-provoking, and frustrating. When you recognize that these are a normal part of your experiences, you may be able to deal with them effectively.
- Meet and get to know members of other cultural groups. Although your professional relationships with individuals may come to an end, you can cherish the personal relationships for the rest of your life.

The underlying theme of these recommendations is to get to know each patient on his or her own terms and to avoid forming an opinion or judgment based on previous knowledge or experience of that patient's culture. Previous knowledge or experience should be drawn on to assist you in asking more constructive questions—*not* to arrive at automatic conclusions about the patient! If you automatically assume certain qualities or form conclusions about a patient simply because they belong to a particular cultural group, you risk stereotyping the patient, which you must always avoid. Your view of a given patient should evolve from your experiences with and information gained from that patient.

You must also realize that you need to understand both yourself and your own cultural background before you can fully appreciate other cultural differences. If you do not understand what you bring to the patient interaction or relationship (i.e., your beliefs, values, and attitudes), then you increase the probability of stereotyping the patient. To practice quality pharmaceutical care, you must be a "cultural student" of your patient and accept his or her differences without prejudice or judgment.

Self-Assessment Questions

1. Compare and contrast culture, ethnocentrism, prejudice, and stereotypes.
2. What are the three most common variables that affect patient assessment?
3. What are the best ways to enhance cultural sensitivity when interacting with patients of different backgrounds?

Critical Thinking Question

1. J.B. is a 58 year-old Native American male who is newly diagnosed with Type 2 diabetes. He has been referred to you for diabetes education. How would you handle this situation, while being sensitive to cultural considerations?

Bibliography

Bates MS. Biocultural dimensions of chronic pain: implications for treatment of multiethnic populations. Albany, NY: State University of New York Press, 1996.

Bates MS, Rankin-Hill L, Sanchez-Ayendez M. The effects of the cultural context of health care on treatment of and response to chronic pain and Illness. Soc Sci Med 1997;45:1433–1447.

Cookfair JN, ed. Nursing process and practice in the community. St. Louis: Mosby–Year Book, 1990.

Davis C. Patient practitioner interaction: An experiential manual for developing the art of health care. Thorofare, NJ: Slack, 1994.

Downes N. Ethnic Americans: for the health professional. Dubuque, IA: Kendall/Hunt Publishing, 1994.

Jamerson K, Dequattro V. The impact of ethnicity on response to antihypertensive therapy. Am J Med 1996;101(suppl 3A):22S–32S.

Kavanagh K, Kennedy P. Promoting cultural diversity: strategies for health care professionals. Thousand Oaks, CA: Sage Publications, 1992.

Kreps G, Kunimoto E. Effective communication in multicultural health care settings. Thousand Oaks, CA: Sage Publications, 1994.

Lindsay J, Narayan MC, Rea K. Nursing across cultures: the Vietnamese client. Home Healthcare Nurse 1998;16:693–700.

Lipson JG, Dibble SL, Minarik PA, eds. Culture and nursing care: a pocket guide. San Francisco: UCSF Nursing Press, 1996.

Ludwig-Beymer PA. Transcultural aspects of pain. In Andrews MM, Boyle JS, eds. Transcultural concepts in nursing care. 3rd ed. Philadelphia: JB Lippincott, 1999.

Lynch E, Hanson J. Developing cross-cultural competence. York, PA: Paul H. Brookes Publishing, 1992.

Narayan MC. Cultural assessment in home healthcare. Home Healthcare Nurse 1997;15:663–672.

Nieto S. Affirming diversity: the sociopolitical context of multicultural education. White Plains, NY: Longman Publishing Group, 1992.

Northouse G, Northouse L. Health communication strategies for health professionals. Stamford, CT: Appleton and Lange, 1992.

Paniagua FA, ed. Assessing and treating culturally diverse clients. Thousand Oaks, CA: Sage Publications, 1994.

Siganga WW, Huynh TC. Barriers to the use of pharmacy services: the case of ethnic populations. J Am Pharm Assoc 1997;NS37:335–340.

Spector R. Cultural diversity in health and illness. Stamford, CT: Appleton and Lange, 1996.

CHAPTER 3

Health and Medication History

Rhonda M. Jones

GLOSSARY TERMS

- Adverse drug reaction
- Allergic reaction
- Chief complaint
- Closed-ended questions
- Health history
- History of present illness
- Open-ended questions
- Past medical history
- Review of systems

With the incorporation of pharmaceutical care principles into pharmacy practice activities, pharmacists now routinely talk to patients on a daily basis. Because this is such an integral part of current pharmacy practice, the pharmacist must be able to communicate well with patients as well as with other health care professionals.

BASIC PATIENT INTERVIEWING SKILLS

The focal point of a pharmacist's assessment of the patient involves asking the patient questions. To elicit useful information, the pharmacist must utilize appropriate interviewing skills.

The Environment

Before a pharmacist talks to a patient or obtains any physical assessment data (e.g., blood pressure), the environment in which the interaction will take place should be prepared. The interaction may occur in a variety of settings, such as a community pharmacy, hospital room, or clinic examination room. However, basic environmental characteristics should be consistent from setting to setting to assist with ensuring a smooth and productive pharmacist–patient interaction. As illustrated in Figure 3-1, appropriate environmental characteristics include:

- Comfortable room temperature.
- Sufficient lighting for the pharmacist and patient to see clearly both each other and any written materials that may be used.
- Quiet surroundings, because noise from one or multiple sources is distracting for both the patient and the pharmacist and may cause misinterpretation of important patient information.
- Clean and organized setting, because distracting objects and miscellaneous clutter do not create a professional atmosphere.
- Four to five feet between the pharmacist and the patient, because a closer distance may create anxiety and greater distance imply a general disinterest in the patient.

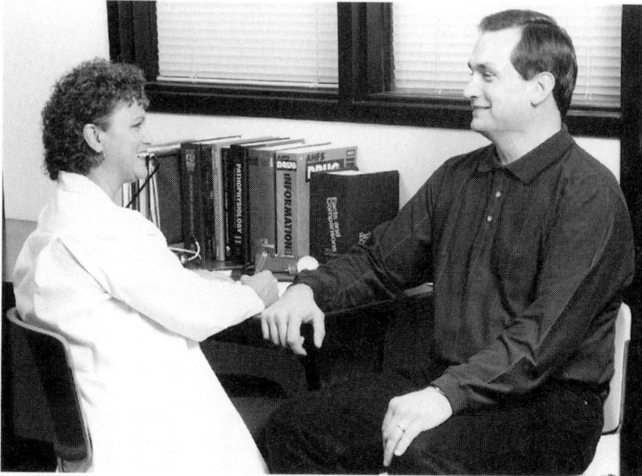

FIGURE 3-1. Pharmacist counseling a patient.

- Privacy, because the patient needs to feel comfortable talking about personal health issues and the pharmacist needs to be able to obtain physical assessment data discreetly.
- Equal-status seating or standing at eye level in a face-to-face position or a 90° angle. All barriers should be removed between the pharmacist and the patient (e.g., prescription counter, glass or plastic safety partitions, shelves, etc.). In the hospital setting, the pharmacist should be seated at eye level with the patient for a face-to-face interaction. Standing over a bedridden patient may imply superiority, possibly causing the patient to feel both inferior and uncomfortable.

Opening Statements

The opening statements between the pharmacist and the patient set the stage for the interaction. The patient should be addressed by his or her surname (if known). If the patient does not already know him/her, the pharmacist should introduce himself or herself and explain the reason for the interaction. In addition, the patient should be told the approximate amount of time that the interaction will take. For example, "Mrs. Smith, I'm Dr. Mark Davis, the pharmacist. I want to talk with you to see how you are doing on your medication. It should only take a few minutes."

Because this type of interaction may be new to some patients, the pharmacist should be prepared for questions (e.g., "Why do you need to talk to me? The other pharmacist doesn't do this."). An additional, brief explanation for the interaction usually resolves any confusion.

Types of Questions

Following the brief introduction, the pharmacist should ask the patient various questions. For an efficient yet productive patient–pharmacist dialogue, these should include a combination of open-ended and closed-ended questions. In general, open-ended questions are used first, to gather general information, and then are followed by closed-ended questions, as appropriate, to gather more specific patient data.

Open-Ended Questions

Open-ended questions require the patient to respond with a narrative or a paragraph format rather than with a simple yes or no. These types of questions elicit open expression, allowing the patient to answer in any way that he or she wishes. They allow the patient to give the pharmacist information from his or her perspective. Open-ended questions are useful in gathering less-structured patient information. For example:

- How are things going for you since the last time I saw you?
- How have you been feeling since you started the new medication?
- What medications are you currently taking?
- How do you take your medications?

Open-ended questions may provide more detail than is needed, however, or they may not provide enough. They are most useful in beginning a patient interview, introducing a new section of questions, and switching to a new topic.

Closed-Ended Questions

Closed-ended questions, or direct questions, ask for specific information and details. They elicit short, one- or two-word answers (e.g., yes or no). Closed-ended questions decrease the patient's options in answering. In addition, they make the patient passive during the interaction, because he or she is forced to answer questions from the pharmacist's perspective. For example:

- Does the chest pain occur when you are sitting down?
- Do you experience any light-headedness or dizziness when you take your Hytrin?
- Did you take your blood pressure medication this morning?
- Have you ever had an allergic reaction to a medication?

Closed-ended questions are most useful after the patient has answered an open-ended question and the pharmacist needs specific details to evaluate the patient's situation appropriately. They also may be useful in speeding up the interaction, because several minutes—or even hours—may be needed when asking only open-ended questions, which fail to provide needed details. Overusing closed-ended questions, however, may lead to an air of interrogation and impersonality, which displays a negative attitude toward the patient. In addition, overuse of closed-ended questions may limit the data obtained and result in an inaccurate assessment. Thus, a combination of open-ended and closed-ended questions is usually the most efficient and productive way of obtaining needed patient information, as shown by the sample interaction between a pharmacist and a patient in Box 3-1.

Verification of Patient Information

While the patient is answering the pharmacist's questions, the pharmacist must respond appropriately to continue the dialogue. Frequently, the pharmacist also needs to verify certain patient details to ensure that he or she is interpreting correctly what the patient is saying. Several feedback techniques can be

Box 3-1

SAMPLE INTERACTION BETWEEN A PHARMACIST AND A PATIENT

Pharmacist: Hi, Mr. Jones. My name is Monica Smith, the pharmacist. I want to talk to you about your medications. It should only take a few minutes.
Patient: Okay.
Pharmacist: How have you been feeling since Dr. Adams prescribed that new medication?
Patient: Oh, I guess alright. Some days I feel lousy, and some days I feel good.
Pharmacist: What do you mean by feeling lousy?
Patient: It's hard for me to get my work done outside. I like to mow the lawn and piddle around in the garden, but lately I just can't get it done.
Pharmacist: Why can't you? Do you feel weak or tired?
Patient: I guess I get short-winded while I'm mowing the lawn, and that wears me out.
Pharmacist: Do you have any chest pain while you're mowing?
Patient: No chest pain, but it's hard for me to breathe.
Pharmacist: Do you have any difficulty breathing at other times during the day or when you lie down at night?
Patient: Just if I try to work outside or go for a walk, and at night, I'm usually okay if I sleep with two pillows.

useful in assisting the pharmacist with both these processes. These techniques include: (1) clarification, (2) reflection, (3) empathy, (4) facilitation, (5) silence, and (6) summary.

Clarification

Clarification is useful if the patient provides confusing or ambiguous information. It can also help in providing the pharmacist with more specific details. For example, "Do you mean that the medication gives you an upset stomach when you say that it makes you sick?"

Reflection

Reflection involves repeating part or all of a patient's response. It acts in a way similar to a mirror, reflecting the patient's words or feelings back to him or her. For example, "What you're telling me is that your baby had diarrhea three times a day after you gave him amoxicillin for 2 days."

Empathy

Frequently, information that the patient relays to the pharmacist also involves feelings or emotions concerning their medications, medical condition, or life situation. If the pharmacist responds with an empathetic statement, illustrating to the patient that he or she understands these feelings, an accepting and trusting rapport can be established. An empathic response identifies a feeling, which is then reflected back to the patient in an understanding, caring, and nonjudgmental way. For example, a patient may state to the pharmacist, "I think I'm going to switch to a different doctor. My current doctor always seems too busy to talk to me!" An empathic response from the pharmacist might be "That must be frustrating for you, when you have a lot of questions about your heart disease."

Facilitation

Facilitation encourages the patient to continue communicating more information. It shows that the pharmacist is interested in what the patient is saying and wants the patient to continue. The conversation can be facilitated both verbally (e.g., "Yes, go on," "Mm-hmm," or "Please continue.") and nonverbally (e.g., maintaining eye contact or nodding yes).

Silence

When being questioned, occasionally the patient will need time to think and to organize what he or she wants to say. The pharmacist should become comfortable with these pauses as a necessary part of the communication process. By interrupting the silence, the pharmacist can destroy the patient's thought process, and valuable information may not be relayed. A long pause, however, could be caused by the patient not understanding or hearing the question; in this case, the pharmacist may need to repeat the question.

Summary

A summary is a review of what the patient has communicated. A summary statement is a verbalization of the pharmacist's understanding of the patient's information, and it can be used at any time during or at the end of the interview. It also allows the patient to agree or disagree and, if needed, to correct the pharmacist's interpretation.

Nonverbal Communication

Appropriate communication involves not only verbal but also nonverbal skills, in which the medium of exchange is something other than vocalized words. Nonverbal communication reflects the person's inner thoughts and feelings and is constantly at work, even if the person is unaware of it. Elements of nonverbal communication include: (1) distance, (2) body posture, (3) eye contact, (4) facial expressions, and (5) gestures. For a successful pharmacist–patient encounter, the verbal and the nonverbal communication must be in congruence. This is very important in establishing rapport with the patient.

Distance

The distance between the pharmacist and the patient plays an important role in a successful interaction. The most comfortable distance is approximately 18 to 48 inches apart. The 18 inches surrounding the body is the most protected space, so a distance closer than this may cause the patient to feel both nervous and uncomfortable. The pharmacist who continually invades a patient's personal space also risks appearing to be bullish and inconsiderate. The pharmacist should, however, maintain a distance close enough to ensure the patient's privacy, especially when discussing personal issues. Frequently, patients will communicate nonverbally their comfort level with the distance (e.g., by stepping back or leaning forward). The pharmacist should note this and adjust his or her distance accordingly.

Body Posture

An "open" body posture, in which the pharmacist is standing or sitting in a relaxed manner and presenting a full frontal appearance to the patient, relays both respect and sincere interest. The legs should be comfortably apart, not crossed, and the arms should be at the side.

In a "closed" body posture, the arms are crossed in front of the chest, the legs are crossed at the knees, the head is facing downward, and the eyes are looking at the floor. This type of posture may shorten or discontinue productive communication between the pharmacist and the patient and, thus, should be avoided.

Eye Contact

Appropriate eye contact does not mean continuously staring at the patient. Instead, the pharmacist should spend most of the interaction looking directly at the patient and only occasionally looking away. This is a very important aspect of good patient interviewing skills. Not looking at the patient may send a message of disinterest and lack of caring. In addition, lack of eye contact may inhibit the pharmacist's ability to identify and to evaluate the patient's nonverbal communication.

Facial Expressions

The pharmacist's facial expressions should be consistent with his or her verbal expressions. If the two do not match, the patient will tend to believe the facial message more than the spoken words. For example, if the pharmacist asks, "What adverse effects are you experiencing from this medication?" and then appears to be bored or distracted, the patient may perceive that the pharmacist is not sincerely interested in what he or she has to say—and any rapport will disintegrate. Appropriate facial expressions should reflect an attentive, sincere, and caring interest in the patient.

Gestures

Gestures also send nonverbal messages regarding emotional feelings or physical symptoms. For example, continuous wringing of the hands or tapping of the fingers often indicates anxiety or nervousness. As with other nonverbal communication, the gestures should match the verbal message. The pharmacist should always be conscientious regarding any gestures that may be distracting to the patient.

Closing Statements

Bringing the interview to an appropriate close is a crucial part of the communication process. Many times, the patient will evaluate the entire interaction based on the final statements; therefore, the pharmacist should not end the interview abruptly. An effective way to close the interaction is to provide a brief summary. This allows both the pharmacist and the patient an opportunity to review what has been discussed and to clarify any misinformation. Once both parties have determined that the information is correct, the pharmacist can conclude with a simple, closed-ended question (e.g., "Do you have any questions?") or a sincere statement (e.g., "Thank you for your time. If you have any questions when you get home, please call me."). Nonverbal cues (e.g., organizing paperwork for the patient's medical record or standing up from the chair) also can be helpful when combined with a summary or a closing question or statement.

Common Errors of Patient Interviewing

When talking to patients, it is easy to fall into nonproductive communication techniques, which may restrict the patient's communication with the pharmacist. These errors may decrease the amount of data obtained from the patient and hinder the development of rapport. Because of their defeating nature, such responses should be avoided when obtaining information from the patient. These include: (1) changing the subject, (2) giving advice, (3) providing false reassurance, (4) asking leading or biased questions, and (5) using professional terminology.

Changing the Subject

Many times, the pharmacist may encounter a situation in which he or she is unsure of how to respond. In this case, the easiest way out is to change the subject (e.g., by introducing a new topic). In such a situation, however, patients are likely to feel as if their concerns were not heard or understood. The pharmacist also should avoid using this response when rushed for time or anxious to obtain specific patient information. Changing the subject should be used only when all appropriate patient information has been gathered concerning one topic and it is time to move on to the next.

Giving Advice

Patients frequently will ask the pharmacist for advice concerning medications or various health problems. For example, "My baby has a rash on her bottom. Do you think it is diaper rash or an allergic reaction to the antibiotic she started yesterday?" In this instance, the patient is directly asking for the pharmacist's professional advice, and an appropriate response would be "Tell me more about the rash." The pharmacist, however, should avoid giving a personal opinion or telling the patient what to do (e.g., "I think using cloth diapers is crazy. That's probably why your baby has a diaper rash. You should quit using them.") These types of statements may be offensive and cause the patient to feel incapable of making his or her own decision. When appropriate, the pharmacist should provide patients with sufficient medical information (e.g., common symptoms associated with a specific medical problem, medication side effects, risks and benefits of taking certain medications, etc.) and make professional recommendations based on the specific patient information.

Providing False Reassurance

When discussing anxiety-inducing health concerns with a patient (e.g., a chronic disease or terminal illness), it may be tempting for the pharmacist to falsely reassure the patient (e.g., "Everything will be all right," or "I'm sure that you will be fine within a short time.") This falsely comforting response may make the pharmacist feel better; however, it may make the patient feel as if he or she should not be upset, worried, scared, frustrated, and so on. Such false reassurances trivialize the patient's feelings by trying to change them rather than trying to understand and accept them. This falsely reassuring response also may close off further communication between the pharmacist and the patient.

Asking Leading or Biased Questions

Leading or biased questions make assumptions regarding the patient's behavior or feelings, and they imply that one answer is better than another. For example, "You take your medications every day, don't you?" This type of question may make the patient feel that he or she should answer yes simply to please the pharmacist rather than risk disapproval by admitting to frequently forgetting to take his or her medications. Leading or biased questioning also conveys a negative judgment, and it leads the patient to answer in a way that corresponds to the pharmacist's assumptions, which decreases the chance of obtaining accurate patient information.

Using Professional Terminology

Many patients do not understand commonly used pharmaceutical and medical terms (e.g., inflammation, decongestant, diuretic) and, thus, may have interpretations of these words that differ from those of the pharmacist. For effective communication, the pharmacist should use words with which the patient is familiar. For example, the patient may have heard of the "blood thinner" Coumadin® but not know what the "anticoagulant" warfarin is, or a patient may refer to antihypertensive medications as "high blood pressure" pills. To ensure that the patient understands what is being said, the pharmacist needs to adjust his or her vocabulary to the patient's level (but without sounding condescending).

HEALTH HISTORY

The **health history** is a concise summary of the patient's current and past medical problems, medication history, family history, social history, and review of systems. The purpose of the health history is to obtain subjective patient information or, in other words, what the patient says about his or her own health, medications, and so on. Usually, these subjective data are then combined with the objective physical examination and laboratory data to evaluate the patient's current health status. In the institutional setting (e.g., hospital or long-term care), the health history usually is obtained by a physician or a nurse and is documented in the patient's medical record. In the ambulatory or community setting, the pharmacist may obtain the health history. For the pharmacist, the primary purpose of the health history is to evaluate the patient's drug therapy (e.g., screening for abnormal symptoms that may be caused by medications).

The patient usually provides his or her own health history. If the patient cannot provide reliable information, however, then a family member, friend, caregiver, or interpreter can be used as the source.

Patient Demographics

Patient demographics include the patient's name, address, phone number, birthdate, sex, race, marital status, and pharmacy. Other items that may be included are the patient's birthplace, ethnic origin, and occupation.

Chief Complaint

The **chief complaint (CC)** is a brief statement of why the patient is seeking care. Typically, it includes one or two primary symptoms, along with their duration, and is recorded in the patient's own words. The best way to elicit the CC is by using an open-ended question (e.g., "What can I do for you today?")

Occasionally, the patient may not have a CC. For example, the patient may be unable to speak (e.g., comatose or a stroke), in which case a family member may be able to describe the patient's problems. The patient also may present to the pharmacist for a medication refill and not identify any particular medical problems; however, on review of the patient's medication profile, the pharmacist may identify a drug-related problem and then question the patient regarding specific symptoms. Through this process, a hidden CC may be discovered.

History of Present Illness

The **history of present illness (HPI)** is a thorough description and expansion of the CC. Specific characteristics should be obtained regarding all the presenting symptoms. These characteristics include:

- Timing: onset, duration, and frequency of symptoms.
- Location: precise area of symptoms.
- Quality or character: specific descriptive terms of symptoms (e.g., sharp pain, black tarry stools).
- Quantity or severity: mild, moderate, or severe.
- Setting: what the patient was doing when the symptoms occurred.
- Aggravating and relieving factors: things that cause or make the symptoms worse and that relieve or make the symptoms better.
- Associated symptoms: other symptoms that occur with the primary symptoms.

The description of the patient's symptoms is recorded in a precise and chronologic sequence. Enough details regarding symptoms need to be obtained, without being excessive and redundant, to evaluate the patient appropriately. In addition, the HPI should include any pertinent "negative" information, which includes secondary symptoms that the patient is *not* experiencing (e.g., patient has a sore throat, stuffy nose, and sneezing but does not have a fever or productive cough).

Past Medical History

The **past medical history (PMH)** includes a brief description of the patient's past medical problems, which may or may not relate to the patient's current medical condition. Hospitalizations, surgical procedures, accidents, injuries, and obstetrical history (for women) also are included, along with the approximate dates and duration (if known). A common abbreviation used in the PMH is S/P, which stands for *S*tatus *P*ost and indicates a past event. For example, a documentation in the PMH might be "S/P hysterectomy in 1987," meaning that the patient had surgery to remove her uterus in 1987.

Family History

The family history is a brief synopsis of the presence or absence of illnesses in the patient's first-degree relatives (i.e., parents, siblings, and children). These data typically include status (i.e., dead or alive), cause of death, age at death, and current health problems of living family members. Specifically, a family history of heart disease, high blood pressure, high cholesterol, diabetes, cancer, osteoporosis, alcoholism, and mental illness should be documented, because it may affect the patient's risk of future illnesses or influence the physician's diagnosis of the patient's current medical problem.

Common abbreviations found in the family history include F for *F*ather, M for *M*other, B for *B*rother, and S for *S*ister. A deceased family member can be indicated with an arrow pointing down (↓) and a living family member with an arrow pointing up (↑). For example, a patient's father who died from a cerebral vascular accident (i.e., stroke) at the age of 67 years can be documented as F↓67(CVA).

Social History

The patient's lifestyle is documented in the social history, which contains his or her use of alcohol, tobacco, and illicit drugs as well as nutrition and exercise. The patient's education, employment, marital status, and living conditions also may be included.

Alcohol consumption is documented as the type, amount, pattern, and duration of alcohol use (e.g., a six-pack of beer daily for 10 years). To describe the drinking habits of patients who drink only when dining out or at social gatherings, the term *social drinking* is sometimes used. This term is open to wide interpretation, however, and should be clarified regarding the specific type, amount, pattern, and duration of alcohol ingestion. For patients who drink regularly, the date and time of the last drink also should be documented.

Tobacco use is quantified by the type of tobacco consumed (i.e., cigarettes, cigars, pipe, or chewing tobacco), number of packs smoked per day (ppd), and pack-years. A *pack-year* is calculated by multiplying the number of packs smoked per day by the number of years that the patient has been smoking. For example, a 20 pack-year smoking history may mean that the patient has smoked 1 ppd for 20 years or 2 ppd for 10 years. Because a given pack-year measurement can include a wide variation in actual smoking habits, the pharmacist should record both the pack-year and the packs per day (e.g., "20 pack-year smoking history, 2 ppd for 10 years").

A history of illicit drug use, also known as recreational or street drugs, may be difficult to obtain from the patient. The pharmacist should use professional, nonjudgmental communication techniques when asking these questions. As with alcohol and tobacco use, illicit drug use also is documented as the type, amount, pattern, and duration of use. The date of the last drug use also should be recorded.

The patient's dietary and exercise habits are particularly useful information if he or she is at high risk of developing heart disease, because a high-fat diet and sedentary lifestyle can contribute to obesity, high cholesterol, diabetes, and hypertension. The number of meals and snacks typically consumed on a daily basis, as well as the type and quantity of food, should be documented. In particular, the percentage of red meat, fat, fiber, and salt consumed on a daily basis should be obtained. Exercise should be recorded as the type, frequency, and duration of activity.

Information regarding the patient's education, employment, marital status, and living conditions is important as well, because these factors can influence the patient's health and medication use. The pharmacist should consider these factors for both diagnostic decision-making and pharmacotherapeutic planning. For example, an unemployed patient may be at high risk for noncompliance if he or she cannot afford an expensive medication.

Review of Systems

The **review of systems (ROS)** is a general description of patient symptoms per body system. The questions to elicit this information typically are closed-ended and ask about the occurrence of common symptoms regarding each system. The order of questioning typically follows a head-to-toe format. The purpose of the ROS is to identify any additional symptoms or medical problems not yet revealed by the patient during the the CC, HPI, or PMH. Both the presence and the absence of symptoms should be noted. The most common symptoms for each body system are:

- General health: fatigue, weakness, fever, and significant weight gain or loss.
- Skin, hair, and nails: changes in color, lesions, dryness, hair loss, and changes in nail texture.
- Eyes: changes in vision, use of glasses, cataracts, and glaucoma.
- Ears: changes in hearing, ringing in the ears, and vertigo.

- Nose and throat: nasal discharge or stuffiness, sneezing, sore throat, and difficulty swallowing.
- Head and neck: lumps or swelling, tenderness, and pain with movement.
- Respiratory system: difficulty breathing, cough, and wheezing.
- Cardiovascular system: chest pain, palpitations, high blood pressure, and high cholesterol.
- Peripheral vascular system: edema, leg pain when walking, and discoloration of lower legs, ankles, or feet.
- Gastrointestinal system: nausea, vomiting, abdominal pain, heartburn, poor appetite, constipation, diarrhea, and change in stool color.
- Hepatic system: nausea, loss of appetite, protruding abdomen, and yellowish eye or skin color.
- Renal system: changes in urination, frequency, urgency, blood in urine, painful urination, incontinence, and frequent urination at night.
- Musculoskeletal system: cramping, pain, stiffness, swelling, and limitation of movement.
- Nervous system: tremors, seizures, imbalance, and paralysis.
- Mental status: anxiety, disorientation, changes in memory, hallucinations, and changes in mood.
- Endocrine system: diabetes and thyroid disease.
- Male reproductive system: problems with sexual function, painful intercourse, genital pain, lesions, and lumps.
- Female reproductive system: menstrual problems, vaginal discharge, vaginal itching, breast tenderness, lumps, dimpling, and discharge.

More detailed questioning is discussed within the chapters for each body system in Part 2 of this book.

Identification of abnormal symptoms through the ROS will lead the practitioner to further patient evaluation during the physical examination, laboratory testing, and diagnostic testing.

MEDICATION HISTORY

In the past, physicians or nurses typically have obtained the medication history, because they have a high amount of direct involvement in patient care. Unfortunately, these medication histories can be incomplete (e.g., lack information concerning allergies, adverse effects, and compliance). Because pharmacists are becoming more involved with direct patient care via pharmaceutical care responsibilities, the medication history now is being obtained increasingly by the pharmacist. Information obtained through the medication history is vital to the pharmacist's evaluation of the effectiveness and tolerability of the patient's medication regimen. The medication history identifies not only what medications the patient is taking but also the patient's compliance, adverse drug reactions, allergies, and understanding of the role the medication plays in treating his or her disease. Data that should be obtained by the pharmacist for the medication history include current and past prescription and nonprescription medications, allergies, adverse drug reactions, and medication compliance.

Current Prescription Medications

The pharmacist should ask the patient what prescription medications he or she is currently taking. In addition to the names of these medications, obtain the dosage, dosing schedule, duration of therapy, reason for taking the medicine, and outcome of therapy. It is best to use an open-ended question to elicit the most accurate patient information. A leading question (e.g., "You're taking captopril, 25 mg three times a day, right, Mrs. Smith?") may encourage the patient to say yes rather than risk embarrassment by admitting that she stopped taking the medication several weeks ago because she ran out.

Some patients may not know the names of their current medications. If this happens, have the patient describe what the medicine looks like, with as much detail as possible. This description should include the dosage form; the size, shape, and color; and the numbers, letters, or words on the dosage form. When documenting this information, the pharmacist should include the patient's detailed description and, if a list of prescribed medications is available, note if it is consistent with the medication that he or she should be taking.

The pharmacist also must obtain the prescribed dosing schedule (e.g., twice a day, once a day), the actual dosing schedule the patient uses, and the approximate times at which the patient takes the medication. If the patient is not taking the medication as prescribed (e.g., the patient takes the medication once a day when it should be three times a day), determine the reason for this discrepancy. Both the prescribed and the actual dosing schedules should be documented along with the reason for future assessment of the patient's medication compliance.

If the patient is taking a "prn" medication on an "as needed" basis, it is important to quantify how often the patient actually takes the medication, because the term *occasionally* could mean one dose a day—or one dose a month. One way to obtain this information is to ask the patient how many doses he or she consumes in a day, a week, or a month. Asking the patient how often he or she has to obtain a new supply of medication may be useful as well.

The pharmacist also should determine when the patient started taking the medication, the reason for taking it, and the outcome of taking it from the patient's perspective. If possible, the exact starting date should be identified, especially if an adverse or allergic reaction is thought to be caused by a particular medication. It is important to obtain the patient's reason for taking the medication as well, because some patients may misunderstand—or not even know—why it was prescribed. Consequently, the patient may take the medication for problems or conditions not treated with that particular medication. In addition, the pharmacist should assess the patient's opinion of how well the medication is treating or controlling the specific condition.

Current Nonprescription Medications

Because nonprescription medications can interact with prescription medications, cause adverse reactions, and be used by patients to treat an adverse reaction caused by a prescription medication, the pharmacist should obtain information concerning any nonprescription medications, including herbal products and vitamins, that the patient may be taking. This information should include the drug name and dosage, actual dosing schedule, duration of therapy, reason for taking the drug, and outcome of therapy. Because many nonprescription medications are taken on a "prn" or "as needed" basis, always quantify the exact use of the medication. Asking how many times in a day, a week, or a month the patient takes the medication, or how often the patient must purchase a new supply, may help the pharmacist to quantify drug usage.

Past Prescription and Nonprescription Medications

Before making current recommendations, the pharmacist should obtain as much information as possible concerning past prescription and nonprescription medications. This information includes the name, dosage, and prescribed as well as actual dosing schedule of the drug, the reason for taking the medication, the duration and outcome of therapy, and why the patient stopped taking it. This information helps the pharmacist to understand what medications successfully (and unsuccessfully) treated past as well as current medical problems.

Allergies

An **allergic reaction** is a hypersensitivity to a particular antigen or allergen, which provokes characteristic symptoms whenever it is encountered. To prevent the recurrence of an allergic reaction, the pharmacist should ask if the patient has allergies to any medication or food (e.g., some vaccines are derived from egg products). Because an adverse drug reaction can be identified mistakenly as an allergy, it is very important to ask the patient what type of reaction was experienced (e.g., rash, breathing problems, etc.). If a drug allergy is identified, the pharmacist should ask the patient the date of the reaction, what was used to treat it, the outcome of the treatment, and whether the patient experiences a reaction with other medications from similar drug classes.

Adverse Drug Reactions

Unlike an allergic reaction, an **adverse drug reaction,** which also commonly is termed a *side effect,* is an unwanted pharmacologic effect that is associated with the medication. One way to elicit information regarding possible current and past adverse drug reactions is to ask whether the patient has ever taken medication that made him or her feel "sick" or that he or she would rather not have taken. Some patients may not associate the symptoms they experience with the medications they are taking (e.g., a cough with angiotensin-converting enzyme inhibitors). Thus, asking whether the patient has experienced a certain side effect that is commonly associated with the medication is helpful. If an adverse drug reaction is identified, the pharmacist should obtain the name of the medication, the dosage, the frequency, the reason for taking the medication, the details of the adverse reaction, and how the adverse reaction was managed (e.g., dosage was decreased, drug was discontinued).

Medication Compliance

Determining patient medication compliance or adherence is one of the primary goals of the medication history. Noncompliance with medications may lead to worsening of patient symptoms, unnecessary diagnostic testing, hospitalizations, and use of additional medications, especially if the noncompliance is not identified and the physician believes the patient is taking the medications as prescribed.

Questioning the patient regarding compliance can be difficult, because most patients know they should be compliant and may feel guilty or ashamed if confronted on this subject by an authoritative health care professional. Some patients may say they are compliant even when they are not. Therefore, the pharmacist should use open-ended questions to find out exactly what medications the patient is taking and how often he or she is taking them. Again, be careful to avoid asking leading questions in which the patient only has to answer yes (e.g., "Mr. Smith, you are taking metoprolol, 100 mg twice a day, aren't you?"). To establish and maintain a good rapport with the patient, it is extremely important for the pharmacist to remain nonjudgmental when questioning the patient regarding compliance. A nonjudgmental attitude encourages the patient to trust the pharmacist, which allows him or her to be more truthful about adherence to the prescribed medication regimen.

Another way to assess compliance is to have patients describe their daily routine for taking their medications. Patients who describe their routine with great detail are more likely to be compliant than those who provide a very vague description or have no routine at all. Empathic statements also may help the pharmacist to obtain more information concerning compliance; such statements may include acknowledging that a medication regimen can be difficult to follow, that it is easy to forget to take medications, and that medications are costly when following a tight budget. If noncompliance is identified, the pharmacist should determine the reason for the noncompliance so that it can be corrected, if possible (e.g., the patient cannot afford an expensive antihypertensive medication, so the pharmacist recommends a more economical alternative to the physician).

Medication compliance also can be assessed by asking the patient how often he or she needs to refill the medication or how long a single bottle of medicine usually lasts before a new supply is needed. If the patient's computerized pharmacy records are accessible, the pharmacist also may review the refill pattern of the patient.

Documentation of the Medication History

The details of the medication history need to be documented in the patient's medical record and communicated to the health care team. Some institutions use a standardized form (Fig. 3-2), but the information may be recorded in a free-text format as well. The standardized form is well-organized, easy to record, and allows specific patient information to be found quickly; however, it does not provide flexibility or needed space for patients who may be taking a large number of medications. In contrast, a free-text format allows a great deal of flexibility from pharmacist to pharmacist, but it also makes it much more diffi-

Patient: *Michael Smith* Date: *10/12/99*

Date of Admission: *10/11/99* Room: *1234* I.D. Number: *123456789*

Address: *9999 Snowy Road*
Anytown, NE 11111 Phone: *555-0000*

Pharmacy: *Bob's Pharmacy* Insurance: *none*

DOB: *4-21-30* Gender: *M* Height: *6'* Weight: *180 lbs*

Current Prescription Medications

Generic (trade) name	Dose	Schedule	Indication	Start Date	Adverse Effects	Compliance
Furosemide (Lasix)	*40 mg*	*Q a.m.*	*leg swelling*	*2/'97*	*none*	*yes*
Captopril (Capoten)	*25 mg*	*TID*	*heart*	*2/'97*	*cough*	*forgets 1/d*
Digoxin (Lanoxin)	*0.125 mg*	*Q a.m.*	*heart*	*'95*	*none*	*yes*
Metformin (Glucophage)	*850 mg*	*TID*	*blood sugar*	*5/'96*	*bloating*	*forgets 1/d*

Current Nonprescription Medications (including herbal and vitamin products)

Generic (trade) name	Dose	Schedule	Indication	Start Date	Adverse Effects	Compliance
Acetaminophen (Tylenol)	*500 mg*	*2 prn (1-2x/wk)*	*pain*	*'80s*	*none*	*yes*
Milk of magnesia	*2 TBS*	*prn (2-3x/mn)*	*constipation*	*'90s*	*none*	*yes*
Ginkgo	*1 tab*	*before meals*		*?*	*none*	*takes PRN*

Past Prescription Medications

Generic (trade) name	Dose	Schedule	Indication	Start Date	Stop Date	Adverse Effects	Treatment
Hydrochlorothiazide	*50mg*	*Q a.m.*	*leg swelling*	*'94*	*2/'97*	*gout*	*d/c by M.D.*
Glyburide	*10mg*	*Q a.m.*	*blood sugar*	*'94*	*5/'96*	*none*	*d/c by M.D.*

Past Nonprescription Medications

Generic (trade) name	Dose	Schedule	Indication	Start Date	Stop Date	Adverse Effects	Treatment
Ibuprofen (Advil)	*200mg*	*prn (Q a.m.)*	*arthritis*	*80s*	*'80s*	*stomach pain*	*d/c by self*

Allergies

Generic (trade) name	Dose	Schedule	Indication	Start Date	Type of Reaction	Treatment
Penicillin	*250 mg*	*QID*	*infections*	*5/'95*	*rash*	*d/c by M.D.*

Pharmacist: *Jane Doe, Pharm.D.*

FIGURE 3-2. Medication history form.

cult to find specific information. In addition, the free-text format may make it easier for a pharmacist to forget to ask patients for certain information (e.g., allergies) and is more time-consuming to use.

Regardless of the format, all components of the medication history must be included in an organized manner, and handwriting must be neat and legible. If the pharmacist follows these guidelines, good communication with other members of the health care team is more likely to occur.

SPECIAL CONSIDERATIONS

Pediatric Patients

The health and medication history for pediatric patients follows the same format as that for adult patients, but several differences in obtaining the information should be noted. One of the major differences is that the information usually comes from the child's parent or guardian. Because the child may not yet be able to communicate what symptoms he or she is experiencing, the parent may describe a change in the child's behavior in relation to activities, eating, and body posture (e.g., the child is not playing and is tugging at his ear).

In addition to the health history, the pharmacist should ask the parent about the child's growth and development. Is the child's height and weight increasing at a steady rate? Has there been any rapid weight gain or weight loss? The pharmacist also should ask the parent at what age the child's immunizations were administered and if the child had any reactions following them.

Geriatric Patients

The format of the health and medication history for geriatric patients also is similar to that for adult patients; however, elderly patients have unique qualities that the pharmacist should keep in mind. First, these patients frequently have lengthy histories, with several interacting illnesses, and these diseases may present as a general functional decline (e.g., he or she can no longer prepare meals, weight loss) rather than as typical symptoms. Second, because of the normal aging process (e.g., hearing loss), it may be difficult for elderly patients to communicate effectively with the pharmacist. If the patient cannot provide an adequate history, the pharmacist should ask the spouse, child, or caregiver for information. Many elderly patients also may disregard certain symptoms, because they think these symptoms are simply part of "growing old." Thus, elderly patients tend to underreport illness. In addition, elderly persons are more sensitive to adverse effects of medications, and they commonly ask their pharmacist about symptoms that actually may be caused by the medications that he or she is taking. Therefore, the pharmacist should always review the patient's medication history when assessing the patient's symptoms.

Elderly patients are more prone to certain types of medical problems (e.g., falls, malnutrition, incontinence, and noncompliance with taking medications), so the pharmacist should assess the patient's activities of daily living, which are crucial to the older person's ability to live alone. Ask the patient if he or she is able to get out of bed, go to the bathroom, bathe, eat, dress, manage household chores, and take medications independently.

Pregnant Patients

The health and medication history for pregnant patients follows the same format as the adult patient. However, the primary focus should be evaluating the teratogenic (fetal) effect of the medications (prescription and nonprescription) that she is taking.

Self-Assessment Questions

1. What are the most appropriate environmental characteristics for a productive pharmacist–patient communication?
2. When are open-ended versus closed-ended questions appropriate in communicating with a patient?
3. When conducting a health history, what characteristics should be obtained regarding all patient symptoms?
4. When obtaining a medication history, how can the pharmacist evaluate the patient's compliance with medications?

Critical Thinking Questions

1. A patient in your pharmacy complains of stomach pains and thinks that a new medicine is causing it. What questions would you ask the patient to determine if this is correct?
2. A 78-year-old woman with a history of congestive heart failure is admitted to the hospital with complaints of shortness of breath, peripheral edema, and difficulty sleeping at night. She is diagnosed with an exacerbation of her congestive heart failure, and the physician increases her furosemide to 80 mg BID. You suspect that she might have been noncompliant with her medications. What questions would you ask this patient to assess her medication profile?

Bibliography

Cassell EJ, Coulehan JL, Putnam SM. Making good interview skills better. Patient Care 1989;23:145–16.

Coulehan JL, Block JR. The medical interview: mastering skills for clinical practice. 3rd ed. Philadelphia: FA Davis, 1997.

Fields AD. History-taking in the elderly: obtaining useful information. Geriatrics 1991;46(8):26–35.

Kaplan CB, Siegel B, Madill JM, et al. Communication and the medical interview: strategies for learning and teaching, J Gen Intern Med 1997;12(suppl 2):S49–S55.

Kassam R, Farris KB, Cox CE, et al. Tools used to help community pharmacists implement comprehensive pharmaceutical care. J Am Pharm Assoc 1999;39:843–856.

McDonough RP. Interventions to improve patient pharmaceutical care outcomes. J Am Pharm Assoc 1996;NS36:453–464.

McDonough RP. Pharmaceutical care interventions—a closer look, J Am Pharm Assoc 1999;39:703–704.

Morley JE. Aspects of the medical history unique to older persons. JAMA 1993;269:675–678.

Otto BJ. The interview. Nursing 1999;29(8):77.

Tietze KJ. Communication skills for the pharmacist. In: Clinical skills for pharmacists: a patient-focused approach. St. Louis: Mosby–Year Book, 1997:17–38.

Tindall WN, Beardsley RS, Kimberlin CL. Communication skills in pharmacy practice. 3rd ed. Baltimore: Lea & Febiger, 1994.

CHAPTER

4

Principles and Methods of the Basic Physical Examination

Jean DeMartinis

GLOSSARY TERMS

- Auscultation
- Inspection
- Palpation
- Percussion

The complete health assessment of an individual has three major components: the interview and health history, the general survey and measurement of vital signs, and the physical examination, which includes diagnostic evaluation, interpretation of findings and diagnosis, treatment, and follow-up. Typically, pharmacists do not perform a complete physical examination, unlike other health care professionals (i.e., physicians, physician assistants, nurse practitioners). It is important, however, for pharmacists to be familiar with the physical examination in terms of the principles, methods, and data that are obtained, because pharmacists routinely utilize the patient data during pharmaceutical care activities.

This chapter introduces the physical examination, which is the primary objective component of the complete health assessment. Because it is unnecessary for pharmacists to become highly skilled in all physical examination techniques, the discussion within this chapter focuses on the basic principles of the examination, the setting, general methods, and equipment. Finally, special considerations for the physical examination of individuals from special populations (e.g., pediatric, geriatric, and pregnant patients) are discussed.

BASIC PRINCIPLES OF THE PHYSICAL EXAMINATION

The overall objective of the physical examination is to obtain valid information concerning the health status of the patient. The definitive purpose of the physical examination is to identify first the "normal" state and then any variations from that state through validation of the patient's complaints and symptoms, screening of the patient's general well-being, and monitoring of the patient's current health problems. This information becomes part of the patient's medical record, forming a baseline of findings that is updated and added to over time.

As discussed in Chapter 3, the medical record consists of both *subjective* and *objective* information. New subjective information is acquired during the patient interview and from the health history. This information alerts the examiner regarding the areas on which to concentrate during the current examination. Corroborating objective information is then obtained through the physical examination. It is important to note, however, that the dividing line between the patient history and the physical examination is abstract. For example, the objective findings do amplify, verify, and clarify the subjective data that are acquired during the initial inquiry, but at the same time, the physical findings continually stimulate the examiner to ask further questions during the examination.

There are no absolutes when discussing what methods and systems to include in a comprehensive physical examination. The choice depends on the patient's age, symptoms, other physical or laboratory data, and the purpose of the examination itself (e.g., a general screening physical, a work or school physical, or a symptom analysis). A return or follow-up visit is one that is scheduled to assess the progress or resolution of identified abnormalities or problems.

Health assessments have often been thought of as isolated incidents. Today, however, it is widely accepted that age-related health screening/monitoring, if the patient is asymptomatic, should be done on a regular basis. Adolescents (age, 12–19 years) should have a complete physical examination every 2 years. Adults (age, 20–59 years) should have a complete physical examination every 5 to 6 years. Other screening examinations, such as mammography, pap test, stool guaiac, and sigmoidoscopy, should be performed on a more regular basis, as suggested by the American Cancer Society's *Guidelines for Periodic Screening*. Older adults (age, >60 years) should have a complete physical examination every 2 years, including the same compilation of screening examinations.

Because pharmaceutical care includes the prevention of health problems, the pharmacist should routinely ask patients when they had their last physical examination. Such questioning should focus on specific screening and monitoring guidelines (e.g., mammography, pap test, stool guaiac, cholesterol, etc.) The pharmacist should encourage patients to see their physician for a complete physical examination if they have not had one within the last 2 years (for patients >60 years). The pharmacist should educate patients about current screening and monitoring guidelines as well.

Regular screening examinations are important, but in reality, few patient encounters are exclusively for health screening. Most interactions are shaped by the patient's complaints. Examinations performed in response to complaints or symptoms are directed at uncovering or preventing a potential health problem and are a focused interaction. In providing pharmaceutical care, the pharmacist can play a vital role in the focused patient encounter by evaluating and identifying patient complaints and symptoms that are medication-related effects.

METHODS OF ASSESSMENT

Four assessment techniques are universally accepted for use during the physical examination: inspection, palpation, percussion, and auscultation. These techniques are used as an organizing framework to bring the senses of sight, hearing, touch, and smell into focus. Data are accumulated using all these senses simultaneously to form a coherent whole. Together, these techniques are referred to as *observation*, and they should always be accomplished in the order given above, with each technique amplifying the results obtained from the previous one. Two exceptions to this rule, however, are when a patient's age or severity of symptoms demand extemporaneous examination and when the abdomen is being assessed (see Chapter 14).

Inspection

The first step in the examination of a patient is **inspection,** which is the visual looking at and evaluating of a person and is probably the oldest method of assessing patients. As individuals, we "size-up" others each day, forming impressions of them, deciding if we like or dislike them, and generally bonding—or staying away—from them. What we do not realize, however, is that we are performing the age-old practice of inspection.

Formally, the examiner uses the sense of sight to concentrate attention on the thorough, persistent, and unhurried visualization of the patient from the moment of first meeting through obtaining the patient history and, especially, throughout the entire physical examination. Inspection also involves using the senses of hearing and smell to corroborate, illuminate, or validate what the eyes are seeing in relation to any sounds or odors originating from the patient. The examiner catalogues the information received by the senses, both consciously and subconsciously, and forms opinions, both subjective and objective, about the patient that will assist in decision-making regarding diagnoses and treatments. Examiners who have practiced observation for years (i.e., expert observers) report they frequently have intuitive perceptions about patients shortly after "laying eyes on them" concerning what could be the source of their problems. Because inspection is commonly used in day-to-day interactions with patients in various pharmacy settings, it may be the single most important method to master early in practice.

Novice examiners can benefit from consciously practicing observation on a daily basis. Try to view patients, the environment, and patient–environment transactions with a critical eye, as if looking through the lens of a camera and taking mental pictures, to build a database structured around lived experiences. Later, these experiences will trigger subconscious perceptions that may prove to be quite beneficial during assessment of a perplexing or complex patient.

In the pharmacy setting, you will use your power of observation to note the way in which your patient walks, talks, dresses, grooms, and behaves toward you as well as others. You will also look more closely at the patient's body for symmetry and at the trunk or limbs for the presence of lesions and, if present, their color, size, shape, and so on. All this—and more—will come naturally to you over time as you practice "observing" in your daily life.

Palpation

Palpation, which is touching or feeling with the hand, is the second step in the examination of a patient and is used to augment the data gathered through inspection. Palpating individual structures on the surface and within the body cavities, particularly the abdomen, elicits important information regarding the position, size, shape, consistency, and mobility of the normal anatomic components, and it uncovers crucial clues to the presence of abnormalities such as enlarged organs and palpable masses. Palpation also may be effective in assessing fluid within a space.

Figure 4-1 shows the areas of the hands that are used for palpation to discriminate findings. The skilled examiner will use the most sensitive parts of the hand for each type of palpation. The pads of the fingers (i.e., the fingertip to the distal interphalangeal joint) are best used for "general" palpation, because nerve endings specific for the sense of touch are clustered very close together on the pads, thus enhancing discrimination and interpretation of what is being touched. Rough measures of temperature are best assessed with the dorsum of the hand. The position, size, and consistency of a structure may be determined most effectively by using the hands to grasp or to

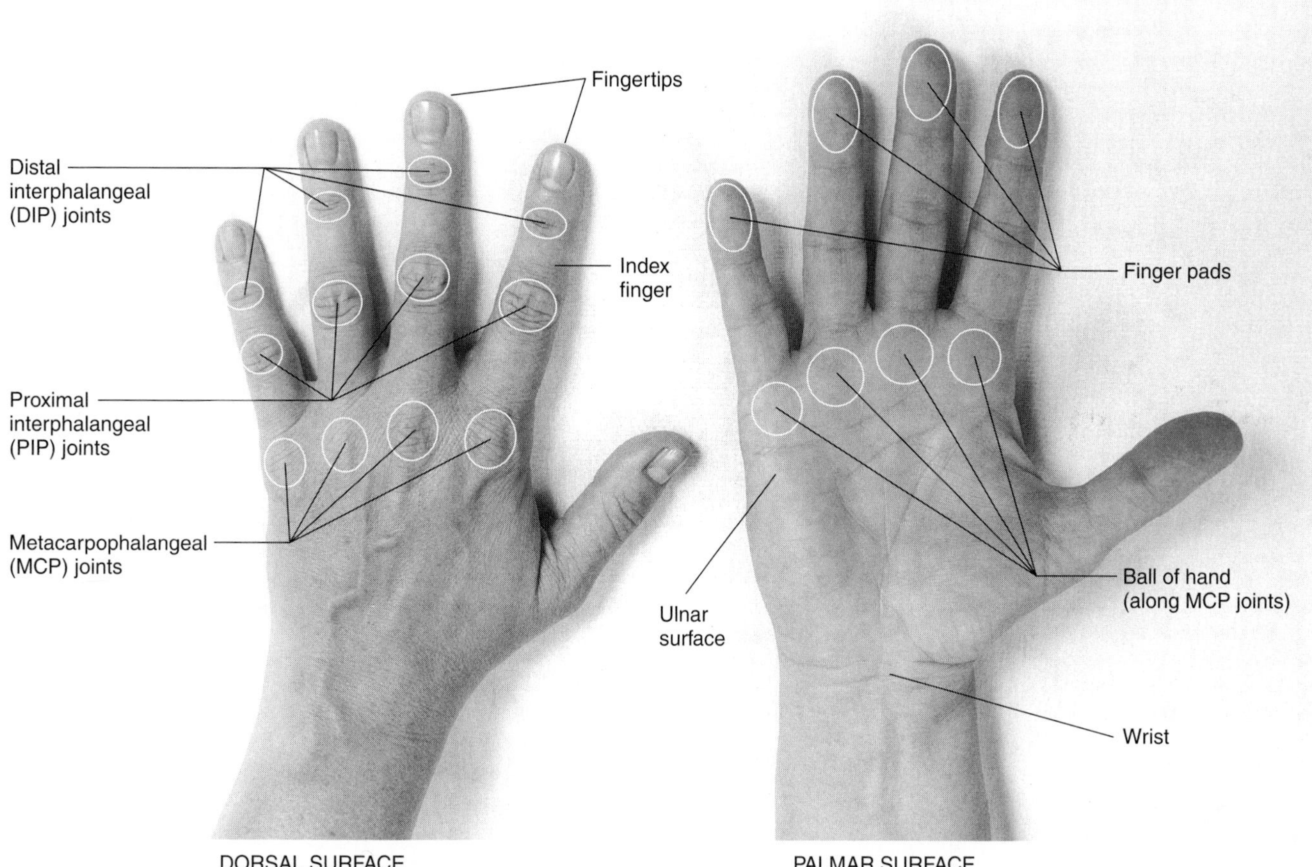

FIGURE 4-1 ■ Areas of the hands used for palpation.

hold. Individual structures within the body cavities, particularly the abdomen, may be palpated for position, size, shape, consistency, and mobility. The examining hand also may be used to detect masses or to evaluate abnormal collections of fluid. Vibration is detected most readily with the palmar surface of the hand, along the bony metacarpophalangeal (MCP) joints or ulnar aspect of the fifth digit from the wrist to the MCP joint. These areas detect vibration well, because sound passes readily through bone. It is most advantageous to use light, medium, and deep palpation for any and all areas being assessed.

Light palpation is always used first, with the strength of palpation advancing as the assessment and the patient's tolerance allow (Fig. 4-2). If you initially palpate too deeply, you will miss surface lesions and may cause unnecessary pain. Light palpation is superficial, gentle, and useful in assessing for lesions on the surface or within muscles. It also serves to relax the patient in preparation for medium and deep palpation. It is performed by pressing the pads of the fingers lightly into the patient's skin, usually in a circular motion.

Medium palpation assesses for mid-level lesions of the peritoneum and for masses, tenderness, pulsations, and pain in most structures of the body. It is performed by pressing the palmar surface of the fingers 1 to 2 cm into the patient's body, again using a circular motion.

Deep palpation assesses organs deep within the body cavities, and it may be performed with one or two hands (Fig. 4-2). In the latter case, the top hand presses the bottom hand down 2 to 4 cm in a circular pattern. Areas of tenderness or discomfort are always palpated last. At times, it may be necessary to cause the patient some discomfort or pain to fully assess a symptom.

Percussion

Percussion, the third step in the examination of a patient, involves striking the body's surface lightly, but sharply, to determine the position, size, and density of the underlying structures as well as to detect fluid or air in a cavity. Striking the surface creates a sound wave that travels 2 to 3 inches (5–7 cm) toward the underlying areas. Sound reverberations assume different characteristics depending on the features of the underlying structures. Table 4-1 describes the quality and character of the sounds elicited by percussion according to the type and density of the tissue and the underlying features. The five percussion notes are identified and characterized as follows:

- *Pitch* (also known as frequency) is the number of vibrations or cycles per second (cps). Rapid vibrations produce a higher-pitched tone, whereas slower vibrations produce a lower-pitched tone.

TABLE 4-1 ➤ PERCUSSION SOUNDS

SOUND	PITCH	INTENSITY	DURATION	QUALITY	LOCATION
Flatness	High	Soft	Short Dullness	Absolute Abnormal: atelectactic lung; dense mass	Normal: sternum, thigh
Dullness	Medium	Medium	Moderate	Muffled thud Abnormal: pleural effusion, ascites	Normal: liver; other organs; full bladder
Resonance	Low	Loud	Moderate/long	Hollow	Normal: lung
Hyperresonance	Very low	Very loud	Long	Booming	Abnormal: emphysematous lung
Tympany	High	Loud	Long	Drum-like Abnormal: air-distended abdomen	Normal: gastric air-bubble

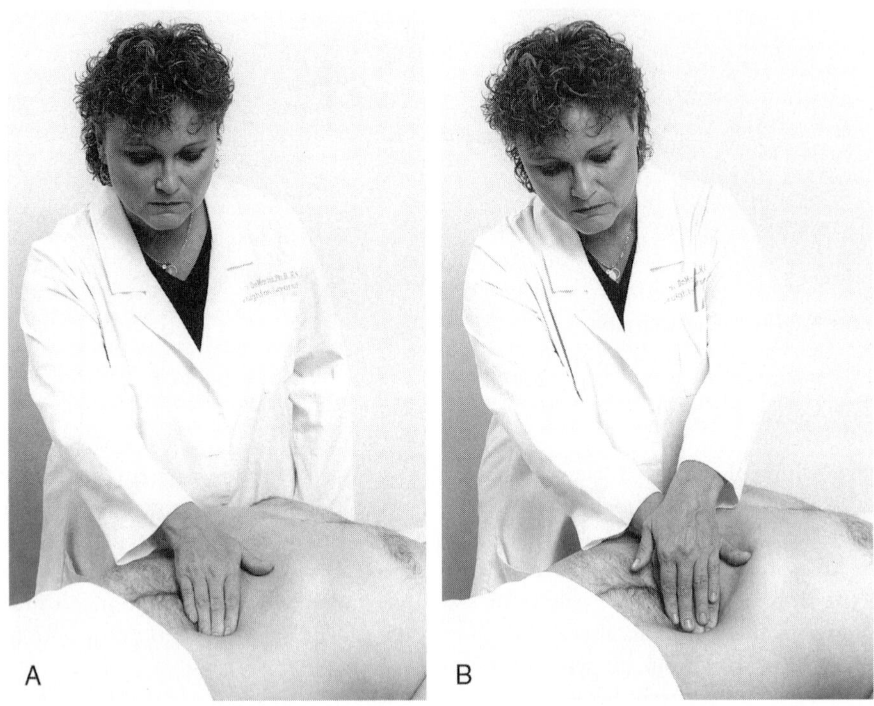

FIGURE 4-2 ■ Techniques used for palpation. **(A)** Light. **(B)** Deep.

- *Amplitude* (also known as intensity) determines the loudness of the sound. The greater the intensity, the louder the sound.
- *Duration* is the length of time that the note lingers.
- *Quality* (also known as timbre, harmonics, or overtone) is a subjective concept used to describe the variance secondary to a sound's distinctive overtones.

A basic principle to understand is that a structure housing more air (e.g., the lungs) produces a louder, lower, longer sound than a denser, more solid structure (e.g., the thigh muscle), which produces a softer, higher, shorter sound. The density of a thick tissue or mass absorbs the sound and blunts the tone, much like acoustic protection absorbs sound in a "soundproof" room.

Direct (i.e., immediate) and indirect (i.e., mediate) are the two methods of percussion. The term *mediate* (indirect) percussion describes the method of using instruments called *pleximeters* and *plessimeters* to invoke a percussion note. Historically, the pleximeter has been small rubber hammer, and it was used to strike a blow against the plessimeter, which is a small, solid object (often made of ivory), that was held firmly against the body's surface. This was the preferred method of percussion for nearly 100 years, but examiners found it cumbersome to carry around the extra equipment. Thus, indirect percussion, using either the index and middle finger or just the middle finger of one hand as the pleximeter, which strikes against the middle finger of the other hand as the plessimeter, has evolved as the current method of choice (Fig. 4-3).

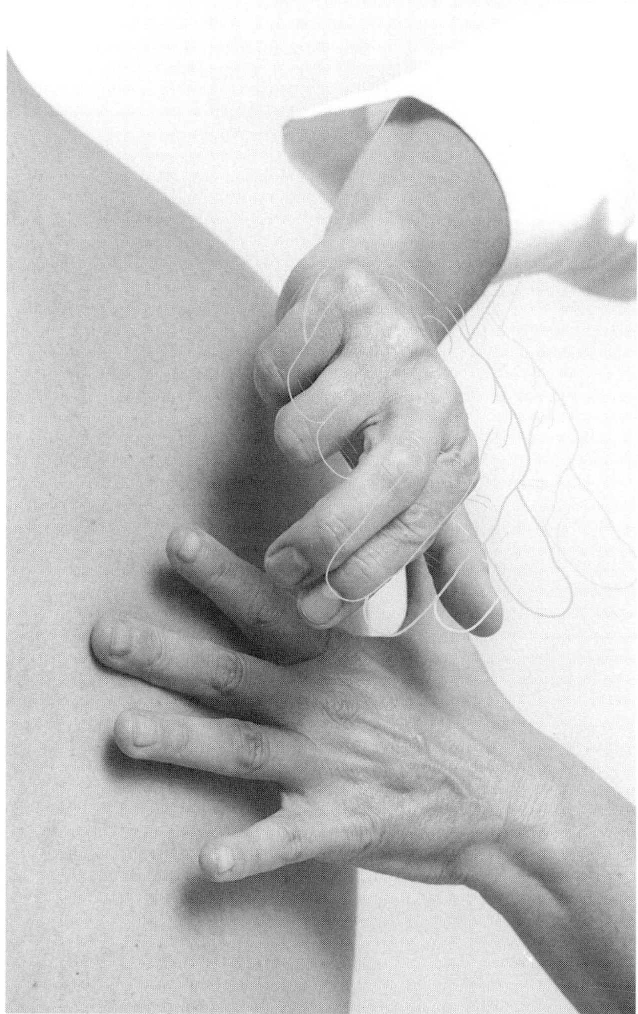

FIGURE 4-3 ■ Indirect finger percussion.

Today, the passive finger (plessimeter) is placed gently and firmly against the body's surface, with the rest of the fingers of that hand slightly raised off the surface of the body to avoid dampening the sound. The pleximeter sharply and crisply, with strong wrist action, strikes the plessimeter between the distal and proximal interphalangeal joints. The hand is flexed back on the forearm and brought forward with a clean, snapping motion that allows a fast strike and rapid removal of the finger, once again so that the sound is not dampened.

Direct and indirect percussion can also be accomplished with the fist (Fig. 4-4). Direct fist percussion involves making a fist with the dominant hand and then striking the body's surface directly. Direct fist percussion may be useful over the posterior thorax, particularly if finger percussion is not successful. During indirect fist percussion, the plessimeter becomes the opposite (or passive) hand, which is placed firmly on the body while the pleximeter (the fist of the dominant hand) does the striking. Both methods of fist percussion are useful in assessing, for example, costovertebral angle tenderness of the kidneys.

Auscultation

Auscultation is the skill of listening to body sounds created in the lungs, heart, blood vessels, and abdominal viscera. Generally, auscultation is the last technique used during the examination. The sounds of particular importance that are heard during auscultation are those that are produced by the movement of air in the lungs, by the thoracic and abdominal viscera, and by the flow of blood through the cardiovascular system. Auscultated sounds are described in terms of frequency (pitch), intensity (loudness), duration, quality (timbre), and timing. Examiners auscultate for heart sounds, blood pressure sounds (i.e., Karotkoff sounds), airflow through the lungs, bowel sounds, and organ sounds.

Auscultation is completed with a stethoscope (Fig. 4-5). Regular stethoscopes do not amplify sound. Instead, they channel sound through an endpiece, tubing, and earpieces to the ear, curtailing any external distraction and thereby singling out and augmenting the sound. Special stethoscopes that do amplify sound, however, are available for examiners with decreased auditory acuity. Regardless, fit and quality of a stethoscope are important. Earpieces must be placed forward into the ears, and the tubing should be no longer than 12 to 18 inches.

The endpiece should have both a diaphragm and a bell (Fig. 4-5). The diaphragm is used to amplify high-pitched sounds, such as the breath sounds heard across the lungs and the bowel sounds heard over the abdomen and when listening to regular heart sounds (S_1 and S_2). The bell is reserved for low-pitched sounds and amplifies exceptionally those sounds made by heart murmurs, arterial (bruits) or venous (hums) turbulence, and organ friction rubs. Because blood flow is a low-pitched sound, the bell is also used when measuring blood pressure; however, proper placement of the bell can be very difficult in some patients. Thus, the diaphragm is also commonly used to measure blood pressure.

Many examiners, both novices and experts alike, tend to place the stethoscope on the chest as soon as the patient has undressed and without having percussed the patient first. If this poor practice becomes habit, then the examiner is sure to miss important clues regarding symptom analysis. It is essential to follow the methods of assessment and to restrain from auscultating the patient until endeavors to evoke responses with the other three methods have been exhausted. (As discussed previously, assessment of the abdomen is the only true exception to this rule. Auscultation of the abdomen must precede palpation and percussion; otherwise, mechanical sounds created in the abdomen from pushing around the bowel contents may produce false "bowel sounds.")

Auscultation is a skill that is easy to learn but difficult to master. First, the wide range of normal sounds must be adequately learned before abnormal and extra sounds can be distinguished. When using the stethoscope, reduce external and extemporaneous artifacts or distracting sounds. Closing your mouth and, once the endpiece is in place, then closing your eyes and concentrating helps immeasurably. By doing this, you eliminate sound transmitted through the open mouth, which can function rather like a megaphone, and distractions created from continuous visual stimulation.

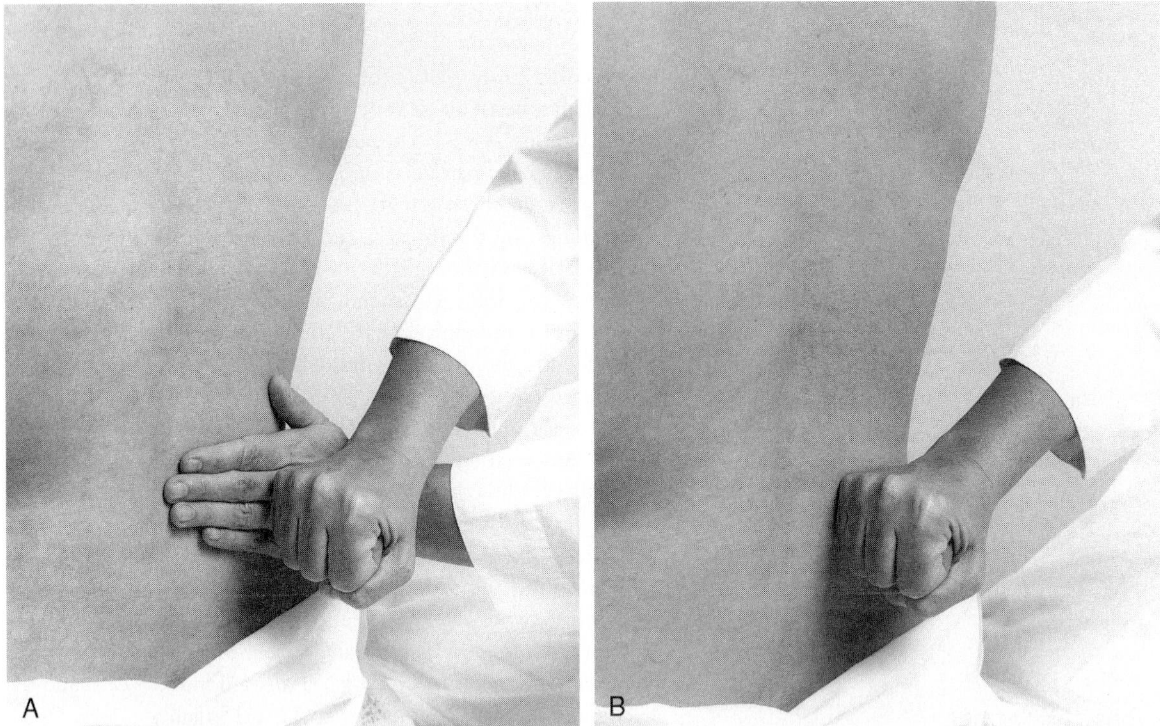

FIGURE 4-4 ■ Fist percussion. **(A)** Indirect percussion over the costovertebral angle (CVA) area. **(B)** Direct percussion over the CVA area.

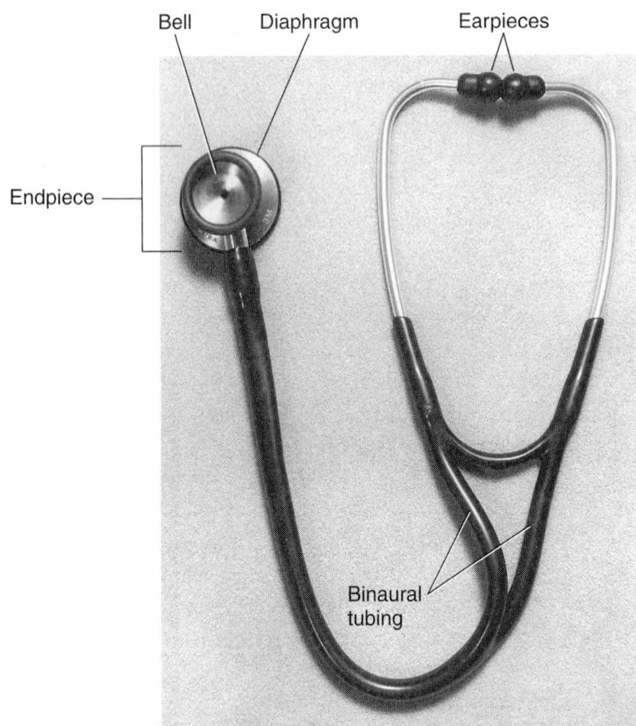

FIGURE 4-5 ■ Binaural stethoscope.

PREPARING FOR THE EXAMINATION

For an efficient and smooth patient interaction, it is important that the examiner prepare before the encounter. Important steps in this preparation include gathering the equipment, preparing the setting, and ensuring the patient's safety.

Gathering the Equipment

The equipment necessary for a comprehensive physical examination performed by a general practitioner is shown in Figure 4-6. It will never be necessary for the pharmacist to use all the equipment shown; nevertheless, it is beneficial to be aware of and familiar with the general equipment used for a complete physical examination. The instruments necessary for a comprehensive physical examination are:

- Penlight or flashlight to check skin and pupillary response to light and to use as a tangential light source to view across the chest and abdomen from the side.
- Ruler or tape measure, preferably marked in centimeters, to measure the size of moles or other skin abnormalities, abdomen girth, fundal height, and circumference of extremities.
- Gloves and a mask with shield or safety goggles to comply with Centers for Disease Control (CDC) guidelines as the situation warrants.
- Otoscope and ophthalmoscope to examine the ears and eyes. (If the otoscope does not include a short, wide speculum, then a nasal speculum is required.)

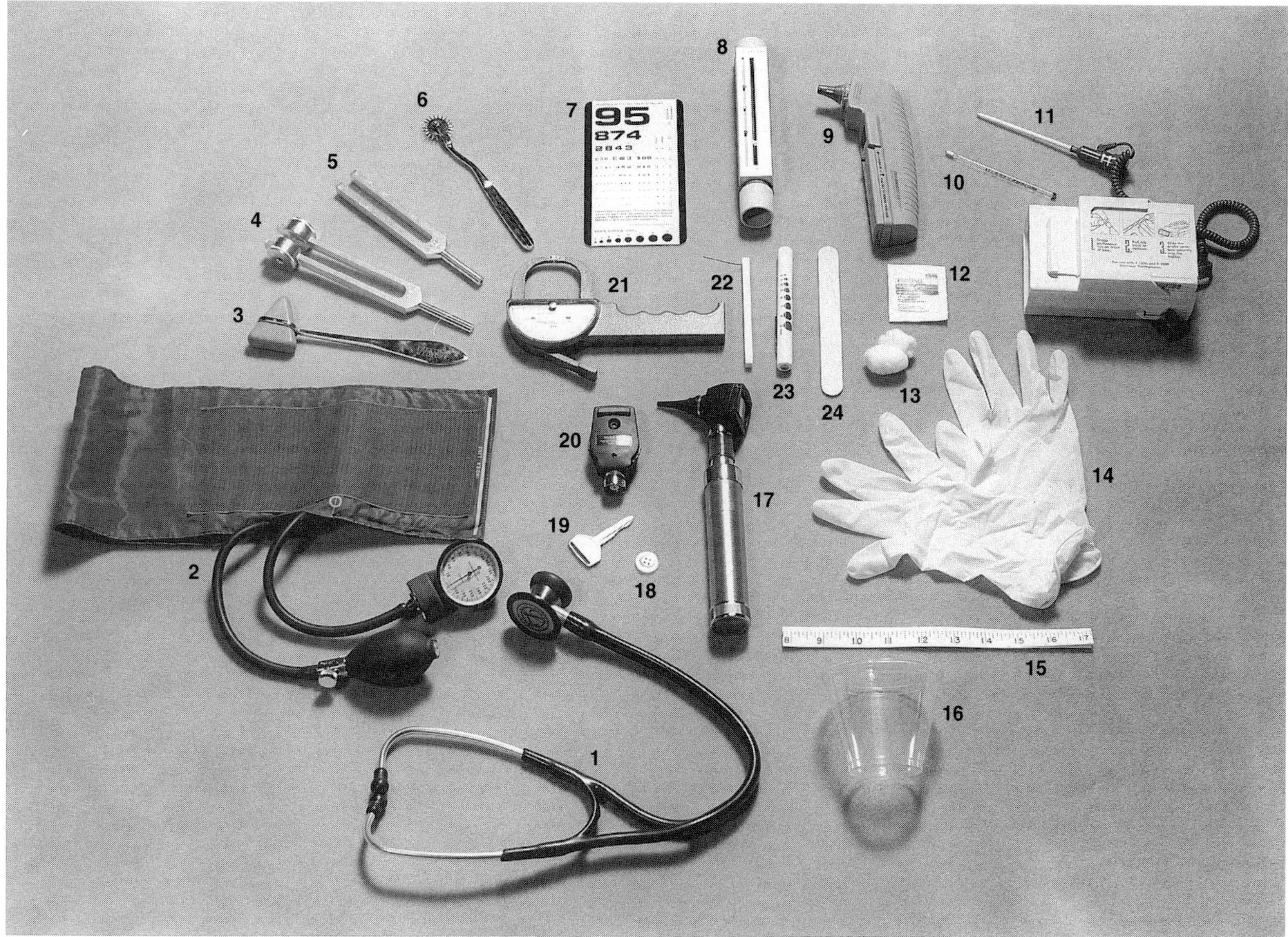

FIGURE 4-6 ■ Equipment used during a comprehensive physical examination: 1, stethoscope; 2, sphygmomanometer; 3, reflex hammer; 4, tuning fork; 5, tuning fork; 6, sensory examination wheel; 7, pocket vision-screening chart; 8, peak flow meter; 9, tympanic membrane thermometer; 10, mercury thermometer; 11, electronic thermometer; 12, alcohol pad; 13, cotton balls; 14, disposable gloves; 15, tape measure; 16, specimen cup; 17, otoscope; 18, button (dull object for sensory examination); 19, key (sharp object for sensory examination); 20, ophthalmoscope endpiece (may be exchanged with the otoscope endpiece); 21, triceps skinfold caliper; 22, monofilament; 23, penlight; 24, tongue depressor.

- Tongue depressor to move or to hold the tongue out of the way as the oropharynx is viewed.
- Stethoscope (with bell and diaphragm endpieces) to auscultate the lungs, heart, and bowels.
- Reflex hammer to assess deep tendon reflexes.
- Various items to test cranial nerves (e.g., coins, pins, buttons, etc.), if applicable.

Additional instruments necessary for the assessment of vital signs (as discussed in Chapter 5) include:

- Thermometer to assess temperature.
- Sphygmomanometer to assess blood pressure.
- Watch with a second-hand or comparable digital screen to assess heart rate and respiration.
- Scale to measure the patient's weight.

Most of the equipment is listed above. Because you must be prepared to conduct a focused examination without interruption, you should have the basic equipment (e.g., sphygmomanometer and stethoscope) readily available in the room and at easy reach. Careful and consistent arrangement of the instruments before beginning will enhance the effectiveness and efficiency of the examination and ensure that the proper sequence of the examination is maintained.

Preparing the Setting

A separate examination room or area with adequate screening should be provided to ensure privacy and confidentiality. The room should be comfortably warm. Good lighting and a quiet environment are important, although sometimes remarkably difficult, to achieve. An effort to effect optimal lighting from either daylight or an artificial source is essential. If overhead fluorescent lighting is the best light source available, then tangential or side lighting also must be used. This is because fluorescent lighting eliminates most surface shadows, which is good if you are working at a desk but hampers your ability to visualize the body's surface characteristics. Using a tangential light source is

Box 4-1

STANDARD PRECAUTIONS FOR INFECTION CONTROL

- Wash hands thoroughly before beginning the examination and after the examination has been completed (before leaving the room).
- If cuts, abrasions, or other lesions are present on the hand(s), wear gloves to protect the patient.
- Routinely wear gloves when contact with bodily fluids is likely:
  - During oral examination.
  - When examining skin lesions.
  - When collecting specimens.
  - When contact with contaminated or soiled surfaces or equipment is necessary.
- Change gloves between tasks and procedures:
  - If wearing gloves, wash hands immediately after the gloves are removed and between patient contacts.
  - Wear mask and eye protection/face shield and/or gown to protect the skin, mucous membranes, and clothing if splashes or sprays of bodily fluids are likely.
  - Follow clinic or facility procedures for routine care and disposal of equipment, linen, and so on.
  - Clearly label all specimen containers to indicate the necessary body fluid precautions.

Based on information from the Centers for Disease Control. Recommendations for preventing transmission of human immunodeficiency virus and hepatitis B virus to patients during exposure-prone invasive procedures. AORN-J, 1991;54(3):576–582.

key to achieving a better view of all the body's curving anatomy for any lumps or bumps, pulsations, or skin lesions. A penlight, gooseneck lamp, or flashlight is most often used to visualize across the body.

Ensuring the Patient's Safety

Standard Precautions

During the physical examination, take standard precautions to ensure the patient's—and your own—safety from transmission of blood-borne diseases and to prevent cross-contamination. Bodily fluids considered to be infectious or potentially infectious include saliva, blood, semen, vaginal fluids, cerebrospinal fluid, and amniotic, pericardial, peritoneal, pleural, and synovial fluids. The CDC have established precautionary guidelines that should be followed to help prevent the spread of infectious agents during a physical examination. See Box 4-1 for a review of the standard precautions.

Latex Allergy

In addition to the standard precautions when gathering physical assessment data, other precautions are important to keep in mind, especially because of the recent surprising and significant increase in the incidence of serious allergic reactions to natural rubber latex products. Pharmacists, in compliance with standard precautions, frequently wear gloves, so it is important for you to be aware of the potential for developing a latex allergy. Also, your patients are exposed to the latex during the examination and could have an allergic reaction. Latex allergies also can occur through the use of equipment and supplies other than gloves that are made of or include latex. The National Institute for Occupational Safety and Health has released recommendations for the prevention of natural rubber latex allergy. See Box 4-2 for a summary of these recommendations.

THE EXAMINATION

Tips for the Novice Examiner

Most errors in physical assessment and diagnosis do not result from ignorance but, rather, from haste and carelessness. The three most common types of errors that are made by novice examiners are: errors of technique, errors of detection and interpretation, and errors of recording. Thoroughness in performing the examination leads to more correct diagnoses than will following sudden hunches.

Box 4-2

RECOMMENDATIONS FOR LATEX ALLERGY PREVENTION

- Use nonlatex gloves when possible (i.e., if contact with bodily fluids or infectious materials is not likely).
- Use hypoallergenic gloves when possible and feasible, if allergy has already developed, or if the patient has known latex sensitivity or allergy. (These gloves are not latex-free, but they may reduce the potential for an allergic reaction.)
- When using latex gloves, choose a powder-free type to reduce protein content in glove.
  - Do not use oil-based hand creams or lotions unless they have been shown to reduce latex problems.
  - Some individuals have benefited from using a silicone-based foam or liquid skin protectant before donning latex gloves.
- After using latex gloves, immediately and gently wash hands with a mild soap, and dry thoroughly.
- Examiners should apprise themselves and their patients regarding available latex allergy education and training.
- If signs and symptoms of allergy develop, avoid contact with latex products, and seek medical attention from a qualified provider who is experienced in dealing with latex allergy.

Based on information from National Institute of Occupational Safety and Health. Recommendations for the prevention of natural rubber latex allergy. Cincinnati, OH: National Institute of Occupational Safety and Health, 1997.

Memorizing the specific examination routine and learning how to "read" symptoms and to assess findings can eliminate two of the three types of errors. In addition, you can improve quickly by watching others perform examinations, by practicing maneuvers, and by obtaining feedback on your technique. It is also helpful to review the patient's medical record, focusing primarily on previous history and physical examinations. The physical findings and subsequent interpretations made by the medical team and other pharmacists that are included in these records will assist you in seeing what common techniques are related to specific symptoms and what these findings mean to other health care professionals.

Novice examiners are often worried about their technical skill, about forgetting significant steps in the examination sequence, or about missing an important finding secondary to omission or lack of knowledge. Many may be embarrassed about seeing a partially undressed patient or about touching patients. All these fears are natural and common; however, your disposition should overtly demonstrate self-confidence, patience, courtesy, consideration, and gentleness. Your face may spontaneously register surprise, worry, alarm, distaste, or even frustration in certain situations, but try to remain aware of the potential for these emotions to appear and work to avoid showing them. Again, this is a matter of remaining sensitive to the feelings and responses of the patient.

Sequence of and Positioning for the Examination

A cephalocaudal, or head-to-toe, approach is considered by experts to be the most logical and consistent sequence for the physical examination. Following the cephalocaudal sequence, you should choose to progress from the least invasive or intrusive to the more invasive or intrusive techniques. You must become compulsive about the routine of the examination, practicing until a consistent pattern of performing the examination has been learned. Initially, it is essential to practice—and to learn—the most comprehensive examination sequence possible. This will prevent omission of a step, which could lead to potentially vital information being missed. Box 4-3 summarizes the suggested sequence and positions for a logical cephalocaudal physical examination; keep in mind that the sequence listed has been revised for a pharmacist who would be examining the patient.

In addition, Figure 4-7 depicts the positions described in Box 4-3 and shows other positions commonly used to assess the different body parts. The most common positions that a pharmacist examiner will use include the seated, Fowler's, semi-Fowler's, supine, side-lying, and standing positions. While assisting the patient into the most appropriate positions for best assessing the selected areas of the body, keep in mind that you should aid the patient to also become as physically relaxed as possible. Awkward positioning, improper technique, or a tense patient contaminates the findings and skews your perceptions. Plan the cephalocaudal examination sequence so that the patient is put through a minimum of position changes, both to help protect the patient's energy and to save time.

Box 4-3

SUGGESTED SEQUENCE OF AND POSITIONING FOR COMPLETE PHYSICAL EXAMINATION OF THE ADULT PATIENT[a]

STANDING AND WALKING INTO THE EXAMINATION ROOM

Begin general survey
Complete health history and medication history
Leave room while the patient undresses (if needed), unless the patient requires assistance and a family member is not present

SEATED ON EXAMINATION TABLE

Wash hands
General survey
Vital signs
Skin, hair, nails, and cranium
Head and neck (including assessment of cranial nerves)
Thorax and lungs
Cardiovascular

LYING SUPINE

Finish cardiovascular assessment
Abdomen (gastrointestinal, renal, endocrine)
Begin musculoskeletal and neurological assessment of the extremities

SEATED AGAIN

Finish musculoskeletal and neurological assessment of the extremities
Finish health teaching

STANDING

Finish musculoskeletal examination of the spine and weight bearing joints
Finish neurological examination
Leave the room while the patient dresses, unless assistance is required. Return for final explanations, teaching, prescriptions, and follow-up instructions.

[a]The techniques/sequence of examination have been modified for applicability to the pharmacist examiner. Further modifications regarding exactly which systems to assess and how many of the assessment techniques to employ for each system will depend on the reason for the patient's visit and on his or her condition.

Performing a Comprehensive Physical Examination

A patient typically presents to a physician, physician assistant, or nurse practitioner with a reason for the visit, such as a request for an assessment and interpretation of a symptom or set of symptoms. Alternatively, a patient may request a health-screening physical. The physician will meet the patient in either a

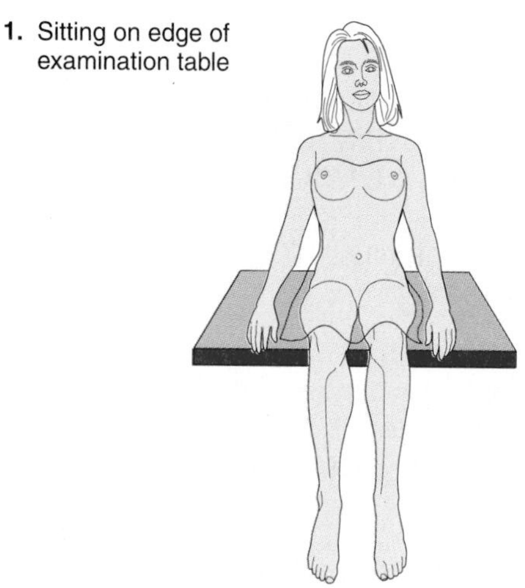

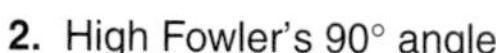

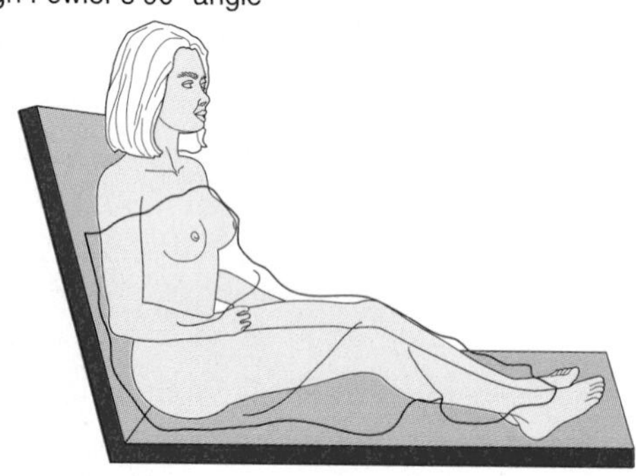

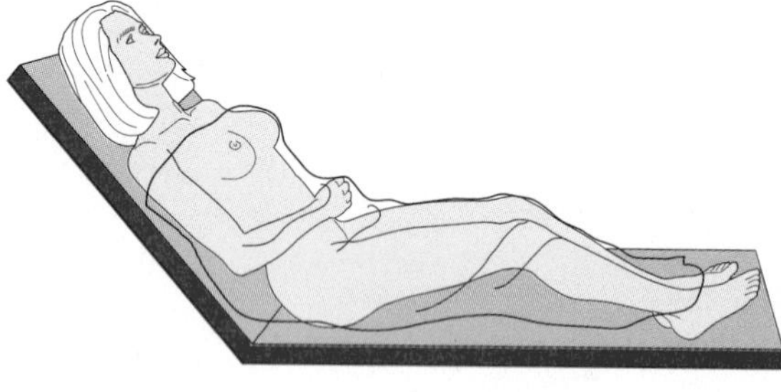

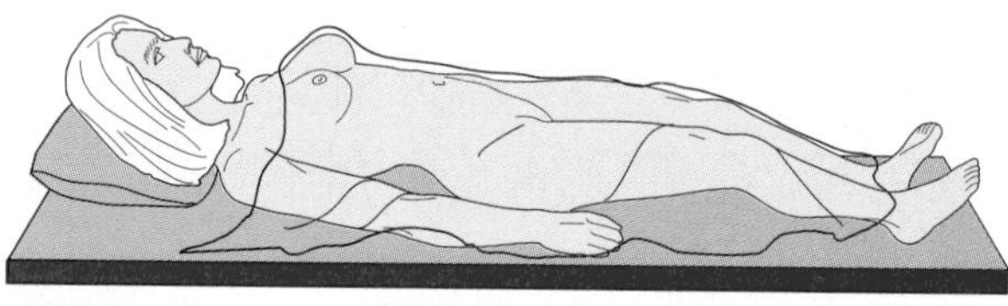

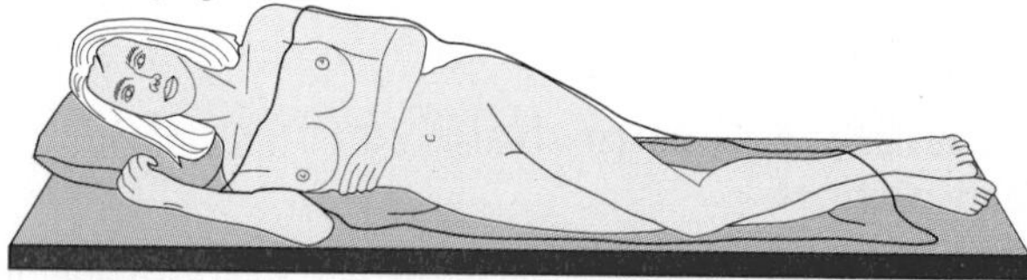

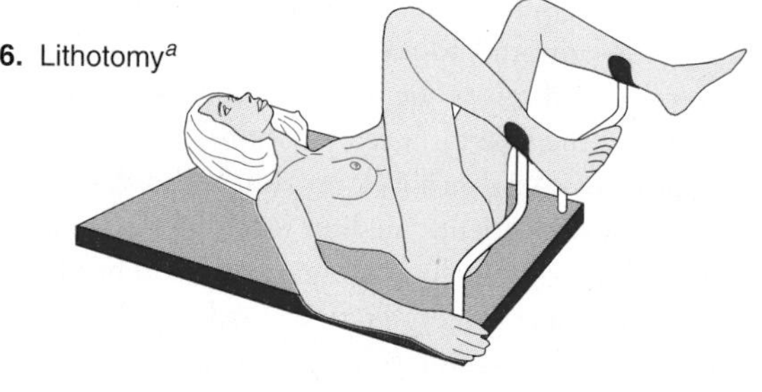

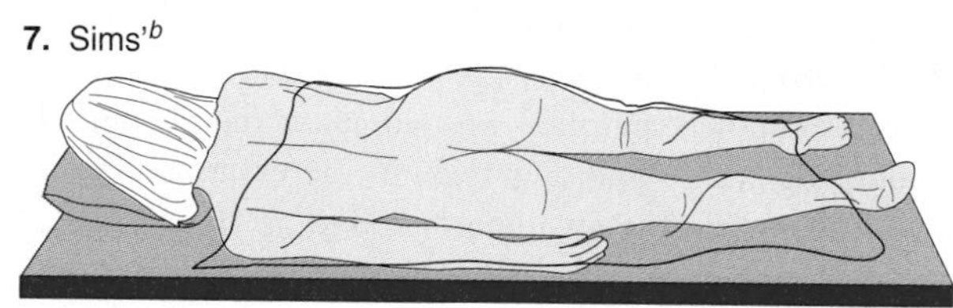

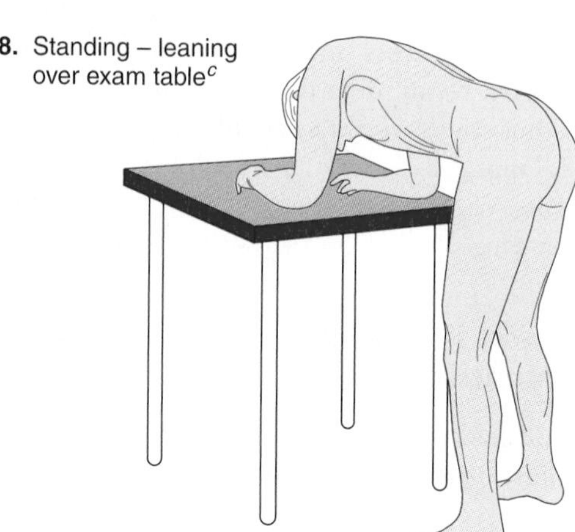

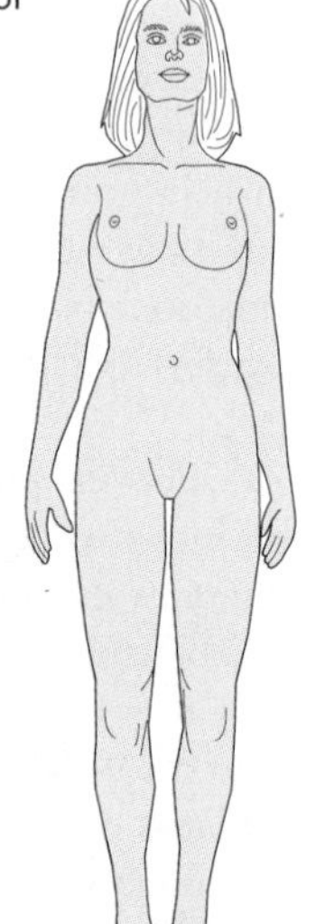

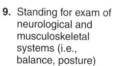

FIGURE 4-7 ■ Most common positions used during the physical examination. [a]For female pelvic and rectal examination, [b]for male rectal/prostate and/or female rectal examination, [c]for male rectal/prostate examination.

clinic (or similar type) room or a hospital room. After the patient history, the vital signs typically are obtained next. This commences the "laying on of the hands" that helps to bridge the gap between talking with the patient and touching the patient during the physical examination. It eases tension, because both the patient and the examiner have a chance to relax and to begin evolving trust. The practitioner should wash his or her hands in the patient's presence if possible. Patients feel better when they see examiners wash their hands, because they perceive it as protection and consideration of their well-being.

The examination begins with the practitioner positioned on or toward the patient's right side. The patient is in the sitting, Fowler's, or semi-Fowler's position, depending on the type of examination table or hospital bed being used and on the patient's condition. Considering patient privacy and modesty, the examiner must be discreet yet fully expose each area to be examined to ensure accurate findings without important omissions. Throughout the entire physical examination, the right and left sides of the body are continually compared while each method of examination is performed.

The examination should proceed in a methodical, slow, and deliberate manner, with the practitioner asking questions—and encouraging the patient to ask questions—to elaborate on evidence given in the health history. The examiner follows the trail of the each change or variation from the "norm" to its end, just as a detective follows every clue in unraveling a mystery. In fact, the methods of the examiner and of the detective are similar in many ways, because the examiner seeks to explain a symptom and the detective to solve a crime.

Each step should be explained as the examination proceeds, giving advance warning if a maneuver may produce discomfort. Brief teaching tips about the patient's body, self-screening methods, signs or symptoms of potential problems, and so on should be provided to the patient. Such sharing of information builds rapport. Remember, however, that when one is nervous, one sometimes becomes nearly mute or overly verbose. Idle chitchat is distracting to the patient and does not build a therapeutic relationship. It may even irritate the patient and shut off further communication. Therefore, you should continually monitor your level of anxiety and concentrate on achieving effective therapeutic communication.

At the end of the examination, summarize the findings, and share the necessary information with the patient. Thank the person for the time spent, and reinforce your teaching regarding medications and home care or follow-up visits.

SPECIAL CONSIDERATIONS

The age of the patient can affect the way in which you should proceed with the examination, especially if the patient is very young or very old.

Pediatric Patients

The physical examination of a child is conducted in an organized and systematic manner, but the preferred cephalocaudal sequence employed with adults should not be expected to be completely successful. For older children and adolescents, the adult examination sequence and methods may work; however, the younger the child, the more probable that an "opportunistic" approach to obtaining vital assessment data will prevail. In other words, the order of the examination may need to be adjusted to accommodate the child's behavior.

Infants are ordinarily less of a challenge, because they are less fearful of strangers, can be distracted while important assessment data are collected, and can be held by the parent for much of the examination. If the infant is asleep or sleepy, then the thorax, lungs, and cardiovascular assessments are completed first, before the infant becomes agitated. If the infant is in an active, playful mood, then an examination of the extremities is performed first. Examination of the head and neck, however, usually causes an infant distress, so this area is assessed last.

Infants closer to 1 year of age, toddlers, and preschoolers are a challenge to even the most experienced examiner. These children have developed, to varying degrees, a normal mistrust of strangers. They may even have had a frightening experience with a health care practitioner and, thus, have developed an intense fear of anyone in an "office" setting or wearing a white coat. For this reason, it is generally helpful to wear plain clothes when interacting with children. Also, it may be advantageous to demonstrate examination techniques on the parent, a doll, or a stuffed animal first. It can be beneficial for the child to play with the equipment and to set the tone of the exam. It is almost always necessary to perform most of the examination while the parent is holding the child; however, the child should not be hampered from getting up and wandering around the examination room. A lot can be assessed while the child is up and about! Otherwise, much data will be missed, and whole systems may have to be omitted from the examination.

For details regarding similarities and differences between the sequencing and techniques of the physical examination for pediatric versus adult patients, refer to the pediatric portion of each chapter in Part 2 of this book.

Geriatric Patients

Assessment of geriatric patients is complicated and, depending on the multiplicity, chronicity, and complexity of underlying physical problems, may be quite time-consuming. The general physical examination is the same as that for adult patients; however, position changes typically are held to a minimum. The room should be kept a little warmer as well, or additional covers may be used. Sometimes, a patient's inability to reach and to hold the optimal positions will require the examiner to assume awkward and uncomfortable positions to complete the assessments adequately.

An elderly patient's energy level and endurance also are observed closely, and the examination typically is tailored accordingly. Older patients may need extra time and assistance with mobility. Furthermore, they may take longer to respond to questions. If a patient does take longer than usual to respond, do not automatically assume that he or she did not hear the question and repeat it louder! Unless the patient has been diagnosed with decreased auditory acuity, you should articulate clearly and in a normal tone of voice. If the patient truly does have decreased auditory acuity, refrain from shouting, because this obscures the consonant sounds and makes it difficult for the patient to understand the communication. Speaking lower in pitch and slightly louder in tone may help.

For details regarding similarities and differences between the sequencing and techniques of the physical examination for geriatric versus adult patients, refer to the geriatric portion of each chapter in Part 2 of this book.

Pregnant Patients

Although pharmacists are not responsible for the examination of pregnant patients, it is important to be aware of the theory and the practice involved. Assessment of pregnant patients builds on the methods learned for nonpregnant patients. A complete physical examination should be performed during the first prenatal visit to establish a current baseline against which changes that occur later during pregnancy can be compared. Also, the first prenatal visit is a key time at which to uncover underlying problems that may affect the pregnancy in particular or the patient's health during the stresses of pregnancy in general.

The initial general physical examination of pregnant patients is the same as that for other adult patients; however, special attention is paid to diagnosis of the pregnancy, assessment of pelvic adequacy, and assessment of fetal growth and well-being. Prenatal assessment always includes an evaluation of both the mother and the developing fetus. After the initial assessment, scheduled re-examinations are performed at regular intervals, which vary according to the mother's condition and fetal development.

For details regarding sequencing and techniques of the physical examination for system assessment of pregnant women, refer to the portion focusing on pregnant patients within each chapter in Part 2 of this book.

Self-Assessment Questions

1. What are the four universally accepted assessment techniques that are used during the physical examination? Briefly describe each one.
2. When physically assessing a patient, what are the standard precautions that you should always follow to prevent the spread of infection?
3. What are the steps in physically assessing a patient following the cephalocaudal approach?
4. What are the key points to keep in mind when physically assessing elderly patients?

Critical Thinking Question

1. You are a pharmacist who is responsible for providing pharmaceutical care to patients in a diabetes clinic. Because diabetes can cause complications that involve various body systems, you routinely perform physical assessments for signs of these complications. RK is a 68-year-old female whom you have worked with for the past 4 years. She is seeing you today for a medication refill and her quarterly diabetes assessment. She typically sees her physician annually for a comprehensive physical examination, and her next appointment is in 6 months. Using the cephalocaudal approach, describe what you would physically examine in this patient.

Bibliography

American Cancer Society. Summary of the American Cancer Society Recommendations for the Early Detection of Cancer in Asymptomatic People. Atlanta, GA: American Cancer Society, 1994.

Barkauskas V, Stoltenberg-Allen K, Baumann L, Darling-Fisher C. Health and physical assessment. 2nd ed. St. Louis: Mosby–Year Book, 1998.

Centers for Disease Control. Recommendations for preventing transmission of human immunodeficiency virus and hepatitis B virus to patients during exposure-prone invasive procedures. AORN-J 1991;54(3):576–582.

Goodfellow L. Physical assessment: a vital nursing tool in both developing and developed countries. Crit Care Nurs Q 1997;20(2):6–8.

Harris R, Wilson-Barnett J, Griffiths P, Evans A. Patient assessment: validation of a nursing instrument. Int J Nurs Stud 1998;35:303–313.

National Institute of Occupational Safety and Health. Recommendations for the prevention of natural rubber latex allergy. Cincinnati, OH: National Institute of Occupational Safety and Health, 1997.

Partial assessment: not a good move. Nursing 1998;3.

Pomeranz A. Physical assessment. Pediatr Clin North Am1998;45:xi,1.

Seidel H, Ball J, Dains J, Benedict GW. Mosby's guide to physical examination. 4th ed. St. Louis: Mosby–Year Book, 1999.

U.S. Department of Health and Human Services. Healthy people 2010: national health promotion and disease prevention objectives. Washington, DC: Public Health Services, 1999.

CHAPTER

5

General Assessment and Vital Signs

Rhonda M. Jones

GLOSSARY TERMS

- Arrhythmia
- Ataxia
- Blood pressure
- Bradycardia
- Bradypnea
- Cachectic
- Coma
- Cyanosis
- Diastolic blood pressure
- Eclampsia
- Hypertension
- Isolated systolic hypertension
- Jaundice
- Kyphosis
- Lesion
- Lethargic
- Lordosis
- Pallor
- Preeclampsia
- Stupor
- Systolic blood pressure
- Tachycardia
- Tachypnea

The *general assessment* (also known as the *general survey*) is a quick assessment of the patient as a whole, including the patient's physical appearance, behavior, mobility, and certain physical parameters (i.e., height, weight, and vital signs). The general assessment should provide an overall impression of the patient's health status. The physical parameters that are measured help to evaluate the whole person, because they apply to several body systems rather than to one specific organ system.

PHYSICAL APPEARANCE, BEHAVIOR, AND MOBILITY

Begin the general survey with a quick observation of the patient's physical appearance. What leaves an immediate impression? Note the following characteristics: (1) age, (2) skin color, (3) facial features, (4) level of consciousness, (5) signs of acute distress, (6) nutrition, (7) body structure, (8) dress and grooming, (9) behavior, and (10) mobility. If you identify abnormalities in any of these areas, document your findings, and then investigate further using specific questions and physical assessment techniques (see Chapters 8–22).

Age

The patient's facial features and body structure should match his or her stated age. If the person looks much older than the stated age, it could be a sign of chronic illness or chronic alcoholism.

Skin Color

Cyanotic changes can be seen most easily in the lips and oral cavity, whereas pallor and jaundice are detected most easily in the nail beds and conjunctiva of the eye. The patient's skin tone should be even, and pigmentation should be consistent with the patient's genetic background. A **lesion** is an area of tissue with impaired function resulting from disease or physical trauma. **Cyanosis** is a bluish discoloration resulting from an inadequate amount of oxygen in the blood; it can be associated with shortness of breath (i.e., difficulty in breathing), lung disease, heart failure, or suffocation. **Pallor** is an abnormal paleness of the skin resulting from reduced blood flow or decreased hemoglobin level, and it can be associated with a wide range of diseases (e.g., anemia, shock, cancer). **Jaundice** is a yellowing of the skin resulting from excessive bilirubin (a bile pigment) in the blood. It can be an indication of liver disease or bile duct obstruction by gallstones.

Facial Features

Facial movements should be symmetric, and the facial expressions should match what the patient is saying (e.g., the patient is telling you that he was just diagnosed with cancer, and he appears to be shocked and sad). If one side of the face is paralyzed (i.e., not moving), the patient may have suffered a stroke or physical trauma or may have a form of temporary facial paralysis called *Bell's palsy.* A flat affect or mask-like expression, in which the patient shows no facial emotion, can be associated with Parkinson's disease and depression. Inappropriate affect, in which the facial expression does not match what the patient is saying, may be a sign of psychiatric illness.

Level of Consciousness

The patient should be alert and oriented to time, place, and person. Disorientation occurs with organic brain disorders (e.g., delirium, dementia), stroke, and physical trauma. A **lethargic** patient typically drifts off to sleep easily, looks drowsy, and responds to questions very slowly. A patient in a **stupor** responds only to persistent and vigorous shaking and answers questions only with a mumble. A completely unconscious patient (i.e., a patient in a **coma**) does not respond to any external stimuli or pain.

Signs of Acute Stress

Signs of acute respiratory distress include shortness of breath, wheezing, or use of accessory muscles to assist in breathing. Facial grimacing or holding a body part are signs of severe pain.

Nutrition

The patient's weight should be appropriate for his or her height and build, and body fat should be distributed evenly. Truncal obesity, in which fat is located primarily in the face, neck, and trunk regions of the body and the extremities are thin, can be caused by Cushing's syndrome (i.e., hyperadrenalism) or by taking corticosteroid medication. If the patient's waist is wider than the hips, then he or she is at increased risk of developing obesity-related diseases (e.g., diabetes, hypertension). A **cachectic** appearance, in which the patient looks emaciated or very thin and has sunken eyes and hollowed cheeks, is associated with chronic wasting diseases (e.g., cancer, starvation, dehydration).

Body Structure

Both sides of the patient's body should look and move the same. The person should stand comfortably erect as appropriate for his or her age. A tripod position, in which the seated patient leans forward with arms braced on the chair arms or on the knees, occurs with chronic respiratory disease. Note any obvious physical deformities, such as **kyphosis** (Fig. 5-1), which is a hunched back, and **lordosis** (Fig. 5-2), which is an inward curvature of the spine typically located in the lower back. Kyphosis and lordosis are commonly associated with osteoporosis (i.e., loss of bone density).

Dress and Grooming

The patient's clothing should correspond with the climate, be clean, and fit appropriately. The patient should appear clean and be groomed appropriately for his or her age, gender, occupation, socioeconomic group, and cultural background.

Behavior

The patient should be cooperative and interact pleasantly and appropriately with others. Speech should be clear and understandable, with appropriate word choice for the patient's educational level and culture.

Mobility

The patient's gait (or walk) should be smooth, even, and well balanced, with the feet approximately shoulder-width apart. A shuffling gait, in which the person hesitates to start walking, takes short and shuffled steps, and has difficulty stopping suddenly, is associated with Parkinson's disease. **Ataxia** is a staggering, unsteady gait that can occur with excessive alcohol or drug ingestion (e.g., barbiturates, benzodiazepines, central nervous system stimulants).

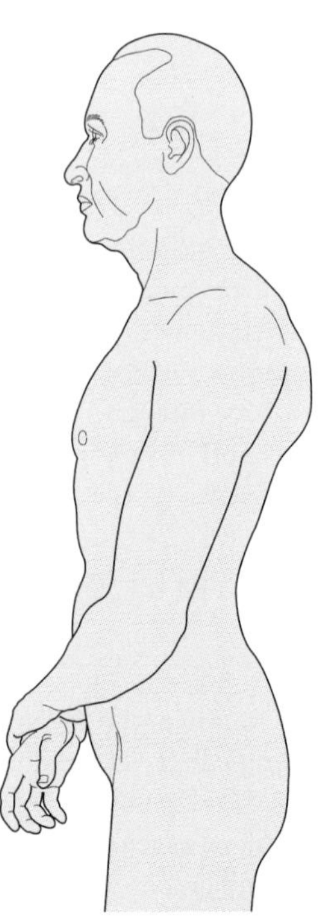
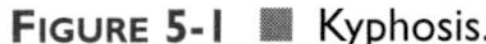

FIGURE 5-1 ■ Kyphosis.

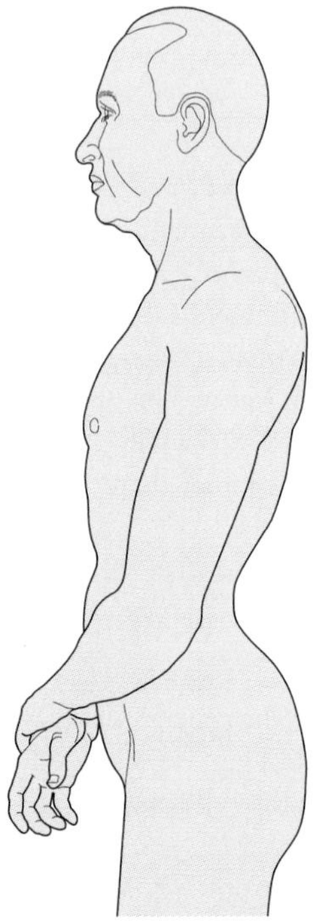

FIGURE 5-2 ■ Lordosis.

PHYSICAL PARAMETERS

Physical parameters that are measured as part of the general assessment reflect the patient's overall health status and include (1) height, (2) weight, and (3) vital signs.

Height

A person's height reflects his or her genetic background and is routinely used to evaluate body proportion. Height can also be compared to previous measurements to assess decreasing bone density or osteoporosis, in which height declines as the disease progresses.

Measure height by having the patient stand erect, without shoes, against a flat and vertical measuring surface, such as the measuring pole on a balance scale. Place the headpiece on the crown of the head, and identify the line where the headpiece intersects the height scale. Height can be recorded in centimeters or inches.

Weight

A person's weight reflects his or her nutritional and overall health status and is best measured with a standardized balance-beam scale. The patient should remove his or her shoes and heavy outer clothing before standing on the scale. If a series of weights is needed, it is best to obtain the measurements at approximately the same time each day and with the patient wearing similar clothing. Weight can be recorded in pounds or kilograms.

To assess the patient's weight, it is best to utilize the patient's body mass index (BMI), which describes the relative weight for height. The BMI is calculated using either of the following equations:

Metric: $\text{BMI} = \text{Weight (kg)}/\text{Height (m}^2\text{)}$
Nonmetric: $\text{BMI} = (\text{Weight [pounds]})/(\text{Height [inches}^2\text{]}) \times 703$

In addition, various tables and nomograms can be useful in determining the BMI. Figure 5-3 shows a nomogram from the U.S. Department of Health and Human Services' *Nutrition and Your Health: Dietary Guidelines for Americans.* In this case, the BMI (kg/m^2) is classified as:

- *Underweight:* BMI, <18.5
- *Healthy Weight:* BMI, 18.5–24.9
- *Overweight:* BMI, 25–29.9
- *Obesity Class I:* BMI, 30–34.9
- *Obesity Class II:* BMI, 35–39.9
- *Obesity Class III:* BMI, ≥40

Patients who are overweight or obese are at a higher risk of morbidity from hypertension, type 2 diabetes, dyslipidemia, coronary heart disease, stroke, gallbladder disease, osteoarthritis, respiratory problems, and certain types of cancer (i.e., endometrial, breast, prostate, and colon).

Unintended weight loss may be a sign of short-term illness (e.g., infection) or of long-term disease (e.g., hyperthyroidism, cancer). Keep in mind that several medications can decrease the patient's appetite or cause nausea or gastritis (e.g., decongestants, SSRI antidepressants, nonsteroidal anti-inflammatory drugs), and in turn, these adverse effects can cause the patient to eat less and, thus, to lose weight. In contrast, disease processes such as hypothyroidism and depression and medications such as corticosteroids can cause weight gain; however, weight gain more commonly reflects excessive caloric intake and a sedentary lifestyle.

Vital Signs

Measurements of vital signs provide valuable information concerning a patient's general state of health. Vital signs include (1) temperature, (2) pulse, (3) respiratory rate, and (4) blood pressure. These measurements should be compared to the normal range for the patient's age and to the patient's previous measurements, if available.

Temperature

To maintain normal metabolic function, the core temperature of the body is regulated by the hypothalamus to stay within a very narrow range. Heat production, which occurs primarily through metabolism and exercise, is balanced with heat loss, which occurs mainly through evaporation of sweat. The normal temperature range for adults is 36.4 to 37.2°C (97.5–99.0°F). Normal body temperature can be affected by biological rhythms, hormones, exercise, and age. Diurnal fluctuations of roughly 1°C normally occur, with the lowest temperature in the early morning and the highest in the late afternoon to early evening. In females, progesterone secretion at ovulation causes a 0.5°C increase in temperature that typically continues until menses. Moderate to heavy exercise also increases body temperature.

In children, wider normal variations of temperature occur because of immature heat-control mechanisms. As a person ages, the mean normal body temperature declines from 37.2°C (99.0°F) in young children to 37°C (98.6°F) in adults to 36°C (96.8°F) in elderly people.

Measurement of body temperature is a routine part of nearly all clinical assessments, because it provides useful insight regarding the severity of illness (e.g., infections). Temperature is recorded in degrees Celsius or degrees Fahrenheit, and the following conversion can be used:

$$C = 5/9 \times (°F - 32)$$
$$F = (9/5 \times °C) + 32$$

Thus, for example,

$$37°C = (9/5 \times 37) + 32 = 66.6 + 32 = 98.6F$$

Temperature can be measured by a variety of thermometers (i.e., glass, electronic, tympanic) and by a variety of routes (i.e., oral, rectal, axillary, tympanic). Figure 5-4 shows several types of thermometers.

ARE YOU AT A HEALTHY WEIGHT?

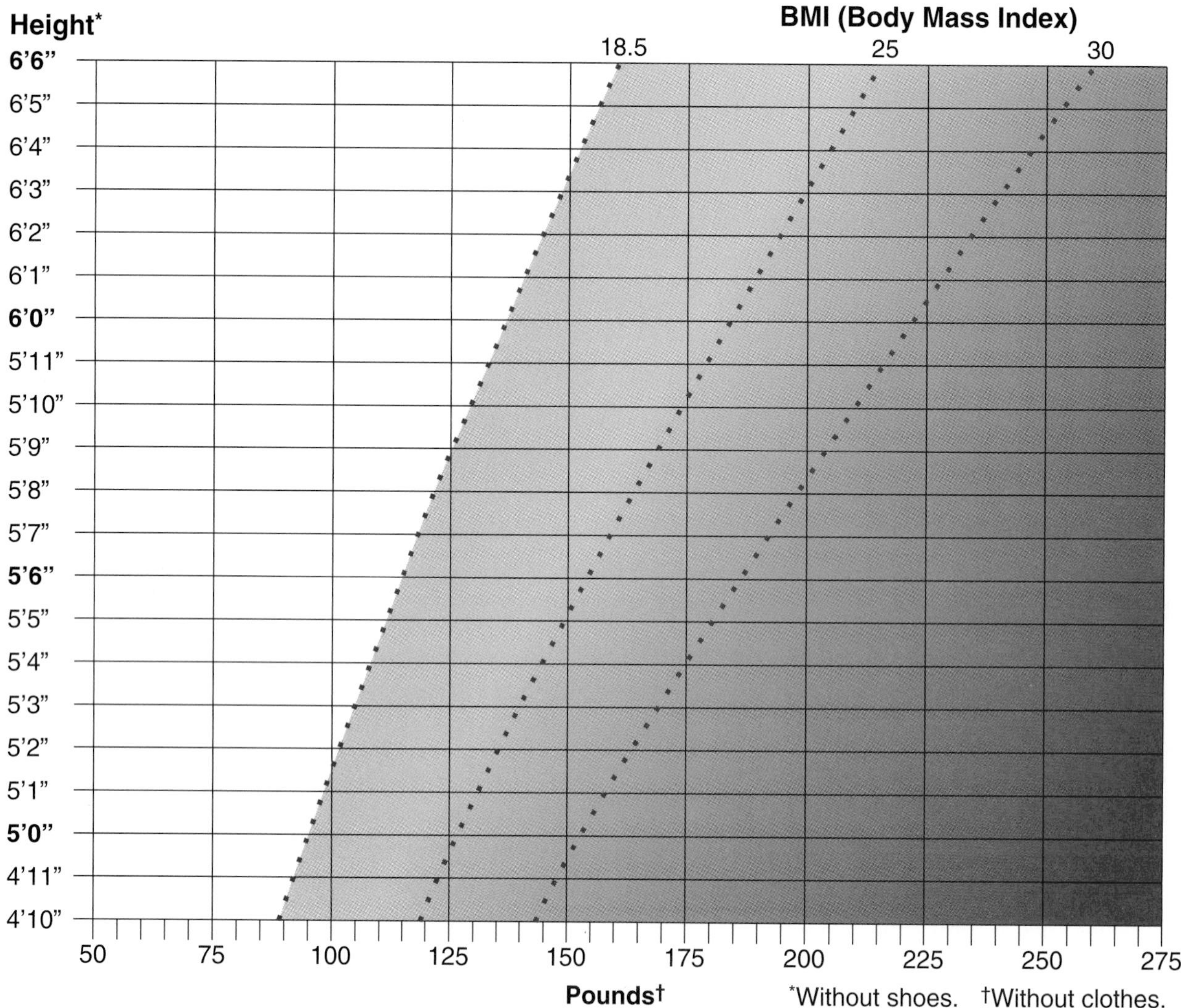

BMI measures weight in relation to height. The BMI ranges shown above are for adults. They are not exact ranges of healthy and unhealthy weights. However, they show that health risk increases at higher levels of overweight and obesity. Even within the healthy BMI range, weight gains can carry health risks for adults.

Directions: Find your weight on the bottom of the graph. Go straight up from that point until you come to the line that matches your height. Then look to find your weight group.

- **Healthy weight** BMI from 18.5 up to 25 refers to healthy weight.
- **Overweight** BMI from 25 up to 30 refers to overweight.
- **Obese** BMI 30 or higher refers to obesity. Obese persons are also overweight.

Source: Report of the Dietary Guidelines Advisory Committee on the Dietary Guidelines for Americans, 2000, page 3.

FIGURE 5-3 ■ Example nomogram for determining body mass index (BMI). (Reprinted from U.S. Department of Agriculture, U.S. Department of Health and Human Services. Nutrition and your health: dietary guidelines for Americans. 5th ed. 2000, pg. 7.)

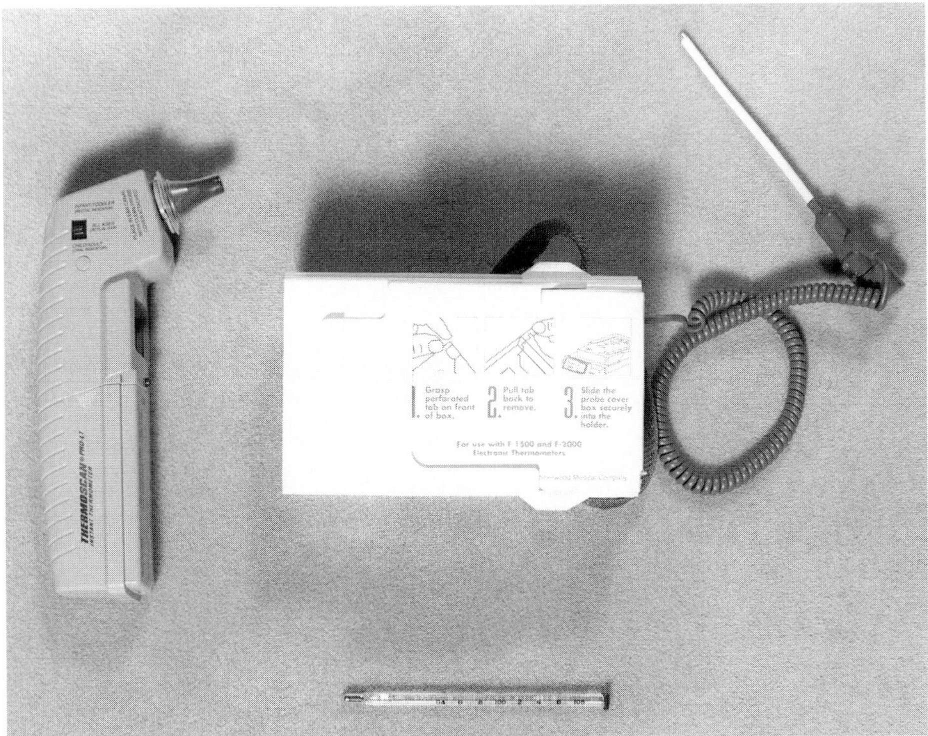

FIGURE 5-4 ■ Types of thermometers.

Oral Route

The oral route is both accurate and convenient for measuring body temperature in an alert patient. Normal body temperature in adults as measured by the oral route is 37°C (98.6°F).

To measure body temperature using the oral route:

- Shake the glass mercury thermometer down to 35.5°C (96°F).
- Place the thermometer tip gently under the patient's tongue in either of the posterior sublingual pockets, not in front of the tongue.
- Instruct the patient to keep his or her lips closed.
- Keep the thermometer in place for 3 to 5 min.
- Gently remove the thermometer from the patient's mouth, and rotate the thermometer to clearly see the mercury level.
- An electronic thermometer uses disposable plastic probe covers and registers a temperature in 20 to 30 sec.

Rectal Route

The rectal route is preferred in patients who are confused, comatose, or unable to close their mouth because of intubation, wired mandible, facial surgery, and so on. It also is commonly used to obtain an infant's temperature (see *Pediatric Patients* later in this chapter). The rectal route is the most accurate way to measure the core body temperature. Normal temperature in adults as measured by the rectal route is 37.5°C (99.5°F), which is approximately 0.5°C (1°F) higher than with the oral route.

To measure body temperature using the rectal route:

- Assist the patient into a lateral position with the upper legs flexed.
- Wear gloves.
- Lubricate a rectal, blunt-tipped thermometer.
- Insert the thermometer 2 to 3 cm (1 inch) into the rectum.
- Leave in place for at least 2 min.

Axillary Route

The axillary route is used in adults only when the oral and rectal routes are not accessible; however, it can be a safe and accurate method in both infants and small children. Normal temperature in adults as measured by the axillary route is 36.5°C (97.7°F), which is approximately 0.5°C (1°F) lower than with the oral route.

To measure body temperature using the axillary route:

- Place the thermometer under the arm into the center of the axilla.
- Lower the patient's arm over the thermometer.
- Fold the patient's arm over his or her chest to keep the thermometer in place.
- Leave the thermometer in place for 5 min in children and 10 min in adults.

Tympanic Route

The tympanic route uses a thermometer with a probe tip that is placed into the ear. This thermometer has an infrared sensor to detect the temperature of blood flowing through the eardrum. This method is noninvasive, quick, and efficient.

To measure body temperature using the tympanic route:

- Place a new, disposable cover on the probe tip.
- Gently place the probe into the person's ear canal (Fig. 5-5).

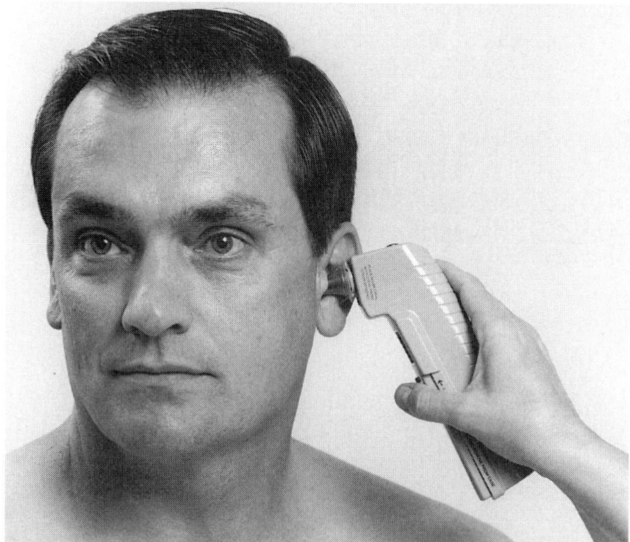

FIGURE 5-5 ■ Tympanic temperature measurement.

- Be careful not to force the probe and not to occlude the canal.
- Activate the instrument by pressing the appropriate button.
- Read the temperature in 2 to 3 sec.

Pulse

When the heart beats, it pushes blood through the aorta and peripheral vasculature. This pumping action causes the blood to pound against the artery walls, creating a pressure wave with each heart beat that is felt in the periphery as the *pulse.* The *peripheral pulse* is palpated to assess the heart rate, rhythm, and function. Because it is easily accessible, the *radial pulse* is most commonly used; it is palpated over the radial artery on the anterior wrist. (Other peripheral pulse measurements are discussed in Chapter 13.)

To measure the radial pulse:

- Place the pads of the first and second fingers on the palmar surface of the patient's wrist medial to the radius bone (Fig. 5-6).
- Press down until pulsation is felt, but be careful not to occlude the artery (in which case no pulse will be felt).
- Count the number of beats in 30 sec, and if the rhythm is regular, multiply that number by two.
- Avoid using only a 15-sec counting interval, because a one- to two-beat error will result in a four- to eight-beat error for the patient's heart rate evaluation. Also, it is easier to multiply the number of beats by two than it is by four.
- If the rhythm is irregular, count the number of beats in 1 min.
- Record the finding as beats per minute (bpm).

Normal heart rates for various ages are listed in Table 5-1. In an adult, a heart rate of less than 60 bpm is called **bradycardia,** and a heart rate of greater than 100 bpm is called **tachycardia.** A well-conditioned athlete, however, can have a normal, resting heart rate of less than 60 bpm, and heart rates greater than 100 bpm can normally occur in patients who are exercising or anxious.

In addition to the pulse rate, the *pulse rhythm* should be evaluated. Normally, the rhythm of the pulse is steady and even. If an irregular rhythm, called an **arrhythmia,** is identified, then the heart sounds should be auscultated with a stethoscope for a more accurate assessment (see Chapter 12 for a full discussion of arrhythmias).

The force of each heart contraction, as reflected in the heart's stroke volume, can also be evaluated by palpating the pulse. Typically, a normal pulse is easily palpated, does not fade in and out, and is not easily obstructed. The force of the pulse generally is described using a fairly subjective four-point scale:

- 0 absent
- 1+ weak, thready
- 2+ normal
- 3+ full or bounding

Respiratory Rate

Inspection is used to evaluate the patient's respiratory rate. Because most people are unaware of their breathing and sudden

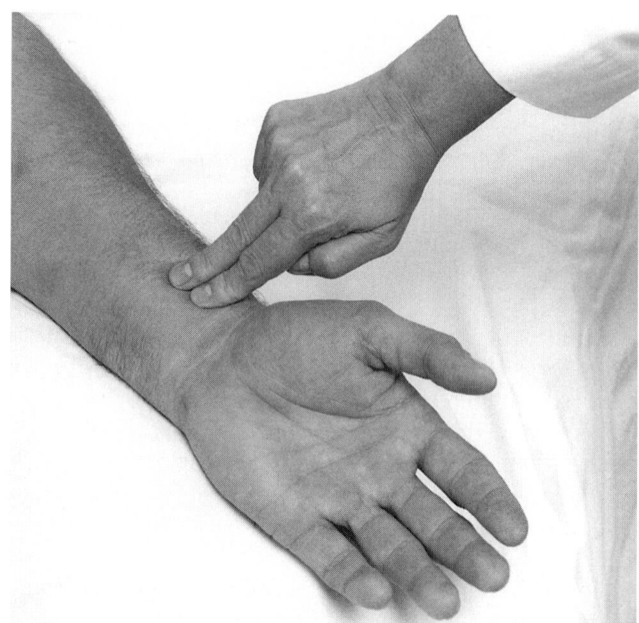

FIGURE 5-6 ■ Radial pulse measurement.

TABLE 5-1 ➤ NORMAL HEART RATES FOR VARIOUS AGE GROUPS

AGE	HEART RATE (BPM)
Newborn	70–170
1–6 years	75–160
6–12 years	80–120
Adult	60–100
Elderly	60–100
Conditioned athlete	50–100

Adapted from Cipolle RJ, et al., and Tomechko MA, et al.

awareness may alter the normal pattern, do not tell the patient that his or her respiratory rate is being measured.

To measure the respiratory rate:

- Maintain the position for a radial pulse measurement.
- Observe the patient's chest or abdomen for respirations.
- Count the number of respirations (inhalation and exhalation are counted as one respiration) in 30 sec, and if the rhythm is regular, multiply this number by two.
- If the rhythm is irregular, count the number of respirations for 1 min.
- Record the value as respirations per minute (rpm).

Normal respiratory rates for various ages are listed in Table 5-2. For adults, a respiratory rate of less than 12 rpm is called **bradypnea,** and a respiratory rate of greater than 20 rpm is called **tachypnea.** (For a more detailed assessment of the respiratory system, see Chapter 11.)

Blood Pressure

Blood pressure is the force of the blood as it pushes against the arterial walls. It is dependent on cardiac output, the volume of blood ejected by the ventricles per minute, and the peripheral vascular resistance. Heart rate, contractility, and total blood volume, which is primarily dependent on the sodium content, influence the cardiac output. Arterial blood viscosity and wall elasticity influence the peripheral vascular resistance.

Blood pressure has two components: *systolic,* and *diastolic.* The **systolic blood pressure** represents the maximum pressure that is felt on the arteries during left ventricular contraction (or *systole*), and it is regulated by the stroke volume (i.e., the volume of blood ejected with each heartbeat). The **diastolic blood pressure** is the resting pressure that the blood exerts between each ventricular contraction.

The primary objective of identifying, treating, and monitoring the patient's blood pressure is to reduce the risk of cardiovascular disease and its associated morbidity and mortality. Therefore, correct measurement of the blood pressure is very important, because this measurement provides the basis for vital clinical decisions, such as the adjustment of antihypertensive medication.

Methods of Measurement

The most common method of blood pressure measurement is the indirect, auscultatory method using a stethoscope and a sphygmomanometer. (For a detailed description of the stethoscope, see Chapter 4.) The blood pressure cuff contains an inflatable rubber bladder within a cloth cover. The bladder is connected to the manometer, which is either a mercury or an aneroid type (Fig. 5-7). The mercury manometer is the most accurate; however, the aneroid manometer is more portable. Because the aneroid manometer is susceptible to drift, it should be calibrated annually against a reliable mercury manometer. To accommodate the wide range of arm circumferences, various cuff sizes are available (e.g., pediatric, adult, large adult). To determine the appropriate cuff size for a given patient, compare the length of the bladder with the circumference of the patient's arm. (You will have to feel the bladder inside the cuff.) For the most accurate measurement, the bladder length should be at least 80% of the arm circumference (Fig. 5-8).

Blood pressure measurement is considered to be *indirect,* because the pressure within the blood vessel is indirectly measured by measuring the pressure in the cuff. As air is pumped into the cuff, the pressure within the cuff increases. When the pressure within the cuff exceeds the pressure within the patient's brachial

TABLE 5-2 ➤ NORMAL RESPIRATORY RATES FOR VARIOUS AGES

AGE	RESPIRATIONS (RPM)
2–6 years	21–30
6–10 years	20–26
12–14 years	18–22
Adult	12–20
Elderly	12–20

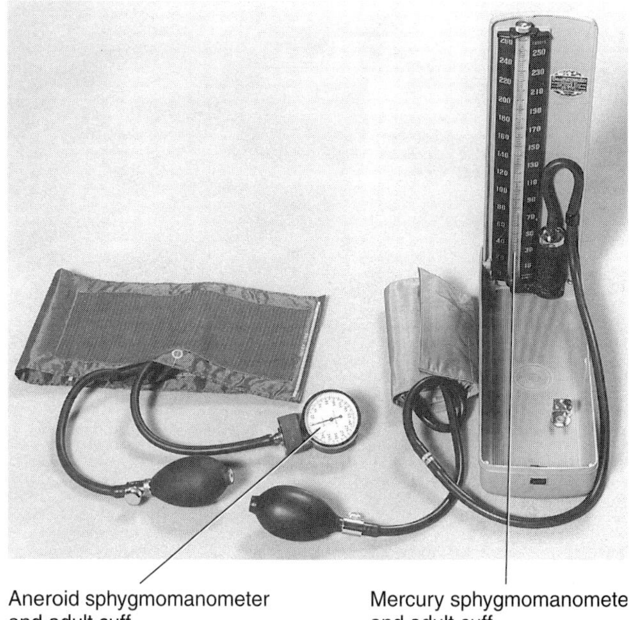

FIGURE 5-7 ■ Blood pressure cuff and sphygmomanometer.

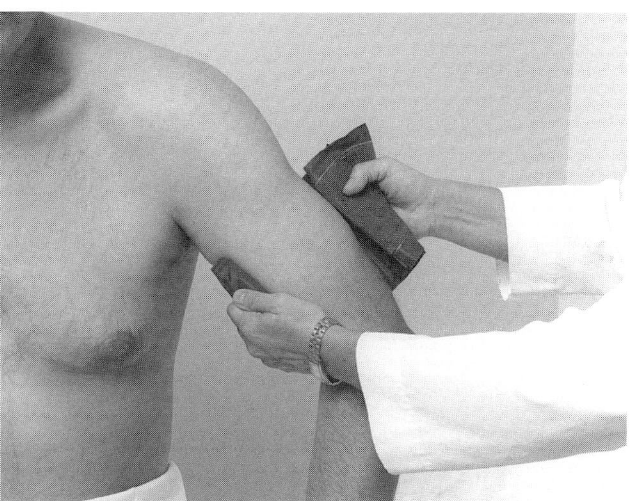

FIGURE 5-8 ■ Determination of appropriate cuff size for blood pressure measurement.

artery, the artery is compressed, and the blood flow diminishes and, ultimately, stops. As air is released from the cuff, the bladder deflates, and the pressure within the cuff decreases. When the pressure within the cuff matches the pressure within the artery, blood begins to flow through the artery once again (Fig. 5-9).

Blood flow within the artery produces distinct sounds, which are called *Korotkoff sounds* that occur in five phases:

- *Phase I:* faint, clear, tapping (the systolic pressure).
- *Phase II:* swooshing.

Phase	Description	Rationale
Cuff correctly inflated	No sound	Cuff inflation compresses brachial artery. Cuff pressure exceeds heart's systolic pressure, occluding brachial artery blood flow.
I	Soft, clear tapping, increasing in intensity	The SYSTOLIC pressure. As the cuff pressure lowers to reach intraluminal systolic pressure, the artery opens, and blood first spurts into the brachial artery.
II	Swooshing	Turbulent blood flow through still partially occluded artery.
III	Tapping	Artery closes just briefly during late diastole.
IV	Muffling	Artery no longer closes in any part of cardiac cycle. Change in quality, not intensity.
V	No sound	Decreased velocity of blood flow. Streamlined blood flow is silent. The last audible sound (marking the disappearance of sounds) is adult DIASTOLIC pressure.

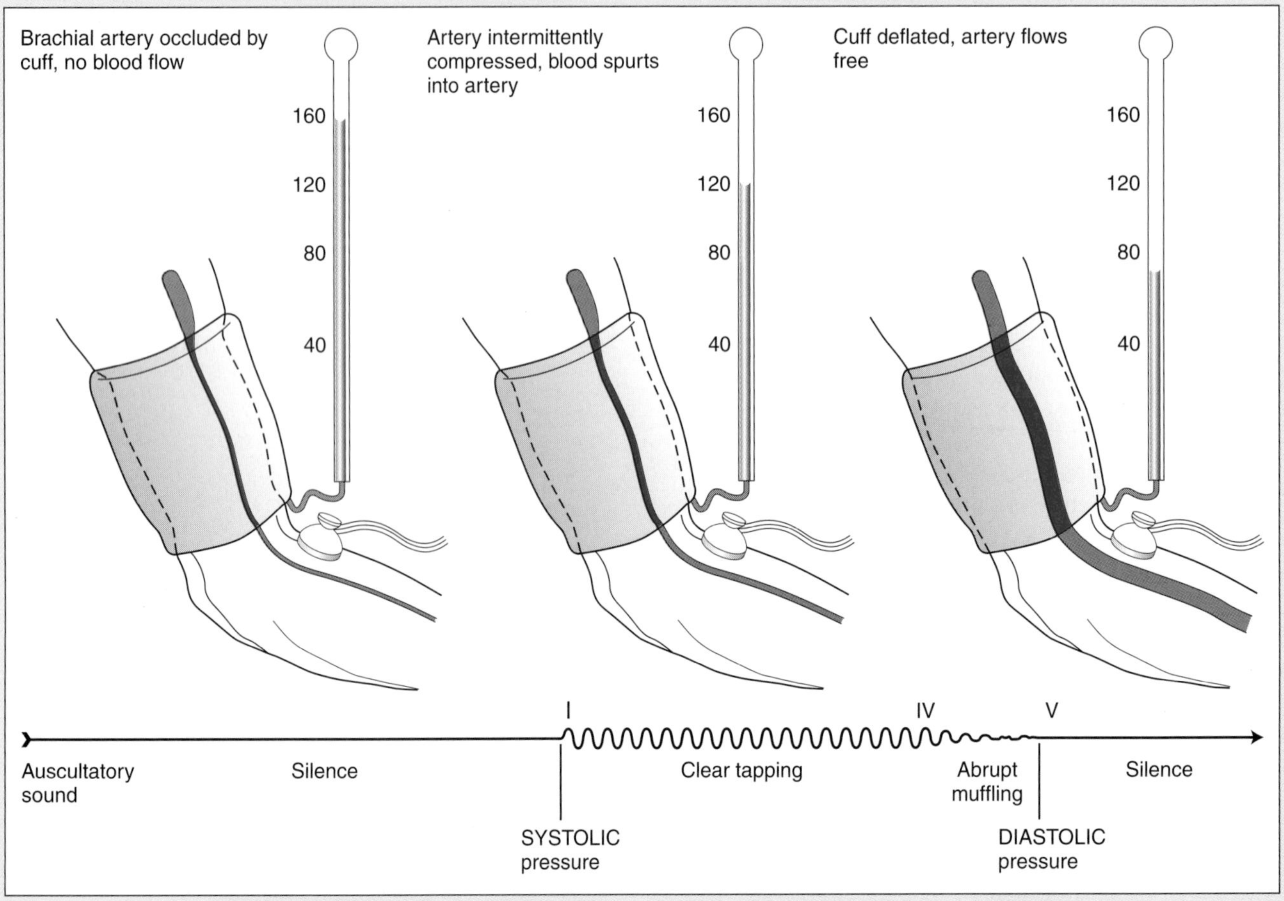

FIGURE 5-9 ■ Korotkoff sounds and blood pressure measurement. (Adapted with permission from Jarvis C. Physical examination and health assessment. 3rd ed. Philadelphia: WB Saunders, 2000;192.)

- *Phase III:* crisp, more intense (tapping).
- *Phase IV:* muffling (in adults, this reflects a hyperkinetic state if it remains throughout cuff deflation).
- *Phase V:* cessation of sound (in adults, diastolic pressure).

These sounds are used to identify the systolic and diastolic blood pressure. For the most accurate measurement, follow these steps:

- Ask the patient if he or she has smoked or ingested caffeine within the previous 30 min. If the patient has, document this information.
- The patient should be seated in a chair with his or her back supported and arm bared and supported at heart level.
- Measurement should begin after at least 5 min of rest.
- Determine the appropriate cuff size (see Fig. 5-8).
- Palpate the brachial artery along the inner upper arm.
- Center the bladder of the cuff over the brachial artery, and wrap the cuff smoothly and snugly around the arm, placing the lower edge of the cuff approximately 1 inch above the antecubital space (Fig. 5-10).
- Position the mercury manometer with the meniscus at eye level (or the aneroid manometer in direct line of sight).
- Instruct the patient not to talk during the measurement.
- Determine the maximum inflation level. (While palpating the radial pulse, inflate the cuff to the point at which the radial pulse can no longer be felt, then add 30 mm Hg to this reading.)
- Rapidly deflate the cuff, and wait 30 sec before reinflating.

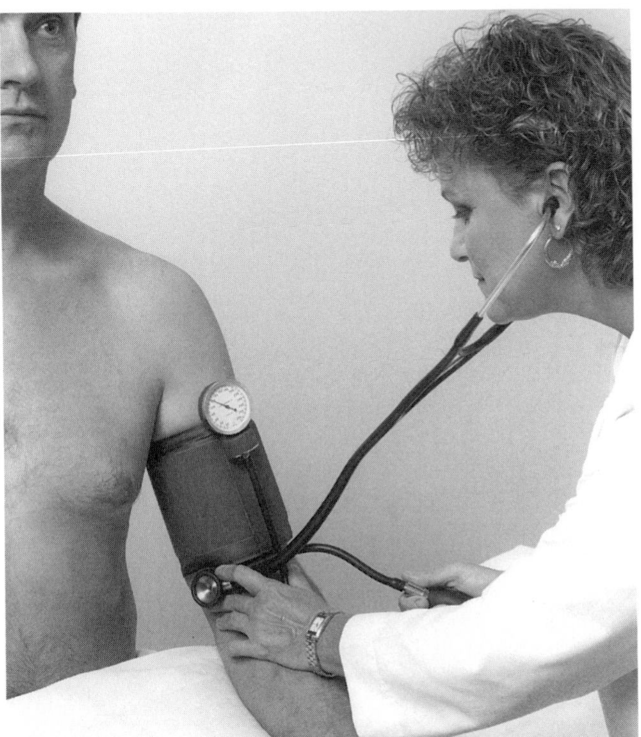

FIGURE 5-10 ■ Proper cuff and stethoscope placement for blood pressure measurement.

- Insert the stethoscope earpieces; make sure that they point forward when in place.
- Place the bell of the stethoscope lightly, but with an airtight seal, over the palpable brachial artery (see Fig. 5-10). Note that the diaphragm of the stethoscope also may be used; however, the bell is designed to pick up low-frequency (i.e., blood pressure) sounds and should be used, if possible. When you are first learning to measure blood pressure, it may be easier to use the diaphragm rather than the bell side of the stethoscope.
- Rapidly inflate the cuff to the maximum inflation level (determined previously).
- Slowly release the air, allowing the pressure to fall steadily at 2 to 3 mm Hg/sec.
- Note the pressure at which the first of two consecutive sounds is heard (Korotkoff Phase I). This is the systolic blood pressure.
- Note the pressure at which the last sound is heard (Korotkoff Phase V). This is the diastolic pressure.
- Continue listening until 20 mm Hg below the diastolic pressure, then rapidly and completely deflate cuff.
- Record the patient's blood pressure in even numbers, along with the patient's position (e.g., sitting, standing, lying), cuff size, and the arm used for measurement.
- Wait 1 to 2 min before repeating the pressure measurement in the same arm.

For the most accurate measurement, two or more readings, each separated by 2 min, should be averaged. If the first two readings differ by more than 5 mm Hg, additional readings should be obtained and averaged. Normal blood pressure for adults is less than 130 mm Hg systolic and less than 85 mm Hg diastolic.

Classification of Measurements

Blood pressure readings are classified according to criteria from the *Sixth Report of the Joint National Committee on Prevention, Detection, Evaluation, and Treatment of High Blood Pressure (JNC-VI)* (Table 5-3). **Hypertension** is defined as a systolic blood pressure of 140 mm Hg or greater or a diastolic blood pressure of 90 mm Hg or greater and is classified (according to its severity) as stage 1, 2, or 3. **Isolated systolic hypertension** is defined as a systolic blood pressure of 140 mm Hg or greater and a diastolic blood pressure of 90 mm Hg or lower and should be staged appropriately (e.g., 170/82 mm Hg is stage 2 isolated systolic hypertension). In addition to the classification of hypertension, the JNC-VI also contains specific recommendations for blood pressure measurement as well as for prevention and treatment of hypertension (Table 5-4).

Common Errors of Measurement

As you learn to measure blood pressure accurately, keep in mind that it will take a fair amount of practice for it to become a comfortable process. In addition, because the measurement process involves several steps, many errors can occur. To prevent these, you should be aware of common mistakes.

Incorrect cuff size is a major source of equipment-related error, especially with obese patients who have large upper arms. Using a cuff that is too small for the patient's arm can produce

TABLE 5-3 ➤ CLASSIFICATION OF BLOOD PRESSURE FOR ADULTS 18 YEARS OF AGE AND OLDER[a]

CATEGORY	SYSTOLIC BLOOD PRESSURE (mm Hg)		DIASTOLIC BLOOD PRESSURE (mm Hg)
Optimal[b]	<120		<80
Normal	<130		<85
High-normal	130–139	or	85–89
Hypertension[c]			
Stage 1	140–159	or	90–99
Stage 2	160–179	or	100–109
Stage 3	≥180	or	≥110

Joint National Committee on Prevention, Detection, Evaluation, and Treatment of High Blood Pressure. The sixth report of the Joint National Committee on Prevention, Detection, Evaluation, and Treatment of High Blood Pressure (JNC-VI). Arch Intern Med 1997;157:2413–2446.

[a]Patients who are not taking antihypertensive drugs and not acutely ill. When systolic and diastolic measurements fall in different categories, select the higher category to classify the individual's blood pressure. For example, a blood pressure of 160/92 mm Hg should be classified as stage 2 hypertension.

[b]Optimal blood pressure with respect to cardiovascular risk. Unusually low readings, however, should be evaluated for clinical significance.

[c]Based on the average of two or more readings taken at each of two or more visits after an initial screening.

a falsely high reading. In contrast, using a cuff that is too large for an extremely thin patient's arm can produce a falsely low reading. Thus, always check for the appropriate cuff size.

Because of isometric muscle contraction, hydrostatic pressure, and gravitational pull, failing to position and support the patient's arm properly can also lead to false readings. If the patient's arm is above heart level, a falsely low reading will be obtained. Conversely, a falsely high reading will occur if the arm is below heart level. Always make sure that the patient's arm is well supported and at heart level.

Anxiety, pain, discomfort, or strenuous activity can cause sympathetic nervous system stimulation and, thus, a falsely high measurement. Therefore, allow the patient at least 5 min to rest and relax before you obtain a reading. In addition, halting during deflation and reinflating the cuff too soon to recheck the systolic blood pressure can cause forearm venous congestion and a falsely high diastolic reading. If a measurement (systolic or diastolic) needs to be rechecked, completely deflate the cuff, and obtain a new reading after waiting for at least 1 to 2 min.

TABLE 5-4 ➤ THE JNC VI GUIDE TO PREVENTION AND TREATMENT OF HYPERTENSION RECOMMENDATIONS

Blood Pressure Measurement	Patient should: • Rest for 5 minutes before measurement. • Refrain from smoking or ingesting caffeine for 30 minutes prior to measurement. • Be seated with feet flat on floor, back and arm supported, arm at heart level. Clinician should: • Use the appropriate size cuff for the patient; the bladder should encircle at least 80 percent of the upper arm. • Use calibrated or mercury manometer. • Average two or more readings, separated by at least 2 minutes.
Primary Prevention	Encourage patients to make healthy lifestyle choices: • Quit smoking to reduce cardiovascular risk. • Lose weight, if needed. • Restrict sodium intake to no more than 100 mmol per day. • Limit alcohol intake to no more than 1-2 drinks per day. • Get at least 30-45 minutes of aerobic activity on most days. • Maintain adequate potassium intake—about 90 mmol per day. • Maintain adequate intakes of calcium and magnesium.
Goal	Set a clear goal of therapy based on patient's risk. Control blood pressure to below: • 140/90 mm hg for patients with uncomplicated hypertension; set a lower goal for those with target organ damage or clinical cardiovascular disease. • 130/85 mm Hg for patients with diabetes. • 125/75 mm Hg for patients with renal insufficiency with proteinuria greater than 1 gram per 24 hours.
Treatment	Begin with lifestyle modifications (see primary prevention box) for all patients. Be supportive! • Add pharmacologic therapy if blood pressure remains uncontrolled. • Start with diuretic or beta-blocker unless there are compelling indications to use other agents. Use low dose and titrate upward. Consider low dose combinations. • If no response, try a drug from another class or add a second agent from a different class (diuretic if not already used).
Adherence	• Encourage lifestyle modifications. Be supportive! • Educate patient and family about disease. Involve them in measurement and treatment. • Maintain communications with patient. • Discuss how to integrate treatment into daily activities. • Keep care inexpensive and simple. • Favor once-daily, long-acting formulations. • Use combination tablets, when needed. • Consider using generic formulas or larger tablets that can be divided. This may be less expensive. • Be willing to stop unsuccessful therapy and try a different approach. • Consider using nurse case management.

Joint National Committee on Prevention, Detection, Evaluation, and Treatment of High Blood Pressure. The sixth report of the Joint National Committee on Prevention, Detection, Evaluation, and Treatment of High Blood Pressure (JNC-VI). Arch Intern Med 1997;157:2413–2446.

Deflating the cuff too quickly (faster than 2 mm Hg/sec) does not allow enough time to hear the possibly faint tapping of the systolic pressure and, thus, can cause a falsely low systolic and/or a falsely high diastolic reading. On the other hand, deflating the cuff too slowly can cause venous forearm congestion and a falsely high diastolic reading. Always deflate the cuff at an appropriate speed (~2 mm Hg/sec).

Factors Affecting Blood Pressure

As mentioned, normal blood pressure is less than 130/85 mm Hg. However, blood pressure can vary with many factors. These factors include:

- *Age:* Blood pressure gradually rises throughout childhood until adulthood.
- *Race:* Hypertension occurs twice as often in African-Americans as in Caucasians.
- *Diurnal Rhythm:* Blood pressure is lowest during the early morning and highest during the late afternoon or early evening.
- *Weight:* Excess body weight closely correlates with increased blood pressure.
- *Exercise:* Increased activity increases blood pressure, which should return to baseline after 5 min of rest.
- *Emotions:* Blood pressure increases with pain, fear, anxiety, anger, and stress.
- *Medications:* An unwanted side effect of some medications (e.g., cyclosporine, corticosteroids, nasal decongestants) is increased blood pressure.

When evaluating your readings, note if any of these factors may be contributing to the patient's blood pressure.

SPECIAL CONSIDERATIONS

Pediatric Patients

Height, weight, and vital signs are routinely measured during the assessment of pediatric patients. For the child younger than 3 years, routine growth measurements include (1) recumbent length, (2) body weight, and (3) head circumference. These measurements are commonly recorded on a physical growth chart (Fig. 5-11) and compared to national statistics based on large, nationally representative samples of children. Children whose measurements fall between the 5th and 95th percentiles are considered to be growing normally (e.g., a height measurement in the 75th percentile means the child is taller than 75% of all children at that age).

Temperature

The child's temperature can be measured using all the same routes as in the adult (i.e., oral, axillary, rectal, tympanic). The oral route can be used when the child is old enough to keep his or her mouth closed and not bite on the glass thermometer (usually 4–5 years of age). The axillary route is preferable to the rectal route in toddlers and preschool children, because it is not intrusive. However, an accurate reading typically takes 4 to 5 minutes to register. The tympanic route can be used with children at any age and provides a reading within a few seconds.

The rectal route is commonly used with infants or older children when the other routes are not feasible. To measure the infant's temperature rectally, place infant in a supine or side-lying position, and flex his or her knees onto the abdomen. The infant also may be placed in a prone position across the examiner's lap as the examiner separates the buttocks. Insert the lubricated rectal thermometer no farther than 1 inch into the rectum (a deeper insertion may cause rectal perforation). Hold the thermometer in place for approximately 2 to 3 min. Normally, rectal temperatures measure slightly higher in children than in adults.

Temperature regulation is less precise in children than in adults, with the average temperature being greater than 37.2°C (99.0°F) until 3 years of age. Normal temperatures in children 3 years and older range from 37.2 to 37.5°C (99.0–99.4°F). Keep in mind that a child's temperature normally is slightly elevated during the late afternoon, after vigorous activity, and after eating. As the child matures, the normal temperature lowers slightly. In older children (5–11 years of age), the normal temperature is 36.7 to 37.0°C (98.0–98.6°F).

Pulse

A child's heart rate normally fluctuates more than an adult's in response to activity, apprehension, crying, and illness. It also is normal for a child's heart rhythm to be irregular at times. Therefore, measure the pulse for 1 min rather than for 30 sec. (Table 5-1 lists normal heart rates according to age.)

Respiratory Rate

An infant's respiratory movements usually are diaphragmatic and, thus, are measured by observing abdominal rather than chest movements. These movements should be counted for 1 min, because the respiratory pattern is very irregular in infants. Similar to the heart rate, the respiratory rate normally lowers as the child ages. (Table 5-2 lists normal respiratory rates according to age.)

Blood Pressure

Blood pressure (both systolic and diastolic) gradually rises during childhood, with a wide variation normally found on measurement. The National Task Force on Blood Pressure Control in Children recommends that children 3 years and older have their blood pressure measured annually as part of the routine physical examination. For accurate measurement, the cuff bladder width should cover approximately 40% of the upper arm circumference. When in place, the bladder should encircle 80 to 100% of the upper arm. Also, a pediatric-sized endpiece should be used on the stethoscope. As in adults, Korotkoff Phase I is used for the systolic pressure. In the past, Korotkoff Phase IV was used for the diastolic pressure in children; however, the National Task Force recommends that Korotkoff Phase V be used to define diastolic blood pressure in children as well as in adolescents and adults.

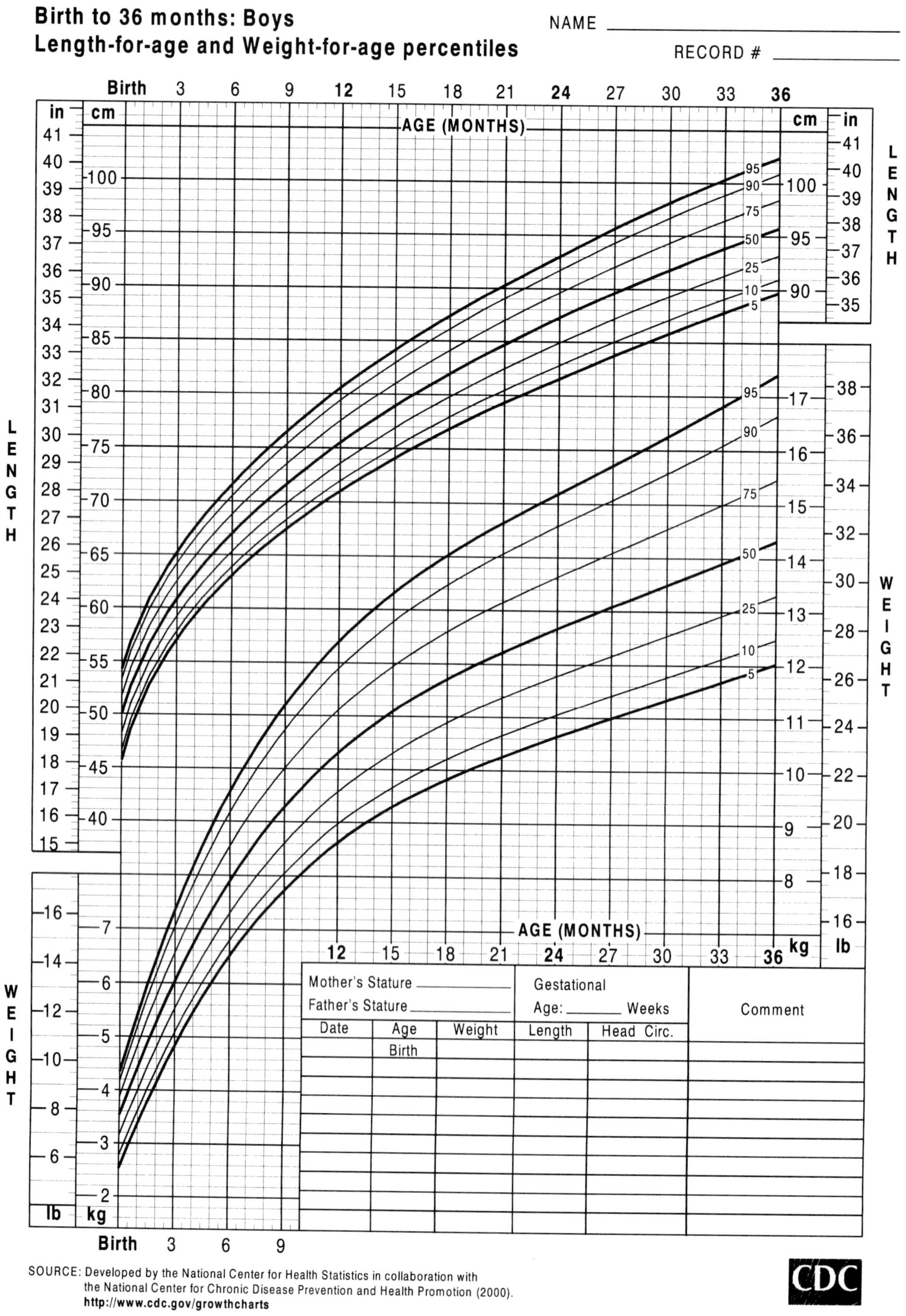

Birth to 36 months: Boys
Length-for-age and Weight-for-age percentiles

NAME ______________________

RECORD # ______________

AGE (MONTHS)

Birth 3 6 9 12 15 18 21 24 27 30 33 36

LENGTH (in / cm)

WEIGHT (lb / kg)

Percentiles: 95, 90, 75, 50, 25, 10, 5

Mother's Stature ______________

Father's Stature ______________

Gestational Age: ________ Weeks

Date	Age	Weight	Length	Head Circ.	Comment
	Birth				

SOURCE: Developed by the National Center for Health Statistics in collaboration with the National Center for Chronic Disease Prevention and Health Promotion (2000). http://www.cdc.gov/growthcharts

FIGURE 5-11 ■ Sample physical growth chart for children.

Birth to 36 months: Girls
Length-for-age and Weight-for-age percentiles

NAME ______________________

RECORD # ______________

AGE (MONTHS)

Birth 3 6 9 12 15 18 21 24 27 30 33 36

LENGTH

WEIGHT

Mother's Stature ______ Father's Stature ______			Gestational Age: ______ Weeks		Comment
Date	Age	Weight	Length	Head Circ.	
	Birth				

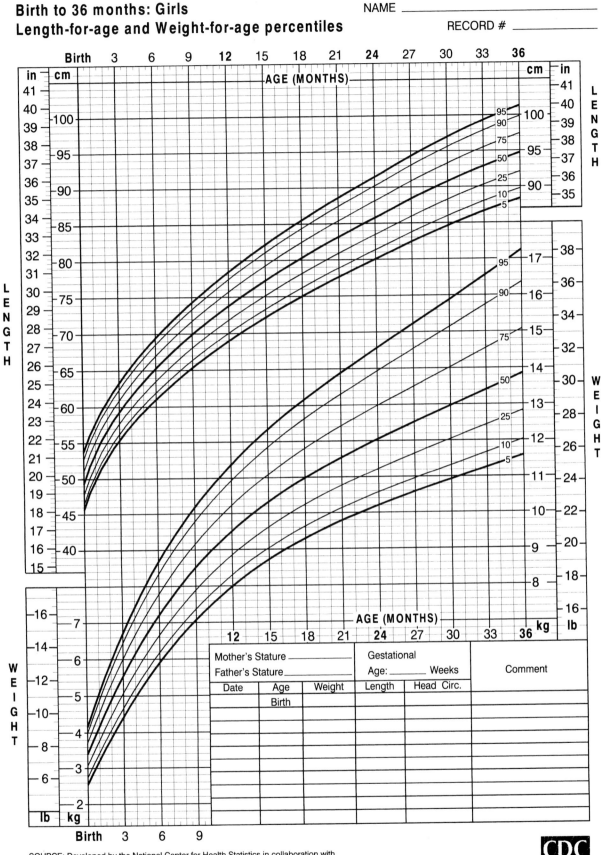

SOURCE: Developed by the National Center for Health Statistics in collaboration with the National Center for Chronic Disease Prevention and Health Promotion (2000).
http://www.cdc.gov/growthcharts

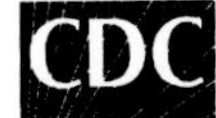

FIGURE 5-11 ■ *continued*

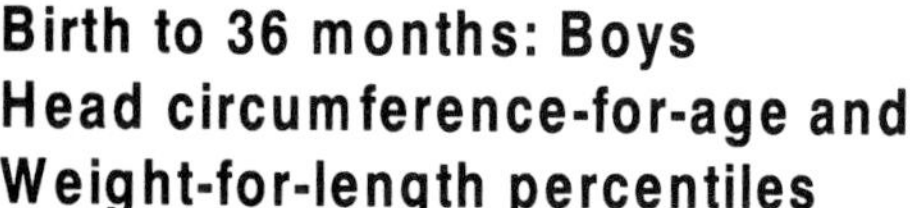

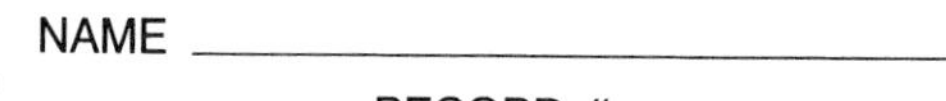

Date	Age	Weight	Length	Head Circ.	Comment

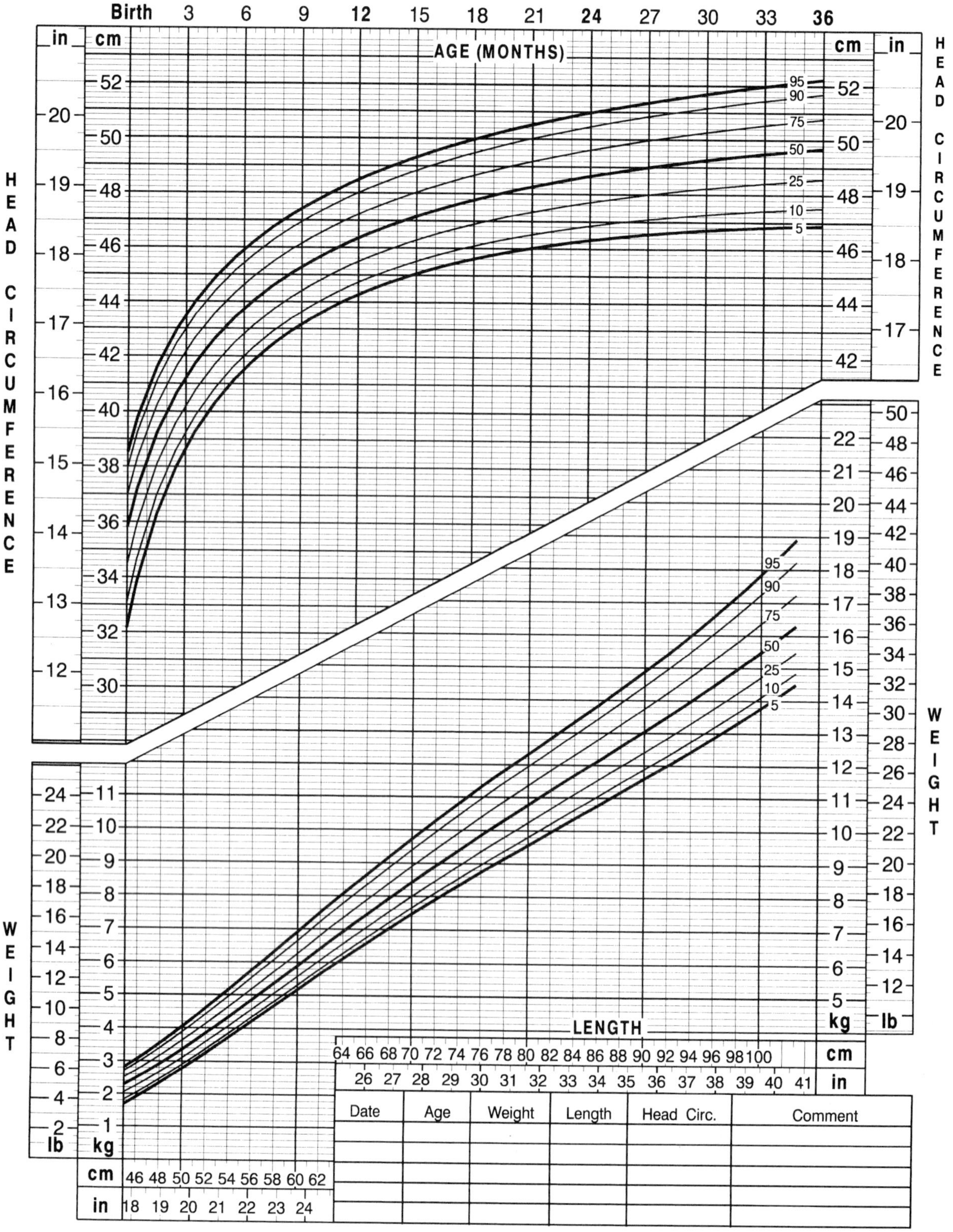

SOURCE: Developed by the National Center for Health Statistics in collaboration with the National Center for Chronic Disease Prevention and Health Promotion (2000). http://www.cdc.gov/growthcharts

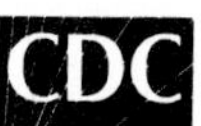

FIGURE 5-11 ■ *continued*

Birth to 36 months: Girls
Head circumference-for-age and
Weight-for-length percentiles

NAME ______________________

RECORD # ______________

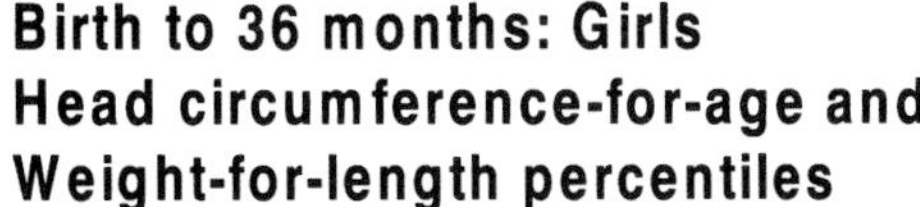

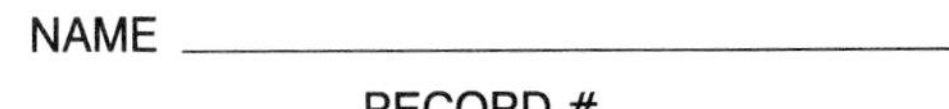

Birth 3 6 9 12 15 18 21 24 27 30 33 36
AGE (MONTHS)
HEAD CIRCUMFERENCE
in
cm
95
90
75
50
25
10
5
WEIGHT
kg
lb
LENGTH
cm 46 48 50 52 54 56 58 60 62
in 18 19 20 21 22 23 24
64 66 68 70 72 74 76 78 80 82 84 86 88 90 92 94 96 98 100 cm
26 27 28 29 30 31 32 33 34 35 36 37 38 39 40 41 in
Date
Age
Weight
Length
Head Circ.
Comment

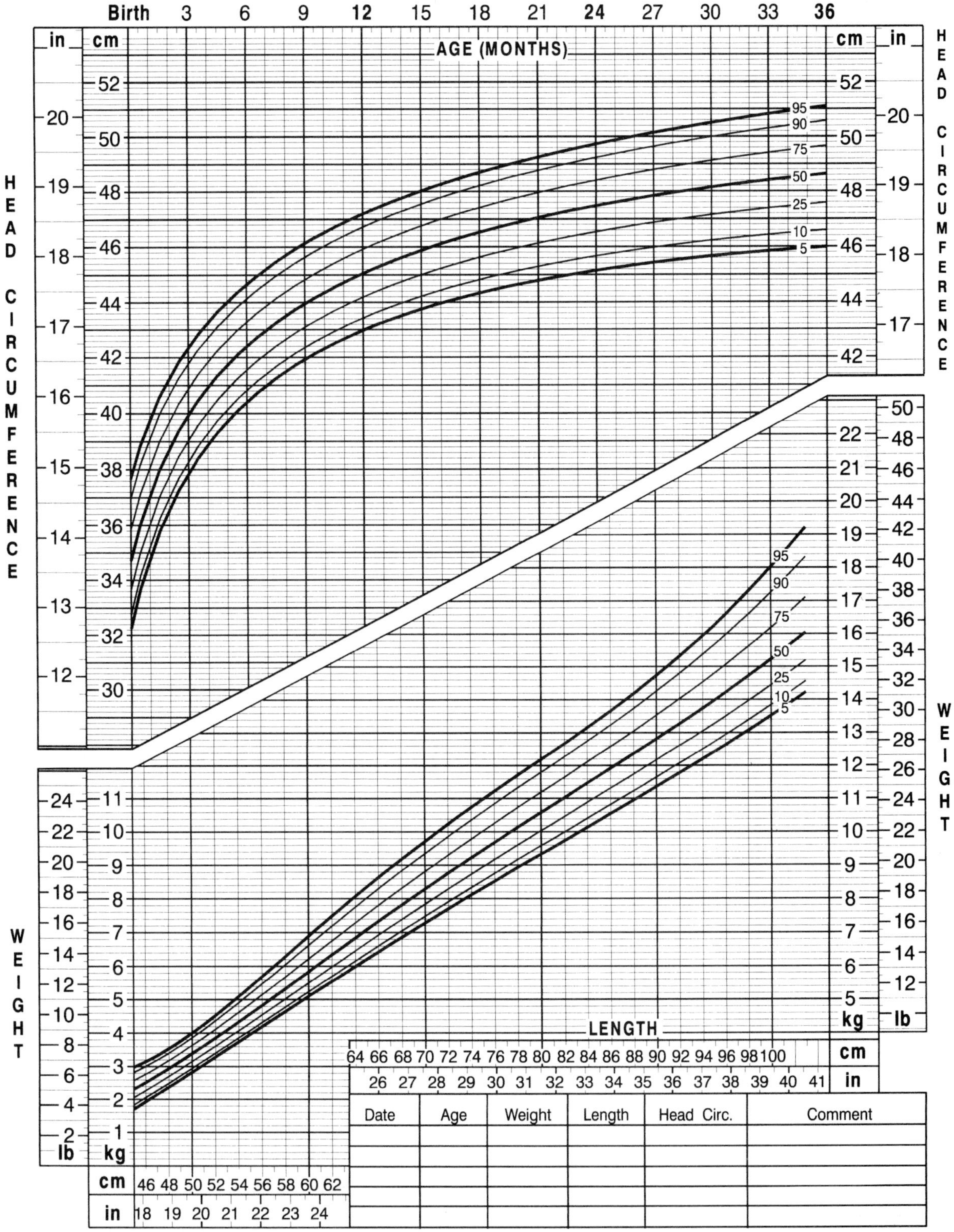

SOURCE: Developed by the National Center for Health Statistics in collaboration with the National Center for Chronic Disease Prevention and Health Promotion (2000).
http://www.cdc.gov/growthcharts

CDC

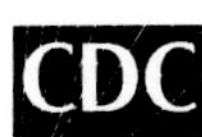

FIGURE 5-11 ■ *continued*

Blood pressure measurements according to the child's sex, age, and height are listed in Tables 5-5 and 5-6. The child's systolic and diastolic blood pressure measurements are compared with the numbers listed in the tables for the appropriate age and height percentiles. The height percentile in these tables is determined from a standard growth chart. The child is considered to have normal blood pressure if both the systolic and diastolic pressures are less than the 90th percentile. If the blood pressure is between the 90th and the 95th percentiles, it is considered to be high-normal and should be evaluated further. If the blood pressure is greater than the 95th percentile, the child may be hypertensive, and measurements should be repeated at future visits. *Hypertension* is diagnosed when the average of repeated blood pressure readings, taken for weeks to months, exceeds the 95th percentile. With repeated blood pressure measurements obtained using the correct techniques, only approximately 1% of children and adolescents will be diagnosed with hypertension.

Geriatric Patients

The aging process causes several changes in a person's physical appearance, mobility, and behavior. By the eighth and ninth decades of life, height may decrease from 2.5 to 10 cm (1–4 inches) from that in young adulthood as the posture changes because of kyphosis (Fig. 5-1) in the upper back and lordosis (Fig. 5-2) in the lower back. Body fat decreases in the extremities and increases in the trunk area. In addition, older adults may use a wider base to walk with shorter, uneven steps.

The aging process also causes minor changes in the vital signs. Older patients experience a decrease in thermal regulation and, thus, are less likely to develop a fever but are more likely to

TABLE 5-5 ➤ BLOOD PRESSURE LEVELS FOR THE 90TH AND 95TH PERCENTILES OF BLOOD PRESSURE FOR BOYS AGED 1 TO 17 YEARS BY PERCENTILES OF HEIGHT

		SYSTOLIC BP (mm HG)							DIASTOLIC BP (mm HG)						
AGE	HEIGHT PERCENTILES* → BP† ↓	5%	10%	25%	50%	75%	90%	95%	5%	10%	25%	50%	75%	90%	95%
1	**90th**	94	95	97	98	100	102	102	50	51	52	53	54	54	55
	95th	98	99	101	102	104	106	106	55	55	56	57	58	59	59
2	**90th**	98	99	100	102	104	105	106	55	55	56	57	58	59	59
	95th	101	102	104	106	108	109	110	59	59	60	61	62	63	63
3	**90th**	100	101	103	105	107	108	109	59	59	60	61	62	63	63
	95th	104	105	107	109	111	112	113	63	63	64	65	66	67	67
4	**90th**	102	103	105	107	109	110	111	62	62	63	64	65	66	66
	95th	106	107	109	111	113	114	115	66	67	67	68	69	70	71
5	**90th**	104	105	106	108	110	112	112	65	65	66	67	68	69	69
	95th	108	109	110	112	114	115	116	69	70	70	71	72	73	74
6	**90th**	105	106	108	110	111	113	114	67	68	69	70	70	71	72
	95th	109	110	112	114	115	117	117	72	72	73	74	75	76	76
7	**90th**	106	107	109	111	113	114	115	69	70	71	72	72	73	74
	95th	110	111	113	115	116	118	119	74	74	75	76	77	78	78
8	**90th**	107	108	110	112	114	115	116	71	71	72	73	74	75	75
	95th	111	112	114	116	118	119	120	75	76	76	77	78	79	80
9	**90th**	109	110	112	113	115	117	117	72	73	73	74	75	76	77
	95th	113	114	116	117	119	121	121	76	77	78	79	80	80	81
10	**90th**	110	112	113	115	117	118	119	73	74	74	75	76	77	78
	95th	114	115	117	119	121	122	123	77	78	79	80	80	81	82
11	**90th**	112	113	115	117	119	120	121	74	74	75	76	77	78	78
	95th	116	117	119	121	123	124	125	78	79	79	80	81	82	83
12	**90th**	115	116	117	119	121	123	123	75	75	76	77	78	78	79
	95th	119	120	121	123	125	126	127	79	79	80	81	82	83	83
13	**90th**	117	118	120	122	124	125	126	75	76	76	77	78	79	80
	95th	121	122	124	126	128	129	130	79	80	81	82	83	83	84
14	**90th**	120	121	123	125	126	128	128	76	76	77	78	79	80	80
	95th	124	125	127	128	130	132	132	80	81	81	82	83	84	85
15	**90th**	123	124	125	127	139	131	131	77	77	78	79	80	81	81
	95th	127	128	129	131	133	134	135	81	82	83	83	84	85	86
16	**90th**	125	126	128	130	132	133	134	79	79	80	81	82	82	83
	95th	129	130	132	134	136	137	138	83	83	84	85	86	87	87
17	**90th**	128	129	131	133	134	136	136	81	81	82	83	84	85	85
	95th	132	133	135	136	138	140	140	85	85	86	87	88	89	89

*Height percentile determined by standard growth curves.
†Blood pressure percentile determined by a single measurement.

National High Blood Pressure Education Program Working Group on Hypertension Control in Children and Adolescents. *Update on the 1987 task force report on high blood pressure in children and adolescents: a working group report from the national high blood pressure education program.* NIH publication no. 96-3790 1996.

TABLE 5-6 ➤ BLOOD PRESSURE LEVELS FOR THE 90TH AND 95TH PERCENTILES FOR GIRLS 1 TO 17 YEARS OF AGE BY PERCENTILES OF HEIGHT

		Systolic BP (mm HG)							Diastolic BP (mm Hg)						
Age	Height Percentiles* → BP† ↓	5%	10%	25%	50%	75%	90%	95%	5%	10%	25%	50%	75%	90%	95%
1	**90th**	97	98	99	100	102	103	104	53	53	53	54	55	56	56
	95th	101	102	103	104	105	107	107	57	57	57	58	59	60	60
2	**90th**	99	99	100	102	103	104	105	57	57	58	58	59	60	61
	95th	102	103	104	105	107	108	109	61	61	62	62	63	64	65
3	**90th**	100	100	102	103	104	105	106	61	61	61	62	63	63	64
	95th	104	104	105	107	108	109	110	65	65	65	66	67	67	68
4	**90th**	101	102	103	104	106	107	108	63	63	64	65	65	66	67
	95th	105	106	107	108	109	111	111	67	67	68	69	69	70	71
5	**90th**	103	103	104	106	107	108	109	65	66	66	67	68	68	69
	95th	107	107	108	110	111	112	113	69	70	70	71	72	72	73
6	**90th**	104	105	106	107	109	110	111	67	67	68	69	69	70	71
	95th	108	109	110	111	112	114	114	71	71	72	73	73	74	75
7	**90th**	106	107	108	109	110	112	112	69	69	69	70	71	72	72
	95th	110	110	112	113	114	115	116	73	73	73	74	75	76	76
8	**90th**	108	109	110	111	112	113	114	70	70	71	71	72	73	74
	95th	112	112	113	115	116	117	118	74	74	75	75	76	77	78
9	**90th**	110	110	112	113	114	115	116	71	72	72	73	74	74	75
	95th	114	114	115	117	118	119	120	75	76	76	77	78	78	79
10	**90th**	112	112	114	115	116	117	118	73	73	73	74	75	76	76
	95th	116	116	117	119	120	121	122	77	77	77	78	79	80	80
11	**90th**	114	114	116	117	118	119	120	74	74	75	75	76	77	77
	95th	118	118	119	121	122	123	124	78	78	79	79	80	81	81
12	**90th**	116	116	118	119	120	121	122	75	75	76	76	77	78	78
	95th	120	120	121	123	124	125	126	79	79	80	80	81	82	82
13	**90th**	118	118	119	121	122	123	124	76	76	77	78	78	79	80
	95th	121	122	123	125	126	127	128	80	80	81	82	83	83	84
14	**90th**	119	120	121	122	124	125	126	77	77	78	79	79	80	81
	95th	123	124	125	126	128	139	130	81	81	82	83	83	84	85
15	**90th**	121	121	122	124	125	126	127	78	78	79	79	80	81	82
	95th	124	125	126	128	129	130	131	82	82	83	83	84	85	86
16	**90th**	122	122	123	125	126	127	128	79	79	79	80	81	82	82
	95th	125	126	127	128	130	131	132	83	83	83	84	85	86	86
17	**90th**	122	123	124	125	126	128	128	79	79	79	80	81	82	82
	95th	126	126	127	129	130	131	132	83	83	83	84	85	86	87

*Height percentile determined by standard growth curves.
†Blood pressure percentile determined by a single measurement.

National High Blood Pressure Education Program Working Group on Hypertension Control in Children and Adolescents. *Update on the 1987 task force report on high blood pressure in children and adolescents: a working group report from the national high blood pressure education program.* NIH publication no. 96-3790 1996.

develop hypothermia. The normal body temperature usually is between 35.5 and 35.8°C (96–97°F). The heart rate remains in the adult normal range (60–100 bpm); however, the rhythm may be slightly irregular. Respirations may be more shallow, with a slightly increased respiratory rate to make up for decreased vital capacity and tidal volume.

Hypertension is very common in older patients. The blood vessels lose elasticity and stiffen with age, and these changes cause decreased vessel compliance as well as increased peripheral resistance. Consequently, the systolic blood pressure increases significantly, causing isolated systolic hypertension. Both the systolic and the diastolic blood pressure, however, increase in many elderly patients. Criteria for the diagnosis of hypertension in elderly patients are the same as those for younger adults.

Pregnant Patients

A pregnant woman's physical appearance changes as her uterus expands with the growing fetus. The trunk area enlarges, which causes the woman's weight to thrust forward. To compensate, the back muscles assume a new balance and posture: The shoulders are back, the head and neck are straight; and the lower back is hyperextended (i.e., lordosis). A pregnant woman also has a "waddling" gait and unsteady balance.

Weight gain typically is approximately 4 pounds during the first trimester and 0.5 to 1 pound per week during the second and third trimesters, with an average total weight gain of between 20 and 40 pounds at term. The heart rate increases by 10 to 15 bpm, and the respiratory rate increases slightly. Respirations also become deeper, and shortness of breath occurs more frequently.

Blood pressure typically remains unchanged during the first trimester, may decrease slightly during the second trimester, and returns to or slightly exceeds prepregnancy levels during the third trimester. Hypertension, however, is one of the major causes of maternal and fetal morbidity and mortality and occurs during approximately 6 to 8% of all pregnancies. Because of the seriousness of hypertension during pregnancy, a pregnant patient's blood pressure should be measured frequently. According to the *Working Group Report on High Blood Pressure in Pregnancy*, women with increased blood pressure during pregnancy are classified according to the following groups: (1) chronic hypertension, (2) preeclampsia-eclampsia, (3) preeclampsia superimposed on chronic hypertension, and (4) gestational hypertension.

Hypertension is defined as a systolic blood pressure of 140 mm Hg or greater or a diastolic blood pressure of 90 mm Hg or greater. *Chronic hypertension* is defined as hypertension that is present and observable before pregnancy or that is diagnosed before 20 weeks of gestation. If hypertension is diagnosed for the first time during pregnancy and does not resolve postpartum, it is also classified as chronic hypertension.

Preeclampsia is a pregnancy-specific syndrome of reduced organ perfusion secondary to vasospasm and activation of the coagulation cascade. It always presents a potential danger to both the mother and the baby. Preeclampsia is determined by increased blood pressure (>140 mm Hg systolic or >90 mm Hg diastolic in a woman who was normotensive before 20 weeks of gestation) and proteinuria. The hypertension that accompanies preeclampsia is primarily a sign of an underlying disorder rather than a primary pathophysiologic feature (as in chronic hypertension). *Proteinuria* is defined as the urinary excretion of 0.3 g or more of protein within 24 h. In a random urine determination (i.e., "dipstick" test), this amount of protein usually correlates with 30 mg/dL (i.e., 1+ dipstick), with no evidence of urinary tract infection. Box 5-1 lists other signs and symptoms that may be associated with a moderate-to-severe form of preeclampsia. **Eclampsia** is the occurrence of seizures that cannot be attributed to other causes in a woman with preeclampsia.

Preeclampsia superimposed on chronic hypertension is highly likely in patients with the following findings:

- New-onset proteinuria (urinary excretion ≥0.3 g of protein within 24 h) in a woman with chronic hypertension but who had no proteinuria early during pregnancy (<20 weeks of gestation).
- Chronic hypertension and proteinuria before 20 weeks of gestation.
- Sudden increase in proteinuria.
- Sudden increase in blood pressure in a woman with previously well-controlled hypertension.
- Thrombocytopenia (platelet count <100,000 cells/mm^3).
- An increase in alanine aminotransferase or aspartate aminotransferase to abnormal levels.

Gestational hypertension is defined as high blood pressure that occurs for the first time after 20 weeks of gestation and without proteinuria. This nonspecific term includes women with preeclampsia who have not yet manifested proteinuria as well as women who do not have preeclampsia.

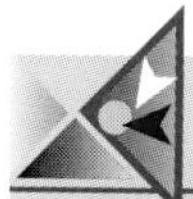

Box 5-1

SIGNS AND SYMPTOMS ASSOCIATED WITH MODERATE TO SEVERE PREECLAMPSIA

- Blood pressure ≥160 mm Hg systolic or ≥110 mm Hg diastolic
- Proteinuria ≥2.0 g in 24 h (i.e., 2+ or 3+ dipstick)
- Increased serum creatinine (>1.2 mg/dL, unless known to be previously elevated)
- Platelet count <100,000 cells/mm^3 and/or evidence of microangiopathic hemolytic anemia
- Elevated hepatic enzymes (alanine aminotransferase or aspartate aminotransferase)
- Persistent headache or other cerebral or visual disturbances
- Persistent epigastric pain

Adapted National High Blood Pressure Education Program. Working group report on high blood pressure in pregnancy. NIH publication 00-3029. 2000.

Self-Assessment Questions

1. You are counseling a 58-year-old woman with hypertension about losing weight to improve her blood pressure control. She is 5 feet, 9 inches tall and weighs 225 pounds. What is her BMI? Would her weight be classified as healthy, overweight, or obese?
2. What are the appropriate steps to measure the radial pulse?
3. What are the appropriate steps to measure the blood pressure?
4. Several common errors can occur during blood pressure measurement. What can you do to avoid making these errors?

Critical Thinking Questions

1. A 78-year-old patient comes to your pharmacy for a refill of his antihypertensive medication and a check of his blood pressure. The blood pressure readings that you obtain are 188/84, 186/88, and 184/80 mm Hg. Is this patient hypertensive? If yes, what stage hypertension does the patient have? How would you explain to this patient what these values mean?
2. A 31-year-old pregnant woman calls your pharmacy and states that her feet and hands are very swollen. She would like to know if she can take any over-the-counter diuretics to get rid of the extra fluid. How would you respond to her question?

Bibliography

American Pharmaceutical Association Comprehensive Weight Management Protocol Panel. APHA drug treatment protocols: comprehensive weight management in adults. J Am Pharm Assoc 2001;41:25–31.

Anderson FD, Maloney JP. Taking blood pressure correctly: it's no off-the-cuff matter. Nursing 1994;November:34–39.

Ebersole P, Hess P: Toward healthy aging: human needs and nursing response. 5th ed. St. Louis: Mosby–Year Book, 1998.

Joint National Committee on Prevention, Detection, Evaluation, and Treatment of High Blood Pressure. The sixth report of the Joint National Committee on Prevention, Detection, Evaluation, and Treatment of High Blood Pressure (JNC-VI). Arch Intern Med 1997;157:2413–2446.

Metropolitan Life Insurance Company. Height and weight tables (http://www.metlife.com). New York, 1999.

National Heart, Lung, and Blood Institute. Clinical guidelines on the identification, evaluation, and treatment of overweight and obesity in adults. 2000.

National High Blood Pressure Education Program. Working group report on high blood pressure in pregnancy. NIH publication 00-3029. 2000.

National High Blood Pressure Education Program Working Group on Hypertension Control in Children and Adolescents. Update on the 1987 task force report on high blood pressure in children and adolescents: a working group report from the national high blood pressure education program. NIH publication 96-3790. Bethesda, MD: NIH 1996.

Perloff D, Grim C, Flack J, et al. Human blood pressure determination by sphygmomanometry. Circulation 1993;88:2460–2467.

Talo H, Macknin ML, Medendorp SV Tympanic membrane temperatures compared to rectal and oral temperatures. Clin Pediatr 1991;30(suppl 4):30–33.

U.S. Department of Agriculture, U.S. Department of Health and Human Services. Nutrition and your health: dietary guidelines for Americans. 5th ed. 2000.

Whaley LF, Wong DL: Nursing care of infants and children. 6th ed. St. Louis: Mosby–Year Book, 1999.

CHAPTER 6

Nutritional Assessment

Raylene M. Rospond

GLOSSARY TERMS

- Anorexia nervosa
- Body mass index
- Bulimia nervosa
- Enteral
- Kwashiorkor
- Macronutrients
- Marasmus
- Micronutrients
- Nutrition
- Obesity
- Parenteral

NUTRITIONAL REQUIREMENTS

Nutrition can be defined as the sum total of the processes involved with the taking in and utilization of food substances. Adequate nutrition is needed for growth, repair, and maintenance of activities in the body. Several functions (or stages) are involved in the process of gaining nourishment: (1) ingestion, (2) digestion, (3) absorption, (4) assimilation, and (5) excretion.

Essential materials, called *nutrients,* must be provided by the diet to maintain these functions. Nutrient requirements vary with a person's age, sex, size, disease state, clinical condition, nutritional status, and level of physical activity, but regardless of individual variation, all people have nutritional requirements for energy, protein, fluid, and micronutrients. The U.S. recommended dietary allowances (RDAs) of standard nutrients should be used as a general guide when assessing a patient's nutritional status. Remember, however, that the RDAs are intended to represent the nutritional needs of *healthy* individuals.

Energy

Energy (or calorie) requirements can be supplied through the ingestion of carbohydrates, fat, and/or protein in the diet. Energy requirements can be calculated based on calories per body weight or by use of the Harris-Benedict equation (Box 6-1).

Box 6-1

HARRIS-BENEDICT EQUATION (KCAL/D)

Females: BEE = 655 + 9.6(wt) + 1.8(ht [in cm]) − 4.7(age)

Males: BEE = 66 + 13.7(wt) + 5(ht [in cm]) − 6.8(age)

Females >60 years: BEE = 9.2(wt) + 637 (ht [in m]) − 302

Males >60 years: BEE = 8.8(wt) + 1,128(ht [in m]) − 1,071

BEE, basal energy expenditure; *ht,* height; *wt,* weight (kg).

The simplest—and probably the most common—method to determine energy requirements is based on a standard number of calories required per kilogram of body weight. This method utilizes lean body weight and does not account for age- or sex-related differences of energy metabolism in adults. Recommended energy requirements using this method are presented in Table 6-1.

The Harris-Benedict equation calculates the basal energy expenditure (BEE), which must then be modified based on a "stress" or "activity" factor. Stress factors include conditions such as minor surgery, fracture, trauma, sepsis, and severe burns. Activity factors involve whether an individual is or is not confined to bed. In the presence of a stress factor, energy requirements as calculated by the Harris-Benedict equation are increased by as little as 30% (e.g., with minor surgery or fracture) or as high as 80 to 130% (e.g., with severe burns). An individual who is not confined to bed has an energy requirement 30% greater than that calculated by the Harris-Benedict equation.

Caloric or energy intake in excess of the energy expended is stored in body reserves. Carbohydrate is stored primarily as liver and muscle glycogen. Fat, which is stored as triglycerides in the adipose tissue, comprises the body's largest fuel reserve.

Protein

Protein requirements in adults vary based on nutritional status, disease state, and clinical condition. Protein requirements are expressed as grams per kilogram of body weight. Protein metabolism is dependent on both kidney and liver function; therefore, requirements will change during disease states that affect these two organ systems (see Table 6-1). After metabolization, protein is excreted as nitrogen. Measuring the amount of nitrogen excreted in the urine during 24 hours is an alternate method for determining individual protein requirements.

Excess protein is stored as visceral or somatic protein. *Visceral protein* stores include plasma proteins, hemoglobin, several clotting components, hormones, and antibodies. *Somatic proteins* stores include skeletal and smooth muscle stores. Stored protein is essential for numerous basic physiological functions; therefore, loss of protein stores results in loss of essential body functions.

TABLE 6-1 ➤ MACRONUTRIENT REQUIREMENTS FOR ADULTS

NUTRIENT	DAILY REQUIREMENT
Energy	
Healthy, normal nutrition status	~25 kcal/kg
Malnourished or mildly metabolically stressed	~30 kcal/kg
Critically ill, hypermetabolic	~30–35 kcal/kg
Major burn injury	40+ kcal/kg
Protein	
Recommended daily allowance	0.8–1.0 gm/kg
Low stress	
Maintenance	1.0–1.2 gm/kg
Anabolic	1.3–1.7 gm/kg
Hypermetabolic stress	1.5–2.5 gm/kg
Renal failure	
No dialysis	0.6–1.0 gm/kg
With dialysis	1.2–2.7 gm/kg
Severe hepatic failure	0.5–1.5 gm/kg
Fluid	
Healthy, normal nutritional status	30 mL/kg or 1 mL/kcal
Fever, excessive sweating, hyperthyroidism, vomiting, diarrhea, high-output fistula	↑ Fluid requirements
Renal failure, congestive heart failure, hypoproteinemia	↓ Fluid requirements

Fluid

Daily adult fluid requirements can be determined based on body weight or on energy requirements (see Table 6-1). Increased fluid requirements occur with increased insensible losses via the skin or metabolism or with increased gastrointestinal losses. Fluid requirements decrease in patients with renal failure, expanded extracellular volume, or hypoproteinemia. When estimating fluid requirements, pharmacists must consider *all* routes of fluid intake or loss. For example, nonnutritional sources of fluid intake (e.g., the amount of volume in intravenous medications) must be considered.

Micronutrients

Nutrients such as carbohydrates, protein, and fat are considered to be **macronutrients.** However, **micronutrients,** such as electrolytes, vitamins, and trace minerals, also are required to maintain adequate nutrition. Recommended daily maintenance doses for micronutrients are outlined in Table 6-2.

Micronutrients are required for the proper use of macronutrients and are involved in a wide variety of physiological functions. Variability in the absorption of various nutrients accounts for the difference between **enteral** (i.e., oral) and **parenteral** (i.e., intravenous) requirements. Poorly absorbed micronutrients will require large doses when ingested through the gastrointestinal tract. Water-soluble micronutrients are given in larger doses parenterally because of more rapid renal excretion when administered via this route. Other factors that can affect micronutrient requirements include gastrointestinal losses (e.g., diarrhea, vomiting, high-output fistula, hypermetabolism), renal function (especially sodium, potassium, magnesium, and phosphorus), and refeeding syndrome (electrolytes).

PATHOLOGY OVERVIEW

Inadequate nutrition can result from lack of food. More commonly, however, malnutrition results from insufficient utilization of nutrients because of an acute or chronic disease and/or its treatment. As a result of malnutrition, individuals are exposed to increased risks of morbidity and mortality from alterations in end-organ function (Table 6-3). In general, states of nutritional deficiency can be categorized as those involving protein-calorie malnutrition or those resulting from a lack of micronutrients (e.g., vitamins, trace minerals).

TABLE 6-2 ➤ RECOMMENDED ADULT DAILY MAINTENANCE DOSES FOR ELECTROLYTES, VITAMINS, AND TRACE MINERALS

NUTRIENT	ENTERAL	PARENTERAL
Electrolytes		
Calcium	800–1200 mg	10–15 mEq
Chloride	1,700–5,100 mg	—
Fluoride	1.5–4.0 mg	—
Magnesium	280–350 mg	10–20 mEq
Phosphorus	800–1,200 mg	20–45 mmol
Potassium	1,875–5,625 mg	60–100 mEq
Sodium	1,100–3,300 mg	60–100 mEq
Vitamins		
Biotin	30–100 μg	60 μg
Cyanocobalamin (B_{12})	2.0 μg	5.0 μg
Folic acid	200 μg	400 μg
Niacin	13–19 mg NE	40 mg NE
Pantothenic acid (B_3)	4.7 mg	15 mg
Pyridoxine (B_6)	1.6–2.0 mg	4 mg
Riboflavin (B_2)	1.2–1.7 mg	3.6 mg
Thiamine (B_1)	1.0–1.5 mg	3 mg
Vitamin A	800–100 μg RE	600 μg RE (3300 IU)
Vitamin C	60 mg	100 mg
Vitamin D	5–10 ug	5 ug (200 IU)
Vitamin E	8–10 mg TE	10 mg TE (10 IU)
Vitamin K	60–80 μg	0.7–2.5 mg
Trace minerals		
Chromium	50–200 ug	10–15 μg[a]
Copper	1.5–3 mg	0.5–1.5 mg
Iodine	150 μg	70–140 μg
Iron	10–15 mg	0.5 mg
Manganese	2–5 mg	0.15–0.8 mg
Molybdenum	75–250 ug	100–200 μg
Selenium	55–70 μg	40–80 μg
Zinc	12–15 mg	2.5–4.0 mg[b]

From Teasley-Strausburg KM, Anderson JD. Assessment of nutrition status and nutrition requirements. In: DePiro JT, Talbert RL, Yee GC, et al., eds. Pharmacotherapy: a pathophysiologic approach. 4th ed. Stamford, CT: Appleton & Lange, 1999:2233; with permission.

NE, niacin equivalents; *RE,* retinol equivalents; *TE,* tocopherol equivalent.

[a]An additional 20 μg/day is recommended in patients with intestinal losses

[b]An additional 12.2 mg/L of small-bowel fluid lost and 17.1 mg/kg of stool or ileostomy output is recommended; an additional 2.0 mg/day for acute catabolic stress.

Protein-Calorie Malnutrition

The three types of protein-calorie malnutrition are (1) marasmus, (2) kwashiorkor, and (3) mixed marasmus-kwashiorkor. Obesity also may be considered to be a form of protein-calorie malnutrition that results from excessive rather than deficient intake of macronutrients. Table 6-4 contrasts these four conditions in terms of their primary nutritional deficit, the time required for the deficit to develop, and the physical, laboratory, and immune parameters that are affected. In addition, anorexia nervosa and bulimia nervosa are eating disorders that can result in serious medical consequences, one of which is malnutrition.

Marasmus

Marasmus is a chronic condition resulting from a deficiency in the total energy intake. Wasting of both somatic protein (i.e., skeletal muscle) and adipose stores is observed, but visceral protein production (e.g., serum albumin and transferrin

TABLE 6-3 ➤ END-ORGAN RESPONSES IN MALNUTRITION

Organ	Anatomical Response	Physiological Response
Body composition	Increase in extracellular water compartment; loss of adipose stores, loss of lean body mass	
Heart	Four-chamber dilation; atrophic degeneration with necrosis and fibrosis; myofibrillar disruption	QT prolongations, low voltage, bradycardia; arterial hypotension, decreased central venous pressure, oxygen consumption, cardiac output, stroke volume, and contractility; preload intolerance; diminished responsiveness to drugs
Lung	Emphysematous changes; pulmonary infarcts; reduced bacterial clearance; muscle atrophy, decrease in diaphragmatic muscle mass and respiratory muscle strength	Pneumonia; decreased in functional residual capacity, vital capacity, and maximum breathing capacity; depressed hypoxic/hypercarbic drives
Hematological system	Failure of stem-cell production; depressed erythropoietin synthesis; decreased PMN chemotaxis; decreased lymphocytes count with reduced helper T and increased suppressor T and killer cells; decreased blastogenesis to phytohemagglutinin	Anemia; anergy; decreased granuloma formation; impaired response to chemotherapy; increased infection rate
Renal system	Epithelial swelling; atrophy; mild cortical calcification	Reduced glomerular filtration rate and inability to handle sodium loads; polyuria; metabolic acidosis
Gastrointestinal system	Disproportionate mass loss; hypoplastic and atrophic changes; decrease in total mucosal height	Depressed enzymatic activity; shortened transit time; impaired motility; propensity for bacterial overgrowth; maldigestion and malabsorption
Liver	Mass loss; periportal fat accumulation	Decreased visceral protein synthesis; depressed microsomal activity; eventual hepatic insufficiency
Pancreas	Fibrosis and acinar atrophy	Exocrine pancreatic insufficiency
Immune System	Decreased total lymphocyte count, CD4+, CD8+, and T-helper:suppressor ratio, secretory immunoglobulin, and serum complement	Decreased delayed cutaneous hypersensitivity, lymphocyte transformation, PMN leukocyte response (phagocytosis, metabolism, bactericidal capacity, chemotaxis)

Adapted from Cerra FB (ed.) Manual of Surgical Nutrition. St. Louis, MO: Mosby–Year Book, 1984:6. 4th ed. Stamford, CT: Appleton & Lange, 1999:2238; with permission.
PMN, polymorphonuclear granulocytes (neutrophils); *QT*, interval on an electrocardiogram from the start of the QRS complex to the end of the T wave.

concentration) is preserved. With severe marasmus, cell-mediated immunity and muscle function are impaired. Patients with wasting diseases (e.g., cancer) commonly have marasmus and a starved, cachectic, or cadaverous appearance. The relative weight-loss threshold for marasmus is 85% of the ideal body weight.

Kwashiorkor

Kwashiorkor results from a deficiency of protein during infancy or early childhood. It is common in patients with an adequate calorie intake but a relative protein deficiency. These patients are often catabolic, usually secondary to trauma, infection, or burns. It involves a depletion of visceral (and, to some degree, somatic) protein pools, with relative preservation of the adipose tissue. Hypoalbuminemia and edema classically characterize kwashiorkor, which can rapidly develop in response to protein deprivation during metabolic stress and may be accompanied by impaired immune function.

Mixed Marasmus-Kwashiorkor

Mixed marasmus-kwashiorkor occurs in chronically ill, starved patients who are undergoing hypermetabolic stress. It manifests as a reduced visceral protein synthesis superimposed on a wasting of somatic protein and energy (i.e., adipose tissue) stores. Immunocompetence is lowered, and the incidence of infection is increased. Poor wound-healing is observed in these patients.

Obesity

In contrast to marasmus, kwashiorkor, and mixed marasmus-kwashiorkor, obesity results from an excessive caloric intake. Nevertheless, it can still be considered a form of malnutrition.

Obesity should not be used interchangeably with the term *overweight.* Many athletes may have above-average muscle development and weigh more than usual for their height, but they do not have excess fat. An overweight person has a body weight 10 to 20% greater than the standard as defined in relation to his or her height. In contrast, **obesity** is defined as an excessive accumulation of body fat. Specifically, a male obese person has an amount of body fat greater than 22 and 25% of men younger than and older than 35 years of age, respectively. For women, these amounts are 32 and 35% for those younger than and older than 35. The normal percentage of body fat is between 15 and 22% in men and between 18 and 32% in women. Morbid obesity, or more than 100 pounds of excess weight, carries a greater level of morbidity and mortality.

TABLE 6-4 ➤ CLASSIFICATION OF MALNUTRITION

CONDITION	PRIMARY DEFICIT	TIME COURSE TO DEVELOP	PHYSICAL EXAMINATION	BODY WEIGHT
Obesity	Energy excess	Months to years	Increased fat deposition, especially abdomen and pelvis	Increased
Marasmus	Energy	Months to years	Cachetic, fat depletion, muscle wasting	Decreased
Kwashiorkor	Protein	Weeks to months	May look well-nourished	Decreased
Mixed marasmus/ kwashiorkor	Protein and energy	Weeks	Cachetic, may have edema, giving more of a normal appearance	Decreased

WNL, within normal limits.

Whether obesity is a symptom of a disease or a disease itself remains under debate. However, obesity appears to be a complex disorder of appetite regulation and energy metabolism. Consequences include psychological and social afflictions as well as medical complications (Box 6-2).

Box 6-2

MEDICAL COMPLICATIONS ASSOCIATED WITH OBESITY

- Gastrointestinal
  - Cholecystitis
  - Cholelithiasis
  - Hepatic steatosis
  - Delayed orocecal transit time
- Endocrine/reproductive
  - Type 2 diabetes mellitus
  - Hirsutism
  - Dyslipidemias
  - Menstrual disorders
  - Preeclampsia
  - Endometrial disorders
- Respiratory
  - Sleep apnea
  - Obesity hypoventilation syndrome
  - Erythrocytosis
  - Respiratory tract infections
- Cardiovascular
  - Coronary artery disease
  - Congestive heart failure
  - Systemic hypertension
- Malignancy
  - Colon
  - Prostate
  - Endometrium
  - Gallbladder
  - Cervical
  - Ovarian
- Musculoskeletal
  - Osteoarthritis
  - Gout

Reprinted from Apovian CM, Jensen GL. Overnutrition and obesity management In: Kirby DF, Dudrick SJ, eds. Practical handbook of nutrition in clinical practice. Boca Raton: CRC Press, 1994:33; with permission.

Anorexia Nervosa and Bulimia Nervosa

Anorexia nervosa and bulimia nervosa are eating disorders that occur predominantly in females. **Anorexia nervosa** is characterized by self-starvation, extreme weight loss, disturbance of body image, and intense fear of becoming obese. Bulimia is characterized by binge eating, which is usually followed by some form of purging (e.g., self-induced vomiting, laxative abuse, or associated behaviors such as diuretic use, diet pill use, or compulsive exercising). The majority of patients present with these disorders, which have a number of overlapping symptoms, during late adolescence or early adulthood. In addition, patients may present initially with either anorexia nervosa or bulimia nervosa but then fluctuate from one to the other. Signs and symptoms of these eating disorders are presented in Figure 6-1.

Single-Nutrient Deficiencies

Malnutrition also may result from micronutrient deficiencies. These may occur in isolation, in combination, or with the macronutrient deficiencies previously discussed. Signs and symptoms of micronutrient deficiencies are outlined in Table 6-5.

Underlying Pathology with Nutritional Effects

Acute and chronic disease may play a role in altering the intake or utilization of nutrients. Malnutrition seldom exists as an isolated disease state; usually, it is found in patients with other, preexisting illnesses (Box 6-3). Disease states specific to children can place the child at high risk for nutritional deficiencies (Table 6-6).

Special Considerations

Pediatric Patients

Daily macronutrient requirements for children vary by age; Table 6-7 outlines the RDAs for energy, protein, and fluid. Caloric requirements in children also vary by age, concurrent disease or symptoms, and developmental status. Energy requirements decrease from birth to adulthood.

Developmental disabilities, such as altered ambulation, cerebral palsy, and Down syndrome, will change a child's caloric requirements; the degree to which a child can ambulate is a critical factor in adjusting calculated energy needs. Protein requirements in children are altered by factors similar to those affecting adults. In general, children require higher amounts of daily pro-

TABLE 6-4 ➤ CLASSIFICATION OF MALNUTRITION—cont.

BODY FAT	ANTHROPOMETRIC MEASUREMENTS	SOMATIC PROTEIN	VISCERAL PROTEIN	IMMUNE FUNCTION
Increased	Increased	WNL	WNL	Normal
Decreased	Decreased	Decreased	Slightly decreased or WNL	Normal or depressed
WNL	Normal	WNL	Decreased	Depressed
Decreased	Variable	Decreased	Decreased	Depressed

tein because of developing muscle mass. Their higher percentage of body water and higher basal metabolic rate means that children also have higher fluid requirements per kilogram of body weight; this requirement is even larger in premature neonates because of large insensible losses and organ immaturity. Fluid status is assessed by monitoring urine output, specific gravity, serum electrolytes, and weight changes; a urine output of 1.0 to 2.0 mL/kg/h (or more) is adequate.

Therapeutic supplementation of vitamins and minerals usually is required only during certain disease states and conditions. Pathologic states (e.g., necrotizing enterocolitis, peritonitis, prematurity, renal and hepatic dysfunction) and drug therapy (e.g., diuretics, amphotericin B, corticosteroids) can alter the normal electrolyte requirements of children. Trace element requirements may be decreased in children with renal disease (zinc, selenium, chromium), cholestatic liver disease (copper, manganese), high ostomy and stool output (zinc, selenium), burns (zinc), prematurity (selenium), and acute illness (selenium).

Geriatric Patients

The decreases in basal metabolic rate, lean body mass, and physical activity that occur in elderly people result in the potential for lower total caloric needs. The BEE can be estimated for individuals older than 60 years using the equations contained in Box 6-1. For active elderly patients, the results of the calculation should be multiplied by 1.2 to 1.5.

Protein requirements, in contrast, do not decrease with age. Adequate protein intake is essential to help decrease the loss that occurs in lean body mass.

Elderly patients are more prone to dehydration because of increased fluid losses from compromised urine-concentrating ability, increased insensible losses via fragile skin, and decreased thirst response. Fluid requirements are estimated to be 30 mL/kg, or 1.5 to 2.0 L/day.

Because of the decreasing total caloric requirements, elderly patients require less thiamine, riboflavin, and niacin in their diet. Iron requirements also decrease for postmenopausal

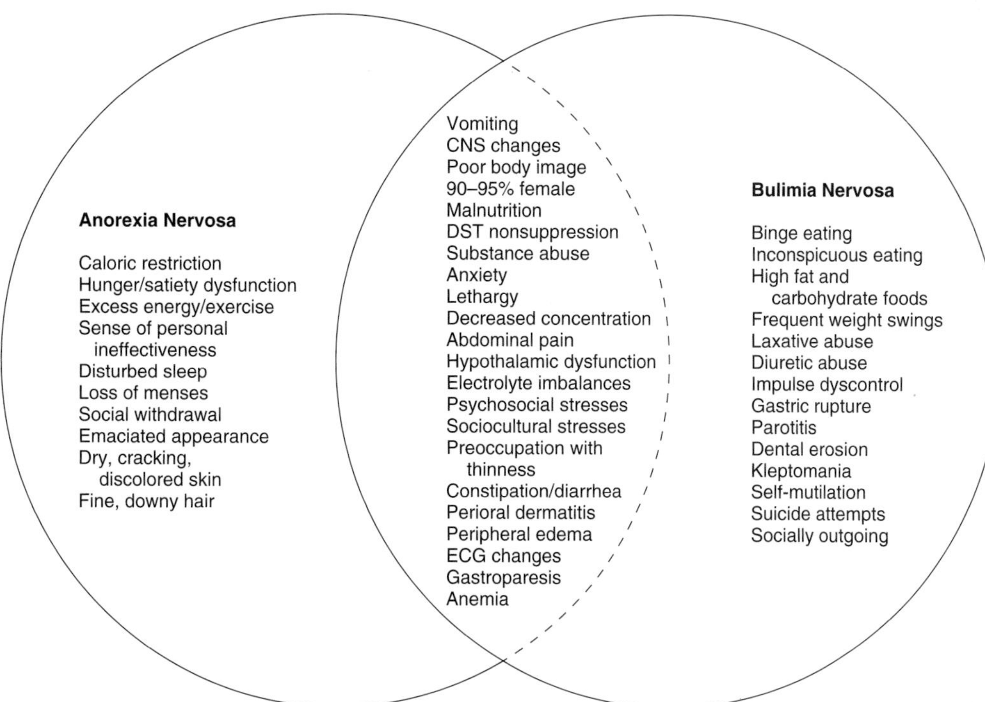

FIGURE 6-1 ■ Signs and symptoms of anorexia and bulimia nervosa. *CNS,* central nervous system; *DST,* dexamethasone suppression test; *ECG,* electrocardiographic. (Reprinted with permission from Marken PA, Sommi RW. Eating Disorders. In DePiro JT, Talbert RL, Yee GC, et al., eds. Pharmacotherapy: a pathophysiological approach. 4th ed. Stamford, CT: Appleton & Lange, 1999:1057.)

TABLE 6-5 ➤ MICRONUTRIENT DEFICIENCIES

MICRONUTRIENT DEFICIENCY	CLINICAL SIGN	SUPPORTIVE OBJECTIVE FINDINGS
Vitamin A	Dry, flaking, scaly skin Follicular hyperkeratosis (dry bumpy skin) Bitot's spots (foamy plaques in eyes) Xerophthalmia (dry eyes) Keratomalacia (softening of corneas) "Night blindness"	Triene/tetraene ratio > 0.4 Decreased plasma retinol
B-complex vitamins	Dry, flaking, scaly skin Glossitis (beefy red tongue)	
Pyridoxine (B_6)	Nasolabial seborrhea Acneiform forehead rash Angular stomatitis (red cracks at sides of mouth) Peripheral neuropathy Convulsive seizures Depression Microcytic anemia	Decreased plasma pyridoxal phosphate
Vitamin B	Disorientation Irritability	
Thiamine (B_1)	Pain in calves and thighs Peripheral neuropathy Wernicke's encephalopathy Hyporeflexia Mental confusion	Decreased RBC transketolase
Riboflavin (B_2)	Nasolabial seborrhea Red conjunctivae Cheilosis (vertical cracks in lips) Angular stomatitis	Decreased RBC glutathione reductase
(B_5)	Magenta/purplish colored tongue	
Niacin (B_3)	Glossitis Cracks in skin Lesions on the hands, legs, face or neck Pellagrous dermatosis (hyperpigmentation of skin exposed to sunlight) Pellegra Peripheral neuropathy Myelopathy Encephalopathy Cheilosis Angular stomatitis Atrophic papillae	Decreased plasma tryptophan Decreased urinary *N*-methyl nicotinamide
Folic acid	Pale conjunctivae secondary to macrocytic anemia	Decreased serum folic acid Decreased RBC folic acid Macrocytosis on RBC smear
Pantothenic acid	"Burning feet" syndrome	
Cyanocobalamin (B_{12})	Pale conjunctivae secondary to macrocytic anemia Peripheral paresthesias Spinal cord symptoms	Decreased serum B_{12} Macrocytosis on RBC smear
Vitamin K	Petechiae and ecchymoses of the skin	Prolonged prothrombin time
Vitamin C	Petechiae and ecchymoses of the skin Bleeding gums Prominent hair follicles Corkscrew hair Splinter hemorrhages of the nails Joint pain Muscle weakness Scurvy Tenderness of extremities Hemorrhages under periosteum of long bones Enlargement of costochondral junction Cessation of osteogenesis of long bones	Decreased serum ascorbic acid Long bone films

LDLs, low-density lipoproteins; *RBC*, red blood cells; *VLDLs*, very low-density lipoproteins.

(Continued)

TABLE 6-5 ➤ *(Continued)*

MICRONUTRIENT DEFICIENCY	CLINICAL SIGN	SUPPORTIVE OBJECTIVE FINDINGS
Vitamin E	Tachycardia secondary to hemolytic anemia (in premature infants) Pallor secondary to hemolytic anemia (in premature infants)	Decreased serum vitamin E Increased peroxide hemolysis Evidence of hemolysis on blood smear
Linoleic Acid	Dry, flaking, scaly skin Follicular hyperkeratosis Eczema Dull, dry, sparse hair Petechia, ecchymoses, bleeding from thrombocytopenia	
Tryptophan	Cracks in skin Lesions on the hands, legs, face or neck	
Excessive serum lipids of LDLs or VLDLs	Xanthomas (excessive deposits of cholesterol)	
Vitamin D	Craniotabes (thinning of the inner table of skull) Palpable enlargement of costochondral junctions Thickening of wrists and ankles Rickets Tetany Osteomalacia	Decreased 25-OH-vitamin D Increased alkaline phosphatase, Decreased calcium Decreased phosphorous Long bone films
Calcium	Osteoporosis Osteomalacia	Decreased serum calcium levels Long bone films Bone densitometry
Copper	Color changes in hair Corkscrew hair Pale conjunctivae secondary to microcytic, hypochromic anemia Skeletal lesions Pale secondary to sideroblastic anemia Neutropenia Dermatitis Anorexia Diarrhea	Decreased serum copper Film changes similar to scurvy
Chromium	Glucose intolerance Peripheral neuropathy Ataxia Increased free fatty acid levels Low respiratory quotient	Decreased serum chromium
Iodine	Cretinism Thyroid enlargement (goiter), myxedema	Decreased total serum iodine: inorganic, protein-bound iodine
Iron	Pale conjunctivae secondary to microcytic, hypochromic anemia Koilonychia (brittle, ridged, or spoon-shaped nails) Tachycardia secondary to anemia	Decreased serum iron; increased total iron-binding capacity
Magnesium	Tremor, spasm Irritability Lack of coordination, convulsions	Decreased serum magnesium
Manganese	Nausea, vomiting Dermatitis, color changes in hair Hypocholesterolemia Growth retardation	Decreased serum manganese
Molybdenum	Tachycardia Tachypnea Altered mental status Visual changes Headache Nausea, vomiting	Decreased serum molybdenum
Potassium	Sore, weak, or painful muscles	Decreased serum potassium
Selenium	Muscle weakness and pain (thigh) Cardiomyopathy	Decreased serum selenium

LDLs, low-density lipoproteins; *RBC*, red blood cells; *VLDLs*, very low-density lipoproteins.

TABLE 6-5 ➤ (Continued)

MICRONUTRIENT DEFICIENCY	CLINICAL SIGN	SUPPORTIVE OBJECTIVE FINDINGS
Sodium	Diarrhea Weakness Mental confusion Nausea Lethargy Muscle cramping	Decreased serum sodium
Zinc	Dull, dry, sparse hair, alopecia Parakeratosis Hepatosplenomegaly Hypogonadism Anorexia Hypogeusia Diarrhea Apathy Depression	Decreased serum zinc
Multiple nutrients	Papillary hypertrophy on tongue	

LDLs, low-density lipoproteins; *RBC*, red blood cells; *VLDLs*, very low-density lipoproteins.

Box 6-3

SELECTED DISORDERS THAT CAN RESULT IN NUTRITIONAL DEFICIENCIES

- Chronic infections
  - Acquired immunodeficiency syndrome
  - Cystic fibrosis
- Inflammatory states
- Neoplastic diseases
- Endocrine disorders
  - Diabetes mellitus
  - Hyperlipidemia
- Chronic illnesses
  - Pulmonary disease
  - Cirrhosis
  - Renal failure
- Hypermetabolic states
  - Trauma
  - Burns
  - Sepsis
- Digestive or absorptive diseases
  - Inflammatory bowel disease
  - Chronic intestinal pseudoobstruction
  - Short bowel syndrome
  - Necrotizing enterocolitis (pediatric patients)
  - Chronic protracted diarrhea

women. Decreased renal and hepatic function may lead to a decreased need for vitamin A in the diet. Vitamin requirements that may be increased include vitamin D (in those with decreased exposure to the sun) as well as vitamins B_6 and B_{12} (to compensate for decreased ability to digest protein).

Pregnant Patients

Pregnancy places additional demands on the body. Sufficient calories and protein must be consumed to support the synthesis of maternal and fetal tissues. Pregnant women require an additional 300 kcal/day before childbirth and an additional 500 to 800 kcal/day while breastfeeding. Additional protein is recommended during pregnancy (30 g) as well as postpartum (20 g) to maintain lactation. Pregnant women also should consume increased amounts of iron, B-complex vitamins, folic acid, calcium, and numerous other vitamins and minerals.

SYSTEM ASSESSMENT

Nutritional assessment is defined by the American Society of Enteral and Parenteral Nutrition as "a comprehensive evaluation to define nutrition status, including medical history, dietary history, physical examination, anthropometric measurements and laboratory data." The purposes of nutritional assessment are (1) to provide data for designing a nutritional care plan that will prevent and/or minimize the development of malnutrition, (2) to establish baseline data for evaluating the efficacy of nutritional care, and (3) to identify individuals who are malnourished or at risk of developing malnutrition.

The first step in evaluating a patient's nutritional status is screening to determine whether any potential for nutritional risk exists. Minimal nutritional screening involves taking a health history regarding conditions that might interfere with adequate food intake, measurement of both height and weight, and routine laboratory tests. Table 6-8 outlines specific signs and symptoms of patients who might be at high risk for malnutrition. Use of a standard form can minimize the time required for you to complete a nutritional screening. In addition to the risks of morbidity and mortality, a patient's drug therapy can be compromised because of malnutrition-induced changes in how the body metabolizes certain drugs (Box 6-4). A comprehensive nu-

TABLE 6-6 ➤ EXAMPLES OF NUTRITIONAL RISK FACTORS ASSOCIATED WITH SELECTED CHILDHOOD DISORDERS

CONDITION	UNDERWEIGHT	OVERWEIGHT	SHORT STATURE	LOW ENERGY NEEDS	HIGH ENERGY NEEDS	FEEDING PROBLEMS	CONSTIPATION	CHRONIC MEDICATIONS
Autism	✓[a]					✓		✓
Bronchopulmonary dysplasia	✓				✓			✓
Cerebral palsy	✓	✓	✓	✓	✓	✓	✓	✓
Cystic fibrosis	✓		✓		✓			
Down syndrome		✓		✓		✓		
Fetal alcohol syndrome	✓		✓					
Heart disease (congenital)	✓				✓			
HIV/AIDS	✓				✓			✓
Prader-Willi syndrome		✓	✓	✓				
Premature birth	✓		✓		✓	✓		
Seizure disorder								✓
Spina bifida	✓	✓	✓	✓		✓	✓	

From Baer MT, Harris AB. Pediatric nutrition assessment: identifying children at risk. J Am Diet Assoc 1997;97(suppl 2):S108, with permission.
AIDS, acquired immunodeficiency syndrome; *HIV*, human immunodeficiency virus.
[a]May be present.

TABLE 6-7 ➤ MACRONUTRIENT REQUIREMENTS FOR CHILDREN

NUTRIENT	DAILY REQUIREMENT
Energy	
Premature	120–150 kcal/kg/day
0–1 years	~100 kcal/kg/day
1–7 years	75–90 kcal/kg/day
7–12 years	60–75 kcal/kg/day
12–18 years	30–60 kcal/kg/day
Protein	
Recommended daily allowance	Infants: 1.6–2.2 gm/kg/day
	Children 1–10: 1.0–2 gm/kg/day
	Children >10: 0.8–1.0 gm/kg/day
Fluid	
Term Infant	Days 1–2: 70 mL/kg/day
	Day 3: 80 mL/kg/day
	Day 15–20: 90–100 ml/kg/day

tritional assessment is recommended for all individuals with confirmed nutritional risk factors. Such a comprehensive assessment extends beyond the information gathered during screening and includes dietary history and intake information, physical examination of clinical signs, anthropometrical measure, and laboratory tests. This level of nutritional assessment is not routinely performed by pharmacists; however, the results are commonly interpreted by hospital pharmacists on nutrition services.

Subjective Information

Clinical evaluation with a medical and dietary history remains the oldest, simplest, and probably the most widely used method of evaluating a patient's nutritional status. Information obtained from the medical and dietary history correlates well with objective evaluations. The medical and dietary history provides information regarding factors that predispose the patient to developing malnutrition. Box 6-5 outlines areas for the pharmacist to focus on while obtaining the medical and dietary history.

Typical questions in the medical and dietary history include:

- What are your typical eating patterns?
- What is your usual weight?
- Have you experienced any changes in appetite, taste, or smell or in your ability to chew or swallow? If so, please describe them.
- How would you describe your current stress level?
- Have you had any recent surgery, trauma, burns, or infection?
- Do you have any chronic illnesses? If so, which ones?
- Are you currently having any problems with vomiting, diarrhea, or constipation? Have you had any in the past?
- Have you ever experienced any food allergies or intolerance? How would you describe these?
- What medications do you currently take? Prescription? Over-the-counter?
- Do you use any vitamin, mineral, or nutritional supplements? If so, what type(s)? How much? For how long?
- What facilities are available for meal preparation? Who prepares your meals?
- Is your income adequate to buy sufficient food? Who does the shopping? What transportation is available for you to travel to the market?
- Do you use alcohol or illegal drugs? When did you have your last drink of alcohol? How much did you drink at that episode? How much do you drink each day? How much each week?
- What are your exercise and activity patterns? Please describe the type and amount per day.

A complete dietary assessment is composed of four stages: (1) measurement of food consumption, (2) calculation of the

TABLE 6-8 ➤ SIGNS AND SYMPTOMS INDICATIVE OF PATIENTS AT RISK FOR MALNUTRITION

PATIENT POPULATION	HIGH-RISK SITUATIONS
Adults	Anemia
	Diabetes mellitus
	Obesity
	Hyperlipidemia
Pregnant women, postpartum, and lactating women	Age <17 years
	Economic deprivation
	Eating disorders/unsound dietary practices/vegetarians
	On special diet for systemic disease
	Hyperemesis gravidarum
	Preeclampsia
	Multiple gestation
	Heavy cigarette smoking
	Vegetarian
	Alcohol abuse
	Iron deficiency anemia
	Weight <85% of that suggested for height
	Rapid weight loss
	Poor weight gain with pregnancy resulting in low-birth-weight infant
	Pregnancy while lactating
Children (infants to school-age)	Obesity
	Failure to thrive
	Vegetarian children
	Multiple food allergies
	Parent with eating disorder
	Selected disease states (see Box 6-3)
Adolescents	Eating disorders
	Obesity
	Vegetarian
	Pregnant adolescent
Elderly	SCALES scale
	Sadness
	Cholesterol
	Albumin
	Loss of weight
	Eating problems
	Shopping and food preparation
	DETERMINE scale
	Disease
	Eating poorly
	Tooth loss/mouth pain
	Economic hardship
	Reduced social contact
	Medications/drugs
	Involuntary weight loss/gain
	Need assistance with self-care
	Age >80 years

nutrient content of the food eaten, (3) assessment of absorbed intakes, and (4) evaluation of nutrient intakes in relation to recommendations. The final two stages are best left to a dietician or a board-certified nutrition specialist.

Quantitative Dietary Assessment

Quantitative dietary assessment can be completed via a 24-h recall or a 3-day food record. The 24-h recall is completed via an interview. The interviewer should ask neutral questions. For example, "I would like you to tell me what you had to eat or drink after you woke up yesterday morning. What was the time? Did you eat that food at home? What did you have next, and when was that?" The interviewer then proceeds through the day, repeating these questions as necessary while recording each food and drink that the patient consumed. While reviewing the patient's responses, the interviewer should probe for more specific descriptions of all the foods and drinks consumed, including the cooking methods and brand names, if possible.

Advantages of the 24-h recall method include low respondent burden (i.e., does not require a lot of additional action by the patient), high compliance, low cost, ease and speed of use, a standardized interview, an element of surprise (i.e., respondents are less likely to modify their eating habits), and suitability for illiterate patients. Disadvantages of this method include its reliance on memory, which makes it unsuitable for young children and elderly patients; errors in the estimation of portion size; overestimation or underestimation of intake; and omission of infrequently consumed foods.

Box 6-4

DRUGS WITH MALNUTRITION-INDUCED CHANGES IN PHARMACOKINETIC PARAMETERS

- Acetaminophen
- Cefoxitin
- Chloramphenicol
- Digoxin
- Estradiol
- Ferrous sulfate
- Gentamicin
- Isoniazid
- (para) Aminosalicylic acid (PASA)
- Penicillin G
- Phenobarbital
- Phenylbutazone
- Phenytoin
- Salicylates
- Sulfadiazine
- Sulfisoxazole
- Tetracycline
- Thiopentyl
- Tobramycin
- Warfarin

Box 6-5

COMPONENTS OF THE MEDICAL AND DIETARY HISTORY

- Eating patterns
- Usual weight; changes in weight
- Changes in appetite, taste, chewing, and swallowing
- Recent surgery, trauma, burns, and infections
- Chronic illnesses
- Vomiting, diarrhea, and constipation
- Food allergies and intolerances
- Medications and/or nutritional supplements
- Use of alcohol and illegal drugs
- Socioeconomic factors
- Usual activity; exercise patterns

The 3-day food record is a prospective rather than a retrospective dietary assessment. Two weekdays and one weekend day should be included to account differences in patterns of food consumption. The patient records the information as the 3 days progress. Therefore, in contrast to the 24-h recall method, patients completing a 3-day food record must be numerate, literate, and highly motivated.

Qualitative Dietary Assessment

Qualitative dietary assessment may be completed using the semiquantitative food frequency questionnaire or by completing a dietary history. A food frequency questionnaire is designed to obtain qualitative or semiquantitative descriptive information regarding usual patterns of food consumption. This method assesses the frequency with which certain food items or food groups are consumed during a specified period of time, such as daily, weekly, monthly, or yearly. Advantages to this method include high response rate, low patient burden, speed, and lack of expense. The questionnaire can be either administered by nonprofessionals or self-administered.

A dietary history is a retrospective review of a patient's usual food intake and meal patterns over varying periods of time. Usually conducted by a nutritionist during a personal interview, a dietary history has three sections: (1) a 24-h recall of actual intake, (2) a questionnaire regarding the frequency of consumption of specific food items, and (3) a 3-day food record using household measures. Advantages of the dietary history include its ability to provide information regarding habitual dietary intake and its relatively low patient burden. Disadvantages of this method include its reliance on memory and ability to estimate portion sizes; therefore, a dietary history would be unreliable in children younger than 14 years, in elderly patients, and in patients with erratic meal patterns.

Objective Information

Physical Examination

A focused physical examination for nutritional assessment should concentrate on measuring lean body mass and adipose tissue distribution as well as on physical findings of vitamin, trace mineral, and essential fatty acid deficiency (see Table 6-5). General physical findings that are suggestive of malnutrition include pallor, edema, cachexia, obesity, ascites, and dehydration. Other physical findings that may be found during a review of systems are outlined in Table 6-9.

Anthropometrical Measurements

Anthropometrical measurements are gross measurements of body cell mass and include measures of growth and measures of body composition. Weight, height, and weight:height ratios are mostly commonly used to assess growth. Additional measures of growth include head circumference as well as recumbent length and stature (in children), knee height, and elbow breadth and frame index (i.e., size of body frame).

Weight

An evaluation of body weight is the initial step in the anthropometrical assessment of an adult. (See Chapter 5 for the proper technique to obtain a weight measurement.) In addition, any visible signs of edema should be recorded to help assess the patient's fluid status.

ABNORMALITIES An unintentional weight loss of ≥10% over any time period should be considered clinically significant.

TABLE 6-9 ➤ SIGNS CONSISTENT WITH MALNUTRITION

General Appearance	Skin and Mucous Membranes	Mucous Membranes	Ocular	Musculoskeletal	Neurologic	Other
Pale Edema Cachexia Obesity Ascites Dehydration	Thin, shiny, scaling skin Decubitus ulcers Ecchymoses Perifollicular petechiae Hyperkeratosis Plaques around hair follicles Poorly healing wounds Easily plucked; dyspigmented, lackluster hair Thin, brittle, and/or spoon-shaped nails Splinter hemorrhages of nails	Pallor or redness of gums Edema of tongue and tongue fissures Glossitis (inflammation of the tongue) Magenta tongue Angular stomatitis (inflammation at corners of mouth) Cheilosis (reddened lips with fissures at angles)	Pale conjunctivae Bitot's spots (grayish, yellow, or white foamy spots on the whites of the eye) Conjunctival or corneal xerosis Keratomalacia (softening of part or all of cornea)	Retarded growth Bone pain or tenderness Epiphyseal swelling Muscle mass less than expected Poor muscle tone Osteomalacia Pain in calves and thighs Carniotabes (thinning of the inner table of the skull) Palpable enlargement of costochondral angles (rachitic rosary) Thickening of wrists and ankles Scurvy Skeletal lesions	Ataxia Positive Romberg test Decreased vibratory or position sense Nystagmus Peripheral neuropathy Hyporeflexia Disorientation Irritability Convulsions Paralysis Encephalopathy	Cardiovascular Beriberi Tachycardia secondary to anemia Glandular Thyroid enlargement **Hepatic** Jaundice Hepatomegaly

Alternatively, body weight as a percentage of the ideal body weight also can be calculated. The ideal body weight can be estimated using the formulas in Box 6-6. An assessment of body weight alone, however, is fairly limiting if the pharmacist is trying to assess a change in nutritional status. Evaluating the change in body weight over time is a more accurate reflection of changing nutritional status. Acute changes may reflect shifts in fluid status. Interpretation of any actual body weight measurements must take into consideration the ideal weight for height, usual body weight, fluid status, and age.

ABNORMALITIES Mild malnutrition may be defined as a current weight 80–90% of the ideal body weight, moderate malnutrition as a current weight 70–80% of ideal, and severe malnutrition as current a weight <70% of ideal.

Despite its limitations, a history of weight over time is one of the easiest—and least expensive—measures of nutritional status.

Height

Height (or stature) generally is measured in the standing position for children older than 2 years and for adults. (See Chapter 5 for the proper technique to obtain a height measurement.)

Body Mass Index

A **body mass index** (BMI) is an alternate way to determine the appropriateness of an individual's weight:height ratio. The BMI may be more objective in the presence of obesity, but it cannot distinguish between excessive weight produced by adipose tissue, muscularity, or edema. The BMI may be calculated by dividing an individual's weight (kg) by his or her height (m^2). (See Chapter 5 for the BMI values associated with appropriate weight.)

Elbow Breadth

The measurement of elbow breadth can be used as an index of frame size. To properly utilize the Metropolitan Life Insurance Table, you need be able to determine whether the patient's frame size is small, medium, or large.

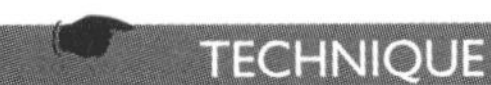

Measurement of Elbow Breadth

- Stand in front of the subject
- Raise the subject's right arm forward and to the horizontal.
- Flex the subject's elbow to 90°, with the back of the hand facing the examiner.
- Locate the lateral and medical epicondyles of the humerus.
- Place the blades of a flat-bladed sliding caliper to the epicondyles, with the blades pointing upward to bisect the right angle formed at the elbow.
- Read the distance between the condyles.
- Record the measurement (cm) to the nearest millimeter.
- Compare the value to the norm.

Box 6-6

BODY WEIGHT CALCULATIONS

IDEAL BODY WEIGHT

Female: 100 pounds (45.5 kg) for first 5 feet + 5 pounds (2.27 kg) for each 1 inch greater than 5 feet ± 10%

Male: 105 pounds (47.6 kg) for first 5 feet + 6 pounds (2.73 kg) for each 1 inch greater than 5 feet ± 10%

WEIGHT AS A PERCENTAGE OF IDEAL BODY WEIGHT

% Ideal body weight = Current weight/Ideal weight × 100

CURRENT WEIGHT AS A PERCENTAGE OF USUAL WEIGHT

% Usual body weight = Current weight/Usual weight × 100

RECENT WEIGHT CHANGE

Usual weight − Current weight/Usual weight × 100

CAUTION The caliper must be held at a slight angle to the epicondyles, and firm pressure must be exerted to minimize the influence of soft tissue on the measurement.

For a man, normal elbow breadth ranges from less than 6.6 up to 6.7 cm for a small frame, from 6.7 to 8.1 cm for a medium frame, and from 7.8 to 8.1 cm or more for a large frame. For a woman, normal elbow breadth ranges from less than 5.6 up to 5.8 cm for a small frame, from 5.7 to 7.1 cm for a medium frame, and from 6.6 to 7.2 cm or more for a large frame.

Skinfold Thickness

In contrast to the anthropometrical measures of growth previously discussed, measurements of skinfold thickness provide an estimate of body fat stores. Skinfolds that can be measured for nutritional assessment include the biceps, triceps, subcapsular, and suprailiac folds. Easy accessibility tends to make the triceps skinfold (TSF) the most commonly used method of estimating subcutaneous fat (Fig. 6-2).

TECHNIQUE

Measurement of TSF

- Extend the patient's arm so that it hangs loosely by his or her side.
- Locate and mark the tip of the acromion process of the shoulder blade at the outermost edge of the shoulder and the tip of the olecranon process of the ulna (Fig. 6-3).

- Measure the distance between these two points using a measuring tape, and mark the midpoint with a soft pen or indelible pencil.
- Grasp a vertical fold of skin, plus the underlying fat, 1 cm above the marked midpoint using your thumb and forefinger.
- Gently pull the skinfold from the underlying muscle tissue.
- Apply the caliper jaws at right angles exactly at the marked midpoint.
- Hold the skinfold between the fingers while the measurement is taken.
- Repeat the measurement three times, and then average the results.
- Record the measurements to the nearest 5 mm (0.5 cm).
- Compare the person's measurements with the standards for his or her age and sex (Table 6-10).

ABNORMALITIES TSF values 10% below or above the appropriate standard are suggestive of under- or overnutrition, respectively. Edema can produce falsely high readings. Examiner error, plastic calibers, or instrument malfunction can lead to unreproducible results.

CAUTION Nonambulatory persons should lie on one side. The uppermost arm should be fully extended, with the palm of the hand resting on the thigh.

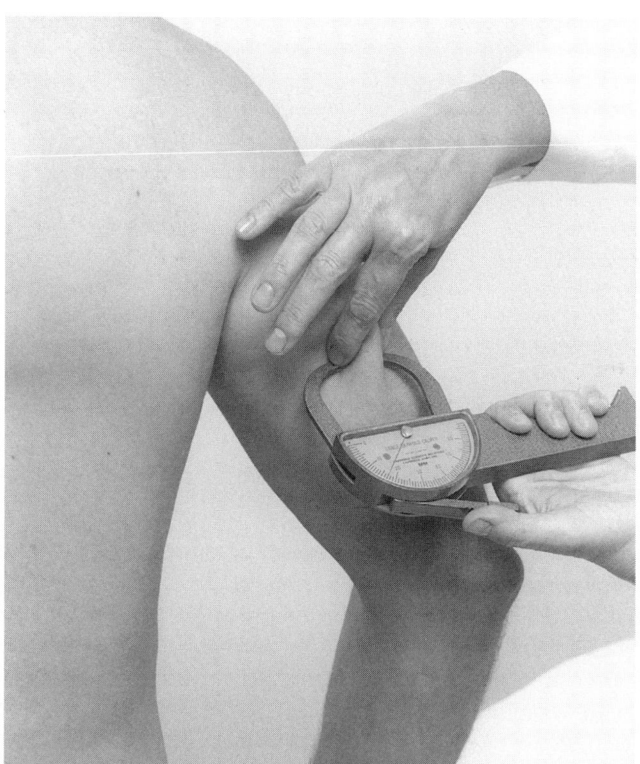

FIGURE 6-2 ■ Measurement of triceps skinfold.

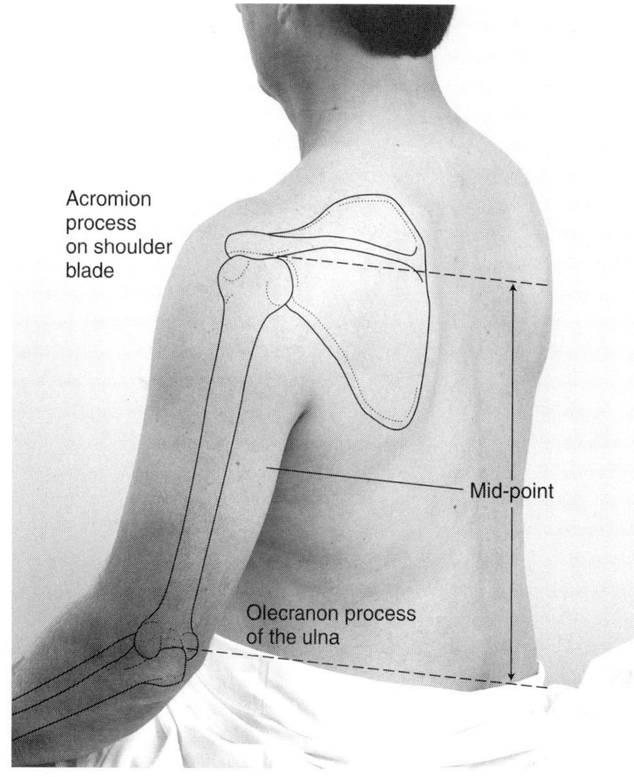

FIGURE 6-3 ■ Location of midpoint of the upper arm.

Determination of the TSF is helpful in establishing evidence of depleted fat stores. In obese patients or in those with extracellular fluid accumulation, however, you may not be able to measure the TSF because of the inability of the calipers to accommodate the skinfolds.

Mid-Upper Arm Circumference

The mid-upper arm circumference is a measure of subcutaneous tissue and skeletal muscle (Fig. 6-4). These measurements should be taken with a flexible, nonstretch tape made of fiberglass or steel; alternatively, a fiberglass insertion tape can be used.

TECHNIQUE

Measurement of Mid-Upper Arm Circumference

- Have the subject stand erect or sit, sideways to the measurer, with his or her arms relaxed and legs apart.
- Locate and mark the measurement point at the midpoint of the upper left arm, midway between the acromion process and the tip of the olecranon (see Fig 6-3).
- Extend the left arm of the subject so that it hangs loosely by his or her side, with the palm facing inward.
- Wrap the tape gently but firmly around the arm at the midpoint.
- Take the measurement (cm) to the nearest millimeter.
- Compare the person's measurements with the appropriate standard for his or her age and sex (Table 6-11).

TABLE 6-10 ➤ 50TH PERCENTILE OF TRICEPS SKINFOLD THICKNESS (CM) BY HEIGHT IN U.S. MEN AND WOMEN AGED 25 TO 54 YEARS WITH SMALL, MEDIUM, AND LARGE FRAMES

HEIGHT (INCHES)	SMALL FRAME	MEDIUM FRAME	LARGE FRAME
60	M: No reference F: 21	M: No reference F: 26	M: No reference F: 38
61	M: No reference F: 21	M: No reference F: 25	M: No reference F: 36
62	M: 11 F: 20	M: 15 F: 24	M: No reference F: 34
63	M: 10 F: 20	M: 11 F: 24	M: No reference F: 34
64	M: 10 F: 20	M: 12 F: 23	M: No reference F: 32
65	M: 11 F: 22	M: 12 F: 22	M: 14 F: 31
66	M: 11 F: 19	M: 11 F: 22	M: 14 F: 27
67	M: 11 F: 19	M: 13 F: 21	M: 11 F: 30
68	M: 10 F: 20	M: 11 F: 22	M: 14 F: 30
69	M: 11 F: No reference	M: 12 F: 19	M: 15 F: 30
70	M: 10 F: No reference	M: 12 F: 19	M: 14 F: 20
71	M: 20 F: No reference	M: 12 F: No reference	M: 15 F: No reference
72	M: 10 F: No reference	M: 12 F: No reference	M: 12 F: No reference

Adapted from Frisancho AR. New standards of weight and body composition by frame size and height for assessment of nutritional status of adults and the elderly. Am J Clin Nutr Assoc 1984;40:808–819.

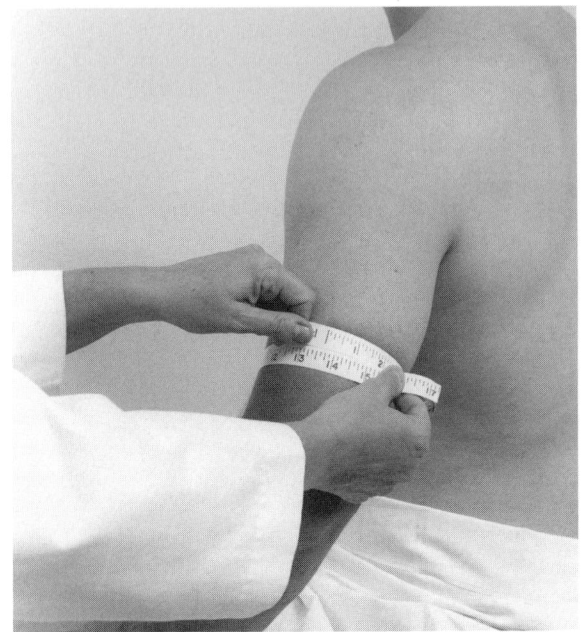

FIGURE 6-4 ■ Measurement of mid-upper arm circumference.

➤ ABNORMALITIES Patients with mid-upper arm circumference measurements less than the 10th percentile or greater than the 95th percentile should be referred for further medical evaluation. Very high or very low readings may be due to examiner error.

CAUTION Sleeved garments should be removed or the sleeves rolled up before completing the measurement. Do not tighten the tape such that skin contour indentations or pinching occurs.

Laboratory Measurements

Laboratory or biochemical assessment is primarily used to detect nutritional deficiencies that have not yet caused symptoms (i.e., subclinical deficiencies) or to confirm current subjective findings. Biochemical assessment of nutritional status may include serum protein status, hematological indices, iron status, mineral status, vitamin status, and lipid status. The results of biochemical tests are evaluated by comparing them to reference values. When interpreting abnormal values, however, always exclude the possibility of laboratory error or other causes of an abnormal value (Box 6-7).

TABLE 6-11 ➤ 50TH PERCENTILE OF UPPER ARM CIRCUMFERENCE (mm) FOR SELECTED AGE GROUPS

AGE GROUP (YEARS)	50TH PERCENTILE
1–1.9	M: 159 F: 156
5–5.9	M: 175 F: 175
10–10.9	M: 210 F: 210
15–15.9	M: 264 F: 254
19–24.9	M: 308 F: 265
25–34.9	M: 319 F: 277
35–44.9	M: 326 F: 290
45–54.9	M: 322 F: 299
55–64.9	M: 317 F: 303
65–74.9	M: 307 F: 299

Adapted from Frisancho AR: New norms of upper limb fat and muscle areas for assessment of nutritional status. Am J Clin Nutr Assoc 1981;30:2540–2548.

Protein Status

The majority of body protein is concentrated in skeletal muscle (i.e., somatic protein pool), with the remainder in visceral protein pools. Visceral protein is found in serum proteins, erythrocytes, granulocytes, lymphocytes, liver, kidney, pancreas, and the heart.

Measures of visceral protein status are most commonly obtained, and these include total serum protein, albumin, transferrin, retinol-binding protein, transthyretin, fibronectin, and somatomedin C. Serum albumin and transferrin are the most frequently used assessment indices and are best employed to monitor long-term changes in nutritional status. Measures of retinol-binding protein and transthyretin in the serum are better suited to monitor short-term changes in visceral protein status, because they have a small total body pool, shorter half-life, and relatively high specificity. Somatomedin C or insulin-like growth factor I is even more sensitive to acute changes in protein status.

The most commonly employed measure to assess somatic protein status is based on the creatinine level. Creatinine is excreted unchanged in the urine as a byproduct of creatine metabolism. Creatine is primarily concentrated in body muscle. The creatinine-height index (CHI), which may be calculated after collection of a 24-h urine sample, is the percentage that the actual 24-h creatinine measure represents of the expected value:

$$\text{CHI} = (\text{Actual 24-h creatinine excretion/Ideal 24-h creatinine excretion}) \times 100\%$$

Ideal creatinine excretion for adults, however, varies by height. The lower the CHI, the more severe the somatic protein depletion. Renal dysfunction, dehydration, high dietary protein intake, steroid use, age, stress, accuracy of the 24-h collection, and appropriateness of ideal weight-for-height standards can all affect the accuracy with which the CHI reflects the muscle mass in a subject.

Determination of nitrogen balance also can be used as an index of total protein nutritional status. Catabolism of amino acids results in the release of nitrogen, which is excreted in the urine as urea. The concentration of urea-nitrogen in the urine is dependent on the amount of protein intake in the diet, the subject's renal function, and the urine volume. The normal range for urinary urea-nitrogen excretion is 9.3 to 16.2 g/day. Nitrogen balance indicates the net change in total body protein mass and, therefore, can provide evidence to determine whether a person is anabolic (i.e., positive nitrogen balance) or catabolic (i.e., negative nitrogen balance). The nitrogen balance can be calculated using the following formula:

$$\text{Balance} = \text{Protein intake (g)}/6.25 - \text{Urinary urea-nitrogen (g)} + 4\text{ g}$$

Hematological Indices

The hematological parameters used most frequently in nutritional assessment are included in a complete blood count, which consists of a hemoglobin, hematocrit, red-cell count, platelet count, number and type of white blood cells (WBC; i.e., differential), and three red-cell indices: (1) mean cell volume, (2) mean cell hemoglobin, and (3) mean cell hemoglobin concentration. In special, comprehensive assessments, indices such as erythrocyte sedimentation rate, reticulocyte count, osmotic fragility, blood coagulation, and bone marrow characteristics also may be used. The indices most commonly

Box 6-7

FACTORS THAT CAN AFFECT BIOCHEMICAL TESTS

- Homeostatic regulation
- Diurnal variation
- Sample contamination
- Physiological state
- Infections
- Hormonal status
- Physical exercise
- Age, sex, and ethnic group
- Recent dietary intake
- Hemolysis (for serum/plasma)
- Drugs
- Disease states
- Nutrient interactions
- Inflammatory stress
- Weight loss
- Sampling and collection procedures
- Accuracy and precision of the analytical method
- Sensitivity and specificity of the analytical method

Adapted from Gibson RS. Nutritional assessment: a laboratory manual. New York: Oxford University Press, 1993:104; with permission.

examined for nutritional assessment are the hemoglobin and hematocrit.

Hemoglobin values vary by age, sex, and race. African Americans have slightly lower hemoglobin values than Caucasians. The normal hemoglobin level ranges from 13 to 18 g/dL in men and from 12 to 16 g/dL in women. Increased hemoglobin levels may occur in dehydration; decreased levels may indicate anemia, recent bleeding, or dilution caused by fluid overload.

Hematocrit values also vary by age and sex. The normal hematocrit value ranges from 37 to 53% in men and from 36 to 46% in women. An elevated hematocrit may occur in dehydration. A decreased value is more common, however, and can occur in several conditions, including chronic infection, chronic inflammation, bleeding, pregnancy, and overhydration.

Iron Status

Once screening has occurred for iron status using the hematological indices, more specific testing may be conducted to isolate the causative factor of an anemia. Serum iron, serum unsaturated iron-binding capacity, and serum ferritin are common biochemical tests for assessing a patient's iron status.

The serum iron count reflects the number of atoms of iron bound to transferrin. Normal serum iron values vary between males (50–160 μg/dL) and females (40–150 μg/dL). Low serum iron values can result from iron deficiency anemia, infection, inflammation, malignancy, and increased erythropoiesis. High serum iron values may result from decreased erythropoiesis, hemochromatosis, hemolytic anemia, acute liver damage, excessive absorption of iron from the gut, transfusions, and iron therapy. In contrast to the serum iron concentration, the total iron-binding capacity is less affected by other disease states, and the serum ferritin value usually is low only in patients with iron deficiency.

Mineral Status

The major mineral components of the human body are calcium, phosphorus, and magnesium. These minerals function in maintaining bone and soft tissue, and they act as regulatory agents in body fluids. The normal serum concentrations for calcium, phosphorus, and magnesium are 8.8 to 10.3 mg/dL (2.2–2.6 mmol/L), 2.5 to 5 mg/dL (0.8–1.6 mmol/L), and 1.6 to 2.4 mEq/L (0.8–1.2 mmol/L), respectively. Trace minerals occur in the body in very small (i.e., "trace") amounts and generally constitute less than 0.01% of body mass. Although as many as 10 trace minerals have been determined to be essential in humans, deficiency states have been identified for zinc, copper, manganese, selenium, chromium, iodine, molybdenum, and iron. (Clinical signs of mineral deficiency and the biochemical assays used to confirm these states are outlined in Table 6-5.)

An evaluation of a patient's medication therapy plays an important role in assessing mineral deficiencies. Many medications have altered efficacy or side effects in the presence of mineral deficiency or excess (Table 6-12). Clinical deficiencies of trace minerals result in patients with abnormal mineral losses. Zinc deficiency occurs most frequently in patients with Crohn's disease, malabsorption syndromes, or fistula losses. Patients with malabsorption states, protein-losing enteropathies, or nephrotic syndrome may be predisposed to copper deficiency. Similarly, molybdenum deficiency may occur in patients with excessive loss via the gastrointestinal tract (e.g., with short-bowel syndrome). Long-term enteral and parenteral nutrition may predispose patients to zinc, copper, chromium, manganese, selenium, and/or molybdenum deficiencies.

Vitamin Status

Vitamin status is the balance of vitamin supply and need in a given patient at a given point in time. A vitamin deficiency is the

TABLE 6-12 ➤ MEDICATION-MINERAL INTERACTIONS

MEDICATION	HYPONATREMIA	HYPOKALEMIA	HYPERKALEMIA	HYPOMAGNESEMIA	HYPOCALCEMIA	HYPERCALCEMIA
Diuretics	✓	✓		✓	✓	✓
Antihypertensives	✓		✓			
Psychotropics	✓					
Corticosteroids		✓				
Analgesics		✓				
Laxatives		✓				
Lithium		✓				
NSAIDs			✓			
Antituberculars			✓		✓	
Heparin			✓			
Alcohol				✓		
Aldosterone				✓		
Amphotericin B				✓		
Neomycin				✓		
Calcium Salts				✓		
Insulin				✓		
Sequestering agents					✓	
Vitamin D and metabolites						✓
Anticonvulsants					✓	
Antiarrhythmics			✓			

NSAIDs, nonsteroidal anti-inflammatory drugs.

shortage of a vitamin relative to its need by a particular subject. A primary vitamin deficiency results from failure to ingest the vitamin in sufficient amounts. Potential causes of primary deficiencies include poor food habits, poverty, ignorance, lack of total food, lack of vitamin-rich foods, anorexia (e.g., homebound elderly, infirm patients, people with dental problems), food taboos and fads (e.g., fasting), and apathy. In contrast, a secondary deficiency results from failure to absorb or otherwise utilize the vitamin. Potential causes of secondary deficiencies include poor digestion (e.g., achlorhydria), malabsorption (e.g., diarrhea, intestinal infection), impaired utilization (e.g., drug therapy), increased requirements (e.g., pregnancy, lactation, infection, rapid growth), vitamin destruction (e.g., storage, cooking), and increased vitamin excretion (e.g., excessive sweating, diuresis, lactation).

Similar to mineral deficiency, clinical signs of most vitamin deficiencies are not very specific. Table 6-5 summarizes the clinical signs associated with deficiency states of various vitamins as well as the biochemical assays that can be utilized to confirm the diagnosis. Some of the most common manifestations of vitamin deficiencies include anemias (e.g., vitamin B_6, vitamin B_{12}, folic acid), peripheral neuropathies (e.g., vitamin B_6, vitamin B_{12}), changes in the skin and mucous membranes (e.g., vitamin B_2 [Fig. 6-5], niacin [Fig. 6-6], vitamin A [Fig. 6-7], vitamin C [Fig 6-8]), alterations in bone formation or composition (vitamins C and D [Fig. 6-9]). Vitamin A deficiencies can present with various changes in the eye, including Bitot's spots (Fig. 6-10), exophthalmia (i.e., dry eyes), keratomalacia (i.e., corneal softening), and night blindness.

Discussions of nutritional status usually highlight the presentation of deficiencies; however, in today's health-conscious society, you also need to recognize the physical presentation of vitamin excess (Table 6-13). Vitamins A and D are considered to have the greatest potential for producing adverse reactions when consumed at levels above the RDA. Niacin has a moderate potential for toxicity, and vitamin E, vitamin C, thiamin, riboflavin, and pyridoxine are classified as having a low toxic potential. Those vitamins with negligible toxicity include vitamin K, pantothenic acid, biotin, folate, and vitamin B_{12}.

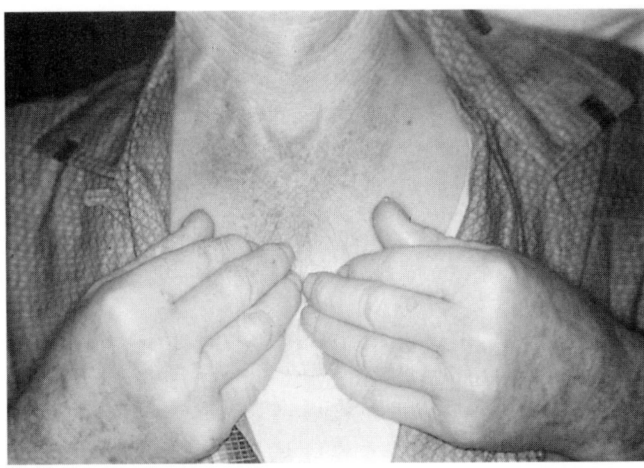

FIGURE 6-6 ■ Pellegra. (See Color Plate 2; Reprinted with permission from Neville BW, Damm DD, White DK, et al. Color Atlas of Clinical Pathology. 2nd ed. Baltimore: Williams & Wilkins, 1999.)

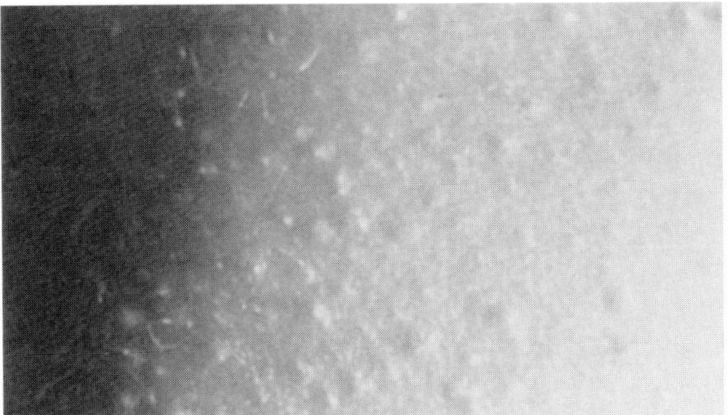

FIGURE 6-7 ■ Follicular hyperkeratosis. (See Color Plate 3; Reprinted with permission from Taylor KB, Anthony LE. Clinical Nutrition. New York: McGraw-Hill, 1983; copyright by Harold H. Sandstead, MD.)

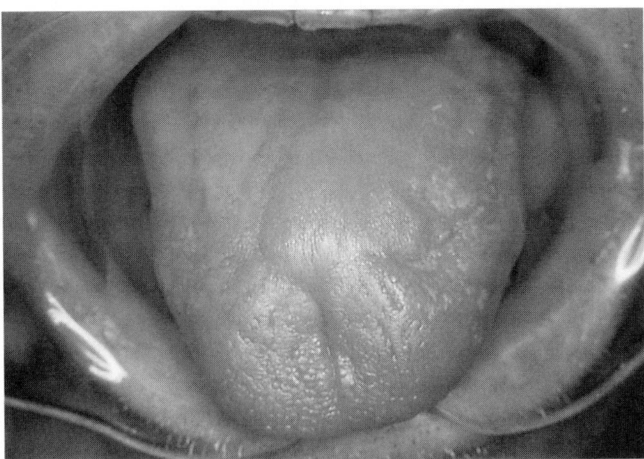

FIGURE 6-5 ■ Atrophic "bald" tongue. (See Color Plate 1; Reprinted with permission from Neville BW, Damm DD, White DK, et al. Color Atlas of Clinical Pathology. 2nd ed. Baltimore: Williams & Wilkins, 1999.)

Measuring the serum concentration can complete the confirmation of a vitamin deficiency or excess. Also, be aware that interactions can occur between medications and different vitamins that can result in decreased efficacy or increased side effects (Table 6-14).

Lipid Status

Assessment of blood lipid status can provide an evaluation of fat metabolism. Total serum cholesterol and serum triglyceride levels most commonly are used to screen for nutritional status as well as cardiovascular risk. This chapter focuses on assessment of nutritional status; for a more complete discussion of cardiovascular assessment, see Chapter 12.

Cholesterol is a precursor for the synthesis of bile acids and steroid hormones. The normal cholesterol concentration varies by age and sex, ranging from 120 to 200 mg/dL. Cholesterol values tend to increase with age and are slightly lower in women until menopause, after which they surpass the

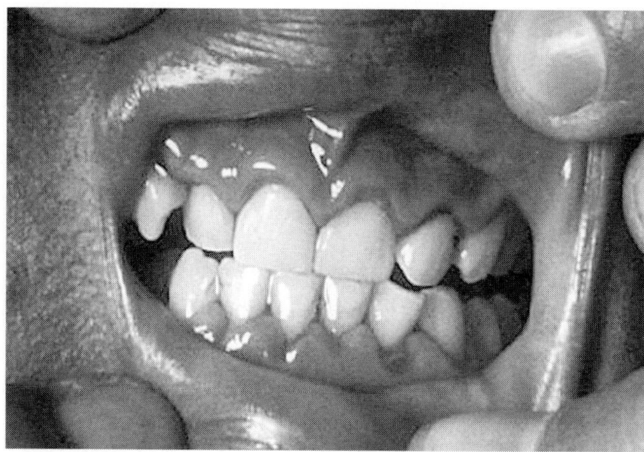

FIGURE 6-8 ■ Scorbutic gums. (Reprinted from the Public Health Image Library, Centers for Disease Control and Prevention.)

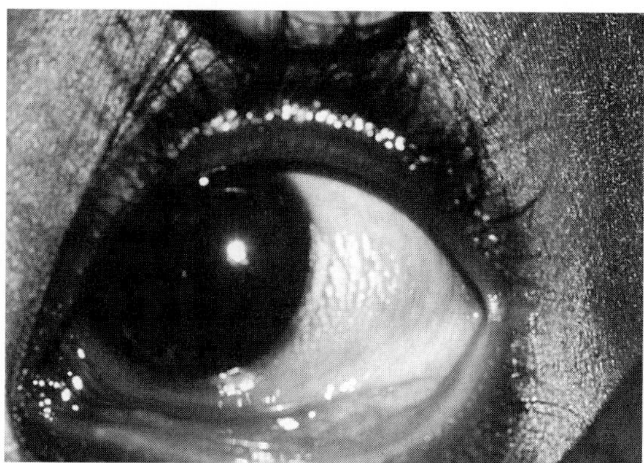

FIGURE 6-10 ■ Bitot's Spots. (See Color Plate 4: Courtesy of D.E. Silverstone, MD, New Haven, CT.)

normal value for men. Fasting blood samples should be used when determining cholesterol values because of the wide variations (≤20%) caused by fatty acid composition and cholesterol content of the diet.

A serum triglyceride level is used to screen for hyperlipidemia and to determine a patient's risk of coronary artery disease. This measure also can help to determine the specific type of hyperlipidemia that is present. Triglyceride concentrations reach normal adult levels by the third day of life, and they gradually increase after 30 years of age. Women tend to have higher serum triglyceride levels than men. The normal triglyceride level ranges from 10 to 190 mg/dL. Patients with diabetes mellitus, chronic renal disease, and certain primary hyperlipidemias often have high serum triglyceride levels.

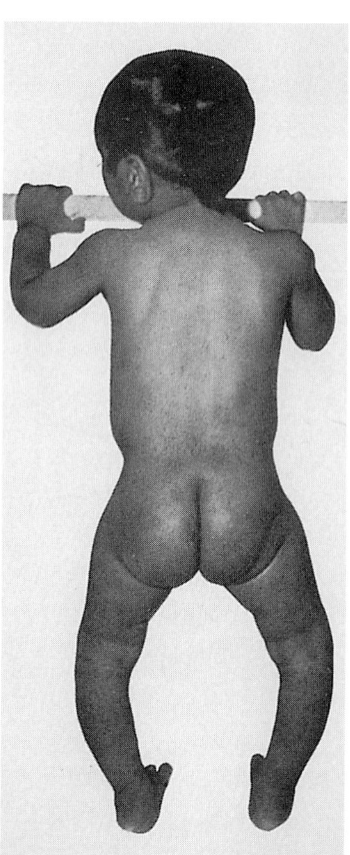

FIGURE 6-9 ■ Rickets. (Reprinted with permission from Latham MC, McGandy RB, McCann MD, et al. Scope manual on nutrition. Kalamazoo, MI. The Upjohn Company, 1980; copyright by Rosa Lee Nemir, MD.)

Indices of Immune Function

The tests of immune function most commonly used in nutritional status are the total lymphocyte count (TLC) and skin testing. A loss of immunocompetence is strongly correlated with malnutrition.

The TLC reflects the total number of circulating lymphocytes, the majority of which are T cells. It can be calculated from the WBC and the WBC differential:

$$\text{TLC (cell/mm}^3\text{)} = \text{WBC} \times (\text{\% Lymphocytes}/100)$$

Mild malnutrition would be considered as between 1,200 and 2,000 cells/mm^3, moderate malnutrition as between 800 and 1,200 cells/mm^3, and severe malnutrition as less than 800 cells/mm^3.

Delayed cutaneous hypersensitivity testing (i.e., skin testing) requires that an antigen be injected intradermally into the forearm of the subject. The response to the antigen, which is measured by the area of redness and/or induration, is noted at 24 and 48 h. A response of 5 mm or greater is generally considered to be a positive reaction. The antigens used in nutritional assessment are mumps, *Candida albicans,* streptokinase-streptodornase, *Trichophyton sp.,* coccidioidin, and purified protein derivative. If a subject does not respond to three out of five tests, they are considered to be anergic, which is correlated with malnutrition.

Both TLC and skin testing may be affected by a number of nonnutritional factors, including age, race, immune system diseases, infectious and inflammatory states, and various malignancies. Immunosuppressive medications (e.g., corticosteroids, chemotherapeutic agents, cyclosporine) also can affect immune responses.

TABLE 6-13 ➤ CLINICAL PRESENTATION OF MICRONUTRIENT EXCESS IN ADULTS

MICRONUTRIENT	CLINICAL PRESENTATION
Vitamins	
Thiamine (B_1)	Headache, muscular weakness, paralysis, cardiac arrhythmia, convulsions, allergic reactions (parenteral administration only)
Riboflavin (B_2)	None described
Niacin (B_3)	Transient flushing of skin and tingling sensations, headache, dizziness, nausea, GI upset, PUD, liver toxicity, hyperuricemia, glucose intolerance, cardiac arrhythmia, anorexia
Pyridoxine (B_6)	Lower serum lipids, peripheral sensory neuropathy, ataxia, skin lesions
Panthothenic acid	Diarrhea observed in only a few cases
Biotin	None described
Folic acid	Allergic reactions in only a few cases
Cyanocobalamin (B_{12})	Allergic reactions in only a few cases
Ascorbic acid (Vitamin C)	Possible kidney stones, diarrhea with 4–15 g/day, gout, lower serum cholesterol, rebound scurvy, increased absorption of iron, interference with oral anticoagulants, treatment of pressure sores Impaired bacterial activity
Vitamin A	***Acute:*** fatigue, cheilitis, abdominal pain, anorexia, blurred vision, lethargy, headache, hypercalcemia, dizziness, nausea and vomiting, irritability, skin desquamation, muscular weakness, peripheral neuritis ***Chronic:*** Alopecia, anorexia, ataxia, bone pain, cheilitis, conjunctivitis, diarrhea, diplopia, dry mucous membranes, dysuria, edema, high CSF pressure, fever, headache, hepatomegaly, hyperostosis, irritability, lethargy, menstrual abnormalities, muscular pain and weakness, nausea, vomiting, polydipsia, pruritis, skin desquamation, erythema, splenomegaly, weight loss.
Vitamin D	Anorexia, bone demineralization, constipation, hypercalcemia, muscular weakness and pain, nausea, vomiting, proteinuria, vague aches, metallic or bad taste, renal failure, hypertension
Vitamin E	Mild GI distress, some nausea, increases the effects of oral anticoagulants
Vitamin K	Vomiting, neonatal jaundice, block the effects of oral anticoagulants (menadione)
Trace minerals	
Selenium	Loss of hair, brittle fingernails, fatigue, irritability, garlic odor or breath
Zinc	Anorexia, nausea, lethargy, dizziness, diarrhea, vomiting (>2 g dose)

CSF, cerebrospinal fluid; *GI,* gastrointestinal; *PUD,* peptic ulcer disease.

TABLE 6-14 ➤ MEDICATION-VITAMIN INTERACTIONS

VITAMIN	DRUG	INTERACTION
Folic acid	Phenytoin	Decreased phenytoin effect; decreased dietary folate absorption
	Sulfasalazine	Decreased dietary folate absorption
	Triamterene	Decreased utilization of dietary folate
	Zinc	Decreased zinc availability
Niacin	Isoniazid	Niacin requirement may be increased
Pyridoxine	Barbiturates	Decreased barbiturate effect
	Oral contraceptives	May increase pyridoxine requirements
	Hydralazine	May increase pyridoxine requirements
	Isoniazid	May increase pyridoxine requirements
	Levodopa	Decreased levodopa effect (not carbidopa)
	Penicillamine	May increase pyridoxine requirements
	Phenytoin	Decreased phenytoin effect
	Oral anticoagulants	Increased anticoagulant effect with large doses of Vitamin A
Vitamin C	Oral anticoagulants	Occasional decreased anticoagulant effect
	Oral contraceptives	Increased serum concentration and possible adverse effects
Vitamin K	Oral anticoagulants	Decreased anticoagulant effect

Special Considerations

Pediatric Patients

Subjective assessment of nutritional status in young children is dependent on obtaining a dietary history from the child's parents, guardian, baby-sitter, or day care center. Certain nutritional problems in children, however, can be predicted from general family characteristics. For example, the incidence of malnutrition appears to increase as family income decreases. In contrast, the higher the educational level of the family members who purchase the food, the better the nutritional status of the family members younger than 17 years. Additional questions that may be pertinent when taking a history related to an infant or child include:

- Is your child willing to eat what you prepare?
- Does the child have any special likes or dislikes?

- How much will the child eat?
- How do you control snack foods?

Obtaining an accurate dietary history from an adolescent poses its own unique problems. The ever-increasing incidences of obesity, anorexia nervosa, and bulimia nervosa in this age group, however, reinforce the importance of broaching this issue, especially with adolescent girls. Pertinent questions for these patients include:

- What is your present weight?
- What would you like to weigh?
- Are you on any special diet to lose weight?
- Have you been on other diets to lose weight? What was involved? If so, were they successful? How often, if ever, do you think about "feeling fat"?
- Do you intentionally vomit or use laxatives or diuretics after eating?
- What snacks or fast foods do you like to eat? When do you eat them? How much do you eat?
- (For girls:) When did you first start menstruating? What is your menstrual flow like?

ABNORMALITIES Menarche is usually delayed if malnutrition is present. Amenorrhea or scant menstrual flow is associated with nutritional deficiency.

Before completing an objective nutritional assessment on children, the invasiveness of the method must be weighed against the potential benefit. Weight, length or height, head circumference, skinfold thickness, and arm muscle circumference are all noninvasive measures for determining body composition. Age-related nomograms have been developed for arm circumference and TSF. Assessments of weight, length or height, and head circumference can be evaluated by use of growth charts and compared graphically to age- and sex-related standards.

Methods to determine weight and stature are different in small children. Significant changes in the apparent weight of a small neonate or infant can be related to a change in scales, addition/deletion of dressings, armboards, diapers, or changes in the caregiver making the assessment. To minimize the effect of these external factors, weights should be assessed over several days. In children and adolescents, weight can be obtained less frequently.

Serum albumin, transferrin, transthyretin (i.e., prealbumin), and retinol-binding protein concentrations are related to age. These values are frequently used to assess visceral protein status in children.

Nitrogen balance in small children and preterm infants must be interpreted with caution. Collecting urine for 24 h in uncatheterized infants is very difficult. In addition, the urinary urea-nitrogen fraction of the total urinary nitrogen is unpredictable in infants.

Assessments of immune function may be less helpful in assessing nutritional status in children than in adults. The lack of an immunological response to a specific challenge may not indicate malnutrition but, rather, be secondary to immaturity or a lack of antigenic experience.

Geriatric Patients

Nutritional assessment is highly dependent on obtaining accurate information during the medical and health history. Special considerations for completing a health and medication history with an elderly patient are outlined in Chapter 3. Additional questions to ask aging patients include:

- How does your diet differ from when you were younger? Why?
- What factors affect the way you eat?

These questions will help to elucidate those physical changes that have caused the patient to modify his or her eating habits. Factors that affect the way an aging individual eats may include socioeconomic status (e.g., living on a fixed income), isolation that results in decreased interest in eating, decreased mobility that affects his or her ability to prepare meals, psychological changes (e.g., depression), concomitant disease states, and medications. Because of the large number of medications that one individual may be prescribed, elderly patients are at high risk for side effects, drug-drug interactions, and drug-nutrient interactions. Undernutrition is more dangerous than overweight in elderly patients.

Malnutrition in elderly people occurs frequently. Identification and early intervention, however, can improve the patient's functional outcome. No single factor adequately screens for malnutrition in this group. Weight adjusted for height, gender, and age remains the cornerstone of nutritional evaluation. Mid-arm circumference is useful to determine accurately the somatic nutritional status in patients with edema; however; this is hard to implement clinically because of difficulties in measuring the skinfold accurately. Visceral protein status is best measured by albumin, and risk should be identified in patients with albumin concentrations closer to 4 rather than to 3.5 g/dL. A cholesterol level of approximately 160 mg/dL or less indicates serious undernutrition in older patients.

Psychosocial factors play a very important role in the development of malnutrition among this patient group. Therefore, pay close attention to identifying factors that may place an elder at risk.

Pregnant Patients

Subjective assessment of nutrition in pregnant patients builds on that which would be conducted in a normal adult. Additional questions to ask pregnant patients include:

- How many times have you been pregnant? When?
- Were any problems encountered during previous pregnancies? During this pregnancy?
- Were any of your children underweight when they were born? If so, what was the weight? Why did your previous doctor feel this happened? Were they born with any other nutrition-related difficulties?
- What foods do you prefer when you are pregnant? What foods do you avoid? Do you crave any particular foods?
- Are you having any problems with this pregnancy so far? Any nausea? Vomiting? Are you taking any medications? Vitamin supplements? Calcium? Folic acid?

These questions will help you to identify any additional risk factors that might be detrimental to a successful pregnancy. When pregnancies occur less than 1 year apart, the nutritional status of the mother needs additional attention, because her nutritional reserves are still depleted. Previously experienced complications (e.g., excessive vomiting, indigestion, constipation) may be anticipated in a subsequent pregnancy to minimize the nutritional impact on the mother and the fetus. A past history of giving birth to a low-birth-weight infant is suggestive of past nutritional difficulties. Giving birth to an infant of more than 10 pounds may be a sign of latent diabetes in the mother.

Weight is an objective measure of nutrition that is used extensively in monitoring a woman during pregnancy. An expectant mother should be considered at risk nutritionally if her weight is 10% or more below the ideal, or 20% or more above the norm, for her height and age group. Fluid status also must be monitored carefully by examining the patient for signs of edema. Excessive edema may increase the weight of the patient and also affect laboratory values (e.g., hemoglobin, hematocrit). Diluted hemoglobin and hematocrit values may lead to unnecessary iron supplementation, which can further inhibit the patient's nutrition by increasing the severity of constipation.

Self-Assessment Questions

1. Name the three macronutrients.
2. Calculate the calorie, protein, and fluid requirements for a 70-kg man.
3. What nutrients are classified as micronutrients?
4. List the three types of protein-calorie malnutrition.
5. Name the major nutritional deficit present in each type of protein-calorie malnutrition.
6. Define anorexia nervosa.
7. Define bulimia nervosa.
8. For each of the following patient groups, list at least two risk factors for poor nutrition: adults, pregnant women, children, adolescents, and the elderly.
9. List at least five components of the medical and dietary history that are important to a nutritional assessment.
10. What methods can be used to perform a quantitative dietary history?
11. What methods can be used to perform a qualitative dietary history?
12. What is the most commonly used anthropometrical measure of growth?
13. Skinfold thickness is a measurement of what?
14. What is the most common laboratory measurement of protein status?
15. Low serum iron values can be found in which medical conditions?
16. What signs found on the skin and mucous membranes are consistent with malnutrition?
17. Excessive niacin in the diet can lead to what signs and symptoms?
18. How would you measure the TSF in a bedridden patient?

Critical Thinking Questions

1. KM is a 65-year-old man who was recently placed on captopril for his blood pressure. He comes to your pharmacy complaining of a racing heart and palpitations. Explain the medication side effect responsible for these symptoms.
2. JJ is a 45-year-old white woman who presents to your pharmacy complaining of right leg pain below the knee. On examination, the leg is warm and erythematous. JJ says that these symptoms are similar to when she has had blood clots in her leg. Her profile reveals she is on warfarin to prevent recurrent deep-vein thrombosis. On questioning, JJ states that she has been eating salads for the last 3 months in an attempt to lose weight. Explain the probable cause of JJ's recurrent deep-vein thrombosis.

Bibliography

Apovian CM, Jensen GL. Overnutrition and obesity management. In: Kirby DF, Dudrick SJ. eds. Practical handbook of nutrition in clinical practice. Boca Raton, FL: CRC Press, 1994:33.

ASPEN Board of Directors. Revised definition of terms used in ASPEN guidelines and standards. Nutr Clin Pract 1995;10:1–3.

Baer MT, Harris AB. Pediatric nutrition assessment: Identifying children at risk. J Am Diet Assoc 1997;97(suppl 2):S107–S115.

Baumgartner TG, ed. Clinical guide to parenteral micronutrition. 2nd ed. Melrose Park, L: Fujisawa, 1991.

Baumgartner TG. Micronutrients. In: Nutrition support pharmacy practice review course. Silver Spring, MD: ASPEN, 1996:38–65.

Baumgartner TG. Trace elements in clinical nutrition. Nutr Clin Pract 1993;8:252–263.

Blackburn GL, Bistrian RB, Maini BS, et al. Nutritional and metabolic assessment of the hospitalized patient. J Parenter Enter Nutr 1977;1:11–22.

Chernoff R. Physiologic aging and nutritional status. Nutr Clin Pract 1990;5:8–13.

Chessman KH, Anderson JD. Pediatric and Geriatric Nutrition Support. In: DePiro JT, Talbert RL, Yee GC, et al., eds. Pharmacotherapy: a pathophysiologic approach. 4th ed. Stamford, CT: Appleton & Lange, 1999:2293–2309.

Duerksen DR, Yeo TA, Siemens JL, O'Connor MP. The validity and reproducibility of clinical assessment of nutritional status in the elderly. Nutrition 2000;16:740–744.

Edington J. Problems of nutritional assessment in the community. Proc Nutr Soc 1999;58:47–51.

Elia M, Ward LC. New techniques in nutritional assessment: body composition methods. Proc Nutr Soc 1999;58:33–38.

Frisancho AR. Anthropometric standards for the assessment of growth and nutritional status. Ann Arbor, MI: University of Michigan Press, 1990.

Frisancho AR: New norms of upper limb fat and muscle areas for assessment of nutritional status. Am J Clin Nutr 1981;30:2540–2548.

Frisancho AR. New standards of weight and body composition by frame size and height for assessment of nutritional status of adults and the elderly. Am J Clin Nutr Assoc 1984;40:808–819.

Gibson RS. Nutritional assessment: a laboratory manual. New York: Oxford University Press, 1993.

Guigoz Y, Vellas B, Garry PJ. Assessing the nutrition status of the elderly: the mini-nutritional assessment as part of the geriatric evaluation. Nutr Rev 1996;54:S59–S65.

Gorstein J, Sullivan K, Yip R, et al. Issues in the assessment of nutritional status using anthropometry. Bull World Health Organ 1994;72:273–283.

Hamaoui E, Hamaoui M. Nutritional assessment and support during pregnancy. Gastroenterol Clin North Am 1998;27:89–121.

Hammond KA. The nutritional dimension of physical assessment. Nutr 1999;15(5):411–419.

Hopkins B: Assessment of nutritional status. In Gottschlich MM, Matarese LE, Shronts EP, eds: Nutrition support dietetics core curriculum. 2nd ed. Silver Spring, MD: ASPEN Publishers, 1993.

Jaffe M. Geriatric nutrition and diet therapy. 2nd ed. El Paso, TX: Skidmore-Roth Publishing, 1995.

Jeejeebhoy KN. Nutritional assessment. Nutrition 2000;16:585–590.

Kirby DF, Didrick SJ. Practical handbook of nutrition in clinical practice. Boca Raton, FL: CRC Press, 1994.

Lee RG, Foerster J, Lukens J, Wintrob MM, eds. Wintrobe's Clinical Hematology, 10th Edition. Philadelphia: Lippincott Williams & Wilkins, 1999.

Lipkin EW, Bell S. Assessment of nutritional status: the clinician's perspective. Clin Lab Med 1993;13:329–352.

Lukaski HC. Methods for assessment of human body composition: traditional and new. Am J Clin Nutr 1987;46:537–556.

Mandt JM, Teasley-Strausburg KM, Shronts EP. Nutritional requirements. In: Teasley-Strausburg KM, ed. Nutrition support handbook: a compendium of products with guidelines for usage. Cincinnati: Harvey Whitney Books, 1992:19–36.

Marken PA, Sommi RW. Eating disorders. In: DePiro JT, Talbert RL, Yee GC, et al., eds. Pharmacotherapy: a pathophysiologic approach. 4th ed. Stamford, CT: Appleton & Lange, 1999:1056–1064.

Mascarenhas MR, Zemel B, Stallings VA. Nutritional assessment in pediatrics. Nutrition 1998;14:105–115.

Metropolitan Life Insurance Company. Statistical bulletin, new weights and standards for men and women. Chicago, Metropolitan Life, 1983;64:2–9

Miller DK, Kaiser FE. Assessment of the older woman. Clin Geriatr Med 1993;9:1–31.

Shronts EP, Lacey JA. Metabolic support. In: Gottschlich MM, Matarese LE, Shronts EP, eds. Metabolic stress—core curriculum. 2nd ed. Silver Spring, MD: ASPEN, 1993;351–366.

Spiekerman AM. Proteins used in nutritional assessment. Clin Lab Med 1993;13:353–369.

Sproat TT. Anemias. In: DePiro JT, Talbert RL, Yee GC, et al., eds. Pharmacotherapy: a pathophysiologic approach. 4th ed. Stamford, CT: Appleton & Lange, 1999:1531–1548.

Teasley-Strausburg KM. Prevalence and significance of malnutrition. In: DePiro JT, Talbert RL, Yee GC, et al., eds. Pharmacotherapy: a pathophysiologic approach. 4th ed. Stamford, CT: Appleton & Lange, 1999:2237–2246.

Teasley-Strausburg KM, Anderson JD. Assessment of nutrition status and nutrition requirements. In: DePiro JT, Talbert RL, Yee GC, et al., eds. Pharmacotherapy: a pathophysiologic approach. 4th ed. Stamford, CT: Appleton & Lange, 1999:2221–2236.

Ulijaszek SJ, Kerr DA. Anthropometric measurement error and the assessment of nutritional status. Br J Nutr 1999;82:165–177.

Williams SR. Basic nutrition and diet therapy. 9th ed. St. Louis: Mosby–Year Book, 1992.

Zeman FJ. Clinical nutrition and dietetics. Lexington, KY: The Collamore Press, 1983.

CHAPTER

7

Pain Assessment

Raylene M. Rospond

GLOSSARY TERMS

- Acute pain
- Chronic pain
- Dysesthetic pain
- Evoked pain
- Malignant pain
- Musculoskeletal pain
- Neuropathic pain
- Nonmalignant pain
- "PQRST" mnemonic
- Referred pain
- Sensitization
- Somatic pain
- Visceral pain

ANATOMY AND PHYSIOLOGY OVERVIEW

Pain is one of the most important senses of the body. Sensations of sight, hearing, smell, taste, touch, and pain result from the stimulation of sensory receptors. Provocation of the sensory pain nerves produces a reaction of discomfort, distress, or suffering. The classic pain pathway consists of a three-neuron chain that transmits pain signals from the periphery to the cerebral cortex: (1) a first-order neuron, (2) a second-order neuron, and (3) a third-order neuron (Fig. 7-1). A pain sensation begins with stimulation of the free nerve endings of a first-order neuron.

Peripheral Pain System

The free nerve endings (or nociceptors) of first-order neurons are the main component of the peripheral pain system. Pain fibers are also involved.

Nociceptors

Nociceptors constitute the peripheral axons of a first-order neuron. Such pain receptors are common in the superficial portions of the skin, in joint capsules, within the periosteum of bones, and around the walls of blood vessels. Deep tissues and most visceral organs have fewer nociceptors. Nociceptors are activated by exposure to extremes of temperature, mechanical damage, or dissolved chemicals. Nociceptive activation leads to impulse conduction to the central nervous system over two types of pain fibers: A-delta fibers, and C fibers (Fig. 7-2).

Pain Fibers

A-delta fibers are small, myelinated fibers that are recruited first in response to noxious stimuli. Myelin is a fat-like substance that forms a sheath around the axons of certain nerves and allows for an enhanced transmission of stimuli. This first response (or "fast" pain) normally presents as a well-localized, discrete sensation. It is often described as a sharp, stinging, or prickling pain, and it lasts only while the stimulus is causing tissue damage. The pain threshold for this type of "first" pain is uniform from one person to another.

Sensations of diffuse, slow, burning, or aching pain result from stimuli transmitted by unmyelinated C fibers. This "second" pain results from the same type of injuries as fast pain sensations; however, it begins later and persists for a longer period

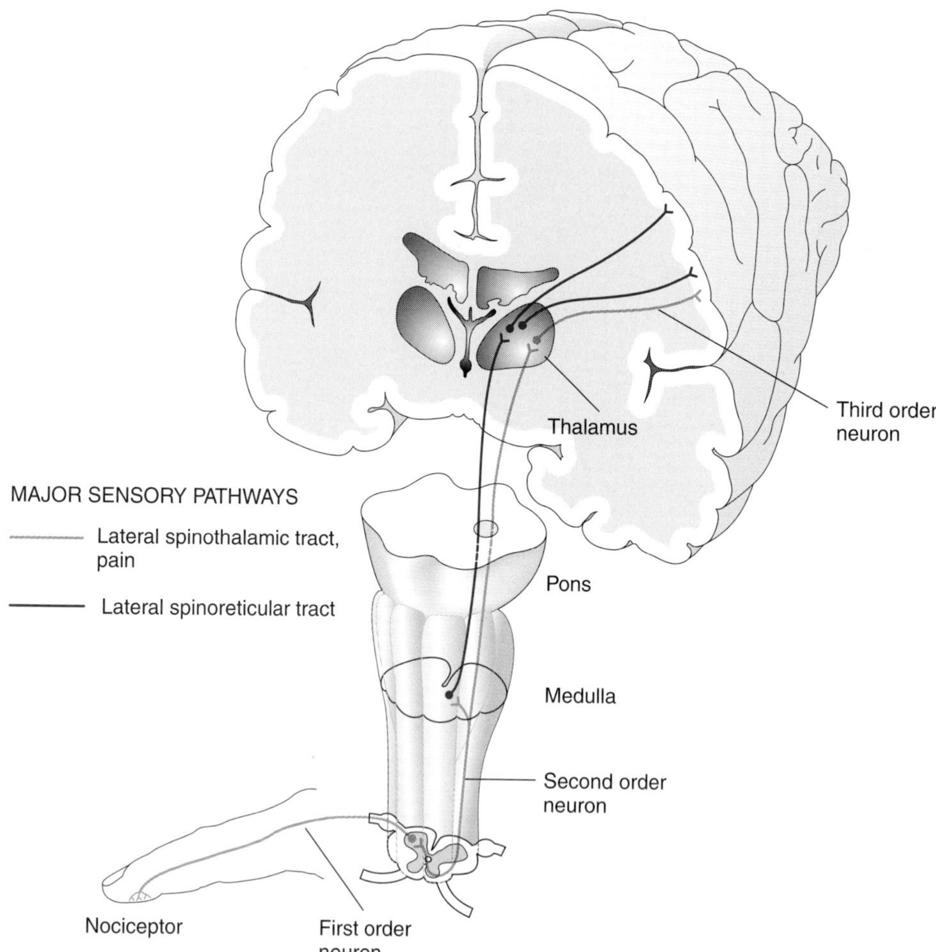

FIGURE 7-1 ■ The classic pain pathway. Discriminative pain impulses travel from the nociceptors along the first-order neurons to the second-order neurons of the spinothalamic tract. From there, they travel through the third-order neurons to the cortex. Similarly, affective pain impulses travel from the nociceptors along the first-order neurons to the second-order neurons of the spinoreticular tract. From there, they travel through the third-order neurons to the brainstem.

of time (see Fig. 7-2). Patients suffering from this type of pain sensation are aware of the pain but are less precise in identifying the discrete area of the body that is affected. These patients will often palpate an area in an attempt to locate the source of the pain. The pain threshold for "second" pain varies between individuals.

Both A-delta and C fibers have the property of **sensitization,** which is an increased sensitivity of the receptors following repeated application of a noxious stimulus. A classic demonstration of sensitization is repeatedly placing the palm of your hand over a candle flame. With each repeated exposure, the time to the sensation of pain decreases (because of sensitization of the fibers).

In addition to a direct effect on pain fibers, injury or trauma to tissue results in the release of chemical mediators such as bradykinin and histamine. These chemicals lead to vasodilation at the site of injury, and this vasodilation is followed rapidly by edema (i.e., a wheal) and a secondary vasodilation that produces reddening (i.e., a flare), which spreads into adjacent, uninjured skin. This tissue reaction also can result in sensitization of the adjacent nerve fibers.

Ascending Pain Pathways

On stimulation of the nociceptors by noxious stimuli, the peripheral axons of first-order neurons transmit the sensory data to their cell body in the dorsal root ganglion. The sensation is then transmitted into the gray matter of the dorsal horn of the spinal cord. Second-order neurons have cell bodies in the dorsal horn, and these neurons ascend the spinal cord through one of two major pathways: the spinothalamic tract, or the spinoreticular tract (see Fig. 7-1).

Spinothalamic Tract

The spinothalamic tract projects from the spine to the thalamus. Pain sensations that originate from small, discrete receptor fields in the periphery travel via a third-order neuron to the cortex (see Fig. 7-1). These sensations result in perception of the discriminative aspects of pain (e.g., nature, location, intensity, duration). Large receptive fields in the periphery also project sensations to the cortex, and these sensations result in perception of the affective or emotional aspect of pain (e.g., suffering).

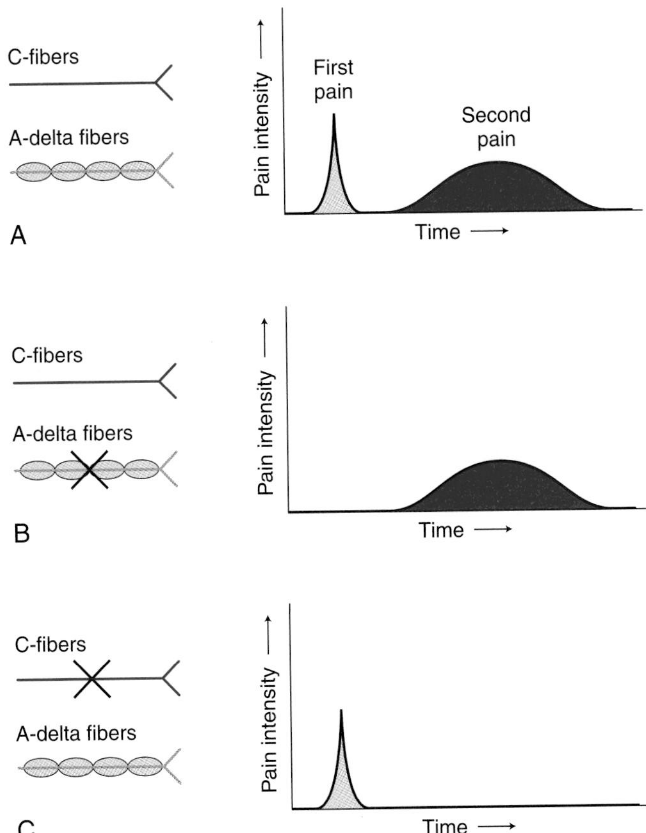

FIGURE 7-2 ■ Pain fiber transmission. **A.** Simultaneous stimulation of A-delta and C fibers result in the initial, acute, severe, "first" pain, followed by a constant and prolonged "second" pain. **B.** Isolated "second" pain in the presence of inhibition (X) of A-delta fibers. **C.** Isolated "first" pain in the presence of inhibition (X) of C fibers.

Spinoreticular Tract

Second-order neurons that ascend through the spinoreticular tract travel to the brainstem. Spinoreticular neurons provide elucidation of the emotional aspects of the sensation of pain.

Descending Pain Pathways

Descending fibers from the cortex, thalamus, or brainstem may inhibit impulses traveling along the ascending pain pathways. These descending fibers terminate in the dorsal gray column of the spinal cord. Neurotransmitters (e.g., epinephrine, norepinephrine, serotonin, various endogenous opioids) are involved in modulation of the pain sensation. The descending pain pathways are responsible for inhibition of pain transmissions from the spinal cord.

Pain-Mediating Substances

Various chemicals in the body are involved in the recognition or the inhibition of pain within the body.

Pain-Producing Substances

Chemicals involved in the recognition of pain may be leaked from damaged cells, synthesized by cells via enzymes induced through tissue damage, or be products of the nociceptors themselves (Table 7-1). Histamine and potassium released from cells after tissue damage can activate and/or sensitize nociceptors. In low concentrations, bradykinin, a polypeptide cleaved from plasma proteins, can produce vasodilation and edema, resulting in hyperalgesia (i.e., excessive sensitivity to pain); in high concentrations, it can directly stimulate nociceptors to fire. Prostaglandins and leukotrienes are compounds that are synthesized in areas of tissue damage and that can produce hyperalgesia by direct action on the nociceptor or by sensitizing nociceptors to other substances. Substance P, a neurotransmitter released from C fibers, also leads to the release of histamine and acts as a potent vasodilator.

TABLE 7-1 ➤ CHEMICALS ACTIVE IN NOCICEPTIVE TRANSDUCTION

SUBSTANCE	SOURCE	POTENCY IN PRODUCING PAIN[a]
Histamine	Release from mast cells	+
Potassium	Release from damaged cells	++
Bradykinin	Plasma proteins	+++
Prostaglandins	Arachidonic acid released from damaged cells	+/–
Leukotrienes	Arachidonic acid released from damaged cells	+/–
Substance P	Primary afferent neurons	+/–

Adapted from Fields HL. Pain. New York: McGraw-Hill, 1987:32.
[a]+, Pain-producing substance; –, pain-mitigating substance.

Pain-Mitigating Substances

Endogenous opioids are a family of peptides widely distributed through the body that influence the reaction to pain. Enkephalins, endorphins, and dynorphins stimulate opioid receptors in the periphery, dorsal horn, and brainstem. Each class of endogenous opioids has a demonstrated preference for a particular type of opioid receptor.

Neurotransmitters such as norepinephrine, serotonin, acetylcholine, and γ-aminobutyric acid are all involved in the inhibition of pain through varying mechanisms. Norepinephrine and serotonin reduce pain by modulating descending impulses from the brain. Acetylcholine and γ-aminobutyric acid inhibit firing of nociceptors (Table 7-2).

Special Considerations

Pediatric Patients

The neurological system of an infant is not fully developed at birth. The major portion of brain growth, along with myelinization of the central and peripheral nervous system, occurs during the first year of life. Several primitive reflexes are pres-ent at birth, however, including withdrawal from painful stimuli. Newborns often require a strong stimulus to respond—and then respond by crying and whole-body movements. The ability to localize the site of the stimulus and to produce a specific motor response develops concurrently with the level of myelinization.

Geriatric Patients

A steady loss of neurons in the brain and spinal cord occurs as part of the normal aging process. This leads to changes in adults older than 65 years that would often be interpreted as abnormal in younger individuals. The velocity of nerve conduction decreases between 5 and 10% as a result of aging. In turn, this can result in decreased reaction time and delayed impulse transmission, thereby diminishing the sensory perceptions of touch and pain.

Pregnant Patients

As the majority of pregnancies occur during the adult years, the transmission of pain either during the pregnancy or labor is similar to that previously described.

TABLE 7-2 ➤ RECEPTORS INVOLVED IN MODULATION OF PAIN

RECEPTOR	ACTION	AGONIST
Opioid	Analgesia	Morphine
Adrenergic	Reduction in sympathetic nervous system output	α_2: Clonidine α & β: Norepinephrine
Serotonergic	Modulation	Tricyclic antidepressants
Cholinergic	Inhibit nociception	Acetylcholine
GABA-ergic	Inhibits firing of nociceptors	Baclofen

Adapted from Reisner-Keller LA. Pain management. In: Herfindal ET, Gourley DR. Textbook of therapeutics: drug and disease management. 6th ed. Baltimore: Williams & Wilkins, 1996; 885.
GABA, γ-aminobutyric acid.

PATHOLOGY OVERVIEW

Acute Pain Syndromes

Acute pain is pain that arises from injury, trauma, spasm, or disease of the skin, muscles, somatic structures, or viscera of the body. The intensity of pain is proportional to the degree of injury, and it decreases as the tissue damage heals. Signs of autonomic nervous system activity (e.g., tachycardia, hypertension, sweating, prolonged dilation of the pupils, pallor) often accompany the sensation of acute pain. Usually, acute pain is associated with an event, is linear in nature (i.e., has a beginning and an end), has a positive meaning or purpose, and often is associated with physical signs. The two major types of acute pain syndromes are somatic pain and visceral pain.

Somatic Pain

Somatic pain results from activation of nociceptors in cutaneous and deep tissues.

Superficial Somatic Pain

Superficial somatic pain results from stimulation of nociceptors in the skin or the underlying subcutaneous and mucous tissue. It is characterized by throbbing, burning, or prickling sensations, and it may be associated with tenderness, pain caused by a stimulus that does not normally cause pain (i.e., allodynia), and hyperalgesia. This type of pain usually is constant in nature and well localized. Superficial pain is experienced most commonly in response to cuts, bruises, and superficial burns.

Deep Somatic Pain

Deep somatic pain results from injury to structures of the body wall (e.g., skeletal muscles). In contrast to the dull, aching pain that is related to the viscera, somatic pain can be localized to a particular area of the body; however, some radiation to adjacent areas may occur. Postoperative pain has a component of deep somatic pain because of trauma and injury to skeletal muscles.

Visceral Pain

Visceral pain results from injury to sympathetically innervated organs. It may be caused by abnormal distention or contraction of the smooth muscle walls, rapid stretch of the surrounding capsule of an organ (e.g., liver), ischemia of visceral muscle, serosal or mucosal irritation, swelling or twisting of tissue attaching organs to the peritoneal cavity, and organ necrosis. Pain attributed to abdominal or pelvic viscera usually is characterized as vague in distribution and quality. It often is described as a deep, dull, aching, dragging, squeezing, or pressure-like pain that is hard to localize. When extreme, it can be described as paroxysmal and colicky and can be associated with nausea, vomiting, sweating, and altered blood pressure and heart rate. Visceral pain often is noticed at the onset or early stages of disease. Pain sensations from visceral organs often are perceived as originating in more superficial regions, usually regions innervated by the same spinal nerves; this localization of pain to superficial or deep tissues distant from the source of pathology is called **referred pain.** Acute myocardial infarction and acute pancreatitis are examples of visceral pain.

Treatment

Treatment of an acute pain syndrome is directed toward the underlying cause and involves use of agents that produce short-term symptomatic relief. The goal is to mollify the pain impulses during the period of tissue healing. Nonsteroidal anti-inflammatory agents (e.g., ibuprofen, naproxen, ketoprofen) can be used "as needed" to reduce swelling and edema. Along with opiates (e.g., morphine, hydromorphone), these agents also can limit pain during the period of healing.

Chronic Pain Syndromes

Chronic pain is pain that persists for a minimum of 6 months and has distinct characteristics when compared to acute pain. For example, acute pain can be traced to an isolated event, but chronic pain usually is part of a more complex situation. Acute pain has a beginning and an end. Chronic pain, however, tends to be circular in nature; the beginning is quickly forgotten in the never-ending cycle of the pain. Acute pain has a positive connotation in that it warns the body of injury, whereas chronic pain serves no physiological purpose. Finally, chronic pain usually is devoid of physical signs and symptoms, so the underlying pathophysiology generally is not detected on physical or radiological examination. Chronic pain can arise from visceral locations, from myofascial tissue, or from neurological causes, and it usually is separated into **malignant (or cancer) pain** and **non-malignant** (or benign) **pain.**

Cancer Pain

Chronic malignant pain can have a combination of acute, intermittent, and chronic pain components. Cancer pain may arise at the primary site of the cancer as a result of tumor expansion, nerve compression, or infiltration by the tumor, malignant obstruction, or infections in a malignant ulcer. Pain also may arise at distant metastatic sites. Furthermore, cancer treatment with surgery, chemotherapy, and radiation therapy may lead to mucositis, gastroenteritis, skin irritation, and subsequent pain. Cancer pain most commonly arises from the musculoskeletal tissue, nervous system, and bone.

Nonmalignant Pain

Noncancer chronic pain can be subdivided into two major subtypes: **neuropathic pain,** and **musculoskeletal pain.**

Neuropathic Pain

Neuropathic pain can be idiopathic in nature or arise from discrete or generalized sites of nerve injury. Onset may occur immediately after an injury or after a variable interval. Neuropathic pain can produce dysesthesia, which is discomfort and altered sensations that are distinct from the usual sensation of pain. This type of **dysesthetic pain** is variously described as burning, tingling, numbing, pressing, squeezing, and itching and often is described as being extremely unpleasant or even intolerable. Neuropathic pain can be constant and steady in nature. In addition to continuous pain, superimposed, intermittent, shock-like pain can occur and often is characterized as sharp, lacinating, electrical, shocking, searing, or jolting. Patients with neuropathic pain also may present with sensory loss, evoked pain, sympathetic dysfunction, and motor and reflex abnormalities. Patients with **evoked pain** have altered sensory thresholds and may suffer from hyperalgesia, allodynia, hyperethesia (i.e., an increased sensitivity to stimulation), and hyperpathia (i.e., a painful syndrome characterized by increased, often explosive reaction to a stimulus). Examples of chronic neuropathic pain syndromes are postherpetic neuralgia, diabetic neuropathy, trigeminal neuralgia, poststroke pain, and phantom pain (i.e., feeling of pain in the area of an amputated limb).

Musculoskeletal Pain

Musculoskeletal pain arises from the muscles, bones, joints, or connective tissue. It may result from injury or be idiopathic or iatrogenic in nature. Common chronic musculoskeletal pain syndromes include pain related to inflammatory diseases of muscle such as polymyositis (a disease of connective tissue characterized by edema, inflammation, and degeneration of muscles) and dermatitis as well as pain related to joint diseases such as arthritis. Diseases of other organ systems (e.g., sickle-cell disease) also may cause musculoskeletal pain. Medications such as zidovudine, amphetamine, phancyclidine, and L-tryptophan may result in chronic musculoskeletal pain.

Treatment

Treatment of chronic pain must focus not only on amelioration of symptoms but also of the resultant suffering and disability. Regular administration of analgesics is recommended to prevent the occurrence of pain rather than to relieve pain after it has already occurred. Use of adjuvant analgesics (e.g., anticonvulsants for neuropathic pain, benzodiazepines for anxiety, antidepressants for depression) is common.

SYSTEM ASSESSMENT

Pain control remains a significant problem in health care worldwide. Problems related to health care professionals, patients, and the health care system as a whole have been identified as barriers to achieving appropriate pain management. Poor assessment techniques on the part of health care professionals and reluctance on the part of patients to report pain are two such problems. Effective pain management depends on careful assessment of both subjective and objective information.

Subjective Information

Subjective, patient-specific information (or self-reported information) is the primary tool in the evaluation of pain. Self-reported information, however, may be influenced by a patient's age, cognitive status, physical disabilities, drug use, and expectations regarding treatment by both the patient and the health care professional. Pharmacists must consider these factors when interpreting the information provided. Self-reported information may be gathered through a detailed interview and/or the use of single-dimension or multidimensional assessment tools.

Pain Interview

The approach to obtaining a detailed history from a patient with pain does not differ significantly from that outlined in Chapter 3. The pharmacist should use a combination of open-ended and closed-ended questions to obtain the type of information required to address the patient's problem. In addition, attention to factors such as identifying a private location of the interview, conveying a supportive and nonjudgmental attitude, particular attention to verbal and nonverbal cues, and setting aside an adequate amount of time to conduct the interview is essential. Use of a simple **"PQRST" mnemonic** also can aid the pharmacist in gathering vital information related to the patient's pain process (Table 7-3). A sample interaction between a pharmacist and a patient in pain is outlined in Box 7-1; the following interview questions focus on use of the "PRSQT" mnemonic in a pharmacist interview:

- What brought on the pain? Injury? Physical exertion? Stress?
- What worsens the pain? Diet? Stress? Physical exertion?
- What relieves the pain? Rest? Quiet? Medications?
- Describe the pain. Is it sharp? Dull? Burning? Aching? Constant? Intermittent?
- Where is the pain? Can you put your finger on it? Do you feel pain in any other areas of your body? Does the pain feel like it spreads out to other areas of the body?
- How severe is the pain? Mild? Moderate? Severe?
- Has the pain changed your lifestyle? How?
- Does the pain wake you up in the night? Do you have trouble getting to sleep?
- Has the pain affected your appetite?
- Do you have any other symptoms? Nausea/vomiting? Diarrhea/constipation? Sweating? Shortness of breath? Light-headedness? Palpitations?
- When does the pain occur? Evenings? Mornings? Daily? Monthly?
- When is the pain worse?
- How long have you been experiencing the pain?

TABLE 7-3 ➤ "PQRST" MNEMONIC FOR EVALUATING PAIN

P	Palliative or precipitating factors associated with the pain
Q	Quality of the pain
R	Region where the pain is located or radiation of the pain
S	Subjective description of severity of the pain
T	Temporal or time-related nature of the pain

Pain Assessment Instruments

Self-reported information also may be gathered using a pain assessment instrument. Note, however, that the depth and complexity of these assessment tools vary considerably. The ideal instrument would be simple to administer, be easily understood by patients, and be valid, sensitive, and reliable. Measurements geared at determining the physical location and severity of the pain are the most common. In some cases, five additional dimensions of information also may be necessary to make an appropriate measurement of a patient's pain and its effect on his or her life:

1. Functional disability caused by the pain, such as changes in activities of daily living or ability to perform self-care.
2. Behavioral/cognitive aspects of the pain, such as the amount of medications needed, number of physician visits, assessment of nonverbal observable behavior, and identification of neurotic symptoms.
3. Emotional responses to the pain, such as depression and anxiety, which can lower the pain threshold and make patients report higher levels of pain.
4. Economic impact of the pain, such as change in ability to work or to afford pain treatment.
5. Sociocultural information on issues such as litigation, patient independence, quality of life, family dynamics, and patient goals.

Assessment tools are available to assist the pharmacist in measuring the impact of pain on one or more of these dimensions.

Single-Dimension Instruments

The visual analog scale (VAS) is one of the most commonly used instruments for pain assessment (Fig. 7-3). This linear scale is a visual representation of the gradation of pain severity that a patient might experience. The range of pain is represented by a 10-cm line, with or without marks at each centimeter. Anchors at each end may be numerical or descriptive. One end represents *no pain,* whereas the other represents *the worst pain imaginable.* The scale may be either vertical or horizontal in orientation.

The major advantages of the VAS are its simplicity and ease of application. A pharmacist can readily use this as a quick assessment tool in any practice situation. During the postoperative period, however, use of the VAS may be limited because of the need for visual and motor coordination as well as the ability to concentrate. The VAS also can be adapted into a pain relief scale by using the anchors *no relief* and *complete relief.*

An alternative to the VAS is the verbal numerical scale (see Fig. 7-3). This scale uses numbers from 0 to 10 to represent the level of pain. The same anchors are used as on the VAS or the pain relief scale. The verbal numerical scale may be more useful during the postoperative period, because its verbal nature eliminates the need for visual and motor coordination.

A verbal rating scale uses words rather than a line or numbers as descriptors for the level of pain (see Fig. 7-3). Scales may

Box 7-1

SAMPLE INTERACTION BETWEEN A PHARMACIST AND A PATIENT WITH PAIN

Pharmacist: Hi. I'm Jessica Howard, the pharmacist. I notice you have been looking at the over-the-counter pain medications. I would be happy to take a few minutes to help you.
Patient: Thanks. I would like that.
Pharmacist: What exactly are you looking for?
Patient: My shoulder has been hurting, and I wanted to get some medication for it.
Pharmacist: When did your shoulder begin hurting?
Patient: Yesterday. I spent the day raking leaves in my yard. I noticed that my shoulder was stiff last night, and when I woke up this morning, it was not only stiff but hurt as well.
Pharmacist: On a scale of 0 to 10, where 0 is "no pain" and 10 is "the worst pain imaginable," how would you rate the pain that you are experiencing now?
Patient: Probably a three.
Pharmacist: Where in your shoulder does it hurt?
Patient: I don't know, just all over.
Pharmacist: Can you point to the area where it hurts?
Patient: Here. Ouch, that really hurts when I press on this area.
Pharmacist: Do you have any other areas of pain in your body?
Patient: My legs hurt a little bit from squatting down to pick up the leaves and put them into the bag.
Pharmacist: How would you describe your pain?
Patient: I'm not sure.
Pharmacist: Does the pain feel sharp, or is it dull and aching?
Patient: I would say it is a combination. Most of the time it is a dull, aching pain, but when I pressed on this area, it was a sharp, cutting type of pain.
Pharmacist: You have mentioned that pressing on this area makes the pain worse. Does anything else make the pain worse?
Patient: When I try to lift or reach with my arms and when I bend my legs it increases the pain.
Pharmacist: Does anything make the pain better?
Patient: Last night I put heat on my shoulder, and it felt slightly better afterward.
Pharmacist: Have you done anything else to treat the pain?
Patient: No.
Pharmacist: Have you taken any medications?
Patient: No.
Pharmacist: Do you have any allergies to medications?
Patient: No.
Pharmacist: Have you had success with any pain medication in the past?
Patient: I really have never taken anything, except a Tylenol for headache.
Pharmacist: This sounds like pain from your muscles. Let's look at the products in the next aisle. If this pain continues for longer than 3 days, if it continues to worsen, or you can no longer move your shoulder, you should see your physician.

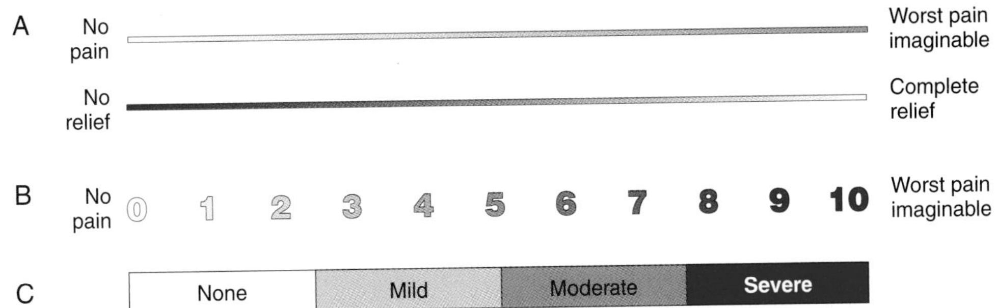

Figure 7-3 ■ Single-dimension assessment tools. **A.** Visual analog scale. **B.** Verbal numerical scale. **C.** Verbal rating Scale.

include descriptors such as *no pain, mild, moderate* and *severe.* Pain relief also may be defined as *none, slight, moderate,* or *good.* Because it restricts the patient's choice of words, this scale does not allow for fine discrimination of pain.

The various single-dimension instruments are compared in Table 7-4.

Multidimensional Instruments

Multidimensional instruments, like single-dimension instruments, assess the level of pain endured by the patient. However, these instruments also provide some measure of the other aspects of pain (e.g., behavioral and emotional responses). Examples of multidimensional assessment tools include a pain

TABLE 7-4 ➤ SINGLE-DIMENSION PAIN ASSESSMENT INSTRUMENTS

INSTRUMENT	TYPE OF PATIENT	TYPE OF PAIN	ADVANTAGES	DISADVANTAGES
Visual analog scale (VAS)	Children ≥7 years Adults	Current pain	Simple Independent of language Easily understood Reproducible	Monodimensional Scale imposes limits Visual and motor coordination required
Verbal numerical scale	Adults	Current pain	Same as VAS Eliminates need for visual and motor coordination May be easier to use than VAS	Monodimensional Scale imposes limits
Verbal rating scale	Adults	Current pain	Simple, easy to administer Sensitive to dosage, sex, and ethnic differences Superior to VAS in assessing on acute pain	Restricted choice of words that represent pain Does not allow for finer pain assessment Assumes equal distance between word descriptors the effects of analgesics

TABLE 7-5 ➤ MULTIDIMENSIONAL PAIN ASSESSMENT INSTRUMENTS

INSTRUMENT	TYPE OF PATIENT	TYPE OF PAIN	ADVANTAGES	DISADVANTAGES
Pain diary	Adults	Previous pain	Reliable More accurate than memory recall for actual drug ingestion	Dependent on accurate recording Dependent on verbal or motor skills
Pain drawings	Children ≥8 years Adults	Current pain	Used by nonexpert assessors High degree of reliability over time Discriminatory ability	Do not measure actual intensity of pain Inadequate for measurement of pain in discrete areas
Faces pain scale	Children ≥3 years Varies with specific scale	Current pain	Full development of verbal facility and conceptual understanding not required Simple, easy to use Minimal instruction required	All faces pain scales are not appropriate for all audiences Differentiation between middle faces on the scale often difficult
Wisconsin Brief Pain Questionnaire	Adults	Cancer pain Noncancer pain	Reliable Valid Easy to administer Interviewer may administer	Does not address emotional significance of pain or situational influences of pain behavior
McGill Pain Questionnaire	Adults	Cancer pain Noncancer pain	Reliable Valid Widely applicable	Construct of the Pain Rating Index Requirement of intellectual capacity and sufficient vocabulary May not be applicable in patients of different cultures or language

diary, pain drawings, the faces pain scales, the Wisconsin Brief Pain Questionnaire, and the McGill Pain Questionnaire. These tools are compared in Table 7-5.

A pain diary is an oral or a written account of a patient's day-to-day experiences and behavior. This type of report is helpful in monitoring daily variations in disease states and in the patient's response to therapy. Patients record their pain intensity as it relates to behaviors such as activities of daily living, sleep, sexual activity, when pain medication is taken, meals, housekeeping, and recreational activities.

Pain drawings are figures of the human body on which a patient is asked to shade in the areas where they are having pain (Fig. 7-4). Such drawings can be used to assess the location and distribution of pain, but they are not helpful in assessing the intensity of pain. Pain drawings can be compared over time to assess changes in response to treatment. Pain within small, confined areas (e.g., the head) cannot be adequately assessed with use of pain drawings.

The faces pain scales were developed in response to the need for an assessment instrument that could be used with children. Verbal and conceptual development limits use of the previously mentioned assessment tools to children older than 7 years. Using a faces pain scale, however, children grade their pain by choosing the picture that best matches their level of pain. The choice is then scored by assigning the number that corresponds with the face selected. The Whaley and Wong faces pain rating

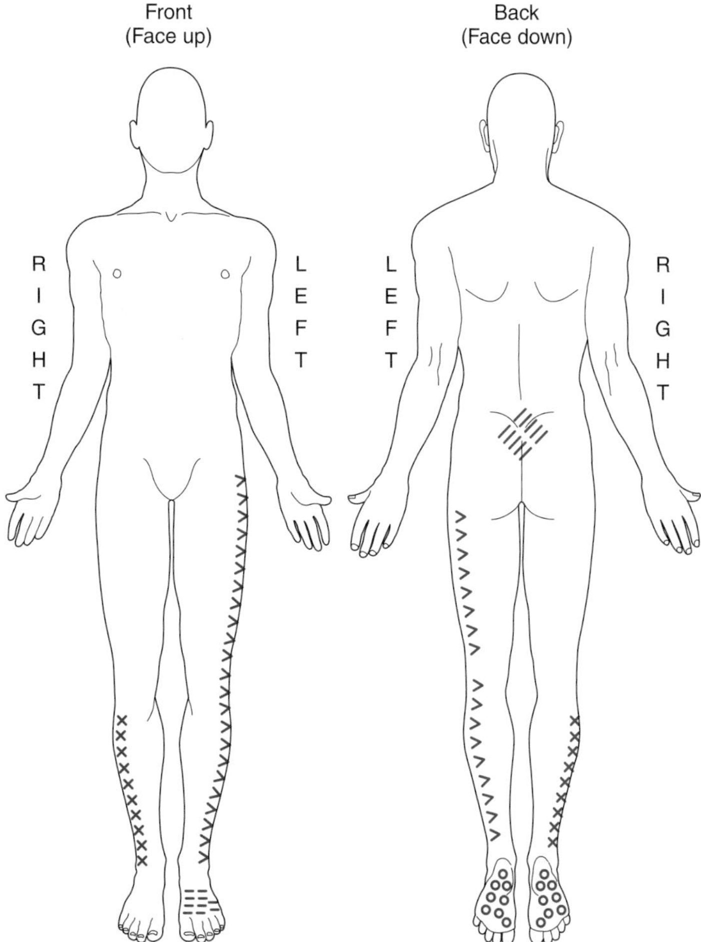

Figure 7-4 ■ Pain drawings. Areas of pain are indicated using various symbols or shadings: = = = for numbness, ooo for pins/needles, xxx for burning, (/ / /) for stabbing, and >>> for aching.

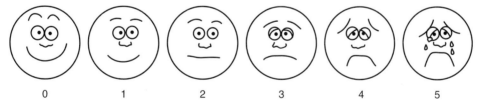

Figure 7-5 ■ The Whaley and Wong faces rating scale. (Reprinted with permission from Whaley LF, Wong DL. Nursing care of infants and children. 4th ed. St. Louis: Mosby–Year Book, 1991.)

scale (Fig. 7-5) uses six cartoon faces, ranging from a smiling face to a sad, crying face, with each face labeled from zero to five.

The Whaley and Wong scale also illustrates two limitations that occur with many of these scales: First, use of a smiling face at the *no pain* end of the spectrum assumes that pain exists on a continuum from pleasure to pain (i.e., that *no pain* is equivalent to pleasure or happiness). A number of researchers oppose this position. The scale developed by Bieri and associates (Fig. 7-6) has eliminated this concern. Second, the best scale realizes equal intervals of change in the severity of pain displayed on the faces that are used, but this has not been established for a number of the faces pain scales. Several of these scales also use photographs of children in increasing levels of pain; an additional limitation exists in these particular scales, in that the pictures have not been tested with children from culturally diverse populations.

The Wisconsin Brief Pain Questionnaire contains 17 questions directed toward assessing pain history, intensity, location, quality, interference with daily activities, effect on

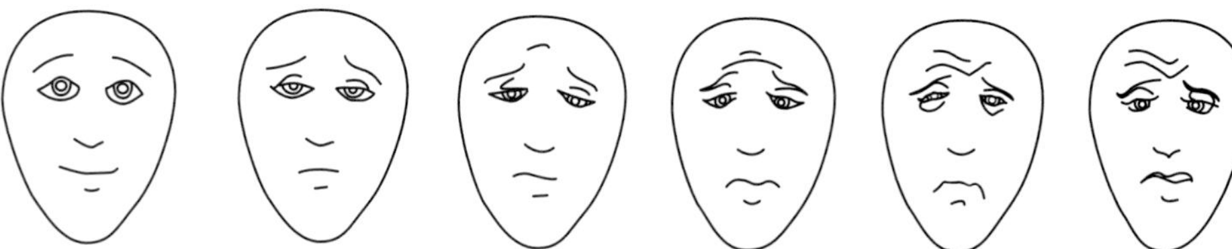

Figure 7-6 ■ Bieri and associates faces pain scale. (Reprinted with permission from Bieri D, Reeve RA, Champion CD, et al. The faces pain scale for the self-assessment of the severity of pain experienced by children: development, initial validation, and preliminary investigation for ratio scale properties. Pain 1990;41:139-150.)

mood, and overall enjoyment of life. This test can be self-administered, or it can be administered by an interviewer with equivalent results.

The McGill Pain Questionnaire (MPQ) (Fig. 7-7) consists of four parts: (1) a pain drawing, (2) a pain rating index (PRI), (3) questions about previous pain experience and location of pain; and (4) the present pain intensity index. The PRI consists of 78 adjectives, which are divided into 20 groups. Each set contains as many as six of these words in ascending order of quality. Groups 1 to 10 describe sensory qualities of the pain (e.g., temporal, spatial, thermal). Groups 11 to 15 describe affective qualities of the pain (e.g., tension, fear, autonomic properties). Group 16 describes the evaluative dimension, and Groups 17 to 20 are miscellaneous and include words specific for certain conditions. A numerical rating is achieved by assigning a number to each adjective and then summing those numbers based on the words chosen to find a total (i.e., the PRI[T]).

Although the words of the PRI are grouped appropriately, criticism revolves around the lack of equidistance between words within each subset; the unequal number of descriptors within each subset; the imbalance between the number of sensory, affective, and evaluative components; and the mode by which the tests are analyzed. Despite this controversy, the MPQ is one of the most widely used assessment instruments. The major limitation of the MPQ is the requirement that the patient understand the words that are utilized in the test. Thus, any intellectual and verbal limitations on the part of the patient would make this instrument an inappropriate choice. The MPQ also may have limited use in patients from different cultures or whose first language is not English.

This discussion has focused only on a few of the available pain assessment instruments. Pharmacists should evaluate their patient population and choose the one or two instruments that seem most appropriate. Individual patient situations may warrant the use of a particular assessment tool. Note that these tools are directed at assessing the character of pain and its impact on the patient and his or her quality of life; use of a pain assessment tool cannot replace the patient interview and medication history. Most important, pharmacists should regularly assess pain, and this assessment should be documented.

Objective Information

Currently, pain cannot be measured directly. Therefore, to augment the information obtained through self-reports or in cases when self-reports cannot be obtained, pharmacists must rely on observations of pain behaviors and/or physiological changes associated with pain. Most important, a lack of objective information does not rule out the presence of pain in a patient.

Behavioral Observations

Pharmacists often must rely on observing displays of behaviors that are associated with pain (Box 7-2). Identification of pain behaviors also may be obtained from a family member or caregiver. Objective measurement of pain behaviors can be affected by many factors, such as the pharmacist's effect on the patient's behavior, the environment in which the behavior is observed (e.g., pharmacy, clinic), the financial resources available to the patient, and the role of parents, spouses, or significant others. Remember that even though these behaviors are identified as objective measures of pain, they do not directly measure the pain stimulus—or the psychological suffering that occurs.

Physiological Indicators

In acute pain syndromes, physiological changes in response to pain are common. Tachycardia, tachypnea, sweating, pallor, and extreme anxiety can be measured. Traumatized areas may be red and swollen in appearance; Chapters 4 and 5 review appropriate physical assessment techniques for these symptoms. Physiological changes are uncommon in chronic pain syndromes, however, because the body has time to compensate or adjust to the pain sensation and its physical impact. In specific syndromes (e.g., headache, low back pain), more complex physiological measures (e.g., electromyography, which records the contraction of a muscle as a result of electrical stimulation) may be appropriate. In general, physiological assessment has the most value in the assessment of acute pain and of pain in newborns and infants.

Special Considerations

Pediatric Patients

Undermedication of pain in children is a significant problem. In the past, a contributing factor to undermedication was the lack of an appropriate assessment device. Recent advancements in our understanding of pain in children, however, along with development of age-appropriate assessment tools, have increased our success in medicating pediatric pain. Nevertheless, use of the

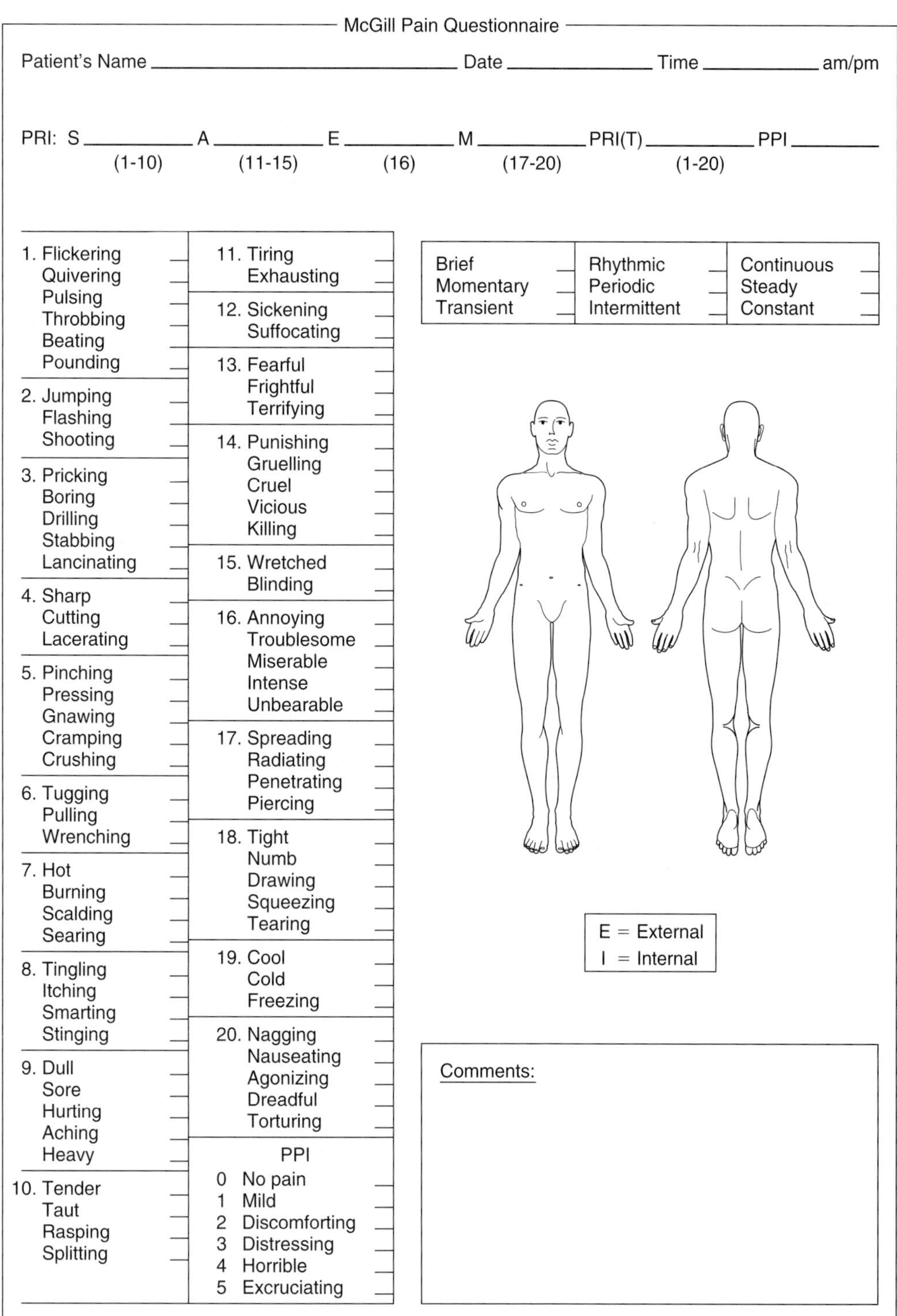

McGill Pain Questionnaire

Patient's Name ______ Date ______ Time ______ am/pm

PRI: S ______ (1-10) A ______ (11-15) E ______ (16) M ______ (17-20) PRI(T) ______ (1-20) PPI ______

1. Flickering, Quivering, Pulsing, Throbbing, Beating, Pounding	11. Tiring, Exhausting
2. Jumping, Flashing, Shooting	12. Sickening, Suffocating
3. Pricking, Boring, Drilling, Stabbing, Lancinating	13. Fearful, Frightful, Terrifying
4. Sharp, Cutting, Lacerating	14. Punishing, Gruelling, Cruel, Vicious, Killing
5. Pinching, Pressing, Gnawing, Cramping, Crushing	15. Wretched, Blinding
6. Tugging, Pulling, Wrenching	16. Annoying, Troublesome, Miserable, Intense, Unbearable
7. Hot, Burning, Scalding, Searing	17. Spreading, Radiating, Penetrating, Piercing
8. Tingling, Itching, Smarting, Stinging	18. Tight, Numb, Drawing, Squeezing, Tearing
9. Dull, Sore, Hurting, Aching, Heavy	19. Cool, Cold, Freezing
10. Tender, Taut, Rasping, Splitting	20. Nagging, Nauseating, Agonizing, Dreadful, Torturing
	PPI: 0 No pain, 1 Mild, 2 Discomforting, 3 Distressing, 4 Horrible, 5 Excruciating

Brief	Rhythmic	Continuous
Momentary	Periodic	Steady
Transient	Intermittent	Constant

E = External
I = Internal

Comments:

Figure 7-7 ■ McGill Pain Questionnaire. (Adapted with permission from Wall PD, Melzack R, eds. Textbook of pain. London: Churchill Livingstone, 1984:199.)

Box 7-2

PAIN BEHAVIORS[a]

- Verbal complaints of pain
- Taking of medicine
- Seeking treatment
- Impaired or changed physical or social functioning
  - Withdrawal
  - Refusal to eat or play
  - Restlessness
  - Agitation
  - Shortened attention span
  - Confusion
  - Irritability
  - Dizziness
  - Sweating
  - Fatigue
- Facial expressions
  - Grimacing
  - Wrinkled forehead
  - Tightly closed or widely opened eyes or mouth
  - Other distorted expressions
- Body movements
  - Guarding
  - Rocking
  - Pulling legs into the abdomen
  - Increased head/finger movements
  - Rubbing painful areas
  - Inability to keep still
  - Pacing
  - Change in gait
  - Protective posturing
  - Flailing of limbs
  - Lack of usual movement
- Vocalizations
  - Crying
  - Whimpering
  - Fussing
  - Grunting
  - Groaning
  - Moaning
  - Screaming

[a]In the context of the text, all the items in this box would be objective signs of pain when observed by a health care professional, family member, or caregiver. If the patient reported one of these behaviors during the pain interview, it would be classified as a subjective symptom.

assessment techniques outlined earlier is limited in children by development of their cognitive skills.

Subjective Assessment

The pharmacist should be able to conduct a pain interview with a child as young as 3 to 4 years of age. Special effort should be made to create a nonthreatening environment for the interview. Although self-report assessment techniques can be used in young children, their verbal communication about pain will be limited by their vocabulary; children may use only words such as *hurt* or *owie* or *booboo* to describe pain. The parent or caregiver, however, often can provide supplemental information. Behavioral or physiological signs of pain are useful in older as well as younger children.

The VAS is best used with children older than 7 years; however, it has been used with those as young as 5 years. Self-report scales based on numbers of objects (e.g., poker chips), increasing color intensity, or a series of faces or photographs are more appropriate for children between 4 and 7 years of age (Figs. 7-5 and 7-6). In children younger than 3 to 4 years, the pharmacist must rely more on behavioral or physiological measures of pain.

Objective Assessment

Objective assessment of pain in children will vary depending on their age and level of development. Pain assessment in newborns and preverbal infants relies on behavioral measurements (e.g., facial expression). Crying is useful in determining the urgency of the required response, but it is not helpful in quantifying pain. Infants in pain may withdraw, exhibit eating and sleeping disturbances, and have difficulty establishing relationships (see Box 7-2). Physiological assessment such as cardiovascular parameters (e.g., heart rate, rhythm, cardiac output) provide immediate feedback in newborns and infants, but these cannot be used in premature infants. Preschool children may be able to provide minimal self-reporting of pain; however, these children may become clingy, immobile, and lose motor skills, verbal abilities, and sphincter control in response to pain. Children younger than 5 years may start to deny pain because the caregivers' responses (e.g., dressing changes, intramuscular injections) often produce more pain; often, these children also may interpret pain as a punishment for a wrongdoing. School-aged children may exhibit more subtle behavioral changes. Pain may result in aggressiveness, extreme shame (more frequent in patients with burns), and nightmares, which may cause them to withdraw. The feeling that they are losing control and concern over the reaction of their peers may result in increased levels of anxiety. Adolescents often respond to chronic pain with extreme oppositional behavior and depression.

Behavioral and physiological measures of pain (e.g., crying, facial expression, verbal complaints, motion, touch) may be quantified using several assessment instruments. Regardless of the scale used, consistency, ease of use, and time required to complete the tool are essential characteristics to consider. In cases where self-report is inappropriate and behavioral changes are absent or inconclusive, the Agency for Health Care Policy and Research notes that an analgesic trial can be diagnostic as well as therapeutic.

Geriatric Patients

Pain is a common compliant in elderly patients, but they may not report pain for numerous reasons (Box 7-3). Assessment of pain in these patients should be preceded by an evaluation of hearing, vision, speech, and sensory ability. Impairments in any of these areas may significantly affect the mode and manner in which pain is assessed.

Subjective Assessment

The method in which an interview with an elderly patient is conducted is dependent on recognizing and accommodating any physical or mental impairment. Alterations in hearing, vision, psychomotor function (e.g., finger dexterity, fine motor skills), verbal language, and cognitive skills (e.g., memory, conceptualization)—either as a normal part of aging or as a result of disease—will affect a patient's ability to identify and to communicate pain when it occurs.

Table 7-6 outlines numerous techniques that the pharmacist can use to maximize the outcome of a pain assessment interview. Asking the patient to describe the pain or to read an assessment tool may provide the pharmacist with an indication of the patient's sensory ability. Other simple screening tools (e.g., the Mini-Mental Status Questionnaire) may be useful in identifying impaired mental processes.

Elderly patients with cognitive and/or verbal impairment are the most difficult to assess. In this case, observations of pain behaviors by the pharmacist or a caregiver become the primary mode for assessing pain. Behaviors that may be displayed in elderly patients suffering from pain are discussed below.

Use of single-dimension instruments such as the VAS may be preferred with elderly patients, because these instruments are quick and less fatiguing. However, in patients with acute pain, lower levels of education, impaired cognition, or impaired motor coordination, the VAS may be too abstract. Furthermore, the normal horizontal presentation of the VAS may be less appropriate as the ability to think abstractly declines. In this case, the vertical presentation of the VAS, which often is referred to as the "pain thermometer," may be more effective. In this presentation, the 0 constitutes the bottom of the thermometer, with the numbers increasing to 10 at the top (much like the increasing degrees on a thermometer).

Multidimensional instruments such as the MPQ are complex and time-consuming. The vocabulary may be hard for elderly patients to understand, and the number of word choices may be overwhelming. Reading competency also must be determined before administering this instrument. In addition, elderly patients may not be able to concentrate long enough to complete the MPQ. In this case, the one-page, short-form MPQ may be an alternative. Pain diaries can provide much useful information; however, some elderly patients may have trouble completing a diary because of deficiencies in fine motor skills or cognitive ability. Pain drawings are effective methods for determining pain location in elderly patients who cannot describe their pain verbally. They are also helpful because elderly patients often have more than one site of pain. The faces pain scales, which were developed for pain assessment in children, may be useful in elderly patients with difficulties in language or mental capacity.

TABLE 7-6 ➤ RECOMMENDATIONS FOR COMMUNICATION WITH IMPAIRED ELDERLY PATIENTS

IMPAIRMENT	INTERVENTION
Hearing	Position the patient facing the interviewer Minimize extraneous noise Use adequate lighting Monitor tone, pacing, and speed of voice Minimize verbal questions and instructions (severely impaired) Use written questions (severely impaired)
Vision	Increase lighting with nonglare bulbs Use buff, orange, or yellow nonglare paper Use large, simple lettering with both upper- and lower-case letters Ensure adequate spacing between lines Avoid italics Minimize decorative or inappropriate drawings Use line drawings with thick outlines rather than full-color photographs
Psychomotor	Use quicker and less fatiguing methods of assessment Graduate page width Number pages Print only on one side of the paper
Verbal	Use written questions or written responses to verbal questions (if no cognitive impairment) Observe behaviors (if cognitive impairment present)
Cognitive	Maintain patient's attention Confirm understanding of questions Keep content simple Explain medical terminology Use examples and demonstrations Observe for behaviors associated with pain

Box 7-3

REASONS WHY ELDERLY PATIENTS DO NOT REPORT PAIN

- Belief that pain is something they must live with
- Fear of the consequences (e.g., hospitalization)
- Fear that their pain is a forecast of serious illness or impending health
- Inability to understand the medical terminology used by health care providers
- Belief that showing pain is unacceptable
- Misunderstanding that symptoms may be a result of the pain

Objective Assessment

As with children, behavioral observation of elderly patients is an important component of the pain assessment process. An acceptance that pain must simply be endured, fear that reporting pain may result in loss of autonomy, and fear that pain is a sign of serious illness—or even impending death—all contribute to a failure to report pain in this age group (see Box 7-3). Signs of physical pain that pharmacists or family members may observe or changes in a patient's normal presentation are extremely important when assessing patients who are confused or lack verbal skills (see Box 7-2). Patients suffering from chronic brain diseases (e.g., Alzheimer's, hydrocephalus, encephalopathy) are totally dependent on the observational skill of health care professionals, family members, and caregivers for recognition of pain. The following are examples of changes in baseline behavior when a patient experiences pain:

- Quiet, withdrawn behavior in a patient who normally moans and rocks.
- Rapid blinking, with slight facial grimacing, in a quiet, nonverbal elder.
- Agitation and combative behavior in a normally friendly, outgoing individual.
- Accurate description of the location of pain in a patient who normally has extremely disjointed verbalization.

Elderly patients may also have atypical presentations of normal clinical pain syndromes. A significant number of myocardial infarctions in this age group occur without pain. Peptic ulcer disease, appendicitis, and pneumonia may elicit behavioral change while the patient only complains of mild discomfort. Abdominal emergencies may present as chest pain.

Behavioral and physiological changes in elderly patients also can be quantified using assessment tools. Adaptation of tools developed for children who are unable to communicate pain verbally (e.g., the faces pain scales, color tools) can be useful in the impaired elder.

Gender and ethnic differences in patients should be considered as well when assessing any patient in pain. In general, African-American, Mexican-American, and Caucasian women tend to express pain more openly than men of the same ethnicities. Variations among ethnic groups regarding the expression of pain also could dramatically affect self-reported modes of pain assessment. Regardless of variations in patient demographics and diseases, effective pain assessment is crucial in the quest to provide optimal pain management to all patients.

Pregnant Patients

Although any pain syndrome can be experienced during pregnancy, the experience of labor pain is unique to this subgroup of patients.

Subjective Assessment

The experience of labor pain involves both a sensory and affective dimension which varies throughout the phases of labor. Therefore routine assessment should occur through the labor process.

In response to questions by the caregivers, women may experience uterine pain as well as referred pain that they may identify as being in their abdomen, lower back, hip bones (iliac crests), gluteal area, or thighs. Labor pain may be described as widespread or localized.

Descriptors used for sensory pain include cramping, sharp, aching, stabbing, heavy, pulling, throbbing, hot, or shooting. Emotionally, women may describe their pain as being exhaustive, intense, and troublesome.

Women experiencing back pain during labor describe those sensations as pressing, pulling, stinging, heavy, hot, aching, or taut. Emotionally they describe the pain as tiring, sickening, and annoying.

Variations in labor pain can occur if a woman has a history of dysmenorrhea (↑ pain) and menstruation related back pain (↑ back pain in labor).

Although ethnicity itself does not appear to vary the pain response, accepted cultural norms may impact a woman's perception of pain.

Objective Assessment

Pain assessment tools used during labor pain should include a sensory and an affective component such as the McGill Pain Questionnaire. Assessment should be completed frequently as the pain experience varies with the phase of labor.

The wider the cultural difference between the patient and the caregiver, the less accurate the caregiver's assessment of the patient's pain.

Self-Assessment Questions

1. Compare and contrast the characteristics of acute and chronic pain.
2. Compare and contrast the words that patients commonly use to describe somatic versus visceral pain.
3. What are common words used to characterize neuropathic pain?
4. What is the primary method used for assessing a patient in pain?
5. The "PQRST" mnemonic is used in completing a pain interview. What does each letter in the mnemonic stand for?
6. What single-dimension assessment instruments are available for use in assessing a patient undergoing treatment of pain?
7. What multidimensional assessment instruments are available for use in assessing a patient undergoing treatment of pain?
8. What pain assessment instruments are most appropriate for use with children?
9. What two types of objective information can be gathered during a pain assessment?
10. What type of behavioral manifestations of pain might be seen in children? How does this compare with behavioral manifestations in elderly patients?
11. What type of physiological changes might represent a pain response?

Critical Thinking Questions

1. You have decided to assess pain in all patients receiving a new prescription for an analgesic as well as with each additional refill. What assessment technique or instrument would you use, and why?
2. A 65-year-old woman with degenerative joint disease is taking chronic nonsteroidal anti-inflammatory

agents for the management of pain. During the last 6 months, she has had four different agents prescribed. What questions would you ask this patient during a pain assessment?

3. A 37-year-old female was admitted to your hospital with a new diagnosis of breast cancer that has metastasized to the bone. She indicates that her pain is a 10 on the VAS. While completing a medication history, she indicates that she has a history of substance abuse. How would this information affect your method of pain assessment?

Bibliography

Acute Pain Management Guideline Panel. Acute pain management: operative or medical procedures and trauma. Clinical practice guideline. AHCPR Publication 92-0032. Rockville, MD: Agency for Health Care Policy and Research, Public Health Service, U.S. Department of Health and Human Services, 1992.

Bieri D, Reeve RA, Champion CD, et al. The faces pain scale for the self-assessment of the severity of pain experienced by children: development, initial validation, and preliminary investigation for ratio scale properties. Pain 1990;41:139–150.

Eland JM. Pain in children. Nurs Clin North Am 1990;25:871–884.

Fields HL: Pain. New York: McGraw-Hill, 1987:32.

Foley KM. The treatment of cancer pain. N Engl J Med 1985;313:84–95.

Hamers JPH. Factors influencing nurses' pain assessment and interventions in children. J Adv Nurs 1994;20:853–860.

Herr KA, Mobily PR. Complexities of pain assessment in the elderly: clinical considerations. J Gerontol Nurs 1991:17:12–19.

Jacox A, Carr DB, Payne R, et al. Management of cancer pain. Clinical Practice Guideline 9. AHCPR Publication 94-0592. Rockville, MD: Agency for Health Care Policy and Research, U.S. Department of Health and Human Services, Public Health Service, 1994.

Koo PJS. Pain. In: Young LY, Koda-Kimble MA, eds. Applied therapeutics: the clinical use of drugs. 6th ed. Vancouver, Canada: Applied Therapeutics, 1995:1–28.

Lloyd-Thomas A. Assessment and control of pain in children. Anaesthesia 1995;50:753–755.

Lowe NK. The nature of labor pain. Am J Obstet Gynecol 2002;186:S16–24.

Mackenna BR, Callander R. Illustrated physiology. 6th ed. New York: Churchill Livingstone, 1997.

Martini FH, Timmons MJ: Human anatomy. 2nd ed. Upper Saddle River, NJ: Prentice Hall, 1997.

Marzinski LR. The tragedy of dementia: clinically assessing pain in the confused, nonverbal elderly. J Gerontol Nurs 1991;17:25–28.

Reisner-Keller LA. Pain management. In: Herfindal ET, Gourley DR. Textbook of therapeutics: drug and disease management. 6th ed. Baltimore: Williams & Wilkins, 1996:1047–1072.

Schnabel GA, Powrie JD. Pain assessment: the pharmacist's challenge in alternative health care environments. The Consultant Pharmacist 1998;7:816–822.

Simons W, Malabar R. Assessing pain in elderly patients who cannot respond verbally. J Adv Nurs 1995;22:663–669.

Van Keuren K, Eland JA. Perioperative pain management in children. Nurs Clin North Am 1997;32:31–44.

Villarruel AM, Denyes MJ. Pain assessment in children: theoretical and empirical validity. Adv Nurs Sci 1991;14:32–41.

Vo Roenn JH, Cleeland CS, Gonin R, et al. Physician attitudes and practice in cancer pain management: a survey from the Eastern Cooperative Oncology Group. Ann Intern Med 1993;119:121–126.

White P. Pain measurement. In: Warfield CA, ed. Principles and practice of pain management. New York: McGraw-Hill, 1993:27–41.

PART *Two*

ASSESSMENT OF BODY SYSTEMS

CHAPTER

8

Skin, Hair, and Nails

Edward M. DeSimone II

GLOSSARY TERMS

- Acne
- Alopecia
- Candidiasis
- Carbuncle
- Chickenpox (varicella)
- Chloasma
- Diaper rash
- Eczema
- Furuncle
- Folliculitis
- Impetigo
- Linea nigra
- Measles
- Onychomycosis
- Pediculosis
- Purpura
- Stevens-Johnson syndrome
- Striae
- Xerosis

ANATOMY AND PHYSIOLOGY OVERVIEW

The skin, also known as the integumentary system, is the largest organ of the body. The nails and hair are considered to be appendages of the skin rather than independent anatomic entities.

Skin

The skin functions as a two-way barrier: It helps to contain body fluids and prevent dehydration of the internal body components while keeping out infectious organisms and toxic substances. It also protects internal structures from mechanical injury, such as external trauma and damage caused by less obvious sources (e.g., ultraviolet radiation). Skin serves as the medium for blood flow and for waste excretion through the sweat glands. These two functions are also tied into the maintenance of body temperature and hydration. In addition to these more commonly understood functions, however, the massive sensory innervation of the skin allows one to sense the environment's texture, temperature, and moisture. The skin also plays a valuable role in expressing emotions, mediated by the brain, through movement of the underlying musculature and dilation or constriction of the underlying blood vessels to reveal embarrassment, fear, anger, shock, and many others.

The skin is divided into three main layers: (1) the epidermis, (2) the dermis, and (3) the hypodermis (subcutaneous tissue) (Fig. 8-1). The *epidermis* is actually composed of five layers of squamous epithelial cells, the most common of which are keratinocytes. Keratinocytes are the cells responsible for production of keratin, the structural protein of the skin, hair, and nails. These cells are believed to be involved in the immune process by first releasing immunoglobulin A and then interleukin-1, which triggers the activation of T cells. The innermost layer, the *stratum germinativum,* is also referred to as the basal cell layer. Approximately half of the keratinocytes move from the basal cell

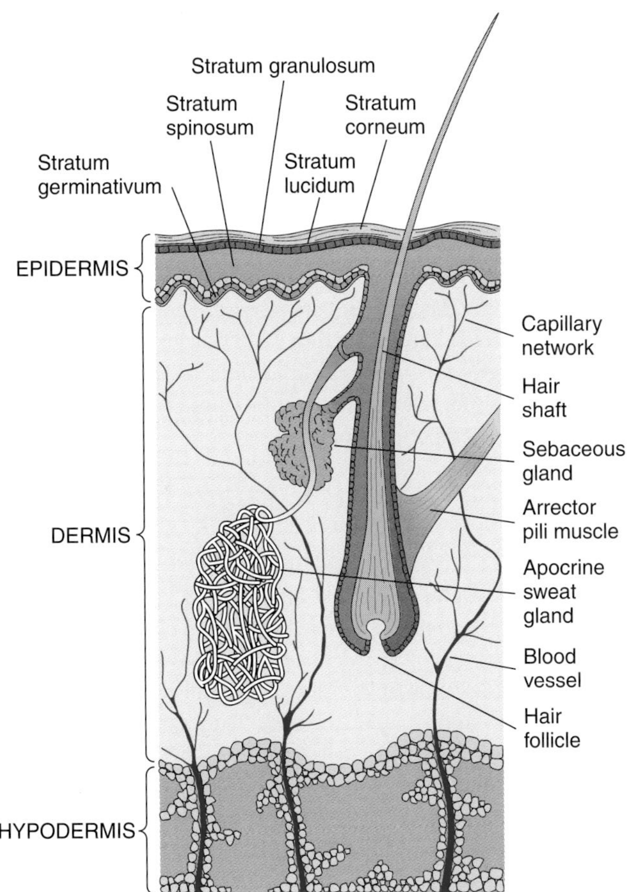

FIGURE 8-1 ■ Skin.

layer up through all the other epidermal layers. Along this journey, their structure changes: They flatten, lose their nuclei, and dry out. When these cells reach the outermost layer, the *stratum corneum,* they become known as horn cells. This is why the stratum corneum is also called the horny layer. These dead horn cells are then shed. This regeneration cycle takes approximately 1 month. Generally, the moisture content of the epidermis ranges from 10% to 20%. If it falls too low, then dry skin, cracks, and fissures can develop.

The second major cell type of the epidermis, the melanocyte, is found in the basal layer. The ratio of keratinocytes to melanocytes is 10:1. Although the number of melanocytes is fairly constant (despite racial origins), the variation in skin color is determined by the size and the number of melanosomes, or pigment granules, produced by these cells. Both the size and the number are higher in individuals with naturally darker skin. Melanosomes migrate throughout the keratinocytes of the epidermis and produce the color pigment, melanin. Individuals with naturally darker skin have a greater amount of melanin than those with lighter skin.

The Langerhans cell is the third major cell type of the epidermis. These cells are found in the stratum spinosum, just above the basal layer. Representing less than 5% of the cells in this layer, they are still involved in several significant activities, including production of interleukin-1 as part of an immune response, induction of graft rejection, and development of allergic contact dermatitis.

The second layer of the skin, the *dermis,* is normally 40-fold thicker than the epidermis and is composed of a mucopolysaccharide substance. Within the dermis are mast cells and fibroblasts. Mast cells have receptor sites for immunoglobulin E and contain a number of important compounds, such as slow-reacting substance of anaphylaxis, prostaglandin E_2, and histamine. Fibroblasts synthesize the structural support components of the skin (i.e., elastic fibers, collagen, and reticulum fibers).

Elastic fibers (elastic tissue) are so named because they give skin its elasticity. The primary component of these fibers is elastin, an amorphous protein. Collagen, a fibrous protein, is the major component of the skin, accounting for more than 70% of its total weight. Known as connective tissue, collagen gives ligaments and tendons the strength they need to hold muscles and bones to their sites of attachment. This also provides the skeleton with its ability to function. In addition, collagen is responsible for giving skin its resistance to injury from external forces. Reticulum fibers, which are also part of the connective tissue system, are smaller than collagen but function in much the same way.

Vascularization of the skin ends in the dermis. Arterioles and lymphatic vessels coming from the subcutaneous tissue supply the entire dermis, and these arterioles become the capillaries that supply the upper level (papillary area). In addition to blood vessels, the dermis contains a massive number of nerves that contribute to the sensations of pain, temperature, itch, touch, and pressure.

The third layer of skin, the *hypodermis* (or subcutis), is composed of fat cells (adipose tissue), collagen, and larger blood vessels. The fatty tissue affects the regulation of body heat and provides a cushioning effect from external pressure and injury.

Several additional structures are also found in the dermis. These are referred to as epidermal appendages (or adnexa), because they terminate at the epidermal surface even though they exist within the dermis. They include two different types of sweat glands: the eccrine units, and the apocrine units. The function of the apocrine units in humans is not well understood, but the eccrine units are responsible for the composition and excretion of sweat. Eccrine units supply all areas of the skin, but they are found in greater numbers in the axillae, on the forehead, and on the soles of the feet and palms of the hands. The sebaceous glands, another appendage, are found on all areas of the body except for the soles of the feet and palms of the hands. The largest concentration of these glands is on the scalp, face, and back. These glands grow in size and become active at puberty with the increased production of androgenic hormones. Sebaceous glands are almost always attached to a hair follicle; the exceptions are around the areolas of women, the prepuce, the border of the lips, and the eyelids. The sebaceous glands produce sebum, a waxy mixture that hydrates the skin and hair.

The thickness of the stratum corneum is the same in both dark- and fair-skinned people, but the densities of these layers are different. The significance of this difference, however, is not known. The difference in skin pigmentation, which is caused by the amount of melanin, affects the amount of ultraviolet (UV) radiation that penetrates the skin. This reduces damage to the skin from both UVA and UVB radiation. People with dark skin have a greater likelihood of hypo- and hyperpigmentation disorders and of diseases such as bullous lupus erythematosus. Without doubt, differences exist in the skin structure of dark-skinned individuals compared to light-skinned individuals. Certain disorders have a different presentation in dark-skinned individuals, and other disorders are almost unique to these same individuals. The most important point is that racially based differences do occur, and that this possibility must be considered when assessing the patient.

Hair

A hair follicle is an insertion into the dermis of epidermal cells that form the outer root sheath of a single hair (Fig. 8-2). (Thus, a hair follicle is also an epidermal appendage.) Medial to the outer root sheath is an inner root sheath that surrounds the hair shaft itself. Moving vertically down the hair follicle, a number of anatomic structures are found. The opening in the epidermis, called the hair canal, is followed by the sebaceous gland duct. Below this is the arrector pili muscle. The hair follicle lies at an angle to the skin, and when the skin is subjected to cold temperature, the arrector pili muscle pulls on the follicle, causing it to move vertically. This piloerection (or "goose bump") increases the relative thickness of the skin, further protecting the skin against injury from cold. At the base of the follicle is the papilla, within which cell growth occurs.

Hair follicles do not produce hair in a nonstop fashion. Rather, they go through cycles of growth, degeneration, and rest. Except for beard and scalp follicles, a typical cycle lasts several months; scalp follicles go through a cycle lasting, on average, 1100 days. Although the number varies by approximately 10% depending on hair color, the average scalp contains approximately 100,000 follicles. Approximately 100 hairs are lost from the scalp each day. Scalp hair grows at a rate of approximately 35 to 37 mm/day, but this growth can be affected by a variety of drugs, such as male and female sex hormones, thyroid hormones, and corticosteroids.

Each individual hair is composed of keratinized epithelial cells, which are held together by a variety of specialized proteins. Ethnic background produces differences in the structure and texture of scalp hair, but this effect of ethnicity is not seen with hair on other parts of the body.

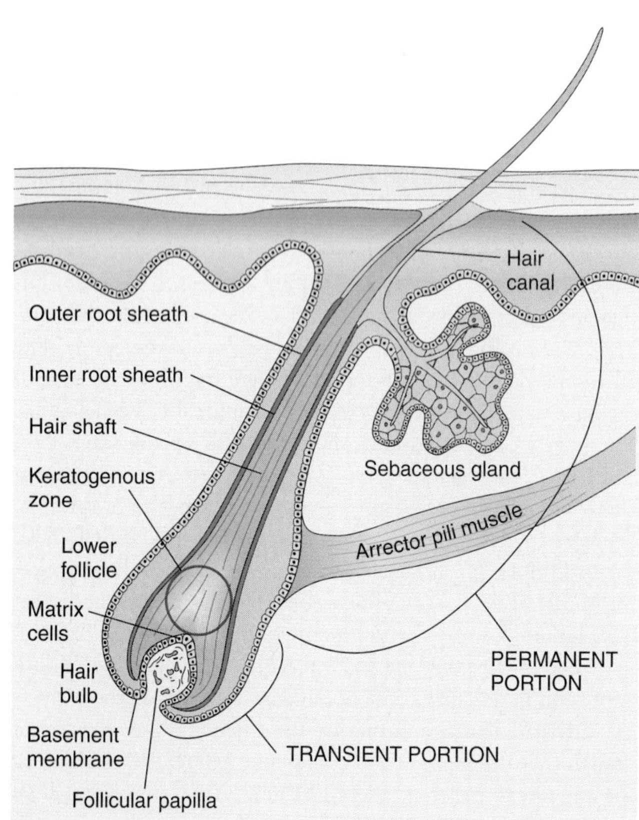

Figure 8-2 ■ Hair.

Nails

The nails, which are composed of keratinized cells, have several key anatomic segments (Fig. 8-3). The first is the nail root or matrix, which begins at the base of the nail. The most proximal part is covered by epidermal tissue (nail fold) and is not visible to the eye. The tissue at the end of the nail fold is the cuticle, which adheres to the nail plate, moves with it a short distance as the plate grows, and then falls off. The light, crescent-shaped area that projects from under the nail fold of the thumbs is the part of the matrix that can be seen. It is called the lunula (little moon) and generally is not seen in the other nails of the fingers or the toes.

The main part of the nail is the nail plate, which forms as cells of the matrix change and become horny flat cells with a high degree of adherence. Underneath the nail plate is the nail bed, which grows out of the basal cell layer of the epidermis. The nail bed does not extend to the end of the nail plate. The area from the end of the nail bed to the distal groove of the nail is called the hyponychium. This area is important, because many different medical conditions arise from this location.

Toenails grow at a slower rate than fingernails. In addition, fingernails of the same individual grow at different rates. Several factors affect the rate of nail growth; these include genetics, age (growth rate begins to slow during the third decade of life), and weather (growth rate increases during the warmer times of the year).

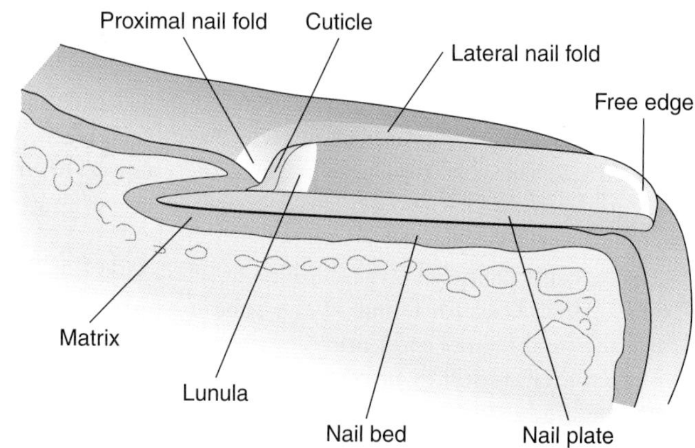

Figure 8-3 ■ Nails.

Special Considerations

Pediatric Patients

It is well accepted that the anatomy and physiology of human skin begins to change during the fetal growth period, and that these changes continue throughout an individual's life. For example, hair follicles are first seen in the fetus at approximately 9 weeks of gestation, with their distribution being limited to the face. The major development of hair follicles, however, begins around the fourth month of gestation. The density of scalp hair (follicles/cm^2) is actually highest at birth and then declines throughout one's life. The distribution and growth of hair (e.g., facial, axillary, and pubic) is regulated by a variety of hormones that become active at puberty. The same is true for sebaceous gland disorders such as acne. In many cases, acne is an early sign that puberty is beginning, but in some cases, the mother's hormone levels may cause a baby to be born with mild acne.

For pediatric patients, two considerations are important. First, certain dermatologic conditions, such as atopic dermatitis, are most likely to occur in children. Second, in children younger than 6 months, the absorptive characteristics of the skin differ from those of adults and are not very well understood. In addition, infants may not be able to safely metabolize or excrete topically absorbed drugs because of the immature status of their systems.

Geriatric Patients

Gross changes in aging skin include wrinkling, dryness (causing the skin to feel rough), changes or unevenness in skin pigmentation, senile lentigines (brown color, age or liver spots), reduced number of moles on the skin, and shiny, thin skin caused by atrophy within all three skin layers. These changes predispose the elderly to skin injuries, especially those resulting from shearing forces (e.g., decubitus ulcers). Aging skin is also likely to heal more slowly, and the 50% decrease in Langerhans cells in geriatric patients indicates a possible reduction in their immunity to skin cancer. Because of the slow development of skin cancers, elderly patients are more likely to have actinic keratoses, which are premalignant lesions on areas of the skin that have had significant exposure to the sun (e.g., the face and hands). In addition, a variety of skin disorders or complaints are more likely in older patients, including pruritis, psoriasis, candidiasis, herpes zoster, seborrheic dermatitis, bullous pemphigoid, and tinea pedis (athlete's foot). As people get older, the vascularity of the skin is also reduced. Because of this, older patients may exhibit pallor (pale appearance) of the skin, feel cold, and suffer a greater degree of bruising.

Changes also occur to the hair and nails with age. Older patients are more likely to exhibit thinning or graying hair (or both) as well as varying degrees of baldness. Decreasing estrogen levels may cause women to develop facial hair. Older patients also have a greater likelihood of splitting nails and of change in nail color. Both the size of the lunula and the thickness of the nail plate are reduced. Elderly individuals are also more likely to have dystrophic toenails, longitudinal ridges, onycholysis, and slowed nail growth.

Pregnant Patients

Pregnancy produces many hormonal changes in the mother, such as elevated levels of progesterone and estrogen, as well as in those hormones produced by the placenta, such as human chorionic gonadotropin. The roles of maternal and placental hormones in the development of dermatologic disorders are not well understood, but many skin changes are seen during pregnancy. For example, hyperpigmentation of the skin may occur around the areolae, genitalia, and thighs. Hyperpigmentation of the face is known as chloasma or melasma ("the mask of pregnancy"). Hair may become thicker or thinner, change in texture and become straighter or curlier, or even fall out. Most pregnant women develop striae gravidarum (stretch marks) around the hips, abdomen, buttocks, or breasts, the exact cause of which is unknown. A variety of skin disorders are also directly associated with pregnancy, including pruritic urticarial papules and plaques of pregnancy and herpes gestationis. Most of these conditions resolve after birth or the termination of lactation.

PATHOLOGY OVERVIEW

Skin

An effective assessment of patient complaints regarding the integumentary system requires an understanding of the clinical presentation (morphology) of rashes, lesions, and disorders of the hair and nails. Skin lesions are categorized as one of three basic types: (1) primary, (2) secondary, and (3) miscellaneous (Table 8-1). Primary lesions may arise from previously normal skin, and they include circumscribed, flat, nonpalpable changes in skin color, such as a macule or patch; palpable, elevated solid masses, such as papules, plaques, nodules, tumor, and wheals; and circumscribed, superficial elevations of the skin formed by free fluid in a cavity within the skin layers, such as vesicles, bulla, and pustules. Secondary lesions result from changes in primary lesions, and they include lesions that produce a loss of skin surface, such as an ulcer or fissure, as well as those that involve materials appearing on the skin surface, such as a crust or scale. Miscellaneous lesions include lichenification, scars, atrophy, excoriations, burrows, comedo, telangiectasias, and nevi.

Because the skin is the largest organ of the body, a vast number of pathologic conditions involve the skin. Many of these conditions may cause a patient to consult with a pharmacist for medical care or over-the-counter treatment. Pathologic conditions in this section are divided into five major categories: (1) inflammatory conditions, (2) infectious conditions, (3) adverse cutaneous drug reactions, (4) infestations, and (5) skin cancer.

Inflammatory Conditions

Contact Dermatitis

Contact dermatitis refers to any rash caused by a substance that contacts the skin. It is generally an inflammatory condition, may be acute or chronic, and is divided into two types, irritant (nonallergic) and allergic contact dermatitis. The irritant type may be caused by soap, detergent, or an organic substance, such as

	Term	Description	Illustration
Primary Lesions	Macule	A flat lesion, flush with the skin with a color different from the surrounding tissue.	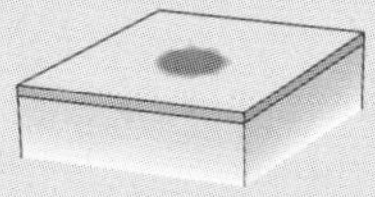
Primary Lesions	Patch	A macule which exhibits some scale or fine wrinkles.	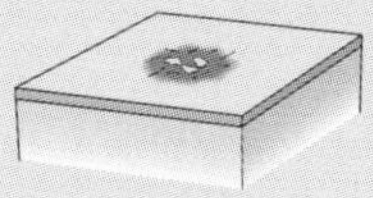
Primary Lesions	Papule	A solid, elevated lesion less than 0.5 cm in diameter.	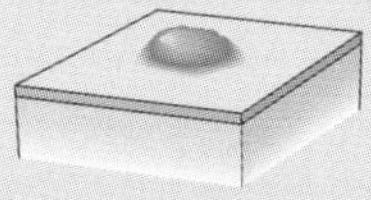
Primary Lesions	Plaque	A lesion greater than 0.5 in diameter but with marginal depth.	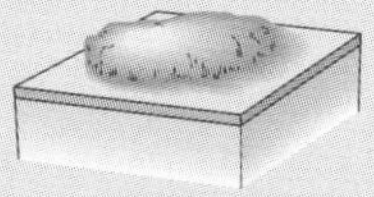
Primary Lesions	Lichenification	Thickening of the skin which can be seen as well as palpated and which has ridged skin markings.	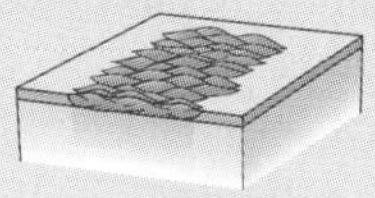
Primary Lesions	Nodule	A lesion greater than 0.5 cm in both width and depth.	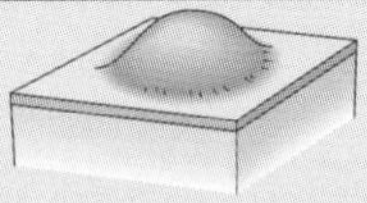
Primary Lesions	Wheal	A transitory papule or plaque arising out of the edema of the dermis which almost always produces pruritis. Also known as hives or urticaria.	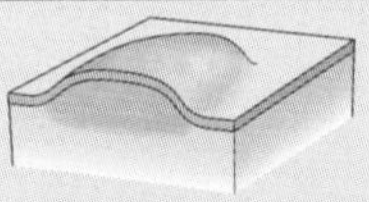
Primary Lesions	Cyst	A nodule containing a liquid or semisolid which can be expressed.	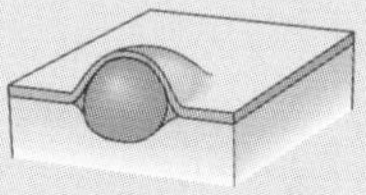
Primary Lesions	Vesicle	A blister less than 0.5 cm in diameter filled with clear liquid.	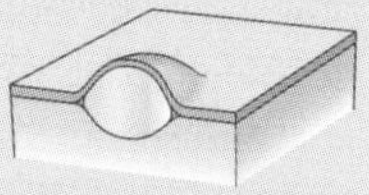
Primary Lesions	Bulla	A blister more than 0.5 cm in diameter filled with clear liquid.	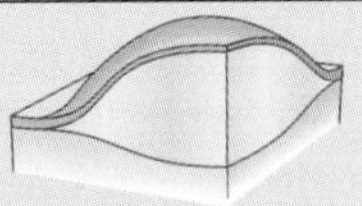
Primary Lesions	Pustule	A vesicle filled with a purulent liquid.	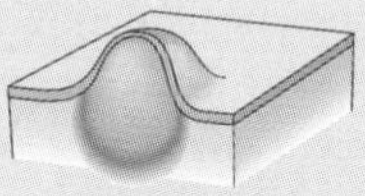
Secondary Lesions	Crust (scab)	Exudate from a lesion which has dried on the skin.	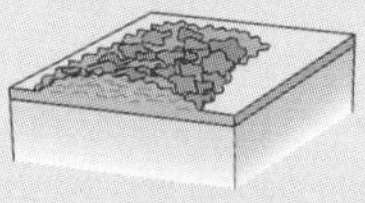
Secondary Lesions	Scale	Aggregation of loose, hyperkeratotic cells of the stratum corneum. They normally are dry and appear to be white in color.	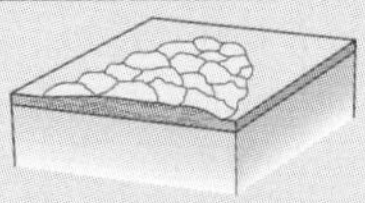
Secondary Lesions	Fissure	A thin tear of the epidermis which may extend to the dermis.	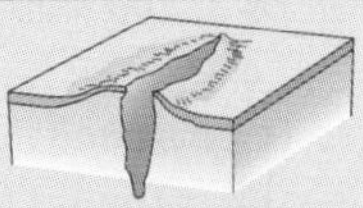
Secondary Lesions	Erosion	Wider than a fissure but limited to the epidermis.	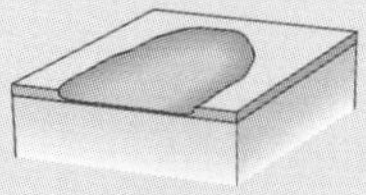
Secondary Lesions	Ulcer	Destruction of the epidermis (with or without dermal injury) which exposes the dermis.	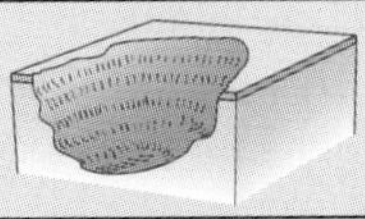

kerosene (Fig. 8-4). Allergic contact dermatitis is immunologic in nature and results when a substance acts as a hapten. The antigenic substance is picked up by the Langerhans cells, which then forward the modified substance to the T cells, triggering the reaction.

Risk factors for the irritant type include:

- Acid, mild or strong
- Alkali, mild or strong
- Soaps
- Detergents
- Cosmetics
- Solvents
- Any substance that can irritate the skin

Risk factors for the allergic type include:

- Plant resins, such as in poison ivy and poison oak
- Metals, such as nickel and cobalt, found in jewelry
- Cement that contains chromium
- Latex and rubber
- Cigarette smoke
- Local anesthetics, especially of the "caine" type
- Neomycin
- Aminobenzoic acid (formerly PABA)

The irritant form usually presents within a few hours of exposure, but the allergic form can take several days, depending on the sensitivity of the exposed individual. Contact dermatitis is generally confined to the area of contact; however, in a highly sensitive person, a widespread or even generalized eruption may occur. Contact with plant resins may produce lesions in a linear streak. The serous fluid within vesicles is nonimmunogenic. Common signs and symptoms of contact dermatitis are listed in Box 8-1.

The first step in treatment is to remove the offending agent. Because contact dermatitis is a self-limiting disorder that clears in a week to 10 days, treatment is symptomatic. Weeping vesicles may be treated with wet dressings using Burow's solution every 2 to 3 hours. Itching may be treated with nonprescription hydrocortisone cream; spray topical anesthetic products (usually containing benzocaine [up to 20%]) may also be used with caution (because of their sensitizing potential). For persistent itching, oral antihistamines may be tried, but their primary mechanism of action is their soporific effect. If these treatments do not reduce the symptoms or if the symptoms are widespread, systemic corticosteroids such as prednisone may be helpful.

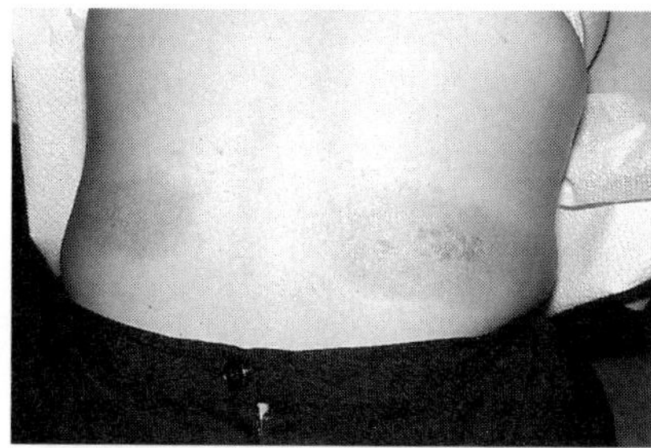

FIGURE 8-4 ■ Contact dermatitis. (See Color Plate 5; reprinted with permission from Goodheart HP. A photoguide of common skin disorders: diagnosis and management. Philadelphia: Lippincott Williams & Wilkins, 1999:44.)

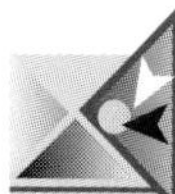

Box 8-1

SIGNS AND SYMPTOMS OF CONTACT DERMATITIS

IRRITANT TYPE

Signs
- Erythema with dull skin
- Vesicles
- Crusts
- Scaling

Symptoms
- Pruritis

ALLERGIC TYPE

Signs
- Erythema
- Papules
- Vesicles
- Erosions
- Crusts
- Scaling
- Blackheads
- Whiteheads (pimples)
- Papules
- Pustules
- Nodules
- Cysts

Symptoms
- Pruritis

Acne

Acne is a self-limiting inflammation of the pilosebaceous unit that presents as pimples, blackheads, cysts, and pustules (Fig. 8-5). It generally appears at puberty because of the emergence of androgenic hormones. Exacerbations may result from occlusion or pressure on the skin (acne mechanica) or from emotional stress. In most cases, the disorder wanes at 18 to 25 years of age.

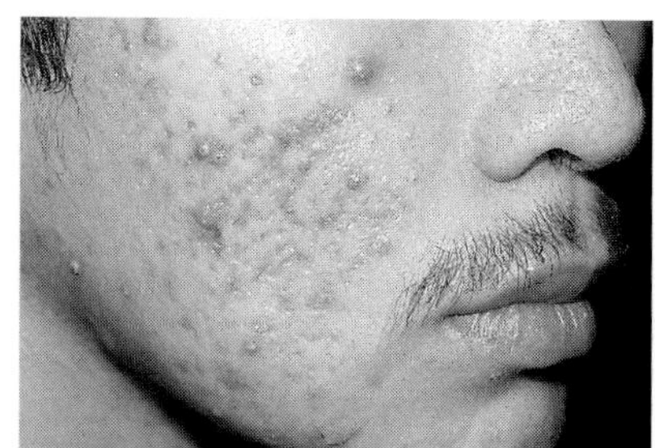

FIGURE 8-5 ■ Acne. (See Color Plate 6; reprinted with permission from Goodheart HP. A photoguide of common skin disorders: diagnosis and management. Philadelphia: Lippincott Williams & Wilkins, 1999:17.)

Lesions are most often found on the face and upper trunk. Signs and symptoms of acne are listed in Box 8-2.

Treatment involves daily washing of the skin to remove excess sebum, which clogs the pores. Depending on the severity of the condition, drug treatment includes topical benzoyl peroxide, topical erythromycin, oral tetracycline or erythromycin, and topical isotretinoin.

Eczema

Eczema is actually a catch-all term for a variety of inflammatory skin conditions. Atopic dermatitis is a chronic, inflammatory disorder of the dermis and epidermis (Fig. 8-6). It often appears during infancy or early childhood (becoming apparent by the age of 1 year in 60% of patients). More than two-thirds of patients have risk factors, which include a personal or family history of allergic rhinitis, hay fever, asthma, and atopic dermatitis. Signs and symptoms of atopic dermatitis are listed in Box 8-3.

Management begins by getting the patient to stop scratching. Wet dressings, skin hydration, topical glucocorticoids, and oral antihistamines help to reduce the pruritis. Oral antistaphylococcal antibiotics, such as erythromycin, azithromycin, clarithromycin, or a penicillinase-resistant penicillin, may be used. Topical mupirocin may also be effective.

Diaper Rash

Diaper rash is an acute, inflammatory condition in the area of the buttocks, genitalia, perineum, and abdomen (Fig. 8-7). It is most often seen in infants because of the occlusive properties of diapers, which hold moisture and fecal materials against the skin in a warm environment. This condition is also seen in adults who must wear adult-type diapers. Signs and symptoms of diaper dermatitis include erythematous patches, erosion of the skin, pain, vesicles, and possibly, ulceration.

Treatment primarily involves frequent diaper changes to keep the area dry. Talcum powder or cornstarch is also used to keep the area dry; in severe cases, the area can be exposed to the air to facilitate drying of the skin, during which time the baby does not wear a diaper. Other treatments include washing the skin with plain water, avoiding friction when drying the skin, and using a skin protectant (e.g., zinc oxide).

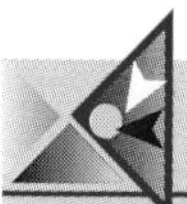

Box 8-2

SIGNS AND SYMPTOMS OF ACNE

SIGNS
- Open comedones (blackheads)
- Closed comedones (whiteheads)
- Papules
- Pustules
- Nodules

SYMPTOMS
- None

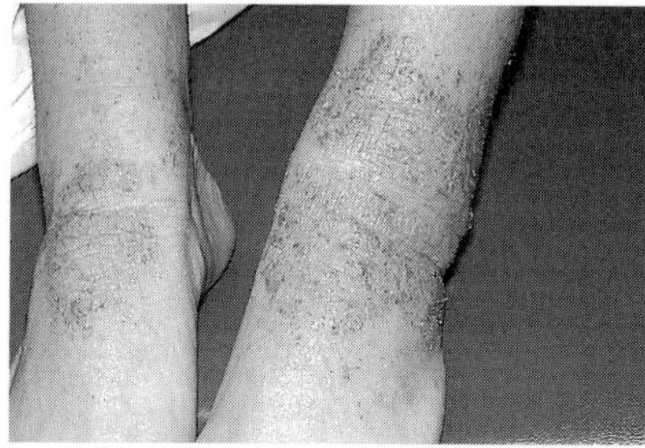

FIGURE 8-6 ■ Atopic dermatitis (eczema). (See Color Plate 7; reprinted with permission from Goodheart HP. A photoguide of common skin disorders: diagnosis and management. Philadelphia: Lippincott Williams & Wilkins, 1999:31.)

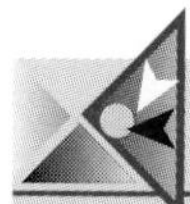

Box 8-3

SIGNS AND SYMPTOMS OF ATOPIC DERMATITIS (ECZEMA)

- Pruritis, in conjunction with:
  - Hay fever
  - Asthma
  - Allergic rhinitis
- Erythematous patches, plaques, or papules
- Lichenification (caused by chronic scratching)

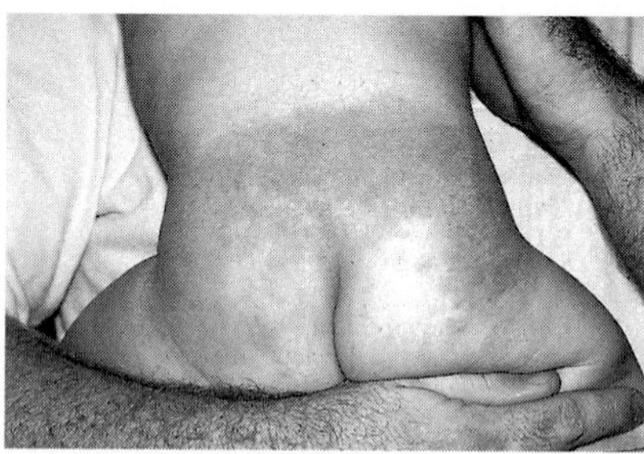

FIGURE 8-7 ■ Diaper rash. (See Color Plate 8; reprinted with permission from Goodheart HP. A photoguide of common skin disorders: diagnosis and management. Philadelphia: Lippincott Williams & Wilkins, 1999:84.)

Infectious Conditions

Measles

Measles is a highly infectious, childhood viral disease that can be fatal. The causative organism has been categorized as a paramyxovirus. Because of mandatory measles vaccination, the incidence of measles in the United States is only approximately 500 cases per year. The single risk factor is not being vaccinated. The virus is transmitted in the air, in blood, and through sexual contact. Signs and symptoms include:

- A prodrome of fever, malaise, sore throat, headache, conjunctivitis, cough, and other constitutional symptoms.
- Disseminated, erythematous rash (subsides in 5–6 days).

- Koplik's spots (small, red spots on the buccal mucosa with a small, white center; considered to be pathognomic for measles) (Fig. 8-8).

Treatment is symptomatic only. Antibiotics are only used for bacterial complications.

Chickenpox

Chickenpox (varicella) is a highly infectious, childhood disease caused by the varicella-zoster virus. Approximately 3 to 4 million cases are reported each year in the United States, with approximately 100 deaths. The incidence is expected to decrease, however, with the release of the varicella-zoster virus vaccine in 1995. Chickenpox is transmitted by direct contact or airborne droplets. The primary risk factor is exposure to a child with a known varicella infection. Children are considered to be infectious from 2 days before onset of the rash until all the vesicles have crusted (typically 4-6 days after onset of the rash). Exposure to the disease appears to generate immunity to additional episodes. Signs and symptoms include:

- A prodrome of malaise, headache, aches, and pains (uncommon or minor).
- Disseminated (although concentrated on trunk and face), erythematous rash that progresses rapidly from papules to vesicles (elliptical dewdrops), pustules, and crusts (Fig. 8-9).

Treatment generally includes oral antihistamines for the pruritis. Oral acetaminophen is preferred over aspirin in children to reduce the risk of Reye's syndrome. Oral antiviral agents, such as acyclovir, famciclovir, and valacyclovir, may be used in severe cases. Topical mupirocin and oral erythromycin and penicillinase-resistant antibiotics may be used to treat secondary skin infections.

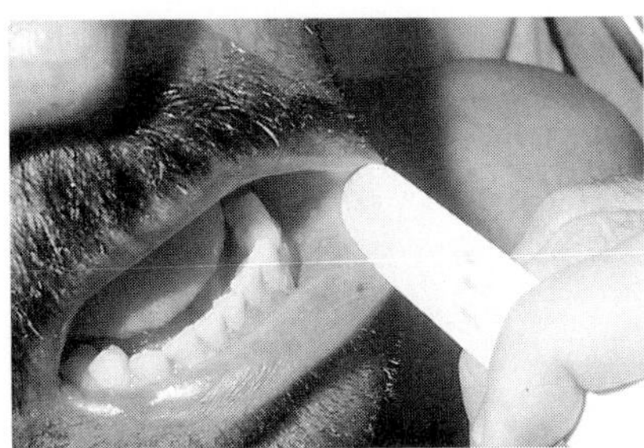

FIGURE 8-8 ■ Koplik's spots with measles. (See Color Plate 9; reprinted with permission from Goodheart HP. A photoguide of common skin disorders: diagnosis and management. Philadelphia: Lippincott Williams & Wilkins, 1999:290.)

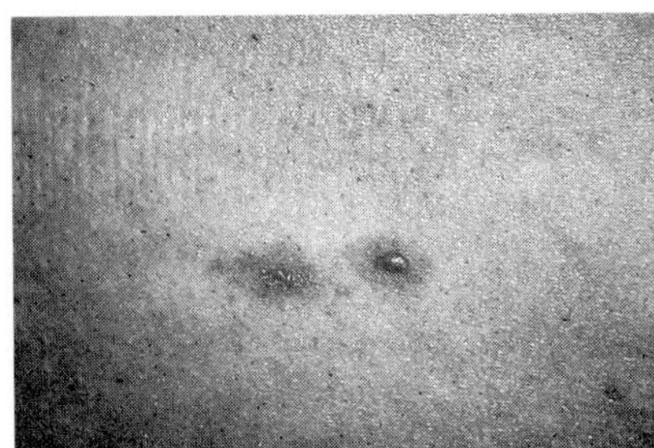

FIGURE 8-9 ■ Varicella (chickenpox). (See Color Plate 10; reprinted with permission from Goodheart HP. A photoguide of common skin disorders: diagnosis and management. Philadelphia: Lippincott Williams & Wilkins, 1999:288.)

Impetigo

Impetigo is a cutaneous bacterial infection caused by *Staphylococcus aureus* and group A β-hemolytic *Streptococcus pyogenes.* Impetigo refers to infection in the epidermis, whereas ecthyma (ulcerative impetigo) involves the dermis as well. Both can be either primary (caused by a loss of skin integrity) or secondary infections resulting from other dermatologic disorders. Primary infection is usually seen in young children. The serous fluid or purulent exudate from lesions can cause autoinoculation and formation of satellite lesions on other parts of the body. The exudate dries and forms crusts. Impetigo is most often found on the face, extremities, and buttocks, whereas ecthyma occurs on the ankles, dorsa of the feet, thighs, and buttocks (Fig. 8-10). Ecthyma may produce pain and tenderness on palpation. In children, impetigo is often found around the mouth because of colonization of the nose by the staph or strep organisms. These lesions can be pruritic, and they can become confluent and form large crusts. Untreated, these infections can lead to glomerulonephritis. Impetigo may last several weeks, whereas ecthyma may last several months. Risk factors for developing impetigo and ecthyma include:

- Warm temperature with high humidity
- Any breakage in the skin
- Preexisting skin disorders (e.g., atopic dermatitis)
- Poor hygiene
- Crowded living conditions
- Neglected minor trauma in the skin

The drug of choice for topical treatment is mupirocin ointment. Numerous oral antibiotics are used depending on the causative organism. Among the drugs recommended are penicillin VK, cephalexin, macrolide antibiotics, amoxicillin/clavulanic acid, trimethoprim/sulfamethoxazole (TMP/SMZ), dicloxacillin, and ciprofloxacin.

Fungal Infections

Fungal infections represent the most common disorder of the skin. A fungal infection of keratinized cells is caused by dermatophytes and is referred to as dermatophytosis. The term *tinea* refers to infections caused by dermatophytes and is usually

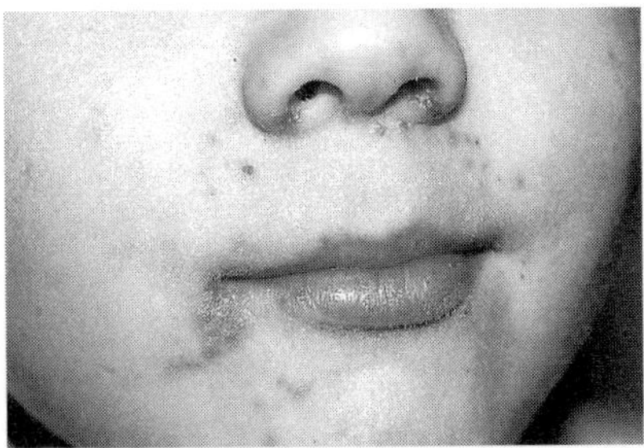

FIGURE 8-10 ■ Impetigo. (See Color Plate 11; reprinted with permission from Goodheart HP. A photoguide of common skin disorders: diagnosis and management. Philadelphia: Lippincott Williams & Wilkins, 1999:292.)

paired with the anatomic site of the infection. **Candidiasis** refers to fungal infections caused by *Candida albicans.*

The most common causes of dermatophytosis are *Epidermophyton, Microsporum,* and *Trichophyton* sp. These dermatophytes can be transmitted by fomites (inanimate objects), by animals (especially cats and dogs), and from soil. The three most common types of dermatophytosis are tinea pedis (athletes foot) (Fig. 8-11), tinea corporis (ringworm) (Fig. 8-12), and tinea cruris (jock itch). The signs and symptoms of these three infections are listed in Box 8-4. Risk factors for dermatophytosis include:

- Warm, intertriginous areas (folds in the skin) of the body, which are almost always moist, causing maceration of the skin and allowing the organism to enter
- Immunosuppressed patients
- Atopic dermatitis
- Corticosteroid use
- Living in climates with high humidity
- Occlusive clothing or footwear
- Obesity

Dermatophytosis can be successfully treated in most cases with topical antifungal agents, many of which are available without a prescription. Some of the more popular include miconazole, clotrimazole, tolnaftate, oxiconazole, naftifine, terbinafine, and ciclopiroxalamine. It normally takes about 4 weeks of topical treatment to clear the infection. In resistant cases or those with concomitant fungal infection of another part of the body, oral antifungal therapy with griseofulvin may be required.

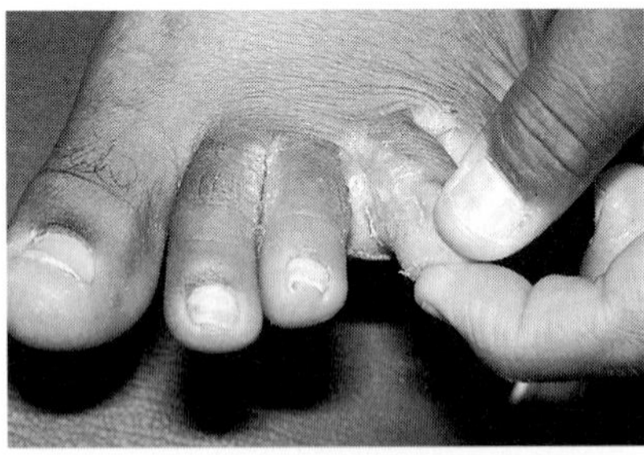

FIGURE 8-11 ■ Tinea pedis (athlete's foot). (See Color Plate 12; reprinted with permission from Goodheart HP. A photoguide of common skin disorders: diagnosis and management. Philadelphia: Lippincott Williams & Wilkins, 1999:120.)

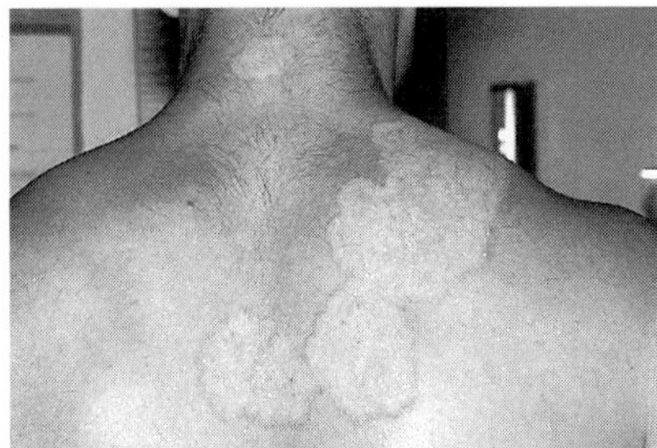

FIGURE 8-12 ■ Tinea corporis (ringworm). (See Color Plate 13; reprinted with permission from Goodheart HP. A photoguide of common skin disorders: diagnosis and management. Philadelphia: Lippincott Williams & Wilkins, 1999:106.)

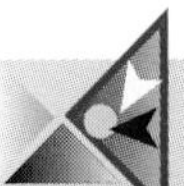

Box 8-4

SIGNS AND SYMPTOMS OF COMMON DERMATOPHYTOSIS

TINEA PEDIS

Signs
- Erythema
- Maceration
- Scaling
- Erosion
- Vesicles
- Pustules

Symptoms
- Pruritis

TINEA CORPORIS

Signs
- Erythema
- Scales
- Plaques, circular and hyperpigmented (red to brown)
- Vesicles (present or absent, at margin)
- Pustules (present or absent, at margin)

Symptoms
- Pruritis

TINEA CRURIS

Signs
- Tend to be bilateral
- Scales
- Plaques, hyperpigmented (red to brown)
- Papules (at margin)
- Pustules (at margin)

Symptoms
- Pruritis (present or absent)

Candidiasis usually occurs in intertriginous areas that are warm and moist, such as between the toes, in the groin and axillae, and under the breasts (Fig. 8-13). Signs and symptoms of candidiasis are listed in Box 8-5.The lesions can become confluent, forming large plaques enveloping the entire groin, axillary area, or skin under the breasts. Risk factors for candidiasis include:

- Warm, intertriginous areas (folds in the skin) of the body, which are almost always moist, causing maceration of the skin and allowing the organism to enter
- Antibiotics
- Steroids, oral and topical
- Diabetes
- Obesity
- Any occupation causing a person's hands to be immersed in water for long periods of time
- Diaper rash

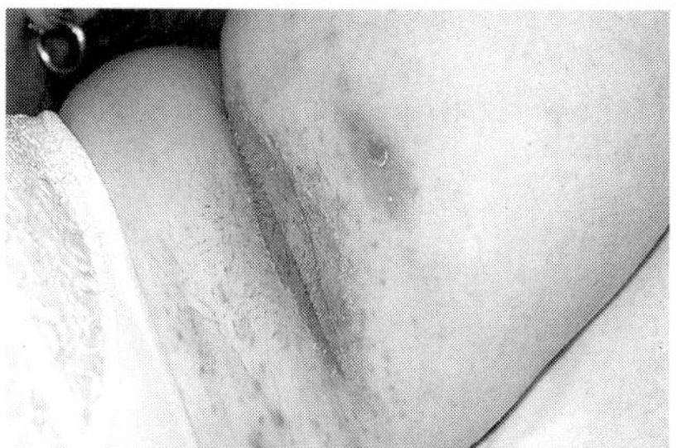

FIGURE 8-13 ■ Candidiasis. (See Color Plate 14; reprinted with permission from Goodheart HP. A photoguide of common skin disorders: diagnosis and management. Philadelphia: Lippincott Williams & Wilkins, 1999:210.)

Treatment is topical and includes use of clotrimazole, miconazole, and nystatin for the infection and corticosteroids to relieve the symptoms.

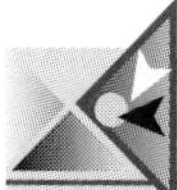

Box 8-5

SIGNS AND SYMPTOMS OF CUTANEOUS CANDIDIASIS

SIGNS
- Erythema
- Papules
- Pustules
- Satellite pustules
- Erosions caused by skin maceration
- Fissures
- Dry skin with scaling (some cases)

SYMPTOMS
- Itching
- Burning sensation

Adverse Cutaneous Drug Reactions

Almost every commonly used drug has been reported to produce adverse cutaneous drug reactions, with the incidence being in the range of 2% to 3% of hospitalized patients. These reactions can occur from any route of administration, but topically applied substances are the most likely to do so. Most often, these are immunologic hypersensitivity reactions (e.g., urticaria, angioedema, fixed drug eruptions, Stevens-Johnson syndrome, and toxic epidermal necrolysis), but some are nonallergic in nature (e.g., drug hypersensitivity syndrome). The reaction is generally unpredictable and can range in effect from mild and self-limiting to severe and life-threatening.

Drug-Induced Urticaria, Angioedema, and Anaphylaxis

Most reactions in this category are allergic in nature, but some are caused by actions of the drug that are unrelated to the immune system. These reactions are referred to as anaphylactoid. Risk factors (not inclusive) for allergic urticaria and angioedema include:

- Antibiotics (especially penicillin, cephalosporins, and sulfonamides)
- Angiotensin-converting enzyme inhibitors
- Aspirin
- Calcium-channel blockers
- Contraceptives, oral
- Cytostatic agents
- Drugs that cause the release of histamine (e.g., amphetamine, atropine, opiates, and hydralazine)

Risk factors (not inclusive) for nonallergic urticaria (anaphylactoid reactions) include:

- Angiotensin-converting enzyme inhibitors
- Calcium-channel blockers
- Nonsteroidal anti-inflammatory drugs
- Drugs that cause the release of histamine
- Radiographic contrast media

Signs and symptoms may vary depending on the causative agent and its mechanism of action. Common symptoms are listed in Box 8-6.

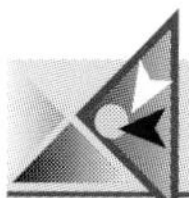

Box 8-6

SIGNS AND SYMPTOMS OF DRUG-INDUCED URTICARIA, ANGIOEDEMA, AND ANAPHYLAXIS

SIGNS
- Difficulty breathing
- Flushing
- Hypotension
- Laryngeal edema
- Large wheals

SYMPTOMS
- Abdominal pain
- Burning sensation, especially of the palms and soles
- Dizziness
- Fatigue
- Headache
- Nausea and vomiting
- Pruritis

The first step in treatment is discontinuing the agent responsible for the reaction. The reaction generally subsides in a matter of hours to several days. Urticarial lesions usually disappear within a few hours and generally do not last for more than 24 hours after the agent is discontinued. In mild cases, no additional treatment is necessary. When the reaction is severe, however, epinephrine, antihistamines, intravenous corticosteroids, or oral prednisone may be needed.

Exanthematous Drug Eruption

An exanthematous drug eruption is one of two types of maculopapular drug eruptions. This type has the highest incidence among adverse cutaneous drug reactions. It is referred to as morbilliform, because it presents as a measles-like rash. Fever may or may not be present. The macules and papules are symmetrically distributed on the extremities and trunk, and they often coalesce to give a very diffuse presentation (Fig. 8-14). This condition most often results from oral or parenteral drug administration. The exact mechanism is unknown, but it is believed to involve a delayed hypersensitivity to a drug. More than 50% of patients infected with the human immunodeficiency virus who are given sulfonamides—and virtually 100% of patients infected with Epstein-Barr virus who are given penicillin—will experience this eruption. Depending on whether a patient has been previously sensitized, the onset of the eruption can vary from as early as 2 days to as long as 3 weeks after taking the drug. In certain cases, a diagnostic problem occurs, because the eruption caused by certain drugs, particularly penicillin, may not present for several weeks after the drug has been discontinued. To further complicate the patient's history, not every drug will cause the eruption to recur when the patient is challenged again with that same drug. Risk factors for exanthematous drug reactions are listed in Box 8-7.

Primary treatment is discontinuation of the drug suspected to be responsible. In some cases, the eruption will slowly subside even if the drug is not discontinued. Itching may be attenuated with use of oral antihistamines.

Fixed Drug Eruption

A fixed drug eruption is a reaction in which the lesions tend to appear at the same anatomic site, most notably the genitalia and the face. Commonly, such eruptions are believed to always be caused by a drug, but some question exists about the ability of certain legumes and food colorings to trigger this reaction. This condition is believed to be an allergic reaction, but the exact mechanism is not well understood. Depending on the sensitivity of the patient, the lesion (only one lesion normally develops) usually appears within 8 hours after taking the drug. The condition presents with erythema and the progression from macules to bullae, which are painful to the touch. Erythema occurs with or without pruritis. Risk factors for fixed-drug reactions are listed in Box 8-8.

Discontinuation of the offending drug is most important, because unlike other types of cutaneous drug reactions, the lesion remains as long as the patient takes the drug. The lesion is inflammatory in nature, so a high-potency topical corticosteroid

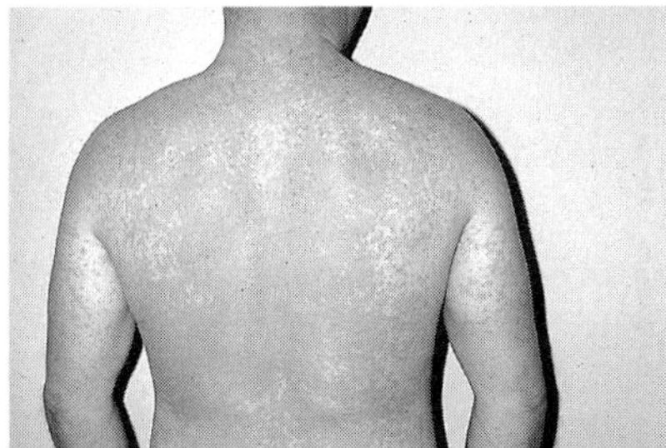

FIGURE 8-14 ■ Drug reaction. (See Color Plate 15; reprinted with permission from Goodheart HP. A photoguide of common skin disorders: diagnosis and management. Philadelphia: Lippincott Williams & Wilkins, 1999:124.)

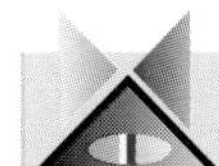

Box 8-7

RISK FACTORS FOR EXANTHEMATOUS DRUG REACTIONS

DRUGS[a]

- Allopurinol
- Barbiturates
- Benzodiazepines
- Carbamazepine
- Cephalosporins
- Erythromycin
- Gold salts (highest incidence)
- Hydantoins
- Nonsteroidal anti-inflammatory drugs
- Penicillins
- Phenothiazines
- Streptomycin
- Sulfonamides
- Tetracyclines

OTHER FACTORS

- Cytomegalovirus mononucleosis
- Epstein-Barr virus
- Human immunodeficiency virus
- Previous exanthematous drug eruption (same drug)

[a]Not all-inclusive.

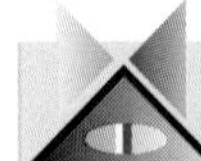

Box 8-8

RISK FACTORS FOR FIXED DRUG REACTIONS

RISK FACTORS[a]

- Acetaminophen
- Amphetamines
- Aspirin and other salicylates
- Barbiturates
- Gold salts
- Hydralazine
- Metronidazole
- Nonsteroidal anti-inflammatory drugs
- Oral contraceptives
- Penicillins
- Quinine
- Sulfonamides
- Tetracyclines

[a]Not all-inclusive.

may be applied. Bacitracin or Silvadene may be applied on vesicles that have lost their integrity. The condition takes several weeks to resolve, but the hyperpigmentation may last for several months.

Stevens-Johnson Syndrome

Stevens-Johnson syndrome (SJS) is one of the most serious drug-related cutaneous diseases. The cause is not always easy to discern, but more than half of all cases are believed to be caused by drugs. The lesions are widespread and cover most of the body, including the mucous membranes. A more severe variant of SJS is toxic epidermal necrolysis. In SJS, a prodromal rash eventually leads to sloughing of large areas of epidermal tissue. At its worst, the patient appears to have received a serious and extensive burn over a large part of the body. Mortality (5% to 18% of patients) most often results from systemic damage, such as that to the respiratory or gastrointestinal tract or to the kidneys. Eruption of the cutaneous lesions is preceded by several days of a prodromal phase, which includes flu-like symptoms. The signs and symptoms of SJS are listed in Box 8-9, and risk factors for SJS are listed in Box 8-10.

Patient care includes discontinuation of the offending drug, third-degree burn procedures (including fluid and electrolyte replacement), prevention and treatment of septic infections, and application of erythromycin ointment to the eyes.

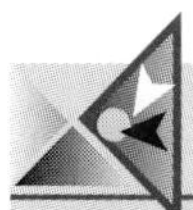

Box 8-9

SIGNS AND SYMPTOMS OF STEVENS-JOHNSON SYNDROME AND TOXIC EPIDERMAL NECROLYSIS

SIGNS

- Erythema
- Macules
- Papules
- Vesicles
- Crinkling of the skin
- Detachment of large areas of the epidermis (greater in toxic epidermal necrolysis than in Stevens-Johnson syndrome)
- Mucous membrane lesions
- Ocular hyperemia
- Renal failure

SYMPTOMS

- Prodrome
  - Conjunctival pruritis
  - Fever
  - Malaise
- Skin tenderness and pain
- Joint pain
- Pain from mucous membrane lesions

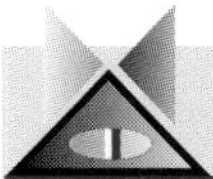

Box 8-10

RISK FACTORS FOR DEVELOPING STEVENS-JOHNSON SYNDROME

DRUGS

- Allopurinol
- Barbiturates
- Cephalosporins
- Hydantoins
- Nonsteroidal anti-inflammatory drugs
- Penicillins
- Sulfonamides

OTHER FACTORS

- Human immunodeficiency virus
- Infections
- Neoplasms
- Pregnancy
- Systemic lupus erythematosus

Drug-Induced Photosensitivity

Drug-induced photosensitivity is a cutaneous adverse reaction to systemic or topical drugs (or chemicals) in which UV radiation strikes the skin and converts drugs in the tissues into either toxic or allergic substances (i.e., haptens). Most often, the cause is UVA (320–400 nm), but it can also be produced by UVB (280–320 nm) and visible light. Photoallergy, which usually follows topical application of a drug, occurs in only 5% of cases, is immunologically mediated, and requires previous sensitization.

Signs and symptoms of photosensitivity reactions are listed in Box 8-11. Photosensitivity presents as a eczema-like condition; phototoxicity presents as an exaggerated sunburn and is dose-related. A phototoxic reaction is fairly well demarcated along the area of exposure, but a photoallergic reaction is more likely to spread into unexposed tissue. One interesting variant of this is called phytophotodermatitis, or "weed whacker" dermatitis, which is a phototoxic reaction caused by UV radiation striking the skin after it comes in contact with various plants, including weeds, carrot greens, and celery. Other causative agents are lime juice and perfumes containing begamot oil, a psoralen.

Drugs that may cause photosensitivity are listed in Box 8-12. Discontinuation of the offending drug usually causes the photosensitivity to resolve.

Infestations

Scabies

Scabies is an intensely pruritic disorder of the skin caused by the mite *Sarcoptes scabiei,* which burrows into the skin. The mite is transmitted by skin-to-skin contact (including sexual contact) and by infested clothing or bedding (mites can live for several days on nonliving environments). An important risk factor is living in an institutional setting. Signs and symptoms include

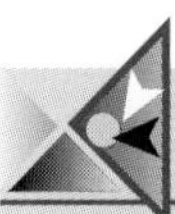

Box 8-11

SIGNS AND SYMPTOMS OF PHOTOSENSITIVITY

PHOTOALLERGY

Signs
- Edema
- Erythema
- Eczema-like, dry, crusted skin
- Scaling
- Lichenification with continuous scratching

Symptoms
- Pruritis

PHOTOTOXICITY

Signs
- Edema
- Erythema
- Vesicles
- Dark red-brown pigmentation (exaggerated sunburn)
- Scaling
- Lichenification, with continuous scratching

Symptoms
- Pruritis

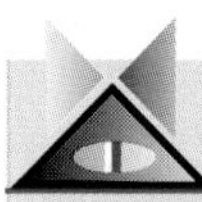

Box 8-12

DRUGS THAT MAY CAUSE PHOTOSENSITIVITY

- Antihistamines
- Antihypertensives
- Chemotherapeutic agents
- Coal tar derivatives
- Estrogens
- Fluoroquinolones
- Monoamine oxidase inhibitors
- Nonsteroidal anti-inflammatory drugs
- Phenothiazines
- Progestins
- Sulfonamides
- Sulfonylureas
- Tetracyclines
- Thiazide diuretics
- Tricyclic antidepressants

pruritis (intense), erythematous papules (in some cases), and intraepidermal burrows (pathognomonic for scabies). Treatment involves either 1% lindane or 5% permethrin cream.

Pediculosis

Pediculosis refers to louse-borne infestations. Three types of lice are common in the United States: (1) head lice (pediculosis capitis), (2) body lice (pediculosis corporis), and (3) pubic lice (pediculosis pubis). Each type of louse is found in its own area of the body, but pubic lice may also be found in other hairy areas, such as the axilla or eyelashes. Risk factors for louse-borne infestations include:

- Sharing infested combs, hats, and brushes, as well as any head-to-head contact (head lice).
- Infested clothing or bedding (body lice, head lice if there is contact with the head).
- Close contact, especially sexual (pubic lice, head lice if there is contact with the head).

Pruritis is the most common symptom of pediculosis. Lice are generally not seen; however, their nits or eggs are often found cemented to hair shafts (Fig. 8.15). Clothing should be washed in hot water and dried hot or dry cleaned. Place anything that cannot be washed in a plastic bag and seal it for 14 days to ensure that all lice and eggs are dead. Drug treatment involves topical lindane (1%), pyrethrins with piperonyl butoxide, permethrins, and malathion (0.5%).

Skin Cancer

The three primary types of skin cancer are basal cell carcinoma (BCC), squamous cell carcinoma (SCC), and melanoma. Approximately 400,000 new cases of BCC, 150,000 new cases of SCC, and 45,000 new cases of melanoma are diagnosed each year in the United States. Risk factors include light skin, excessive exposure to UV radiation (the sun or tanning beds and booths), and patients who take immunosuppressant drugs.

The signs and symptoms of BCC and SCC are similar and include:

- Translucent, shiny papule or nodule (BCC).
- Single ulceration with a rolled border (BCC) (Fig. 8-16).
- Single papule or plaque that continues to grow (SCC) (Fig. 8-17).

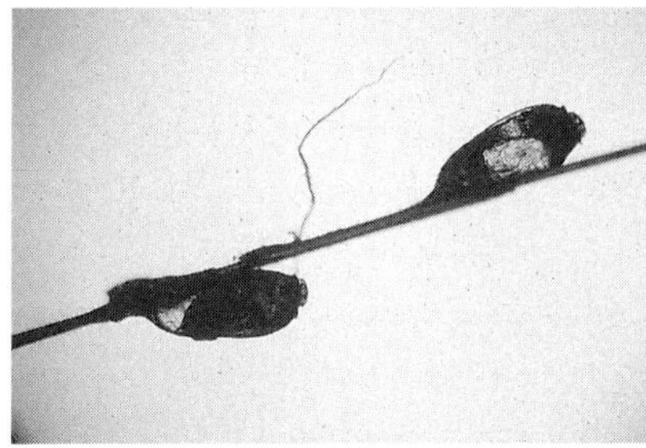

FIGURE 8-15 ■ Pediculosis (lice). (See Color Plate 16; reprinted with permission from Goodheart HP. A photoguide of common skin disorders: diagnosis and management. Philadelphia: Lippincott Williams & Wilkins, 1999:132.)

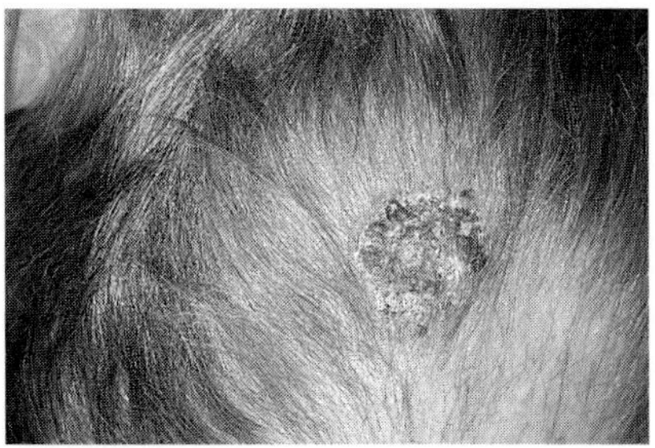

FIGURE 8-16 ■ Basal cell carcinoma. (See Color Plate 17; reprinted with permission from Goodheart HP. A photoguide of common skin disorders: diagnosis and management. Philadelphia: Lippincott Williams & Wilkins, 1999:144.)

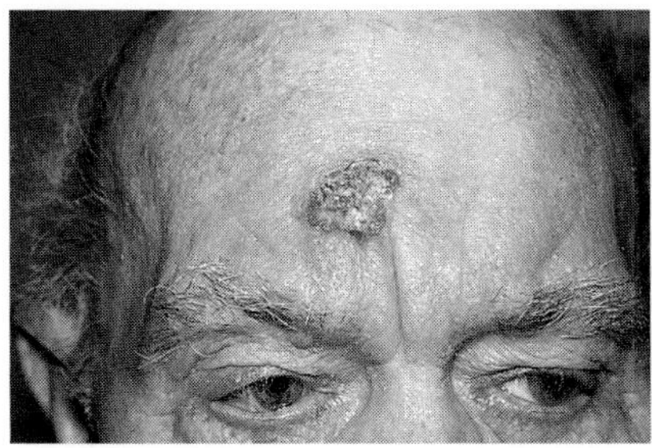

FIGURE 8-17 ■ Squamous cell carcinoma. (See Color Plate 18; reprinted with permission from Goodheart HP. A photoguide of common skin disorders: diagnosis and management. Philadelphia: Lippincott Williams & Wilkins, 1999:152.)

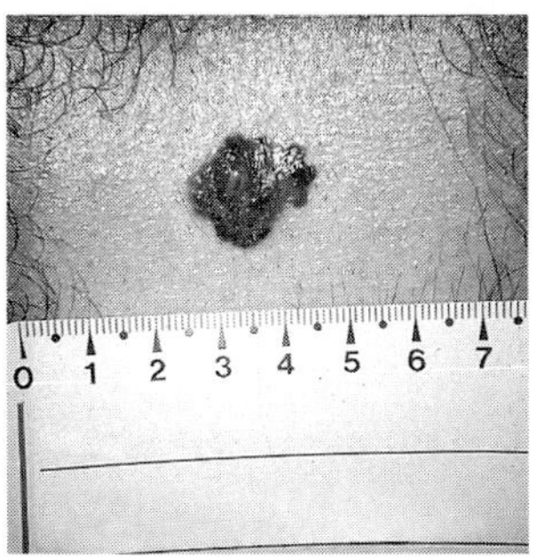

FIGURE 8-18 ■ Melanoma. (See Color Plate 19; reprinted with permission from Goodheart HP. A photoguide of common skin disorders: diagnosis and management. Philadelphia: Lippincott Williams & Wilkins, 1999:250.)

The signs and symptoms for melanoma (Fig. 8-18) create the acronym *ABCDE,* as follows:

- *A*symmetry
- *B*order is irregular
- *C*olor is changed or mottled
- *D*iameter is greater than 6 mm (end of a pencil)
- *E*nlargement of mole over time

Treatment depends on the length of time the lesions have been left untreated. Surgical removal is often the preferred treatment.

Hair

Folliculitis (inflammation of hair follicles) may be caused by bacteria or fungi and usually involves the upper part of the hair follicle (Fig. 8-19).

Infectious Folliculitis

Folliculitis is most likely to occur on areas of the body that are shaved, although it may occur anywhere. Preexisting folliculitis may be aggravated by shaving. Causative organisms include *Staphylococcus aureus* and *Pseudomonas aeruginosa* (hot tub folliculitis, which usually occurs several days after using a hot tub). Common signs and symptoms are listed in Box 8-13. Risk factors include shaving, hair extraction, occlusion of follicles (e.g., by clothing, bandages, or chemicals such as oil), and living in climates with high humidity. In cases of superficial folliculitis, the inflammation clears spontaneously, but topical treatment with mupirocin or triple-antibiotic ointments is effective. If topical treatment does not produce results, oral antibiotics may be used. The choice of antibiotic is determined by the causative organism and can include cephalexin, erythromycin, dicloxacillin, and minocycline.

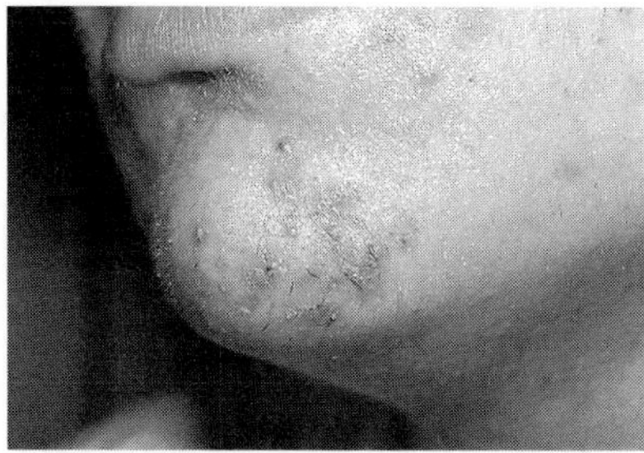

FIGURE 8-19 ■ Folliculitis. (See Color Plate 20; reprinted with permission from Goodheart HP. A photoguide of common skin disorders: diagnosis and management. Philadelphia: Lippincott Williams & Wilkins, 1999:17.)

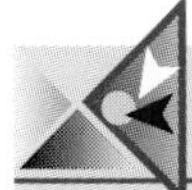

Box 8-13

SIGNS AND SYMPTOMS OF INFECTIOUS FOLLICULITIS (BACTERIAL)

SIGNS

- Occur around each follicle
- Erythema
- Papules
- Pustules (in "hot tub" folliculitis, they appear all over the trunk)
- Crusts

SYMPTOMS

- Pruritis
- Tenderness on palpation

Two of the most common fungal infections affecting hair are tinea capitis (scalp) and tinea barbae (beard). As with the fungal infections of the skin, these are caused by dermatophytes. The spores that transmit tinea capitis are spread by fomites (i.e., objects capable of transmitting a disease-causing organism) from people or animals. Affected patients are more likely to have dark skin, and children are more commonly affected than adults. Tinea capitis has no other true risk factors, except for overcrowding in social environments where the condition is endemic. Common signs and symptoms are listed in Box 8-14. Oral antifungals are the treatment of choice and include itraconazole, terbinafine, ketoconazole, and griseofulvin. Topical therapy is ineffective. If left untreated, scarring alopecia is likely to develop. Tinea barbae occurs in the beard and moustache area, and this condition is seen only in men. Common signs and symptoms are found in Box 8-14, and treatment is the same as for tinea capitis.

Furuncles and Carbuncles

A **furuncle** is a deep-seated folliculitis caused by *Staphylococcus aureus.* A **carbuncle,** or boil, forms from the coalescence of adjacent furuncles and can penetrate beyond the dermis into the subcutaneous layer. These conditions occur more commonly in men than in women. Common signs and symptoms include pain, tenderness, inflammation, erythema, nodules, and pustules. Risk factors include:

- Chronic *S. aureus* carriers
- Diabetes
- Obesity

Treatment in many cases requires only drainage of the lesion. In some cases, systemic antibiotics are also used; these include amoxicillin/clavulanic acid, dicloxacillin, cephalexin, any macrolide antibiotic, ciprofloxacin, minocycline, and TMP-SMZ.

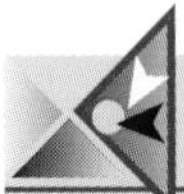

Box 8-14

SIGNS AND SYMPTOMS OF INFECTIOUS FOLLICULITIS (FUNGAL)

TINEA CAPITIS

Signs

- Around the hair follicle
- Inflammation (present or absent)
- Alopecia
- Plaques
- Pustules
- Hair loss
- Hair loss with round, gray patch (gray patch type)
- Hair loss with black dot where hair shaft is broken off at the skin line (black dot type)

Symptoms

- Pain
- Tenderness

TINEA BARBAE

Signs

- Around the hair follicle
- Erythema
- Inflammation
- Papules
- Pustules
- Crusts
- Hair loss
- Red, patchy areas with scaling

Symptoms

- None

Alopecia

The term *defluvium* means loss of hair, and **alopecia,** or baldness, is the condition that results. Alopecia may be localized (areata), involve the entire scalp and eyebrows (totalis), or the entire body (universalis). Alopecia is divided into two basic categories: cicatricial (scarring) alopecia, in which some damage or problem is associated with the hair follicle, resulting in an inability to produce hair; and noncicatricial (nonscarring) alopecia, which produces several effects, including a change in hair texture. The causes of alopecia are many, and the risk factors vary according to the type. Some of the more common causes include anemia, chemical agents (e.g., heavy metals), endocrine diseases (e.g., hypopituitarism), heredity, infections, mechanical trauma, and neoplasms. Some of the risk factors include autoimmune disorders (alopecia areata), inflammatory diseases (scarring alopecia), drugs (drug-induced alopecia), and heredity (androgenic alopecia). Signs and symptoms of alopecia are listed in Box 8-15.

Treatment varies depending on the cause. Topical minoxidil is helpful in some cases of androgenic alopecia. Discontinuation of the offending drug is the treatment for drug-induced alopecia. Treatment of the underlying inflammatory disease may help in cases of scarring alopecia if the damage is not too severe. No treatment is currently effective for alopecia areata.

In contrast to alopecia, hypertrichosis and hirsutism represent increases in body hair. Hirsutism refers to the distribution of hair according to male patterns on women only, and it can be caused by a variety of adrenal, endocrine, and ovarian diseases. Hypertrichosis refers to excessive growth of body hair that is unrelated to androgens and sex. More than 15 disorders, including numerous drugs, can produce hypertrichosis.

Nails

Any change in the normal structure, shape, or color of the nails should be considered suggestive of a potential systemic disease after local infection and trauma have been ruled out. One of the most common primary disorders of the nails is **onychomycosis,** which is an infection of the nail caused by yeasts, molds, fungi, or some combination thereof (Fig. 8-20). Tinea unguium refers to a nail infection caused specifically by a dermatophytic fungus. The infection may invade the nail on any side or even from the nail plate, and most cases occur on

Box 8-15

SIGNS AND SYMPTOMS OF ALOPECIA

AREATA

Signs

- Erythema (present or absent)
- Patches of hair loss
- Areas of spontaneous regrowth
- Visible follicle openings
- Nails show dystrophic changes referred to as "hammered brass"

Symptoms

- None

SCARRING

Signs

- Inflammation
- Loss of hair follicle
- Scarring
- Any other signs related to the cause of the disorder

Symptoms

- None

DRUGS

Signs

- Erythema (present or absent)
- Patches of hair loss (faster and more expansive than in areata)
- Areas of spontaneous regrowth
- Visible follicle openings

Symptoms

- None

HEREDITY

Signs

- Slow thinning of individual hairs
- Slowly receding hair line

Symptoms

- None

the feet (almost always on the big toe). The signs of tinea unguium are white color of the nail plate, thickening and cracking of the nail, and rising of the nail from the nail plate. *Candida* sp. tend to infect the lateral nail folds and produce erythema, edema, and pain to the touch. Risk factors for onychomycosis include:

- Walking barefoot in areas with the potential for heavy contamination (e.g., community pools)
- Occlusive footwear
- Diminished blood flow to the extremity
- Systemic disorders (numerous)

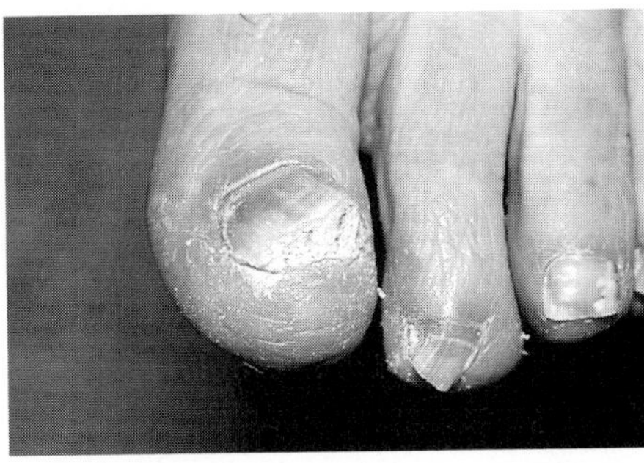

FIGURE 8-20 ■ Onychomycosis. (See Color Plate 21; reprinted with permission from Goodheart HP. A photoguide of common skin disorders: diagnosis and management. Philadelphia: Lippincott Williams & Wilkins, 1999:146.)

Treatment requires use of oral antifungal agents. The preferred agents are fluconazole, itraconazole, ketoconazole, and terbinafine.

SYSTEM ASSESSMENT

Accurate assessment of a dermatologic presentation requires a complete patient history, including past and current medical history, present and recent medications, family history, occupation and hobbies, and possibly, sexual history. Occupation and hobbies are especially important in evaluating dermatologic complaints because of the relationship between chemicals and solvents and a variety of disorders.

Subjective Information

Because of easy accessibility, individuals frequently present skin, hair, and nail complaints to the pharmacist. The most common symptoms include skin rashes, itching (pruritus), and pain/tenderness. Additional symptoms may indicate a skin eruption secondary to a systemic disorder.

Skin Characteristics

? INTERVIEW Tell me more about your skin problem? When did the condition start? Where on the body did the problem first appear? How did it spread? Has the skin condition changed? How have the lesions, rash, or skin color changed? Is there anything that appeared to trigger the reaction? What treatments have you tried, and what were the outcomes of these treatments?

ABNORMALITIES The very appearance of skin lesions, rash, or skin color changes is, by definition, abnormal, but the origins, characteristics, and changes over time are often specific to certain conditions. For example, linear streaking of a papulovesicular rash may indicate poison ivy dermatitis. For dermatologic conditions, asking these questions can jog the memory and assist the patient in providing even more diagnostic information.

Pruritus

? INTERVIEW Does it itch? If yes, where does it itch? When did the itching start? Is it continuous or intermittent? Is the itching mild or intense?

ABNORMALITIES Pruritus is common in most dermatologic conditions. The absence of pruritus is actually more diagnostic, because it helps to rule out (or at least to reduce the probability of) certain disorders.

Tenderness/Pain

? INTERVIEW Do you feel tenderness or pain? If yes, when did the tenderness or pain start? Is it continuous or intermittent? Describe the pain. When does it hurt?

ABNORMALITIES Pain is often secondary to localization of purulent material. When the tissue is intact, such as the lateral nail folds, hair follicles, or in furuncles, the pain may be throbbing. During palpation, the pain may become extreme.

Additional Symptoms

? INTERVIEW Are you experiencing nausea, dizziness, headache, or fatigue? If yes, when does each occur? Is each continuous or intermittent? Describe each symptom you are experiencing. Is the symptom mild or intense?

ABNORMALITIES Any of these symptoms may indicate drug-induced urticaria and angioedema. In general, however, primary skin diseases normally do not produce such symptoms; thus, any of these symptoms may suggest systemic disease.

Objective Information

Objective patient information includes physical assessment as well as laboratory and diagnostic tests. Determining the site of the eruption is important, because certain disorders tend to be found on specific areas of the body. Determining the evolution of the eruption is another important aspect. For example, what started out as a maculopapular rash might not be assessed until it has become an erosion with crusts.

Physical Assessment

An accurate assessment of the skin, hair, and nails differs from the assessment of internal systems, because the visual characteristics of these anatomic areas are often the sole determinant of the patient's problem. Additional symptoms may occur, but they do so infrequently.

Physical assessment should be performed in a room with sufficient light. Natural lighting works well but is often unavailable. Most examining areas have overhead fluorescent lighting, which is bright but tends to make raised lesions look flatter than they actually are. A movable incandescent lamp and penlight are recommended for supplemental lighting; they can be shined from the side to see the elevation of a skin lesion. A penlight can also be helpful in evaluating lesions within the mouth. A magnifying glass and probe can be useful as well.

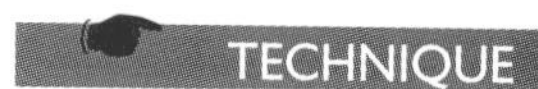

STEP 1 Inspect the Skin (Including the Scalp)

- Note the color of the skin and its uniformity.
- Note the characteristics of the lesion.
- Identify the type of lesion (e.g., macule, papule, pustule, or plaque) as described in Table 8-1.
- Evaluate the shape of the lesions (e.g., round, oval, annular, or irregular).
- If a nevi (mole), note any abnormal characteristics, using elements of the acronym *ABCDE* as warning signs.
  - Determine if the eruption is localized or generalized. Pay particular attention to the location (e.g., on the elbows and knees, in intertriginous areas, only on exposed areas, or where clothing constricts the skin).
  - Identify whether a single or multiple lesions are present.
  - Categorize the lesion arrangement (e.g., solitary, paired, linear, concentric, or confluent).
  - Determine the color of the area (e.g., red, white, tan, gray, brown, or black). Does the color indicate cyanosis, jaundice, or pallor? The specific color may be diagnostic by itself, but it may also serve to confirm a diagnosis. Also, determine if an area is hypo- or hyperpigmented.

STEP 2 Palpate the Skin

- Palpate the area to see if it blanches or is movable, tender, nodular, or moist.
- Note the temperature, texture, and presence of any edema.
- Pinch up a large fold of skin. Note the skin's ease of rising and turgor (i.e., its ability to return to place immediately when released).

ABNORMALITIES Poor turgor (pinched skin recedes slowly or "tents" and stands by itself when released) is present with dehydration or extreme weight loss.

CAUTION

- Palpation should always be conducted while wearing gloves. This is especially true in cases with skin drainage or an open wound.
- Never palpate an inflamed area, because this can cause a potential infection to spread deeper into the tissue. In the presence of infection, palpation may also produce intense pain.

ABNORMALITIES Abnormalities of color include pallor (anemia, arterial insufficiency), erythema, cyanosis (hypoxemia, heart failure, chronic bronchitis), and jaundice (hepatitis, cirrhosis, sickle-cell disease).

TECHNIQUE

STEP 3 Inspect the Hair

- Note the color, texture, and distribution of the hair.
- Evaluate the structure of the hair.

ABNORMALITIES In addition to genetic changes in hair color, changes in hair pigmentation can occur for several medical reasons, including nutritional deficiencies (e.g., kwashiorkor), albinism (10 major types), metabolic disorders (e.g., phenylketonuria), autoimmune diseases (e.g., pernicious anemia and thyroiditis), poliosis (localized loss of hair pigment), diseases of premature aging, and protein or copper deficiencies (often seen as graying of the hair in patches).

ABNORMALITIES Numerous disorders involve the structure or shape of hair shafts. Some of these include increased fragility of the hair and disorders not associated with increased fragility.

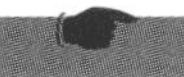
TECHNIQUE

STEP 4

Inspect the Nails

- Inspect the nail for atrophy, hypertrophy, abnormal shape (spoon nails can be caused by iron deficiency or Raynaud's syndrome and can even be inherited without concomitant disease), pitting (seen in psoriasis), or color changes (caused by kidney or pulmonary disease or by certain cancers).
- Evaluate the nail bed for separation from the nail plate (onycholysis) and hemorrhage (caused by many conditions, including trauma, psoriasis, and cirrhosis).
- Evaluate the nail folds for erythema, inflammation, swelling, tenderness, or separation from the nail plate.

ABNORMALITIES Infection of the nail folds by a wide variety of organisms, both bacterial and fungal, is common.

Laboratory and Diagnostic Tests

The following laboratory and diagnostic tests may be useful in assessing certain conditions of the skin, hair, and nails:

- Gram stain and culture of exudates can identify bacteria and yeast as the causative organisms. Skin tissue of the vesicles and scales, or the hair or nails, can be viewed under a microscope after clearing with 10% KOH (20% for nails). The presence of mycelia (the filamentous structures of fungi) indicates a fungal infection. The Tzanck test involves examination of tissue from vesicles, the results of which can help to support a diagnosis of herpes or measles.
- A Wood's lamp produces long-wave UV radiation, also known as "black" light, that in turn produces fluorescence in the presence of certain dermatophytes on hair in cases of tinea capitis and of erythrasma of the skin. This lamp can also help to better define the color distinction between the skin of lesions and normal skin, especially in patients with very light or very dark skin. When the light produces a particular color of urine, it indicates a diagnosis of porphyria, a systemic disorder that produces a variety of skin lesions.
- Diascopy involves firmly placing a glass slide over a skin lesion. It is helpful in differentiating erythema, which blanches under pressure, from **purpura** (hemorrhage into the skin with obvious discoloration), which does not. It is also used to determine the exact color of skin lesions in several systemic disorders.
- Patch testing can be done to determine specific patient allergies. More than a thousand compounds, ranging from dust and mold to chemicals and foods, can be tested with available allergen products.
- Immunofluorescence involves performing a biopsy of skin tissue to identify problems associated with the immune system. It is also useful in establishing the diagnosis of bullous disorders, such as bullous pemphigoid, connective tissue disorders, and various types of skin tumors.
- Laboratory tests are useful in establishing the diagnosis of skin diseases that cause abnormalities in blood and organ function. For example, eosinophilia is common in many adverse cutaneous drug reactions, anemia is found in systemic lupus erythematosus, and a complete blood count with differential is necessary in the diagnosis of cutaneous T-cell lymphoma.

Special Considerations

Pediatric Patients

? INTERVIEW Any problems with diaper rash? Do you use cloth or disposable diapers? How often do you change the diaper? Have you noticed any new rashes? Have you introduced any new foods or formula? Does your child have any allergies? Are the child's immunizations up-to-date? What precautions do you use to protect your child from sunburn? Do you use sunscreens and sunblocks?

ABNORMALITIES Children may develop many of the same conditions that adults do, but a variety of diseases are more commonly seen in pediatric patients. These include diaper rash, chickenpox (varicella), head lice, sunburn, measles, rubella, impetigo, candidiasis, and atopic dermatitis.

Geriatric Patients

? INTERVIEW What changes have you noticed in your skin as you have gotten older? Any problems with dry skin or itching? How often do you evaluate your skin for changes in moles and possible skin cancer?

The history of the presenting problem is most important in geriatric patients, because most persons older than 60 years suffer from some degree of **xerosis** (dryness of the skin), with rough and scaly patches. Because of the normal aging process, dry skin is very common in elderly patients. Therefore, obtaining a thorough understanding of how the new condition compares to the normal skin condition is vital. The dry skin also is usually associated with pruritis, especially at night. This itching can lead to excoriations, lichenification, and infection, which may appear to be the primary problem rather than a result of constant scratching. A reduction in skin elasticity is normal in elderly patients as well, but it can also be a sign of dehydration. Blood tests may be indicated to determine the actual cause of a significant loss in skin elasticity.

Pregnant Patients

? INTERVIEW Any problems with color changes in the skin? Stretch marks? Spider veins?

Pregnancy normally causes many changes in the skin. Specifically, **striae** (silver to pink jagged lines on the skin), which are more commonly known as "stretch marks," frequently appear during the second trimester on the abdomen, breasts, and hips. Striae fade after delivery, but they usually do not completely disappear. Other changes include **chloasma,** a irregular brown patch of hyperpigmentation on the face; **linea nigra,** a brownish-black line down the middle of the abdomen; and spider veins, lesions with tiny red centers and radiating vascular branches on the face, neck, chest, arms, and legs. Pregnancy may also cause the hair to become thicker and more coarse.

APPLICATION TO PATIENT SYMPTOMS

Patients often consult their pharmacist for treatment of skin eruptions. This is especially true for localized conditions, which often produce not much more than annoying pruritus. Some of the most common complaints of patients include a rash with itching.

Rash

The type of lesion is usually the first consideration in making an accurate assessment of the nature of the problem. Table

CASE STUDY

RL is a 55-year-old man with a history of mild hypertension, which is well controlled. He asks the pharmacist to recommend something to stop the itching of a rash.

ASSESSMENT OF THE PATIENT

Subjective Information

55-year-old man complaining of rash with itching

TELL ME MORE ABOUT YOUR RASH. WHERE IS IT? On both of my arms and my face.

DESCRIBE THE ITCHING. It's not real bad, but I feel like scratching all the time. The more I scratch, the worse it feels.

HOW LONG HAS IT BEEN ITCHING? For the past 3 days.

HAVE YOU BEEN WORKING OUTSIDE RECENTLY, SUCH AS IN A GARDEN? No. I just cleaned my garage and put away my lawnmower and tools for the winter.

WHEN WAS THAT? Last weekend, 5 days ago.

HAVE YOU EVER SUFFERED FROM POISON IVY? Yes. I break out if I come in contact with it, but I haven't been near it at all.

WHAT IS YOUR OCCUPATION? I'm an accountant.

DO YOU HAVE ANY HOBBIES THAT INVOLVE WORKING WITH CHEMICALS? Not really.

HAVE YOU USED ANY NEW SOAP OR COLOGNE RECENTLY? No.

HAVE YOU TREATED THE RASH OR ITCHING WITH ANYTHING? Not yet, but I can't stand it anymore. I have to drink a glass of wine just to get to sleep at night.

DO YOU HAVE ANY OTHER SYMPTOMS? No.

WHAT PRESCRIPTION MEDICATIONS DO YOU TAKE? Hydrochlorothiazide and Xanax.

HAVE YOU BEEN TAKING ANY NONPRESCRIPTION MEDICATIONS? Yes, Tums for heartburn. Sometimes I get headaches, and I take a couple of aspirin. I just didn't take anything for the itch, because I can't afford to be sleepy at work.

ARE YOU ALLERGIC TO ANY PRESCRIPTION OR NONPRESCRIPTION MEDICATION? No.

Objective Information

Computerized medication profile:

- Hydrochlorothiazide: 25 mg, one tablet daily with breakfast; No. 60; Refills: 5; Patient obtains refills every 60 days.
- Alprazolam (generic Xanax): 0.5 mg, one-half or one tablet three times a day as needed for anxiety; No. 20; Refills: 2; Patient obtains refills every 15 to 20 days.

Physical Exam

Face: erythematous papules on both cheeks and the forehead with mild edema

Continued

CASE STUDY—continued

Arms and hands: erythematous papules and vesicles with erosions, crusts, and scaling from below the elbow extending to the back of the hands on both arms; no linear streaking; lesions appear in clusters on each arm and hand

DISCUSSION

RL presents with all the signs of acute allergic contact dermatitis. His only complaint is itching; he has no additional symptoms. He claims to have worked indoors without any significant exposure to the sun. His occupation and hobbies do not appear to be involved in this outbreak. His rash is localized to the arms and face and began several days after he worked in the garage. In addition, RL states a history of poison ivy dermatitis.

The most obvious source of inoculation with the poison ivy resin (toxicodendrol) are the tools in the garage. Because no linear streaking is present, RL probably did not rub up against the plant. Rather, the resin remaining on his tools probably came in contact with his hands, which then spread the resin to his arms and face. Sensitive patients must be aware that the resin stays active for many months on tools and equipment. Tools should be cleaned with alcohol or appropriate organic solvent.

Because RL's major problems are itching and oozing vesicles, the pharmacist recommends Burow's solution (aluminum acetate, 1:40). RL should apply cold compresses to the arms three to six times a day for approximately 30 minutes. He should make up a fresh solution each time. Although the cold compresses should reduce the pruritus, use of a benzocaine spray product (up to 20%) may be helpful on his arms. Because RL has no drug allergies, this is a reasonable recommendation even though topical anesthetics can cause sensitization. If an annoying itch remains, chlorpheniramine, 4 mg every 4 to 6 hours orally, may be helpful and will produce less sedation than diphenhydramine. Because there is full involvement of the face, including edema, the pharmacist refers RL to his physician, who supports the pharmacist's recommendations. The physician then prescribes Medrol dose-pack (methylprednisolone). The pharmacist fills the prescription and counsels RL on the proper use of the methylprednisolone and the importance of compliance with the tapering dose.

Figure 8-21 provides a decision tree for rash.

PHARMACEUTICAL CARE PLAN

Patient Name: R.L.

Date: 5/9/02

Medical Problems:

Hypertension
Anxiety

Current Medications:

Hydrochlorothiazide, 25 mg, one tablet QD with breakfast
Alprazolam (generic Xanax), 0.5 mg, one-half or one tablet TID PRN anxiety

S: 55-year-old man complaining of rash and itching on his face and both arms below the elbow. The more he scratches, the worse it feels. Rash began 2 days after he worked in the garage putting away his lawnmower and tools for the winter.
Needs a glass of wine at bedtime to get to sleep. Used no new colognes or soaps recently. Occupation and hobbies are negative for precipitating factors. Denies working in his garden or outdoors at all last week. Has not yet used any medication to treat his problem.
No additional complaints.
Has a history of poison ivy dermatitis.
Takes Tums for heartburn and aspirin for headaches on an infrequent basis.

O: Rash on both arms below the elbow and the face.

Arms: Erythematous papules and vesicles with erosions, crusts, and scaling below the elbows, including the back of the hands. The lesions appear in clusters, with no linear streaking.

Face: Erythematous papules on both cheeks and the forehead with mild edema.

A: Poison ivy dermatitis from contact with toxicodendrol on tools.

P:
1. Recommend cold compresses of Burow's solution for weeping lesions.
2. Recommend topical spray containing benzocaine for itch.
3. Recommend chlorpheniramine, 4 mg orally, for itch, if necessary.
4. Counsel RL about proper use of these three medications.
5. Educate RL about transmission of poison ivy dermatitis.
6. Refer RL to physician for facial edema.
7. New prescription for Medrol dose-pack (methylprednisolone).
8. Counsel RL about the importance of taking all the medication, following the prescribed taper schedule.
9. Follow-up phone call in 5 days to monitor RL's condition and compliance.

Pharmacist: *Thomas Forlenza, Pharm.D.*

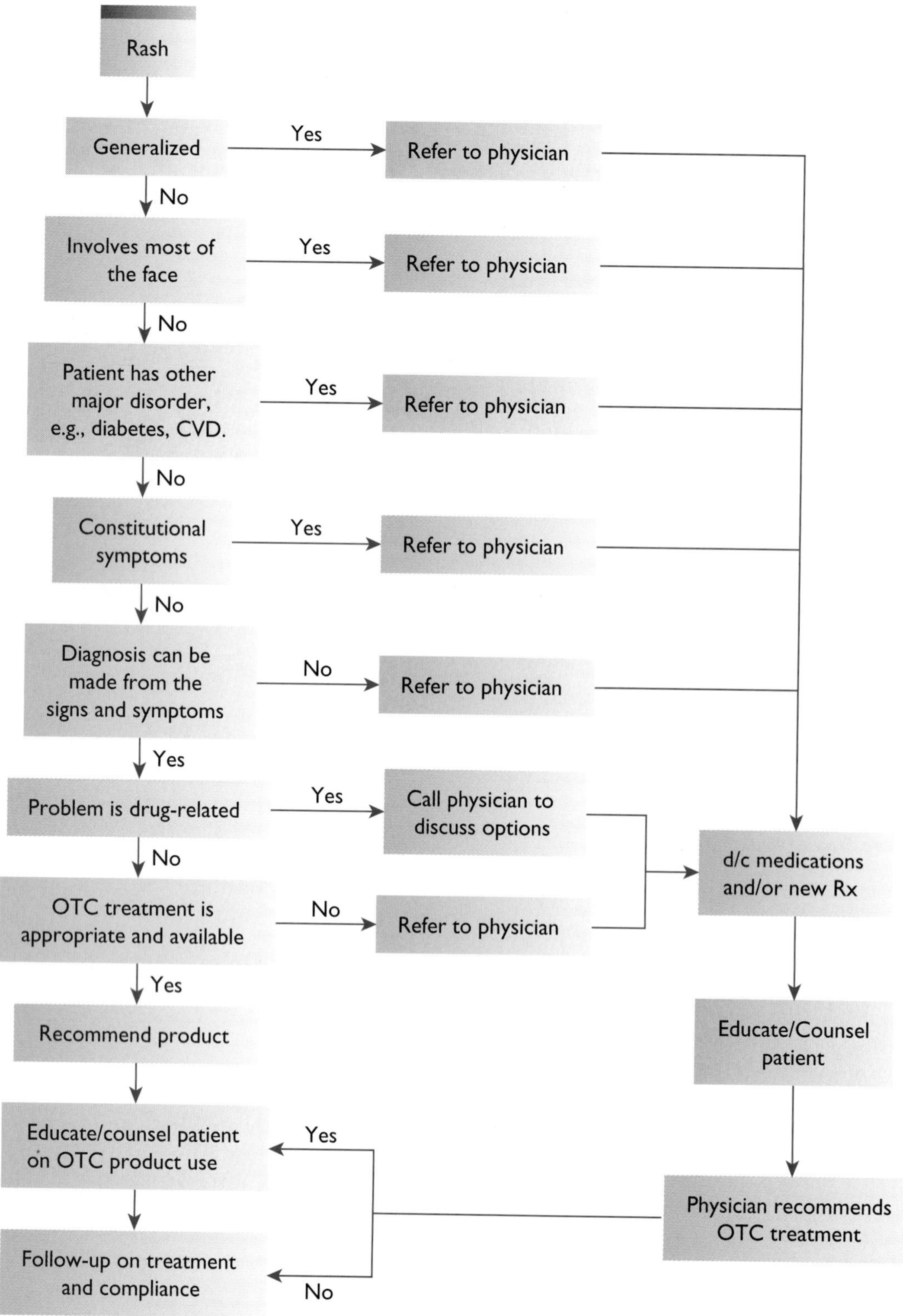

Figure 8-21 ■ Decision tree for rash. *CVD*, cardiovascular disease; *d/c*, discontinue; *OTC*, over the counter; *Rx*, prescription.

8-1 lists the clinical presentation of selected dermatologic disorders.

Self-Assessment Questions

1. What critical aspects of the patient history indicate contact dermatitis rather than some other condition?
2. Aside from direct contact with the plant, how else can poison ivy dermatitis be contracted?

Critical Thinking Questions

1. Would you have referred RL to a physician if the condition appeared on both legs and arms but not on his face?
2. If RL had presented with erythema and vesicles of the entire trunk from the waist up, with a sharp demarcation at the wrists, no involvement of the tops of the hands, no facial involvement, and no constitutional symptoms, what would have been your assessment and plan?

Folliculitis

Folliculitis is an infection of the upper part of a hair follicle and may be either superficial or perifollicular. A furuncle is folliculitis that develops an abscess and becomes nodular. The coalescence of adjacent furuncles is a carbuncle.

CASE STUDY

DD is a 32-year-old man complaining of a painful, red area on his wrist. He asks the pharmacist to recommend something to clear it up.

ASSESSMENT OF THE PATIENT

Subjective Information

32-year old male complaining of a painful, red area on his wrist

TELL ME MORE ABOUT THIS AREA ON YOUR WRIST. Well, it started out as a small pimple on my wrist. It probably broke open while I was working. Then a little pus came out of it.

HOW LONG HAVE YOU HAD IT? It started about 3 days ago.

IS THERE ANY ITCHING? There's no itching in the red area, but it does itch all around it.

DESCRIBE THE INTENSITY OF THE ITCH. The itching just started this morning. It's not too bad yet.

DO YOU HAVE AN INFECTION OR ITCHING ANYWHERE ELSE? No, just on my wrist.

WHAT KIND OF WORK DO YOU DO? I'm an auto mechanic.

HAVE YOU TREATED THE AREA WITH ANYTHING? I washed it out real well the first time, because there was grease all over the area. Then I used this antibiotic ointment we have in our first-aid kit and covered it with a bandage.

HOW OFTEN DID YOU DO THIS? Every morning and evening for the past 3 days.

WHAT'S THE NAME OF THIS OINTMENT? Triple-antibiotic ointment.

HAVE YOU EVER USED THIS PRODUCT BEFORE? About a year ago when I cut my leg.

DO YOU HAVE ANY OTHER SYMPTOMS? It's very painful. It just throbs constantly, and I can't even touch it.

WHAT PRESCRIPTION MEDICATIONS DO YOU TAKE? Flexeril once in awhile for my back, that's all.

HAVE YOU BEEN TAKING ANY NONPRESCRIPTION MEDICATIONS? Sometimes I use Ben-Gay, and I take ibuprofen for minor muscle aches or headaches.

ARE YOU ALLERGIC TO ANY PRESCRIPTION OR NONPRESCRIPTION MEDICATION? Penicillin.

WHAT HAPPENS WHEN YOU TAKE PENICILLIN? I break out in hives real bad.

Objective Information

Computerized medication profile:

- Flexeril (cyclobenzaprine): 10 mg, one tablet three times a day; No. 21; Refills: 3; Patient had prescription refilled once so far last week.

Physical Exam

Wrist: Numerous erythematous papules and pustules in an area approximately 2 cm in diameter; hair follicle in the center of each papule and pustule; one small erosion with a central necrotic plug; a firm, tender nodule is palpable; an area of macules and papules with erythema extending another 1 cm around the primary area of infection; eruption appears to be isolated on the left wrist; no other observable problems

DISCUSSION

DD presents with the signs and symptoms of infectious folliculitis (Box 8-13). He has no constitutional symptoms and complains of pain and itching. His occupation as an auto mechanic may be a significant contributing factor. Occlusive substances like grease can trap microorganisms and facilitate their growth, especially if accompanying cuts or scratches are present. The location of the eruption, on

Continued

CASE STUDY—continued

the top of the wrist, may relate to pressure and moisture associated with the cuffs of a shirt or a watch. This may produce warmth, moisture, and maceration of the skin. The most common cause of infectious folliculitis is *Staphylococcus aureus*. The presence of a single, tender nodule with central necrosis and throbbing pain indicates progression of the folliculitis to a furuncle.

The pruritic macules and papules surrounding the folliculitis indicates the possibility of an allergic contact dermatitis on top of the primary problem. Triple-antibiotic ointment contains neomycin, a known sensitizer. DD states that he used the product about a year ago. Previous sensitization is necessary for such an allergic reaction. His previous use is consistent with the required elements for this problem.

The pharmacist recommends that DD discontinue using the triple-antibiotic ointment. If the itching is bothersome, a cold water compress can be used as needed. The pharmacist contacts DD's physician and recommends mupirocin ointment and erythromycin orally, because DD is allergic to penicillin. The physician prescribes Bactroban (mupirocin) ointment to be applied twice a day to the affected area. He also prescribes erythromycin stearate, 500 mg four times a day for 10 days. The pharmacist fills the prescriptions and counsels DD on the proper use of both medications.

Figure 8-22 shows the decision tree for hair.

PHARMACEUTICAL CARE PLAN

Patient Name: DD

Date: 1/20/02

Medical Problems:

Chronic lower back muscle spasms and pain

Current Medications:

Flexeril (cyclobenzaprine), 10 mg, one tablet three times a day

S: 32-year-old man complaining of infection on his left wrist. Complains of throbbing pain and sharp pain when the eroded area is palpated. Began as a small pimple and developed into a pustule that ruptured during work. Works as an auto mechanic and washed grease out of the infected area.

Applied triple-antibiotic ointment to the infected area and bandaged it twice a day for the past 3 days. Used this product once before about a year ago on a cut.

Has a history of penicillin allergy manifested by hives.

Sometimes uses Ben-Gay and ibuprofen for minor muscle aches and for occasional headaches.

O: Numerous papules and pustules, each with a central hair follicle in an area approximately 2 cm in diameter localized to the top of the left wrist. One small erosion with a central necrotic plug and a firm, tender nodule. Also a small ring of erythematous macules and papules surrounding the folliculitis and extending outward approximately 1 cm beyond the rim.

A: Folliculitis with furunculosis and allergic contact dermatitis caused by neomycin.

P:
1. Recommend discontinuation of triple-antibiotic ointment.
2. Recommend cold compresses for itch.
3. Call physician to discuss the patient's condition, and recommend Bactroban ointment and erythromycin orally.
4. New prescription: Bactroban ointment, apply to affected area three times a day.
5. New prescription: Erythromycin stearate, 500 mg one tablet three times a day for 10 days.
6. Counsel DD about proper use of Bactroban.
7. Counsel DD about how to take erythromycin and the importance of continuing it for 10 days.

Pharmacist: *Lauren Barone, Pharm.D.*

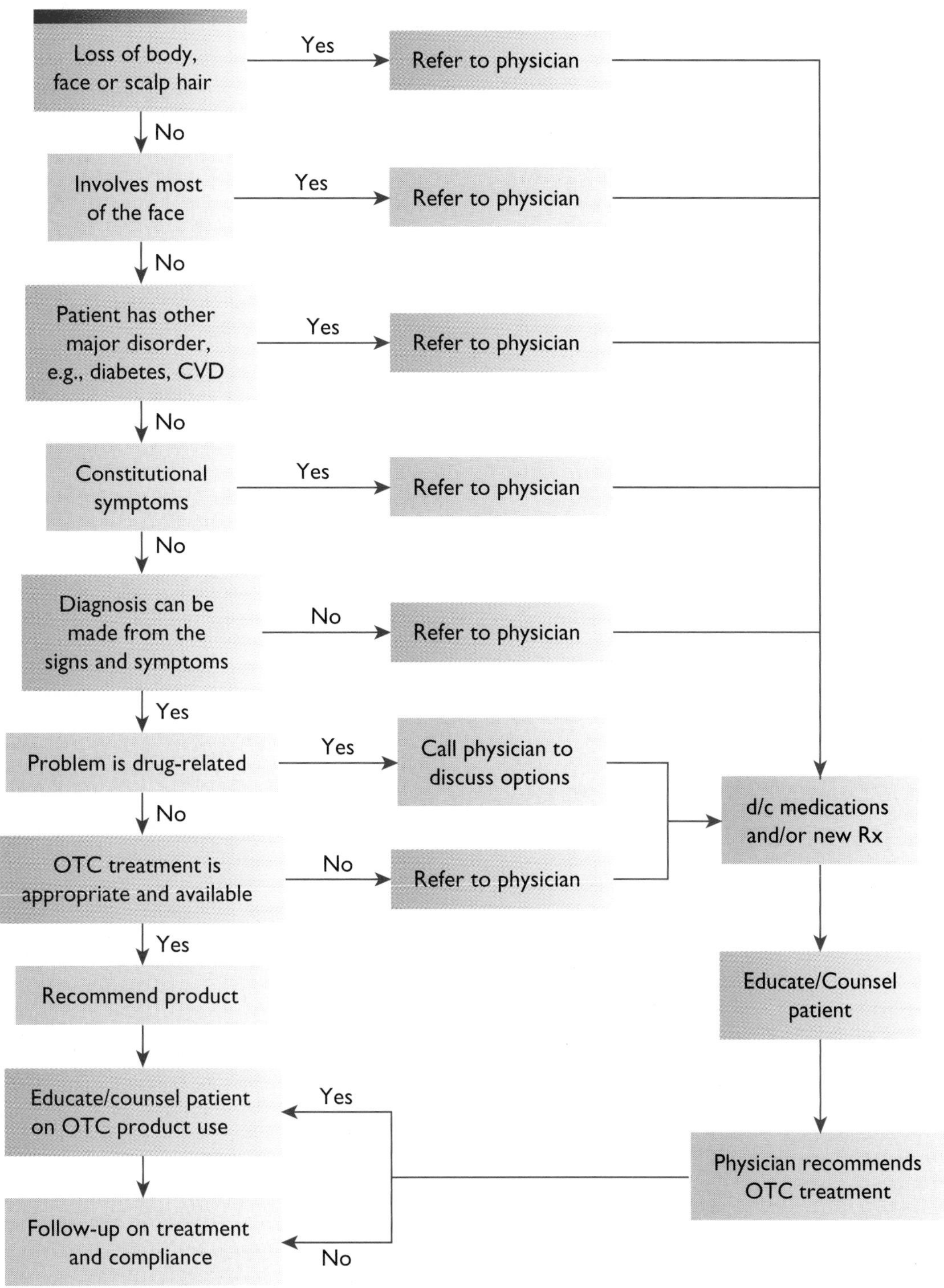

FIGURE 8-22 ■ Decision tree for loss of hair. *CVD,* cardiovascular disease; *d/c,* discontinue; *OTC,* over the counter; *Rx,* prescription.

Self-Assessment Questions

1. Which signs and symptoms indicate furunculosis rather than just folliculitis?
2. Which other information from the patient history suggests a second problem?
3. Which information supports the diagnosis of an allergic condition?

Critical Thinking Questions

1. In the case of DD, would you have referred him to a physician if he only had the folliculitis without the furuncle?
2. If DD had presented with multiple follicular pustules appearing all around the trunk 5 days after sitting in a hot tub, what would have been your assessment and plan?

Nail Infection

Infections can occur in any part of the nail area, especially the lateral skin folds, proximal nail fold, the nail plate, and the nail bed. These infections are most often caused by dermatophytes, *Candida albicans,* and a variety of bacteria, including *Staphylococcus aureus* and *Pseudomonas aeruginosa.*

CASE STUDY

FN is a 23-year-old woman who complains of an infection in the nails of two fingers and asks the pharmacist to recommend something to treat it.

ASSESSMENT OF THE PATIENT

Subjective Information

23-year-old woman female complaining of infected fingernails

WHERE IS THE PROBLEM? On the index finger and middle finger of my right hand.

DESCRIBE THE PROBLEM YOU ARE HAVING. There is a slight throbbing at the tips of these two fingers, and it hurts a lot when I touch or bump the area.

HOW LONG HAVE YOU HAD THIS PROBLEM? I just noticed it yesterday.

HAVE YOU EVER HAD THIS PROBLEM BEFORE? No.

HAVE YOU USED ANYTHING TO TREAT IT? I've just been taking Tylenol for the pain.

HAS IT HELPED? Not really.

WHAT IS YOUR OCCUPATION? I'm a graduate student, but I work part-time as a dishwasher at a local restaurant.

DO YOU HAVE ANY HOBBIES? Between school and work, I don't have any time for hobbies.

DO YOU HAVE ANY OTHER SYMPTOMS? No.

WHAT PRESCRIPTION MEDICATIONS DO YOU TAKE? I don't take anything.

HAVE YOU BEEN TAKING ANY NONPRESCRIPTION MEDICATION? I only take multiple vitamins with iron.

ARE YOU ALLERGIC TO ANY PRESCRIPTION OR NONPRESCRIPTION MEDICATION? Not really, although I've had vaginal infections after taking antibiotics.

Objective Information

Erythema and swelling of the lateral and proximal nail folds
Retraction of the cuticle toward the proximal nail fold
Gentle pressure on the nail causes purulent material to be expressed from the nail folds
Brownish-green discoloration on the lateral margins of the nail

DISCUSSION

FN presents with the signs and symptoms of candida paronychia, which is an inflammation of the nail fold with separation of the skin from the proximal portion of the nail caused by *Candida albicans.* Paronychia can also be caused by a variety of bacteria. She has a purulent exudate with edema and erythema, which indicate an infection. Her medical and drug histories are unremarkable. Her job as a dishwasher, however, supports the diagnosis of *candida paronychia,* because individuals whose hands are often wet or frequently immersed in water are at risk for this condition. The discoloration of the nail also supports this diagnosis. A fungal culture can be done to confirm the presence of *Candida* sp.. A bacterial culture may also be done to be sure that a superinfection, usually *Staphylococcus aureus,* does not exist.

The first thing needed is to eliminate the wet environment. FN may need to change jobs; otherwise, this could develop into a chronic problem that is resistant to treatment. Topical treatment includes the use of either clotrimazole or miconazole solutions or creams. Nystatin cream can also be used but is not as popular as the imidazoles. If the condition does not respond to topical therapy, oral fluconazole or itraconazole is effective.

The pharmacist recommends miconazole cream applied twice a day. The pharmacist also counsels FN on keeping the fingers dry and on proper use of the miconazole cream. If

Continued

CASE STUDY—continued

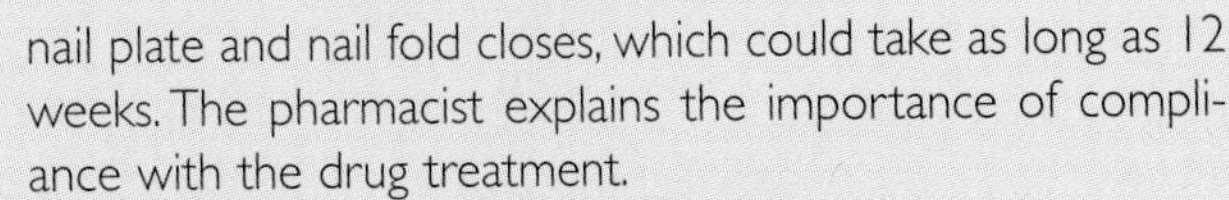

the condition shows no sign of improvement in 2 weeks, the pharmacist will refer the patient to a physician. In this case, the pharmacist would recommend itraconazole, 200 mg daily. Treatment should continue until the space between the nail plate and nail fold closes, which could take as long as 12 weeks. The pharmacist explains the importance of compliance with the drug treatment.

Figure 8-23 shows the decision tree for nails.

PHARMACEUTICAL CARE PLAN

Patient Name: FN

Date: 11/8/02

Medical Problems:
None

Current Medications:
None

S: 23-year-old woman complaining of infection of nails on two fingers. Complains of throbbing in the fingertips with increasing pain when they are touched or bumped. Pain began 1 day ago. Has taken Tylenol for the pain but found it not to be very effective.

Works part-time as a dishwasher. Denies ever having this problem before. Takes a multiple vitamin with iron. Says that she has had vaginal infections in the past from taking antibiotics.

O: Erythema and swelling of the lateral and proximal nail folds. Retraction of the cuticle toward the proximal nail fold. Gentle pressure on the nail causes purulent material to be expressed from the nail folds. Some brownish-green discoloration on the lateral margins of the nail.

A: Candida paronychia.

P:
1. Recommend keeping the fingers dry.
2. Recommend applying miconazole cream to the nail folds twice a day for at least 2 weeks.
3. Counsel FN about the proper use of the cream.
4. If no improvement after 2 weeks, refer patient to physician.
5. Recommend itraconazole, 200 mg daily, to be taken until the space between the nail plate and nail fold closes.
6. Explain the importance of compliance with the drug treatments.

Pharmacist: *Michelle Donato, Pharm.D.*

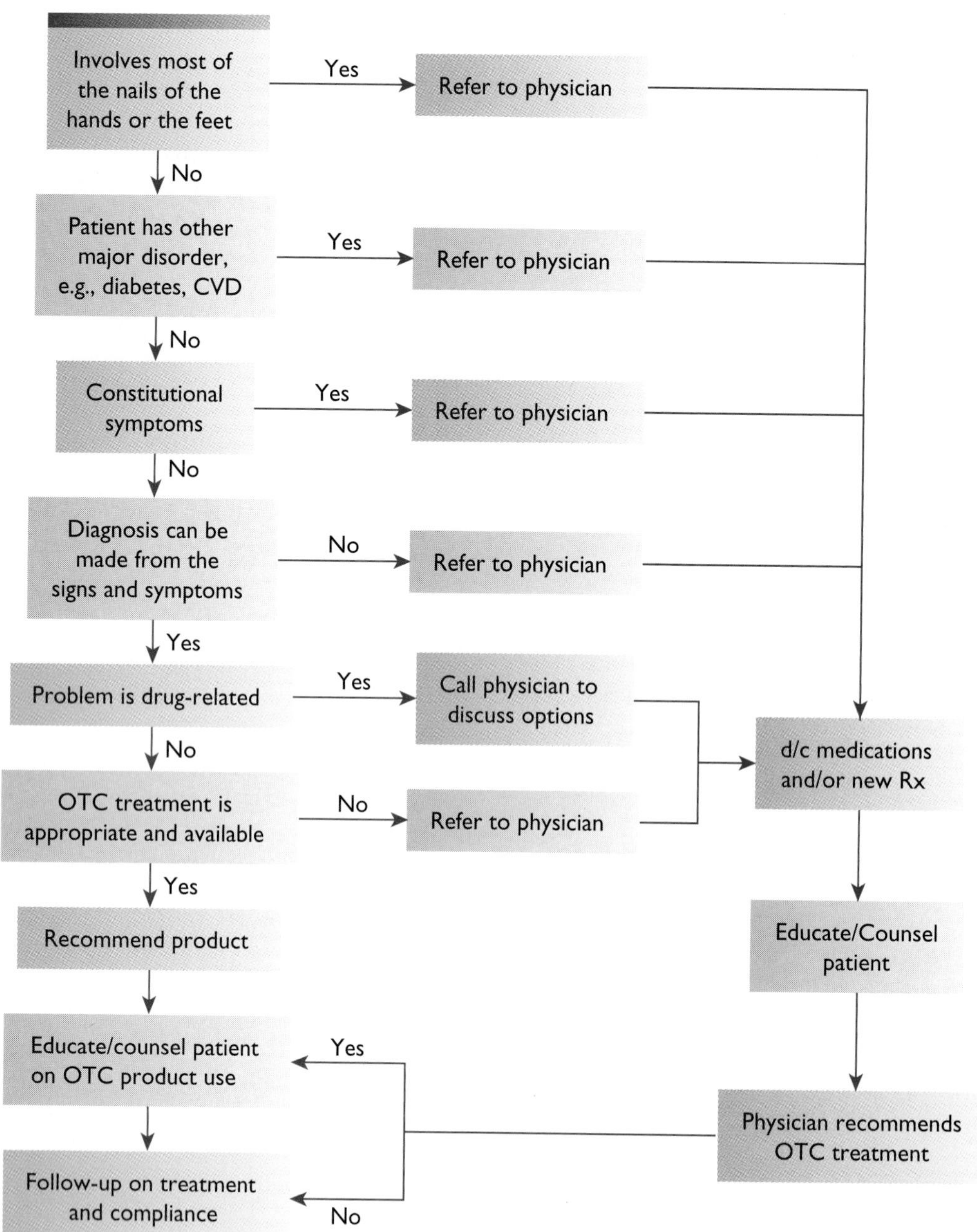

Figure 8-23 ■ Decision tree for nails. *CVD*, cardiovascular disease; *d/c*, discontinue; *OTC*, over the counter; *Rx*, prescription.

Self-Assessment Question

1. What signs and symptoms indicate that the infection is probably caused by *Candida albicans* rather than by a dermatophyte?

Critical Thinking Question

1. If FN presented with all the same signs and symptoms but with fever as well, what would be your recommendation?

Bibliography

Allen LV, Berardi RR, DeSimone EM, et al. Handbook of nonprescription drugs. 12th ed. Washington, DC: American Pharmaceutical Association, 2000.

Arnold HL, Odom RB, James WD. Andrews' diseases of the skin. 8th ed. Philadelphia: W.B. Saunders, 1990.

Fitzpatrick TB, Johnson RA, Wolff K, et al. Color atlas and synopsis of clinical dermatology. 3rd ed. New York: McGraw-Hill, 1997.

Freedberg IM, Fitzpatrick TB, Eisen AZ, et al. Fitzpatrick's dermatology in general medicine. 5th ed. New York: McGraw-Hill, 1999.

Moschella SL, Hurley HJ. Dermatology. 3rd ed. Philadelphia: WB Saunders, 1992.

Newcomer VD, Young EM. Geriatric dermatology: clinical diagnosis and practical therapy. New York: Igaku-Shoin, 1989.

Rassner G. Atlas of dermatology with differential diagnoses. 2nd ed. Baltimore-Munich: Urban & Schwarzenberg, 1983.

Stedman's medical dictionary. 26th ed. Baltimore: Williams & Wilkins, 1995.

Koda-Kimble MA, Young LY, eds. Applied therapeutics: the clinical use of drugs. Baltimore: Lippincott Williams & Wilkins, 2001.

Chapter 9

Eyes and Ears

Raylene M. Rospond

Glossary Terms

- Arcus senilis
- Cataracts
- Conjunctivitis
- Ectropion
- Entropion
- Exophthalmos
- Glaucoma
- Mydriasis
- Nystagmus
- Otalgia
- Otitis media
- Otitis externa
- Presbyopia
- Presbycusis
- Proptosis
- Pseudoptosis
- Scotoma
- Strabismus
- Styes
- Xanthomas
- Xanthelasma

ANATOMY AND PHYSIOLOGY OVERVIEW

The Eye

The eye is a gelatinous sphere that rests within the bony orbit of the skull along with the extrinsic eye muscles, lacrimal gland, cranial nerves and blood vessels, and a layer of protective orbital fat. The wall of the eye is comprised of three layers or tunics: (1) the fibrous tunic, (2) the vascular tunic, and (3) the neural tunic. The two chambers in the center of the eyeball are the posterior chamber (also called the vitreous chamber) and the anterior chamber (Fig. 9-1).

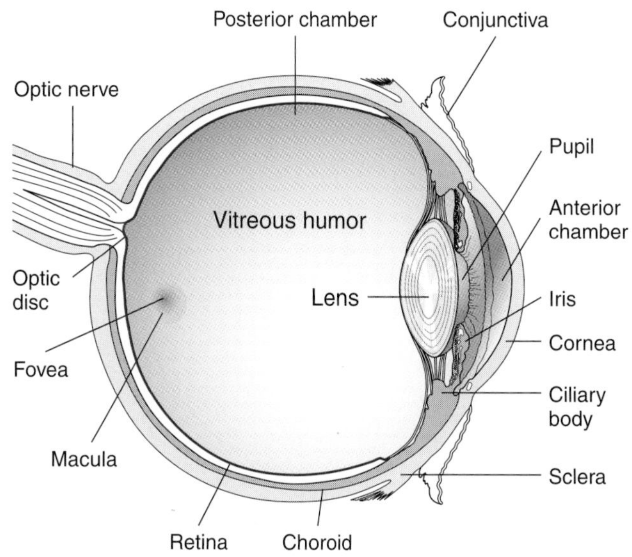

FIGURE 9-1 ■ Layers of the eye.

Layers of the Eye

The fibrous tunic is the outermost wall of the eye, and it consists of the sclera and the cornea. This tunic provides the eye with mechanical support and physical protection, an attachment site for extrinsic eye muscles, and assistance with focusing. The sclera (i.e., "the white of the eye") is contiguous with the cornea, which is clear. The cornea covers the iris and the pupil, and it plays a role in refracting incoming light onto the inner retina. Although the sclera contains blood vessels, the cornea is avascular. The cornea is also the most sensitive portion of the eye and is very sensitive to touch.

The vascular tunic, or uvea, is the middle layer of the eye. It contains blood vessels, lymphatics, and the intrinsic eye muscles, and it includes the iris, ciliary body, and choroid. The iris can be seen through the cornea as a colored ring. It contains blood vessels, pigment cells, and two layers of smooth muscle fibers. These muscles dilate or contract to change the size of the pupil (i.e., the center opening) to regulate the amount of light entering the eye. The pigment cells of the iris determine the eye color. When no pigment cells are present, the eye appears blue. The ciliary body is involved in holding the lens posterior to the iris and centered on the pupil so that any light passing through the pupil will pass through the lens, which then focuses the visual image on the retinal photoreceptors. The choroid is made of capillaries that deliver oxygen and nutrients to the outer portion of the retina.

The neural tunic, or retina, has both an outer pigmented layer and an inner neural retina. The pigmented layer absorbs light after it passes through the retina. The neural retina contains photoreceptors that respond to light, provides preliminary neural processing and integration of visual information, and supplies blood to the tissues lining the posterior cavity. The neural retina contains photoreceptors known as rods and cones. Rods provide black-and-white vision in dim light, whereas cones are involved in providing color vision in bright light.

Chambers of the Eye

The chambers of the eye are the posterior, or vitreous, chamber and the anterior chamber. The posterior chamber contains the gelatinous vitreous body, whereas both the anterior and posterior chambers are filled with aqueous humor. The aqueous humor is similar to cerebrospinal fluid, and it forms a fluid cushion for the eye as well as a route for nutrient and waste transport. The vitreous body, or vitreous humor, helps to maintain the shape of the eye and supports the retina.

The posterior part of the eye, as seen through an ophthalmoscope, is called the fundus. Structures here include the retina, choroid, fovea, macula, optic disc, and retinal vessels (Fig. 9-2). The optic nerve and its retinal vessels enter the eyeball posteriorly at the optic disc. Lateral and slightly inferior to the disc is a darker, pigmented area called the fovea, which surrounds the point of central vision (the area of sharpest vision). The macula is a circular area that surrounds the fovea but has no discernible margins. The macula receives and transduces light from the center of the visual field.

Accessory Structures of the Eye

The accessory structures of the eye include the eyelids, the superficial epithelium of the eye, and the structures associated with the production, secretion, and removal of tears (Fig. 9-3). The eyelids keep the eye surface lubricated and protected from foreign objects. The eyelashes provide additional protection from foreign matter and insects.

Several glands line the margin of the eyelid. The glands of Zeis are large, sebaceous glands associated with the eyelashes. Along the inner margin of the lid are the meibomian glands, which secrete a lipid-rich product that keeps the eyelashes from sticking together.

The epithelium covering the inner surface of the eyelids and the outer surface of the eye is called the conjunctiva. The palpebral conjunctiva covers the inner surface of the eyelids, and the ocular, or bulbar, conjunctiva covers the anterior surface of the eye. The conjunctiva is kept moist by a continuous supply of tears, which wash over the eyeball.

The lacrimal apparatus produces, distributes, and removes tears. Tears reduce friction, remove debris, prevent bacterial infection, and provide nutrients and oxygen to portions of the conjunctiva. Tears that accumulate in the medial canthus of the eye drain down through the lacrimal duct into the nasal cavity.

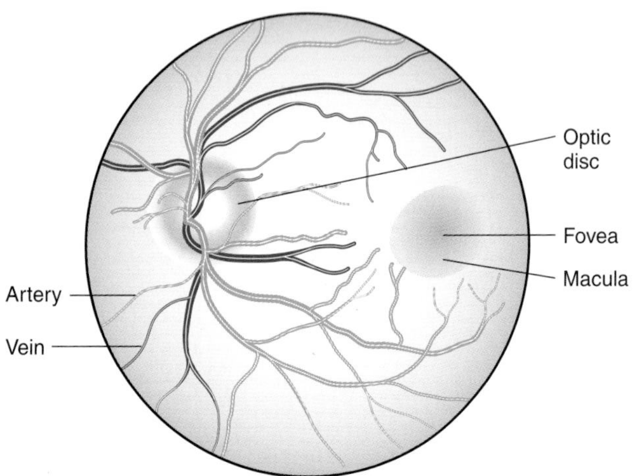

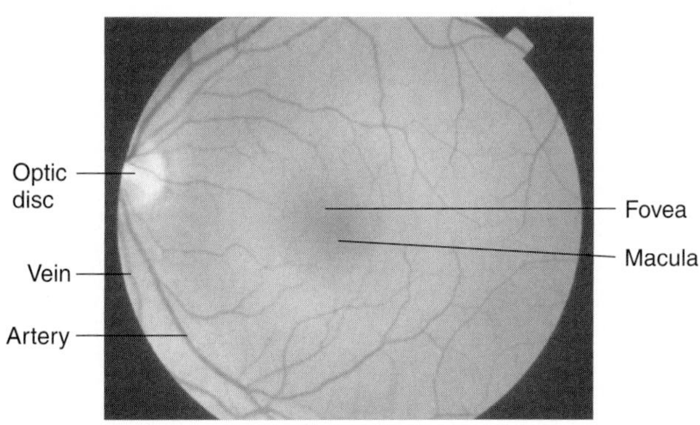

FIGURE 9-2 ■ Fundus of the eye. **(A)** Drawing of the fundus as seen through an opthalmoscope. **(B)** Photograph of the retina. (See Color Plate 22: Photograph from the National Eye Institute, National Institutes of Health.)

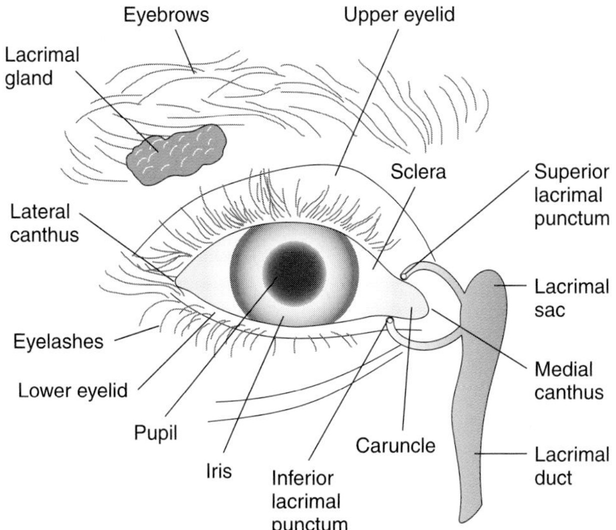

FIGURE 9-3 ■ Accessory structures of the eye.

Visual Fields and Pathways

A visual field is the entire area that is seen when an eye looks at a central point. This area of vision is normally limited by the brows above, by the cheeks below, and by the nose medially. Overlap of the visual fields with simultaneous use of both eyes produces normal binocular vision.

For an image to be seen, light rays reflected from an object must pass through the pupil and be focused on the retina. The image projected onto the retina is upside down, however, and is reversed from its actual appearance. An object viewed in the upper nasal visual field reflects its image onto the lower temporal area of the retina (Fig. 9-4). The retina then transforms the light stimulus into nerve impulses, which are conducted through the optic nerve and the optic tract to the visual cortex of the occipital lobe. Before entering the optic tract, fibers that originated in the nasal portion of the retina cross over to travel in the opposite optic tract. At this point, the left optic tract carries fibers from the left half of each retina, whereas the right optic tract contains fibers only from the right halves (Fig. 9-5).

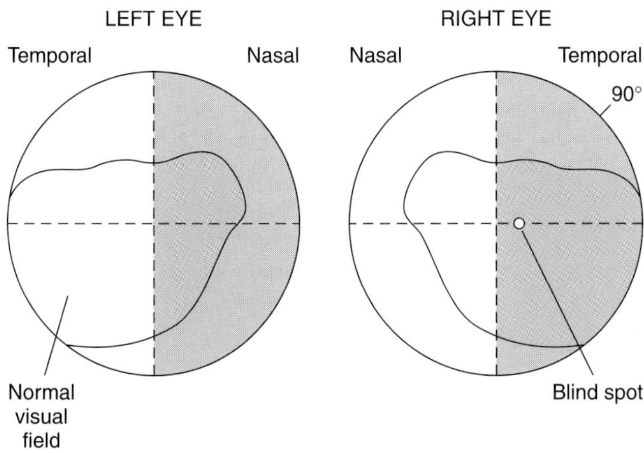

FIGURE 9-4 ■ Visual fields.

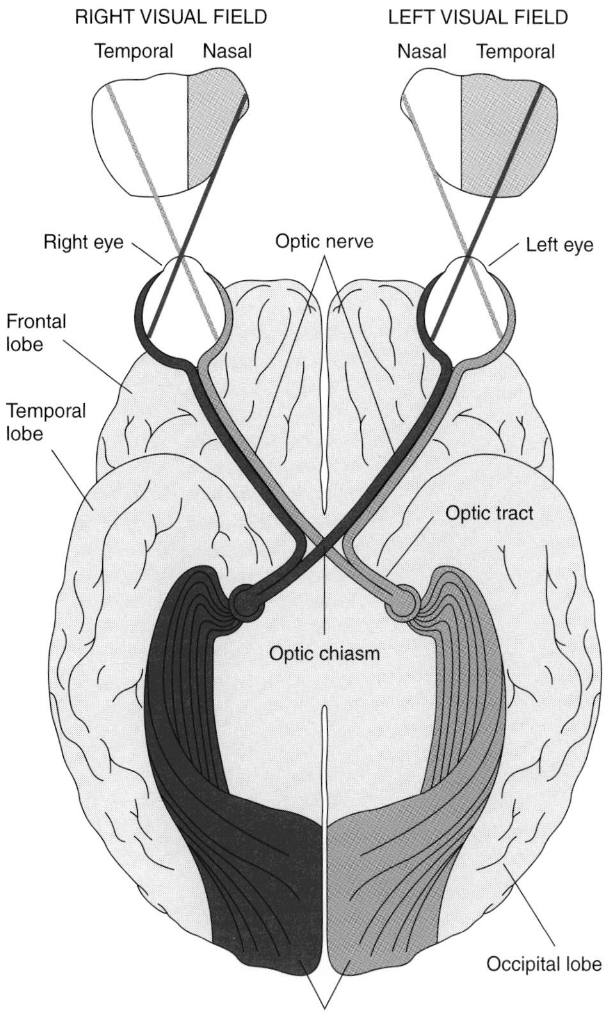

FIGURE 9-5 ■ Visual pathways.

Visual Reflexes

One of the best-known visual reflexes is the pupillary light reflex, which consists of a change in the pupil size in response to light. Two light reflexes occur simultaneously when one eye is exposed to bright light: a direct light reflex (constriction of the pupil of that eye), and a consensual light reflex (constriction of the pupil of the opposite eye). This happens because the optic nerve carries the sensory afferent message (the light) through the optic nerve, which then synapses with both sides of the brain. A motor efferent message (pupillary constriction) is then sent back to the iris of each eye via the oculomotor nerve (Fig. 9-6).

Accommodation is an adaptation of the eye for near vision by increasing the curvature of the lens through movement of the ciliary muscles. Accommodation can be indirectly observed through two separate reflexes: the near reaction, and convergence (Fig. 9-7). The near reaction, or pupillary constriction, occurs when a person shifts gaze from a far object to a near one. Convergence of the eyes (motion toward) occurs as a person continues to focus on an object that is moving toward the center of the eyes from a distance. In lay terms, convergence may be referred to as "crossing your eyes."

Extraocular Movements

Six muscles control and coordinate the movement of each eye. The function of each muscle and of the nerve that innervates it can be tested by asking the patient to move the eye in the direction controlled by that muscle. Because each muscle is coordinated with one in the other eye, the axes of the two eyes remain parallel. Parallel movement of both eyes is called conjugate movement. Movement of the extraocular muscles is stimulated by cranial nerves III, IV, and VI (Fig. 9-8).

The Ear

The ear is comprised of three specific anatomic regions: (1) the external ear, (2) the middle ear, and (3) the inner ear (Fig. 9-9). The external ear is the visible portion of the ear, and it collects and directs sound waves to the eardrum. The middle ear is a chamber located within the temporal bone. Structures within the middle ear amplify sound waves and transmit them to the appropriate portion of the inner ear. The inner ear contains the sensory organs for equilibrium and hearing.

External Ear

The external ear is composed of the auricle, the external auditory canal, and the tympanic membrane. The auricle is the cartilaginous area of the ear that extends from the side of the head (Fig. 9-10). It protects the ear, and it blocks or facilitates passage of sound into the external auditory canal. The earlobe, or the lower end of the auricle, is also called the tragus. The external auditory canal is the passageway that ends at the tympanic membrane (i.e., the eardrum). To protect the tympanic membrane, the canal is lined with numerous small hairs that

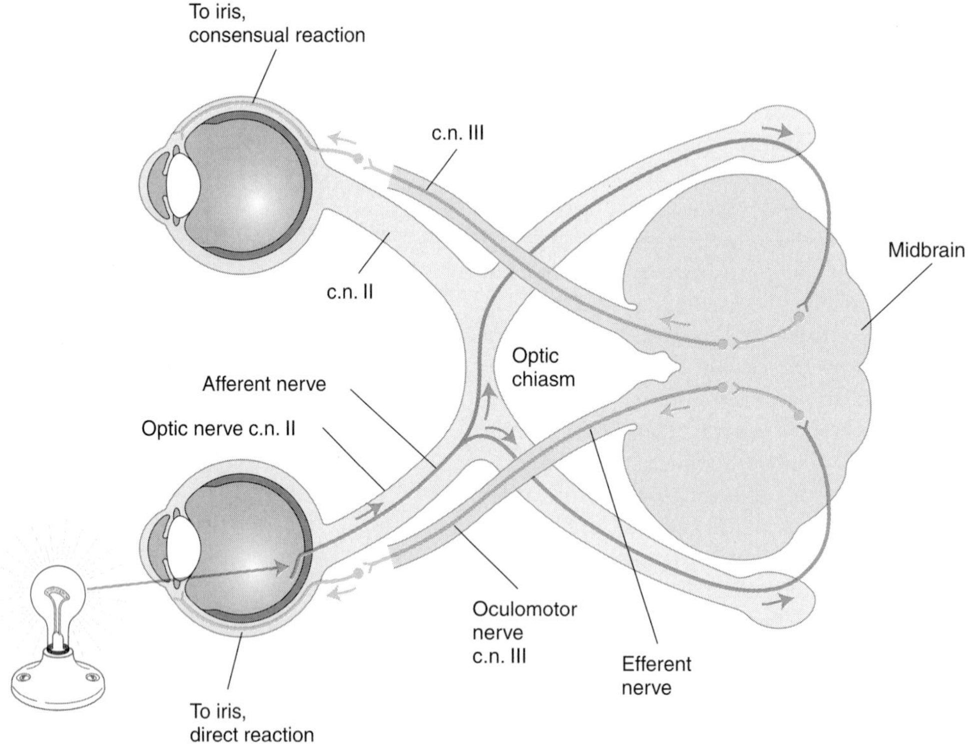

FIGURE 9-6 ■ Visual light reflexes.

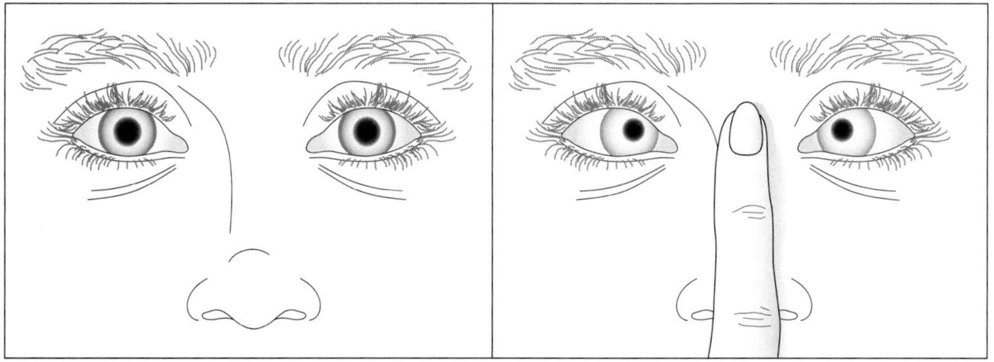

FIGURE 9-7 ■ Accommodation.

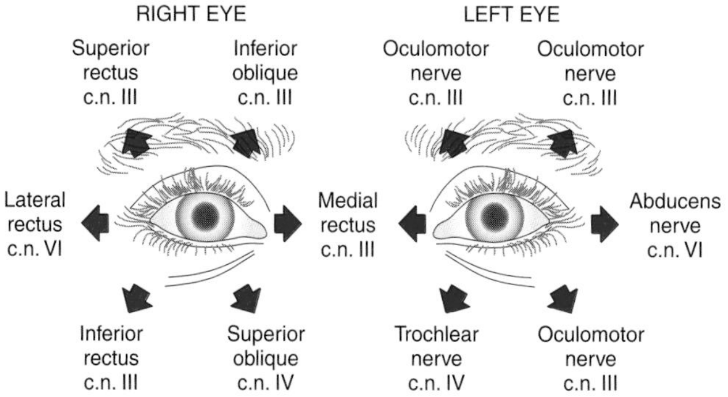

RIGHT EYE
Superior rectus c.n. III
Inferior oblique c.n. III
Lateral rectus c.n. VI
Medial rectus c.n. III
Inferior rectus c.n. III
Superior oblique c.n. IV
LEFT EYE
Oculomotor nerve c.n. III
Oculomotor nerve c.n. III
Abducens nerve c.n. VI
Trochlear nerve c.n. IV
Oculomotor nerve c.n. III

FIGURE 9-8 ■ Extraocular movements. Right eye shows the muscles responsible for movement; left eye shows the cranial nerves responsible for movement.

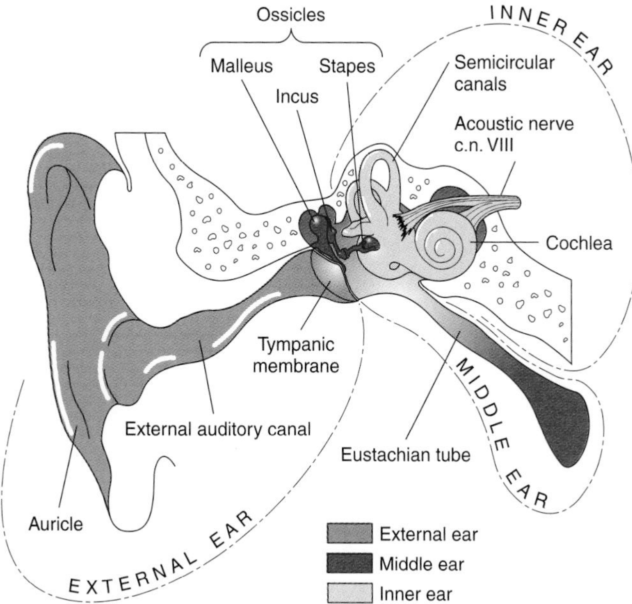

FIGURE 9-9 ■ Anatomic regions of the ear: external ear, middle ear, and inner ear

protrude into the canal. Ceruminous glands secrete a waxy material called cerum. The hairs and cerum protect the ear by restricting the entry of foreign objects and insects. Cerumen also reduces the chances of infection by slowing the growth of microorganisms. Cerumen usually looks wet, sticky, and honey-colored in white and black persons, but more dry and flaky in Asians and Native Americans. The tympanic membrane, as seen at otoscopic examination, is a thin, pearly gray, slightly concave, and semitransparent sheet that separates the external ear from the middle ear. The small, slack, superior portion of the tympanic membrane is called the pars flaccida. The remainder of the eardrum, which is thicker and more taut, is the pars tensa. The annulus is the outer fibrous rim of the eardrum. A cone of light is visible at the five-o'clock position when examining the right ear; this is merely a reflection of the otoscope's light. In the left ear, the cone of light appears at the seven-o'clock position (Fig. 9-11).

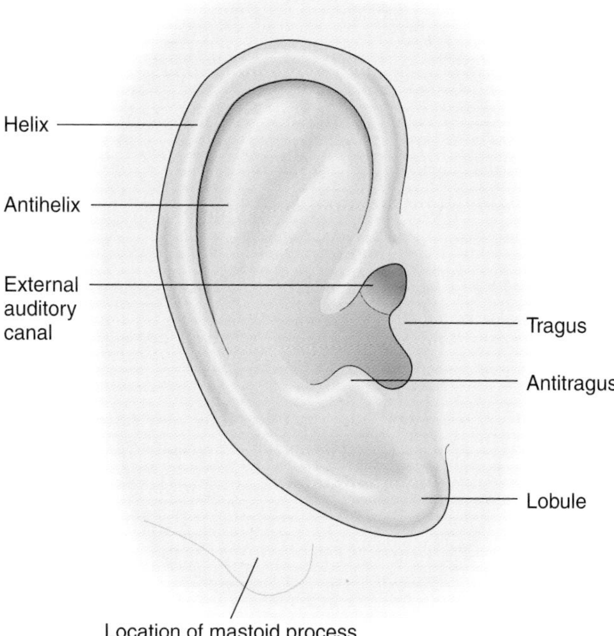

FIGURE 9-10 ■ Auricle of the ear.

Middle Ear

The middle ear is an air-filled cavity that transmits sound via the auditory ossicles. The middle ear is connected to the nasopharynx by the eustachian tube. Approximately 4 cm in length in adults, the eustachian tube equalizes the pressure in the middle ear with the external atmospheric pressure. Unfortunately, the eustachian tube also provides an ideal pathway for microorganisms to travel from the nasopharynx into the middle ear.

The auditory ossicles are three tiny bones in the middle ear through which sound vibration is transferred. The three auditory ossicles are the malleus, the incus, and the stapes. The malleus is attached to the center of the tympanic membrane. Vibrations from the malleus are transmitted through the air to the incus and stapes through a thin membrane to the cochlea of the inner ear. This part of the hearing pathway is known as the conductive phase, and a disorder here causes conductive hearing loss.

At otoscopic examination, the three parts of the malleus as well as the incus may be visible through the tympanic membrane (Fig. 9-11). The malleus is divided into the umbo, the manubrium (handle), and the short process. The incus may be visualized as a whitish haze lateral to the manubrium.

Inner Ear

Vibrations received from the middle ear are coded by the cochlea and then sent to the brain through the cochlear nerve. This second part of the hearing pathway is called the sensorineural phase; a disorder here causes sensorineural hearing loss. Air conduction is the primary path by which the cochlea normally senses vibrations. Bone conduction bypasses the external and middle ear, however, and is used for testing purposes. A vibrating tuning fork, when placed on the patient's head, sets the

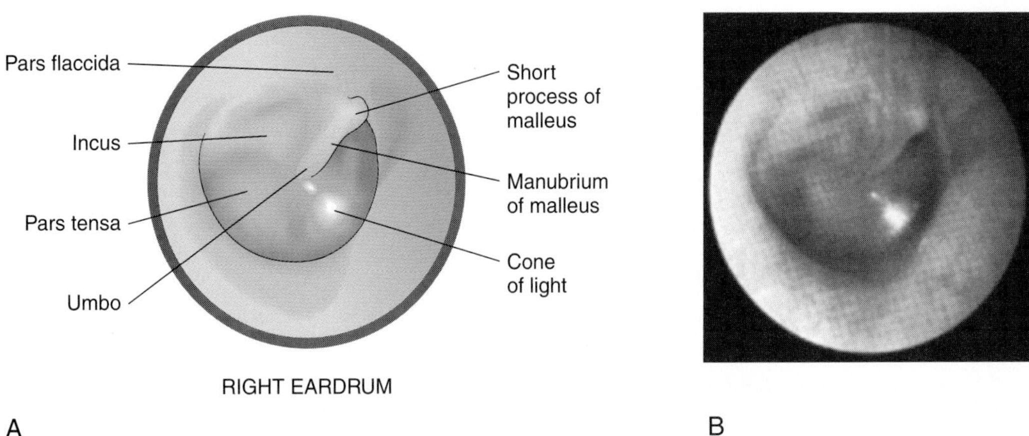

FIGURE 9-11 ■ Otoscopic view of the normal tympanic membrane. **(A)** Drawing. **(B)** Photograph. (See Color Plate 23: Photograph courtesy of Lowell General Hospital, Lowell, MA.)

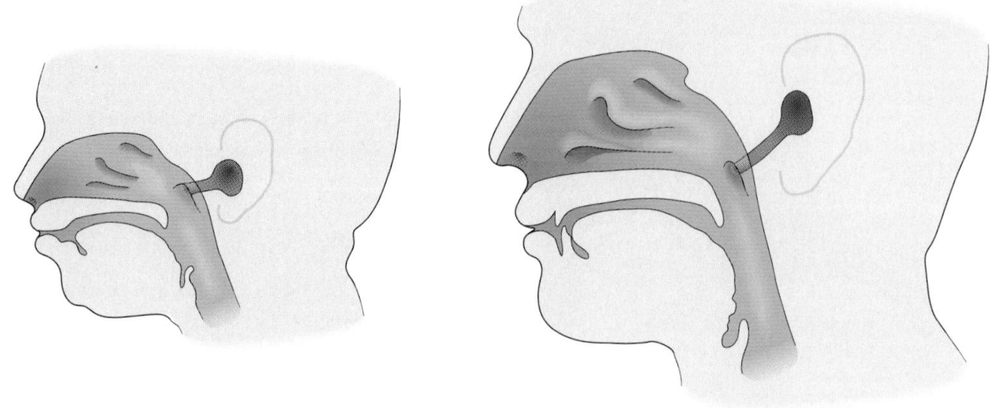

FIGURE 9-12 ■ Eustachian tube of the child and the adult.

bone of the skull into vibration, directly stimulating the cochlea. In normal individuals, air conduction is more sensitive than bone conduction.

In addition to the sense of hearing, the inner ear provides the sense of equilibrium. The vestibule and the semicircular canals provide equilibrium by sensing the position and movement of the head (Fig. 9-9).

Special Considerations

Pediatric Patients

At birth, the pigment of the iris is minimal, and the pupils are small. In addition, eye function is limited, but peripheral vision is fully developed. Eye movements become coordinated by 4 months of age, and central vision matures by 8 months of age. This allows an infant to see a single colored image by 9 months of age. Young children are far-sighted, because the shape of their eyeball is less spherical than in adults. The globe of the eye grows to adult size and shape by 8 years of age, which results in normal adult visual acuity.

The eustachian tube in infants and toddlers is at a 10° angle to the horizontal plane, as compared to a 45° angle in adults (Fig. 9-12). It is also shorter and wider than in adults. These differences account for the higher incidence of acute otitis media in children younger than 6 years.

The external auditory canal is also shorter than in adults and slopes upward. Thus, before otoscopy, the examiner must pull back and down on the tragus to straighten the canal for insertion of the speculum.

Geriatric Patients

As individuals age, physiologic changes occur that affect the eyes and the ears (Table 9-1). The eyes in particular are greatly affected. Loss of subcutaneous fat and muscle tone as well as decreased skin elasticity lead to wrinkling and drooping around the eyes, which often feel dry and as if burning because of involution of the lacrimal glands. Arcus senilis, an infiltration of degenerative lipid material, may become apparent on the cornea. Pupil size decreases, and visual acuity may gradually decline after the age of 50 years, progressing more rapidly after the age of 70. Decreased accommodation in the eye, leading to far-sightedness (i.e., **presbyopia**) may result in blurred vision and difficulty reading. In addition, elderly patients need more light to see because of decreased adaptation to darkness. Eye problems in elderly patients that can lead to morbidity, and disability may be

TABLE 9-1 ➤ PHYSICAL ABNORMALITIES OF THE EYES AND EARS ATTRIBUTABLE TO AGING

ORGAN ASSESSED	PHYSICAL FINDINGS
Eyes	Decreased central and peripheral vision
	Loss of one-third to one-half of outer eyebrow
	Wrinkles around eyes
	Pseudoptosis (upper lid resting on lashes)
	Ectropion (turning outward of the lower lid)
	Entropion (turning inward of the lower lid)
	Dry eyes
	Arcus senilis (gray-white arc or circle around cornea)
	Xanthelasma (soft, raised yellow plaques on lid at inner canthus)
	Small pupils
	Slowed pupillary light reflex
	Opaque lens
	Pale retinal vessels
	Drusen (benign hyaline deposits on retina)
Ears	Pendulous earlobes
	Coarse wiry hairs in external auditory canal
	Tympanic membrane (white, opaque, and thick)
	High-tone frequency hearing loss
	Bony landmarks more prominent

divided into either local degenerative disorders, such as macular degeneration, glaucoma, and cataract, or systemic disorders, such as diabetes, hypertension, and vascular disease.

Hearing loss, especially in the high-frequency range, occurs as the structures of the middle and inner ears degenerate. **Presbycusis** is a type of hearing loss that occurs with aging as the auditory nerve degenerates. With its normal onset among patients during their fifties, this hearing loss begins with difficulty hearing consonants. It slowly progresses until entire words sound garbled. Difficulty localizing sound and background noise add to the resulting communication difficulties experienced by many elderly patients. In addition, the cilia lining the ear canal become coarse and stiff, and the cerumen becomes drier and accumulates at a higher rate.

Pregnant Patients

During pregnancy, hormonal changes can result in a temporary state of far-sightedness. This typically resolves following childbirth.

PATHOLOGY OVERVIEW

The Eye

Patients with ophthalmic conditions commonly present to the pharmacist for consultation. Many symptoms related to the eye are minor and can be managed through general self-care. The potential risk to vision that is inherent with eye complaints, however, requires that a pharmacist understand the most common disorders of the eye as well as the signs and symptoms that require immediate referral to a primary care provider or an emergency room. Conjunctivitis and glaucoma are only two of the many ophthalmic conditions that pharmacists will encounter in their practice, but they are among the most common.

Conjunctivitis

Conjunctivitis refers to any inflammation of the clear mucous membrane of the eye and can be divided in two groups: infectious (bacterial, viral, chlamydial, and gonoccocal), and noninfectious (allergic, dry eye, toxic, contact lens use, neoplasm, foreign body, factitious, and idiopathic). Viral conjunctivitis, most commonly caused by an adenovirus, is probably the most common form and is usually preceded by a recent cold, sore throat, or exposure to someone with the condition. Individuals suffering from viral conjunctivitis often have a "pink eye," with either a watery or, in some cases, an exudative discharge. Viral conjunctivitis is usually self-limiting, with symptoms resolving over 1 to 3 weeks. Treatment is aimed at symptomatic relief using artificial tear preparations and ocular decongestants. Certain forms of viral conjunctivitis are very contagious; therefore, thorough handwashing, not sharing towels, and proper disposal of tissues should be reinforced.

Bacterial conjunctivitis is commonly caused by *Staphylococcus aureus, S. epidermidis, Streptococcus pneumoniae* or *Haemophilus influenzae.* This condition is characterized by a red eye with a purulent discharge (Fig. 9-13). Chlamydial conjunctivitis may have many signs and symptoms in common with both viral and bacterial conjunctivitis and is often misdiagnosed. Infection with *Neisseria* sp. should be ruled out when severe, bilateral, purulent conjunctivitis is present in a sexually active adult or in a neonate 3 to 5 days postpartum. Both chlamydial and gonococcal conjunctivitis require aggressive antibiotic therapy, but conjunctivitis caused by other bacteria is usually self-limiting within 2 weeks.

A noninfectious cause of conjunctivitis is an allergic reaction. Allergic conjunctivitis is characterized by a red eye with a watery discharge. In fact, the hallmark symptom of this condition is copious, clear, watery discharge. Severe forms of allergic conjunctivitis may present with a clear, gel-like form of discharge. Itching is also a common symptom. Allergic conjunctivitis may result from seasonal exposure to allergens such as pollen or from perennial exposure to items such as animal dander. A personal or family history of atopic disease is common in patients suffering from allergic conjunctivitis. Allergic conjunctivitis is generally treated with topical antihistamines, mast-cell stabilizers, or anti-inflammatory agents. Chemical or toxic conjunctivitis can result from an accidental splash of a chemical to the eye.

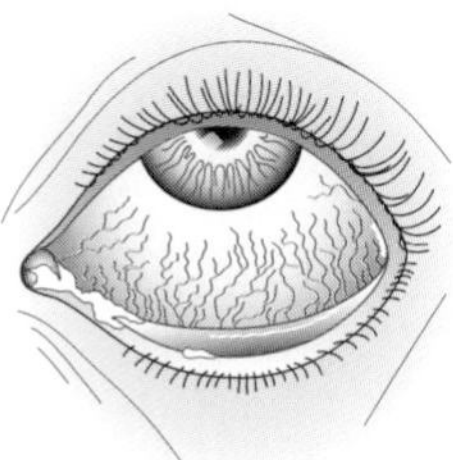

FIGURE 9-13 ■ Bacterial conjunctivitis. Red, inflamed vessels on conjunctiva exudate are common with bacterial infection (seen here at the medical canthus).

For any form of conjunctivitis, the primary presenting symptom is a "red eye." A more extensive list of signs and symptoms can be found in Box 9-1. In patients with chronic signs and symptoms that do not appear to be infectious or allergic in their cause, dry-eye medications or contact lenses should be considered as a cause. Box 9-2 provides a list of common medications that can cause conjunctivitis.

Glaucoma

Glaucoma is actually a group of eye disorders involving optic neuropathy. The disease is characterized by changes in the optic disc and by loss of visual sensitivity and field. The signs and symptoms (listed in Box 9-3) develop and progress in response to several pathologic factors, including increased intraocular pressure (IOP), retinal ischemia, reduced or dysregulated blood flow, and physiologic changes of the extracellular matrix of the optic disc. There are two major types of glaucoma: open angle, and closed angle. Either type may be a primary, inherited disorder; secondary to disease, trauma, or drugs; or congenital.

Primary open-angle glaucoma (POAG) is a bilateral, genetically determined disorder that accounts for 60% to 70% of all glaucoma cases and is usually found in individuals older than 50 years. Treatment is initiated in patients who are at risk for visual field loss with the goal of lowering the IOP to a level associated with decreased risk to the optic nerve (usually 25%–30% reduction). Medications that are used to treat POAG include topical β-blocking agents, parasympathomimetic agents, adrenergic agents (α/β-agonists and α_2-agonists), carbonic anhydrase inhibitors, and prostaglandin analogues.

Overall, POAG accounts for 5% or less of all primary glaucoma cases, but it must be treated as an emergency when it occurs

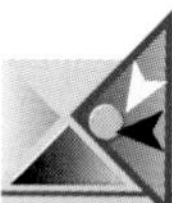

Box 9-1

SIGNS AND SYMPTOMS OF CONJUNCTIVITIS

SIGNS

- Inner aspect of lid more red than white around cornea (usually bilateral)
- Conjunctival swelling
- Eyelid edema
- Normal cornea and pupil
- Periauricular, submandibular lymph adenopathy (viral, chlamydial, toxic, or gonococcal)

SYMPTOMS

- Pink or red eye (viral, bacterial, allergic, chemical, or chlamydial)
- Eye discomfort (viral or sand/grit/foreign-body sensation).
- Blurred vision (should clear with a blink)
- Irritated, burning, or itching eyes (allergic)
- Discharge
  - Serous: viral, allergic, or toxic
  - Mucoid: chlamydial, allergic, or toxic
  - Mucopurlent: chlamydial, bacterial, or toxic
  - Purulent: bacterial or gonococcal
- Crusting on eyelashes (bacterial or viral)
- Eyelids sticking together (bacterial)
- Epiphora (chemical)
- Low-grade fever (viral)

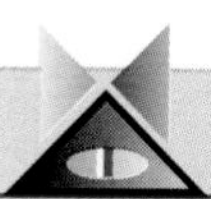

Box 9-2

DRUGS THAT CAN CAUSE CONJUNCTIVITIS

- Neomycin
- Ophthalmic decongestants
  - Naphazoline
  - Tetrahydrozoline
  - Phenylephrine
- Isotretinoin

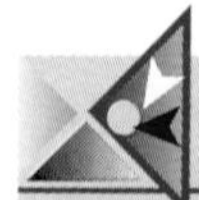

Box 9-3

SIGNS AND SYMPTOMS OF GLAUCOMA

SIGNS

Primary Open-Angle Glaucoma

- Optic disc abnormalities
- Visual field defects
- Increased intraocular pressure (not always present)

Angle-Closure Glaucoma

- Cloudy, edematous cornea
- Closed-angle, narrow anterior chamber
- Hyperemic conjunctiva
- Edematous and hyperemic optic disc
- Increased intraocular pressure

SYMPTOMS

Primary Open-Angle Glaucoma

- Rare until significant damage done
- Loss of peripheral vision
- Blind spots

Angle-Closure Glaucoma

- Blurred or hazy vision
- Halos around lights
- Headache (around the eye)
- Ocular pain or discomfort
- Nausea
- Vomiting
- Diaphoresis
- Abdominal pain

to avoid visual loss. The goal of initial therapy is rapid reduction of the IOP to preserve vision and to avoid surgical or laser iridectomy, which produces a hole in the iris. Acute attacks are treated with a combination of pilocarpine, hyperosmotic agents, and a secretory inhibitor (β-blocker, α_2-agonist, and topical or systemic carbonic anhydrase inhibitors).

Several medications may induce or potentiate glaucoma. The potential for this to occur depends on the type of glaucoma and whether the patient is adequately treated for the condition. Patients with treated, controlled POAG are at minimal risk of increased IOP induced by anticholinergics or vasodilators; however, they are very susceptible to glucocorticoid-induced increases in IOP. In patients with closed-angle glaucoma, any drug that produces **mydriasis** (a long-continued or excessive dilatation of the pupil of the eye) or swelling of the lens may produce angle closure. Topical anticholinergics and sympathomimetics have the highest risk for causing this effect. Drugs associated with potentiation of glaucoma are listed in Box 9-4.

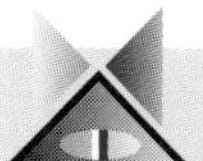

Box 9-4

DRUGS THAT MAY INDUCE OR POTENTIATE GLAUCOMA

OPEN-ANGLE GLAUCOMA

- Ophthalmic corticosteroids (high risk)
- Systemic corticosteroids
- Nasal/inhaled corticosteroids
- Fenoldapam
- Ophthalmic anticholinergics
- Vasodilators (low risk)
- Cimetidine (low risk)

CLOSED-ANGLE GLAUCOMA

- Topical anticholinergics (high risk)
- Topical sympathomimetics (high risk)
- Antihistamines
- Systemic anticholinergics
- Heterocyclic antidepressants
- Phenothiazines
- Ipratropium
- Benzodiazepines
- Theophylline (low risk)
- Vasodilators (low risk)
- Systemic sympathomimetics (low risk)
- Central nervous system stimulants (low risk)
- Tetracyclines (low risk)
- Carbonic anhydrase inhibitors (low risk)
- Monoamine oxidase inhibitors (low risk)
- Topical cholinergics (low risk)

Reprinted with permission from Dipiro JT, Talbert RL, Yee GC, et al., eds. Pharmacotherapy: a pathophysiologic approach. 4th ed. Stamford, CT: Appleton & Lange, 1999:1477.

The Ear

Patients of all ages present to the pharmacist with symptoms related to the ear. Pharmacists familiar with these common pathologic conditions can differentiate between conditions that can be self-treated, such as excessive cerumen, and those that require referral to a physician, such as otitis media and otitis externa.

Otitis Media

Otitis media (OM) is inflammation of the middle ear that is frequently diagnosed in infants and toddlers, primarily because of their short, wide, and minimally sloped eustachian tube. In addition, several risk factors contribute to the higher incidence and increased frequency of OM in children. The frequency appears to parallel the incidence of viral upper respiratory infections; therefore, OM is more frequent during the winter months. Conditions that lead to malformations of the eustachian tube, such as cleft palate, adenoid hypertrophy, and Down's syndrome, can also contribute to the development of acute OM (AOM). A history of recurrent AOM or respiratory tract infections in a sibling doubles a child's risk of developing AOM. Attending day care centers and parental smoking also increases a child's risk of AOM. Finally, the earlier the age of a child's first episode of OM, the greater the risk of developing more severe, persistent, and recurrent episodes.

Different types of OM include AOM, OM with effusion, chronic purulent OM, and OM without effusion. The most common diagnosis is AOM (Fig. 9-14), which involves rapid onset of signs and symptoms of inflammation (Box 9-5). Otitis media with effusion is similar to AOM, except that the patient does not display the signs and symptoms of acute infection but may have nonspecific complaints, such as rhinitis, cough, and diarrhea. The opacity of the tympanic membrane makes the type of effusion (serous, mucous, or purulent) difficult to determine. Chronic purulent OM and OM without effusion are rare.

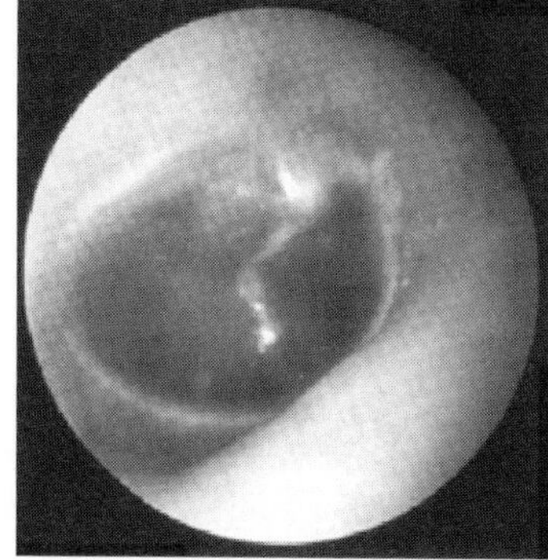

FIGURE 9-14 ■ Acute otitis media. (See Color Plate 24: Photograph courtesy of Lowell General Hospital, Lowell, MA.)

Therapy for AOM includes oral antibiotics, analgesics, antipyretics, and local heat. Antihistamines and decongestants have not been efficacious in resolving effusions or in relieving symptoms. Proper treatment of AOM should provide symptomatic relief within 24 to 72 hours. Patients who present with recurrent signs and symptoms within 1 month of a previous episode are considered to have a resistant infection and should be treated with a different antibiotic. Otitis media with effusion

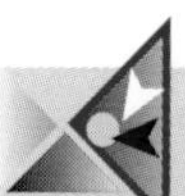

Box 9-5

SIGNS AND SYMPTOMS OF ACUTE OTITIS MEDIA

SIGNS

- Otalgia
- Hearing loss
- Abnormal otoscopic examinatio.
- Redness or opacity of tympanic membrane
- Absence of light reflex
- Bulging and/or immobile tympanic membrane
- Otorrhea

SYMPTOMS

- Fever
- Irritability
- Lethargy
- Anorexia
- Vomiting
- Pain

may be managed with symptomatic therapy; however, it does not require antibiotic therapy. Myringotomy and insertion of tympanostomy tubes may be considered for treatment of persistent middle ear effusions (four episodes in 6 months, or six episodes in 12 months).

Otitis Externa

Otitis externa is an inflammation of the skin lining the external auditory canal (Fig. 9-15). Prolonged exposure of this dark, warm cul-de-sac to moisture results in maceration and fissures in the epithelial lining. In turn, this provides fertile ground for bacterial and fungal growth. Bacterial infection with *Pseudomonas* sp., *Staphylococcus* sp., *Bacillus* sp., or *Proteus* sp. is common and leads to inflammation and epidermal destruction of the tympanic membrane. If uncontrolled, such infection may lead to perforation of the tympanic membrane. Because this area of the body has little subcutaneous tissue, inflammation and swelling result in increased skin tension, which causes pain disproportionate to any visible swelling. As the inflammation progresses, the pain may increase significantly, especially while chewing. Any action that disrupts the skin integrity, such as attempts to clean or scratch the ears with cotton swabs, hairpins, pencils, or other objects, can result in otitis externa.

Types of otitis externa include acute otitis externa (i.e., swimmer's ear), allergic external otitis, dermatitis of the external auditory canal, chronic external otitis, and malignant external otitis. Common signs and symptoms present with external otitis can be found in Box 9-6. Treatment includes antibiotic and hydrocortisone drops applied in the ear canal. Oral antibiotics should be employed if cellulitis and lymphadenopathy are present. Astringents such as Burow's solution (i.e., aluminum acetate

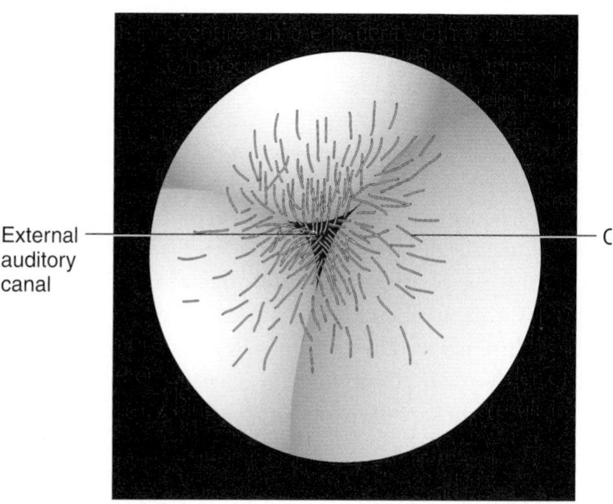

FIGURE 9-15 ■ Otitis externa. This condition involves severe swelling of external auditory canal with erythema, tenderness, and a narrowed canal lumen.

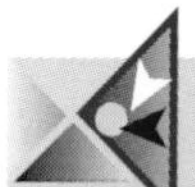

Box 9-6

SIGNS AND SYMPTOMS OF OTITIS EXTERNA

SIGNS

- Increase in ear pain when pulling up on auricle or pressing on tragus
- Lymphadenopathy (chronic)
- Swelling in region of ear and mastoid bone (malignant)
- Swollen inflamed ear canal and tympanic membrane

SYMPTOMS

- Ear pain (more severe in chronic and malignant cases)
- Ear discharge
- Hearing loss
- Itching (swimmer's ear or allergic)
- Burning or stinging (allergic or dermatitis)
- Fever (chronic)

solution) may be used to treat eczematous or weeping skin. Warm water, saline, or Burow's solution soaks may be used to treat crusting and edema of the auricle and surrounding tissue. Burow's solution also may be used to treat fungal otitis externa, because the resulting lower pH retards fungal reproduction and allows the immune system to clear the infection. Cleaning the ear canal with saline or warm water using a soft rubber-bulb syringe can help to clear debris.

SYSTEM ASSESSMENT

Pharmacists rarely assess the eyes and the eyes together. Instead, the patient's primary reason for visiting the pharmacist usually centers on symptoms involving one of these areas, prompting a focused assessment of that area alone.

Subjective Information

When asked questions about the eyes or ears, some patients are reluctant to admit sensory impairments. This reluctance is often due to unspoken fears. For example, some patients may fear that a diagnosis of hearing loss will require them to be fitted for a hearing aid, or that if the extent of their vision loss is discovered, they might lose their right to drive a car. Even impairment in the sense of smell may provoke vague fears of "old age setting in," a brain tumor, or some other serious condition. Thus, great sensitivity and, sometimes, careful investigation are required to determine the true status of a patient's hearing and vision.

The Eye

The first step in triaging the variety of disorders that commonly affect the eye is to conduct a patient interview. By gathering accurate information from the patient or caregiver, the pharmacist can determine whether the patient is suffering from a mild condition such as allergic conjunctivitis or from a more serious, sight-threatening infection. For the benefit of discussion, many interview questions are provided here. The pharmacist should select those that are most appropriate based on the patient's clinical presentation and any answers that he or she provided during the interview.

? INTERVIEW When did the redness in your eye develop? Does it affect one eye or both? What do you think may have caused this redness? Have you recently injured your eye? Have you recently been in an accident or injured your head? What is the nature of your work? Have you been working outside or in an environment that would cause your eyes to water, itch, or burn? Have your eyes been exposed recently to any irritants, such as smog, chemicals, or glare from the sun? Have you recently applied any pesticides or fertilizers?

➤ ABNORMALITIES Ocular redness can result from conjunctivitis, keratitis, uveitis, episcleritis/scleritis, acute glaucoma, eyelid abnormalities, and orbital disorders. These questions are designed to determine whether the potential cause relates to trauma, allergens, chemicals, or some combination thereof.

? INTERVIEW Are you experiencing any difficulty in seeing or blurring of your vision? Did this change come on suddenly or progress slowly? Is this difficulty occurring in one eye or both? Is the difficulty constant, or does it come and go? Do objects appear out of focus? Does it feel like a clouding over of objects is occurring? Does it feel like "grayness" of vision? Do spots move in front of your eyes? If so, one or many? In one or both eyes?

➤ ABNORMALITIES Floaters are common with myopia or after middle age because of condensed vitreous fibers. Usually, they are not significant; however, acute onset of floaters may occur with retinal detachment.

? INTERVIEW Are you seeing any halos/rainbows around objects? Any rings around lights?

➤ ABNORMALITIES Halos around lights occur with acute narrow-angle glaucoma. Digoxin has been reported to cause yellow-green halos around objects when ingested in toxic amounts.

? INTERVIEW Do you have a blind spot? If so, does it move as you shift your gaze? Do you have any loss of peripheral vision?

➤ ABNORMALITIES **Scotoma** is a blind spot in the visual field surrounded by an area of normal or decreased vision. This occurs with glaucoma and with optic nerve and visual pathway disorders.

? INTERVIEW Are you experiencing any night blindness?

➤ ABNORMALITIES Night blindness occurs with optic atrophy, glaucoma, or vitamin A deficiency.

? INTERVIEW Do you have any other eye problems? Any discharge? If so, what color is the discharge? Clear? White? Yellow? Is the discharge stringy? Do you have morning crusting? Difficulty opening eyelids? Does it affect one or both eyes? Itching? Stinging? Blurred vision? Photophobia? Pain? Is the pain sharp or dull? Is it constant or intermittent? How long have these symptoms been present? What were you doing when you noticed them? Have you had a similar problem before?

➤ ABNORMALITIES Symptoms that accompany red eye can help in determining the potential cause. In particular, the type of discharge can help to determine the underlying cause of conjunctival inflammation. Serous or watery discharge is commonly associated with viral or allergic ocular conditions. A mucoid (stringy or ropy) discharge is characteristic of allergy or dry eyes. A mucopurulent discharge (yellow or green) with morning crusting and difficulty opening the eyelids is suggestive of bacterial infection. Itching is a hallmark of allergy. Refer patients with pain, photophobia, and blurred vision that does not clear with a blink to an ophthalmologist to rule out uveitis, keratitis, acute glaucoma, and orbital cellulitis. Unilateral conjunctivitis may indicate keratitis, nasolacrimal duct obstruction, occult foreign body, or neoplasia.

? INTERVIEW Have you recently had a head cold, sinus problem, or influenza? Have you recently been around anyone with "pink eye"?

➤ ABNORMALITIES These questions are directed at determining a viral cause of conjunctivitis.

? INTERVIEW Do you have any allergies? To what are you allergic? What symptoms do you have? Do you wear contact lenses? Are they hard or soft lenses? What contact lens products do you use? Do you use eye cosmetics? Have you changed brands of eye makeup or used a friend's eye makeup? How old are your eye cosmetics? Do you use hair spray, spray deodorants, or perfume?

➤ ABNORMALITIES These questions are directed to identify an allergic or toxic cause of the conjunctivitis. Hypersensitivity to thimerosal and other mercurial compounds can affect contact lens wearers. Eye cosmetics older than 6 months can grow bacteria and produce infection.

? INTERVIEW What medications do you take? Are you currently taking any prescription products? Have you recently used a nonprescription eye product? If so, which one(s) did you use? For what symptoms?

➤ ABNORMALITIES A positive answer can raise questions about a drug-induced cause of the redness. Refer patients with symptoms that have not responded to nonprescription therapy within 72 hours to a physician. Medications may cause conjunctivitis. Ocular decongestants can cause medical problems in patients from systemic hypertension, arteriosclerosis, and hyperthyroidism. Diuretics and antidepressant medications may cause dry eyes.

? INTERVIEW Do you have any chronic disease, such as diabetes, glaucoma, hypertension, or collagen vascular disease? Have you had any conditions in the past that affected your eyes?

➤ ABNORMALITIES Collagen vascular disease may be associated with dry eyes. Chlamydial or gonococcal conjunctivitis may cause red eye.

The Ear

Obviously, when asking questions about the client's ear or hearing, be aware that certain conditions, including the presence of a foreign body, excessive cerumen, refractory OM, and normal changes of aging, can reduce acuity of hearing. Thus, you may be required to speak more slowly than usual or to increase your volume.

? INTERVIEW When did the pain in your ear begin? Is the pain sharp and localized or dull and generalized? Is it constant or made worse by pulling on the ears, chewing, sneezing, or swallowing? How did the pain start? Was it sudden, gradual, or insidious? How long has it lasted?

➤ ABNORMALITY Ear pain may be caused by disorders of the ear or the periotic area. The most probable causes of ear pain are OM, otitis externa, and temporomandibular joint arthralgia (see Chapter 17). Serious disorders that may cause ear pain are cancer of the external ear, tongue, and throat; herpes zoster; and cholesteatoma (a cyst-like sac filled with epithelial cells and cholesterol that can erode and destroy the auditory ossicles). Pain that becomes more severe by pulling upward on the auricle or pushing on the lobe is associated with otitis externa. Both OM and otitis externa may cause pain on chewing, swallowing, or sneezing. The patient's description of the pain, its pattern of onset, and its duration can provide clues regarding the cause (Table 9-2).

? INTERVIEW Is there liquid coming out of your ear? What does it look like? How much comes out? Does it flow all the time? Do your ears feel congested? Do your ears itch?

➤ ABNORMALITY Symptoms of itching, pain, discharge, and deafness are often associated with external ear disorders. Pain, discharge, and deafness are symptoms often associated with middle ear disorders.

? INTERVIEW Are you experiencing any hearing loss? When did it start? Did the loss come on slowly or all at once? Is it on one side or both? Has your hearing decreased overall or just with certain sounds? In what situations do you notice the loss? Do people seem to shout at you? Have you recently traveled by airplane? Any family history of hearing loss? Have you tried anything to help your hearing? How does the loss affect your daily life? Any problems with your job? How do your family and friends react?

TABLE 9-2 ➤ CHARACTERISTICS OF EAR PAIN

Description of Pain	Onset	Duration	Disease/Disorder
Excruciating pressure	Sudden	30 min to several hours	Acute otitis media, chronic otitis media
Fullness	Insidious, sporadic	Hours to days	Serous otitis media
Dull	Gradual	Days	Otitis externa
Pressure	Insidious	Days to weeks	Temporomandibular joint disorder
Fullness, aching	Gradually progressive	Weeks to months	Tumors of pharynx or larynx
Burning	Gradual	Hours	Hematoma, frostbite
Pressure	Insidious	Days to weeks	Chronic mastoiditis (inflammation of the mastoid bone)
Excruciating	Sudden	Hours	Myringitis

ABNORMALITIES Presbycusis has a gradual onset over years, as compared to hearing loss from trauma, which is often sudden. Any sudden hearing loss in one or both ears not associated with an upper respiratory infection warrants a referral. Hearing loss may be apparent when competition from background noise is present, such as at a party, and may cause social isolation. Medications may also cause hearing loss that may be reversible or irreversible. A list of potentially ototoxic medications can be found in Box 9-7.

INTERVIEW Are you dizzy? Do you feel like you are going to fall down? Does the room feel like it is spinning? Do you hear clicking or popping sounds? Do you hear a constant tone or noise? Is it high or low in pitch? Do ordinary sounds seem hollow, as if you're hearing them in a barrel or underwater? How long have these symptoms been present? What were you doing when you noticed them? Have you had a similar problem before? Have you taken any aspirin or other drugs?

ABNORMALITIES Deafness, dizziness, and tinnitus indicate an inner ear problem. Aspirin and other medications may cause tinnitus or hearing loss (Box 9-7). "Barrel" or underwater sounds can result from a cerumen impaction, especially after water exposure or fluid accumulation in the middle ear. Pain and barrel sounds associated with air pressure changes, such as during air travel, suggest barotrauma or barotitis.

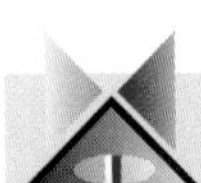

Box 9-7

POTENTIALLY OTOTOXIC DRUGS[a]

- Acetylsalicylic acid
- Amikacin
- Amphotericin B
- Bumetanide
- Capreomycin
- Carboplatin
- Chloroquine
- Cisplatin
- Ethacrynic acid
- Furosemide
- Gentamicin sulfate
- Hydroxychloroquine
- Kanamycin sulfate
- Mechlorethamine
- Neomycin sulfate
- Oral contraceptives
- Oil of wintergreen
- Quinine or synthetic substitutes
- Salicylates
- Streptomycin sulfate
- Tobramycin sulfate
- Vancomycin HCl
- Viomycin

[a]Not all inclusive.

INTERVIEW Do you have, or have you recently had, a cold or the flu? Do you have a fever? Runny nose? Sore throat?

ABNORMALITIES The risk for OM increases with upper respiratory infections. Fever is more prevalent with OM. Discharge from the ear may result from a perforated eardrum. Change in hearing can occur from either OM or otitis externa.

INTERVIEW Have you been swimming during the past few days? Have you attempted to clear your ears recently to remove earwax? What method did you use? Are your ear canals dry and flaky or wet and sticky? Do you use ear plugs or a hearing aid? Under what conditions?

ABNORMALITIES These questions are directed toward identifying whether trauma to the external auditory canal has occurred. Trauma combined with a warm, most environment is likely to result in infection.

INTERVIEW Have you had similar problems in the past? How long ago? What have you already done to treat your earache? Do you wear dentures or have any dental problems? What is your occupation?

ABNORMALITIES If it recurs less than 1 month from previous treatment, OM indicates a resistant infection. Patients with ill-fitting dentures or poor dentition may suffer from ear infections caused by blockage of the eustachian tube where it drains into the oropharynx. Occupations in which the patient is exposed to loud, repeated noise might result in hearing loss.

Objective Information

Objective patient data pertaining to the eye and the ear include inspection and palpation of both as well as otoscopic, ophthalmologic, hearing, and visual acuity examinations.

Physical Assessment

The Eye

Pharmacists are often presented with symptoms related to the eye. In evaluating these symptoms, the ability to inspect the outer eye and conjunctiva is extremely valuable. This allows pharmacists to differentiate problems that can be safely self-treated from those that should be referred to a primary care provider. A pharmacist rarely—if ever—completes a full ophthalmologic examination. In specialized practice environments, however, a pharmacist might complete this examination in monitoring treatment of chronic diseases that may present with eye complications, such as diabetes and hypertension.

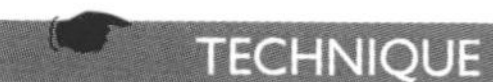

TECHNIQUE

STEP 1

Inspection of the Eyes

- Inspect the eyes, eyelids, and eyebrows for position, shape, symmetry, and movement. The eyes, eyelids, and eyebrows should be symmetrical in shape and position and freely mobile. The eyes should align with the top of the auricle. The skin of the eyelids should be loose, thin, and elastic.
- Inspect for bulging eyes (i.e., **proptosis**).
- Check the upper and lower eyelid margins for integrity, color, texture, and position. Edges of the eyelids should frame the upper and lower margins of the irises when the eyes are open.
- Ask the patient to close his or her eyes. The eyelids should completely cover the eyes.
- Inspect the orientation of the eyelids and eyelashes. Note whether they turn inward or outward.
- Observe the patient blinking.
- Gently pull down on the lower eyelid, and ask the patient to look up (Fig. 9-16).
- Examine the exposed palpebral conjunctiva for clarity, discharge, and inflammation. Conjunctiva should be transparent and free of discharge or hyperemia.
- Inspect the sclera. Normally, the sclera is white and translucent.
- To check the lacrimal apparatus, ask the patient to look down. With your thumb, slide the outer part of the upper eyelid up along the bony orbit, and inspect for any redness or swelling.

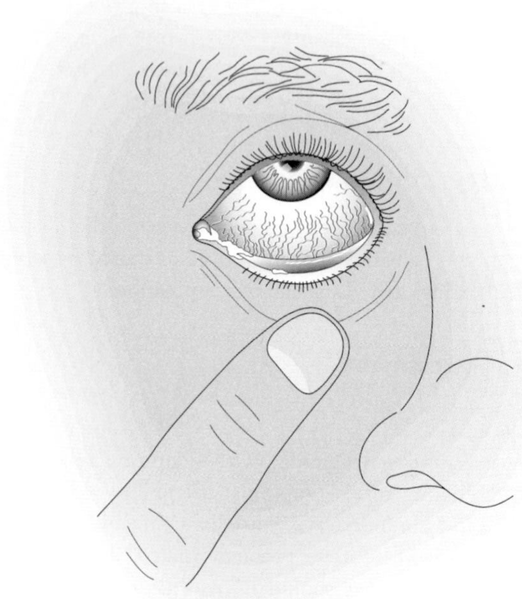

FIGURE 9-16 ■ Inspection of the conjunctiva.

- Shine your penlight at an oblique angle onto the cornea from the temporal side of the eye. Note any clouding, opacity, or injury.
- Shine your penlight on the bridge of the patient's nose, and note where the spots of light fall and whether the light falls on the same spot on each eye. This checks for **strabismus** (i.e., deviation of one eye).
- Inspect the iris, noting its shape and pigmentation. Irises should be flat, circular, and have similar pigmentation in both eyes.

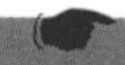

ABNORMALITIES Bilateral proptosis or **exophthalmos** is commonly associated with thyroid disease (see Chapter 20). Unilateral proptosis may indicate a tumor. Incomplete eye closure may occur with exophthalmos or cranial nerve VII weakness (see Chapter 18). Conjunctival scarring can result in inversion of the eyelids. Red eyelid margins with dried mucus on lashes suggests blepharitis. Inflammation and dilation of conjunctival blood vessels is typical of conjunctivitis. **Styes** are acute pustular infections of an eyelash follicle or sebaceous glands of the eye. **Xanthomas** are soft, yellowish, raised waxy lesions either on or beneath the eyelid, and they may be associated with hyperlipidemia. Corneal haziness or cloudiness with edema may indicate increased IOP.

TECHNIQUE

STEP 2

Examination of the Pupil

- With normal room light, measure your patient's pupils using a small ruler. Document the result in millimeters, and compare the measurements of both eyes. Pupils are normally 3 to 5 mm in size. A slight difference of less than 1 mm is common.
- Assess pupil shape. Normally, pupils are round.
- To test the pupillary light reflex, darken the room, stand to one side, and ask the patient to gaze into the distance.
- Next, advance a light in from the side, and note the response of the pupil in the eye on the same side. Constriction of the pupil on the same side is a normal direct light reflex (Fig. 9-6).
- Advance the light in from the side again, and note the response of the pupil in the eye on the opposite side. Constriction of the pupil on the opposite side is a normal consensual light reflex (Fig. 9-6).
- Repeat this procedure on the patient's other side.
- To test for accommodation, hold your finger approximately 3 inches from the patient's nose. Ask the patient to focus on a distant object, such as the corner of the room. Then, have the patient shift his or her gaze to your finger. A normal response includes constriction of the pupils and convergence of the eyes (Fig. 9-7).

ABNORMALITIES Irregularly shaped pupils may result from previous surgery or iris inflammation. Unequal pupil diameter can result from a congenital disorder or cranial nerve palsy. Pinpoint or dilated pupils may result from various medications, such as narcotic analgesic and inhaled ipratropium, respectively.

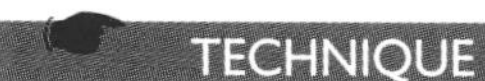

TECHNIQUE

STEP 3

Assessment of Extraocular Muscles

To test the extraocular muscles, check the "six cardinal positions of gaze" by completing the following steps (Fig. 9-17):

- Instruct the patient to move only the eyes and not the head when following the movement of your finger.
- Ask the patient to report any diplopia (double vision) or blurred vision during the test.
- Hold your finger approximately 12 to 18 inches directly in front of the patient at a high level.
- Move your finger from the midline to the patient's right side (first position).
- Move your finger upward, staying to the right of the midline (second position).
- Move your finger downward, staying to the right of the midline (third position).
- Move your finger left, across the midline (fourth position).
- Move your finger upward, staying to the left of the midline (fifth position).
- Move your finger straight down, staying to the left of the midline (sixth position).
- Observe the patient's eyes for parallel movement and for **nystagmus** (involuntary oscillating eye movements)

ABNORMALITIES Lack of parallel eye movement (deviation of one eye) would indicate an abnormality. Nystagmus may result from disorders of the labyrinth, vestibular portion of cranial nerve VII, metabolic disorders, medications (such as phenytoin), and cerebellar disease.

TECHNIQUE

STEP 4

Testing Visual Acuity

A visual acuity test should be completed if the patient presents with an eye complaint, especially vision loss. Visual acuity is tested with a vision-screening card, such as a Rosenbaum pocket vision screener or a Snellen vision chart (see Fig. 4-6).

To test far vision:

- Have the patient stand 20 feet away from a Snellen eye chart. If the patient wears glasses or contact lens, conduct the test with them on.
- Hand the patient an opaque card, and instruct the patient to place the card over one eye.
- Ask the patient to read through the smallest line of print possible. Encourage the patient to try the next smallest line as well.
- Note the line on the chart at which the patient can identify more than half the letters.
- Record the numeric fraction that is to the left of that line, along with the use of glasses, if any.
- Repeat with the opposite eye.

To test near vision:

- Hold a pocket card 14 inches from the patient.
- Hand the patient an opaque card, and instruct the patient to place the card over one eye.
- Ask the patient to read through the smallest line of print possible. Encourage the patient to try the next smallest line as well.
- Note the line on the chart at which the patient can identify more than half the letters.
- Record the numeric fraction that is to the right of that line, along with the use of glasses, if any.
- Repeat with the opposite eye.

ABNORMALITIES Vision of 20/40 or less with corrective lenses may be caused by opacities in the corneas, such as those seen with glaucoma. In this example, the numerator indicates the distance that the patient is standing from the chart (20 feet), whereas the denominator gives the distance at which a normal eye could have read that particular line. Therefore, 20/40 means that the patient can read at 20 feet what the normal eye could read at 40 feet.

TECHNIQUE

STEP 5

Testing Visual Fields

To evaluate the patient's visual fields and peripheral vision, conduct the confrontation test as follows:

- Have the patient stand.
- Place yourself, also standing, 3 to 4 feet directly in front of the patient.
- Ask the patient to stare straight ahead and meet your gaze.
- Ask the patient to cover the left eye while you cover your right eye.
- Slowly bring your fingers from beyond the limits of the visual fields in one quadrant at a time.

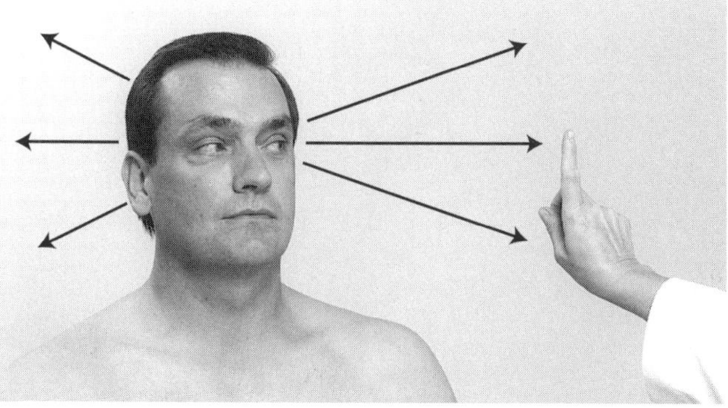

FIGURE 9-17 ■ Extraocular muscle movements.

- Ask the patient to tell you when he or she can first see your fingers.
- Repeat the test with the left eye. In other words, the patient covers the right eye while you cover your left eye.
- Again, test the visual fields.

ABNORMALITIES If you see your fingers before the patient does, he or she may have restricted visual fields.

TECHNIQUE

STEP 6

Palpation of the Eye

- Have the patient sit comfortably.
- Using your thumb and index finger, gently palpate the eyelid and orbital rim. The eyeball should feel firm, smooth, and yielding to slight pressure.
- Apply gentle pressure on the punctum (the opening of either the upper or the lower lacrimal duct at the inner canthus of the eye).

ABNORMALITIES Eyelid edema can result from sinusitis. Purulent discharge from the punctum indicates infection of the lacrimal duct.

TECHNIQUE

STEP 7

Ophthalmoscopic Examination

An ophthalmoscopic examination must be completed to evaluate the retina and the optic disc. This technique is difficult to complete, and differentiating the presence of abnormalities requires significant experience. An ophthalmoscopic examination is indicated as part of an initial physical examination or for suspected or known disorders of the retina, macula, or optic disc. Ophthalmologists are the most skilled at performing this examination, which is easiest to conduct when the patient's pupils are dilated. The procedure for completing this examination is included here for completeness.

- Darken the room to help dilate the pupils.
- Ask the patient to remove any eyeglasses. Remove yours as well.
- Select the large, round aperture on the ophthalmoscope with the white light for routine examination.
- Instruct the patient to look at a point on the wall behind you and across the room. Instruct the patient to keep looking at it even though your head may get in the way.
- Match sides with the person. Hold the ophthalmoscope in your right hand and up to your right eye to view the patient's right eye.
- Use your thumb to anchor the upper lid of the patient and to prevent any blinking.
- Begin approximately 10 inches away from the person, at an angle approximately 15° lateral to the person's line of vision (Fig. 9-18).
- Note the red reflex (the red glow filling the patient's pupil), which is caused by reflection of the ophthalmoscope light off the inner retina.
- Keeping the red reflex in sight, move closer to the eye.
- As you advance, adjust the lens to +6, and note any opacities in the media.
- Progress toward the patient until your foreheads almost touch (Fig. 9-18).
- Adjust the diopter setting to bring the ocular fundus into sharp focus. Use the red lenses for near-sighted eyes and the black lenses for far-sighted eyes.
- Locate the optic disc on the nasal side of the retina. The disc should appear creamy yellow-orange to pink, round or oval, as well as distinct and sharply demarcated.
- Locate the retinal vessels. Follow a paired artery and vein out to the periphery in the four quadrants.
- Locate the macula by looking temporal to the optic nerve. The macula may appear darker and slightly yellow compared to the retina.
- View the fovea (the depression in the center of the macula). You should observe a pinpoint white light reflected back to the ophthalmoscope.

A
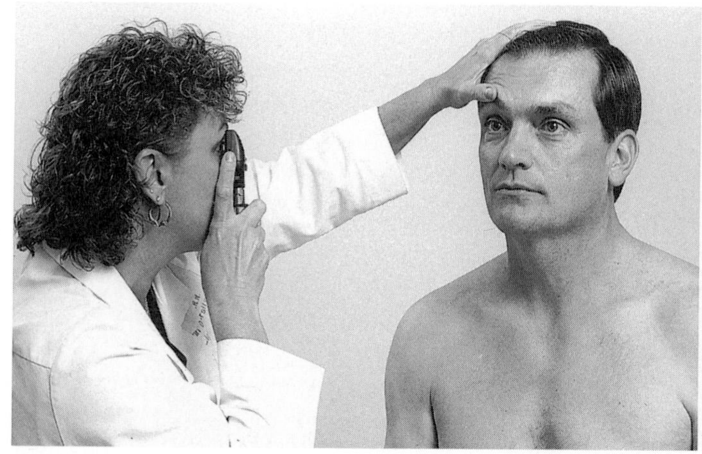
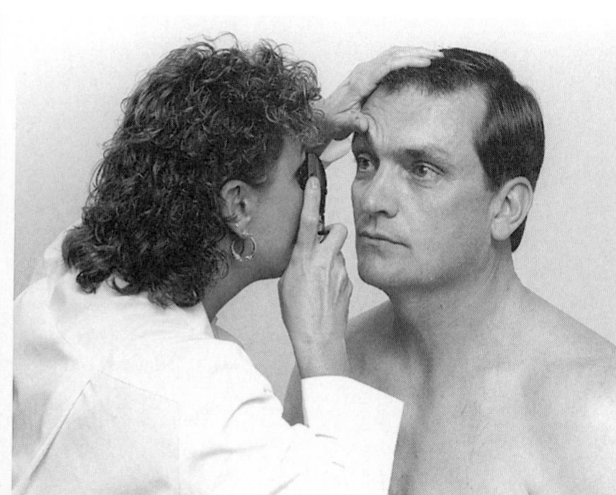
B

FIGURE 9-18 ■ Approach to ophthalmologic examination. **(A)** Distant. **(B)** Close.

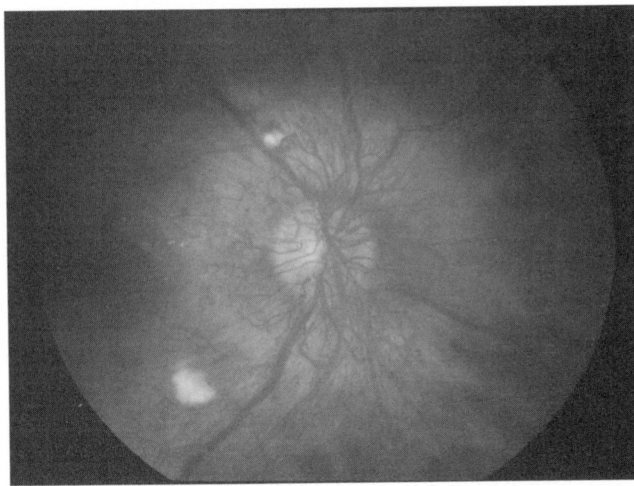

FIGURE 9-19 ■ Diabetic retinopathy. (See Color Plate 25: Photograph from the National Eye Institute, National Institutes of Health.)

ABNORMALITIES **Cataracts** produce opacity of the lens. Retinal abnormalities, such as detachment, hemorrhages, and exudates, can be seen in diabetic retinopathy (a noninflammatory disorder of the retina from diabetes that may cause blindness) (Fig. 9-19). Bulging of the optic disc can result from increased IOP. Systemic diseases such as hypertension can affect the retinal vessels, resulting in abnormalities such as nicking or pinching of the underlying vessel (A-V nicking [arteriovenous, nicking at the junction where the artery & veins meet in the eye].).

The Ear

Similar to the pharmacist's limited role concerning the eye, physical examination of the ear by a pharmacist currently centers around inspection of the outer ear and, possibly, unaided inspection of the external auditory canal. In contrast to an ophthalmologic examination, an otoscopic examination is not difficult and, in the future, may be within the realm of the pharmacist. Hearing assessments also are fairly simple to complete and could extend the pharmacist's ability to monitor medications that can cause hearing loss as an adverse effect; however, this is not commonly done in practice today.

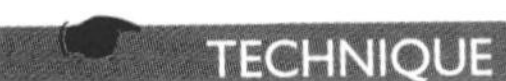

STEP 1

Inspection of the Ear

- Observe ear size and placement. Auricles should be equal in size and placement, symmetrically positioned, and freely mobile.
- Assess the skin color, texture, and integrity. Skin should be clean, dry, and the same color as other skin. Skin should also be free of scales, redness, and inflammation.
- Inspect the auricle.
- Inspect the external auditory canal. The size of the opening should not be swollen, red, or have discharge. Cerumen should be present but not excessive.

ABNORMALITIES Dry, scaly skin on the external ear may indicate psoriasis or seborrhea. Painful, crusted lesions on the helix (the inward curved rim of the external ear) may be seen in squamous cell carcinoma. Hard nodules or calculi on the auricle rim or outside the opening of the external auditory canal may represent gouty deposits.

TECHNIQUE

STEP 2

Palpation of the Ear

- Palpate the auricle, checking for freedom of movement, tenderness, and lesions.
- Palpate behind the external ear for lesions and tenderness.
- Palpate the preauricular and postauricular lymph nodes for tenderness and enlargement. These nodes should be nonpalpable or small, soft, and nontender. (See Chapter 10 for a more detailed discussion of lymph node examination.)

ABNORMALITIES Tenderness and pain on movement of the auricle or earlobe indicates acute otitis externa, not OM. Otitis media may cause tenderness behind the ear.

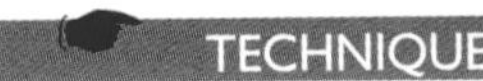

STEP 3

Otoscopic Examination

- Choose the largest speculum that will fit comfortably in the patient's ear canal.
- Tilt the patient's head slightly away from you, toward the opposite shoulder.
- Inspect the auditory canal with the otoscope penlight. Note any redness, swelling, lesions, foreign bodies, or discharge.
- Pull the auricle up and back on an adult or older child. Pull the auricle down on an infant or child younger than 3 years.
- Hold the auricle gently but firmly throughout the examination.
- Hold the otoscope by the handle, and rest the back of your hand along the person's cheek to stabilize the instrument.
- Insert the speculum slowly and carefully along the axis of the canal. Watch the insertion, then put your eye up to the otoscope. Avoid touching the canal wall (Fig. 9-20).
- Rotate the otoscope to visualize all the tympanic membrane. Note the membrane's color, position, and integrity. The normal eardrum is a shiny and translucent pearly-gray color, flat, and intact. Visualize the cone of light and the bony landmarks (Fig. 9-11).

ABNORMALITIES Redness and swelling of the external auditory canal occur with otitis externa, and the canal may be swollen completely shut. A reddened tympanic membrane with purulent, foul-smelling ear drainage suggests otitis externa. A bulging, reddened, or perforated

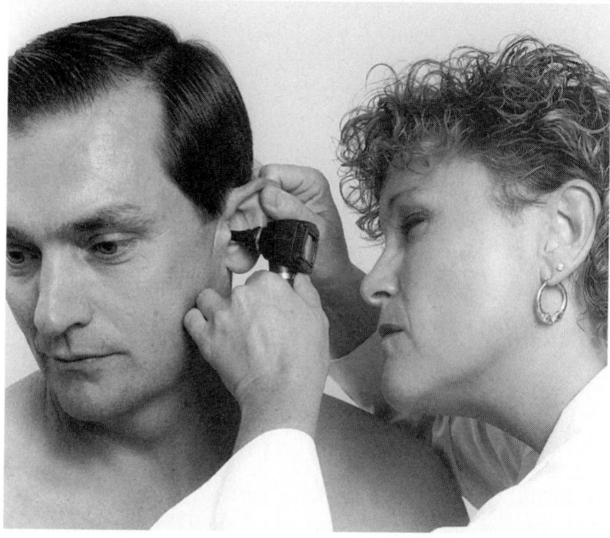

FIGURE 9-20 ■ Speculum placement for otoscopic examination.

tympanic membrane with an absent cone of light and loss of bony landmarks is usual with OM. A perforated eardrum appears as a hole in the center of the tympanic membrane. Scarring of the eardrum appears as opacities.

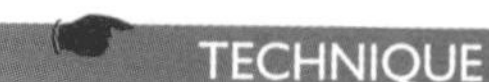
TECHNIQUE

STEP 4

Testing Auditory Acuity

- Occlude one of the patient's ears with your gloved finger.
- Stand 1 or 2 feet away from the patient.
- Exhale fully, and whisper softly toward the unoccluded ear. Choose numbers or words with two equally accented syllables.
- If necessary, increase your voice to a medium volume, followed by a loud whisper and then by a soft, medium, and loud voice.
- Make sure the patient cannot read your lips by covering your mouth or obstructing the patient's vision.
- Repeat with the opposite ear.

ABNORMALITIES Chronic OM, aging, and medications can result in hearing loss.

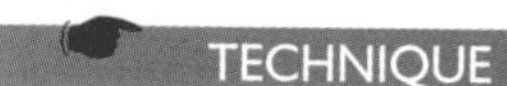
TECHNIQUE

STEP 5

Testing Air and Bone Conduction of Sound

If hearing is decreased, the pharmacist should try to distinguish between conductive and sensorineural hearing loss. Air and bone conduction should be evaluated in a quiet room with a tuning fork (preferably of 512 Hz).

For the Weber test:

- Stand to the side of the patient.
- Instruct the patient to indicate if the tone sounds the same in both ears or sounds better in one.
- Hold the tuning fork by the stem, and strike the tines softly on the back of your hand.
- Place the base of the vibrating tuning fork firmly on top of the patient's head (Fig. 9-21).
- Record the findings. A normal Weber test is negative for lateralization.

For the Rinne test:

- Stand to the side and back of the patient. Instruct the patient to tell you when the sound can no longer be heard.
- Hold the tuning fork by the stem, and strike the tines softly on the back of your hand.
- Place the base of the vibrating tuning fork on the mastoid bone behind the patient's ear and level with the ear canal.
- When the patient indicates the sound is gone, quickly place the fork close to the ear canal with the "U" facing forward (Fig. 9-21).
- Ask the patient to tell you if he or she can hear the sound. The patient should be able to hear the vibration through the air after they could not hear it any longer through the bone.
- Instruct the patient to tell you when the sound can no longer be heard.
- Repeat with the opposite ear.
- Document the results. A normal Rinne test is positive, which is when sound is usually heard twice as long by air conduction (AC) as by bone conduction (BC). It is documented as "AC > BC," indicating that air conduction of sound next to the ear canal is greater than bone conduction of sound through the mastoid process.

ABNORMALITIES Lateralization of sound during the Weber test (hearing the sound only on one side) is abnormal. During conductive hearing loss, sound lateralizes or is heard in the "bad" ear. The ear with conductive hearing loss has a better chance to hear bone-conducted sound, because it is not distracted by background noise. During sensorineural hearing loss, sound lateralizes to the "good" or unaffected ear. The ear with nerve-based hearing loss is unable to perceive the sound. Abnormal Rinne test results occur when air conduction is not greater than bone conduction. When conductive hearing loss is present, the patient should have a negative Rinne test: air conduction less than or equal to bone conduction (AC = BC; AC < BC). A patient suffering from sensorineural hearing loss hears poorly both ways, but the normal ratio (AC > BC) is maintained (Fig. 9-21).

Laboratory and Diagnostic Tests

Clinically, no laboratory tests are used to assess function of the eyes and the ears. Patients suffering from vision changes, such as decreased vision, blurred vision, or other defects, should be referred to an ophthalmologist for a dilated funduscopic examination. Specialized equipment, such as a tonometer (measures pressure inside the eye), slit lamp (allows a view of the front of the eye), phoro-optometer (detects refractive errors), and indirect ophthalmoscope (wider view of the retina), is used by op-

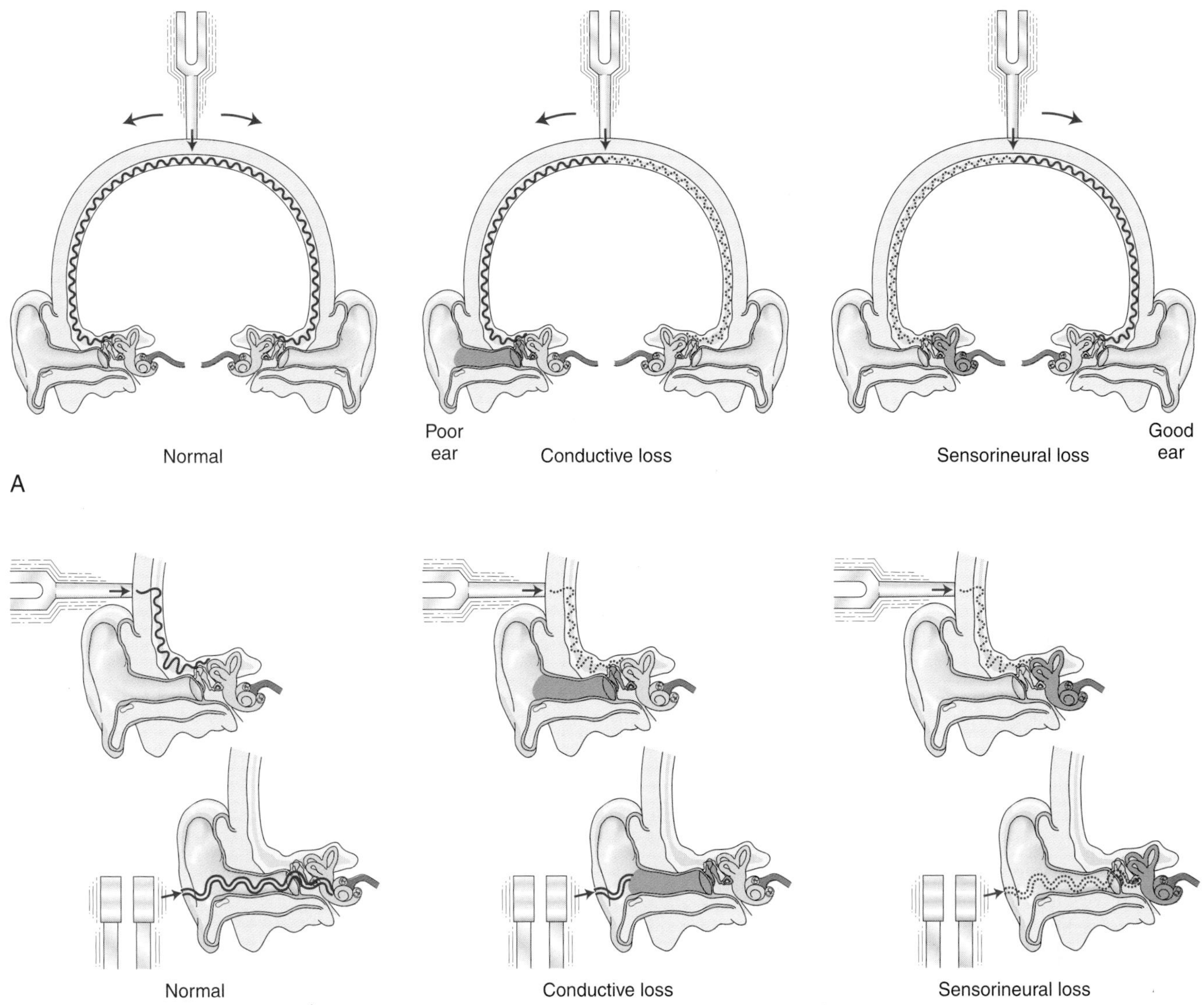

FIGURE 9-21 ■ Hearing acuity. **(A)** Weber test. A normal result is when sound is heard equally in both ears. Conductive loss is indicated when sound lateralizes to the impaired ear. Sensorineural loss is indicated when sound lateralizes to the good ear. **(B)** Rinne test. A normal result is when air conduction is greater than bone conduction (AC > BC). Conductive loss is indicated when bone conduction is greater than or equal to air conduction (BC > AC or BC = AC). Sensorineural loss is indicated when the patient hears poorly in both ears but air conduction is greater than bone conduction (AC > BC).

tometrists and ophthalmologists for the diagnosis of eye diseases and disorders. Systemic diseases also may result in changes in vision, and in these cases, other radiologic tests, such as computed tomography and magnetic resonance imaging, may be indicated.

When further evaluation on the ear is required, specialized equipment is again employed. When a more detailed evaluation of the tympanic membrane is indicated, a tympanometer is used to determine how well the eardrum moves when a soft sound and air pressure are introduced into the ear canal. A "flat" line on a tympanogram may indicate that the eardrum is not mobile; a "peaked" pattern often indicates normal function.

Techniques to evaluate hearing acuity were outlined earlier in this chapter. If deficits are found, however, further evaluation is usually required. Audiologists are professionals who specialize in evaluating hearing loss and in conducting hearing tests. Test results are recorded on an audiogram, which is a graph showing hearing sensitivity. The degree of hearing loss is determined by measuring the hearing threshold (the levels in decibels [dB] at which a signal is just barely heard). In other words, thresholds are measured at several frequencies (pitches) and are graphed on the audiogram. The frequencies tested are those that are important for hearing and understanding speech and other environmental sounds. Frequency is noted in Hertz (Hz). The louder the sounds must be before they are heard, the greater the degree of hearing loss. Thus, when the hearing test is completed, the patient should be able to tell how well he or she hears at low, medium, and high pitches. If hearing loss is present, the patient should also be able to tell which part of the hearing mechanism (the outside, middle, or inner ear) is causing the loss. Ranges have been established to help a person identify how much difficulty should be expected from a given hearing loss. The typical ranges for adults are:

- −10 to 25 dB = normal range.
- 26 to 40 dB = mild hearing loss.
- 41 to 55 dB = moderate hearing loss.
- 56 to 70 dB = moderately severe hearing loss.
- 71 to 90 dB = severe hearing loss.

Special Considerations

Pediatric Patients

When evaluating the eyes and ears of infants and children, several additional questions may be appropriate depending on the age of the child. Asking about the mother's history of vaginal infections and whether she had an infection at the time of delivery is important for ascertaining the risk to the infant of acquiring such an infection at birth. Certain forms of vaginitis, such as gonorrhea and genital herpes, may result in ocular sequelae in the newborn. Depending on the age of the child, interview questions related to vision development, routine vision testing at school, and safety measures for protection of the eye from trauma might be relevant.

Children have a high incidence of upper respiratory infections, which can predispose them to OM. Pharmacists should focus on subjective questioning related to the incidence and duration of previous infections, evidence of hearing loss, and potential effect of any infections and hearing loss on normal development. Pharmacists should also be cognizant of the increased risk of foreign bodies in both the ears and the nose when interviewing or examining children.

Visual acuity develops for months after birth. The examination techniques used to screen visual acuity should be based on the child's age. Pupillary light reflexes such as the blink reflex (the neonate blinks in response to bright light) and the direct pupillary reaction will be intact in neonates; however, this does not mean that an infant can see. The developmental benchmarks for visual acuity in an infant are outlined in Table 9-3.For children between 2.5 and 3 years of age, the Allen test (picture cards) can be substituted for the Snellen E chart. For intermediate ages (3–6 years), the child can point a finger in the direction of the "table legs" on the Snellen E chart. By the age of 7 or 8 years, the standard Snellen alphabet chart can be used. Normally, a child achieves 20/20 acuity by the age of 6 or 7 years. In addition, children should be assessed for color blindness and strabismus (squint or crossed eye), because this may affect their visual acuity.

TABLE 9-3 ➤ DEVELOPMENTAL BENCHMARKS FOR VISUAL ACUITY IN INFANTS

AGE	BENCHMARK
Birth to 2 weeks	Refuse to open eyes after exposure to bright light Increasing alertness to an object in line of vision May fixate on an object in line of vision
2 to 4 weeks	Fixate on an object in line of vision
1 month	Fixate and follow a light or bright toy
3 to 4 months	Fixate, follow, and reach for the toy
6 to 10 months	Fixate and follow the toy in all directions

TABLE 9-4 ➤ NORMAL PHYSICAL ABNORMALITIES OF THE EYES AND EARS IN INFANTS AND CHILDREN

ORGAN ASSESSED	PHYSICAL FINDINGS
Eyes	Corneal light reflex: some asymmetry before age of 6 months Doll's eye reflex: as you turn baby's body, the eyes will look in same direction; when turning stops eyes shift to opposite direction after few beats of nystagmus; disappears by 2 months of age Setting sun sign: eyes appear to deviate down, exposing the white rim of the sclera over the iris. Epicanthal fold (excess skinfold extending over the inner corner of the eye) Sclera: blue appearance because of thinness at birth Lacrimal glands: nonfunctional at birth Iris: permanent color not differentiated until 6 to 9 months
Ears	Tympanic membrane: first few days after birth, may appear thickened, opaque, and mildly red; may look injected in infants after crying

Similar to visual acuity, hearing acuity also develops over the first few months of life. Newborns should startle and blink in response to a loud, sudden noise. Infants 3 to 4 months of age should blink and stop their movement, appearing to "listen." Other behaviors that should be observed in response to a loud, sudden noise are cessation of sucking, becoming quiet if crying, or starting to cry if quiet. By 6 to 8 months, infants should turn their heads to "find" the sound and respond to their own name. Preschool and school-aged children may be screened with audiometry.

Because of the anatomic differences in the external auditory canal and eustachian tubes of infants and toddlers, the pharmacist should begin an examination by pulling down on the auricle rather than up (as in adults). Additional abnormalities found on examination of the eye and ear that are normal in infants and children are summarized in Table 9-4.

Physical examination techniques used for the eyes and ears vary substantially in children compared to adults and are summarized in Table 9-5.

Geriatric Patients

Many changes normally occur in the eyes and ears as a result of aging. Subjective questioning of the elderly patient by the pharmacist should be directed at obtaining information about the impact of these changes on the patient's functional status. For example, ask if the patient has experienced any decrease in normal activities, such as reading, sewing, or any occupation or hobbies that require keen vision. More specifically, ask whether the patient has noticed any visual difficulty with climbing stairs or driving. This will help to determine if a loss of depth perception is occurring and allow the pharmacist to provide education on how to prevent falls and accidents. Because decreased tear

TABLE 9-5 ➤ PHYSICAL EXAMINATION OF THE EYES AND EARS IN CHILDREN

ORGAN	ALTERATIONS IN PHYSICAL EXAMINATION TECHNIQUE
Eyes	Inspection: • Perform examination in dimly lit room, hold infant upright, suspended under its arms or have parent hold infant over shoulder (all actions encourage an infant to open his or her eyes). • Draw a line across center of eyes to detect appropriate placement. This should be horizontal. Ophthalmoscopic examination: • Deferred until 2 to 6 months of age, but can elicit red reflex in newborns. • Children should be positioned supine on examination table with the head near one end. • Do not hold eyelids forcibly open, because it will elicit resistance. • May have child sit on parent's lap as an alternative.
Ears	Inspection: • Observe position and alignment of the ears. The top of the auricle should be level with the corner of the eye and positioned within 10° of vertical. Otoscopic examination: • Complete otoscopic examination at the end of the physical examination. • Infant should be propped up against parent. Toddler may lie on examining table. Stabilize head to avoid movement against the otoscope. • Pull auricle back and straight down in children under 3 years of age.

production occurs with age, questions related to the eyes feeling dry or burning are also appropriate.

The physical examination techniques used for eyes and ears in geriatric patients are the same as those described previously. Abnormalities found on examination of the eye and ear that can be attributed to aging are summarized in Table 9-1.

Pregnant Patients

The method of subjective questioning used for adults does not need to be varied when interviewing a pregnant woman. Direct special attention, however, toward identifying symptoms that may result from complications related to the pregnancy. As previously mentioned, hormonal changes during pregnancy may alter the curvature of the eye and result in complaints of decreased vision. Women in their third trimester should be questioned carefully about visual changes, such as new onset of blurred vision or spots before their eyes, because these may be signs of preeclampsia.

Pregnancy-induced hypertension may be a problem for some women. To differentiate chronic hypertension from pregnancy-induced hypertension, a retinal examination may be indicated. Patients with pregnancy-induced hypertension present with segmental arteriolar narrowing and a glistening appearance consistent with edema. Hemorrhages and exudates that are often present in patients with long-standing chronic hypertension, however, are absent.

APPLICATION TO PATIENT SYMPTOMS

Symptoms related to disorders of the eyes and ears commonly prompt patients to ask a pharmacist for advice. Many of these clinical situations can be managed with over-the-counter products, but others may result in serious patient outcomes, such as vision and hearing loss, without immediate referral to a primary care provider. Application of the subjective and objective assessment techniques previously presented should allow the pharmacist to differentiate those situations that can be self-treated from those that require referral to a physician.

Red Eye

Minor irritation of the eye is a common cause of redness. Pollutants, chlorine, and smoke can be incorporated into tears and irritate the surface of the eye. Infectious diseases and glaucoma, however, can also result in inflammation of the eye. Therefore, pharmacists must gain a more detailed understanding of how to assess patients who present with this condition.

CASE STUDY

MY is a 31-year-old woman who presents to St. Luke's Clinic with complaints of red eyes that burn, feel irritated, and have discharge. The clinic pharmacist performs the initial patient interview and medication history. The pharmacist notes that MY has a young boy with her.

ASSESSMENT OF THE PATIENT

Subjective Information

31-year-old woman complaining of red eyes that burn, feel irritated, and have discharge

GOOD MORNING, I AM THE CLINIC'S PHARMACIST, DR. MYERS. CAN YOU TELL ME WHAT PROBLEMS YOU ARE CURRENTLY HAVING? Well, as I told the receptionist, my eyes started getting red yesterday and feeling slightly irritated. I woke up this morning with my eyes crusted shut. Today, they look redder, and I'm always carrying a tissue because they are tearing. I was afraid of this happening. My son had a similar infection 4 or 5 days ago.

ARE YOU HAVING ANY OTHER PROBLEMS WITH YOUR EYES? Well, during the day I often have to wipe this whitish-yellow "junk" out of my eyes.

DO YOUR EYES ITCH? Only a little.

ARE YOU HAVING ANY PAIN OR SWELLING IN YOUR EYES? They feel dry and a little irritated but not really painful. Although I can't really see any difference, they kind of "feel" swollen.

HAVE YOU INJURED YOUR EYE AT ALL IN THE LAST COUPLE OF DAYS? No.

HAVE YOU NOTICED ANY CHANGES IN YOUR VISION? No.

DO YOU WEAR GLASSES OR CONTACTS? Yes, I wear both. I had been wearing my contacts until this morning, but I am really faithful to only wearing them while I am at work and I clean them every day.

WHEN WAS YOUR LAST EYE EXAMINATION? It was October of this year. Everything was fine. I didn't need any new glasses or contacts.

HAS YOUR DAILY ROUTINE BEEN THE SAME AS USUAL THE LAST FEW DAYS? Yes.

HAVE YOU DONE ANYTHING NEW? Well, I started working in the day care center where my son is cared for about 2 weeks ago.

HAVE YOU USED ANY NEW PRODUCTS SUCH AS COSMETICS OR FACIAL CLEANSERS? No.

DOES ANYTHING MAKE YOUR EYES WORSE? Sunlight makes them tear more.

DOES ANYTHING MAKE YOUR EYES BETTER? No, although keeping them closed feels the best.

HAVE YOU TRIED TO TREAT YOUR EYE PROBLEMS WITH ANYTHING? Yes. I tried Visine drops yesterday, but it burned a little and did not make them feel any better.

YOU MENTIONED THAT YOUR SON HAD SIMILAR PROBLEMS A FEW DAYS AGO. HAVE YOU EVER EXPERIENCED SYMPTOMS LIKE THIS BEFORE? Yes, once before when my son was about 3, we both had something like this.

DID YOU SEE A DOCTOR THE LAST TIME YOU HAD THESE PROBLEMS? Yes.

HOW HAS IT BEEN TREATED? The doctor gave me eye drops.

DO YOU REMEMBER THE NAME OF THE EYE DROPS? No.

DID YOU SEE A DOCTOR ABOUT YOUR SON'S SYMPTOMS A FEW DAYS AGO? Yes.

DID THE DOCTOR PRESCRIBE SOME MEDICINE FOR YOUR SON? Yes.

DO YOU REMEMBER THE NAME OF THE MEDICINE? Yes. In fact, I have some left. It was Ilotycin ointment.

BESIDES THE MEDICATION, DID THE DOCTOR TALK TO YOU ABOUT ANY OTHER WAYS TO TREAT YOUR SYMPTOMS? No.

HOW DO YOU REMOVE THE "WHITISH-YELLOWISH" JUNK FROM YOUR EYES? I just wipe it out with my fingers.

DO YOU WASH YOUR HANDS AFTER YOU WIPE IT OUT OF YOUR EYES? No.

DID YOU USE A WASHCLOTH TO WASH OUT YOUR SON'S EYES WHEN HE HAD THIS PROBLEM? Yes.

WHAT DID YOU DO WITH THE WASHCLOTH WHEN YOU WERE DONE WITH IT? I just left it hanging in the bathroom.

OKAY, JUST A FEW MORE QUESTIONS. DO YOU HAVE ANY OTHER PROBLEMS ANYWHERE ELSE? No.

HAVE YOU HAD ANY OTHER SYMPTOMS, SUCH AS FEVER, SWOLLEN GLANDS, OR HEADACHE? No.

HAVE YOU HAD ANY RECENT ILLNESSES? I had a cold about 5 days ago, but it's gone now.

DO YOU HAVE ANY OTHER MEDICAL CONDITIONS? No.

ARE YOU TAKING ANY MEDICATIONS CURRENTLY? No.

DO YOU HAVE ANY ALLERGIES? Penicillin.

WHAT HAPPENS WHEN YOU TAKE PENICILLIN? I break out in hives all over my body.

DO YOU HAVE ANY OTHER ALLERGIES, SUCH AS TO FOOD OR TO THINGS IN THE ENVIRONMENT? No.

Objective Information

MY is a 31-year-old, well-nourished, well-developed, healthy woman in no apparent distress. Posture and gait are normal.

Continued

CASE STUDY—continued

Speech is clear. Her affect is appropriate to her mood, which is concerned about her problem.

Pulse: 72 bpm, regular

Respirations: 15 rpm, easy and nonlabored

Temperature: 98.4°F

Blood pressure: 120/78 mm Hg, sitting in left arm

Height: 5'7"

Weight: 132 lbs

Skin: uniformly tan, with no lesions present

Eyes: Vision is 20/30 in each eye with glasses. Sclera is mildly injected bilaterally; conjunctiva is red and slightly swollen, with small amount of yellowish material bilaterally. Pupils are equal, round, and reactive to light and accommodation (PERRLA). Extraocular muscles are intact (EOMI).

Remainder of physical examination: within normal limits

DISCUSSION

The major issue in this case is differentiating between viral, bacterial, and allergic conjunctivitis. Itching is often considered to be a hallmark symptom of allergic conjunctivitis, but in MY's case, the history of her son's bacterial infection coupled with the yellowish exudates and a past history of similar symptoms lend support to bacterial conjunctivitis. Discharge from an allergic conjunctivitis would be serous or mucoid in nature. MY's handling of the discharge and the washcloth also indicates a mode by which she could have contracted her son's bacterial conjunctivitis. Using contaminated washcloths left in the bathroom, either at home or at the day care center, would be a prime way for her to have obtained a similar infection. On examination, the injection of her sclera is consistent with her complaint of red, irritated eyes. In addition, her conjunctiva is inflamed, and a discharge is noted. MY's vision is normal with her corrective lenses, which supports her claim that her vision has not been affected. Her cranial nerves II, III, IV, and VI are all intact based on her normal findings. This would help to rule out a neurologic cause of her symptoms. Figure 9-22 provides a decision tree for the symptom of red eye.

■ PHARMACEUTICAL CARE PLAN ■

Patient Name: MY

Date: **1/12/02**

Medical Problems:
None

Current Medications:
None

S: MY is a 31-year-old woman who presents with complaints of red, burning eyes with yellowish exudates for 2 days. MY reports her son had a similar eye infection 4–5 days ago. She tried Visine yesterday with no relief; otherwise, she has taken no medication for her condition. MY has a stated allergy to penicillin that results in hives.

O: MY is a 31-year-old, well-nourished, well-developed, healthy woman in no apparent distress. Posture and gait are normal. Speech is clear. Her affect is appropriate to her mood, which is concerned about her problem.

Pulse: 72 bpm, regular

Respirations: 15 rpm, easy and nonlabored

Temperature: 98.4°F

Blood pressure: 120/78 mm Hg, sitting in left arm

Height: 5'7"

Weight: 132 lbs

Skin: Uniformly tan, with no lesions present

Eyes: Vision is 20/30 in each eye with glasses. Sclera is mildly injected bilaterally; conjunctiva is red and slightly swollen, with small amount of yellowish material bilaterally. PERRLA. EOMI.

Remainder of physical examination: Within normal limits

A: Physician diagnosed bacterial conjunctivitis

P:
1. Recommend Ilotycin ophthalmic ointment, because she already has this medication on hand. Apply to both eyes twice daily for 5 days.
2. Educate MY on the proper self-care management of conjunctivitis to avoid transmission among family members and children in day care.
3. Check MY's understanding of the proper way to apply Ilotycin ointment.
4. F/U with MY in 3 days to evaluate improvement in symptoms and identify any potential side effects.

Pharmacist: Robert Myers, Pharm.D.

Self-Assessment Questions

1. What is the most common form of conjunctivitis?
2. What are the signs and symptoms of POAG?
3. What is the hallmark sign of allergic conjunctivitis?
4. What signs or symptoms indicate that a patient should be referred to a primary care provider for further assessment?
5. What items should be assessed when inspecting the eye?
6. Define PERRLA and EMOI.

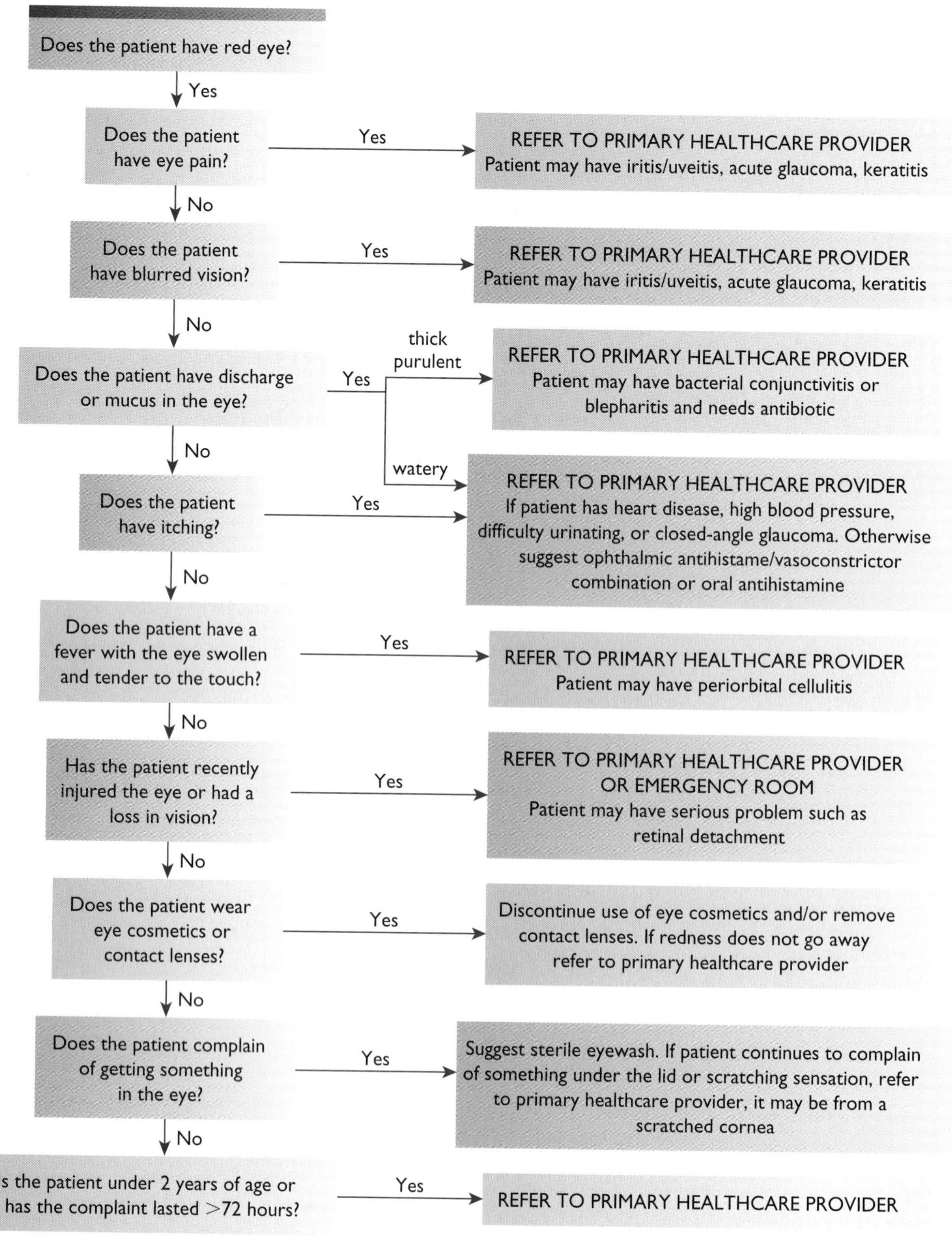

FIGURE 9-22 ■ Decision tree for red eye.

Critical Thinking Question

1. TS is a 75-year-old man who presents to the pharmacy with a prescription for prednisone, 30 mg by mouth every day for 10 days, for an acute exacerbation of his asthma. On review of his medication profile, the pharmacist notes TS is also on the following medications: albuterol, two puffs every 4 hours as needed for wheezing; Intal, two puffs twice daily; and Pilocarpine 0.5%, one drop in both eyes three times daily. What questions would you ask this patient? What are the potential drug-therapy problems? Would you fill this prescription? Why, or why not?

Ear Pain

Ear pain, or **otalgia,** is the most common complaint in adults presenting with problems involving the ear. The type, pattern of onset, and duration of the pain can provide the pharmacist with clues regarding the potential cause and, thereby, the need for referral to a physician.

CASE STUDY

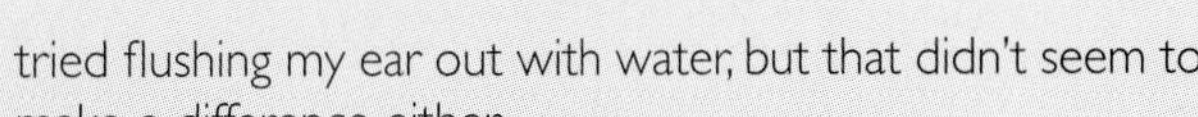

AR is a 37-year-old man who approaches the pharmacist complaining of pain in his ear. Concerned about the cause, the pharmacist asks AR to step into the patient care room to discuss his ear pain.

ASSESSMENT OF THE PATIENT

Subjective Information

37-year-old man complaining of ear pain

TELL ME MORE ABOUT THE EAR PAIN YOU HAVE BEEN HAVING. Well, about 2 weeks ago, I started having pain in my right ear, but now my jaw hurts as well.

DO YOU HAVE PAIN ANYWHERE ELSE BESIDES YOUR RIGHT EAR AND JAW? No.

DO YOU HAVE ANY PAIN IN YOUR LEFT EAR? No.

HOW DID THE PAIN START? After I returned from vacation, I noticed that it kind of hurt, and it has slowly gotten worse over the last couple of weeks.

DID YOU INJURE YOUR RIGHT EAR AT ALL DURING VACATION? No, not that I can think of.

WHAT DID YOU DO ON VACATION? My family went to Florida. We spent most of the time at the beach.

DID YOU FLY TO FLORIDA? Yes.

HOW WOULD YOU DESCRIBE THE PAIN? My right ear kind of aches all the time.

IS THERE ANY TIME DURING THE DAY THAT IT DOESN'T HURT? No.

DOES ANYTHING MAKE THE PAIN WORSE? My jaw hurts more when I try to eat.

DOES IT HURT TO TOUCH YOUR RIGHT EAR? Yes! My wife accidentally bumped it this morning, and I thought I would fall off my chair. I also cannot sleep with the right side of my head on the pillow.

DOES ANYTHING MAKE THE PAIN BETTER? Not that I can think of.

HAVE YOU TRIED TO TREAT THE PAIN WITH ANYTHING? Well, I tried Tylenol, and it really does not seem to help. When it first started, I thought I might have a lot of earwax, so I tried to clean my ear with cotton swabs, but that hurt more. I also tried flushing my ear out with water, but that didn't seem to make a difference either.

WHAT DOSE OF TYLENOL DID YOU TAKE? I took two pills.

WAS THAT REGULAR STRENGTH OR EXTRA-STRENGTH? I think it was regular.

HOW MANY TIMES A DAY DID YOU TAKE THE TYLENOL? Three to four times a day.

WHEN DID YOU LAST TAKE TYLENOL? Yesterday.

ARE YOU HAVING ANY OTHER PROBLEMS WITH YOUR EARS? No.

SO YOUR EAR OR EARS DO NOT ITCH? No.

HAVE YOU NOTICED ANY DRAINAGE FROM YOUR RIGHT EAR? No.

HOW IS YOUR HEARING? Fine.

ARE YOU HAVING ANY TROUBLE WITH RINGING IN YOUR EARS? No.

ARE YOU HAVING ANY TROUBLE WITH FEELING DIZZY, UNSTABLE, OR LIKE YOU ARE GOING TO LOSE YOUR BALANCE? No.

HAVE YOU HAD A RECENT ILLNESS? No.

ARE YOU HAVING ANY OTHER PROBLEMS OR SYMPTOMS? No, I don't think so.

HAVE YOU NOTICED ANY FEVER, SWOLLEN GLANDS, COUGH, HEADACHE, SINUS CONGESTION, OR RUNNY NOSE? No.

HAVE YOU EVER HAD EAR PAIN LIKE THIS IN THE PAST? No.

HOW IS YOUR OVERALL HEALTH? Fine.

DO YOU SUFFER FROM ANY CHRONIC ILLNESS? No.

DO YOU SMOKE? Yes.

HOW MUCH DO YOU SMOKE PER DAY? Probably about half a pack.

HOW LONG HAVE YOU BEEN SMOKING? I started when I was in college, so probably 15 years.

DO YOU HAVE ANY ALLERGIES? No.

ARE THERE ANY MEDICATIONS YOU CANNOT TAKE? No.

Continued

CASE STUDY—continued

Objective Information

AR is a well-developed, well-nourished, well-dressed, healthy 34-year-old man who appears his stated age, is oriented × 3, and seems in no apparent distress. AR walks and moves easily and responds quickly to questions. Speech is clear. Mood and affect are appropriate for the situation.

Pulse: 78 bpm, regular

Respirations: 16 rpm, easy and nonlabored

Temperature: 97.3°F

Blood pressure: 124/84 mm Hg, sitting in right arm

Skin: color a uniform, tanned appearance

Ears: Position of auricles are appropriate and symmetric. Color is consistent with skin tone. No lumps or deformities. Right auricle and tragus are tender to palpation. Right ear canal is red and swollen. No cerumen in canal. Right tympanic membrane (TM) is flat, intact, and pearly gray; landmarks identified; and cone of light in five-o'clock position. Left ear canal is without erythema, swelling, discharge, and cerum. Left TM negative. Acuity good (to whispered voice). Weber midline, AC > BC.

Pharynx: light pink with no exudates, swelling, or ulcerations; tonsils 1+ (normal)

Neck: no adenopathy

Lungs: thorax symmetric on inspection, no audible breath sounds, good expansion, all lung fields clear to auscultation (CTA)

DISCUSSION

Ear conditions that can be self-treated include cerumen impaction and water-clogged ears. Conditions such as swimmer's ear (otitis externa), OM, perforated eardrum, foreign objects in the ear, and symptoms such as loss of hearing, ear pain, drainage, and tinnitus must be referred to a physician.

Although cerumen impaction can cause ear discomfort, pain is not usually a symptom, and AR states that his ear hurts when the pharmacist touches it. In addition, during the pharmacist's interview, AR denied other symptoms related to cerumen impaction, such as a feeling of fullness, vertigo, and partial hearing loss of certain tones or tinnitus. Pain when touching the auricle, touching the tragus, or on examination is a classic sign of otitis externa (swimmer's ear), which is associated with damage to the lining of the external auditory canal that makes it ripe for bacterial infection. Because of the duration of AR's ear pain and its current radiation to his jaw, the pharmacist calls AR's physician, who requests that AR come in that day.

Figure 9-23 presents a decision tree for the symptom of ear pain.

PHARMACEUTICAL CARE PLAN

Patient Name: AR

Date: 1/14/01

Medical Problems:
None

Current Medications:
Tylenol, 650 mg, by mouth periodically for ear pain

S: AR presents to the pharmacy complaining of right ear pain for 2 weeks. Pain now radiates into his jaw, making it difficult to eat. Pain did not improve with Tylenol or flushing. AR has no other symptoms or known drug allergies.

O: AR is a well-developed, well-nourished, well-dressed, healthy 34-year-old man who appears his stated age, is oriented × 3, and seems in no apparent distress. AR walks and moves easily and responds quickly to questions. Speech is clear. Mood and affect are appropriate for situation.

Pulse: 78 bpm, regular

Respirations: 16 rpm, easy and nonlabored

Temperature: 97.3°F

Blood pressure: 124/84 mm Hg, sitting in right arm

Skin: Color is a uniform, tanned appearance

Ears: Position of auricles is appropriate and symmetric. Color is consistent with skin tone. No lumps or deformities. Right auricle and tragus are tender to palpation. Right ear canal is red and swollen. No cerumen in canal. Right TM is flat, intact, and pearly gray; landmarks identified; and cone of light in five-o'clock position. Left ear canal is without erythema, swelling, discharge, and cerum. Left TM negative. Acuity good (to whispered voice). Weber midline, AC > BC.

Pharynx: Light pink with no exudates, swelling, or ulcerations; tonsils 1+ (normal)

Neck: No adenopathy

Lungs: Thorax symmetric on inspection, no audible breath sounds, good expansion, all lung fields CTA

A: Possible otitis externa.

P:
1. Call primary care provider, and describe findings.
2. Instruct patient to see primary care provider immediately.
3. Educate patient about the potential harm that can occur if you flush the ear when you have ear pain.
4. Educate patient about how to lower risk of recurrent otitis externa.

Pharmacist: *Josephine Gray, Pharm.D.*

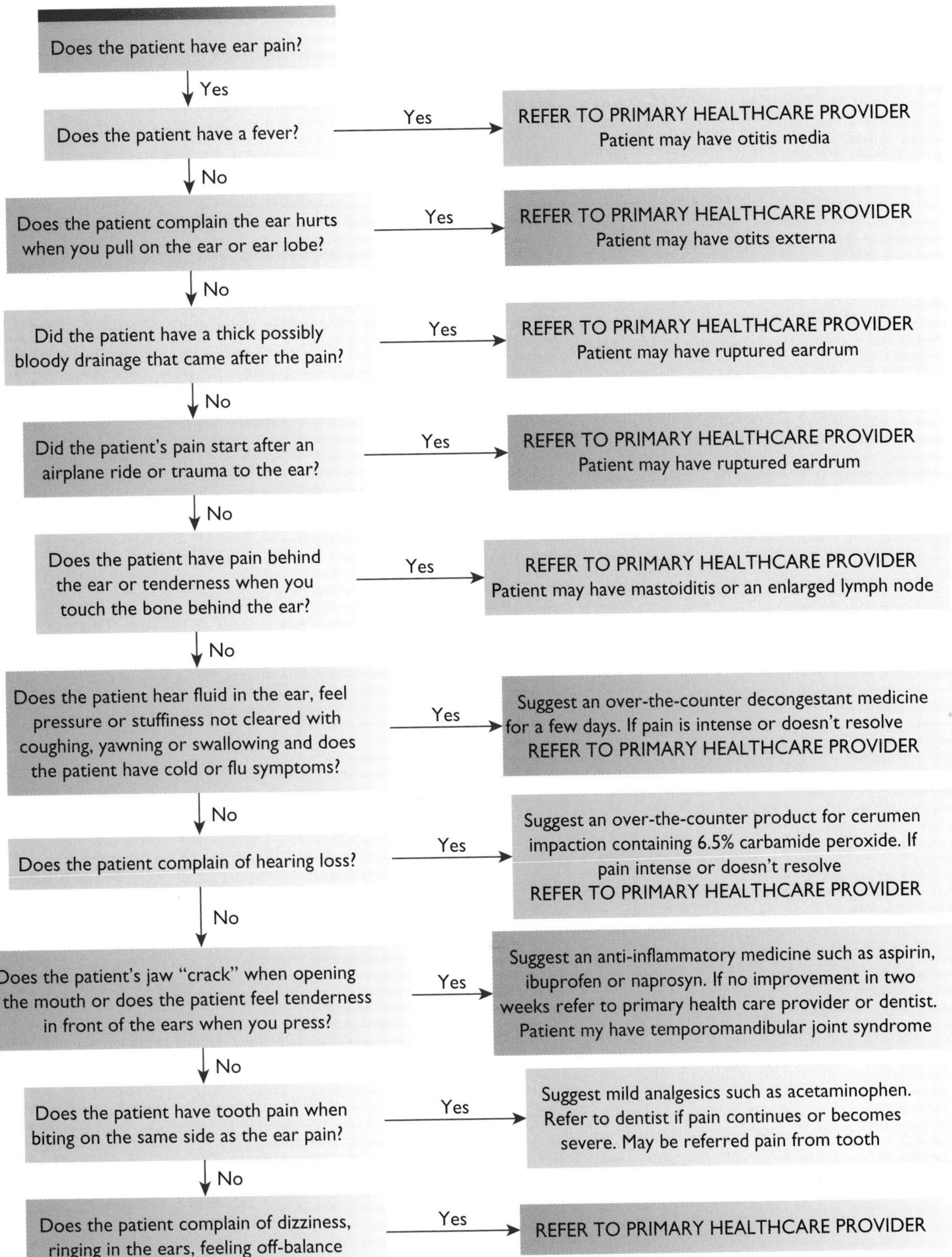

FIGURE 9-23 ■ Decision tree for ear pain.

Self-Assessment Questions

1. Compare and contrast the signs and symptoms of OM and otitis externa.
2. Outline the proper technique for performing an otoscopic examination. How does this technique change when performing the examination on a child?
3. List the landmarks of the inner ear that are visible through the tympanic membrane on a normal otoscopic examination.
4. Outline the proper technique for performing the Weber and the Rinne tests.
5. When performing the Weber test, how does the lateralization of sound differ in unilateral conductive hearing loss compared to unilateral sensorineural hearing loss?
6. When performing the Rinne test, how do air conduction and bone conduction of sound differ in patients with conductive compared to patients with sensorineural hearing loss?

Critical Thinking Questions

1. A 5-year-old girl is brought into the pharmacy with her mother. Her mother states that the girl is complaining of ear pain and requests a refill on the amoxicillin that was filled at the pharmacy 3 weeks ago. The pharmacist notes that the child has cotton balls in her ears. What should the pharmacist do? What questions should the pharmacist ask the child? What questions should the pharmacist ask the mother? Should the pharmacist refill the prescription?
2. A 68-year-old woman presents to your pharmacy complaining of ringing in her ears and dizziness for 2 weeks. Her pharmacy profile indicates she has coronary artery disease (myocardial infarction 3 years ago) and osteoarthritis, for which she takes a baby aspirin daily, Vioxx, and metoprolol. During the patient interview, what questions should the pharmacist ask? What physical examination techniques should be performed? What findings would require a referral to her primary care provider?

Bibliography

Biedlingmaier JF. Two ear problems you may need to refer. Postgrad Med 1994;96(5):141–148.

Cochrane DG, Marlowe FI, Reich JJ., et al. Ear emergencies. Patient Care 1991;August:90–113.

Dowell SF, Butler JC, Glebink GS. Acute otitis media: management and surveillance in an era of pneumococcal resistance—a report from drug-resistance *Steptococcus pneumoniae* Therapeutic Working Group. Pediatr Infect Dis J 1999;18:1–9.

Dowell SF, Marcy SM, Phillips WR, et al. Principles of judicious use of antimicrobial agents for pediatric upper respiratory tract infections. Pediatrics 1998;101:165–171.

Duguid G. Managing ocular flashes and floaters. Practitioner 1998;242:302–304.

Elder M, Rhodri D. Contact lenses and their complications. Practitioner 1993;237:509–512.

Fiscella RG, Jensen MK. Ophthalmic Disorders. In: Berardi RR, DeSimone EM, Newton GD, et al. (eds). Handbook of nonprescription drugs. 13th Edition. Washington, DC: American Pharmaceutical Association, 2002:543–570.

Godrich J. The ageing eye. Practitioner 1993;237:514–518.

Janda AM. Ophthalmic disorders in primary care. Hospital Physician 1993;March:46–50.

King RA. Common ocular signs and symptoms in childhood. Pediatr Clin North Am 1993;40:753–766.

Kruk P, Farber ME. Ocular manifestations of systemic disease: six illustrated cases. Patient Care 1998;April:111–137.

Krypel L. Otic Disorders. In: Berardi RR, DeSimone EM, Newton GD, et al (eds). Handbook of nonprescription drugs. 13th Edition. Washington, DC: American Pharmaceutical Association, 2002: 603–620.

Lesar TS. Glaucoma. In: Dipiro JT, Talbert RL, Yee GC, et al., eds. Pharmacotherapy: a pathophysiologic approach. 4th ed. Stamford, CT: Appleton & Lange, 1999:1466–1488.

MacKenna BR, Callander R. Illustrated physiology. 6th ed. New York: Churchill Livingstone, 1997:265–287.

Management of acute otitis media. Summary, Evidence Report/Technology Assessment: Number 15, June 2000. Rockville, MD: Agency for Healthcare Quality and Research (http://www.ahrq.gov/clinic/otitisum.htm).

Martini FH, Timmons MJ. Human anatomy. 2nd ed. Upper Saddle River, NJ: Prentice-Hall, 1997:455–477.

Matoba AY. Acute bacterial infections of eyelids and tarsal plate. Ophthalmol Clin North Am 1992;5(2):169–176.

Morrow GL, Abbott RL. Conjunctivitis. Am Fam Physician 1998;57:735–746.

Murray S. Ocular emergencies. Practitioner 1993;237:495–498.

Murtagh J. The painful ear. Aust Fam Physician 1991;20:1779–1783.

Olsen KD, Schnidler RA. Earache in adults: sifting the clues. Patient Care 1990;March:94–108.

Panizza F. Tropical ear. Aust Fam Physician 1994;23:2095–2101.

Potsic WP. Office pediatric otology. Otolaryngol Clin North Am 1992;25:781–789.

Richer M, Deschenes M. Upper respiratory tract infections. In: Dipiro JT, Talbert RL, Yee GC, et al., eds. Pharmacotherapy: a pathophysiologic approach. 4th ed. Stamford, CT: Appleton & Lange, 1999:1671–1684.

Scott C, Dhillon B. Conjunctivitis. Practitioner 1998;242:305.

Soparkar CN, Wilhelmus KR, Koch DD, et al. Acute and chronic conjunctivitis due to over-the-counter ophthalmic decongestants. Arch Ophthalmol 1997;115:34–38.

Stool SE, Berg AO, Berman S, et al. Otitis media with effusion in young children. Clinical practice guideline No. 12. Washington, DC: AHCPR Publication 94-0622. July 1994.

Wald ER. Conjunctivitis in infants and children. Pediatr Infect Dis J 1997;16:817–820.

Weber CM, Eichenbaum JW. Acute red eye: differentiating viral conjunctivitis from other, less common causes. Postgrad Med 1997;101:185–196.

Weinberger DG, Andersen PE. Diagnosis and treatment of common ear, nose and throat disorders. Hospital Physician 1996;June:11–23.

Wilson J. Common ENT problems. Practitioner 1994:238:453–460.

Woolford T, Lau M, Farrington T. Avoiding the pitfalls in ENT. Practitioner 1994;238:482–487.

CHAPTER

10

Head and Neck

Raylene M. Rospond and Michele Faulkner

GLOSSARY TERMS

- Acromegaly
- Acute sinusitis
- Chronic sinusitis
- Cushing's disease
- Gingivitis
- Graves' disease
- Hydrocephalus
- Macroencephalopathy
- Microencephalopathy
- Periodontitis
- Pharyngitis
- Phonophobia
- Photophobia
- Rhinitis
- Rhinorrhea

ANATOMY AND PHYSIOLOGY OVERVIEW

The head and neck comprise the skull, related muscles, and internal structures that support the functions of the special senses and the central nervous system. The head and neck also include structures for respiration, digestion, and endocrine function as well as some lymphatic structures. Thus, assessment of this region can be challenging. Because of the systematic approach used in this text, many of the internal structures of the head and neck are covered in other chapters (Box 10-1).

Box 10-1

STRUCTURES OF THE HEAD AND NECK

- Brain[a]
- Cranial nerves[a]
- Ears[b]
- Eyes[b]
- Nose
- Mouth
- Muscles of the head and neck
- Paranasal sinuses
- Pharynx
- Skull

[a]Discussed in detail in Chapter 18.
[b]Discussed in detail in Chapter 9.

Skull

The skull is composed of 22 flat, irregular bones that are tightly adjoined by sutures. The skull houses and protects the brain, and it positions and protects the eyes, ears, and teeth (Fig. 10-1). The cranial bones include the frontal bone of the forehead, the temporal bones above and behind the ears, the occipital bone at the back of the head, and the parietal bones, which join to form the roof of the cranium.

The face, which is generally described as extending from the natural hairline to the chin and from one ear across the front of the head to the other ear, is comprised of a series of bones that are also considered to be part of the skull. The mandible, the only skull bone that is freely moveable, makes up the lower jaw and chin, and it holds the lower set of the teeth. The upper set of teeth are held by the maxilla, which are located on either side of the nasal bones. The maxilla extend upward and form the openings that hold the eyes. On either side of the face are the zy-

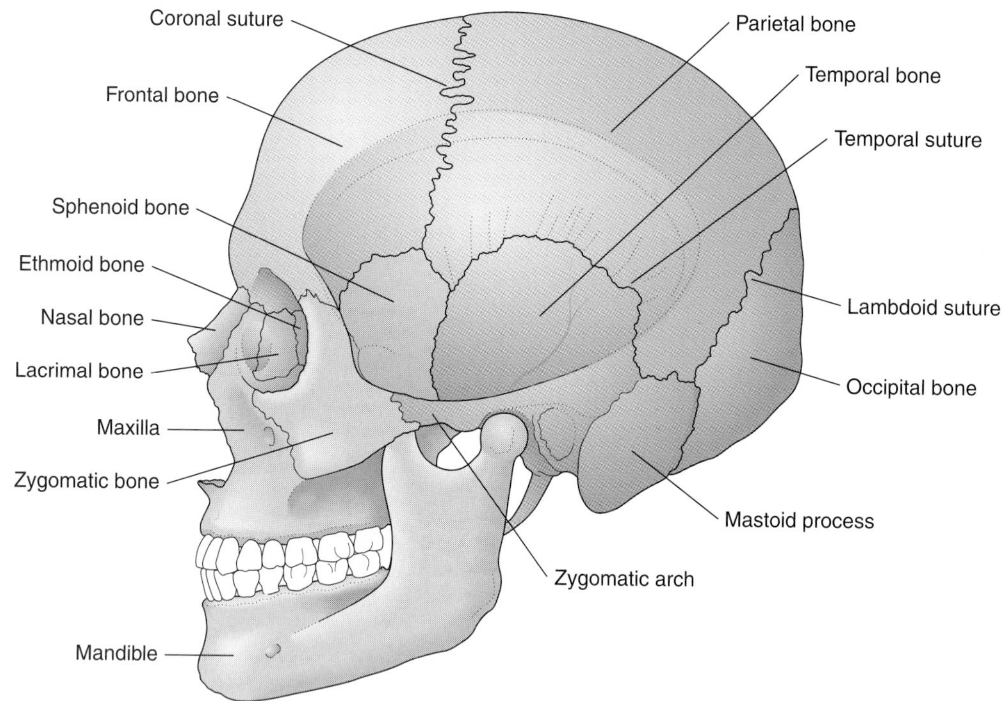

FIGURE 10-1 ■ The skull.

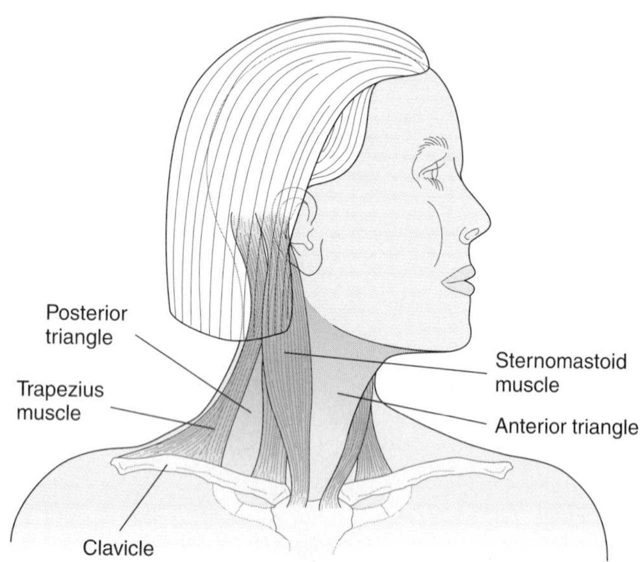

FIGURE 10-2 ■ Muscles of the neck.

gomatic bones, which are commonly referred to as "cheek bones."

Muscles of the Neck

The neck is divided into two triangles by the sternocleidomastoid muscle (Fig. 10-2). The anterior triangle is bounded by the mandible and the sternocleidomastoid muscle, which meet at the body's midline. Midline structures of the neck are located in the anterior triangle. The posterior triangle is bounded by the trapezius muscle, the sternocleidomastoid muscle, and the clavicle.

The muscles of the face that are responsible for creating facial expressions are attached superficially. They include the muscles that close the eye (orbicularis oculi) and that aid in lip movement (orbicularis oris) as well as the buccinator, or "cheek muscle," that helps to hold food stationary in the mouth for adequate chewing. Several other muscles involved in mastication and jaw movement include the lateral pterygoid, which opens the mouth, as well as the temporalis muscle (extending from the side of the skull) and the masseter muscle, which are responsible for closing the mouth. Along with the lateral pterygoid muscle, the medial pterygoid aids in the lateral movement of the jaw. These two muscles are behind the maxilla and lie too deep to be palpated.

Structures of the Head and Neck

The major internal structures of the head and neck include the brain, paranasal sinuses, eyes, ears, nose, mouth, pharynx, trachea, lymph nodes, and the parotid, submandibular, sublingual, and thyroid glands. Internal structures that are discussed in this chapter include the nose, paranasal sinuses, mouth, pharynx, and lymph nodes of the head and neck.

Nose

The nose is the primary passageway for air entering the respiratory system and the main organ involved in the sense of smell (Fig. 10-3). Air enters the nasal cavity through the nares, then passes into the widened area known as the vestibule. The air then continues through the narrow nasal passage to the nasopharynx. The ala is the lateral outside wing of the nose on either side. The collumella divides the two nares and is continuous inside with the nasal septum. The cartilage of the septum

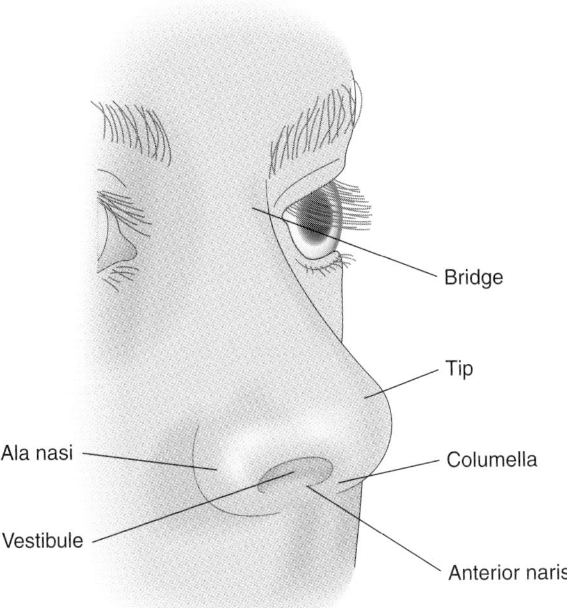

FIGURE 10-3 ■ The nose.

supports the bridge and apex (i.e., the tip) of the nose. The nasal septum is the wall that separates the right and left nasal cavities.

Inside, the nasal cavity extends back over the roof of the mouth (Fig. 10-4). The lateral walls of each nasal cavity contain three parallel bony projects: the superior, middle, and inferior turbinates. The turbinates slow the movement of air by creating swirls and eddies in the airflow pattern. This allows the air to be warmed and humidified and dust to be removed before the air reaches the respiratory tract. Nasal mucosa appears redder than oral mucosa because of the rich blood supply, which is present to warm the inhaled air. Below each turbinate is a cleft, the meatus, that is named according to the turbinate above it. The nasolacrimal duct drains into the interior meatus, whereas the middle meatus drains most of the paranasal sinuses. Their openings are not usually visible. The nasal cavity opens into the nasopharynx at the internal nares. The rhythmic movements of the nasal cilia cause the mucous blanket of the nose to move posteriorly, where it is swallowed. Any foreign particles caught in the cilia or mucus are then removed through the gastrointestinal tract and do not reach the lungs.

Paranasal Sinuses

The paranasal sinuses are air-filled chambers that open into the nasal cavities and are contained within the frontal, sphenoid, ethmoid, and maxillary bones (Fig. 10-5). Sinuses make skull bones lighter, resonate during sound production, and produce mucus, which functions to humidify the air and to trap dust and microorganisms. Mucus is continually released into the nasal cavities and passed back toward the throat, where it is swallowed.

Mouth

The lips are located on the upper and lower margin of the mouth and are made of muscular folds covered by skin on the outside and by a mucous membrane on the inside. The mouth is lined by oral mucosa that forms the gums, or gingivae, that surround the base of each tooth (Fig. 10-6). The gingivae are pale or coral pink in lighter-skinned people and diffusely or partly brown in darker-skinned individuals. The roof of the oral cavity is formed by the hard and soft palates. The hard palate is so named because of the bony process underneath; it makes up the largest section of the roof of the mouth. Muscle, rather than bone, underlies the soft palate, which is located at the back of the mouth. The tongue is a large muscle attached to the floor of the mouth by a thin band of mucous membrane called the frenulum and acts to process food, prepare food for swallowing, and analyze food through touch, temperature, and taste receptors. The teeth (32 in adults) are composed of dentin and lie in bony sockets that expose the enamel-covered crowns. The uvula is a fleshy extension that dangles from the posterior margin of the soft palate and helps to prevent food from entering the pharynx prematurely.

The primary purpose of the salivary glands is to keep the environment of the mouth moist. They also aid in digestion (specifically, the breakdown of starches), but their role is negligible at best. The sublingual gland is located beneath the floor of the mouth. Saliva is secreted from this gland through several small ducts. The submandibular duct, which originates with the submandibular gland in the neck, is adjacent to the frenulum of the tongue.

Pharynx

The nose and mouth connect to each other by a common passageway or chamber called the pharynx (Fig. 10-7). Along with the larynx, or "voice box," the pharynx makes up what is commonly referred to as the throat. This structure is shared by the digestive and respiratory systems. It extends from the internal nares to the entrance of the esophagus, and it is divided into three regions:

- The nasopharynx is the uppermost portion of the pharynx. It extends from the base of the skull to the soft

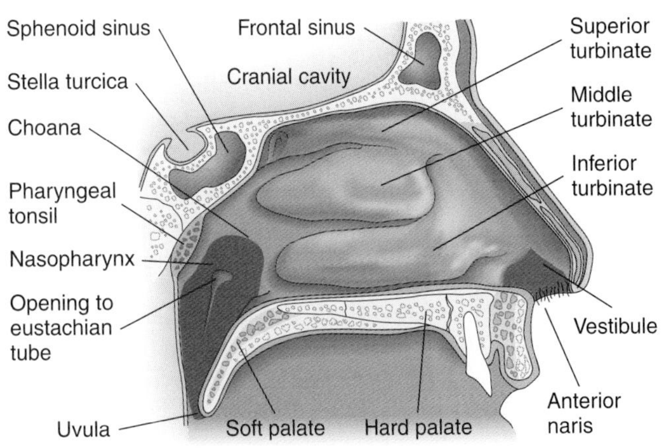

FIGURE 10-4 ■ Turbinates of the nose.

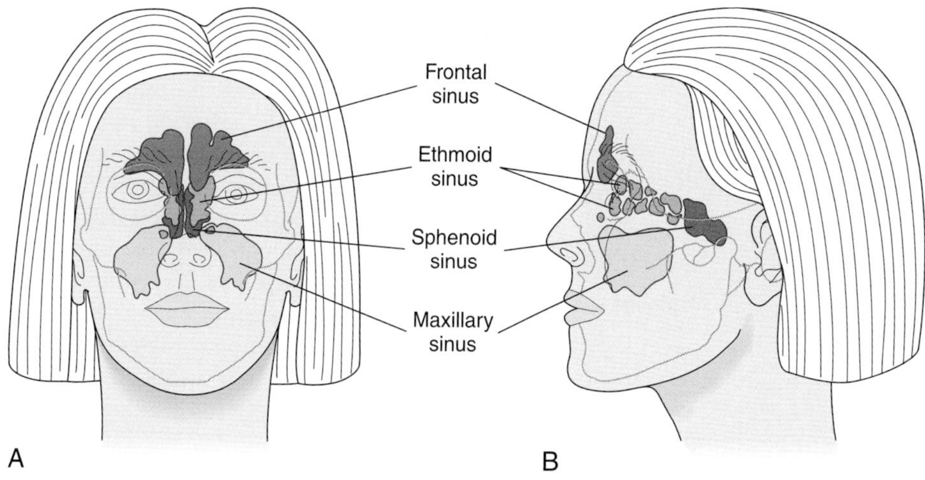

FIGURE 10-5 ■ Paranasal sinuses. **(A)** Frontal view. **(B)** Lateral view.

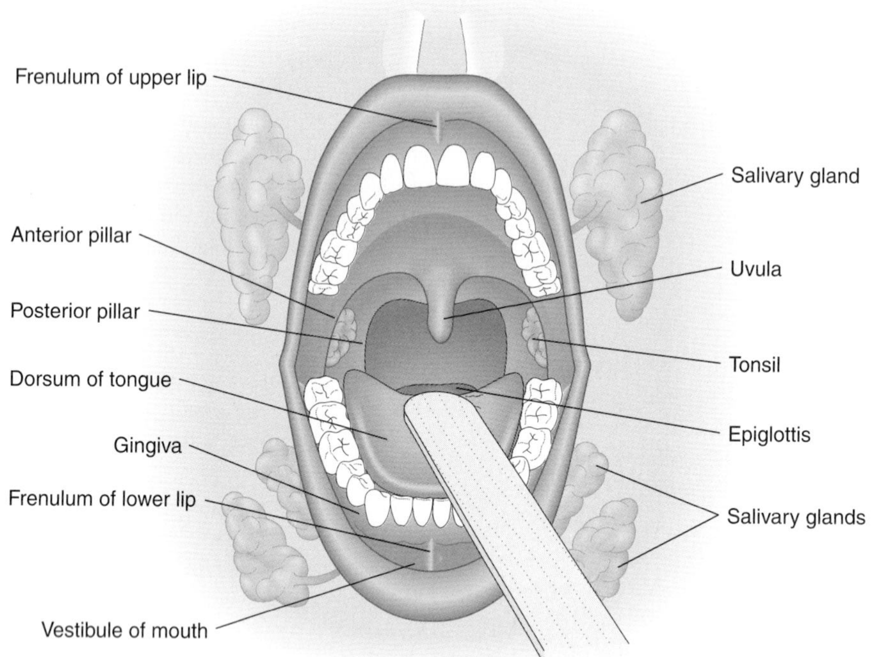

FIGURE 10-6 ■ Structures of the mouth.

palate and is connected to the nasal cavity via the internal nares. The soft palate separates it from the oral cavity. The pharyngeal (adenoid) tonsils and the openings of the auditory tubes are located within this portion.

- The oropharynx extends between the soft palate and the base of the tongue. The palatine tonsils lie just below the palate on either side of the passageway between the oral cavity and the oropharynx. They are made of lymphoid tissue and are housed within epithelium (like that found in the oral cavity). The high incidence of infection at this site is hypothesized to result from two indentations in the epithelial layer that may trap viruses and bacteria.
- The laryngopharynx is between the entrance to the esophagus and the hyoid bone. The hyoid is a small, U-shaped bone in the front of the neck between the larynx and the mandible.

Lymph Nodes

The primary function of the lymphatic system is the production, maintenance, and distribution of lymphocytes. The lymph nodes (also called the lymph glands) are oval lymphoid organs ranging in diameter from 1 to 25 mm. The shape of a typical lymph node resembles that of a lima bean. The location of the lymph nodes in the head and neck are listed in Table 10-1 and can be seen in Figure 10-8. The deep cervical chain is often obscured by the overlying sternocleidomastoid muscle. The tonsillar and supraclavicular nodes may be palpable, however, because they lie at the two extremes of this muscle. Lymph nodes filter and purify

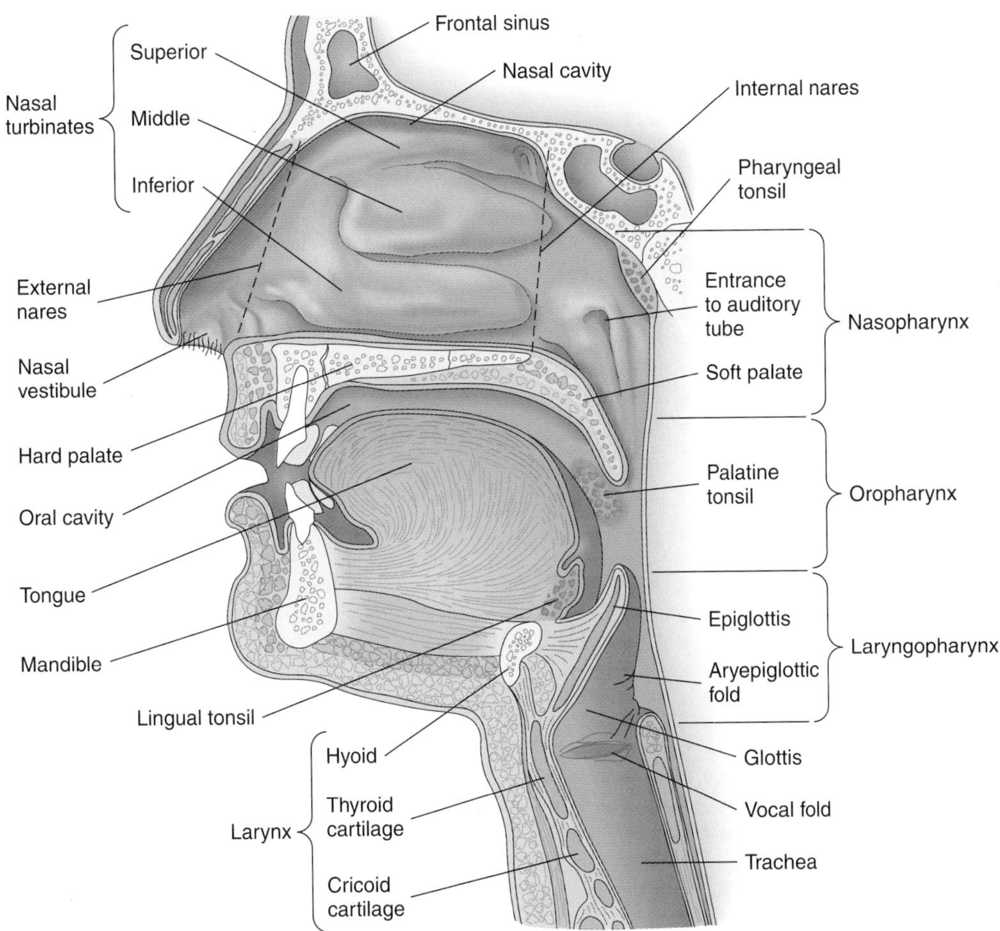

FIGURE 10-7 ■ Pharynx.

TABLE 10-1 ➤ LOCATION OF LYMPH NODES IN THE HEAD AND NECK

LYMPH NODE	LOCATION FOR PALPATION
Preauricular	In front of the ear
Postauricular	Superficial to the mastoid process
Occipital	At the base of the skull posteriorly
Tonsillar	At the angle of the mandible
Submandibular	Midway between the angle and the tip of the mandible
Submental	In the midline, a few centimeters behind the tip of the mandible
Superficial cervical	Superficial to the sternomastoid muscle
Posterior cervical	Along the anterior edge of the trapezius muscle
Deep cervical chain	Under the sternomastoid muscle; often cannot be palpated; hook your thumbs and fingers around either side of the muscle to find them
Supraclavicular	Deep in the angle formed by the clavicle and the sternomastoid muscle

lymph, removing 99% of the antigens present before it reaches the venous system. The largest lymph nodes are found where peripheral lymphatics connect with the trunk, in regions such as the base of the neck, the axillae, and the groin. Lymph nodes are also liberally distributed in areas that are particularly susceptible to injury or invasion. "Swollen glands" usually indicate inflammation or infection of peripheral structures.

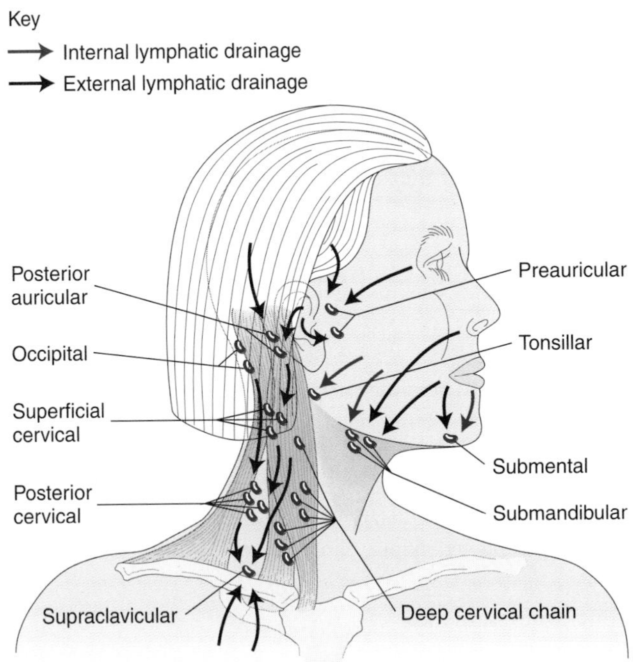

FIGURE 10-8 ■ Lymph nodes and lymphatic drainage of the head and neck.

Special Considerations

Pediatric Patients

The skull of an infant is not completely ossified. Spaces known as fontanelles, or "soft spots," exist between the bone sutures. These spaces leave the infant brain more vulnerable to injury. The anterior fontanelle, which is located on the top of the head, is typically closed by 18 months of age. The posterior fontanelle, which is located at the back of the head, closes by 3 months.

The maxillary and ethmoid sinuses are well developed at birth, whereas the frontal and sphenoid sinuses, which originate from the ethmoid sinuses, are not fully developed until 10 years of age. The palatine tonsils are typically larger in the young. Lymphocytes found here play an important role in early immunity. Lymphoid tissues grow rapidly during late childhood and remain prominent in adolescents. Therefore, cervical lymph nodes are often easily palpable in teenagers.

Geriatric Patients

As an individual ages, the facial bones and orbits appear more prominent, and the facial skin sags because of decreased elasticity, decreased subcutaneous tissue, and decreased moisture in the skin. The lower face may look smaller if teeth have been lost. In the mouth and pharynx, the mucosa atrophies, and the epithelium thins. Because this is most prevalent in the cheek and tongue, loss of taste buds (along with decreased salivary secretions) results in a reduction of taste sensation as well as increased risk of oral ulcerations. Periodontal disease and loss of teeth may also contribute to poor nutrition in the elderly. Tonsils gradually become smaller after the age of 5 years and may be invisible in adults. The ability to palpate cervical lymph nodes diminishes with age, but submandibular glands become easier to feel in older people.

Pregnant Patients

Because of fluctuating changes in hormonal balance during pregnancy, the gingivae often become mildly inflamed, and hyperplasia may be noted. Pregnant women may also experience nasopharyngeal stuffiness or obstruction, with symptoms profound enough that they may seek medical assistance.

PATHOLOGY OVERVIEW

Headache

Headache is a common patient complaint. The pain of a headache may exist on its own, or it may be experienced as a result of a local or systemic illness. Of the multiple headache types, the most common are tension headache, migraine headache, and cluster headache. The diagnosis of headache type frequently can be made simply by taking a thorough patient history.

Tension Headaches

Tension headache pain is typically described as "band-like." Patients may tell of tightness and pressure on both sides of the head. The pain is usually constant as opposed to pulsating, but the intensity may vacillate during a single episode. Most tension headaches are acute; however, a minority of patients may be diagnosed with chronic tension headache if pain occurs on at least 15 occasions during a single month. This chronic type of headache is more prevalent in females. The acute form of tension headache can often be attributed to stressful situations, whereas chronic tension headache exists regardless of the patient's stress level. Anxiety, depression, and related symptoms are often present in those who experience frequent tension headaches. Excessive muscular contraction, brought about by feelings of uneasiness or anxiety, may contribute to headache pain; this contraction is commonly noted in the area of the temporal and masseter muscles. Tension headache is sometimes related to temporomandibular joint syndrome.

Although more common in adults, tension headache may occur in children. Neurologic symptoms seldom are associated with this particular headache type. Mild analgesic medications are frequently employed to control tension headache pain. Chronic use of these agents on a daily basis, however, may lead to headache rebound as the analgesia wears off.

Migraine Headaches

The pain of migraine headache is also noted more frequently in women than in men. Age at onset of the first episode is usually between 15 and 35 years, but these headaches are most frequent between the ages of 35 and 40. Migraine pain is typically felt on one side of the head only and is most often centered in the area of the temple; however, children may experience bifrontal pain. Headache duration can be anywhere from 4 hours to 3 days. Unlike tension headache pain, migraine pain is usually of a pulsating or throbbing nature, and it may be made worse by physical activity. Migraines are sometimes accompanied by nausea and vomiting, **phonophobia** (sensitivity to sound), and **photophobia** (sensitivity to light). Often, patients with a migraine headache will seek out dark, quiet places until the pain is relieved. At least half of migraine sufferers experience a prodrome (a symptom or set of symptoms unique to the patient that warn of an impending headache). Symptoms may be psychologic, neurologic, constitutional, or autonomic in nature. Approximately 10% of patients experience an aura, which usually lasts less than 1 hour. Auras typically manifest as sensory changes. Patients may see flashes of light, smell something that is not really there, or experience tingling or numbness in the extremities.

Migraine headache is believed to result from a combination of vascular and neuronal changes. Initial vasoconstriction eventually leads to distention of the blood vessels in the head. This places pressure on nerve fibers and allows protein leakage that produces a sterile inflammation, causing migraine pain. Changes in hormone levels have been linked to migraine headache, because 60% of women with this type of headache have pain at menstruation. Changes in weather or sleep patterns, occupational exposure to noxious substances, use of vasodilating medications or hormones, drug withdrawal, missing meals, and particular foodstuffs (especially fatty foods and chocolate) have been linked to migraine headache as well.

Most patients headaches are given medication to take at the first sign of a migraine headache. Whether a patient needs prophylactic therapy to prevent migraines depends on the headache severity, frequency, and how significantly the pain affects the patient's quality of life. Mild analgesics usually are employed initially. Ergotamine derivatives and serotonin-receptor stimulants such as sumatriptan are used to offset vascular dilation. Narcotic pain relievers are rarely used for migraine pain, however, because frequent use can lead to rebound headache.

Cluster Headaches

Cluster headaches are usually first noted during the third decade of life. Men are affected more often than women. As with migraine headaches, the pain of cluster headaches is typically unilateral. Cluster headache pain is primarily described as being centered around the eye, and it is constant and severe rather than throbbing. Concomitant symptoms may include tearing of the eye on the affected side, nasal stuffiness, drooping of the eyelid, nausea, vomiting, phonophobia, and photophobia. Cluster headaches can be episodic or chronic, with each cluster of headaches lasting from 2 weeks to 3 months. Individual headaches last anywhere from 15 minutes to 3 hours. Patients are often in remission for as long as 2 years before another cluster of headaches begins.

The mechanism of a cluster headache is similar to that of a migraine headache. Hypoxia also appears to be a factor, because pure oxygen relieves pain in as many as 70% of sufferers. Precipitators of pain are the same as for migraine headache. If prophylaxis is employed, it should continue until the patient has experienced a headache-free period of at least 2 weeks.

Alternative causes of general headache pain include bleeding in the head, tumors, infection, concussion, and uncontrolled high blood pressure. Patients should be questioned about recent traumas and past medical history. If the headache is accompanied by a stiff neck and a fever, meningitis should be suspected. In patients with stiff neck but without fever, a subarachnoid hemorrhage should be ruled out by a physician. Drowsiness and confusion may be signs of a cerebrovascular problem that should be evaluated immediately.

Sinusitis

Sinusitis is classified as acute or chronic based on pathologic findings and duration of infection. Symptomatology like that of a common cold (e.g., purulent nasal discharge, headache, facial pain, fever, cough, and nasal obstruction) that remains for more than 7 to 10 days is classified as **acute sinusitis.** This is a common condition, and it is associated with bacterial and viral infections of the upper respiratory tract. Typical bacterial pathogens in children include *Streptococcus pneumonia, Haemophilus influenzae,* and *Moraxella catarrhalis.* Rhinovirus, influenza virus, adenovirus, and parainfluenza virus are common causes of viral sinusitis. **Chronic sinusitis** may be diagnosed if the disease has been present for 8 weeks, symptoms have been present for periods greater than 10 days on more than four occasions over a 1-year period, or an individual repeatedly fails to respond to medical therapy.

Signs and symptoms of sinusitis are outlined in Box 10-2; however, these may vary between children and adults. In children, halitosis (not related to pharyngitis or poor dental hygiene) or morning periorbital swelling (with or without concomitant pain) may be signs of a sinus infection. Headache pain related to the sinuses is rare in children younger than 5 years, because the frontal sinuses are not yet fully developed.

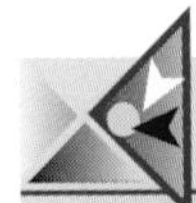

Box 10-2

SIGNS AND SYMPTOMS OF SINUSITIS

SIGNS

- Mucopurulent nasal discharge
- Abnormal transillumination
- Poor response to decongestants
- Headaches that respond poorly to analgesics

SYMPTOMS

- Colored nasal discharge
- Nasal congestion
- Facial pain (particularly unilateral)
- Maxillary toothache
- Fever
- Cough

Many symptoms of sinusitis resolve within 48 hours without medical treatment. Goals of therapy include symptomatic relief, improving sinus function, and preventing intracranial complications by eradicating the causative pathogen. Antibiotics are the primary therapy for bacterial sinusitis, with amoxicillin being the drug of choice. Trimethoprim/sulfamethoxazole is preferred for patients who are allergic to penicillin. Acute sinusitis is usually treated for 10 to 14 days. Nasal spray decongestants, oral decongestants, or both may be used as adjunct therapy. Because of tolerance and possible rebound congestion, nasal decongestants should not be used for more than 72 hours; these topical agents should also be used with caution in children. Because they may inhibit mucus clearance, antihistamines should be avoided in patients without true allergy.

Allergic Rhinitis

Rhinitis is an inflammation of the nasal mucous membrane. Allergic rhinitis is caused by exposure of the mucous membrane to inhaled allergenic materials, and it is one of the most common medical disorders, affecting 20% of the American population. Allergic rhinitis may be seasonal (intermittent symptoms) or perennial (constant symptoms). A family history of allergic rhinitis significantly increases an individual's risk for developing this condition. The peak incidence occurs in childhood and adolescence, but 70% of all individuals at risk for this disease develop symptoms by the age of 30 years. The signs and symptoms of allergic rhinitis are listed in Box 10-3.

Allergic rhinitis must be treated properly to reduce the risk of developing complications. Untreated symptoms may lead to inability to sleep, chronic malaise, fatigue, and poor work or school performance. Other complications may include loss of

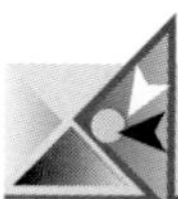

Box 10-3

SIGNS AND SYMPTOMS OF ALLERGIC RHINITIS

SIGNS

- Allergic shiners
- Transverse nasal crease
- Adenoidal breathing
- Pale, bluish, edematous nasal turbinates
- Tearing
- Conjunctival redness and edema
- Periorbital swelling

SYMPTOMS

- Clear rhinorrhea
- Sneezing
- Nasal congestion
- Post-nasal drip
- Itching eyes, ears, nose, or palate

smell or taste, sinusitis, or development of nasal polyps. Patients with allergic rhinitis may also be at risk for development of acute or chronic otitis media with effusion, asthma, recurrent and chronic sinusitis, as well as facial and dental problems. The goal for treatment of allergic rhinitis is to minimize—or to prevent—symptoms. This is best accomplished by allergen avoidance, medications for the prevention or treatment of symptoms, and specific immunotherapy. Suitable medications include antihistamines (systemic, ophthalmic, and intranasal), decongestants (systemic and topical), intranasal corticosteroids, mast cell stablizers, and intranasal anticholinergics.

Gingivitis

Gingivitis, an inflammation of the gingivae, is the most common—and the mildest—form of periodontal disease (Fig. 10-9). The primary cause of periodontal disease is accumulated bacterial plaque. During the early stages, microorganisms in plaque produce harmful products, such as acids, toxins, and enzymes,

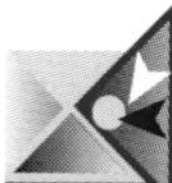

Box 10-4

SIGNS AND SYMPTOMS OF GINGIVITIS

SIGNS

- Erythema of the gums
- Bluish hue to the gums
- Bleeding on probing
- A sulcular depth exceeding 4 mm when measured by a periodontal probe
- Swollen, puffy gingiva

SYMPTOMS

- Bleeding when brushing teeth
- Tender gums
- Red gums

that damage tissues. This tissue damage results in dilatation and proliferation of gingival capillaries, increased flow of gingival fluid, and increased flow of blood, with resultant erythema of the gingivae. Signs and symptoms of gingivitis are outlined in Box 10-4. Removal and control of supragingival plaque is the key to reversing gingivitis. Preventing the development of subgingival plaque is vital to avoid the development of **periodontitis,** an inflammation of the tissue supporting the teeth (Fig. 10-10).

Acute necrotizing ulcerative gingivitis, or "trench mouth," is an acute bacterial infection characterized by necrosis and ulceration of the gingivae with underlying inflammation (Fig. 10-11). It can cause irreversible bone loss. Patients suffering from trench mouth complain of severe pain, bleeding gingivae, halitosis, foul taste, and increased salivation. They may also complain of lymphadenopathy and malaise.

Pharyngitis

Pharyngitis is an inflammation of the pharynx and surrounding lymphoid tissues that is often caused by viruses or bacteria (Fig. 10-12). In children younger than 4 years, viruses are usually the cause. Group A β-hemolytic streptococci is the most common bacterial pathogen and is responsible for 10% of sympto-

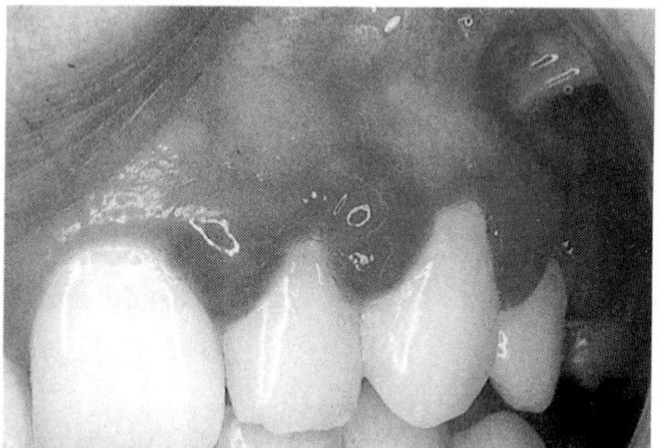

FIGURE 10-9 ■ Gingivitis. (See Color Plate 26; reprinted with permission from Tyldesley WR. A color atlas of orofacial diseases. 2nd ed. London: Wolfe Medical Publications, 1991.)

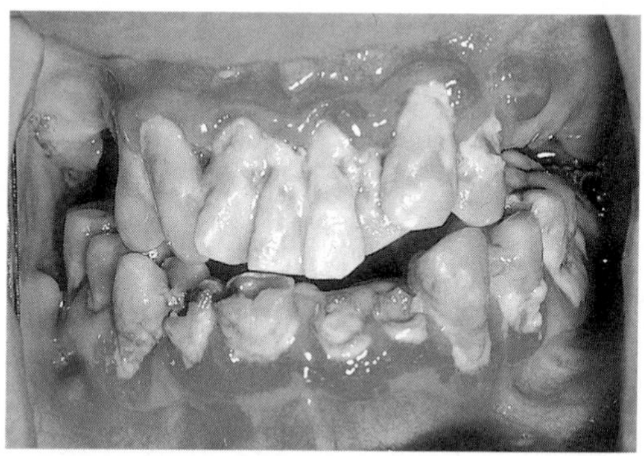

FIGURE 10-10 ■ Periodontitis. (See Color Plate 27; courtesy of Dr. Tom McDavid.)

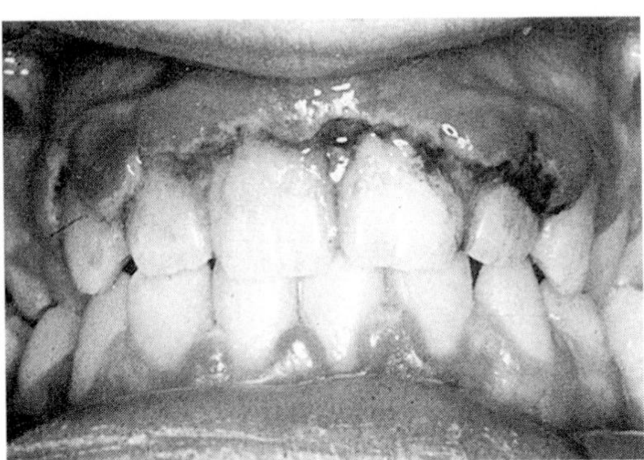

Figure 10-11 ■ Acute necrotizing ulcerative gingivitis. (See Color Plate 28; reprinted with permission from Tyldesley WR. A color atlas of orofacial diseases. 2nd ed. London: Wolfe Medical Publications, 1991.)

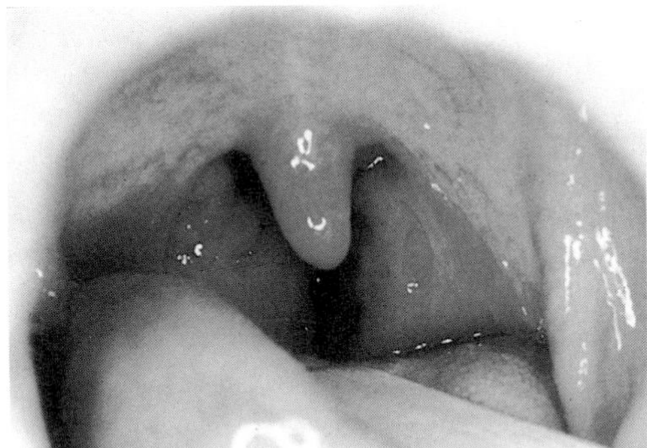

Figure 10-12 ■ Severe pharyngitis. (See Color Plate 29; reprinted with permission from Bickley LS. Bates' guide to physical examination and history taking. 7th ed. Philadelphia: Lippincott Williams & Wilkins, 1999:202.)

matic pharyngitis in adults and for 30% in children. The peak incidence of streptococcal pharyngitis occurs between 4 and 14 years of age. Accurately differentiating between viral and streptococcal pharyngitis is important because of the serious potential sequelae of infection with group A β-hemolytic streptococci, including abscesses, rheumatic fever, and glomerulonephritis.

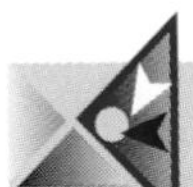

Box 10-5

SIGNS AND SYMPTOMS OF PHARYNGITIS

SIGNS

- Hyperemia of the pharynx
- Hypertrophied tonsils
- Tonsillar exudate
- Swollen, tender anterior cervical lymph nodes

SYMPTOMS

- Sore throat
- Dysphagia
- Fever

Common signs and symptoms associated with pharyngitis are listed in Box 10-5. Treatment of viral pharyngitis focuses on the management of symptoms. Oral antibiotic therapy for at least 10 days should be employed when bacterial pharyngitis is suspected. Penicillin is the drug of choice for pharyngitis caused by group A β-hemolytic streptococci. Ampicillin and amoxicillin offer no therapeutic advantages over penicillin. Macrolide antibiotics, such as erythromycin or azithromycin, may be used in penicillin-allergic patients. Recurrent episodes of streptococcal pharyngitis may be treated with cephalosporins that have activity against β-lactamase-producing bacteria.

Noninfectious causes of pharyngitis should be considered when there is difficulty establishing a diagnosis. Allergies, sinusitis, postnasal drip, and certain malignancies can affect the upper respiratory tract or pharynx directly. Exposure to irritating substances (e.g., cigarette smoke and other environmental pollutants); ingestion of hot foods, liquids, or caustic substances; as well as direct trauma to the pharynx should also be considered.

SYSTEM ASSESSMENT

Subjective Information

When assessing the head and neck, keep in mind that subjective patient data may relate to a number of pathologic states. Thorough subjective assessment helps the pharmacist to determine if the patient has a condition that can be self-treated or that should be referred to a primary care provider. Generally, it is best to avoid leading questions. In the case of headache, however, such questions may be necessary when gathering information about auras, because patients unfamiliar with migraine headaches probably will not connect things such as strange odors to an impending migraine.

Headache Pain

? INTERVIEW Describe your pain as completely as possible. Where is the pain concentrated? Describe what the pain feels like. Is it constant or intermittent? How often do you experience this pain? Does the pain occur at a particular time of day? How long does the pain last? Do you have any other symptoms that accompany the headache? Do you notice any strange sensations, visual changes, or smells before the headache? Describe them. When do these symptoms begin in relation to the beginning of the pain?

ABNORMALITIES Migraine pain usually is centered in the area of the temple, whereas cluster headaches are felt around the eye. Both types also typically are unilateral, as compared to tension headache, which is bilateral. Migraine headache pain is pulsatile, cluster headache pain is constant and sharp, and tension headache pain is associated with pressure and a squeezing sensation. Both cluster and migraine headaches may be accompanied by phonophobia and photophobia, nausea, and vomiting. Auras are not associated with cluster headaches, as they are with migraines.

? INTERVIEW Have you recently started or stopped taking any drugs? Do you work outside the home? What type of work to you do? Have your eating or sleeping habits recently changed? Have you recently experienced any falls or head trauma?

➤ ABNORMALITIES Medication withdrawal or initiation can be responsible for the onset of a headache. Vasodilators and hormonal therapy have been associated with migraine headache pain. Exposure to fumes or chemicals at work or around the home can cause headaches. Oversleeping has also been linked to migraine and cluster headache pain.

? INTERVIEW What relieves your headache pain? Have you been using medication to treat your headache? How often do you take it? Have you noticed any aching muscles during your headache? Where are these muscles located?

➤ ABNORMALITIES Overuse of analgesics for headache can cause rebound when the medication wears off. Tension headaches are often associated with unconscious tensing of muscles in relation to emotional stress, especially those associated with the temple, neck, and jaw.

Facial Pain

? INTERVIEW Tell me about this pain you have been experiencing. Point to the painful area. Do you have any other symptoms? Are you congested? Do you have pain anywhere on or near your face? Have you noticed any swelling? Do you have pain anywhere else? Are any areas painful to the touch?

➤ ABNORMALITIES Pain from sinusitis varies according to the sinus that is involved. Frontal sinus involvement may result in pain on the forehead. Maxillary sinus involvement can cause pain in the upper jaw, teeth, or cheek. Ethmoid sinus involvement can result in pain between the eyes and cause swelling of the eyelid. A sphenoid sinus infection may cause earaches, neck pain, and deep aching at the top of the head. Palpation of the frontal or maxillary sinuses often results in pain when infection is present.

? INTERVIEW Do you now or have you recently had a headache? If so, did it occur at a particular time of day? Describe the pain. Is it continuous, or does it come and go? Does anything make the pain worse?

➤ ABNORMALITIES Headache on awakening in the morning may result from sinus involvement. Sinus headache pain often varies with the position of the head, worsening when the head is lowered. Migraine, cluster, and tension headaches usually present with continuous pain.

? INTERVIEW Do you have any other symptoms anywhere on your body? Do you have a runny nose? If so, describe the color and consistency of the drainage. Do you have a cough? Is it a dry cough? Is there a particular time of day that it gets worse or better? Have you noticed a change in taste or smell? Are you having any difficulties chewing, swallowing, or speaking?

➤ ABNORMALITIES Drainage of mucus from the paranasal sinuses may cause pharyngitis and worsening cough at night. Infection of the teeth may result in facial pain or halitosis.

Rhinorrhea

? INTERVIEW Do you have a nasal discharge? Is it clear or colored? How long have you had it? Have you had it before? Does it impact your daily activities?

➤ ABNORMALITIES Rhinorrhea is a recurrent or chronic, watery nasal discharge. It may be caused by inflammatory or noninflammatory processes. Inflammatory rhinorrhea can be infectious (viral or bacterial) or noninfectious (allergic or nonallergic rhinitis) in nature. Bacterial rhinitis may product a colored discharge.

? INTERVIEW What other symptoms do you have? Are the symptoms present all through the year or only during selected times of the year? What factors aggravate these symptoms? Are the symptoms better or worse at home? At work? At school?

➤ ABNORMALITIES Viral rhinitis is usually caused by the common cold. It can occur at any time and has no pattern. The most common noninfectious cause of rhinorrhea is allergic rhinitis. Individuals suffering from year-round symptoms are more likely to have perennial allergic rhinitis. Symptoms associated with selected times of the year are consistent with seasonal allergic rhinitis. Most patients with vasomotor rhinitis complain of a blocked nose or feeling of nasal congestion. Conditions frequently observed in conjunction with rhinorrhea include purulent sinusitis, nasal polyps, otitis media, loss of hearing, chronic conjunctivitis, and mouth breathing.

? INTERVIEW Do you or anyone in your family have a history of allergies? If so, do your symptoms vary during different times of the year?

➤ ABNORMALITIES Allergic rhinitis is associated with concurrent atopic disease or family history.

? INTERVIEW Do you have a fever, sore throat, cough, vomiting, or diarrhea? Do you have sneezing, nasal congestion, or itching eyes, ears, nose, or palate?

ABNORMALITIES Patients suffering from viral rhinitis may also complain of sore throat, malaise, fatigue, and fever. Fever from infectious rhinitis is more common in children. Patients with allergic rhinitis rarely have fever, sore throat, vomiting, or diarrhea. Sneezing and itching are common with allergic rhinitis.

INTERVIEW What prescription or nonprescription medications are you currently taking? Which have you taken in the past to treat your symptoms? Are you allergic to any medications? Do you have any dietary restrictions?

ABNORMALITIES Rhinitis medicamentosa results from development of tachyphylaxis to topical decongestants.

Bleeding Gums

INTERVIEW How long have your gums been bleeding? Do your gums bleed when you brush or floss your teeth? Is the bleeding only in one area or in several? How long does the bleeding last? Do your gums bleed when you eat? Do your gums ever bleed without an identifiable cause? Do you have a history of problems with your gums or teeth? What medications were you taking around the time your gums began to bleed? What medications are you currently taking?

ABNORMALITIES Bleeding gums may occur with gingivitis. Marginal gingivitis should cause minimal bleeding with stimuli. The number of areas will vary depending on the severity of the gingivitis. As gingivitis progresses, bleeding may become spontaneous and include all areas of the gums. Medications that thin the blood, such as aspirin, heparin derivatives, and warfarin, may cause bleeding from the gums.

INTERVIEW Do you have any other symptoms? Have you noticed an area that is particularly irritated? Do you have a lesion or sore? Is the sore visible? What does it look like? Is there any drainage from the sore? Does the sore cause you discomfort? Have you noticed a change in taste? Have you noticed whether you have bad breath? Are your glands swollen? Have you had a fever? How long have the symptoms been present? Are these symptoms new, or have you had them before?

ABNORMALITIES Aphthous ulcers, or "canker sores," appear as small, round, painful ulcers with a white base surrounded by a red halo (Fig. 10-13). Acute necrotizing ulcerative gingivitis occurs suddenly in adolescents and young adults and is accompanied by fever, malaise, halitosis, and enlarged lymph nodes. Carcinomas of the tongue and mouth (Fig. 10-14) can result in bleeding from the mouth, halitosis, and lymphadenopathy.

INTERVIEW How often do you see your dentist? How often do you brush your teeth? How often do you floss your teeth? Do you use toothpaste? Are any of your teeth loose? Have any of your teeth fallen out? Do you wear dentures or a bridge? Do they fit tightly? Have they ever caused you to have sore places in your mouth?

ABNORMALITIES Gingivitis occurs from inadequate dental hygiene that results in the accumulation of plaque both in and around the gums. A history of tooth loss or any currently loose teeth may indicate severe gingivitis. Loose or malfitted dentures may cause inflammation or bleeding of the gums.

Sore Throat

INTERVIEW Is your throat sore now? Does it hurt to swallow? How long have you had a sore throat? Describe what it feels like. Is there a time of day when it feels worse or better? How often do you get a sore throat? Have you noticed any postnasal drip or sinus congestion?

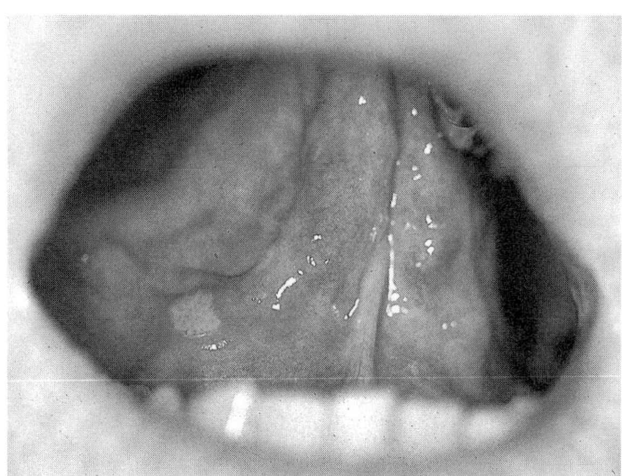

FIGURE 10-13 ■ Aphthous ulcer. (See Color Plate 30; reprinted with permission from Bickley LS. Bates' guide to physical examination and history taking. 7th ed., Philadelphia: Lippincott Williams & Wilkins, 1999:200.)

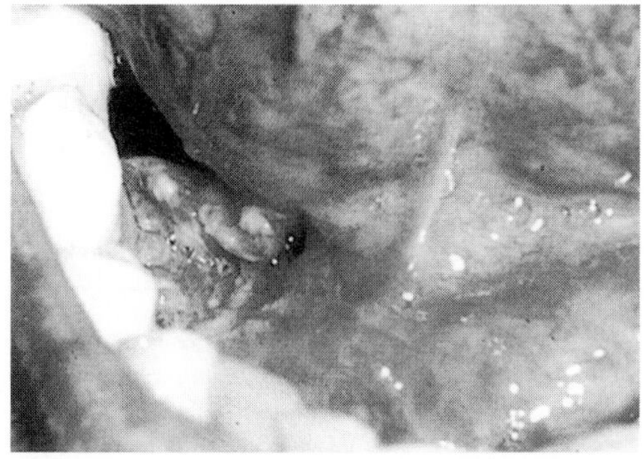

FIGURE 10-14 ■ Carcinoma of the mouth. (See Color Plate 31; reprinted with permission from Robinson HBG, Miller AS. Colby, Kerr, and Robinson's color atlas of oral pathology. Philadelphia: JB Lippincott, 1990.)

ABNORMALITIES Pharyngitis is synonymous with inflammation of the pharynx. Patients with pharyngitis are often referred to as having a "sore throat." Typically, the pain is most intense on swallowing. In mild cases, inflammation may not be readily apparent, and pain may be the only obvious symptom. Patients with postnasal drip often complain of increased pain in the middle of the night or on awakening in the morning because of increased throat contact with sinus or nasal drainage when in a recumbent position.

INTERVIEW Have you recently had a cold? Has anyone in your home recently been ill with a sore throat or a cold? Have you had a fever? When did the symptoms start? Is the sore throat accompanied by any other symptoms? Is the pain isolated to the throat, or do you feel discomfort somewhere else? Have you noticed any discoloration in the back of your throat?

ABNORMALITIES In more severe cases, the inflammation is more obvious and may be accompanied by redness and an exudate. In children, parainfluenza infection is accompanied by a fever in as many as 80% of cases. They often develop a cough concomitantly and may be hoarse. Symptoms accompanying sore throat in adults frequently mimic those seen with the common cold. Hoarseness may be present and may be accompanied by coughing. Tonsillar involvement may cause pain that is felt in the ears, and symptoms may be more extreme, including headache, fatigue, and vomiting.

INTERVIEW Do you inhale dust or fumes at work? Is your home or office dry?

ABNORMALITIES Environmental exposure to irritants or dry air can result in sore throat. Prolonged exposure to the outdoors during the colder seasons may precipitate symptoms. Patients may notice that when they are out of a particular environment for a period of time, their symptoms abate.

Swollen Lymph Nodes

INTERVIEW When did you notice the swelling in your neck? Is the swelling hard or soft? Can you move the swelling up and down easily? What size is the swelling?

ABNORMALITIES Acute enlargement usually indicates a bacterial or viral infection; persistent enlargement is often a characteristic sign of malignancy. Lymph nodes are softer and more movable with infection. Malignant lymph nodes are often hard and fixed. Tender lymph nodes usually indicate infection. Chickenpox and other viral infections often cause lymph nodes to become larger than usual.

INTERVIEW Do you have any other symptoms? Any tenderness? Fever? Sore throat? Fatigue? Rash?

ABNORMALITIES Patients with mononucleosis have large, painful lymph nodes accompanied by sore throat, fever, and fatigue.

INTERVIEW Have you ever smoked or chewed tobacco? If so, for how long? Are you still smoking or chewing? How many packs do you smoke per day? How many dips do you chew per day? Do you drink alcohol? How much do you drink per day? How long have you been drinking alcohol regularly?

ABNORMALITIES Smoking or chewing tobacco or drinking alcohol increases the risk of head and neck cancer.

INTERVIEW What prescription and nonprescription medications are you currently taking?

ABNORMALITIES Drugs such as phenytoin, hydralazine, and allopurinol can cause lymphadenopathy.

Objective Information

Objective information pertaining to the head and neck primarily includes inspection of the skull, scalp, face, mouth, and neck and palpation of the head and neck, mouth, trachea (see Chapter 11), thyroid gland (see Chapter 20), and lymph nodes. Auscultation of the neck vessels may be performed to evaluate for bruits and hums (see Chapter 12). For detailed examination techniques to evaluate function of the cranial nerves, see Chapter 18.

Physical Assessment

The Skull, Scalp, and Face

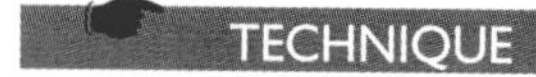

STEP 1

Inspection and Palpation of the Skull and Scalp

- Ask the patient to sit comfortably upright and to remove any wig or hair ornaments.
- Face the patient, and sit or stand at the same level whenever possible.
- Inspect the scalp. Begin at the front of the head and work backward. Note any scales, lesions, open lesions, scabbed areas, lumps, nits, tenderness, indentations, or areas of hair loss.
- Observe the general size and shape of the skull. Note any deformities, swelling, or masses.
- Palpate the skull, and feel for contour, symmetry, and size.
- Palpate any lumps or lesions observed, testing for mobility, tenderness, and consistency.

ABNORMALITIES Birth defects present with deformities in the size of the skull and may include **microencephalopathy** (decreased skull size) and **macroencephalopathy** (enlarged skull size). **Hydrocephalus** (excess fluid in the skull) is seen as an enlargement of the head without a change in the face. Abnormal enlargement of both the facial and skull bones may result from hyperactivity of the pituitary gland and is called **acromegaly.** Deformities or swelling may indicate recent trauma or a space-occupying lesion (e.g., tumor).

TECHNIQUE

STEP 2

Inspection and Palpation of the Face

- Observe the face for symmetry of all individual features.
- Note any involuntary movements of tics.
- Observe the facial skin. Note the color, pigmentation, texture, and distribution of hair. Document the size, shape, and configuration of any lesions.
- Palpate the temporal muscle by placing your middle and index fingers on the patient's temple.
- Ask the patient to clench his or her teeth. Compare the strength of the contractions on each side.
- Move your fingers to the mastoid process.
- Ask the patient to again clench his or her teeth.
- Place the fingertips lightly on the temporomandibular joint on either side of the face.
- Ask the patient to open and close his or her mouth.
- Palpate the temporal pulses, which are located near the temples on either side of the face. Note the strength, amplitude, and rhythm of the pulsations.

ABNORMALITIES Limited mobility, pain, or clicking heard on jaw movement may indicate dysfunction of the temporomandibular joint. Excessive production of adrenocorticotrophic hormone in patients with Cushing's disease may result an abnormal roundness of the face, which is often accompanied by reddened skin and excess hair above the lip and on the chin. Individuals with sunken skin and eyes may be dehydrated, malnourished, or have a wasting disease (e.g., cancer). Excess thyroid hormone, as seen in patients with Graves' disease, may result in a thinning of the face in conjunction with protruding or bulging eyes.

Nose

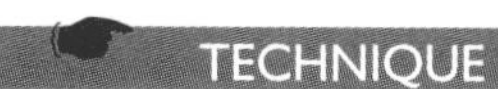

STEP 1

Inspection of the Nose

- Inspect the nose, noting the shape, size, and color. Skin color should blend with that of the face. Nares should be oval and symmetric, with the columella positioned in the midline.
- Note any discharge.
- Palpate the ridge and soft tissues.
- Place one finger on each side of the nasal arch and then gently palpate, moving the fingers from the nasal bridge to the tip.
- Occlude one naris with your finger to check for patency.
- Ask the patient to breathe with his or her mouth closed. Note any noise or discomfort.

ABNORMALITIES Nasal flaring may be present in respiratory distress. Narrowing of the nares may result in chronic nasal obstruction. A transverse crease across the nose may indicate chronic nasal itching and allergies. A malodorous, purulent discharge from the nares may indicate the presence of a foreign body if unilateral or an upper respiratory infection if bilateral. Watery, mucoid discharge may be present in rhinitis or allergies. Fractures of the nose may result in depression of the nasal bridge or displacement of the bone.

TECHNIQUE

STEP 2

Inspection of the Nasal Cavity

- Hold the speculum in the palm of the hand. An otoscope with a clean speculum may be used to perform this technique (Fig. 10-15).
- Slowly insert the speculum into the nasal cavity.
- Note any deviation, inflammation, or perforation of the septem

CAUTION **Do not touch the nasal septum with the speculum, because this can be very painful.**

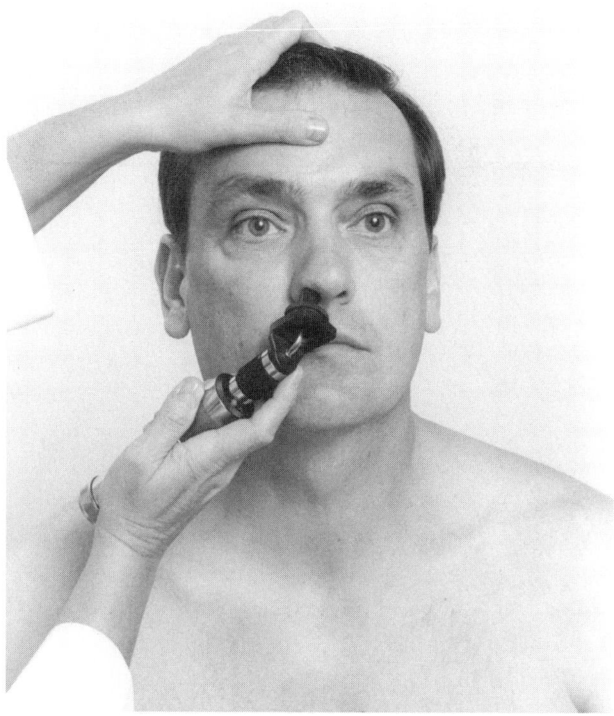

FIGURE 10-15 ■ Inspection of the nasal cavity.

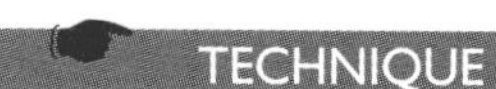
TECHNIQUE

STEP 3

Inspection of the Nasal Mucosa

- Inspect the nasal mucosa for color, hair, discharge, masses, and lesions. The color of the nasal mucosa and septum should be a deeper pink than the oral mucosa.
- Keep the patient's head erect to examine the inferior turbinate.
- Tilt the patient's head back to examine the middle turbinate. The superior turbinate will not be visible.
- Inspect the nasal septum for alignment, perforation, bleeding, and crusting.
- Repeat the procedure in the other naris.

ABNORMALITIES Increased redness of the mucosa may result from infection. Allergies may cause the turbinates to appear bluish-gray or pale pink, with a "boggy" or spongy appearance. A rounded mass projecting into the nasal cavity may be a polyp.

Sinuses

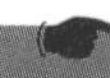
TECHNIQUE

STEP 1

Inspection and Palpation of the Sinuses

- Palpate the frontal and maxillary sinuses for tenderness and injury (Fig. 10-16).
- Place your thumb on the upper inner aspect of the orbit of the eye, and press gently but firmly upward. Note any increase in pain or tenderness as well as any swelling.
- For the maxillary sinus, place your thumb under the zygomatic bone and gently press upward. Note any pain or tenderness.

ABNORMALITIES Local tenderness when palpating the frontal or maxillary sinuses in a patient complaining of pain, fever, or nasal discharge, or any noticeable swelling below or above the eyes, suggests acute sinusitis.

TECHNIQUE

STEP 2

Transillumination of the Sinuses

- Darken the room.
- Ask the patient to close his or her eyes.
- Place the penlight on the supraorbital ring, and direct the light upward. A diffuse, red glow is a normal response in the area of the frontal sinus just above the eyebrow (Fig. 10-17).
- Place the penlight on the patient's cheekbone, just below the eye (i.e., the area of the maxillary sinus).
- Ask the patient to open his or her mouth. You should see a dull glow on the corresponding area of the hard palate. Transillumination of the maxillary sinus may also be done by asking the patient to close his or her mouth around the penlight and then observing for a dull glow in the area of the maxillary sinuses.

ABNORMALITIES Lack of transillumination may occur if inflammation or fluid is present in the sinus. When transilluminating the maxillary sinus, lack of symmetric illumination may be considered to be significant.

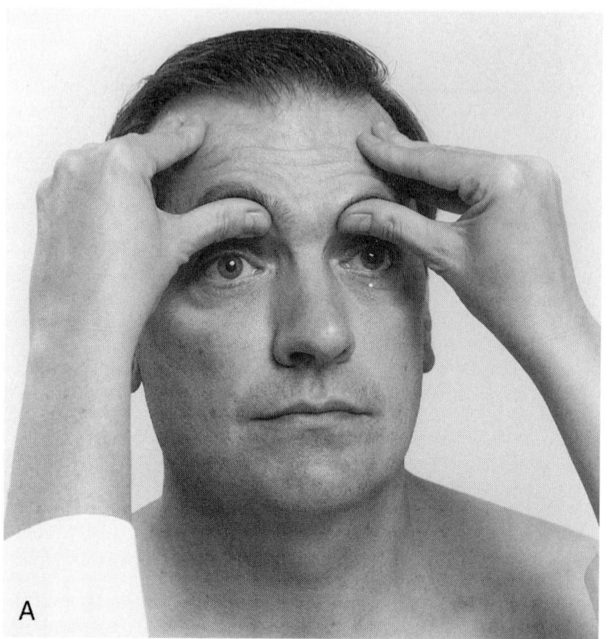

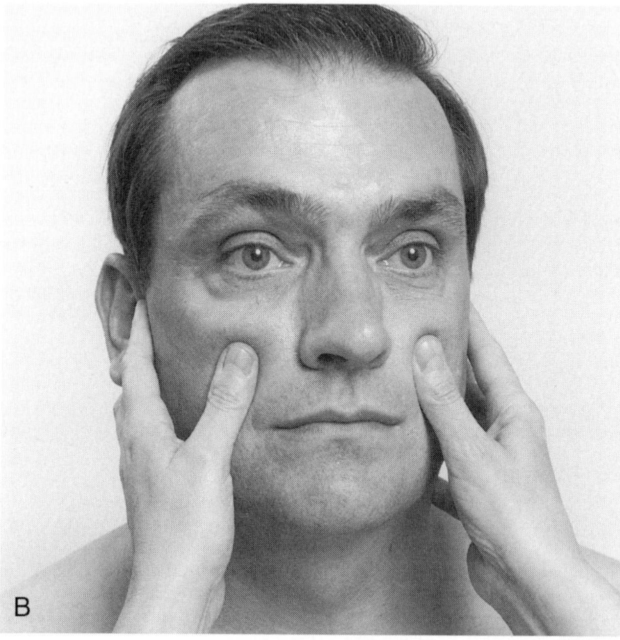

FIGURE 10-16 ■ Palpation of the sinuses. **(A)** Frontal sinuses. **(B)** Maxillary sinuses.

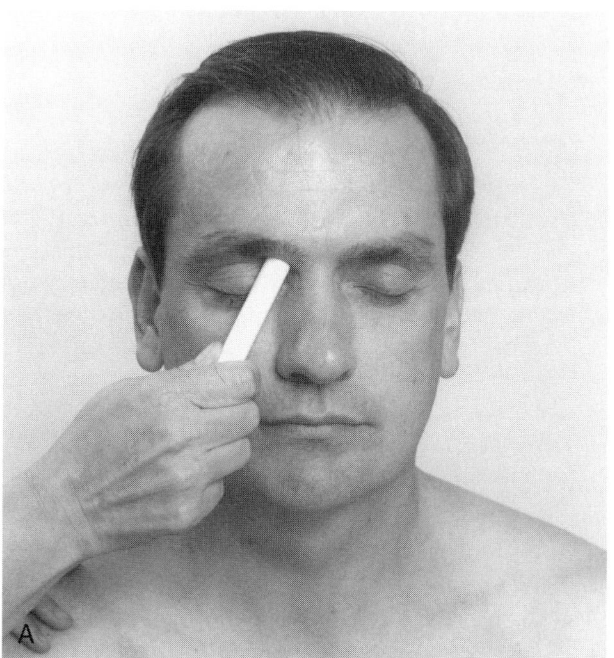

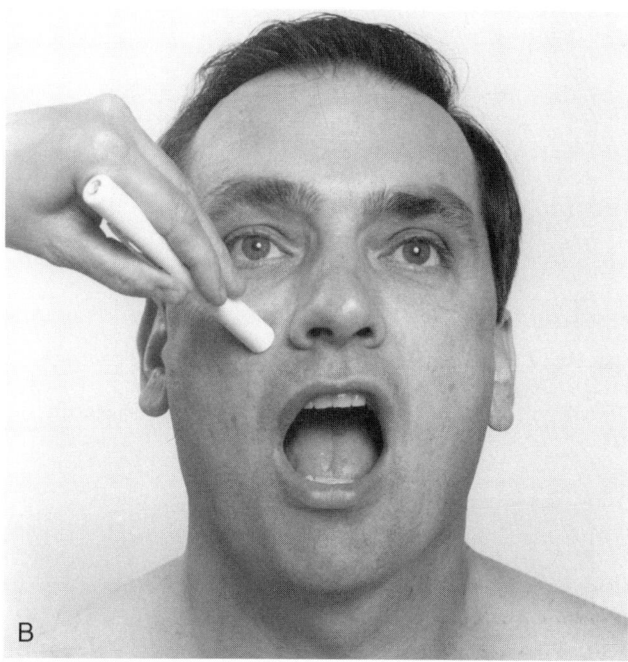

FIGURE 10-17 ■ Transillumination of the sinuses. **(A)** Frontal sinus. **(B)** Maxillary sinus.

Mouth and Pharynx

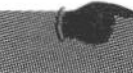
TECHNIQUE

STEP 1

Inspection and Palpation of the Mouth

- Inspect the patient's lips for color, moisture, lesions, and swelling.
- Ask the patient to open his or her mouth wide. Have the patient remove any dentures, if present.
- Using a tongue blade, expose the mucosa on each side of the mouth. Note the color, pigmentation, and overall condition of the mucosa as well as of the other internal structures.
- Inspect the teeth and gums. Note any swelling, bleeding, retraction, or discoloration of the gums. Identify any abnormalities in the position or shape of the teeth and if any teeth are missing.
- Observe the patient's tongue. Note the symmetry, position, size, color, and texture.
- Have the patient move his or her tongue up, down, and from side to side.
- Ask the patient to touch his or her tongue to the roof of the mouth.
- Inspect the underside of the tongue for lesions using a penlight and a tongue blade.
- Ask the patient to protrude his or her tongue.
- With your right hand, grasp the tip of the patient's tongue with a square of gauze, and gently pull it to the patient's left (Fig. 10-18).
- Inspect the side of the tongue.
- Palpate the tongue with your gloved left hand, feeling for any induration.
- Reverse the procedure for the other side.

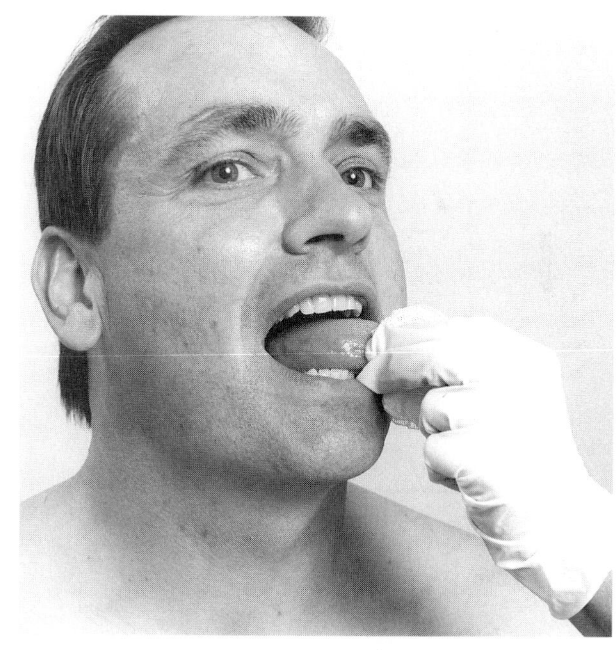

FIGURE 10-18 ■ Inspection of the tongue.

- Inspect the lingual frenulum and the submandibular ducts on either side.
- Palpate any lesions for tenderness and consistency.

ABNORMALITIES Pale or blue-colored lips in light-skinned people can indicate shock, anemia, or cyanosis. White spots on the sides of the mouth, soft palate, or hard palate may indicate candidiasis, which is a fungal infection sometimes called "oral thrush" (Fig. 10-19). Such spots may also indicate leukoplakia (Fig. 10-20), which are whitish lesions often caused by irritation (e.g., from chewing tobacco).

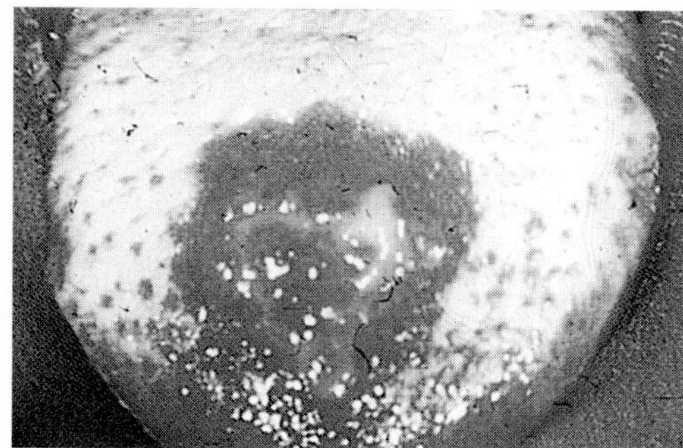

FIGURE 10-19 ■ Candidiasis. (See Color Plate 32; reprinted with permission from Robinson HBG, Miller AS. Colby, Kerr, and Robinson's color atlas of oral pathology. Philadelphia: JB Lippincott, 1990.)

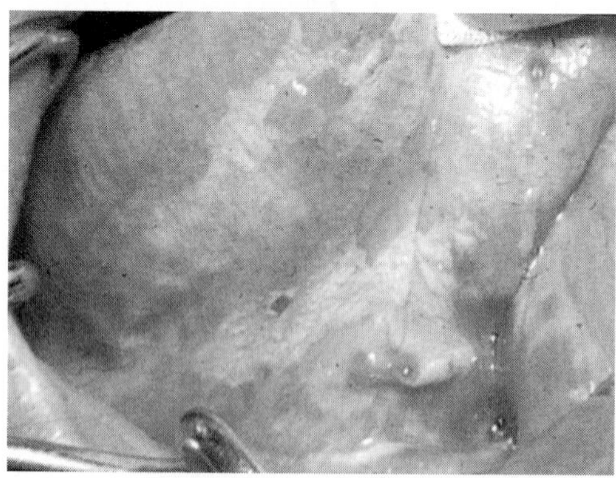

FIGURE 10-20 ■ Leukoplakia. (See Color Plate 33; reprinted with permission from Robinson HBG, Miller AS. Colby, Kerr, and Robinson's color atlas of oral pathology. Philadelphia: JB Lippincott, 1990.)

Gingivitis may present with redness and swelling of the gingival margins as well as with blunting, swelling, and redness of the interdental papillae. Dark-skinned patients routinely present with a dark line along the gum margin; however, this is a normal finding. Gingival hyperplasia presents as swollen gingival masses that may be severe enough to cover the teeth. A persistent red or white nodule or ulcer on the tongue should be suspected of being cancer until proven otherwise. Cancer of the tongue occurs primarily on the side; in most other cases, it appears at the base.

 TECHNIQUE

STEP 2

Inspection of the Pharynx

- Smell the patient's breath from approximately 12 inches away.
- Ask the patient to open the mouth and say "ah" or yawn.
- Press a tongue blade firmly down on the midpoint of the arched tongue, if necessary, to visualize the pharynx (Fig. 10-21). Illuminate the inside of the mouth with a penlight.
- Observe the soft palate, uvula, tonsils, and posterior pharynx. Look for symmetry, color, exudate, swelling, ulceration, and tonsillar enlargement.
- Touch the tongue blade lightly to the back of the tongue. Observe for the gag reflex.
- Discard the tongue blade after use.

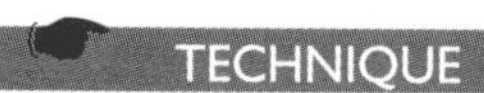 ABNORMALITIES A white exudate on the posterior pharynx or tonsils may indicate an infection such as "strep throat" or "mono." Deviation of the uvula may occur with cranial nerve X palsy (see Chapter 18). Deviation of the uvula to the side or absence of movement may indicate nerve damage. Halitosis may indicate an underlying disorder. Sweet, fruity breath is seen with diabetic ketoacidosis or malnourishment. Patients with end-stage renal failure may have breath that smells of ammonia. A musty odor may indicate liver disease, and a foul odor may indicate dental or respiratory infections. Chemical or alcohol ingestion may be detectable by smelling the breath as well.

Neck and Lymph Nodes

TECHNIQUE

STEP 1

Inspection and Palpation of the Neck

- Have the patient look straight ahead.
- From the front, inspect the neck for symmetry, masses, scars, pulsations, and swelling. (For a thorough evaluation of the carotid arteries and jugular vein, see Chapter 12.)
- From the back, palpate the trapezius muscle, which is attached to the clavicle, and observe for masses and tenderness.
- Ask the patient to place the chin on the chest, and have the patient slowly roll the head in a full circle. Observe for any limitation of movement or discomfort.
- Note the position of the trachea and whether it deviates to one side.

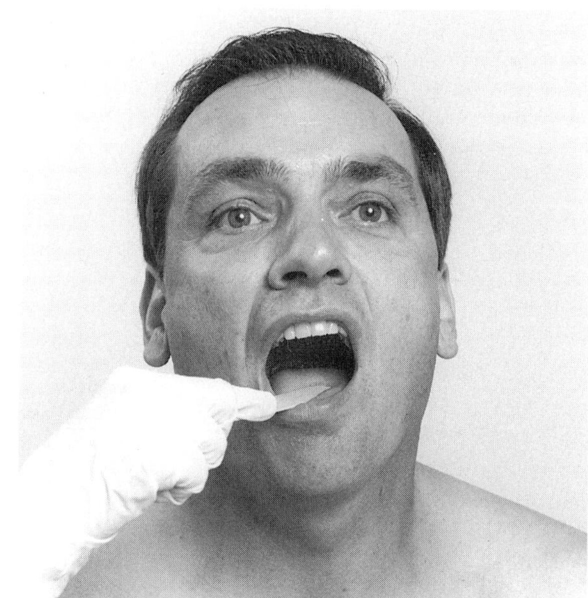

FIGURE 10-21 ■ Inspection of the pharynx.

- Palpate the trachea for any deviation by placing your finger along one side. Note the space between the trachea and the sternocleidomastoid muscle; this space should be the same on either side. Check for masses and tenderness.
- Have the patient slightly extend his or her head. Ask the patient to swallow twice. (You may give the patient a sip of water.) Look for symmetric movement on swallowing. Make sure no masses are identifiable during the swallowing process.
- For a thorough discussion of inspection and palpation of the thyroid gland, see Chapter 20.

ABNORMALITIES Deviations of the trachea indicate a mediastinal shift that can be caused by a mass, lung abnormality, or air in the space surrounding the lungs. A reduced range of motion may be caused by arthritis or by muscle irritation or spasm. Stiffness of the neck is a common symptom of meningitis. Any mass may be indicative of a tumor.

TECHNIQUE

STEP 2

Inspection and Palpation of the Lymph Nodes

- Figure 10-22 depicts palpation of the lymph nodes.
- Ask the patient to relax the muscles of his or her neck and to bend the neck slightly forward toward the side you are palpating. You may want to brace the top of the patient's head with one hand as you palpate with the other.
- Use the pads of your index and middle fingers to gently move the skin over the tissue where the nodes are located (see Fig. 10-8). Feel the nodes in the following sequence: preauricular, posterior auricular, occipital, tonsillar, submandibular, submental, superficial cervical, posterior cervical, deep cervical chain, and supraclavicular (see Table 10-1).
- If you palpate an enlarged node, note its size, consistency, mobility, tenderness, temperature, and location.
- To distinguish a lymph node from a muscle or an artery, try to roll the node in two directions: up and down, and side to side. This cannot be done with a muscle or an artery.
- Ask the patient if the node is tender.

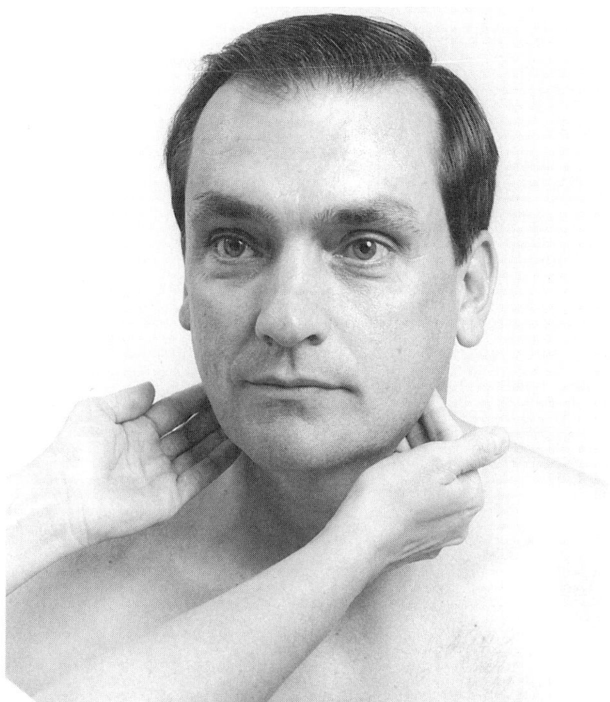

FIGURE 10-22 ■ Palpation of the lymph nodes.

ABNORMALITIES Tender, palpable lymph nodes may result from a recent infection. Infectious mononucleosis may cause enlargement or tenderness of the cervical, inguinal, and axillary lymph nodes. Firm, enlarged, nontender, immobile lymph nodes may suggest malignancy.

Laboratory and Diagnostic Tests

Laboratory and diagnostic testing to evaluate symptoms involving the head and neck include:

- Rapid streptococcus tests are based on rapid detection of the antigens to *Streptococcus* sp. A positive result from an antigen test is considered to be equivalent to a culture; however, because of the rapid test's lower sensitivity, a negative result requires a follow-up culture. The benefit of rapid results from this test may also be offset by the increased cost as compared to a culture.
- Throat culture requires that the tonsils and pharyngeal area of the patient be swabbed and the sample be left to sit in a controlled environment for 24 to 48 hours to allow for adequate growth of a potential pathogen. Throat culture is the gold standard for diagnosis of bacterial pharyngitis, but it requires proper technique by an experienced individual.
- Plain radiography of the sinuses has been used in the past to confirm a diagnosis of chronic sinusitis. Two to three views of the sinuses are usually obtained. Fluid in the maxillary antra and mucosal thickening would potentially confirm the presence of sinusitis. A relatively high occurrence of abnormal radiographic findings can be found in asymptomatic patients, however. Therefore, use of sinus radiography in establishing the diagnosis of acute sinusitis is not warranted.
- Computed tomography, ultrasonography, and magnetic resonance imaging are all radiographic imaging techniques that may be used to assess a patient's condition when the primary care provider is considering chronic sinusitis or malignancy as causative factors or if surgical intervention may be necessary. Underlying disorders resulting in headache can also be identified in this way.

Special Considerations

Pediatric Patients

Pediatric patients require that additional questions be asked of the parent or guardian.

? INTERVIEW Has your child started getting teeth? At what ages did the teeth appear? Has your child been to the dentist? Did you notice any thumb-sucking after the child's permanent teeth came in? Have you noticed your child grinding his or her teeth?

➤ ABNORMALITIES Delayed teeth may impair nutrition. Teeth may be delayed in certain diseases (e.g., Down syndrome). Prolonged thumb-sucking may affect occlusion of the teeth.

Examination of the mouth, head, and neck of a child requires special positioning. An infant should be placed on an examination table, but an older child may sit on the lap of a parent or caregiver. Detection of fontanelles may occur in children older than the expected age when a developmental disability or congenital disease is present. Increased intracranial pressure may be indicated by bulging of the fontanelles.

To examine the mouth, ask a young child to open the mouth "as big as a lion" and to move the tongue in different directions. Alternatively, ask the child to stick out the tongue and to "pant like a dog." Gum hypertrophy may occur normally during puberty. Children with malnutrition or dehydration may present with a sweet, fruity breath odor.

Geriatric Patients

Geriatric patients require additional questions to be asked.

? INTERVIEW Do you experience any problems with dry mouth? Are you taking any medications? Do you have any trouble eating? Do you have loss of teeth? Have you noticed any change in your sense of taste or smell?

➤ ABNORMALITIES The elderly may suffer from xerostomia, which is a dry mouth caused by ingestion of medications (e.g., anticholinergics) that interfere with production of saliva. Xerostomia may also result from systemic diseases (e.g., rheumatoid arthritis and scleroderma), heavy smoking, or exposure of the head and neck to radiation. This, along with changes in the tongue and loss of teeth, may make mastication and swallowing more difficult.

? INTERVIEW Have you ever experienced dizziness with head or neck movement? Have you ever fallen? Have you ever had a head injury? Have you ever experienced weakness or impaired balance?

Geriatric patients may be sensitive to having their oral cavity examined because of the physical changes that occur with age, including tooth loss, gingival recession, and dry mouth. The pharmacist should reassure the client that a full examination of the gums is necessary to ensure that no problems are present.

The onset of headache for the first time in a geriatric patient is more likely to be caused by some other underlying pathology. These patients should be referred to a physician for a thorough evaluation.

Pregnant Patients

Pregnant patients require additional questions to be asked.

? INTERVIEW Are you experiencing any other symptoms? Are you experiencing any changes in your voice?

➤ ABNORMALITIES Elevated estrogen levels, which increase vascularity, may result in nasal stuffiness, decreased sense of smell, and epistaxis. Hoarseness, vocal changes, or persistent cough may result from laryngeal changes that are also hormonally mediated.

Pregnant women are more susceptible to gingivitis because of the increased vascularity of their gums, which results from increased estrogen levels. Gingivitis of pregnancy is characterized by red, swollen gingival tissue that bleeds easily. The condition continues for as long as the woman is breastfeeding but resolves within 1 year of weaning. This increased vascularity may also result in hoarseness, vocal changes, or persistent cough.

Pregnant women may also experience hyperpigmented patches on the face as well as facial edema. Both conditions typically subside after birth of the child.

Alterations in hormone levels are also sometimes responsible for changes in the incidence of headache among pregnant patients. Some women begin to experience headaches for the first time during pregnancy. Patients with a history of headache may find that their headaches become more frequent, whereas others may find themselves in a remission from symptoms that lasts until birth of the child. More than 50% of women with a history of migraine find relief from these symptoms during pregnancy.

APPLICATION TO PATIENT SYMPTOMS

Headache Pain

CASE STUDY

BM is a 21-year-old female who approaches the pharmacy counter seeking help for relief of headache pain. BM is escorted to the patient consultation area for evaluation.

ASSESSMENT OF THE PATIENT

Subjective Information

21-year-old woman complaining of headache pain

TELL ME MORE ABOUT THE SYMPTOMS YOU'VE BEEN HAVING? I have this headache that started earlier today and just won't go away.

DESCRIBE THE PAIN FOR ME. It's like a rubber band is wrapped around my head.

WHERE DO YOU FEEL THE PAIN? It's on both sides of my head.

HAVE YOU EVER EXPERIENCED A HEADACHE LIKE THIS BEFORE? Yes.

TELL ME MORE ABOUT YOUR PAST EXPERIENCE WITH THESE HEADACHES. I always seem to get them when I am stressed, especially around midterm and final exam week.

DOES ANYTHING APPEAR TO TRIGGER THESE HEADACHES? Not that I have noticed.

HAVE YOU BEEN KEEPING TRACK OF WHEN YOU GET THESE HEADACHES? No.

DO THEY OCCUR AT A PARTICULAR TIME OF DAY? Not really.

HOW LONG DOES EACH HEADACHE LAST? It varies a little bit. Usually they last a few hours.

DO YOU EXPERIENCE ANY OTHER SYMPTOMS WHEN YOU HAVE THESE HEADACHES? No.

HAVE YOU EXPERIENCED ANY STRANGE SENSATIONS BEFORE YOU STARTED TO FEEL THE PAIN? Like what?

HAVE YOU NOTICED ANY ODORS THAT DIDN'T HAVE AN OBVIOUS SOURCE OR CHANGES IN YOUR VISION? No.

DO YOU RECALL BEGINNING ANY NEW MEDICATIONS OR HERBAL PRODUCTS BEFORE THE BEGINNING OF YOUR HEADACHES? Nothing that I haven't taken before. I took Tylenol for the headache earlier, but it doesn't seem to be working.

HOW MUCH TYLENOL DID YOU USE? I take it like it says to on the bottle. I took two 365-mg tablets.

HAD YOU RECENTLY STOPPED TAKING ANY MEDICATIONS WHEN YOU FIRST NOTICED THE HEADACHES? No, I've never had to take anything regularly.

DO YOU TAKE BIRTH CONTROL PILLS? No.

HAVE YOU BEEN EATING REGULAR MEALS? Yes, I eat three meals a day. Sometimes I get fast food, but not very often.

DO YOU SLEEP LATER THAN USUAL ON CERTAIN DAYS OF THE WEEK? No. I really can't sleep any longer than about 8 hours. I have class at eight in the morning three days a week, so I have to be up.

DO YOU REMEMBER IF YOU HAD FALLEN OR WERE HIT IN THE HEAD AROUND THE TIME THAT THE HEADACHES STARTED? No, I didn't have any accidents or falls.

DO YOU WORK? Just work-study at the library.

DOES ANYTHING RELIEVE YOUR PAIN? I don't know. I haven't really tried anything but the Tylenol.

Objective Information

Temperature: 98.2°F
Blood pressure: 102/71 mm Hg
Pulse: 64 bpm
Respiration: 18 rpm
HEENT: Unremarkable, except neck muscle extremely tight.
Lungs: Clear to auscultation
Heart: Regular rate and rhythm
Extremities: Within normal limits

DISCUSSION

Tension headache appears to be the likely pathology in this case. Most individuals experience tension headache as a result of stress, anxiety, or muscle tension. In this case, BM is 21 years old. Because she is young and appears to have no other physical or psychologic maladies, her headache is less likely to be secondary to another disease state. BM describes her pain as having a rubber band–like quality. This, too, is consistent with typical tension headache pain, as opposed to the constant pain of a cluster or migraine headache. The diffuse bilateral nature of the pain also makes migraine headache less likely. Most migraines last for anywhere from 4 hours to 3 days. The duration of BM's headaches has been a few hours, and therefore, they do not fit the pattern of migraine. Additional symptoms that accompany a migraine headache

Continued

CASE STUDY—continued

include nausea, vomiting, and photophobia. BM has stated that she has not experienced any other symptoms. Attempts to identify a prodrome or aura were unsuccessful. This does not rule out migraine, however, because only approximately one in two individuals who suffer from migraine headache will experience a prodrome. In addition, only one in 10 individuals who suffer from migraine headache can identify an aura. Medication use, overuse, or withdrawal; alterations in sleep patterns; and occupational chemical exposure all have the potential to exacerbate migraine headache, but each of these was ruled out in the case of BM. In addition, BM has normal blood pressure and is not taking medication to treat hypertension, which makes it an unlikely contributing factor in this case.

Because the onset of BM's headache pain is acute, starting in the last couple of hours, its nature is described as as band-like tightness, and she is currently under stress with examinations and has extreme muscle tightness in her neck, this case would appear to be most consistent with a tension headache. As long as she has no contraindication to salicylates or nonsteroidal anti-inflammatory drugs, the pharmacist should be able to recommend an over-the-counter (OTC) analgesic and advise that this headache should resolve as the stressful period of her life passes.

Figure 10-23 shows a decision tree for headache pain.

PHARMACEUTICAL CARE PLAN

Patient Name: BM

Date: 3/18/01

Medical Problems:
None

Current Medications:
Tylenol (acetaminophen), 650 mg one time

S: BM is a 21-year-old white female who presents to the pharmacy with an acute headache that started within the last 2 hours. The patient describes the headache as rubber band–like in nature. The headache appears to coincide with major examination times and is similar to others experienced in the past. The patient denies medication use except for Tylenol, which she took after the onset of the headache. Her medical history is otherwise negative.

O: The patient looks her stated age. She appears to be in moderate distress.

Temperature: 98.2°F

Blood pressure: 102/71 mm Hg

Pulse: 64 bpm

Respiration: 18 rpm

HEENT: Physical examination of head is unremarkable. Neck muscles are extremely tight.

A: Probable tension headache associated with midterm examinations.

P: 1. Recommend ibuprofen, 400 mg every 6 hours as needed and taken with food.
2. Refer patient to a physician for follow up if headache does not resolve within 24 hours.

Pharmacist: *Sherry Baily, Pharm.D.*

Self-Assessment Questions

1. How would the pain of a tension headache be described?
2. What factors can precipitate a tension headache?

Critical Thinking Questions

1. When evaluating BM for headache, what questions should be asked to help differentiate among migraine, cluster, tension, and other types of headache?
2. What factors would need to be present to conclude that BM may be experiencing chronic tension headaches?

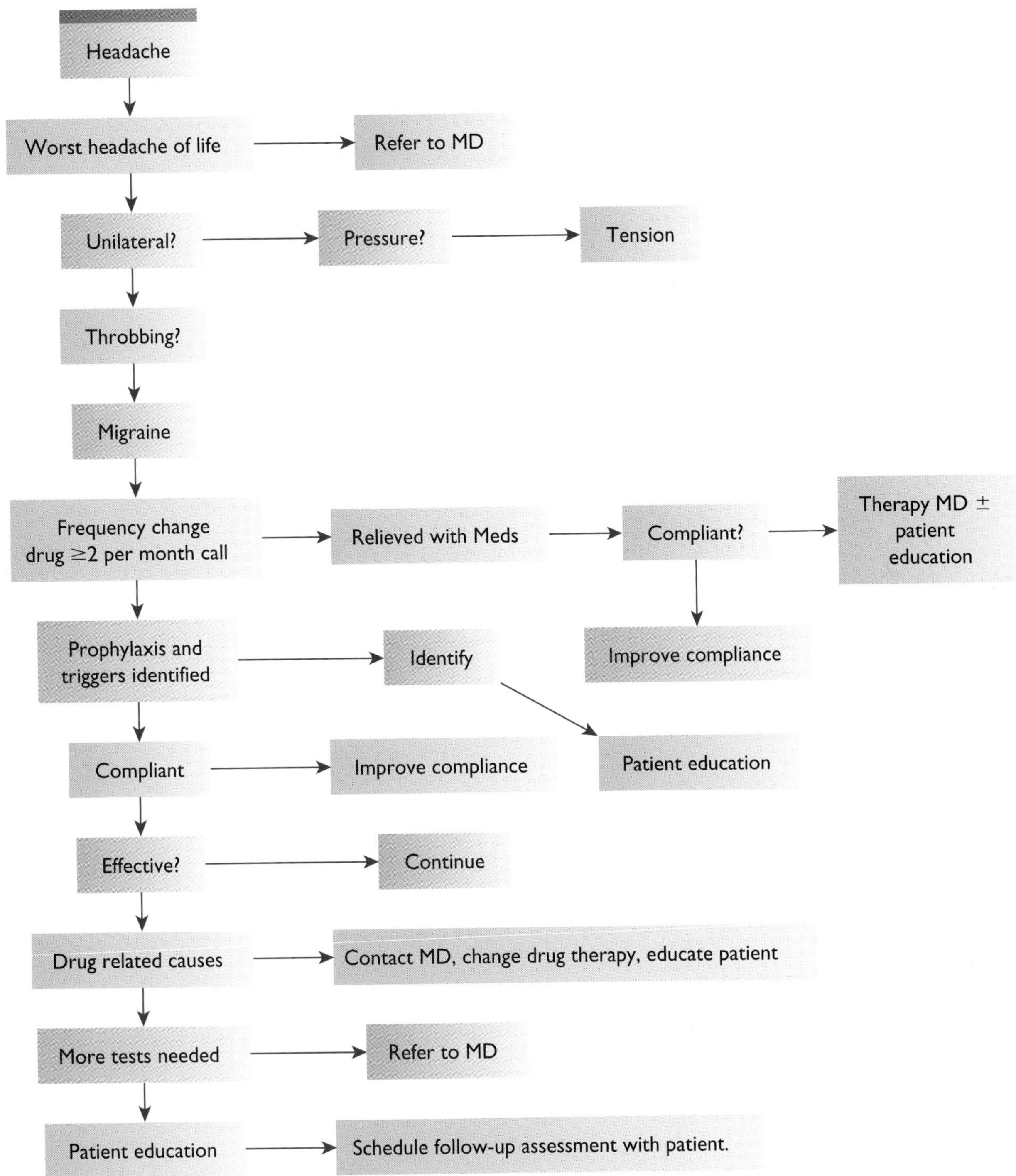

FIGURE 10-23 ■ Decision tree for headache pain.

Facial Pain

CASE STUDY

SS is a 34-year-old woman who presents to the pharmacy with a "bad cold" and asks the pharmacist to recommend a different OTC medication because her current medicine is not working. The pharmacist asks SS to step into the consultation room for a more thorough evaluation of her symptoms.

ASSESSMENT OF THE PATIENT

Subjective Information

34-year-old woman complaining of a "bad cold"

Describe for me this "bad cold" you have been experiencing. I have just felt awful for the last week.

What symptoms are you having? A terribly runny nose, a cough, and pain when I move my head.

What color is the drainage from your nose? It was clear, but in the last couple of days it has become yellowish in color. It is really nasty looking.

Are you having any drainage down your throat? Yes. It really tastes bad and upsets my stomach, so I haven't really been hungry.

Describe your cough for me. My coughing seems to be getting worse. It is really bad at night, and I haven't really been able to get a good night's sleep.

Have you had any other symptoms? When the cold first started, I thought I felt feverish, but that has gone away.

Any other symptoms? Not that I can think of.

Have you had any headaches? No.

Do you have any allergies? No.

What prescription medications do you take? I only take my birth control pills.

What medications have you been taking for your cold? Benadryl and Robitussin DM.

How are you taking the Benadryl? I have been taking 25 mg every 6 hours.

How were you using the Robitussin DM? I was taking one tablespoonful four times a day.

What makes you feel that these medications are not working? Even though I've been taking them regularly, my cough and runny nose seem to be getting worse.

Have you ever had a sinus infection? No.

Do you smoke? No.

Do you use alcohol? Rarely.

Objective Information

Temperature: 97°F
Blood pressure: 96/70 mm Hg
Pulse: 70 bpm
Respiration: 16 rpm
HEENT: Periorbital swelling bilaterally, greater on the left; nose: turbinates red and boggy, with some yellow discharge; left maxillary sinus tender to palpation; frontal sinus nontender bilaterally; pharynx: pink and moist, without exudate or lesions; neck: enlarged periauricular lymph node, mobile and tender to palpation
Lungs: Clear to auscultation

DISCUSSION

Facial pain can result from a number of conditions within the head and neck. Sinusitis, one of the most common causes of facial pain, is a process that is associated with both bacterial and viral infections of the upper respiratory tract. The onset of acute sinusitis usually occurs during or after an upper respiratory tract infection. In this case, SS has been suffering from symptoms of a cold for 5 days before the worsening of her symptoms. She presents with a number of signs and symptoms consistent with sinusitis. She complains of nasal discharge that has changed from clear to yellow-green in color, halitosis, and cough. Persistence of nasal discharge and cough for more than 10 days following a viral infection is often consistent with sinusitis.

On physical examination, SS has facial pain on palpation of her left maxillary sinus. Facial pain and headache are common symptoms associated with sinusitis. The lack of a headache in this case may relate to her frontal sinuses not being painful to palpation. Maxillary sinus involvement may result in pain in the cheek or teeth, whereas ethmoid sinusitis can cause pain deep and medial to the eye.

The primary causative organisms of sinusitis are *Streptococcus pneumoniae* and *Haemophilus influenzae.* Treatment of sinusitis revolves around the use of antibiotics and decongestants. Therefore, SS should be referred to her primary care provider for confirmation of the diagnosis and an antibiotic prescription. During the interim, she should use a decongestant rather than an antihistamine. This is important to aid in decongesting the nose to allow for drainage of the sinus contents through the natural ostia.

Continued

CASE STUDY—continued

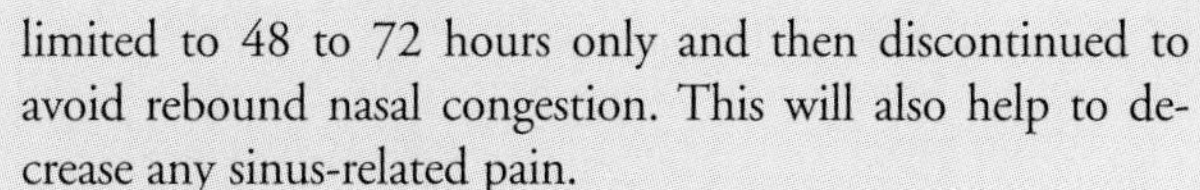

Antihistamines should be avoided, because drying of the mucosal membranes may interfere with clearance of the mucous secretions. SS has been taking Benadryl, an OTC preparation containing diphenhydramine, which is an antihistamine. Topical decongestants may be used; however, they should be limited to 48 to 72 hours only and then discontinued to avoid rebound nasal congestion. This will also help to decrease any sinus-related pain.

Figure 10-24 shows the decision tree for facial pain.

Pharmaceutical Care Plan

Patient Name: SS

Date: 6/24/02

Medical Problems:
None

Current Medications:
Benadryl, 25 mg four times daily
Robitussin DM, one tablespoonful four times daily

S: SS is a 34-year-old woman who presents with a 1-week history of nasal drainage and cough and a 2-day history of worsening nasal drainage (yellowish color), increase in cough (especially at night), postnasal drainage, insomnia, and decrease in appetite. At the start of the cold symptoms, the patient was febrile.

O: Patient appears tired but is in no apparent distress.

Temperature: 97°F

Blood pressure: 96/70 mm Hg

Pulse: 70 bpm

Respiration: 16 rpm

HEENT: Periorbital swelling bilaterally, greater on the left; nose: turbinates red and boggy with some yellow discharge; left maxillary sinus tender to palpation; frontal sinus within normal limits; pharynx: pink and moist without exudates or lesions; neck: enlarged left cervical lymph node, mobile and tender to palpation.

Lungs: Clear to auscultation.

Heart: Regular rate and rhythm.

A: Possible bacterial sinusitis.

P:
1. Refer the patient to her primary care provider for further evaluation and possible antibiotic therapy.
2. Have SS discontinue the antihistamine.
3. Recommend SS take an oral decongestant (e.g., pseudoephedrine, 30 mg PO every 6 hours) until she sees her primary care provider.

Pharmacist: *Christina Geittman, Pharm.D.*

Self-Assessment Questions

1. What are the signs and symptoms of sinusitis?
2. Pain resulting from sinusitis varies depending on which sinus is involved. Which type of pain is expressed by patients with involvement of the frontal, maxillary, and ethmoid sinuses, respectively?
3. What is the role of radiologic procedures in the diagnosis of acute sinusitis?

Critical Thinking Questions

1. If SS reported using nasal decongestants, how would the questions the pharmacist asks her change?
2. What factors in the patient history would need to be present to increase the pharmacist's concern about chronic sinusitis in this case?

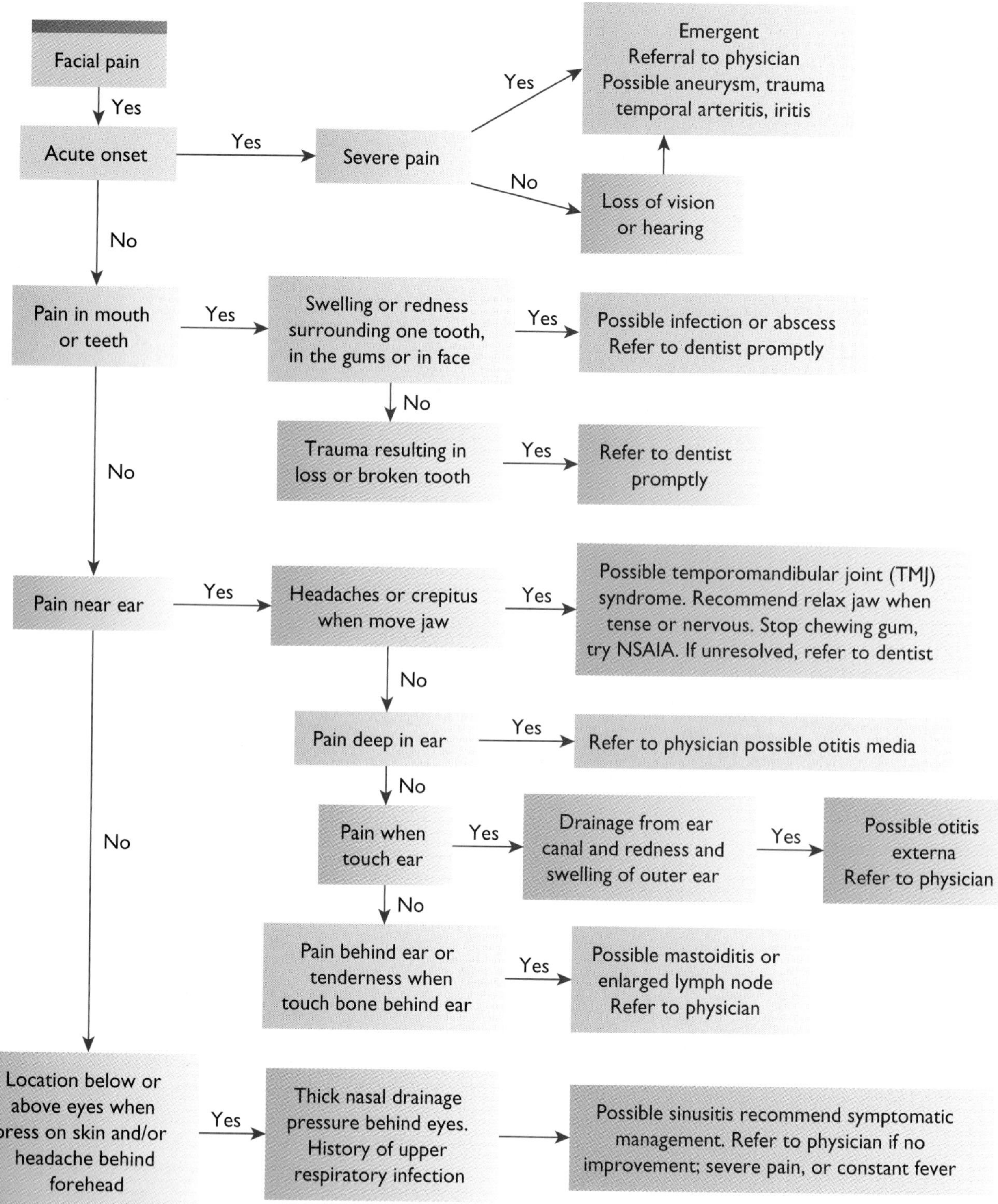

FIGURE 10-24 ■ Decision tree for facial pain.

Sore Throat

CASE STUDY

BJ is a 4-year-old Hispanic boy who is brought by his mother to the local free clinic with the complaint of a sore throat. The pharmacist's responsibilities at this clinic are to prescreen patients by completing a patient interview and medication history and by assessing basic vital signs. The pharmacist calls BJ and his mother into an examination room.

ASSESSMENT OF THE PATIENT

Subjective Information

4-year-old Hispanic boy with sore throat

TELL ME MORE ABOUT BJ'S SYMPTOMS. He has been complaining of a sore throat on and off for the last week.

DOES BJ HAVE ANY OTHER SYMPTOMS? He felt very warm last night, and his cheeks and ears were red, but I don't have a thermometer, so I couldn't take his temperature. He has had a runny nose, and I noticed yesterday he has a bump on his neck.

HOW HAS BJ BEEN ACTING DURING THE PAST 7 DAYS? He is usually very active. When he feels warm he just lies around, but otherwise he plays just like normal. He acts just like he does today.

HOW LONG HAS HE HAD THE SYMPTOMS YOU MENTIONED? He always seems to have a runny nose. I think he has felt warm for the last couple of days.

WHAT COLOR IS THE DRAINAGE FROM HIS NOSE? It's kind of a whitish color.

YOU SAID HE ALWAYS SEEMS TO HAVE A RUNNY NOSE. IS THERE A CERTAIN TIME OF DAY OR SEASON WHEN HIS NOSE SEEMS TO RUN MORE THAN OTHER TIMES? His nose runs a lot when he first gets up in the morning, but it never seems to completely stop. I don't think that it runs at one time of year more than any other. He has a runny nose whenever he gets a cold.

DOES HE HAVE A SORE THROAT AND A FEVER TOGETHER VERY OFTEN? About once a year, but this is the second time this year. He had "strep" last time.

HAS HE BEEN EXPOSED TO ANYONE WITH A SORE THROAT OR A RUNNY NOSE, EITHER AT HOME OR IN A DAY CARE SETTING? Yes, everyone at his day care has a runny nose. They also posted last week that one child has "strep" throat.

WHAT HAVE YOU TRIED AT HOME TO TREAT HIS SYMPTOMS? I gave him some Tylenol, but he still felt warm after that. I used warm tea with lemon for the sore throat. His runny nose never seems to get better, although I usually give him Dimetapp. Nothing seems to help much.

HOW MUCH DIMETAPP AND TYLENOL HAVE YOU BEEN GIVING BJ, AND HOW OFTEN? I gave him three chewable Tylenol every 4 hours, and half a teaspoon of Dimetapp about every 6 hours.

DOES BJ HAVE ANY ALLERGIES TO MEDICATION? He is allergic to penicillin.

Objective Information

Information Obtained from Chart

PMH: Normal pregnancy and vaginal delivery. Born at 39 weeks of gestation; birth weight, 8 pounds, 1 ounce; home with mother in 2 days. No surgeries, serious illnesses, or hospitalizations. Chickenpox at age 2 years. History of infrequent acute otitis media, infrequent colds, and sore throats.

FH: Parents in good health; review of systems negative.

SH: Both parents work outside the home, no siblings, attends day care 4 days per week.

PE: BJ is an alert, active 4-year-old and developmentally appropriate for his age.

Weight: 37 pounds
Height: 41.5 inches
Temperature: 101°F
Pulse: 100 bpm
Respirations: 24 rpm
Blood pressure: 90/60 mm Hg

Complete Physical Examination Performed by Primary Care Provider

Skin: Pink, warm, and dry, with elastic turgor and no lesions.
HEENT: Ears nontender bilaterally to palpation. Tympanic membranes pearly gray and mobile. Conjunctiva red with scant yellow drainage bilaterally. Sclera clear. No photosensitivity. Slightly pink nasal mucosa with white, profuse drainage; inferior and middle turbinates have mild swelling.

Mouth and throat are pink and moist without lesions. Uvula is midline with erythema. Posterior pharynx is very erythematous without exudates. No abnormalities of the hard or soft palate or pharynx, no bulging of the anterior or posterior pillars of the oropharynx, and no drooling. Teeth in good repair; no apparent cavities or halitosis. Gums are pink and moist without erythema or swelling.

Continued

CASE STUDY—continued

Neck: Shotty deep cervical lymph nodes; 2 cm oval; freely mobile superficial cervical node on left side without redness, warmth, or tenderness. No other lymphadenopathy noted. Full range of motion of head and neck.
Heart: Regular rate and rhythm without murmurs
Lungs: Clear to auscultation
ABD: Soft and flat, with active bowel sounds in all four quadrants; no hepatosplenomegaly
Extremities: Radial and pedal pulses +2 and equal bilaterally
Laboratory: Negative rapid strep test

DISCUSSION

Sore throat may result from a number of disease processes. The most common reasons include viral or bacterial infection, ear infection, mouth infection, or dental infection. The history related to the onset of symptoms can aid in differentiating viral and bacterial pharyngitis. Bacterial pharyngitis is more abrupt, whereas viral processes tend to have a more gradual onset of symptoms. In addition, viral causes of pharyngitis are most common in preschoolers, especially when accompanied by nasal symptoms, low-grade fever, and minimal toxicity. School-age children with sore throats will test positive for group A β-hemolytic streptococci (GABHS) in 25% to 50% of cases, but it is uncommon in children younger than 2 years. At 4 years of age, BJ is at risk for GABHS, and although he is currently not in school, he does attend a day care center. The presentation of BJ's symptoms (nasal drainage, mild temperature), however, is consistent with a viral cause. BJ's mother has also described a gradual onset of symptoms spanning the past 7 days, which is more characteristic of a viral infection.

The color of the nasal drainage can also help to differentiate between possible causes of pharyngitis. Allergies tend to result in a clear, watery drainage as opposed to the white, purulent, or green drainage that occurs with infectious processes. Nasal drainage is usually absent in GABHS pharyngitis. Allergic rhinorrhea can result in a sore throat caused by postnasal drip; however, BJ's nasal drainage is not consistent with a seasonal or perennial allergic pattern.

BJ's day care attendance places him at higher risk, because most cases of sore throat are communicable. GABHS is most predominant from December to May. Respiratory viruses are seen primarily in winter as compared to enteroviruses, which predominate in the summer and fall. Five to ten percent of all febrile illness in young children result from adenovirus, with infants and preschool children having the highest rates of infection. Therefore, except for BJ's previous history of strep throat, the large majority of the subjective evidence would appear to support a diagnosis of viral pharyngitis.

As the pharmacist observes the primary care provider's physical examination, the results continue to support the diagnosis of viral pharyngitis. Except for his temperature, BJ's vital signs are within normal limits for a 4 year old; however, temperature is only a nonspecific indicator of an infectious process.

The cervical lymphadenopathy found in BJ is common in children, and it usually results from an infectious process. Inflammation of the lymph nodes can be ruled out, because the node is nontender and less than 3 cm in size. Neoplasms would produce hard, fixed nodes, and retropharyngeal abscesses usually limit the range of motion of the neck.

The normal presentation of the mouth, gums, and teeth would rule out the possibility of dental or mouth infections. The absence of petechiae on the hard or soft palate as well as tonsillar exudates in BJ decreases the likelihood of GABHS.

It is important that the physical examination include a thorough assessment of the heart, lungs, and ears, because children with sore throats may have an associated otitis media or respiratory infection. BJ's tympanic membrane is pearly gray and mobile, his lungs are clear to auscultation, and his heart has a regular rate and rhythm. This would rule out an associated otitis media, respiratory infection, or influenza. Influenza would also be excluded, because BJ is not suffering from decreased activity or generalized aches and pains. Conjunctivitis often presents in association with viral illnesses. Although streptococcal infections sometimes affect the eyes and cause photosensitivity, drainage is not typically noted. BJ has erythematous conjunctivae with a mild yellow drainage that would be consistent with a viral infection.

A rapid strep test was completed for two reasons. First, BJ has had a previous case of strep throat and is currently attending a day care center that has at least one reported case. This increases his risk for GABHS. Second, the potential sequelae of missing a subtle streptococcal pharyngitis are serious and include rheumatic fever and poststreptococcal glomerulonephritis. Controversy exists about whether the improved sensitivity and specificity of current rapid strep tests is sufficient to eliminate the need for follow-up throat culture. Most practitioners, however, still complete a throat culture to confirm negative results from a rapid strep test.

Figure 10-25 shows the decision tree for facial pain.

Continued

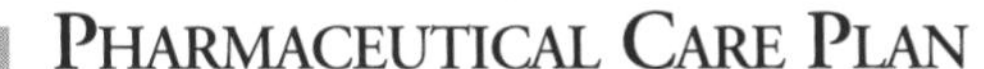

CASE STUDY—continued

PHARMACEUTICAL CARE PLAN

Patient Name: BJ

Date: 6/27/00

Medical Problems:
None

Current Medications:
Chewable Tylenol (acetaminophen), 3 tablets by mouth every four hours for fever
Dimetapp, half-teaspoonful every 6 hours for runny nose

S: BJ is a 4-year-old boy with an approximately 7-day history of sore throat and a 2-day history of a runny nose, temperature, and a lump on his neck. Tylenol and Dimetapp have been used for symptomatic relief with questionable results.

O: Alert, active 4-year-old in no apparent distress

Weight: 37 pounds

Height: 41.5 inches

Temperature: 101°F

Pulse: 100 bpm

Respirations: 24 rpm

Blood pressure: 90/60 mm Hg

Physical examination: Within normal limits except for conjunctiva (red with scant yellow drainage bilaterally); slightly pink mucosa with white, profuse drainage; and mild swelling of the inferior turbinates. Mouth is pink, uvula is midline with erythema, and posterior pharynx is very erythematous without exudates. No petechiae noted on the hard or soft palate or pharynx. No bulging of the anterior or posterior pillars of the oropharynx or drooling.

Neck: Shotty deep cervical lymph nodes; 2 cm oval; freely mobile superficial cervical node on left side without redness, warmth, or tenderness. No other lymphadenopathy noted. Full range of motion of head and neck.

Laboratory: Negative rapid strep test.

A: Viral pharyngitis.

P:
1. Have BJ drink plenty of fluids.
2. Continue chewable acetaminophen for fever.
3. Continue Dimetapp for nasal discharge.
4. Educate mother about when to call the clinic or take BJ to the emergency room.
5. Check throat culture in 24 hours, and call mother with the result.

Pharmacist: *Christina Halfax, Pharm.D.*

Self-Assessment Questions

1. Compare and contrast the signs and symptoms of viral versus bacterial pharyngitis.
2. What are the potential complications of an untreated strep throat?
3. What is the role of a rapid strep test in the physical assessment of pharyngitis?

Critical Thinking Questions

1. What medications could leave white spots in the mouth that might be misinterpreted as exudate?
2. When examining a patient's mouth and throat in a community setting, what findings indicate the need for referral to a physician?

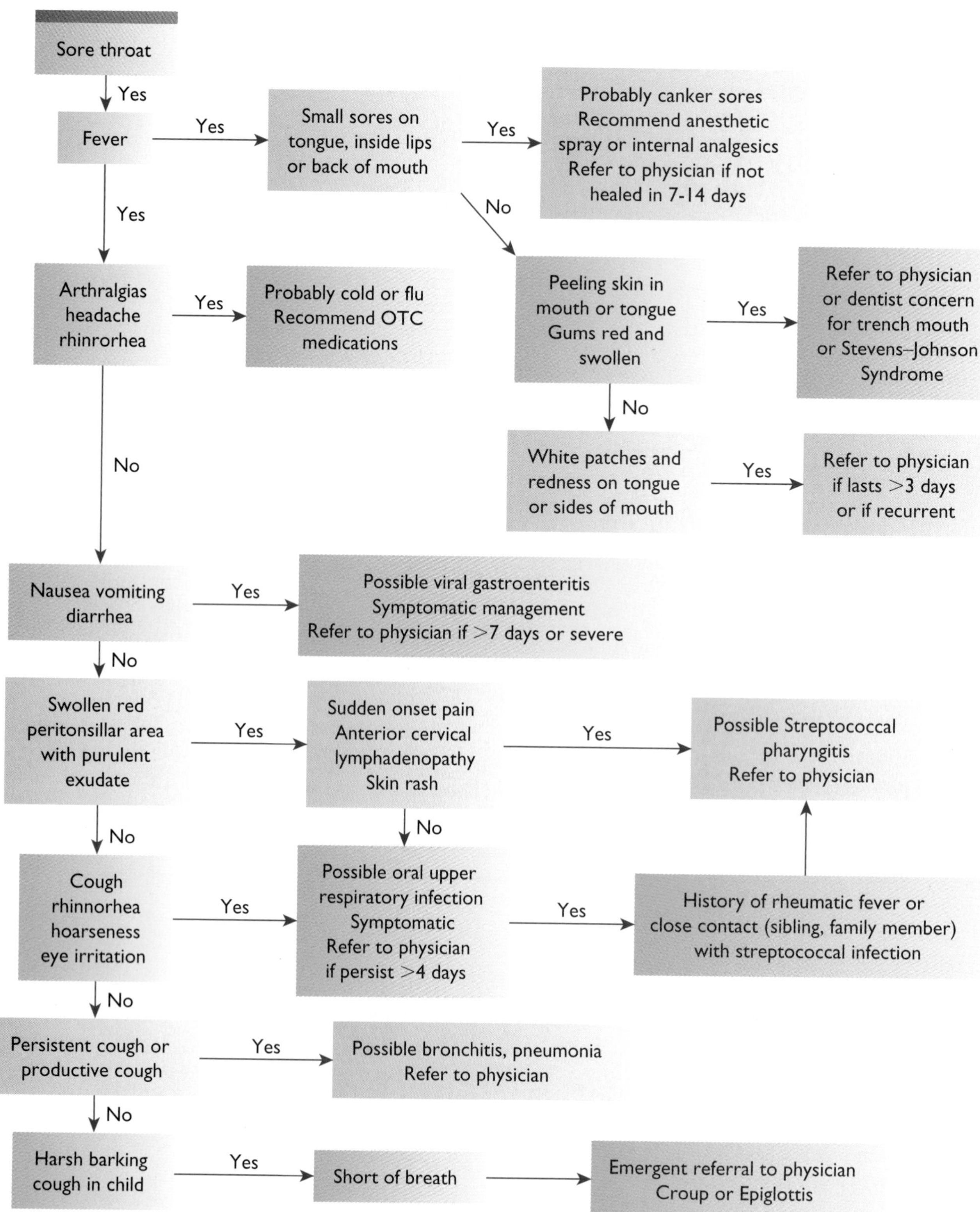

FIGURE 10-25 ■ Decision tree for sore throat.

Bibliography

Attia MW, Zaoutis T. Pharyngitis in children. Del Med J 1999;71:459–465.

Bartlett JC. Respiratory tract infections. 2nd ed. Philadelphia: Lippincott Williams & Wilkins; 1999.

Beers MH, Berkow R, eds. The Merck manual of diagnosis and therapy. 17th ed. Whitehouse Station, NJ: Merck and Co., 2000.

Bisno AL. Acute pharyngitis: etiology and diagnosis. Pediatrics 1996;9:949–954.

Boyd-Monk H. Assessing acquired ocular diseases. Advances in Physical Assessment 1990;25:811–822.

Cauthorne-Burnette T, Estes MEZ. Clinical companion for health assessment and physical examination. Albany, NY: Delmar Publishers, 1998.

Chow JM. The diagnosis and management of sinusitis. Compr Ther 1995;21(2):74–79.

Druce HM. Sinusitis: agents, diagnostic strategies and techniques, treatments, and problems. Immunol Allergy Clin North Am 1993;13:119–132.

Estrada B. GAS pharyngitis: when it doesn't go away. Infect Med 1999;16:822–823.

Hopkins B. Assessment of nutritional status. In: Gottschlich MM, Mantarese LE, Shronts EP, eds. Nutrition support dietetics: core curriculum. 2nd ed. Silver Springs, MD: American Society for Parenteral and Enteral Nutrition, 1993:15–70.

Gwaltney JM. Rational management of sore throat. Patient Care 1996;September:76–93.

Jones NS. Current concepts in the management of pediatric rhinosinusitis. J Laryngol Otol 1999;113:1–9.

Kennedy V, Youngs R. A guide to the management of chronic sinusitis. Practitioner 1998;242:712–717.

Lance JW, Goadsby PJ. Mechanism and management of headache. 6th ed. Oxford: Butterworth-Heinemann; 1998.

Lee JM, Ryan-Wenger N. The "Think-Aloud" seminar for teaching clinical reasoning: a case study of a child with pharyngitis. Pediatr Health Care 1997;11:101–110.

Little DR, Mann BL, Sherk DW. Factors influencing the clinical diagnosis of sinusitis. J Fam Pract 1998;46:147–152.

Little, et al. How family physicians distinguish acute sinusitis from upper respiratory tract infection. J Fam Pract 2000;13(2):101–106.

Martini FH, Timmons MJ. Human anatomy. 2nd ed. Upper Saddle River, NJ. Prentice Hall, 1997:633–638.

McMinn RMH, Gaddum-Rosse P, Hutchings RT, Logan BM. McMinn's functional and clinical anatomy. London: Mosby, 1995.

Noak H, Rothrock JF. Migraine: definitions, mechanisms, and treatment. South Med J 1996;89:762–769.

Perkins A. An approach to diagnosing the acute sore throat. Am Fam Physician 1997;January:131–138.

Poole MD. A focus on acute sinusitis in adults: change in disease management. Am J Med 1999;106(5A):38S–52S.

Pray WS. Plaque-induced diseases: caries and gingivitis. In: Nonprescription product therapeutics. Lippincott Williams & Wilkins, 1999:33–52.

Ratcliff PA, Johnson PW. The relationship between oral malodor, gingivitis and periodontitis. A review. J Periodontol 1999;70:485–489.

Richer M, Deschenes M. Upper respiratory tract infections. In: Dipiro JT, Talbert RL, Yee GC, et al., eds. Pharmacotherapy: a pathophysiologic approach. 4th ed. Stamford, CT: Appleton & Lange, 1999:1671–1684.

Weinberger DG, Andersen PE. Diagnosis and treatment of common ear, nose and throat disorders. Hospital Physician 1996;June:11–23.

Wilson J. Current approaches to sinusitis. Practitioner 1994;238:467–474.

CHAPTER

11

Respiratory System

Rhonda M. Jones

GLOSSARY TERMS

- Asthma
- Bradypnea
- Bronchitis
- Bronchophony
- Chronic obstructive pulmonary disease
- Crackles
- Cyanosis
- Dyspnea
- Egophany
- Emphysema
- Friction rub
- Hyperpnea
- Hyperresonance
- Hypoxemia
- Orthopnea
- Pallor
- Paroxysmal nocturnal dyspnea
- Pneumonia
- Resonance
- Rhonchi
- Tachypnea
- Tactile fremitus
- Wheezes
- Whispered pectoriloquy

ANATOMY AND PHYSIOLOGY OVERVIEW

The primary function of the respiratory system is transporting air into and out of the lungs so that oxygen can be exchanged for carbon dioxide. The upper respiratory system includes the nose, nasal cavity, sinuses, and pharynx. The lower respiratory system includes the trachea, bronchi, and lungs (Fig. 11-1). In this chapter, only the lower respiratory system is discussed. (For a discussion of the upper respiratory system, see Chapter 10.)

The thoracic cage, or the bones of the chest, consists of 12 thoracic vertebrae, 12 pairs of ribs, and the sternum (Fig. 11-2). The ribs and the sternum form the rib cage and support the thoracic cavity. The spaces between the ribs are termed the intercostals spaces and are numbered according to the superior rib above (e.g., the second intercostal space is located below the second rib). The diaphragm is a muscle that separates the thoracic cavity from the abdomen and is used during inspiration.

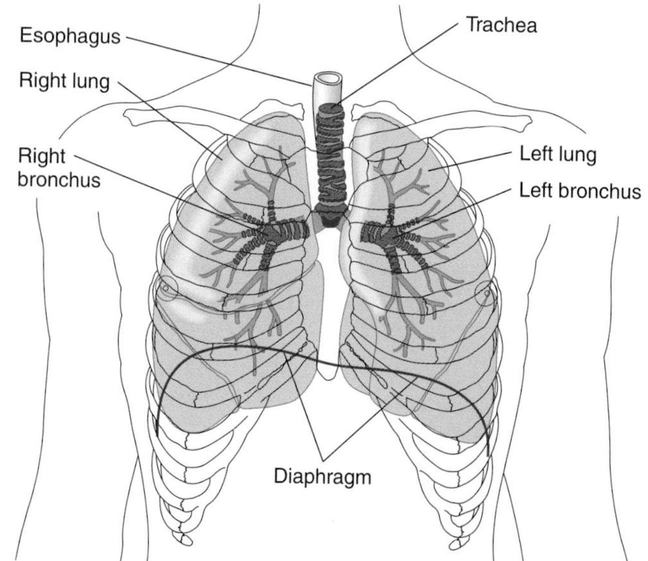

FIGURE 11-1 ■ The lower respiratory system.

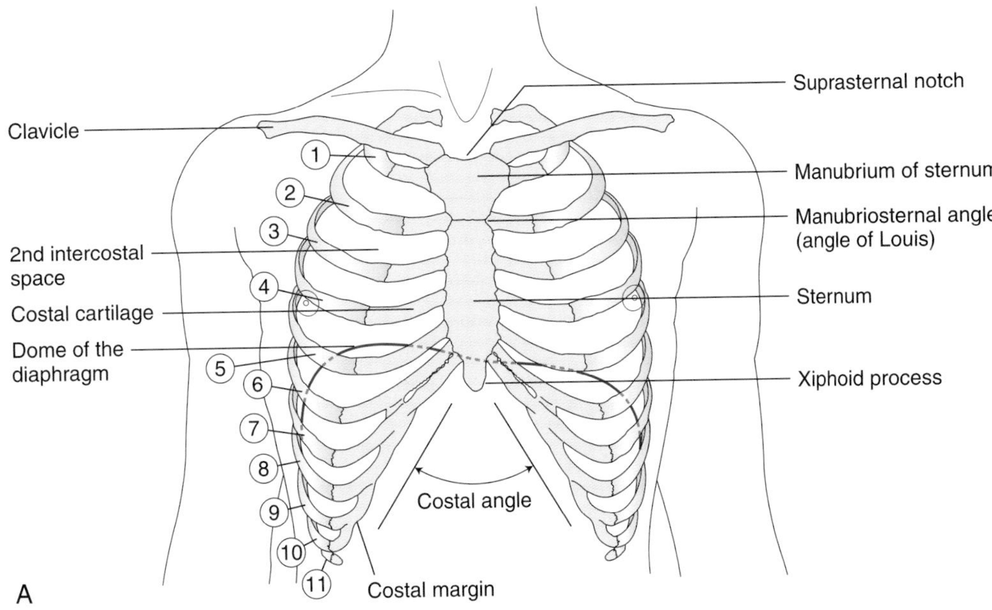

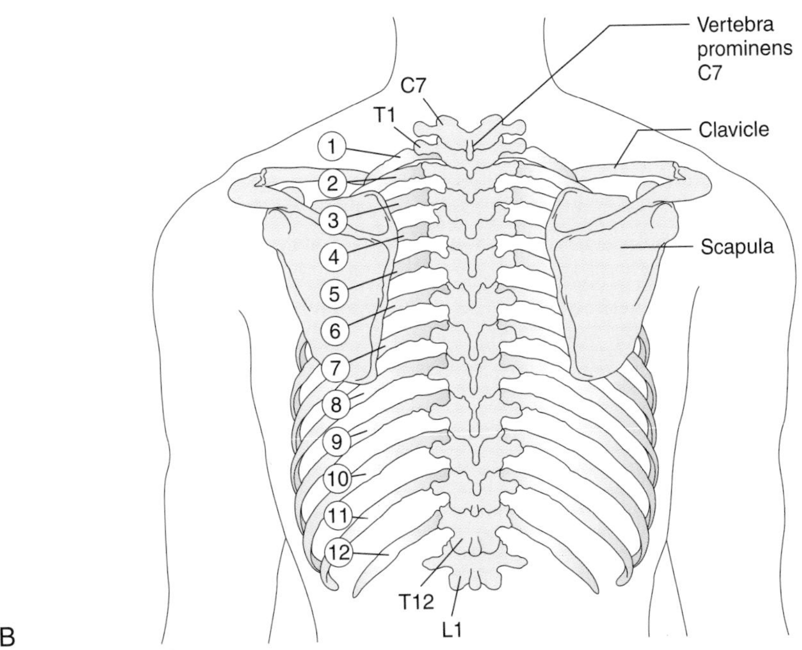

FIGURE 11-2 ■ The thoracic cage (bones of chest, vertebrae, ribs, and sternum). **(A)** Anterior thoracic cage. **(B)** Posterior thoracic cage.

Surface Landmarks

Surface landmarks of the thorax are useful in identifying the underlying internal structures and in describing physical findings. They also facilitate documentation and communication of physical findings to other health care professionals.

Anterior Thoracic Landmarks

Primary anterior thoracic landmarks include the suprasternal notch, sternum, and manubriosternal angle. The suprasternal notch is the U-shaped depression at the top of the sternum between the clavicles. The sternum, or "breastbone," consists of the manubrium, the body, and the xiphoid process. The articulation between the manubrium and the body of the sternum is the manubriosternal angle, which is commonly referred to as the angle of Louis. The angle of Louis is continuous with the second rib and is a useful place to start counting the ribs. It is also useful in locating the underlying structures, because the trachea bifurcates into the right and left main bronchi just under the angle of Louis.

Posterior Thoracic Landmarks

Posterior thoracic landmarks include the vertebra prominens, spinous processes, and scapula. The vertebra prominens is the seventh cervical vertebra and is found as the bony spur that protrudes from the base of the neck when the neck is flexed anteriorly. If two vertebra are observed when the neck is flexed, the superior one is C7, and the inferior one is T1. The spinous processes are the knobs on the vertebrae, which form the spinal column. The scapula, or the "shoulder blades," are located symmetrically on each side of the spinal column. The lower tip of the scapula is usually located at the seventh or eighth rib.

Reference Lines

Reference lines are used to identify and to document findings vertically on the chest. On the anterior chest, these include the midsternal and midclavicular lines (Fig. 11-3). On the posterior chest, these include the vertebral and scapular lines. The lateral chest is divided by the anterior, posterior, and midaxillary lines.

Trachea and Bronchial Tree

Air is inhaled through the mouth and the nose, and it then passes through the pharynx, larynx, and finally, a tough, flexible tube called the trachea (i.e., the windpipe). The trachea is approximately 1 inch in diameter and 4.25 inches in length, and it branches to form the left and right primary bronchi (Fig. 11-4). The left primary bronchus supplies air to the left lung; the right primary bronchus supplies air to the right lung. As the primary bronchi enter the lungs, they divide into smaller passageways, which are called secondary bronchi and bronchioles. The bronchioles are the thinnest segments of the bronchial tree and supply air to the alveoli, which are the exchange surfaces of the lungs. The alveoli are connected to an extensive network of blood vessels, through which oxygen is exchanged for carbon dioxide (Fig. 11-4).

Lungs

The thoracic cavity is composed of the rib cage (as the "walls") and the diaphragm (as the "floor") (Fig. 11-5). The mediastinum separates the two pleural cavities. Each lung is positioned within a single pleural cavity, which is lined with a serous membrane called the pleura. The parietal pleura covers the inner surface of the thoracic wall and extends over the diaphragm and mediastinum. The visceral pleura covers the outer lung surfaces and extends into the fissures between the lobes. The pleural membranes secrete a small amount of pleural fluid, which provides a moist, slippery coating for lubrication during breathing.

The lungs are each divided into distinct lobes. The right lung has three lobes: the superior, the middle, and the inferior. The left lung has only two lobes: the superior, and the inferior. The base of each lung rests on the superior surface of the diaphragm.

Respiration

Respiration is the process of exchanging oxygen and carbon dioxide. Air is brought into the lungs through inspiration and is expelled through expiration. The muscles that assist with respiration are the diaphragm and the external and internal intercostals. During inspiration, downward contraction of the diaphragm increases the volume of the thoracic cavity, causing air to rush into the lungs. The external intercostals assist with inspiration by elevating the ribs. During expiration, the diaphragm relaxes back against the lungs, decreasing the volume of the thoracic cavity and, thereby, forcing air out of the lungs. Simultaneously, the internal intercostals depress the ribs, assisting with expiration.

When the depth and the rate of respiration need to be increased, such as during exercise or with respiratory distress, the

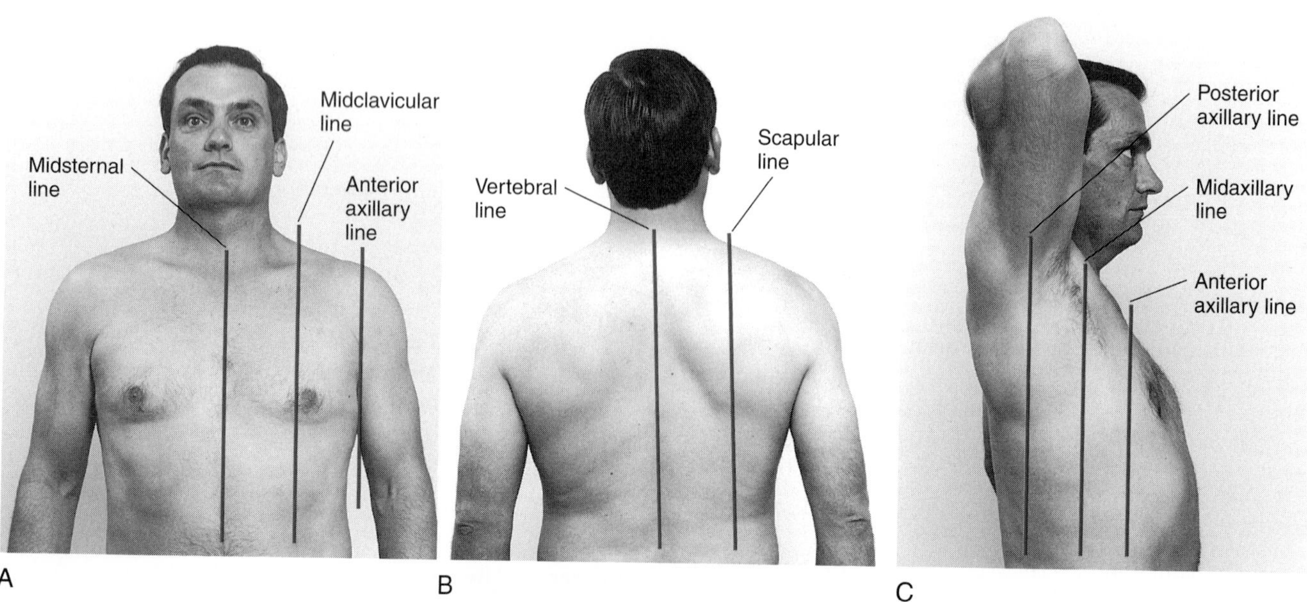

FIGURE 11-3 ■ Reference lines. **(A)** Midsternal and midclavicular lines. **(B)** Vertebral and scapular lines. **(C)** Anterior, posterior, and midaxillary lines.

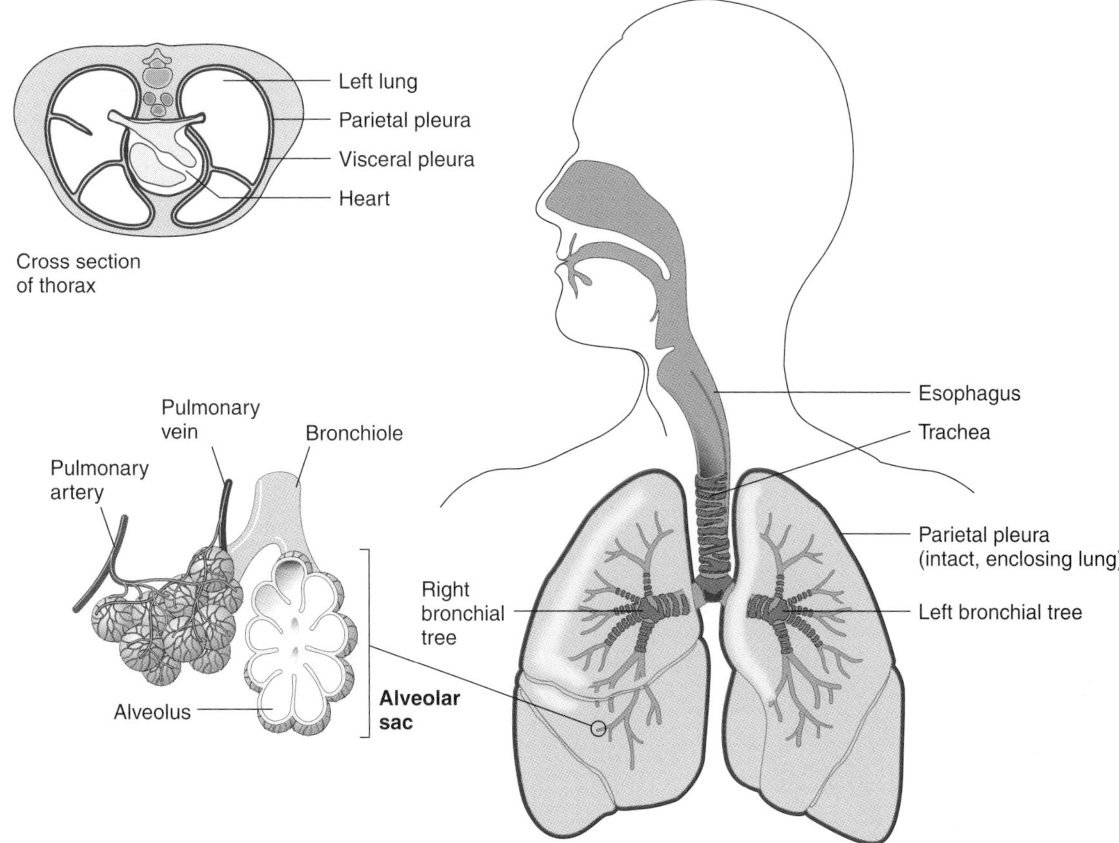

FIGURE 11-4 ■ The trachea and bronchial tree.

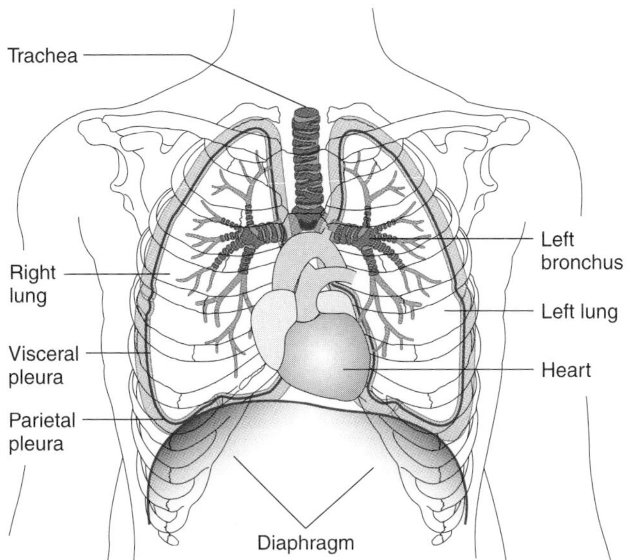

FIGURE 11-5 ■ The thoracic cavity (rib cage and diaphragm).

accessory muscles in the neck elevate the ribs and sternum, allowing a larger volume of air to enter the lungs during inspiration. These muscles include the sternomastoids, scaleni, and the trapezii (Fig. 11-6). In addition, during expiration, the abdominal muscles powerfully contract, forcing the diaphragm further against the lungs.

Special Considerations

Pediatric Patients

All body systems in the child develop in utero. The respiratory system, however, does not function on its own until birth, and it continues to develop throughout childhood. The diameter and length of the airways increase, as do the number and size of the alveoli. In addition, the infant's chest is round, whereas the toddler's chest is more oval, usually reaching the adult shape (i.e., a 1:2 diameter) by the age of 6 years.

Geriatric Patients

Several factors cause a person's respiratory efficiency to decline with increasing age. During aging, elastic tissue, such as the tissue of the lungs, deteriorates throughout the body. Thus, the lungs' ability to inflate and deflate slowly declines. Arthritic changes in the ribs and decreased flexibility of costal cartilage also occur with increasing age. These changes, along with decreasing elasticity, cause stiffening and reduction in chest movement that, in turn, decrease respiratory volume. This volume reduction is a significant cause of the decreased exercise performance that occurs in elderly persons.

Pregnant Patients

As the fetus grows inside the uterus, it elevates the diaphragm by approximately 4 cm. Meanwhile, the mother's higher estro-

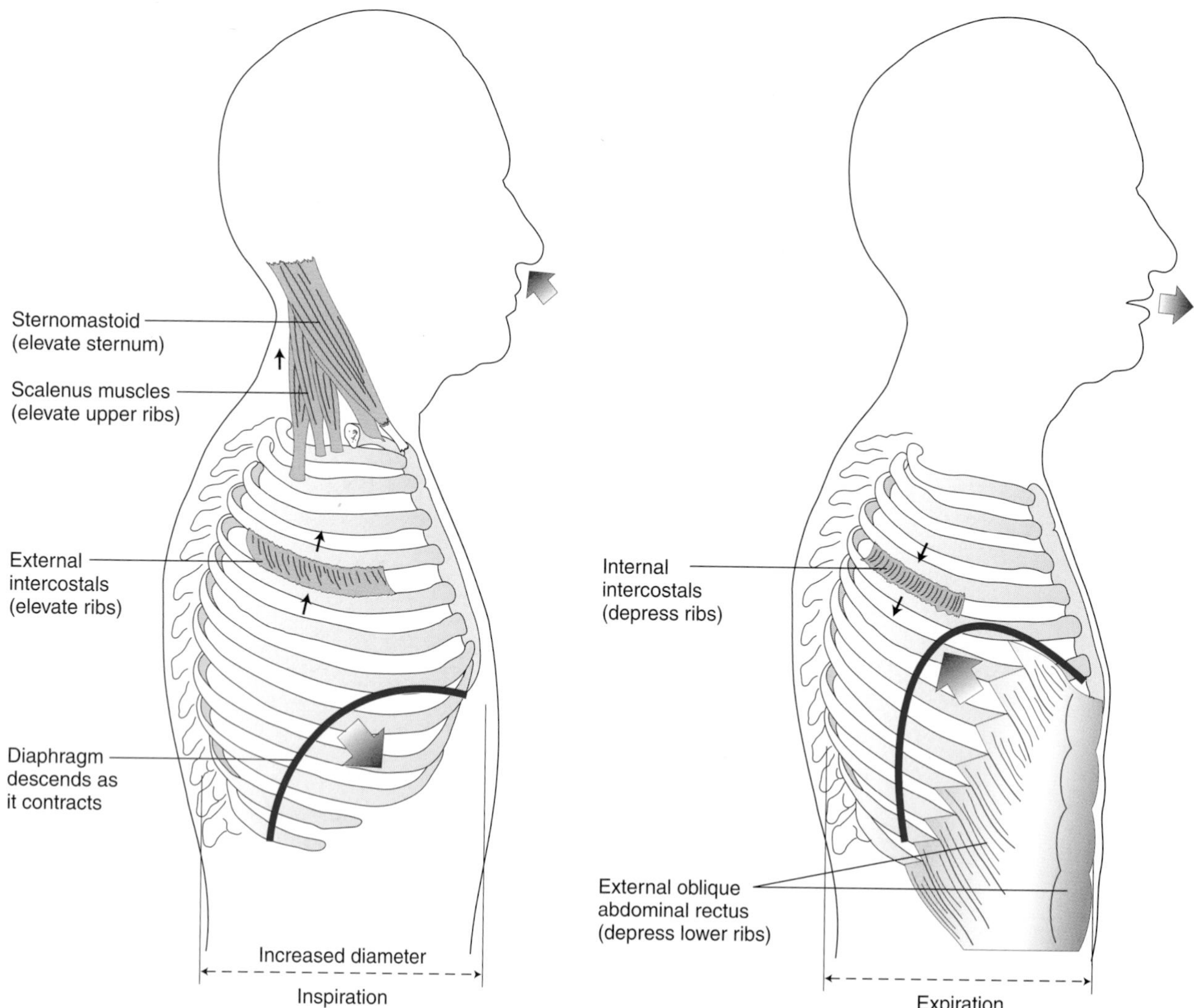

FIGURE 11-6 ■ Muscles of respiration.

gen levels relax the ligaments of the rib cage, increasing the total rib cage circumference by approximately 6 cm. The growing fetus also increases the oxygen demand on the mother's body. Typically, the mother compensates by breathing deeper with each breath while maintaining a fairly consistent respiratory rate. The mother may also experience shortness of breath (SOB).

PATHOLOGY OVERVIEW

Numerous respiratory problems can occur. The pharmacist, however, most commonly encounters asthma, chronic obstructive pulmonary disease (COPD), and pneumonia. Pharmacists not only educate patients about the proper use of medications for these diseases (e.g., metered dose inhalers, spacers, and antibiotics), but many also educate patients about the disease itself (i.e., asthma and COPD), its prevention, and self-treatment. Many pharmacists also assist patients in assessing and monitoring their breathing with peak flow meters (discussed later).

Asthma

Asthma is a chronic inflammatory disorder of the airways in which many different cells (mast cells, eosinophils, T lymphocytes, neutrophils, and epithelial cells) play a role. This inflammation causes recurrent episodes of widespread but variable airflow obstruction, which results from an increased responsiveness of the trachea and bronchi to various stimuli (physical, chemical, immunologic, and pharmacologic irritants). Even emotions such as anxiety and distress can precipitate an episode. Persistent bronchial inflammation, which causes mucus hypersecretion and bronchial smooth muscle hypertrophy, is the primary mechanism causing the hyperreactivity.

Common signs and symptoms associated with asthma are listed in Box 11-1. Because asthma is an obstructive lung disease, airflow limitation primarily occurs during expiration. This causes the classical symptoms of **dyspnea** (i.e., SOB) and expiratory wheezing. **Wheezes** are a whistling respiratory sound caused by turbulent airflow through constricted bronchi.

An asthma attack can last anywhere from one to several hours, and it can subside spontaneously or need medications.

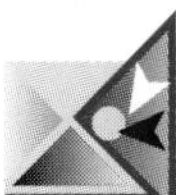

Box 11-1

COMMON SIGNS AND SYMPTOMS OF ASTHMA

SIGNS

- Recurrent and episodic
- Wheezes
- Use of accessory muscles to breathe
- Increased respiratory rate
- Increased heart rate
- Decreased FEV_1/FVC
- Decreased PEF

SYMPTOMS

- Dyspnea (breathlessness)
- Cough (nonproductive)
- Chest tightness/pressure
- Anxiety

FEV_1, forced expiratory volume in 1 second; *FVC*, forced vital capacity; *PEF*, peak expiratory flow.

Asthma severity is classified according to the frequency of symptoms (especially at night) and the lung function (Table 11-1). Factors that contribute to the severity of asthma include rhinitis, sinusitis, gastroesophageal reflux, viral respiratory infections, some medications (sensitivity to aspirin, nonsteroidal anti-inflammatory drugs and sulfites, and β-blockers).

The primary risk factor for asthma is the exposure of sensitive patients to inhalant allergens. When this occurs, patients can experience an increase in airway inflammation, hyperresponsiveness, asthma symptoms, need for medication, and even death caused by asthma. Common allergens include:

- Viral respiratory infections
- Environmental allergens (environmental tobacco smoke, air pollution, animal dander, dust mites, indoor fungi [molds], and pollen)
- Exercise
- Occupational chemicals or allergens
- Environmental changes (new house, workplace, or vacation) and irritants (tobacco smoke, strong odors, air pollutants, and aerosols)
- Emotions (fear, anxiety, and anger)
- Food or food additives
- Endocrine factors (menses, pregnancy, and thyroid disease)

A stepwise approach to pharmacologic therapy is currently recommended, with the specific type and amount of medication being determined by the severity of the asthma and being directed toward the suppression of airway inflammation (Table 11-2). Medications are categorized into two general classes: quick-relief medications to treat acute symptoms and exacerbations, and long-term control medications to treat persistent asthma. High-dose therapy is initiated at the onset of the asthma attack to establish prompt control; the dose is then cautiously tapered down once control has been achieved. Common quick-relief medications used to treat an acute asthma attack include bronchodilators (β-agonists, theophylline, and anticholinergics), which are administered by oral inhalation, nebulization, or intravenously, and corticosteroids, which are administered by oral inhalation or intravenously. Long-term control is best achieved with inhaled corticosteroids. Early intervention with inhaled corticosteroids can improve asthma

TABLE 11-1 ➤ CLASSIFICATION OF ASTHMA SEVERITY

CLINICAL FEATURES BEFORE TREATMENT*

	Symptoms**	Nighttime Symptoms	Lung Function
Step 4 Severe Persistent	• Continual symptoms • Limited physical activity • Frequent exacerbations	Frequent	• FEV_1 or PEF ≤60% predicted • PEF variability >30%
Step 3 Moderate Persistent	• Daily symptoms • Daily use of inhaled short-acting $beta_2$-agonist • Exacerbations affect activity • Exacerbations ≥2 times a week; may last days	>1 time a week	• FEV_1 or PEF >60%-<80% predicted • PEF variability >30%
Step 2 Mild Persistent	• Symptoms >2 times a week but <1 time a day • Exacerbations may affect activity	>2 times a month	• FEV_1 or PEF ≥80% predicted • PEF variability 20-30%
Step 1 Mild Intermittent	• Symptoms ≤2 times a week • Asymptomatic and normal PEF between exacerbations • Exacerbations brief (from a few hours to a few days); intensity may vary	≤2 times a month	• FEV_1 or PEF ≥80% predicted • PEF variability <20%

*The presence of one of the features of severity is sufficient to place a patient in that category. An individual should be assigned to the most severe grade in which any feature occurs. The characteristics noted in this figure are general and may overlap because asthma is highly variable. Furthermore, an individual's classification may change over time.

**Patients at any level of severity can have mild, moderate, or severe exacerbations. Some patients with intermittent asthma experience severe and life-threatening exacerbations separated by long periods of normal lung function and no symptoms.

National Heart, Lung, and Blood Institute, Global strategy for the diagnosis & management of asthma, Expert panel report 2. US Department of Health and Human Services, Public Health Service, NIH Publication NO. 97–4051, 1997.

TABLE 11-2 ➤ STEPWISE APPROACH FOR MANAGING ASTHMA IN ADULTS AND CHILDREN OLDER THAN 5 YEARS OF AGE: TREATMENT

PREFERRED TREATMENTS ARE IN BOLD PRINT.

	LONG-TERM CONTROL	QUICK RELIEF	EDUCATION
STEP 4 Severe Persistent	Daily medications: • **Anti-inflammatory: inhaled corticosteroid (high dose)** AND • Long-acting bronchodilator: either **long-acting inhaled beta$_2$-agonist,** sustained-release theophylline, or long-acting beta$_2$-agonist tablets AND • Corticosteroid tablets or syrup long term (make repeat attempts to reduce systemic steroids and maintain control with high dose inhaled steroids)	• Short-acting bronchodilator: **inhaled beta$_2$-agonists** as needed for symptoms. • Intensity of treatment will depend on severity of exacerbation; see component 3-Managing Exacerbations. • Use of short-acting inhaled beta$_2$-agonists on a daily basis, or increasing use, indicates the need for additional long-term control therapy.	Steps 2 and 3 actions plus: • Refer to individual education/counseling
STEP 3 Moderate Persistent	Daily medication: • Either **Anti-inflammatory: inhaled corticosteroid (medium dose)** OR Inhaled corticosteroid (low-medium dose) and add a long-acting bronchodilator, especially for nighttime symptoms; either **long-acting inhaled beta$_2$-agonist,** sustained-release theophylline, or long-acting beta$_2$-agonist tablets • If needed Anti-inflammatory: **inhaled corticosteroids (medium-high dose)** AND **Long-acting bronchodilator,** especially for nighttime symptoms; either long-acting **inhaled beta$_2$-agonist,** sustained-release theophylline, or long-acting beta$_2$-agonist tablets.	• Short-acting bronchodilator; **inhaled beta$_2$-agonists** as needed for symptoms. • Intensity of treatment will depend on severity of exacerbation; see component 3-Managing Exacerbations • Use of short-acting inhaled beta$_2$-agonists on a daily basis, or increasing use, indicates the need for additional long-term-control therapy.	Step 1 actions plus: • Teach self-monitoring • Refer to group education if available • Review and update self-management plan
STEP 2 Mild Persistent	One daily medication: • **Anti-inflammatory**: either **inhaled corticosteroid** (low doses) or **cromolyn or nedocromil** (children usually begin with a trial of cromolyn or nedocromil). • Sutained-release theophylline to serum concentration of 5-15 mcg/mL is an alternative, but not preferred, therapy. Zafirlukast or zileuton may also be considered for patients >12 years of age, although their position in therapy is not fully established.	• Short-acting bronchodilator; **inhaled beta$_2$-agonists** as needed for symptoms. • Intensity of treatment will depend on severity of exacerbation; see component 3-Managing Exacerbations • Use of short-acting inhaled beta$_2$-agonists on a daily basis, or increasing use, indicates the need for additional long-term-control therapy.	Step 1 actions plus: • Teach self-monitoring • Refer to group education if available • Review and update self-management plan

NHLBI. Global strategy for the diagnosis and management of asthma. Expert panel report 2. US Dept. of Health and Human Services, Public Health Services, NIH Publication No. 97–4051, 1997.

Continued

TABLE 11-2 ➤ *(Continued)*

PREFERRED TREATMENTS ARE IN BOLD PRINT.

	LONG-TERM CONTROL	QUICK RELIEF	EDUCATION
STEP 1 Mild Intermittent	• No daily medication needed.	• Short-acting bronchodilator; **inhaled beta$_2$-agonists** as needed for symptoms. • Intensity of treatment will depend on severity of exacerbation; see component 3-Managing Exacerbations • Use of short-acting inhaled beta$_2$-agonists on a daily basis, or increasing use, indicates the need for additional long-term-control therapy.	• Teach basic facts about asthma • Teach inhaler/spacer/holding chamber technique • Discuss roles of medications • Develop self-management plan • Develop action plan for when and how to take rescue actions, especially for patients with a history of severe exacerbations • Discuss appropriate environment control measures to avoid exposure to known allergens and irritants (See component 4.)

↓ **Step down**
Review treatment every 1 to 6 months; a gradual stepwise reduction in treatment may be possible.

↑ **Step up**
If control is not maintained, consider step up. First, review patient medication technique, adherence, and environment control (avoidance of allergens or other factors that contribute to asthma severity).

NOTE:

- The stepwise approach presents general guidelines to assist clinical decisionmaking; it is not intended to be a specific prescription. Asthma is highly variable; clinicians should tailor specific medication plans to the needs and circumstances of individual patients.
- Gain control as quickly as possible; then decrease treatment to the least medication necessary to maintain control. Gaining control may be accomplished by either starting treatment at the step most appropriate to the initial severity of the condition or starting at a higher level of therapy (e.g., a course of systemic corticosteroids or higher dose of inhaled corticosteroids).
- A rescue course of systemic corticosteroids may be needed at any time and at any step.
- Some patients with intermittent asthma experience severe and life-threatening exacerbations separated by long periods of normal lung function and no symptoms. This may be especially common with exacerbations provoked by respiratory infections. A short course of systemic corticosteroids is recommended.
- At each step, patients should control their environment to avoid or control factors that make their asthma worse (e.g., allergens, irritants); this requires specific diagnosis and education.
- Referral to an asthma specialist for consultation or comanagement is *recommended* if there are difficulties achieving or maintaining control of asthma or if the patient requires step 4 care. Referral may be *considered* if the patient requires step 3 care (see also component 1-Initial Assessment and Diagnosis).

NHLBI. Global strategy for the diagnosis and management of asthma. Expert panel report 2. US Dept. of Health and Human Services, Public Health Services, NIH Publication No. 97–4051, 1997.

control, normalize lung function, and possibly, prevent irreversible airway injury. Scheduled doses of inhaled β-agonists, leukotriene-receptor antagonists, 5-lipoxygenase inhibitors, anticholinergics, and oral theophylline are also used to prevent recurrent asthma attacks.

Patient education is the cornerstone of asthma management and should be incorporated into routine health care, including pharmaceutical care practices. The most effective nonpharmacologic intervention is the identification and avoidance of environmental precipitants or exposures. In other words, environmental control strategies are a key to successful asthma management by decreasing the risk of asthma attacks.

Chronic Obstructive Pulmonary Disease

Chronic obstructive pulmonary disease is characterized by airflow limitation (primarily expiratory flow) that is not fully reversible. The airflow limitation is progressive and associated with an abnormal inflammatory response to noxious particles or gases, primarily cigarette smoke. The chronic inflammation occurs throughout the airways, parenchyma, and pulmonary vasculature. Activated inflammatory cells (macrophages, T lymphocytes, and neutrophils) release a variety of mediators (leukotrienes, interleukin-8, and tumor necrosis factor) that damage the lung structures and that sustain neutrophilic inflammation. In the trachea, bronchi, and larger bronchioles, chronic inflammation leads to enlarged mucus-secreting glands and an increased number of goblet cells, which cause mucus hypersecretion. In the small bronchi and bronchioles, chronic inflammation leads to repeated cycles of injury and repair of the airway wall. This continual repair process structurally changes the airway wall by increasing its collagen content and creating scar tissue, which narrows the lumen and produces fixed airway obstruction.

Patients with COPD experience symptoms of cough, sputum production, and dyspnea; other signs and symptoms are listed in Box 11-2. Chronic cough is usually the first symptom of COPD and initially is intermittent but later is present every day (frequently throughout the day). Tenacious sputum is usually produced with the cough. As lung function deteriorates, breathlessness or dyspnea becomes worse, and this is why most persons seek medical attention. The objective signs of COPD are identified by spirometry (*see Laboratory and Diagnostic Tests*). Specifically, the presence of a forced expiratory volume in 1 second (FEV_1) after bronchodilator therapy less than 80% of the predicted value in combination with an FEV_1/forced vital capacity (FVC) less than 70% illustrates the presence of airflow limitation that is not fully reversible and confirms a diagnosis of COPD.

In addition, COPD is a general term used to describe patients with chronic bronchitis, emphysema, or some combination of both. Chronic **bronchitis** is characterized by inflammation and edema of the bronchioles, which causes excessive mucus production and airway obstruction. Patients with chronic bronchitis have a persistent productive cough on most days for at least 3 months a year in at least two consecutive years. Patients may appear cyanotic (bluish) because of chronic **hypoxemia** (low oxygen concentration in the blood) and are sometimes referred to as "blue bloaters." Other common signs and symptoms associated with chronic bronchitis are listed in Box 11-3.

Emphysema is characterized by an abnormal, permanent enlargement of airspaces distal to the bronchioles. This permanent enlargement destroys the alveolar walls. Consequently, elastic recoil decreases, and bronchiolar collapse results during expiration. Dyspnea is usually the first symptom, whereas a cough (usually nonproductive) is variable from patient to patient. Patients frequently need to use accessory muscles to assist their breathing, which usually has a long expiratory phase. Patients are typically not cyanotic and may occasionally be referred to as "pink puffers." Other signs and symptoms associated with emphysema are listed in Box 11-4.

The classification of COPD is based on the severity of disease (Table 11-3). Stage 0 (at risk) is characterized by chronic cough and sputum production, but the lung function (as measured by spirometry) is still normal. Stage I (mild COPD) is characterized by mild airflow limitation and usually, but not always, by chronic cough and sputum production. Stage II (moderate COPD) is characterized with the progression of symptoms, specifically SOB, which typically occurs on exertion. Most individuals seek medical attention during this stage because of the dyspnea or increasing exacerbations of the disease. As the dyspnea and exacerbations increase, the patient's quality of life begins to be affected. Stage III (severe COPD) is characterized by severe airflow limitation, respiratory failure, or clinical signs of right heart failure. The patient's quality of life is significantly decreased, and exacerbations may be life-threatening.

Risk factors for COPD include both genetic factors (deficiency of a_1-antitrypsin and airway hyperresponsiveness) and environmental exposures. By far, cigarette smoking is the most significant environmental exposure for the development of COPD. Other environmental risk factors include air pollution and heavy exposure to occupational dusts and chemicals (e.g., grain, coal, and asbestos).

The overall approach to stable COPD is a stepwise increase in treatment based on the severity of disease (Table 11-4). Individualized assessment of disease severity as well as response to various therapies is a key management strategy. Pharmacologic therapy is used to prevent and to control symptoms, to reduce the frequency of exacerbations, and to improve exercise/activity tolerance. Unfortunately, no existing medication has been shown to modify the long-term decline in lung function. The primary medications used for symptom management are inhaled bron-

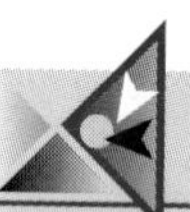

Box 11-2

SIGNS AND SYMPTOMS ASSOCIATED WITH CHRONIC OBSTRUCTIVE PULMONARY DISEASE

SIGNS

- Abnormal spirometry (FEV_1 <80% of predicted value and FEV_1/FVC <70%)
- Gas-exchange abnormalities
- Pulmonary hyperinflation
- Pulmonary hypertension
- Cor pulmonale

SYMPTOMS

- Mucus hypersecretion
- Chronic cough
- Chronic sputum production
- Expiratory airflow limitation/dyspnea
- Chest tightness
- Wheezing

FEV_1, forced expiratory volume in 1 second; FVC, forced vital capacity.

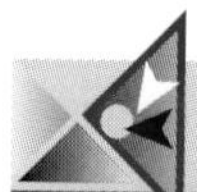

Box 11-3

COMMON SIGNS AND SYMPTOMS OF CHRONIC BRONCHITIS

SIGNS

- Typically obese
- Hypoxia
- Carbon dioxide retention
- Cyanosis
- "Blue bloaters"
- Crackles/rhonchi
- Decreased breath sounds
- Altered pulmonary function tests
- Altered blood gases

SYMPTOMS

- Cough (productive; most days for at least 3 months/year for 2 consecutive years)
- Dyspnea
- Frequent respiratory infections
- History of cigarette smoking

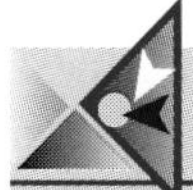

Box 11-4

COMMON SIGNS AND SYMPTOMS OF EMPHYSEMA

SIGNS

- Prolonged expiration
- Thin
- Use of accessory muscles to assist breathing
- Tripod position to assist breathing (sitting forward with hands on hips/knees)
- Usually not cyanotic ("pink puffers")
- Barrel chest
- Decreased breath sounds
- Decreased FEV_1/FVC
- Altered blood gases (advanced stages)

SYMPTOMS

- Dyspnea (usually severe)
- Weight loss
- Cough (variable; nonproductive)

FEV_1, forced expiratory volume in 1 second; *FVC*, forced vital capacity.

TABLE 11-3 ➤ CLASSIFICATION OF CHRONIC OBSTRUCTIVE PULMONARY DISEASE

STAGE	CHARACTERISTICS[a]
0:At risk	Normal spirometry Chronic symptoms (cough, sputum production)
I:Mild COPD	$FEV_1/FVC < 70\%$ $FEV_1 \geq 80\%$ predicted value With or without chronic symptoms (cough, sputum production, dyspnea)
II:Moderate COPD	$FEV_1/FVC < 70\%$ FEV_1 30%–80% predicted value
IIA	FEV_1 50%–80% predicted value
IIB	FEV_1 30%–50% predicted value With or without chronic symptoms (cough, sputum production, dyspnea)
III:Severe COPD	$FEV_1/FVC < 70$ FEV_1 30%–50% predicted value and respiratory failure or clinical signs of right heart failure.

Adapted from National Heart, Lung, and Blood Institute. Global strategy for the diagnosis, management, and prevention of chronic obstructive pulmonary disease. NHLBI/WHO workshop report. U.S. Department of Health and Human Services, Public Health Service, National Institutes of Health publication no. 2701A, 2001. Available from http://www.goldcopd.com

FEV_1, forced expiratory volume in 1 second; *FVC*, forced vital capacity.

[a]All FEV_1 values refer to postbronchodilator therapy.

TABLE 11-4 ➤ THERAPY AT EACH STAGE OF CHRONIC OBSTRUCTIVE PULMONARY DISEASE

STAGE	CHARACTERISTICS	RECOMMENDED TREATMENT[A]	
All		Avoidance of risk factors Influenza vaccination	
0:At risk	Chronic symptoms (cough and sputum production) Exposure to risk factors Normal spirometry		
I:Mild COPD	$FEV_1/FVC < 70\%$ $FEV_1 \geq 80\%$ With or without symptoms	Short-acting bronchodilator when needed	
II:Moderate COPD IIA	$FEV_1/FVC < 70\%$ FEV_1 50%–80% predicted With or without symptoms	Scheduled treatment with one or more bronchodilators	Inhaled glucocorticosteroids if significant symptoms and lung function response
IIB	$FEV_1/FVC < 70\%$ FEV_1 30%–50% predicted With or without symptoms	Scheduled treatment with one or more bronchodilators	Inhaled glucocorticosteroids if significant symptoms and lung function response or if repeated exacerbations
III:Severe COPD	$FEV_1/FVC < 70\%$ $FEV_1 < 30\%$ predicted or presence of respiratory failure or right heart failure	Scheduled treatment with one or more bronchodilators Inhaled glucocorticosteroids if significant symptoms and lung function response or if repeated exacerbations Treatment of complications Long-term oxygen therapy if respiratory failure	

Adapted from National Heart, Lung, and Blood Institute. Global strategy for the diagnosis, management, and prevention of chronic obstructive pulmonary disease. NHLBI/WHO workshop report. U.S. Department of Health and Human Services, Public Health Service, National Institutes of Health publication no. 2701A, 2001. Available from http://www.goldcopd.com

FEV_1, forced expiratory volume in 1 second; *FVC*, forced vital capacity.

[A]Patients must be taught how and when to use their inhalers, oral medications, and oxygen therapy. β-Blocking agents (including eye drop formulations) should be avoided.

chodilators, primarily β_2-agonists, which are used on an as-needed or a scheduled basis. Other bronchodilators include anticholinergics, theophylline, or a combination of one or more of these drugs. Scheduled treatments with inhaled steroids are reserved for symptomatic patients with a documented spirometric response to their use or for those with an FEV_1 less than 50% of the predicted value and repeated exacerbations that require treatment with antibiotics, oral glucocorticosteroids, or both. Chronic treatment with oral glucocorticosteroids is not recommended because of unfavorable side effects and no evidence of long-term benefit from their use. Other pharmacologic agents used for symptom control include antibiotics for infectious exacerbations as well as influenza and pneumococcal vaccines.

Nonpharmacologic prevention and treatment includes patient education, smoking cessation, avoidance of environmental factors, exercise training, and oxygen therapy. Patient education is a key component in the management of COPD. Smoking cessation is the single most effective intervention to reduce the risk of developing COPD and to stop its progression. The numerous products available over the counter (OTC) present pharmacists with an ideal opportunity to have a positive impact on patient care by playing an integral part in smoking cessation.

Pneumonia

Pneumonia is an inflammation of the lungs that is most commonly caused by a community-acquired bacterial infection, *Streptococcus pneumoniae,* which is also generally referred to as pneumococcal pneumonia. Other bacterial pathogens of community- and hospital-acquired pneumonia are listed in Box 11-5. The infection causes interalveolar exudation (slow release of fluid containing proteins and white blood cells) that results in consolidation or solidification of the lungs. Typically, the consolidation is confined to one lobe (e.g., right lower lobe pneumonia). Risk factors for developing pneumonia include:

- Age (elderly and infants)
- Smoking
- Chronic bronchitis
- Chronic illness (e.g., congestive heart failure [CHF], diabetes, and COPD)
- Stroke
- Critical illness
- Alcoholism
- Surgery (ineffective coughing and deep breathing after surgery)

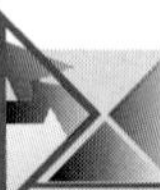

Box 11-5

CAUSES OF BACTERIAL PNEUMONIA

COMMUNITY-ACQUIRED PNEUMONIA

- *Streptococcus pneumoniae*
- *Haemophilus influenzae*
- *Staphylococcus aureus*
- *Klebsiella pneumoniae*
- *Mycoplasma pneumoniae*

HOSPITAL-ACQUIRED (NOSOCOMIAL) PNEUMONIA

- *Pseudomonas aeruginosa*
- *Staphylococcus aureus*
- *Legionella pneumophila*
- *Klebsiella pneumoniae*

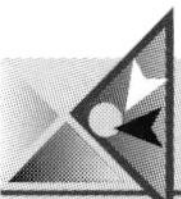

Box 11-6

SIGNS AND SYMPTOMS OF PNEUMONIA

SIGNS

- Tachypnea
- Tachycardia
- Mild hypoxemia
- Decreased breath sounds
- Dullness on chest percussion
- Vowel tone changes with auscultation
- Consolidation on chest radiograph
- Elevated white-blood-cell count with a left shift

SYMPTOMS

- Fever
- Chills
- Productive cough
- Rust-colored, purulent sputum
- Pleuritic (sharp, knife-like) chest pain

Typically, pneumonia follows a viral upper respiratory tract infection, with patients abruptly experiencing high fever; "chills"; productive cough with rust-colored, purulent sputum; and sharp chest pain. Other signs and symptoms associated with pneumonia are listed in Box 11-6. Pneumococcal pneumonia is commonly treated with a penicillin antibiotic. Other alternative antibiotics include a first-generation cephalosporin or erythromycin.

SYSTEM ASSESSMENT

Subjective Information

Patients frequently present to the pharmacist with various subjective respiratory complaints. These patients typically request advice concerning OTC "cough and cold" products. To determine the most probable cause of the respiratory symptoms and the need for a specific OTC product or physician referral, the pharmacist must ask appropriate questions to elicit specific patient data.

Cough

? INTERVIEW How long have you had the cough? What time of the day does it usually occur? Early morning? Does it wake you up at night? Do you cough up any sputum, or is it a dry, hacking cough? What makes the cough worse? What relieves it? Do you have any other symptoms with it? Fever? Chest pain? Runny nose? Nasal congestion? Headache? Swollen glands? Gasping? Any recent illness? Any injury?

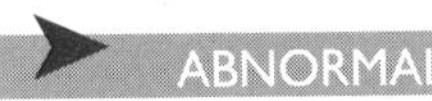

ABNORMALITIES Table 11-5 lists common causes of characteristic coughs.

Sputum

? INTERVIEW How much sputum do you cough up? What color is it? Does it ever have blood in it? What consistency is it? Thick and purulent? Frothy? Fever? Any other symptoms?

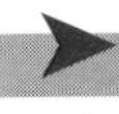

ABNORMALITIES Table 11-6 lists sputum characteristics and possible causes.

Dyspnea

? INTERVIEW When do you become short of breath? Is the onset quick or gradual? What brings it on? Exertion? Rest? Lying down? What relieves it? Does it occur at any specific time of day? At night? If yes, how many pillows do you need to use to sleep comfortably at night? Any other symptoms? Chest pain? Wheezing? Fever? Cough? Any bluish discoloration around the lips, nose, fingers, or toes? Do you smoke? Have you smoked in the past? Have you ever been told you have a respiratory problem such as asthma? Do you use an inhaler? How do you use it? Does anyone in your family have similar problems?

ABNORMALITIES SOB with exertion, commonly termed dyspnea on exertion (DOE), may occur with angina or CHF. In turn, CHF may cause SOB while the patient is lying flat, or **orthopnea,** in which the patient may need more than one pillow to sleep at night. In addition, CHF may cause a sudden gasping for air while sleeping at night, or **paroxysmal nocturnal dyspnea,** during which the patient may need to rush and open a window to get some fresh air. Asthma attacks usually cause wheezing along with SOB and may be associated with a specific allergen (e.g., pollen or dust). Chronic bronchitis typically causes mild to moderate SOB, depending on the extent of disease, along with a productive cough. Emphysema causes severe SOB, usually with a nonproductive cough. Patients with COPD frequently present with a combination of both chronic bronchitis and emphysema symptoms, however. The presence of cyanosis is caused by a significant reduction in arterial oxygenation.

TABLE 11-5 ➤ COUGH CHARACTERISTICS AND ASSOCIATED CAUSES

CHARACTERISTIC	POSSIBLE CAUSE
Continuous throughout the day	Respiratory infection
Nighttime	Postnasal drip, sinusitis, CHF, or ACE inhibitors
Early morning	Chronic bronchitis or smoking
Productive	Chronic bronchitis or pneumonia
Dry, hacking	Viral infection, asthma, mycoplasma pneumonia, or ACE inhibitors
Barking	Croup
Wheezing	Asthma or allergies

ACE, angiotensin-converting enzyme; *CHF*, congestive heart failure.

TABLE 11-6 ➤ SPUTUM CHARACTERISTICS AND ASSOCIATED CAUSES

CHARACTERISTIC	POSSIBLE CAUSE
Mucoid	Viral infections
Purulent	Chronic bronchitis or bacterial infections
Yellow-green	Chronic bronchitis or bacterial infections
Rust-colored	Pneumococcal pneumonia or tuberculosis
Pink, blood-tinged	Pneumococcal or staphylococcal pneumonia
Pink, frothy	Pulmonary edema
Profuse, colorless	Carcinoma
Bloody	Pulmonary emboli, tuberculosis, tumor, or warfarin therapy

Wheezing

? INTERVIEW How often does the wheezing occur? What usually causes it? What usually stops the attack? Are attacks occurring more frequently than they used to? Any other symptoms? Do you use a peak flow meter to assess your breathing? If yes, please show me how you use it. What are the values that you usually get?

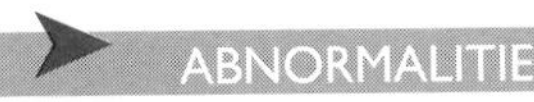

ABNORMALITIES Wheezing may be caused by asthma or heart failure.

Chest Pain with Breathing

For a complete discussion of chest pain, see Chapter 12.

? INTERVIEW Describe the pain. Is it sharp and stabbing? Specifically, where does it hurt? When does it occur? When you breathe in? Any other symptoms?

ABNORMALITIES Pleuritic chest pain is typically a sharp, stabbing pain that is felt on inspiration and is usually localized to one side. It is caused by inflammation of the parietal pleura.

Objective Information

Objective patient data include the physical assessment as well as laboratory and diagnostic tests. Pharmacists most commonly inspect the patient for abnormal respiratory symptoms. The techniques of palpation, percussion, and auscultation are included here for completeness of the respiratory assessment; pharmacists rarely perform these during a physical examination.

Physical Assessment

Physical assessment pertaining to the respiratory system includes inspection of the neck and chest as well as palpation, percussion, and auscultation of the posterior chest.

TECHNIQUE

STEP I

Inspect the Chest

Inspection is useful to assess the chest's shape and symmetry, the pattern and ease of respiration, and the appearance of cyanosis.

- Have the patient sit upright, leaning slightly forward with the arms resting comfortably across his or her lap.
- Inspect the chest's shape and symmetry. Normally, the chest's anteroposterior diameter is less than the transverse or side-to-side diameter.
- Inspect how the chest moves with respiration. Normally, symmetric movement occurs on both sides.

ABNORMALITIES A barrel chest has an anteroposterior diameter equal to or greater than the transverse diameter (Fig. 11-7) and is a sign of "air trapping" in the lungs, which can occur with the normal aging process as the lungs lose their elasticity. A barrel chest can also develop, however, from chronic emphysema caused by hyperinflation of the lungs. Patients may sit with their hands on their knees to support the rib cage and allow the lungs to expand further. This position is commonly called the tripod position.

TECHNIQUE

STEP I (Continued)

- Observe the patient's rate, rhythm, depth, and ease of breathing (see Chapter 5 for a detailed description of measuring the respiratory rate). Normally, the patient's respiratory rate should be between 12 and 20 bpm, the rhythm regular, and the breathing easy and quiet. An occasional sigh is normal.
- Inspect the patient's neck, and note use of accessory muscles (sternomastoid and scalenes) to assist with inspiration.

ABNORMALITIES Use of accessory muscles is a sign of respiratory distress; the patient should be referred immediately to a primary care provider. **Tachypnea** is rapid breathing (usually >20 bpm) and is either shallow or has no change in depth. It can be caused by pain, anxiety, fever, or anemia. **Bradypnea** is slow breathing (usually <12 bpm) and may occur with central nervous system depression induced by oversedation or a cerebral vascular accident (i.e., stroke), elevated intracranial pressure, or hyperkalemia. **Hyperpnea,** also known as Kussmaul respirations, is fast, deep breathing that occurs normally with exercise; however, it can also occur with forms of metabolic acidosis (e.g., diabetic ketoacidosis). Cheyne-Stokes respirations are an irregular increase is rhythm and decrease in depth (deep and fast, then slow and shallow) interrupted by regular episodes of apnea. They can be normal in elderly patients; however, they can also be associated with severe heart failure, uremia, and neurologic disorders.

TECHNIQUE

STEP I (Continued)

- Inspect the patient's skin color and condition, including the lips, nostrils, and mucous membranes. These should be consistent with the patient's genetic background and should not show any signs of **cyanosis** (a bluish color resulting from lack of oxygen in the blood) or **pallor** (a pale color resulting from decreased blood flow.

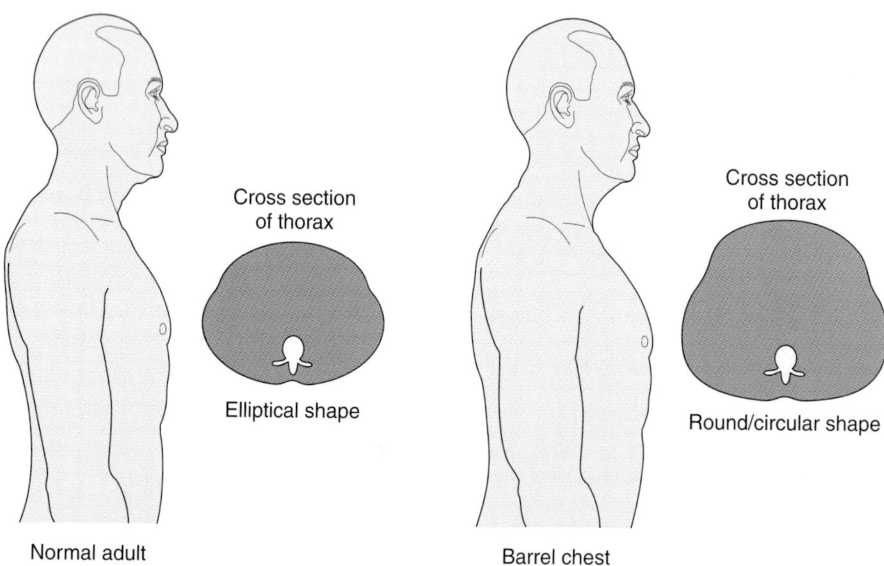

FIGURE 11-7 ■ Comparison of normal chest and barrel chest.

STEP 2

Palpate the Posterior Chest

- Have the patient sit upright, leaning slightly forward with the arms resting comfortably across his or her lap. Ask male patients to disrobe to the waist and female patients to wear a gown with the back open.
- Place your hands on the chest wall with your thumbs at the level of T9 or T10 (Fig. 11-8).
- Slide your hands medially, so that a small fold of skin rests between your thumbs.
- Ask the patient to inhale deeply. As the patient breathes in, your thumbs should move apart symmetrically.

ABNORMALITIES A delay in chest expansion or an asymmetric chest expansion may occur with pneumonia, thoracic trauma, or marked atelectasis (lung obstruction). If pain occurs with inhalation, the pleurae may be inflamed.

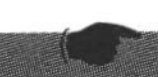
TECHNIQUE

STEP 3

Assess Tactile Fremitus

Tactile fremitus refers to palpable vibrations transmitted through the bronchial tree to the chest wall when a patient speaks.

- Lightly place the balls of your hands on the patient's posterior chest, with one hand on each side of the chest (Fig. 11-9).
- Have the patient repeat the word *ninety-nine.*
- Evaluate the intensity of the vibration.
- Repeat the above steps across the lung fields as shown in Figure 11-11, comparing side to side simultaneously. Normally, the vibrations should feel the same in the corresponding area on each side.

ABNORMALITIES Consolidation or dense tissue conducts sound better than air does; therefore, conditions such as pneumonia intensify the vibrations (increased fremitus). Decreased intensity (decreased fremitus) occurs with obstruction of the vibrations (e.g., pneumothorax, emphysema, and pleural effusion).

TECHNIQUE

STEP 4

Percuss the Posterior Chest

Percussion of the posterior chest helps to evaluate the density of underlying lung tissue to a depth of approximately 5 to 7 cm.

- Starting just above the scapulae, systematically percuss the patient's posterior chest at 3- to 5-cm intervals, moving from side-to-side and downward (Fig. 11-10).
- Avoid the scapulae, spine, and ribs, because bones diminish useful percussion by altering the tone obtained.
- Listen for any differences in volume and pitch, comparing side-to-side.

ABNORMALITIES **Resonance** is a long, low-pitched sound that can usually be heard over all the lung fields; however, it is a subjective term and does not have a set, standard sound. **Hyperresonance** is an abnormally long, low-pitched sound heard with emphysema or a pneumothorax in which a large amount of air is present. Dullness occurs with abnormal, dense tissue in the lungs (e.g., pneumonia, pleural effusion, and atelectasis).

TECHNIQUE

STEP 5

Auscultate the Breath Sounds

Air passing through the tracheobronchial tree creates a char-

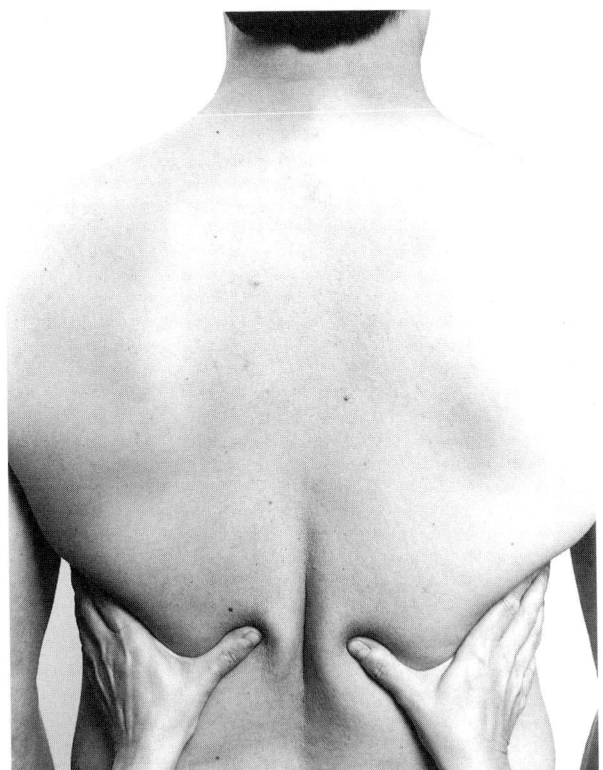

FIGURE 11-8 ■ Palpation of the posterior chest.

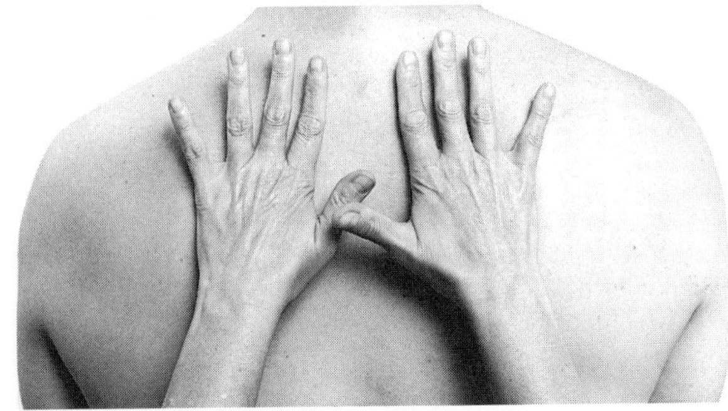

FIGURE 11-9 ■ Assessment of tactile fremitus.

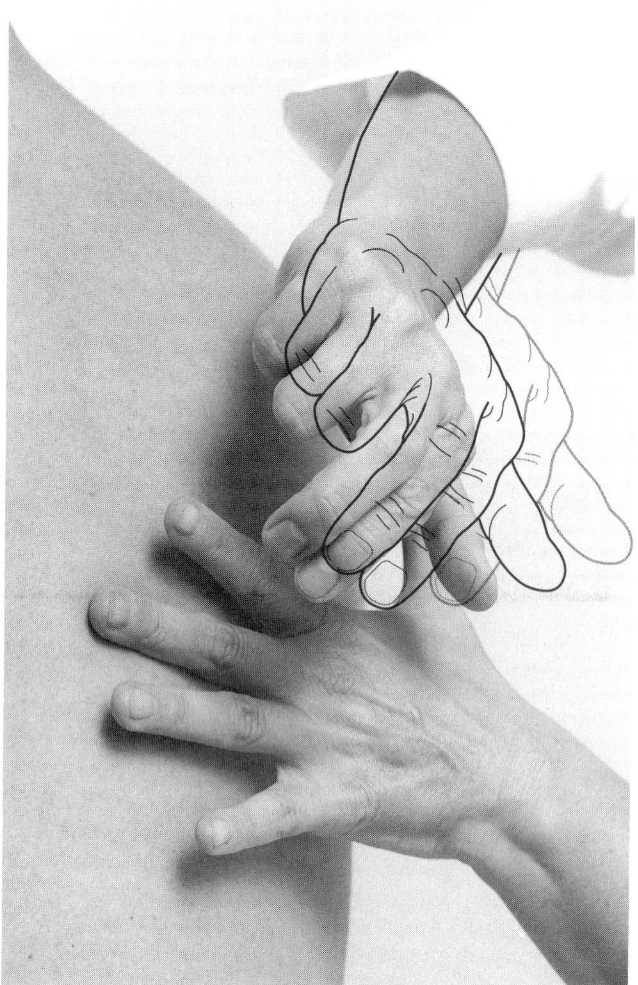

FIGURE 11-10 ■ Palpation of the posterior chest.

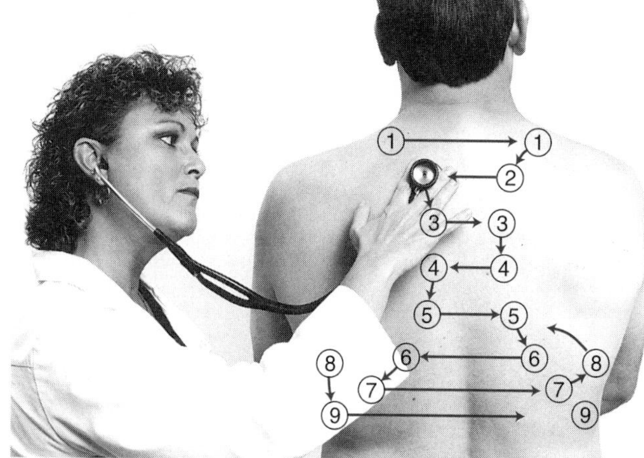

FIGURE 11-11 ■ Auscultation of breath sounds.

acteristic set of sounds that can be heard through the chest wall with a stethoscope. Abnormalities, such as obstruction or parenchyma changes within the lungs, cause these sounds to change.

- Have the patient sit, leaning slightly forward with the arms resting comfortably across his or her lap.
- Instruct the patient to breathe slowly, deeply, and regularly through the mouth.
- Standing behind the patient, firmly place the diaphragm of the stethoscope on the posterior chest, over the upper lobes of the lungs and just above the clavicle (Fig. 11-11).
- Continue across and down the posterior chest in a Z-shaped pattern.
- Listen to at least one full respiration in each location, comparing side-to-side the pitch, intensity, and duration of the breath sound.
- Note the presence of adventitious sounds.

Three different types of breath sounds should be heard, depending on the location. Bronchial sounds are high-pitched and loud, with inspiration shorter than expiration, and are normally heard over the trachea and larynx. Bronchovesicular sounds have a medium pitch and intensity, last equally long during inspiration and expiration, and are normally heard over the major bronchi or between the scapulae. Vesicular sounds are low-pitched and soft, with inspiration longer than expiration, and are normally heard over the smaller bronchioles and alveoli or over most of the peripheral lung fields.

ABNORMALITIES Bronchial or bronchovesicular breath sounds heard over the peripheral lung fields may indicate consolidation (e.g., pneumonia). Diminished or absent breath sounds may occur with obesity, COPD, pneumothorax, or pleural effusion. Adventitious sounds are abnormal sounds that are superimposed or added on top of normal breath sounds. They can be heard over any area of the lungs, during both inspiration and expiration, and include crackles, rhonchi, wheezes, and a friction rub (Table 11-7).

TECHNIQUE

STEP 6

Auscultate the Voice Sounds

If abnormalities are detected during the previous physical examination techniques, eliciting voice sounds may help to determine a specific lung pathology. By listening to voice sounds through the stethoscope, the presence of bronchophony, egophony, and whispered pectoriloquy can be determined.

- Place the stethoscope in the same locations as those for the auscultation of breath sounds (Fig. 11-11).
- Ask the patient to repeat the word *ninety-nine* as you listen through the stethoscope.

ABNORMALITIES Normally, the voice transmission should sound soft and muffled. If the words sound clear and loud (i.e., bronchophony), it may be an indication of consolidation or atelectasis.

- Ask the patient to repeat *ee* as you listen through the stethoscope.

TABLE 11-7 ➤ ADVENTITIOUS SOUNDS

SOUND	CHARACTERISTICS	CAUSE	CLINICAL CONDITION
Crackles or rales	Short, popping sounds. Pitch and intensity vary. Can be heard during inspiration, expiration, or both	Created when air is forced through bronchial passageways narrowed by fluid, mucus, or pus, or by the popping open of previously deflated alveoli	Can be a sign of infection, inflammation, or CHF
Rhonchi	Deep, coarse sounds that have a snoring quality, and are heard primarily during expiration	Usually caused by secretions in the large airways and typically clear after coughing	Bronchitis or pneumonia
Wheezes	High-pitched, musical sounds that can be heard during inspiration or expiration	Airway narrowing	Usually a sign of asthma but can also occur with other causes of airway narrowing, such as COPD and bronchitis
Friction rub	A deep, harsh, grating or creaking sound that is usually heard more often during inspiration than expiration	Occurs when inflamed pleural surfaces lose their normal lubricating fluid and rub together during respiration	Can be associated with any condition that causes pleural irritation, such as pleuritis or pneumonia

➤ ABNORMALITIES Normally, it should sound like ee. If consolidation is present, the word will sound like *ay,* which is termed **egophany.**

- Ask the patient to whisper *one-two-three* as you listen through the stethoscope.

➤ ABNORMALITIES Normally, the words should sound very faint and muffled. Consolidation and pleural effusions can cause these sounds to be more distinctive and clear. This is called **whispered pectoriloquy.**

Laboratory and Diagnostic Tests

Pulmonary function tests include blood gas measurements, oxygen saturation (O_2 sat), and spirometry. Arterial blood gas measurements are the best indicators of overall lung function and include PaO_2, $PaCO_2$, and pH. The adequacy of gas exchange in the lungs determines the values of these gases. Normal values are listed in Table 11-8. Oxygen saturation is the ratio between the actual amount of oxygen bound to hemoglobin and the potential amount of oxygen that could be bound to hemoglobin at a given pressure. Normally, the O_2 sat of arterial blood is 97.5% at a PaO_2 of 100 mm Hg. The O_2 sat is very useful in determining the need for supplemental oxygen therapy.

Spirometry includes tests that measure various lung volumes with a spirometer. The tidal volume is the volume of air that is inhaled or exhaled during normal breathing. The vital capacity is the maximum volume of air that a person can exhale after maximum inhalation. The volume of air that remains in the lungs after maximum exhalation is the residual volume. The total lung capacity is the vital capacity plus the residual volume. Because patients with obstructive lung diseases (e.g., asthma or COPD) have difficulty exhaling, they usually have decreased vital capacity, increased residual volume, and normal total lung capacity. In addition to measuring lung volumes, the spirometer can also be used to assess the patient's ability to move air into and out of the lungs. The forced expiratory volume is the maximal volume of air that is exhaled as forcefully and as completely as possible after maximal inhalation. This volume curve is plotted against time. The FEV_1 of the FVC is commonly used to evaluate the lung's ability to move air; it is usually documented as the percentage of the total volume of air exhaled, or the FEV_1/FVC. Normally, FEV_1 is 80% of the FVC.

The peak expiratory flow (PEF) is the maximal flow rate (L/min) that can be produced during forced expiration. It provides a simple, quantitative, and reproducible measure of the existence and severity of airflow obstruction. Inexpensive, portable, handheld peak flow meters can be used to easily measure the PEF (Fig. 11-12). Peak flow meters are commonly used to assess the effectiveness of bronchodilator therapy and to monitor asthma control at health care facilities, including pharmacies, and by patients at home. In adults, predicted values for the PEF are based on the person's age, height, and sex. In children and adolescents, predicted PEF values are based on height. Predicted values are useful for monitoring new patients; however, chronic asthma is best monitored according to a patient's "personal best" values, which are determined by the patient and his or her physician. The peak flow values are then categorized into green, yellow, and red zones (similar to a traffic light) according to the percentage of the patient's personal-best number (Table 11-9). In addition to the categorized values, Table 11-9 outlines the corresponding asthma management directions in each PEF zone for the patient to follow at home.

TABLE 11-8 ➤ NORMAL VALUES FOR ARTERIAL BLOOD GASES

ARTERIAL BLOOD GASES	NORMAL RANGE
pH	7.36–7.44
PaO_2	90–100 mm Hg
$PaCO_2$	35–45 mm Hg

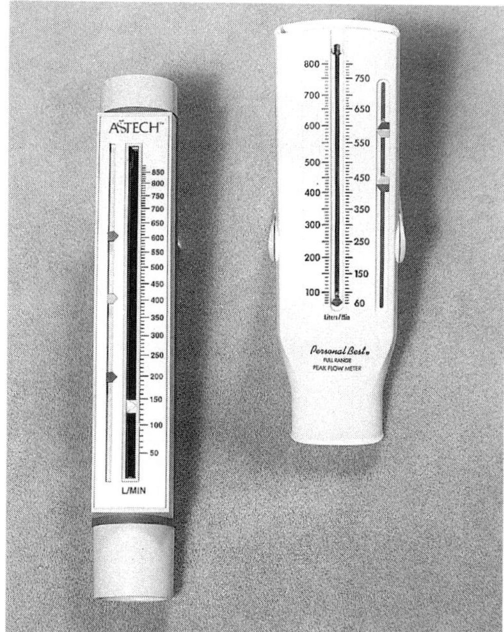

FIGURE 11-12 ■ Peak flow meters.

Many pharmacists are now educating patients about the proper use of peak flow meters as well as the monitoring of asthma and the effectiveness of chronic bronchodilator therapy. When a patient is well educated and monitors his or her asthma control using a peak flow meter, there is great potential for improved health outcomes.

Chest radiography (x-ray) evaluates lung and cardiac structures and is commonly used as a general screening assessment of the respiratory system. It is useful in assessing inflammation, fluid and air accumulation, and tumors in the lung, pleura, and pericardium.

Special Considerations

Pediatric Patients

Pediatric patients require additional questions for the child's parent or guardian.

? INTERVIEW How often does the child have a "head cold?" Are there any smokers in the house? Any history of food, environmental, or drug allergies?

ABNORMALITIES More than four to six colds (upper respiratory infections) per year is considered abnormal. Secondhand smoke increases the risk of upper respiratory infections in children. If an infant or toddler has a history of allergies, consider formula or new foods as possible allergens.

The first respiratory assessment of the newborn is the Apgar Scoring System. The five standard parameters of the Apgar system include heart rate, respiratory effort, muscle tone, reflex irritability, and color, which are scored at 1 minute and again at 5 minutes after birth. A 1-minute total Apgar score of 7 to 10 indicates a newborn in good condition who needs only routine care (e.g., suctioning of the nose and mouth). A 1-minute total Apgar score of three to six indicates a moderately depressed newborn who needs more resuscitation and subsequent close observation. A 1-minute total score of zero to two indicates a severely depressed newborn who needs full resuscitation, ventilatory assistance, and subsequent intensive care.

Newborns normally may breathe rapidly, with interspersed periods of apnea (usually <15 seconds). By 6 weeks of age, however, this irregularity should subside. Irregular breathing after 6 weeks of age is considered to be abnormal and may indicate respiratory distress.

A key component of assessing the child's respiratory function is cooperation of the child. One way to enhance cooperation is to allow the parent to hold the child during the examination. Try to distract younger children by having them play with a toy during the examination—or by making a game of the examination itself. Allow older children to play with the stethoscope, or invite them to listen to their heart and lung sounds.

Because the child's thoracic cage is small, breath sounds may be referred from one lung to another. The examiner should use a pediatric-size stethoscope and the bell side to auscultate a child's breath sounds, because it detects softer, lower-pitched sounds. Breath sounds are usually louder and harsher in children than in adults because of the child's thin chest wall and underdeveloped musculature.

Geriatric Patients

Geriatric patients also require additional questions of the patient or caregiver.

TABLE 11-9 ➤ PEAK EXPIRATORY FLOW RATES

GREEN ZONE	YELLOW ZONE	RED ZONE
Good control PEF >80% of predicted or personal best No wheezing or SOB Take medication as usual	Caution/moderate exacerbation PEF 50%–80% of predicted or personal best Persistent wheezing and SOB Take a short-acting, inhaled β_2-agonist right away; if attacks occur frequently, dosage may need to be increased	Medical alert/severe exacerbation PEF <50% of predicted or personal best Severe wheezing and SOB Take a short-acting, inhaled β_2-agonist right away. Call 911 for emergency assistance.

PEF, peak expiratory flow; *SOB*, shortness of breath.

? INTERVIEW What is your usual amount of activity during the day? If you use an inhaler, please show me how you use it.

➤ ABNORMALITIES Older patients frequently have decreased respiratory efficiency and, thus, may not be able to tolerate many activities. Because of arthritic changes and decreased understanding of instructions resulting from poor hearing or eyesight, elderly patients may not use their inhaler correctly.

Because elderly patients have decreased tissue and cartilage elasticity, the chest does not expand as easily as that of a younger adult. During auscultation, an elderly patient may fatigue easily while breathing deeply. The examiner should be careful so the patient does not hyperventilate or become dizzy; allow brief periods of quiet breathing while auscultating the breath sounds.

Pregnant Patients

During the third trimester, pregnant patients commonly complain of SOB, which is primarily a result of the expanding uterus impinging on the diaphragm's ability to fully expand. Because the fetus increases the oxygen demand on the mother's body, the pregnant patient's respirations may be deeper, but the respiratory rate should remain normal.

APPLICATION TO PATIENT SYMPTOMS

Many times, the pharmacist is the health care professional who identifies a respiratory problem in a patient. For example, the pharmacist may notice that a patient is frequently requesting refills of his or her inhaler, is frequently short of breath when conversing with the pharmacist over the phone or in person, or is complaining of a chronic cough. Therefore, the pharmacist must be able to evaluate common respiratory symptoms, determine possible causes of these symptoms, and take appropriate action to either further assess the symptom or to correct the problem identified. Common respiratory symptoms include dyspnea, wheezing, and cough.

Dyspnea

Patients with dyspnea may report that they "can't get enough air" or complain of "breathlessness." Various causes of dyspnea include:

- *Pulmonary:* COPD, asthma, and emphysema
- *Cardiac:* CHF and coronary artery disease
- *Emotional:* anxiety

CASE STUDY

AL is a 72-year-old woman with a history of COPD and osteoarthritis. She returns to the pharmacy today requesting a refill of her albuterol inhaler. She states that she feels these inhalers are a waste of money, because they hardly hold any medicine and they don't really help her breathing anyway. Based on AL's complaints, the pharmacist suspects she is having respiratory difficulty and asks her to step into the patient care room.

ASSESSMENT OF THE PATIENT

Subjective Information

72 year-old white woman with frequent refills of albuterol inhaler

DO YOU EXPERIENCE SHORTNESS OF BREATH? Yes.

HOW OFTEN DOES THIS HAPPEN? Nearly every day, when I try to do my housework during the day.

DOES IT APPEAR AT NIGHT? No.

HOW LONG HAS IT BEEN GOING ON, OR IS THIS A RECENT CHANGE? It has been getting worse over the past 2 or 3 months.

WHAT MAKES THE SHORTNESS OF BREATH BETTER OR GO AWAY? Well, I use those inhalers, but they don't seem to work very well. I usually have to sit down and rest to catch my breath.

DO YOU EXPERIENCE ANY OTHER SYMPTOMS, SUCH AS CHEST PAIN, LIGHT-HEADEDNESS, DIZZINESS, COUGH, FEVER, OR WHEEZING? No. Oh, I do have to cough up a bunch of "gunk" in the morning when I wake up, but that usually goes away by noon.

WHAT COLOR IS THIS "GUNK" THAT YOU COUGH UP? Clear-colored to a whitish color.

WHAT MEDICATIONS DO YOU TAKE? I use a couple of different inhalers to help me breathe.

WHEN DO YOU USE YOUR INHALERS? Whenever I can't breathe very well.

HOW MANY TIMES A DAY DOES THIS TEND TO BE? Usually six to eight times a day.

DO YOU USE A SPACER WITH YOUR INHALER? No.

SHOW ME HOW YOU USE YOUR INHALERS AT HOME? [Patient demonstrates the following use of her albuterol inhaler: does not shake the canister, does not exhale before placing the inhaler in her mouth, presses down on the canister and inhales, does not hold her breath, and quickly exhales.]

Continued

CASE STUDY—continued

I NOTICED THAT YOU USE BOTH AN ALBUTEROL AND AN AZMACORT INHALER. WHEN YOU USE THESE TOGETHER, WHICH ONE DO YOU USE FIRST? Oh, I don't know. I usually don't pay any attention to it. I just grab whichever one is closest.

DO YOU USE A PEAK FLOW METER TO EVALUATE YOUR BREATHING? No.

DO YOU CURRENTLY SMOKE, OR HAVE YOU SMOKED IN THE PAST? Well, I quit smoking about 5 years ago when I started having problems with my breathing. But I smoked two packs per day for about 50 years before I quit.

Objective Information

Computerized medication profile:

- Albuterol inhaler: two puffs PRN for SOB; No. 1, 17-mg canister; Refills: 5; Patient obtains refills every 2 weeks for the last 2 months.
- Azmacort (triamcinolone) inhaler: two puffs three times daily; No. 1, 20-g canister; Refills: 5; Patient obtains refills every 2 weeks for the last 2 months.
- Ibuprofen: 400 mg, one tablet every 6 hours as needed for arthritis pain; No. 30; Refills: 3; Patient obtains refills once every couple of months.

Patient in no acute distress but currently slightly SOB; no use of accessory muscles; can complete short sentences
Heart rate: 67 bpm
Blood pressure: 138/82 mm Hg
Respiratory rate: 18 rpm
Auscultation: normal breath sounds; no wheezing, crackles, or rhonchi present

DISCUSSION

The concern in this case centers around AL's frequent SOB with her daily activities and frequent refills of inhalers. The pharmacist needs to determine whether the SOB results from progressing COPD or other disease processes (e.g., CHF) or from improper use of her inhalers. AL states that her SOB occurs with daily activities and not at night. (For a complete description of dyspnea caused by CHF, see Chapter 12.) She does not experience any other symptoms and usually needs to sit down and rest for the SOB to improve, because as she states, the inhalers don't work very well. AL uses improper technique with her inhalers and sometimes uses the steroid inhaler before the β-agonist inhaler. In addition, she uses the steroid inhaler as she needs it rather than on a scheduled basis.

Along with identifying possible causes of AL's SOB, the pharmacist must determine the severity of the SOB. AL is not in acute respiratory distress, has a normal respiratory rate, and has normal breath sounds with no adventitious sounds. After evaluating all of AL's subjective and objective information, the pharmacist concludes that she is probably experiencing SOB because of improper use of her inhalers. Figure 11-13 illustrates the pharmacist's decision-making process. Because AL is not in any current distress and her vital signs and breath sounds are normal, the pharmacist educates the patient about proper inhaler technique and using the β-agonist inhaler before the steroid inhaler.

PHARMACEUTICAL CARE PLAN

Patient Name: AL

Date: 7/14/02

Medical Problems:
COPD
Osteoarthritis

Current Medications:

Albuterol inhaler, two puffs PRN for SOB, No. 1, 17-mg canister, Refills: 5, patient obtains refills every 2 weeks for the last several months

Azmacort (triamcinolone) inhaler, two puffs three times daily, No. 1, 20-g canister, Refills: 5, patient obtains refills every 2 weeks for the last several months

Ibuprofen, 400 mg, one tablet every 6 hours as needed for arthritis pain, No. 30, Refills: 3, patient obtains refills once every couple of months

S: 72 year-old woman complaining of frequent SOB that occurs with daily housework. Has little relief from albuterol or steroid inhalers. Chronic, productive cough every morning with clear to white-colored sputum. Improper use (technique and timing) of inhalers.

Frequent request for refills of inhalers.

O: Mild SOB; no use of accessory muscles.

Skin, lips, mucous membranes: Normal color

Heart rate: 67 bpm

Continued

CASE STUDY—continued

PHARMACEUTICAL CARE PLAN

Blood pressure: 138/82 mm Hg

Respiratory rate: 18 bpm

Auscultation: Clear; no wheezes, crackles, or rhonchi

A: SOB and uncontrolled COPD, probably caused by improper use of inhalers.

P: 1. Educate patient about proper techniques for inhaler use and to use the albuterol before the Azmacort inhaler.

2. Discuss with the patient use of a peak flow meter to evaluate her breathing, if she is comfortable doing this at home.
3. Follow-up with a phone call in 2 weeks to monitor the patient's SOB, use of inhalers, and need for refills. If inhaler technique is still difficult for the patient, consider use of a spacer to improve drug delivery.

Pharmacist: *Sonya Garcia, Pharm.D.*

Self-Assessment Questions

1. Compare and contrast the clinical presentation of asthma, COPD, and pneumonia.
2. What are the various causes of dyspnea?
3. What interview questions are the most useful in differentiating possible causes of SOB?
4. When auscultating the chest, which sounds are classified as adventitious sounds?
5. What signs and symptoms are consistent with respiratory distress?

Critical Thinking Questions

1. How would the pharmacist's assessment and plan change if AL had been using accessory muscles, had been leaning forward in a tripod position, and had not been able to complete a full sentence?
2. AL comes back to the pharmacy 2 weeks after being educated about the proper use of her inhalers, and she requests another refill of both inhalers. What questions should the pharmacist ask to assess her current health and medication use?

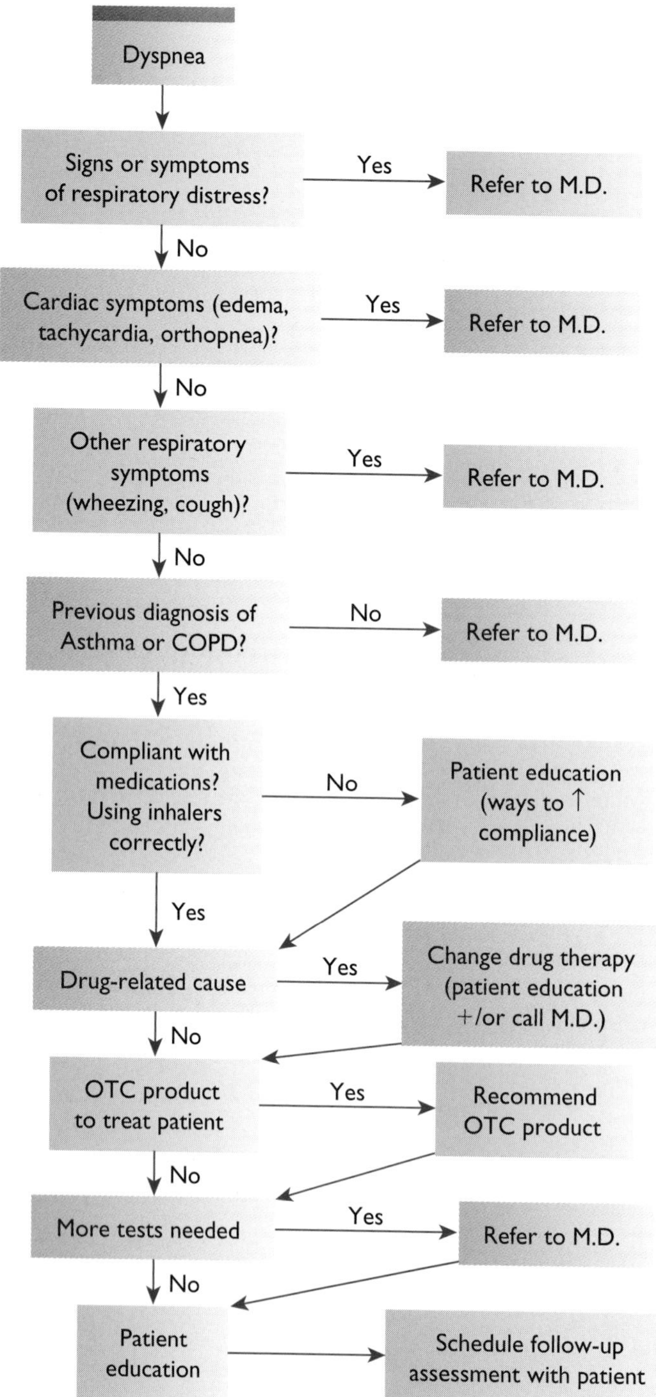

FIGURE 11-13 ■ Decision tree for dyspnea. *OTC*, over-the-counter.

Wheezing

Wheezes are usually heard during expiration, but they can occur throughout inspiration or expiration. Wheezes are commonly associated with asthma; however, they can be caused by other disease states (e.g., COPD). In addition, some medications can also induce wheezing in patients who are sensitive to them (Box 11-7).

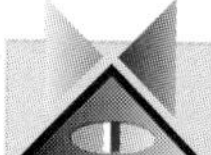

Box 11-7

DRUGS THAT MAY INDUCE WHEEZING

- Aspirin[a]
- Nonsteroidal anti-inflammatory drugs[a]
- β-Adrenergic blockers[b]

[a]In patients older than 40 years with severe asthma as well as nasal polyps.
[b]In patients with preexisting asthma.

CASE STUDY

JB is a 10-year-old boy with a lifelong history of asthma. He and his mother come into the pharmacy with a new prescription for a steroid inhaler. The pharmacist asks JB and his mother to step into the patient care room to discuss the new medication.

ASSESSMENT OF THE PATIENT

Subjective Information

10-year-old boy with a new prescription for a steroid inhaler

SINCE YOU HAVE A NEW PRESCRIPTION TODAY, I ASSUME THAT YOU JUST CAME FROM THE DOCTOR'S OFFICE? Yes, we did.

HAS JB BEEN HAVING PROBLEMS CONTROLLING HIS ASTHMA? Yes. Lately, he has been experiencing wheezing, coughing, and shortness of breath almost every day.

WHAT USUALLY BRINGS ON AN ASTHMA ATTACK? Usually exerting himself, like when he goes outside to play.

WHAT MEDICATIONS HAS JB BEEN USING? Albuterol inhaler, two puffs every 4 to 6 hours when he needs it to help him breathe. Over the past couple of months, he has been using it nearly every day, and it seems to stop the asthma attack.

DOES JB TAKE ANY OTHER PRESCRIPTION OR NONPRESCRIPTION MEDICATIONS? No. Oh, I do give him Tylenol once in awhile for a headache.

JB, SHOW ME HOW YOU USE YOUR INHALER. [JB demonstrates proper technique for using the albuterol inhaler.]

Objective Information

Computerized medication profile:

- Albuterol inhaler: two puffs every 4 to 6 hours as needed for wheezing; No. 1; Refills: 11; Patient obtains refills every 3 to 4 weeks
- AeroBid (flunisolide): two puffs twice a day; No. 1; Refills: 11; new prescription today

Patient in no acute distress
Skin, lips, and mucous membranes: Normal color
Heart rate: 60 bpm
Respiratory rate: 20 rpm
Blood pressure: 112/70 mm Hg
Lung auscultation: Bilateral expiratory wheezes
Peak flow meter: 60% of predicted best

DISCUSSION

JB is a young boy with a long-standing history of asthma. Recently, his asthma has been uncontrolled, with frequent attacks occurring at home when he goes outside to play. JB uses the albuterol inhaler appropriately, which usually relieves the asthma attack, and he is not taking any medications that may induce an attack. Today, he visited his physician, who prescribed a steroid (AeroBid) inhaler. JB's vital signs are within normal limits. JB is not in acute distress but does have expiratory wheezes on lung auscultation and is at 60% of his predicted ability with a peak flow meter.

The pharmacist concludes that JB's asthma attacks probably result from worsening of his asthma, not from improper use of his inhaler or from other medications. Figure 11-14 illustrates the pharmacist's decision process. The pharmacist also agrees that a scheduled steroid inhaler is the most appropriate therapy for JB at this time. The pharmacist educates JB and his mother about the proper use of the new AeroBid inhaler and continued use of the albuterol inhaler. To monitor JB's asthma at home, the pharmacist also educates JB and his mother about the appropriate use of a peak flow meter and initiates a home asthma management plan according to what JB's peak flow meter readings are at home. The pharmacist also schedules a follow-up assessment with JB and his mom in 1 month to evaluate the frequency of asthma attacks, the effectiveness of the new inhaler, any side effects, and the readings from the peak flow meter.

PHARMACEUTICAL CARE PLAN

Patient Name: JB

Date: 10/17/02

Medical Problems:
Asthma

Current Medications:
Albuterol inhaler, two puffs every 4 to 6 hours as needed for wheezing, No. 1, Refills: 11
AeroBid (flunisolide), two puffs twice a day, new prescription today

S: 10-year-old boy with frequent wheezing, SOB, and coughing when playing outside. Relieved with albuterol inhaler. Uses inhaler appropriately. Saw physician today; new prescription: AeroBid inhaler, two puffs BID.

O: Patient in no acute distress.

Heart rate: 60 bpm

Respiratory rate: 20 rpm

Blood pressure: 112/70 mm Hg

Lungs: Bilateral expiratory wheezes

Peak flow meter: 60% of predicted best (yellow zone)

A: Progressive worsening of asthma.

P:
1. Educate patient and mother about proper use of AeroBid inhaler with continued use of albuterol inhaler.
2. Educate patient and mother about proper use of peak flow meter.
3. Institute a home asthma management program to monitor and treat JB's asthma.
4. Follow-up assessment in 1 month to check asthma symptoms, frequency of attacks, efficacy of steroid inhaler, peak flow meter readings, and use of inhalers.

Pharmacist: *Joshua Jones, Pharm.D.*

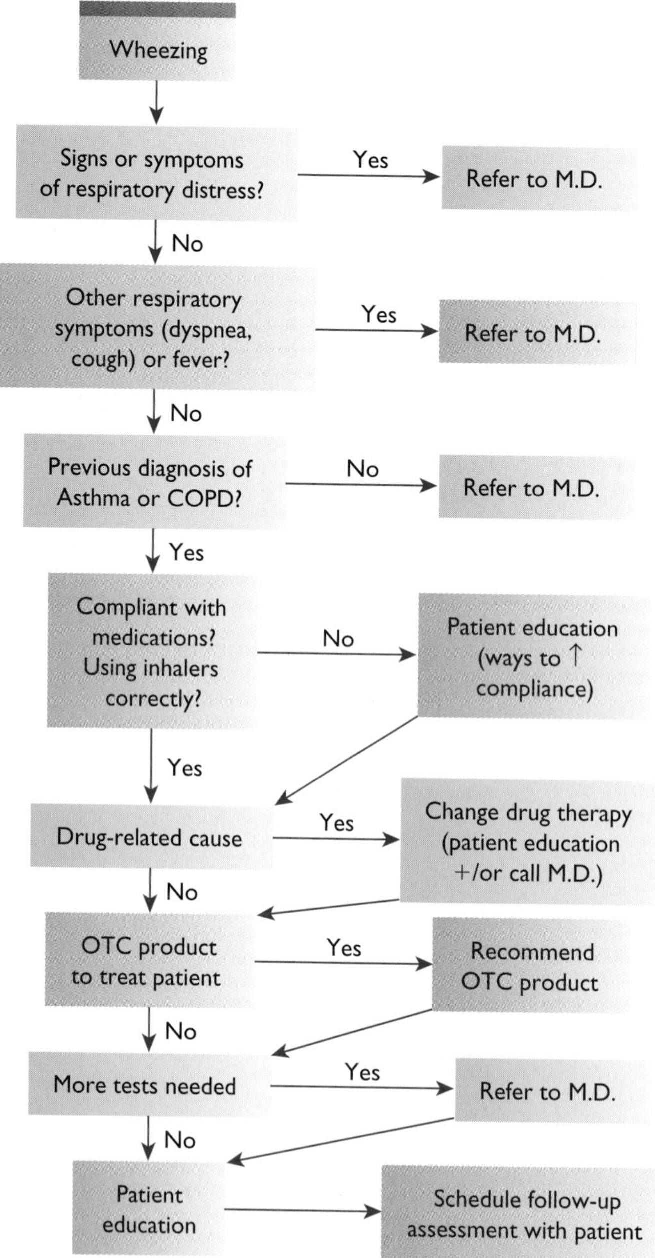

FIGURE 11-14 ■ Decision tree for wheezing. *OTC*, over-the-counter.

Self-Assessment Questions

1. What signs and symptoms are commonly associated with asthma?
2. What factors, including specific medications, may induce wheezing or an acute asthma attack?
3. Besides lung auscultation, what other tests are useful in assessing or monitoring lung function in patients with asthma?
4. Describe the green, yellow, and red zones of a peak flow meter.

Critical Thinking Questions

1. JB comes back 1 month later for his follow-up appointment and states that his PEF values have frequently been in the yellow zone. What does this mean? What questions should the pharmacist ask JB to further assess his asthma management?
2. A 23-year-old college student enters the pharmacy and states that he has been having chest tightness. He is not sure what wheezing is, but he thinks that is what he has been experiencing. He wants to try an OTC product he saw on television that is supposed to help you breathe better, and he asks the pharmacist if it works very well. How should the pharmacist respond to this patient? What questions should the pharmacist ask to further assess his health problem?

Cough

A cough is very forceful expiration of irritant particles in the airways. Patients may describe it as a tickling sensation, a dry cough, a hacking cough, or a productive cough. Patients may also complain of a fever and chills, nasal congestion, runny nose, sore throat, chest tightness, SOB, or sharp chest pain, depending on the cause of the cough. Various causes of a cough include pneumonia, upper respiratory infection (e.g., head cold), asthma/bronchoconstriction, bronchitis, sinusitis, environmental irritants, and CHF. The pharmacist should also keep in mind that angiotensin-converting enzyme (ACE) inhibitors may also cause a cough. Patients usually complain of a persistent (not episodic), dry, nonproductive cough that is usually worse at night. Patients may also describe it as a tickling sensation. In addition, ACE inhibitor-induced coughs are more common in women than in men.

CASE STUDY

BD is a 67-year-old man who comes into the pharmacy and asks the pharmacist to recommend a product for a cough that he has been having. Keeping in mind that there could be several different causes of BD's complaint, the pharmacist asks BD to step into the patient care room so that he can further assess his cough.

ASSESSMENT OF THE PATIENT

Subjective Information

67-year-old man complaining of cough

HOW LONG HAVE YOU HAD THE COUGH? The past week or so. It came on fairly suddenly.

WHAT TYPE OF COUGH IS IT? DRY AND HACKING? PRODUCTIVE? It is productive. I usually cough up a lot of "gunk" from my lungs.

WHAT COLOR IS THE "GUNK" THAT YOU COUGH UP? Sort of rust-colored.

DOES IT OCCUR AT ANY PARTICULAR TIME OF DAY? No. It is all day long.

DO YOU ALSO HAVE THE COUGH DURING THE NIGHT? Once in awhile, but usually not.

WHAT MAKES IT WORSE? Nothing really.

WHAT MAKES IT BETTER? HAVE YOU TRIED ANY MEDICATION TO HELP WITH IT? I haven't tried anything yet. That's why I came here today.

ANY OTHER SYMPTOMS? FEVER? CHILLS? RUNNY NOSE? SHORTNESS OF BREATH? CHEST PAIN? I haven't taken my temperature, so I don't know if I have a fever. I have had the chills the past day or so, but I've been able to breathe okay and I haven't had any chest pain or runny nose.

HAVE YOU BEEN ILL RECENTLY? Yes. With this cough, I just don't feel good.

WHAT MEDICATIONS ARE YOU TAKING? Captopril, 25 mg twice a day, for high blood pressure.

WHEN DID YOU START TAKING THE CAPTOPRIL? A couple of years ago.

WHAT NONPRESCRIPTION MEDICATIONS ARE YOU TAKING? None. I don't like taking pills if I don't need to.

Objective Information

Computerized medication profile:

- Captopril: 25 mg, one tablet twice a day for blood pressure; No. 60; Refills: 11; Patient obtains refills every 25 to 35 days.

Patient frequently coughs (productive, with rust-colored sputum)
Skin, lips, and mucous membranes: Normal color
No use of accessory muscles
Temperature: 102.0°F
Heart rate: 104 bpm
Respiratory rate: 22 rpm
Blood pressure: 124/78 mm Hg
Lung auscultation: Decreased breath sounds in right lower lobe; no rales, crackles, or rhonchi
Voice sounds: Positive for bronchophony, egophony, and whispered pectoriloquy

DISCUSSION

When a patient complains of a cough, the pharmacist must ask several questions to determine a possible cause. In the case of BD, the pharmacist needs to determine if his cough results from a common "cold," a respiratory infection (e.g., pneumonia), a respiratory disease (e.g., asthma, COPD), or the captopril, an ACE inhibitor. BD complains of a productive cough with rust-colored sputum that occurs all day long but usually not at night. He has had chills the last day or two and does not feel well but has not experienced any other symptoms. The only medication BD is taking is captopril, twice a day. The pharmacist witnesses BD coughing and notices that the sputum is slightly rust-colored. On physical examination, the patient has a fever, tachypnea, and tachycardia. His breath sounds are decreased in the right lower lobe of his lungs, and his voice sounds change with auscultation.

After evaluating BD's subjective and objective information, the pharmacist concludes that all his signs and symptoms are consistent with pneumonia. Figure 11-15 illustrates the steps involved with the assessment process. The pharmacist recommends that the patient see his physician today for antibiotic therapy. The pharmacist calls BD's doctor and makes an appointment for him later that morning.

Continued

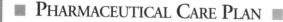

CASE STUDY—continued

PHARMACEUTICAL CARE PLAN

Patient Name: BD

Date: 2/28/02

Medical Problems:
Hypertension

Current Medication:
Captopril, 25 mg, twice a day, No. 60, Refills: 11

S: 67-year-old man complaining of a productive cough with rust-colored sputum that occurs all day long and does not feel well. Came on suddenly about 1 week ago. Has had chills the last day or two. No SOB or chest pain. Has not tried anything to relieve the cough.

O: Patient frequently coughs (productive, with rust-colored sputum).

Temperature: 102.0°F

Heart rate: 104 bpm

Respiratory rate: 22 rpm

Blood pressure: 124/78 mm Hg

Auscultation: Decreased breath sounds in right lower lobe.

Voice sounds: Positive for bronchophony, egophony, and whispered pectoriloquy.

A: 1. Productive cough, probably caused by pneumonia.
2. Hypertension: controlled.

P: 1. Refer patient to physician for antibiotic therapy.
2. Call physician's office, and schedule an appointment for later this morning
3. Follow-up assessment in 2 weeks to monitor patient signs and symptoms of pneumonia.

Pharmacist: *John Davis, Pharm.D.*

Self-Assessment Questions

1. What are useful interview questions to differentiate possible causes of a cough?
2. Differentiate the common characteristics and various causes of a cough and sputum production.
3. What do the terms *bronchophony, egophony,* and *whispered pectotriloquy* mean?

Critical Thinking Questions

1. In the case of BD, how would the pharmacist's assessment and plan change if he had complained of a dry, tickling cough that usually occurred at night and did not have a fever or chills?
2. A 56-year-old woman is taking warfarin, an anticoagulant, and aspirin, a blood "thinner," for her heart and complains that she has been coughing up a lot of sputum every morning. She also has been smoking two packs per day for the last 40 years. What questions should the pharmacist ask to assess this patient's cough and sputum production?

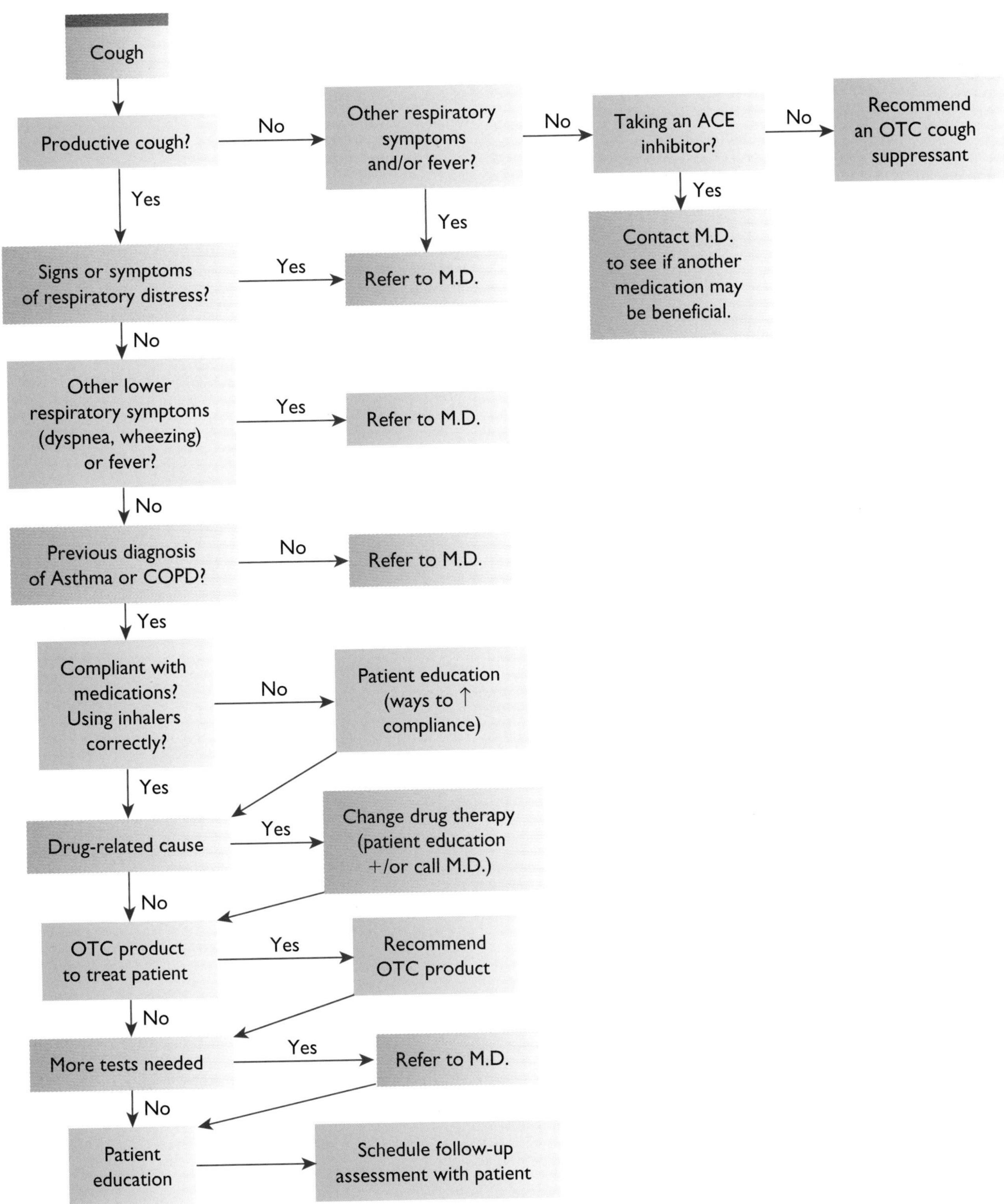

FIGURE 11-15 ■ Decision tree for cough. *ACE*, angiotensin-converting enzyme; *OTC*, over-the-counter.

Bibliography

Carlson KL. Assessing a child's chest. RN 1989;52(11):26–32.

Dorland's pocket medical dictionary. 25th ed. Philadelphia: WB Saunders, 1995.

Finesilver C. Respiratory assessment. RN 1992;55(2):22–30.

Dang-Vu PA, Zerngast W. Drug induced pulmonary disorders. In: The clinical use of drugs. 7th ed. Philadelphia: Lippincott Williams & Wilkins, 2001:24, 1–15.

Kuhn JK, McGovern M. Respiratory assessment of the elderly. J Gerontol Nurs 1992;18(5):40–43.

Kumar V, Cotran RS, Robbins SL. Basic pathology. 6th ed. Philadelphia: WB Saunders, 1997.

Martini FH, Timmons MJ. Human anatomy. 2nd ed. Upper Saddle River, NJ: Prentice-Hall, 1997.

National Heart, Lung, and Blood Institute. Guidelines for the diagnosis and management of asthma. Expert panel report 2. U.S. Department of Health and Human Services, Public Health Service, National Institutes of Health publication no. 97-4051, 1997. Available at http://www.nhlbi.nih.gov/guidelines/asthma

National Heart, Lung, and Blood Institute. Global strategy for the diagnosis, management, and prevention of chronic obstructive pulmonary disease. NHLBI/WHO workshop report. U.S. Department of Health and Human Services, Public Health Service, National Institutes of Health publication no. 2701A, 2001. Available at http://www.goldcopd.com

Pagana KD, Pagana TJ. Mosby's diagnostic and laboratory test reference. 2nd ed. St. Louis, Mosby, 1995.

Self TH. Asthma. In: Applied therapeutics: the clinical use of drugs. 7th ed. Philadelphia: Lippincott Williams & Wilkins, 2001:21.1–46.

Self TH, Strayhorn VA. Long-term management of asthma. J Am Pharm Assoc 1997;NS37:422–438.

Small RE, Kennedy DT. New asthma guidelines: applications for pharmaceutical care. J Am Pharm Assoc 1997;NS37:419–421.

Striesmeyer JK. A four-step approach to pulmonary assessment. Am J Nurs 1993;93(8):22–31.

Kradjan WA, William DM. Chronic obstructive pulmonary disease. In: Applied therapeutics: the clinical use of drugs. 7th ed. Philadelphia: Lippincott Williams & Wilkins, 2001:22.1–32.

CHAPTER

12

Cardiovascular System

Rhonda M. Jones and Maryann Z. Skrabal

GLOSSARY TERMS

- Afterload
- Angina pectoris
- Angioplasty
- Arrhythmia
- Arteriosclerosis
- Blood pressure
- Bradycardia
- Bruit
- Cardiac output
- Congestive heart failure
- Contractility
- Corneal arcus
- Circus senilis
- Coronary heart disease
- Diastole
- First heart sound
- Hepatojugular reflex
- Hypertension
- Murmur
- Myocardial infarction
- Orthopnea
- Paroxysmal nocturnal dyspnea
- Preload
- Prinzmetal angina
- Pulse pressure
- Second heart sound
- Stable angina
- Stroke volume
- Systole
- Tachycardia
- Unstable angina

ANATOMY AND PHYSIOLOGY OVERVIEW

Circulatory System

The circulatory system consists of two types of blood vessels, the arteries and the veins. Arteries carry blood away from the heart, and veins carry blood back to the heart. The blood vessels are arranged in two continuous loops, the pulmonary circulation and the systemic circulation, which are connected by the heart on one end and the various organ systems on the other. The rhythmic pumping of the heart delivers nutrients to and removes waste products from all the organ systems within the body (Fig. 12-1).

Heart

The heart is a combination of cardiac muscles that maintain the circulation of the blood. The heart wall is composed of several layers (Fig. 12-2). The pericardium is a tough, double-walled, fibrous sac that encases and protects the heart. It has two layers that contain a small amount of visceral fluid, which allows friction-free movement of the heart muscle. The myocardium is the muscular wall of the heart and is responsible for most of the ventricular pumping. The endocardium is the thin layer of endothelial tissue that lines the inner surface of the heart chambers and valves.

The heart itself is divided into four chambers: the left and right atria, and the left and right ventricles (Fig. 12-3). The left heart is composed of the left atrium and ventricle; the right heart is composed of the right atrium and ventricle. The atria are thin-walled reservoirs for holding blood, and the ventricles are muscular pumping chambers. The left and right heart are separated by a blood-tight partition called the cardiac septum.

The four chambers are separated by two sets of valves, the main purpose of which is to prevent backflow of blood. The

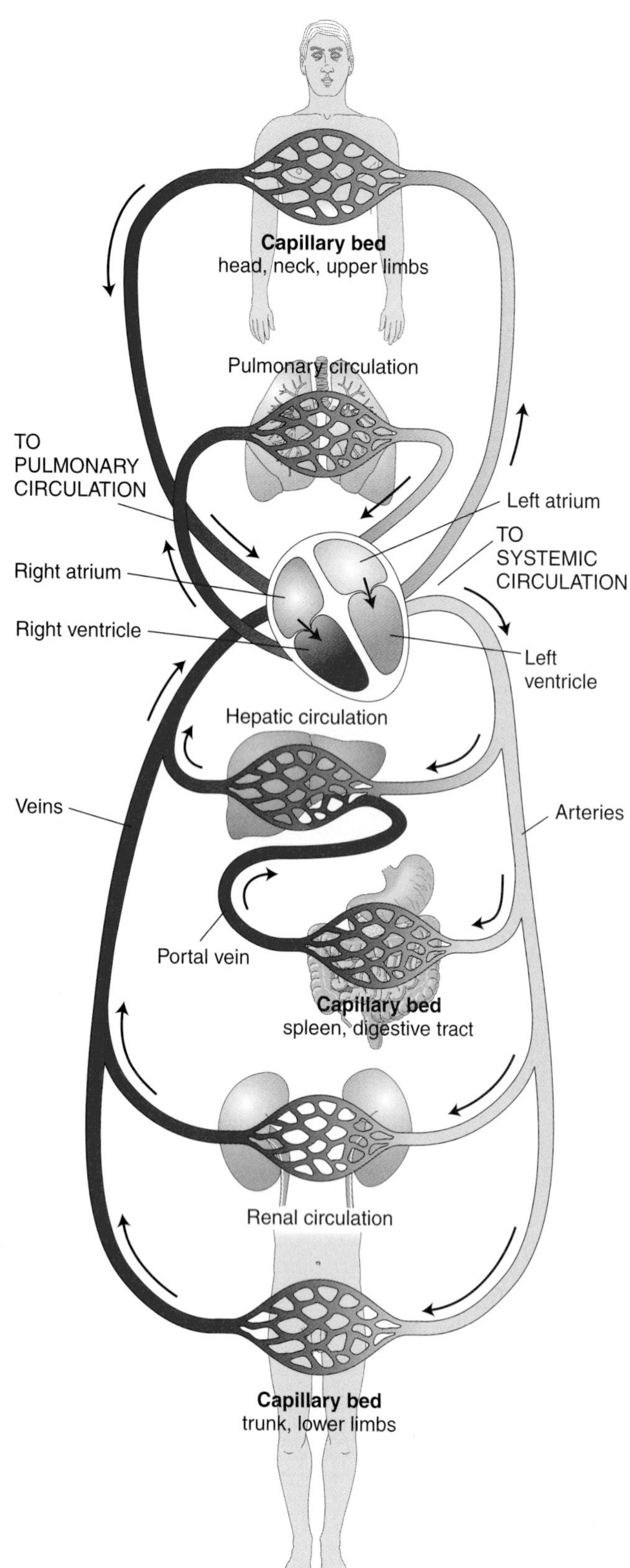

Figure 12-1 ■ The circulatory system.

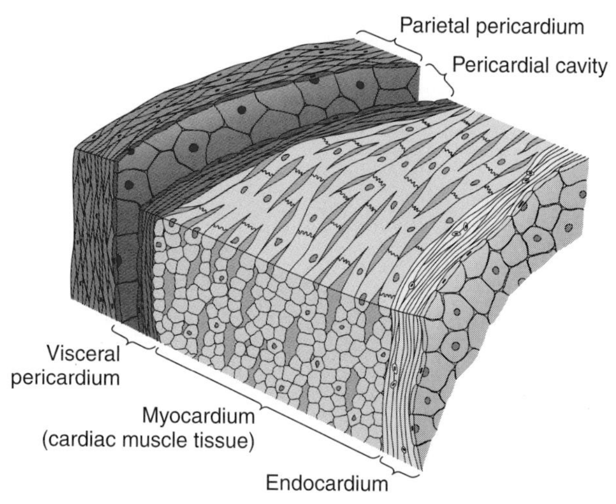

Figure 12-2 ■ The cardiac muscle.

valves open and close passively in response to pressure gradients in the moving blood, and they permit blood flow in only one direction. The two atrioventricular (AV) valves separate the atria and the ventricles. The tricuspid is the right AV valve, and the bicuspid (or mitral) is the left AV valve. The AV valves open during diastole (the heart's filling phase) to allow the ventricles to fill with blood. The semilunar (SL) valves are between the ventricles and the arteries. The SL valves are the pulmonic in the right side of the heart and the aortic in the left side of the heart. The SL valves open during systole (the heart's pumping phase) to allow blood to be ejected from the heart.

The circulation of blood through the body occurs in one continuous loop. Deoxygenated red blood cells (venous blood) are transported from the body's periphery to the right atrium (RA) through the inferior and superior vena cava. From the RA, the venous blood passes through the tricuspid valve into the right ventricle (RV). From the RV, the blood passes through the pulmonic valve into the lungs via the pulmonary artery. The lungs then oxygenate the blood, and the pulmonary veins carry the oxygenated blood back to the left atrium (LA). From the LA, the blood passes through the mitral valve to the left ventricle (LV). The LV ejects the blood through the aortic valve to the aorta, and the aorta then delivers the oxygenated blood to the body.

Conduction System

The heart functions autonomously within the body. An intrinsic electrical conduction system allows it to stimulate and coordinate the sequence of muscular contractions within the cardiac cycle (Fig. 12-4). An electrical current or impulse stimulates each myocardial contraction. This impulse is both generated and paced by the sinoatrial node, which is located at the juncture of the superior vena cava and the RA. From the sinoatrial node, the impulse travels through both atria to the AV node, which is located in the atrial septum. While at the AV node, the impulse is delayed for approximately one-tenth of a second before it passes into the AV bundle (or bundle of His) and then down its left and right branches. The Purkinje fibers spread the

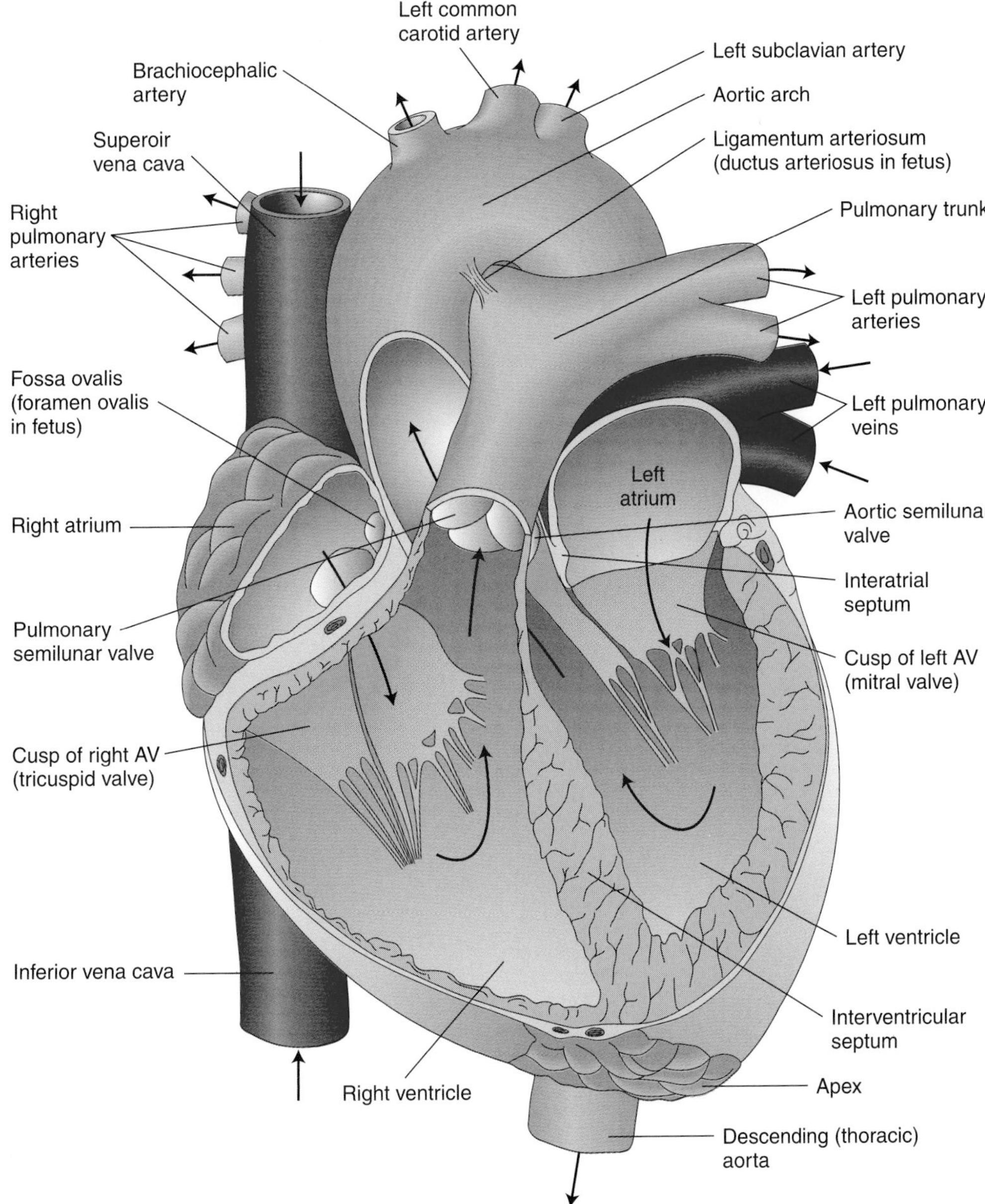

FIGURE 12-3 ■ Anatomy of the heart.

impulse throughout the ventricular myocardium, where it stimulates ventricular contraction.

A small amount of electrical current spreads to the heart's surface, where it can be measured and recorded on an electrocardiogram (ECG). Each electrical impulse produces a series of waves that is recorded on the ECG. The peaks and troughs of these waves are arbitrarily labeled *PQRST* (Fig. 12-5). Their clinical significance is as follows:

- *P wave:* Atrial depolarization (the spread of a stimulus through the atria).
- *PR interval:* The time between initial stimulation of the atria and initial stimulation of the ventricles.
- *QRS complex:* Ventricular depolarization (the spread of a stimulus through the ventricles).
- *T wave:* Ventricular repolarization (the return of stimulated ventricular muscle to a resting state).

The electrical impulse slightly precedes the corresponding myocardial contraction that it stimulates within the heart.

Cardiac Cycle

The cardiac cycle defines the events that are involved in each full heartbeat. It occurs in two phases, diastole and systole (Fig. 12-5). During **diastole,** the ventricles relax, the AV valves open, and blood flows passively from the pressure-filled atria into the low-pressure ventricles. As the ventricles fill with blood, the pressure within them rises. In turn, this rise in pressure causes the AV valves to close, preventing regurgitation of blood into the atria and producing the first heart sound (S_1). Occurrence of the first heart sound signals the beginning of **systole.** Once the pressure in the ventricles exceeds the pressure in the aorta and the pulmonary artery, the ventricles contract, the SL valves open, and blood is ejected into the pulmonary

Sinoatrial node
Bundle of His
Right bundle branch
Atrioventricular node
Left bundle branch
(posterior-superior division)
Left bundle branch
(anterior-superior division)
Purkinje's fibers

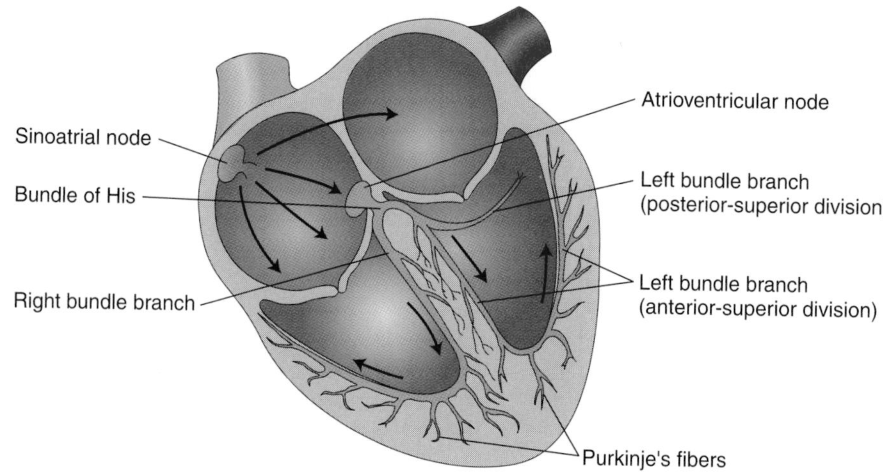

FIGURE 12-4 ■ Cardiac conduction.

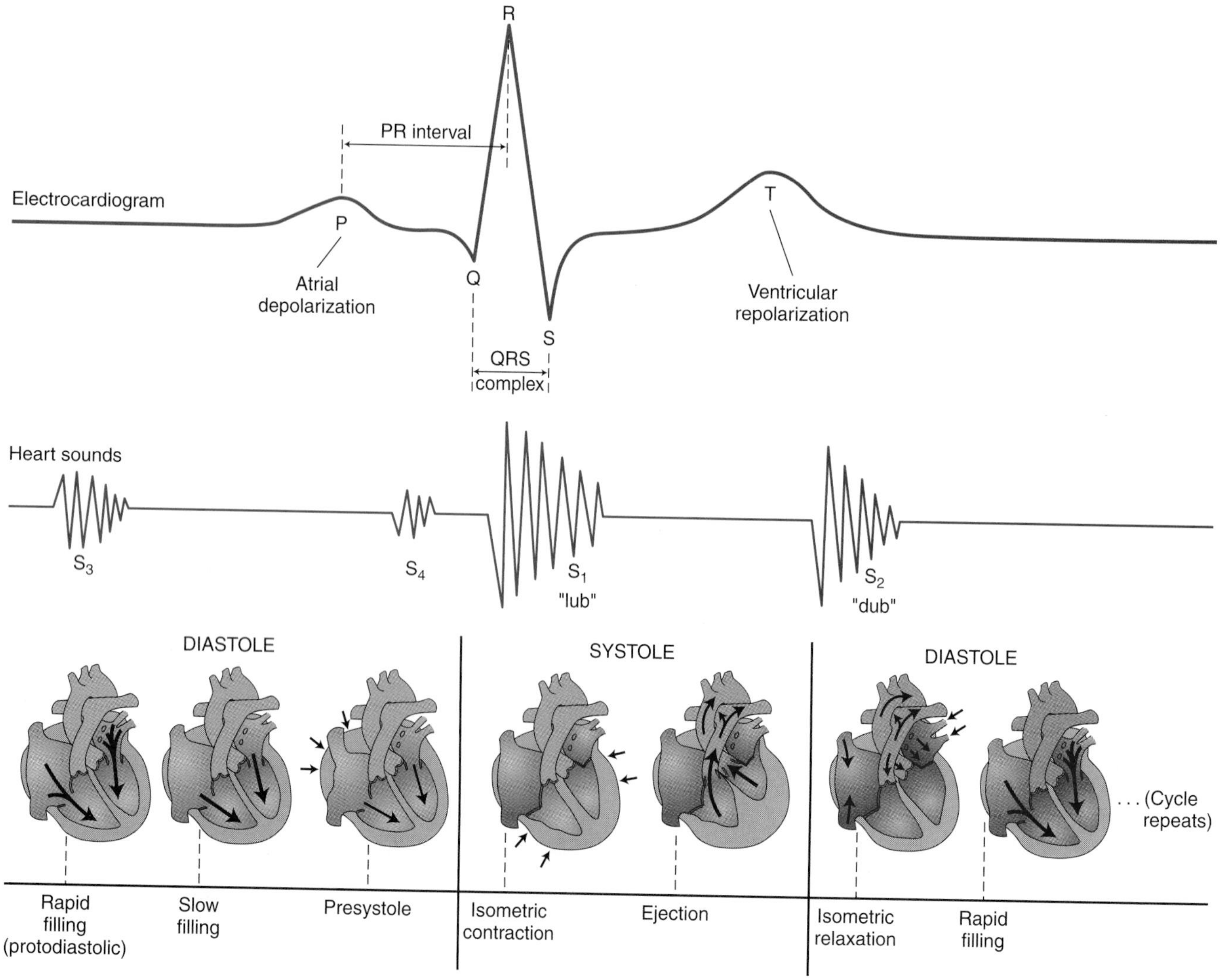

R
PR interval
Electrocardiogram
P
T
Atrial
depolarization
Q
S
Ventricular
repolarization
QRS
complex
Heart sounds
S3
S4
S1
"lub"
S2
"dub"
DIASTOLE
SYSTOLE
DIASTOLE
. . . (Cycle
repeats)
Rapid
filling
(protodiastolic)
Slow
filling
Presystole
Isometric
contraction
Ejection
Isometric
relaxation
Rapid
filling

FIGURE 12-5 ■ The cardiac cycle and electrocardiogram.

and systemic arteries. When the ejection is complete, the pressure in the ventricles drops below that in the aorta and the pulmonary artery, and the SL valves snap shut, causing the second heart sound (S_2) and the end of systole. Once again, the ventricles relax and the atria fill with blood delivered from the lungs and the systemic circulation, which is the start of diastole.

Heart Sounds

As mentioned, events during the cardiac cycle generate sounds that can be heard through a stethoscope placed over the chest wall. These sounds include both normal sounds (S_1 and S_2) and, occasionally, extra heart sounds (S_3 and S_4) (Fig. 12-5).

Normal Heart Sounds

The **first heart sound** (S_1) is produced by closure of the AV valves and signals the beginning of systole. The characteristic description of the first heart sound is "lub," and it is usually loudest over the apex area of the heart. The **second heart sound** (S_2) is produced by closure of the SL valves and signals the ending of systole. The characteristic description of the second heart sound is "dub," and it is usually loudest over the base of the heart.

Extra Heart Sounds

With the opening of the AV valves, rapid filling of the ventricles (diastole) begins. This is normally a passive and quiet interval until ventricular filling is almost complete. Occasionally, however, a third heart sound (S_3) may be heard at the end of the rapid filling interval. An S_3 is normal in children and young adults, but when present in individuals older than 30 years, it represents a volume overload to the ventricle. Conditions that may be responsible for this volume overload include regurgitant valvular lesions and congestive heart failure.

At the end of diastole, a fourth heart sound (S_4) may be heard. Again, this is normal in children and young adults, but when present in those older than 30 years, it typically indicates an increased resistance to filling secondary to a noncompliant ventricle or an increase in volume. Conditions that may be associated with S_4 include hypertension, coronary artery disease, aortic stenosis, severe anemia, or hyperthyroidism.

The presence of an S_3 or S_4 creates a beat or rhythm similar to the gallop of a horse. Therefore, these sounds are commonly called an S_3 or S_4 gallop.

Blood flowing through normal cardiac chambers and valves usually makes no noise. Some conditions, however, cause turbulent blood flow, and a subsequent heart murmur can be heard. A heart **murmur** is a gentle, blowing, swishing sound that can be heard on the chest wall. Often, heart murmurs have no pathologic significance, but they may indicate serious heart disease. Conditions resulting in a heart murmur include structural defects in the valves, unusual openings in the chambers, or increases (e.g., exercise) or decreases (e.g., anemia) in the blood velocity.

Pumping Action of the Heart

On contraction of the left and right ventricles, blood is pumped into the systemic and the pulmonary circulation, respectively. **Stroke volume** is the amount of blood that is ejected in one full heartbeat. It depends on preload, afterload, and myocardial contractility. **Preload** refers to the passive stretching of the ventricular muscle as the volume of blood in the ventricle at the end of diastole increases. **Afterload** refers to the vascular resistance against which the ventricle must contract. Myocardial **contractility** refers to the ability of the cardiac muscle, when given a load, to shorten and contract. The volume of blood that is pumped from each ventricle in 1 minute is the **cardiac output;** this is the product of the heart rate and the stroke volume. To adapt to the body's metabolic needs, the heart can alter its cardiac output.

Blood pressure is the force of the blood as it pushes against the vessel walls. Systolic blood pressure is the maximum pressure felt on the artery during left ventricular contraction or systole. It is regulated by the stroke volume and the compliance of the blood vessels. Diastolic blood pressure is the resting pressure that the blood exerts in between each ventricular contraction. It is dependent on peripheral vascular resistance. The **pulse pressure** is the difference between the systolic and the diastolic pressure, and it reflects the stroke volume. (For a full discussion of blood pressure, see Chapter 5).

Lipid Metabolism

Regulation of serum lipid levels by lipoproteins and apolipoproteins plays an important role in the development of coronary heart disease (CHD), so an understanding of these components is essential. The key components include cholesterol, triglycerides, lipoproteins, and apolipoproteins.

Cholesterol is a cell membrane component and precursor for the formation of steroid hormones and bile acids. Most cholesterol synthesis occurs in the liver and intestinal mucosa, and synthesis is greater during the night than during the day. Total cholesterol is equal to the sum of low-density lipoprotein (LDL) plus high-density lipoprotein (HDL) plus approximately one-fifth of the triglycerides (i.e., very low-density lipoprotein [VLDL]).

Triglycerides consist of free fatty acids and glycerol, and they are an important source of stored energy. Their role in atherosclerosis is controversial, but extremely high levels (>500–1000 mg/dL) can cause pancreatitis. Triglycerides are dependent on dietary fat. When elevated, they tend to be associated with low HDL, which is important in the atherosclerotic process.

Lipoproteins are water-soluble particles that are responsible for the transport of water-insoluble cholesterol and triglycerides in the plasma. The density of the lipoproteins is determined by the relative content of protein and lipid. Lipoproteins include chylomicrons, VLDL, intermediate-density lipoproteins, LDL, HDL, and lipoprotein (a). The LDL is considered to be the "bad cholesterol," and it is the subfraction of cholesterol that lodges into the arterial wall, becomes oxidized, and stimulates development of the atherosclerotic plaque. The HDL is considered to be the "good cholesterol" and is responsible for removal of cholesterol from the arterial wall and peripheral tissues and its transport back to the liver for disposal. Lipoprotein (a) is genetically determined and highly inheritable. It is similar to LDL but, in addition, contains a protein that has an increased tendency to clot.

Apolipoproteins play a major role in the binding, solubilization, and transport of lipids. They are responsible for providing structure to the lipoprotein, activating enzyme systems, and binding with cell receptors. Lipoprotein metabolism includes an exogenous and an endogenous pathway (Fig. 12-6). The exogenous pathway involves the metabolism of dietary fat. Dietary fat is absorbed into the intestinal wall to become chylomicrons, which empty into the peripheral venous system and then travel through the circulation into the arterial system and, eventually, into muscle or adipose tissues. Lipoprotein lipase hydrolyzes the triglycerides to produce fatty acids for energy or storage. The endogenous pathway involves the synthesis of cholesterol in the liver and begins with the production of VLDL. After lipoprotein lipase metabolizes VLDL in the circulation, intermediate-density lipoprotein is produced and, eventually, is used for production of LDL in the liver. Production of LDL is regulated by increasing or decreasing LDL receptors on the liver. Reverse cholesterol transport refers to the activity of HDL, which acts as a cholesterol scavenger by removing cholesterol from peripheral tissues and returning it to the liver.

Special Considerations

Pediatric Patients

Development of the heart and the circulatory system occurs very early in life. By the third week of fetal development, a tubular heart is pumping and circulating blood. The lungs are nonfunctional, however, so the blood is oxygenated through the umbilical vessels of the placenta. Because there is no need for blood to be circulated to the lungs for oxygenation, fetal circulation has two major differences. First, a gap between the two atria, the foramen ovale, allows blood to flow from the RA to the left atrium (Fig. 12-3). Second, the ductus arteriosus provides an external short circuit between the pulmonary and aortic blood vessels (Fig. 12-3). Through these mechanisms, only a small amount of blood enters the pulmonary circulation, and both the right and left ventricles pump blood into the systemic circulation.

At birth, major changes occur. As the baby takes his or her first breath, the lungs and pulmonary blood vessels expand. The foramen ovale closes, separating the left and right atria, and the ductus arteriosus also closes, isolating the pulmonary and systemic blood vessels. The right ventricle now pumps blood to the pulmonary circulation, and the LV pumps blood to the systemic

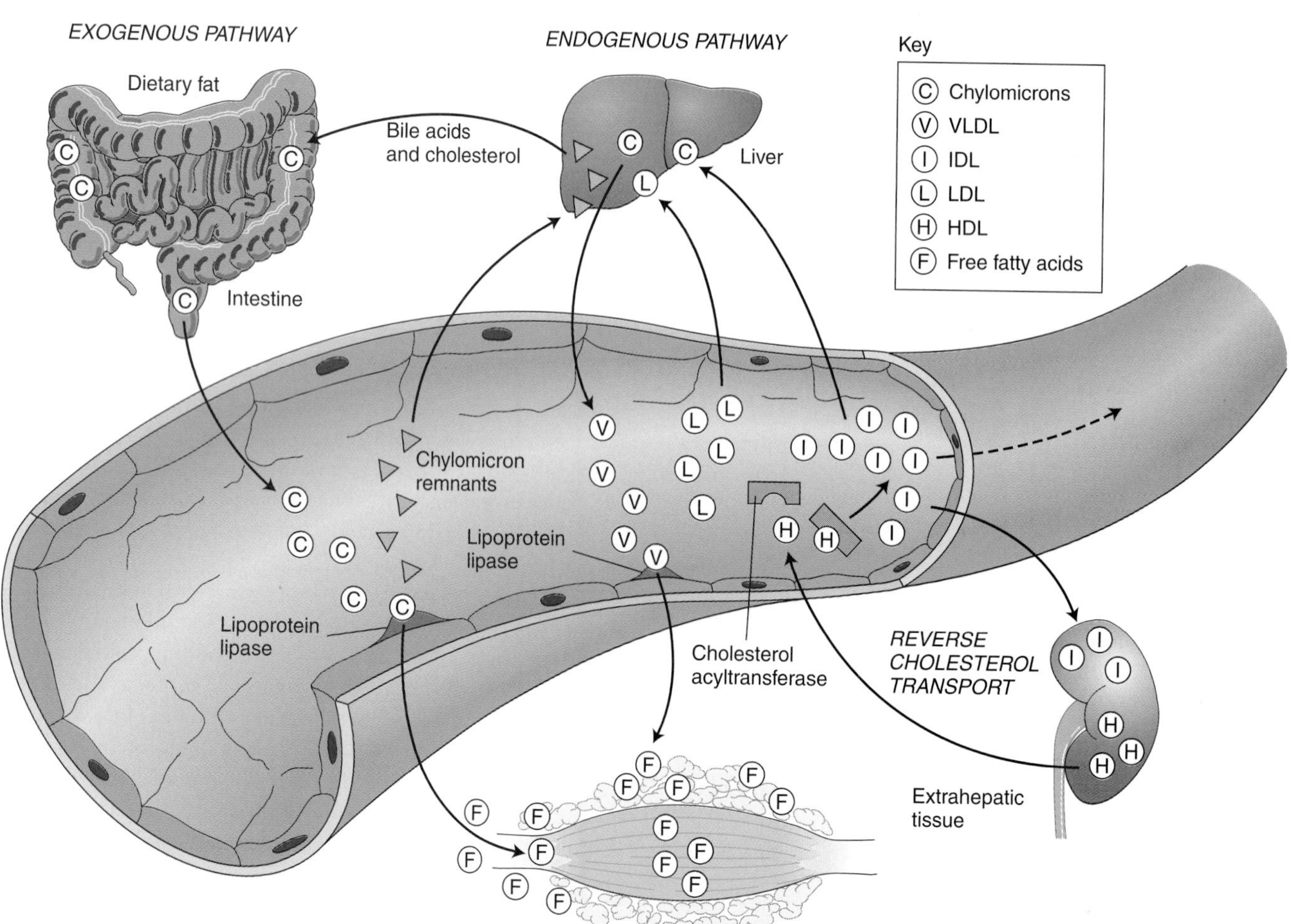

FIGURE 12-6 ■ Lipoprotein metabolism: exogenous and endogenous pathways, and reverse cholesterol transport.

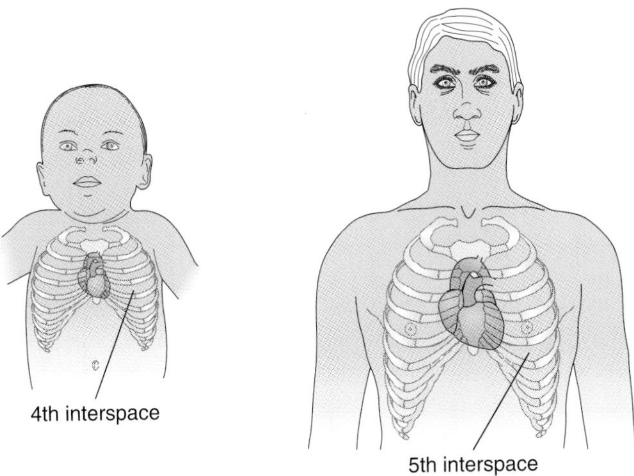

FIGURE 12-7 ■ Location of the heart in pediatric and adult patients.

circulation, just as in the adult heart. The position of the heart, however, is more horizontal in the chest of infants and children than in adults (Fig. 12-7). The adult heart position is usually reached by 7 years of age.

Hyperlipidemia in children is often related to a genetic process. Early detection is important, because the risk for cardiovascular events is greatly increased at a much younger age in this population. All children should be tested early if a family history exists. Dietary therapy is generally recommended after age 2, and drug therapy may be used after age 10, to bring the cholesterol down to desirable levels.

Geriatric Patients

Functioning of the cardiovascular system gradually declines with age. The maximum cardiac output is reduced, and calcification of weakened vessel walls, or **arteriosclerosis,** diminishes their elasticity and vasomotor tone, reducing their ability to adjust to changing body needs. This stiffening of the blood vessels may lead to an aneurysm, which can cause stroke, infarct, or massive hemorrhage, depending on the vessel involved. Coronary circulation can also be restricted by the progression of atherosclerosis. Formation of these atherosclerotic plaques can increase the risk of thrombi formation and, thus, the risk of developing coronary artery disease.

Changes in the ECG occur secondary to histologic changes within the conduction and neurologic systems. Common ECG changes in older adults include P-R interval prolongation (i.e., first-degree AV block); Q-T interval prolongation; left-axis deviation; and bundle-branch block.

Hyperlipidemia in elderly patients carries a higher risk for CHD than in younger patients. Many studies have found that increases in body weight associated with aging (especially central obesity) contribute to abnormal lipid concentrations in elderly people. Central obesity is more strongly associated than lower-body obesity with diabetes, hypertension, altered lipid profiles, and gallbladder disease. Excess upper-body fat associated with insulin resistance leads to increased hepatic production of triglycerides and cholesterol-rich lipoproteins. Levels of HDL cholesterol are higher in women than in men until menopause, but then they are equal. In men, triglycerides increase until age 50 and then decline.

Pregnant Patients

Pregnancy causes several cardiovascular changes. Total blood volume increases by 30% to 40%, with the cellular components increasing approximately 20% and the fluid component increasing approximately 40% to 50%. The heart rate increases by approximately 10 to 15 bpm. The stroke volume also increases, so the total cardiac output increases by approximately 32%. Blood pressure remains constant, however, throughout most normal pregnancies.

Cholesterol levels increase by approximately 30 to 40 mg/dL, and triglyceride levels increase by approximately 150 mg/dL in pregnancy. Dietary therapy is preferred over drug therapy in these patients.

PATHOLOGY OVERVIEW

Cardiac dysfunction is a common cause of morbidity and mortality. Major cardiac diseases include CHD, angina pectoris, myocardial infarction, congestive heart failure, hypertension, and arrhythmias.

Coronary Heart Disease

Coronary heart disease, which is also termed *coronary artery disease* or *ischemic heart disease,* refers to degenerative changes in the coronary circulation resulting from an imbalance between myocardial oxygen demand and the blood supply. The most common cause of CHD is a progressive atherosclerosis of the coronary arteries. This build-up of atherosclerotic plaques (fatty deposits) narrows the vessel lumen, reducing coronary arterial blood supply and causing myocardial ischemia. Risk factors are either directly associated with development of CHD (i.e., causative) or directly affect development of causative risk factors (i.e., predisposing). Causative and predisposing risk factors are listed in Box 12-1, but one of the most common symptoms of CHD is angina pectoris.

Angina Pectoris

Angina pectoris refers to intermittent chest pain caused by temporary oxygen insufficiency and myocardial ischemia. It can be classified into three major variants: (1) stable angina, (2) unstable angina, and (3) Prinzmetal or variant angina.

Stable Angina

Stable angina occurs most commonly when the workload of the heart increases through exertion or stress. It is usually associated with a significant amount of atherosclerotic narrowing in one or more coronary arteries. Because of the large amount of obstruction, the myocardial oxygen supply cannot be increased sufficiently to meet the higher oxygen demands that are required by

Box 12-1

RISK FACTORS FOR CORONARY HEART DISEASE

CAUSATIVE

- Cigarette smoking
- Hypertension
- Low high-density lipoprotein cholesterol (< 40 mg/dL)
- High total and low-density lipoprotein cholesterol
- Type 1 and type 2 diabetes mellitus

PREDISPOSING

- Obesity/overweight
- Physical inactivity
- Family history of premature coronary heart disease (in male first-degree relative < 55 years; in female first-degree relative < 65 years)
- Age (men ≥45 years; women ≥55 years)
- Insulin resistance

Information from National Cholesterol Education Program. Summary of the third report of the national cholesterol education program expert panel on detection, evaluation, and treatment of high blood cholesterol in adults (adult treatment panel III). Bethesda, MD: NIH publication no. 01-3670, 2001; and Trujillo TC, Nolan PE. Ischemic heart disease: anginal syndromes. In: Koda-Kimble MA, Young LY, eds. Applied therapeutics: the clinical use of drugs. Baltimore, MD:. Lippincott Williams & Wilkins, 2001.

exercise or other conditions that stress the heart. Anginal or cardiac chest pain is typically described as a diffuse, heavy pressure or a deep squeezing, crushing, and aching feeling over the sternum area within the chest. The pain may (or may not) radiate to the shoulder, jaw, back, neck, left arm, and occasionally, the right arm. Differentiating characteristics of common types of chest pain are listed in Table 12-1.

Factors that may precipitate angina include:

- Exercise or strenuous activity
- Activity involving use of the arms above the head
- Cold environment
- Emotional stress
- Extreme fear or anger
- Coitus

Anginal pain is usually relieved with rest, which decreases the workload of the heart, or with nitroglycerin. Stable angina can often be controlled with a combination of lifestyle changes and pharmacologic therapy. Lifestyle changes include (1) limiting activities that precipitate the angina, (2) avoiding stressful situations, (3) stopping smoking, (4) consuming a low-fat/low-cholesterol diet, and (5) exercising moderately. Medications that may be used to treat stable angina include nitrates, β-blockers, calcium-channel blockers, and aspirin.

Unstable Angina

Unstable angina is characterized by an increased frequency of anginal pain. Compared to episodes of stable angina, these anginal attacks are usually precipitated by less exertion or may even occur at rest, are more intense, and last longer. This type of angina is sometimes referred to as preinfarction angina, meaning that it is a more serious, potentially irreversible type of myocardial ischemia. Patients with unstable angina are at increased risk of myocardial infarction.

Unstable angina is caused by acute plaque changes with superimposed partial thrombosis, distal embolization of the thrombus, vasospasm, or some combination thereof. These changes are essentially caused by progressive coronary atherosclerosis and its associated lesions. The pain may (or may not) be relieved by rest, depending on the severity of the atherosclerotic disease. Because of the severity of unstable angina, one or more medications are needed to treat it. Useful medications include nitrates, β-blockers, calcium-channel blockers, heparin, and aspirin.

Unstable angina can also be treated with balloon angioplasty or coronary bypass surgery. Balloon **angioplasty** is a nonsurgical method of mechanically dilating a partially obstructed coronary artery. In this procedure, a balloon catheter is pushed through the artery until the obstruction site is reached. Once in place, the balloon is inflated several times, compressing the plaque against the vessel wall and resuming blood flow. A coronary artery bypass graft surgery (CABG) involves taking a section of either the patient's internal thoracic artery or femoral vein and then surgically attaching it to the affected coronary artery. The "graft" then allows blood to flow around the obstructed portion of the native artery. Bypass surgery is usually reserved for cases of severe unstable angina that do not respond to other forms of treatment.

Prinzmetal Angina

Prinzmetal angina (or variant angina) is angina that occurs at rest. It is caused by a coronary artery spasm near an atherosclerotic plaque or in the absence of atherosclerotic disease. Patients with Prinzmetal angina are usually younger than those with

TABLE 12-1 ➤ DIFFERENTIATING CHARACTERISTICS OF CHEST PAIN

CHARACTERISTIC	CARDIAC	GASTROINTESTINAL	MUSCULOSKELETAL
History	Risk factors for coronary heart disease	Gastritis or indigestion	Trauma
Type of pain	Heavy pressure, crushing, or squeezing sensation	Burning sensation	Sore, achy feeling; sharp pain
Precipitating factors	Exertion or stress	Food consumption	Physical movement
Relieved by	Rest or nitroglycerin	Antacids	Rest, heat, or pain medication

chronic stable angina, and they usually do not have risk factors associated with CHD. Treatment includes calcium-channel blockers, nitrates, aspirin, or some combination thereof.

Myocardial Infarction

Myocardial infarction (MI) is the occurrence of myocardial cell death and necrosis caused by local, severe, or prolonged ischemia. It is considered to be a medical emergency. The majority of MIs result from total coronary artery occlusion, which occurs secondary to fissuring and rupture of atherosclerotic plaques. The plaque damage allows blood to be exposed to collagen and fatty acids, and in turn, this activates platelet production, beginning the formation of the thrombus that occludes the artery. Risk factors for MI are the same as those for CHD. Common signs and symptoms are listed in Box 12-2. Treatment of an acute MI has shifted during the last 15 years from prevention and management of complications (i.e., arrhythmias, pain, and blood pressure control) to limiting the extent of myocardial necrosis and preventing reinfarction. Because most acute MIs result from sudden occlusion of a coronary artery due to a thrombus formation, thrombolytic agents are a primary treatment. Agents that are primarily used include streptokinase, anistresplase, alteplase (tPA), and reteplase; other cornerstone therapy includes antiplatelet and anticoagulant drugs (e.g., aspirin, warfarin, and low-molecular-weight heparins), β-blockers, and vasodilators (e.g., angiotensin-converting enzyme [ACE] inhibitors, nitrates, or calcium-channel blockers). Adjunctive therapy includes analgesics (e.g., morphine or meperidine), antiarrhythmics (e.g., lidocaine, procainamide, or amiodarone), stool softeners, and oxygen.

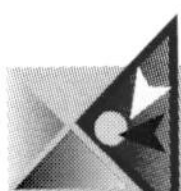

Box 12-2

SIGNS AND SYMPTOMS OF MYOCARDIAL INFARCTION

SIGNS

- Rapid, weak heart rate
- Electrocardiographic changes (i.e., Q waves, ST-segment elevation, and T-wave inversion)
- Rise in creatinine phosphokinase (MB isoenzyme) within 2 days of the anginal attack
- Rise in lactate dehydrogenase (LDH, isoenzyme) within 24 hours of the anginal attack

SYMPTOMS

- Moderate to severe angina not relieved by rest or nitroglycerin (may last several hours) (may radiate to arm(s), neck, jaw, shoulder, or back)
- Shortness of breath
- Nausea, vomiting, or both
- Sweating
- Light-headedness or dizziness
- Fainting

Congestive Heart Failure

Congestive heart failure (CHF) occurs when the heart is unable to pump sufficient blood to meet the metabolic needs of the body. It results primarily from low or insufficient cardiac output, which may be caused by failure of either or both ventricles of the heart. Traditionally, CHF has been classified as either low- or high-output failure, with the vast majority (>90%) of cases being low-output failure.

Low-Output Failure

Low-output failure, the most common type of CHF, is characterized by a diminished volume of blood being pumped by a weakened heart in patients with normal metabolic needs. In other words, the heart is unable to pump all the blood with which it is presented through venous return. The ejection fraction (i.e., the percentage of left ventricular volume pumped during systole) is significantly decreased, which over time causes the ventricles to enlarge as they become congested with retained blood.

Because the traditional classification of low-output failure does not adequately describe the complex nature of heart failure, it is further divided into left or right ventricular dysfunction, with left ventricular dysfunction being the most common form of low-output failure. In left ventricular dysfunction, the LV cannot pump all the blood with which it is presented by the left atrium, causing blood to back up into the pulmonary circulation. Right-sided dysfunction is primarily caused by pulmonary hypertension and cor pulmonale. Consequently, both these conditions cause elevated pulmonary artery pressure, which impedes emptying of the right ventricle and, thus, causes increased workload on the right side of the heart.

Left ventricular dysfunction is further subdivided into systolic and diastolic dysfunction. In both forms, the stroke volume and the subsequent total cardiac output are reduced. The factor differentiating these two disorders is the left ventricular ejection fraction (LVEF). In systolic dysfunction, the LVEF is greatly reduced (<40%), and this reduction is frequently caused by factors that result in the heart failing to pump blood (i.e., in decreased muscle contractility). The LV then becomes enlarged with blood (i.e., dilated) and hypokinetic. Causes of pump failure include:

- Cardiomyopathy secondary to ischemic heart disease
- MI
- Arrhythmias
- Chronic hypertension
- Rheumatic heart disease
- Chronic alcoholism
- Viral infections

In left ventricular diastolic dysfunction, the LVEF remains normal and the cardiac muscle function (i.e., contractility) unimpaired. The LV is stiff (reduced wall compliance) or is unable to relax during diastole, both of which result in an elevated resting pressure within the ventricle despite a relatively low volume of blood. The high pressure impedes left ventricular filling, which normally occurs via a passive inflow against a low-resistance pressure. Because of the end-diastolic ventricular volume being smaller, the stroke volume and the cardiac output are still reduced. In other words, left ventricular diastolic dysfunction causes a high fraction of a low volume to be ejected. Causes of left ventricular diastolic dysfunction include:

- Coronary ischemia
- Hypertension
- MI
- Ventricular wall hypertrophy
- Hypertrophic cardiomyopathy
- Constrictive pericarditis
- Restrictive cardiomyopathy
- Valvular heart disease

High-Output Failure

In contrast, high-output failure is characterized by a healthy, functioning heart with an abnormally high metabolic demand from body tissues. The heart is unable to pump enough blood to meet the increased needs of the tissues and, thus, becomes exhausted from the extra workload placed on it. Causes of high-output failure include hyperthyroidism and severe anemia.

Regardless of the origin, however, several compensatory mechanisms are activated as the heart begins to fail in an attempt to maintain normal cardiac output and oxygenation of vital organs. These mechanisms include:

- Cardiac dilation, which is caused by the residual blood that accumulates in the ventricle. This increase in the end-diastolic volume causes ventricular myocardial fibers to stretch, dilating the ventricle.
- Cardiac hypertrophy, which is also an adaptation to the increased diastolic volume, through which ventricular muscle mass and wall thickness increase.
- Activation of the sympathetic nervous system, which is caused by release of norepinephrine and other catecholamines in response to the decreased cardiac output and, ultimately, decreased tissue perfusion. These catecholamines increase the heart rate and contractility of the ventricle, which maintains the cardiac output and tissue perfusion to major organs.
- Increased stimulation of the renin-angiotensin system in response to release of catecholamines. Although essential in maintaining cardiovascular homeostasis, catecholamines also cause vasoconstriction in the skin, gastrointestinal tract, and renal circulation, thus increasing the workload of the heart by enhancing systemic vascular resistance. The decreased renal perfusion activates the renin-angiotensin system, which stimulates the release of aldosterone and, ultimately, increases the total plasma volume of extracellular fluid through resorption of both sodium and water. The increased intravascular volume worsens the venous pooling of blood caused by the failing ventricle.

All these metabolic effects of the failing right or left ventricle result in several common signs and symptoms, which are listed in Box 12-3.

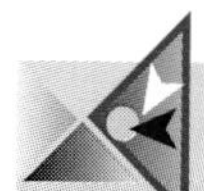

Box 12-3

SIGNS AND SYMPTOMS OF CONGESTIVE HEART FAILURE

SIGNS

- Tachycardia
- S_3 gallop
- Left ventricular hypertrophy
- Rales or crackles
- Ejection fraction < 40%
- Weight gain
- Increased blood urea nitrogen
- Jugular venous distension
- Hepatomegaly
- Hepatojugular reflex

SYMPTOMS

- Shortness of breath
- Dyspnea on exertion
- Orthopnea
- Paroxysmal nocturnal dyspnea
- Peripheral edema
- Cough
- Weakness
- Fatigue

Treatment of CHF primarily involves managing (if possible) the underlying cause (e.g., hypertension), correcting the patient's symptoms, avoiding complications, and improving the patient's quality of life. Treatment modalities include limited-to-moderate physical activity, a sodium-restricted diet (2–4 g NaCl/day), and pharmacologic agents, such as diuretics, ACE inhibitors, digoxin, vasodilators (hydralazine and digoxin), and in severe cases, β-blockers (carvedilol) and inotropic agents.

Hypertension

Hypertension is defined as elevated systolic blood pressure (>140 mm Hg), elevated diastolic blood pressure (>90 mm Hg), or both as measured on at least two separate occasions. *The Sixth Report of the Joint National Committee on Detection, Evaluation, and Treatment of High Blood Pressure* classifies blood pressure based on systolic and diastolic values and categorizes patients into different stages (Table 12-2). (For a detailed discussion of blood pressure measurement, see Chapter 5.)

The vast majority of patients have idiopathic or essential hypertension, in which no cause is identified for the increased blood pressure. Various genetic and environmental factors are thought to play a role in elevating blood pressure through their effects on cardiac output, peripheral resistance, or both. Occasionally, patients have secondary hypertension caused by renal disease, adrenal disorders (e.g., primary aldosteronism,

Cushing's syndrome, or pheochromocytoma), or pregnancy. In addition, several medications can increase a patient's blood pressure and potentially cause secondary hypertension (Box 12-4). Risk factors for developing hypertension include:

- Obesity
- African-American race
- High-sodium diet
- Excessive alcohol consumption
- Family history of hypertension
- Patients with high-normal blood pressure

Hypertension is typically asymptomatic, meaning that patients usually do not experience any subjective symptoms when their blood pressure is elevated. Objective signs of hypertension include elevated blood pressure and, occasionally, an S_4. Because of the relationship between various lifestyle factors and the risk of high blood pressure, lifestyle modifications play an important role in the treatment of hypertension. Lifestyle modifications include restriction of dietary sodium (2–4 g NaCl/day), weight reduction, consistent aerobic physical activity (walking, running, biking, or swimming for 30–45 min, 3–5 days a week), decreasing dietary saturated fats, cessation of smoking, restriction of alcohol consumption to 1 ounce of ethanol or less (≤2 ounces of 100 proof whiskey, 8 ounces of wine, or 24 ounces of beer) per day, and maintaining an adequate intake of dietary potassium, calcium, and magnesium. If lifestyle modifications do not sufficiently lower the patient's blood pressure, several classes of medications are usually effective; routine management includes diuretics, ACE inhibitors, β-blockers, angiotensin II-receptor antagonists, calcium-channel blockers, and peripheral α-antagonists.

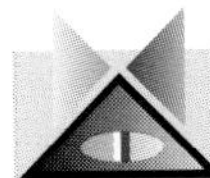

Box 12-4

DRUGS THAT MAY INCREASE BLOOD PRESSURE[a]

Alcohol
Appetite suppressants
Cocaine
Corticosteroids
Cyclosporine
Decongestants
Estrogens
Monoamine oxidase inhibitors
Nonsteroidal anti-inflammatory drugs
Oral contraceptives
Excessive thyroid hormone
Tricyclic antidepressants

[a]Not all inclusive.

Arrhythmia

Cardiac **arrhythmia** is an irregular rate of cardiac contraction. It can result from abnormal electrical impulse formation, conduction, or both. The various forms of arrhythmias are classified according to the location of the malfunctioning electrical current. Supraventricular arrhythmias originate above the AV bundle and include sinus bradycardia and tachycardia, atrial flutter, atrial fibrillation, Wolff-Parkinson-White syndrome, and premature atrial contractions. Ventricular arrhythmias originate below the AV bundle and include premature ventricular contractions, ventricular tachycardia, and ventricular fibrillation. Various cardiac and systemic causes of arrhythmias include:

- Ischemic heart disease
- Cardiomyopathy
- Cardiac surgery
- Mitral valve disease
- Metabolic or electrolyte imbalance
- Chronic pulmonary disease
- Cerebrovascular accident
- Alcohol

Signs and symptoms of arrhythmias are listed in Box 12-5. The primary goals of arrhythmia treatment are (1) to control the ventricular rate, (2) to convert the heart to normal sinus rhythm, and (3) to resolve the patient's symptoms. Medications used to control the ventricular rate include digoxin, β-blockers, calcium-channel blockers, and adenosine. Chemical cardioversion and maintenance of normal sinus rhythm can be accomplished through use of antiarrhythmic agents (quinidine, procainamide, lidocaine, propafenone, β-blockers, calcium-channel blockers, and amiodarone). Patients with atrial fibrillation may also be treated with aspirin or warfarin, because these patients have an increased risk of stroke. Patients who do not convert with drug therapy or who are hemodynamically unstable may be cardioverted by a direct electrical current. An implantable cardioverter/defibrillator may also be used. Electrode pads are surgically placed around the left and right ventricles and function as a defibrillator when an abnormal rhythm is detected.

TABLE 12-2 ➤ CLASSIFICATION OF BLOOD PRESSURE IN PATIENTS 18 YEARS AND OLDER[a]

CATEGORY	SYSTOLIC (MM HG)		DIASTOLIC (MM HG)
Optimal[b]	<120		<80
Normal	<130		<85
High-normal	130–139	or	85–89
Hypertension[c]			
Stage 1	140–159	or	90–99
Stage 2	160–179	or	100–109
Stage 3	≥180	or	≥110

Reprinted with permission from Joint National Committee on Prevention, Detection, Evaluation, and Treatment of High Blood Pressure. The Sixth Report of the Joint National Committee on Detection, Evaluation, and Treatment of High Blood Pressure (JNC VI). Arch Intern Med 1997;157:2413-2446.

[a]Not taking antihypertensive drugs and not acutely ill. When systolic and diastolic blood pressure fall into different categories, select the higher category to classify the individual's blood pressure. For example, 160/92 mm Hg should be classified as stage 2 hypertension.

[b]Optimal blood pressure with respect to cardiovascular risk. Unusually low readings, however, should be evaluated for clinical significance.

[c]Based on the average of two or more readings taken at each of two or more visits after an initial screening.

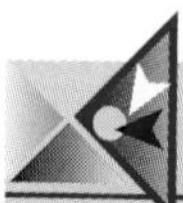

Box 12-5

SIGNS AND SYMPTOMS OF ARRHYTHMIAS

SIGNS

- Irregular heart rhythm
- Normal heart rate, bradycardia, or tachycardia
- Abnormal electrocardiogram

SYMPTOMS

- Palpitations
- Shortness of breath
- Dizziness/light-headedness
- Syncope
- Nervousness
- Anxiety

Lipid Disorders

Hyperlipidemia is an elevation of cholesterol, cholesterol esters, phospholipids, or triglycerides. Hyperlipoproteinemia is an elevation of lipoproteins in the plasma. These lipid disorders result from malfunctions in lipid metabolism that usually involve overproduction or decreased clearance of cholesterol-containing products.

In patients with elevated LDL or cardiovascular risk factors, LDL is deposited in the arterial walls, where it becomes oxidized. In turn, this oxidation stimulates the body to send white blood cells to the area to clean up the arterial wall, which leads to development of fibrosis and calcification. As more white blood cells continue to migrate to the site, the fatty plaque worsens in the arterial wall, and occlusion or rupture may occur, leading to thrombus and possible MI.

The benefit of cholesterol lowering is the reduction of fat in the arterial walls, leading to a process called plaque stabilization. Coronary angiography has shown that cholesterol reduction and plaque stabilization, over a long period of time, can result in improvement in 30% and no progression of blockages in at least 60% of patients with existing plaques.

Secondary causes of hyperlipidemia that need to be ruled out include:

- Hypothyroidism
- Diabetes mellitus
- Ethanol use
- Renal abnormalities
- Liver disease
- Drugs such as β-blockers, thiazide diuretics, and estrogen therapy

Hyperlipidemia is typically asymptomatic, with patients rarely showing any subjective evidence of the disease. Because of the lack of subjective symptoms, risk factors for CHD, lipid laboratory values, and physical signs are important to the pharmacist when evaluating for lipid disorders (Box 12-6).

The goals of therapy, according to the National Cholesterol Education Program Guidelines Adult Treatment Panel III (ATP III), are first to identify the presence of clinical atherosclerotic disease that confers high risk for CHD (i.e., clinical CHD, symptomatic carotid artery disease, peripheral arterial disease, abdominal aortic aneurysm, and diabetes) and then to determine the presence of major risk factors other than LDL (Box 12-7). (Note that LDL is not counted among the risk factors for LDL goal determination, because the purpose of counting those risk factors is to modify the treatment of LDL.) If two or more risk factors (other than LDL) are present without CHD or CHD risk equivalent, then ATP III guidelines recommend assessment of the 10-year CHD risk according to the Framingham Tables for Men and Women (Table 12-3). The patient's LDL goal is then determined based on his or her risk category (Table 12-4). In general, the higher the patient's risk for CHD, the lower the LDL goal and the more aggressive the treatment. For step-by-step assessment and treatment guidelines, the reader is referred to the publication *ATP III Guidelines at-a-Glance Quick Desk Reference* (NIH publication no. 01-3305).

Because of the strong relationship between lifestyle and high cholesterol, lifestyle modifications must be addressed as the cornerstone of therapy. These include nutritional and exercise

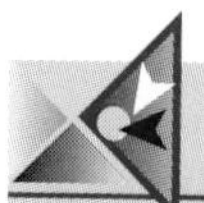

Box 12-6

SIGNS AND SYMPTOMS OF HYPERLIPIDEMIA

SIGNS

- Low-density lipoprotein cholesterol (primary target of therapy):
  - $<$100 mg/dL: Optimal
  - 100–129 mg/dL: near-optimal/above optimal
  - 130–159 mg/dL: borderline high
  - 160–189 mg/dL: high
  - $\geq$190 mg/dL: very high
- Total cholesterol:
  - 200–239 mg/dL: borderline high
  - $\geq$240 mg/dL: high
- High-density lipoprotein cholesterol:
  - 40 mg/dL: low
  - 40–59 mg/dL: normal
  - $\geq$60 mg/dL: high

SYMPTOMS[a]

- Xanthelasmas
- Skin xanthomas
- Tendon xanthomas
- Arcus senilis

Information from National Cholesterol Education Program. Summary of the third report of the national cholesterol education program expert panel on detection, evaluation, and treatment of high blood cholesterol in adults (adult treatment panel III). NIH publication no. 01-3670, 2001.

[a]Rare, except in severe cases.

Box 12-7

MAJOR RISK FACTORS (EXCLUSIVE OF LOW-DENSITY LIPOPROTEIN CHOLESTEROL) THAT MODIFY LDL GOALS[a]

- Cigarette smoking
- Hypertension (blood pressure ≥140/90 mm Hg or on antihypertensive medication)
- Low high-density lipoprotein cholesterol (<40 mg/dL)[b]
- Family history of premature coronary heart disease (in male first-degree relative <55 years; in female first-degree relative <65 years)
- Age (men ≥45 years; women ≥55 years)

Information from National Cholesterol Education Program. Summary of the third report of the national cholesterol education program expert panel on detection, evaluation, and treatment of high blood cholesterol in adults (adult treatment panel III). Bethesda, MD: NIH publication no. 01-3670, 2001;

[a]In Adult Treatment Panel III, diabetes is regarded at a coronary heart disease risk equivalent.

[b]A level ≥ 60 mg/dL counts as a "negative" risk factor; its presence removes one risk factor from the total count.

therapy. Therapeutic lifestyle changes include diet (saturated fat <7% of calories, cholesterol <200 mg/day), weight management, and increased physical activity. Information about recommended dietary changes should be available in the pharmacy. A nutritional regimen allowing for weight loss is important if the patient is overweight. An exercise program is also an important element of therapeutic lifestyle changes and should emphasize aerobic physical activity (walking, running, biking, or swimming for 30–45 min, 3–5 times/week). In addition, names of local dietitians and physical therapists who may be contacted for further assistance should be posted in the pharmacy.

If the goals of therapy are not reached using lifestyle changes, drug therapy may be necessary. The choice of which agent to use depends on the cholesterol profile, the patient's risk (and prevention), and the patient's characteristics. The most commonly used agents include 3-hydroxy-3-methylglutaric coenzyme A reductase inhibitors (statins), bile acid sequestrants, nicotinic acid (niacin), and fibric acids.

SYSTEM ASSESSMENT

Subjective Information

When assessing the cardiovascular system, subjective patient information can be invaluable. It is important for the pharmacist to ask the patient appropriate questions to elicit specific data.

Chest Pain

? INTERVIEW Do you ever have any chest pain or discomfort? If yes,

Onset and duration: When did the pain start? How long did it last? Have you had this type of chest pain before? How often do you experience the chest pain?

Characteristics: Describe the pain. Is it a severe crushing or pressure, or is it a sharp, stabbing pain? Is there a burning sensation?

ABNORMALITIES Angina is typically described as a heavy pressure or a crushing/squeezing sensation. Try to differentiate from other causes of chest pain (Table 12-1).

? INTERVIEW Where is the pain? Does it radiate to any other areas?

ABNORMALITIES A patient who describes the pain by clenching his or her fist over the sternum may have angina. Angina or a progressing MI may cause the pain to radiate to the jaw, shoulder, back, or left or right arm.

? INTERVIEW What brought on the pain? Physical exertion? Cold weather? Intercourse? A stressful situation?

ABNORMALITIES Angina is typically caused by physical exertion, cold weather, intercourse, or an emotionally stressful situation.

? INTERVIEW What relieves the pain? Rest? Nitroglycerin?

ABNORMALITIES Relief of chest pain following sublingual nitroglycerin usually occurs if the pain is cardiac in origin.

? INTERVIEW Do you experience any other symptoms? Nausea/vomiting? Sweating? Shortness of breath? Light-headedness?

ABNORMALITIES Patients experiencing an MI may also have nausea/vomiting, shortness of breath (SOB), sweating, and/or light-headedness in addition to chest pain.

Dyspnea

? INTERVIEW Do you ever experience any shortness of breath? If yes,

Onset and duration: When does it occur? How long does it last? Is it constant, or does it come and go?

Cause: What brings it on? Exertion? Lying flat? Sleeping at night? How many pillows do you need to sleep comfortably at night?

ABNORMALITIES SOB with exertion, commonly termed *dyspnea on exertion,* may occur with angina or CHF. Congestive heart failure may cause SOB while lying flat (i.e., **orthopnea**), in which the patient may need more than one pillow to sleep comfortably at night. CHF may also cause a sudden gasping for air while sleeping at night

TABLE 12-3 ➤ FRAMINGHAM TABLES FOR MEN AND WOMEN

MEN

Estimate of 10-Year Risk for Men
(Framingham Point Scores)

Age	Points
20–34	−9
35–39	−4
40–44	0
45–49	3
50–54	6
55–59	8
60–64	10
65–69	11
70–74	12
75–79	13

Total Cholesterol	Points				
	Age 20–39	Age 40–49	Age 50–59	Age 60–69	Age 70–79
<160	0	0	0	0	0
160–199	4	3	2	1	0
200–239	7	5	3	1	0
240–279	9	6	4	2	1
≥280	11	8	5	3	1

	Points				
	Age 20–39	Age 40–49	Age 50–59	Age 60–69	Age 70–79
Nonsmoker	0	0	0	0	0
Smoker	8	5	3	1	1

HDL (mg/dL)	Points
≥60	−1
50–59	0
40–49	1
<40	2

Systolic BP (mmHg)	If Untreated	If Treated
<120	0	0
120–129	0	1
130–139	1	2
140–159	1	2
≥160	2	3

Point Total	10-Year Risk %
<0	<1
0	1
1	1
2	1
3	1
4	1
5	2
6	2
7	3
8	4
9	5
10	6
11	8
12	10
13	12
14	16
15	20
16	25
≥17	≥30

10-Year risk ______%

WOMEN

Estimate of 10-Year Risk for Women
(Framingham Point Scores)

Age	Points
20–34	−7
35–39	−3
40–44	0
45–49	3
50–54	6
55–59	8
60–64	10
65–69	12
70–74	14
75–79	16

Total Cholesterol	Points				
	Age 20–39	Age 40–49	Age 50–59	Age 60–69	Age 70–79
<160	0	0	0	0	0
160–199	4	3	2	1	1
200–239	8	6	4	2	1
240–279	11	8	5	3	2
≥280	13	10	7	4	2

	Points				
	Age 20–39	Age 40–49	Age 50–59	Age 60–69	Age 70–79
Nonsmoker	0	0	0	0	0
Smoker	9	7	4	2	1

HDL (mg/dL)	Points
≥60	−1
50–59	0
40–49	1
<40	2

Systolic BP (mmHg)	If Untreated	If Treated
<120	0	0
120–129	1	3
130–139	2	4
140–159	3	5
≥160	4	6

Point Total	10-Year Risk %
<9	<1
9	1
10	1
11	1
12	1
13	2
14	2
15	3
16	4
17	5
18	6
19	8
20	11
21	14
22	17
23	22
24	27
≥25	≥30

10-Year risk ______%

U.S. DEPARTMENT OF HEALTH AND HUMAN SERVICES
Public Health Service
National Institutes of Health
National Heart, Lung, and Blood Institute

Bethesda, MD: NIH Publication N. 01-3305
May 2001

TABLE 12-4 ➤ LDL CHOLESTEROL GOALS AND TREATMENT RECOMMENDATIONS

RISK CATEGORY	LDL GOAL (MG/DL)	LDL LEVEL AT WHICH TO INITIATE TLC (MG/DL)	LDL LEVEL AT WHICH TO CONSIDER DRUG THERAPY (MG/DL)
CHD or CHD risk equivalents (10-year risk >20%)	<100	≥100 mg/dL	≥130 (100–139: drug optional[a])
2+ Risk factors (10-year risk ≤20%)	<130	≥130	10-year risk of 10%–20%: ≥130; 10-year risk of <10%: ≥160
0–1 Risk factor[b]	<160	≥160	≥190 (160–189: LDL-lowering drug optional)

National Cholesterol Education Program. Summary of the third report of the national cholesterol education program expert panel on detection, evaluation, and treatment of high blood cholesterol in adults (adult treatment panel III). Bethesda, MD: NIH publication no. 01-3670, 2001.

CHD, coronary heart disease; *LDL*, low-density lipoprotein; *TLC*, therapeutic lifestyle changes.

[a]Some authorities recommend use of LDL-lowering drugs in this category if an LDL level of <100 mg/dL cannot be achieved by TLC. Others prefer use of drugs that primarily modify triglycerides and HDL (e.g., nicotinic acid or fibrate). Clinical judgment may also call for deferring drug therapy in this subcategory.

[b]Almost all people with zero or one risk factor have a 10-year risk of <10%; thus, 10-year risk assessment in people with zero or one risk factor is not necessary.

(i.e., **paroxysmal nocturnal dyspnea** [PND]), during which the patient may need to rush and open a window to get some fresh air.

? INTERVIEW What makes it better or go away? Do you experience any other symptoms? Chest pain? Edema?

➤ ABNORMALITIES Angina may cause SOB along with chest pain. In addition to SOB, CHF may cause edema in the feet, ankles, and lower legs (least severe in the morning on rising and more severe in the evening).

Palpitations

? INTERVIEW Do you ever experience any palpitations or a fluttering feeling in your chest? If yes,

Onset and duration: When do they occur? How long do they last? How frequently do they occur?

Cause: What brings on the palpitations? Emotional stress? Excessive caffeine? Cold medicine?

Relief: What makes them get better or go away?

Symptoms: Do you experience any other symptoms with the palpitations? Light-headedness, dizziness, or fainting? Shortness of breath?

➤ ABNORMALITIES Cardiac arrhythmias may also cause light-headedness, dizziness, fainting, or SOB in addition to the chest palpitations.

? INTERVIEW Patient history: Do you have any history of heart problems? Heart disease? Heart attack? High blood pressure? Irregular heart rhythm? Heart failure? Heart murmur? Rheumatic heart disease? High cholesterol? Diabetes?

Family history: Have any immediate family members had heart disease? Heart attack or angina? High blood pressure? Diabetes?

Medication history: What prescription or nonprescription medications are you currently taking? Do you currently take, or have you taken in the past, any medicine for high blood pressure or chest pain? Digoxin? Water pills or diuretics? Aspirin or warfarin? Nitroglycerin?

Social history: Do you smoke or chew tobacco? If so, how much each day? For how many years? Do you drink alcohol? If so, how much each day or week? For how many years?

Risk Factors for CHD

? INTERVIEW Do you have elevated cholesterol? If so, when did you have your cholesterol tested? Was it a fasting measurement? How high was your total cholesterol? Your HDL? Your LDL?

➤ ABNORMALITIES Box 12-1 lists risk factors for CHD. Box 12-6 lists the desirable levels of total, HDL, and LDL cholesterol. Box 12-7 lists risk factors that modify LDL goals. When fasting is indicated, it should be for at least 12 hours.

? INTERVIEW Have you ever had trouble with your thyroid? Diabetes mellitus? Alcohol use? Kidney problems? Liver disease? What medications do you currently take?

➤ ABNORMALITIES Secondary causes of hyperlipidemia include hypothyroidism, diabetes mellitus, alcohol use, kidney problems, liver problems, and use of medications such as β-blockers, thiazide diuretics, and estrogen therapy.

INTERVIEW Have you ever had a heart attack, stroke, or heart surgery? How old are you? Do you have high blood pressure? Do you smoke? Do you have any relatives who had a stroke, heart attack, or bypass surgery at a young age? Do you have diabetes?

ABNORMALITIES The occurrence of an MI, cerebrovascular accident, transient ischemic attack, CABG, or PVD classify the patient as secondary prevention. Risk factors for CHD include men 45 years and older and women 55 years and older or undergoing premature menopause without estrogen replacement, hypertension or the use of blood pressure medications, smoking, family history of premature CHD, and diabetes mellitus; these warrant assessment in all patients.

Objective Information

Objective patient information pertaining to the cardiovascular system primarily includes the physical assessment and laboratory and diagnostic tests.

Physical Assessment

Physical assessment of the cardiovascular system involves inspection, palpation, and auscultation of the carotid arteries, jugular veins, and heart. Keep in mind that pharmacists rarely perform the physical examination techniques described here; these techniques are included for completeness of the chapter. Pharmacists do, however, commonly use these data when evaluating patient drug therapy.

Carotid Arteries

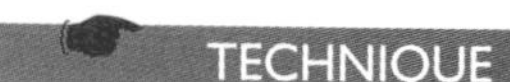

STEP 1

Palpate the Carotid Pulse

Palpation of the carotid arteries is shown in Figure 12-8.

- The patient should be sitting with the examiner behind.
- Palpate each carotid artery medial to the sternocleidomastoid muscle in the neck. Palpate with the first three fingers, positioning them between the larynx and the anterior border of the sternocleidomastoid muscle in the lower third of the neck.

CAUTION **Palpate only one carotid artery at a time to avoid diminishing arterial blood flow to the brain.**

- Press gently, but firmly, until the pulse is felt. Evaluate the pulse's contour and amplitude.
- Normally, the right and left carotid pulses are synchronous, of equal amplitude, and are 2+ on a grade scale of 0 to 4+, with 0 being a very weak pulse and 4+ a very brisk pulse.

ABNORMALITIES A small, weak, or diminished pulse occurs with low cardiac output or severe mitral stenosis. A full, strong, or hyperkinetic pulse may occur with anxiety, anemia, thyrotoxicosis, hypertension, aortic regurgitation, or hypertrophic cardiomyopathy. (For a complete discussion of pulses, see Chapter 13.)

TECHNIQUE

STEP 2

Auscultate the Carotid Arteries

Auscultation of the carotid arteries is shown in Figure 12-9 and should be reserved for patients who are middle-aged, elderly, or have signs and symptoms of cardiovascular disease.

- Lightly place the diaphragm of the stethoscope over the carotid artery in the upper (angle of the jaw), middle (midcervical area), and lower (base of the neck) thirds.
- Ask the patient to hold his or her breath briefly so that the tracheal breath sounds do not interfere. Listen for the presence of a **bruit** (i.e., a blowing, murmur-like sound of vascular rather than cardiac origin).
- Normal heart sounds may be heard. Be careful not to confuse these with a bruit.

ABNORMALITIES A carotid bruit suggests narrowing or partial occlusion of the lumen, most commonly associated with atherosclerosis.

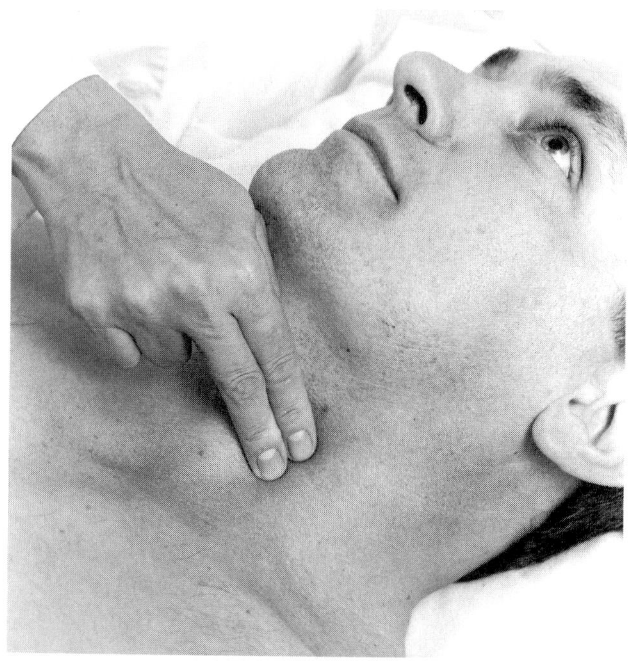

FIGURE 12-8 ■ Palpating the carotid arteries.

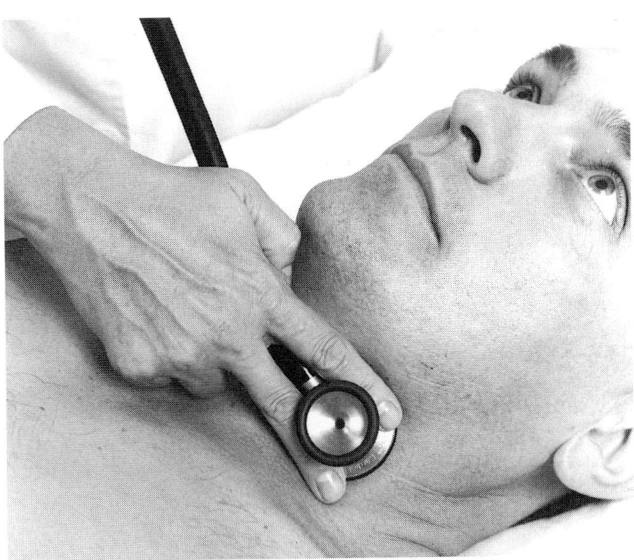

FIGURE 12-9 ■ Auscultating the carotid arteries.

Jugular Veins

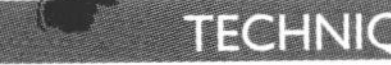

STEP 1

Inspect the Jugular Venous Pulse

Inspection of the jugular venous pulse is shown in Figure 12-10.

- Position the patient in a supine position at a 30° to 40° angle from the horizontal (by placing a pillow under the patient's head and neck) so that the pulsations can best be seen. Generally, the higher the venous pressure, the higher the position that is needed.
- Remove the pillow, and position the patient's head slightly upward or downward and slightly toward the side that is being examined.

CAUTION **Be careful not to turn the head too far, because this will tense the neck muscles and make the observations much more difficult.**

- Shine a penlight horizontally across the side of the neck, and note the external jugular veins overlying the sternocleidomastoid muscle.
- Visibility of the veins varies among patients. In some, they are not visible; in others, they are clearly visible even in the supine position.

STEP 2

Estimate the Jugular Venous Pressure

Estimation of the jugular venous pressure is shown in Figure 12-11. The crest of the jugular vein can be used as a convenient rough estimate of mean right arterial pressure.

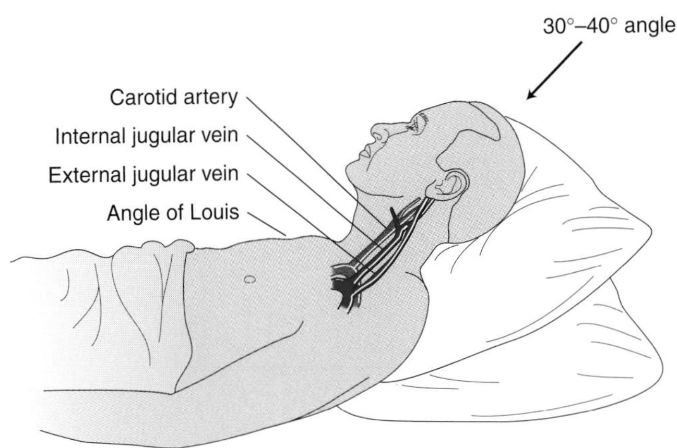

FIGURE 12-10 ■ Inspecting the jugular venous pulse.

- Hold a centimeter ruler vertically on the sternal angle.
- Align a straight edge perpendicular from the crest of the distended jugular vein to the vertical ruler, similar to a T-square.
- Note the level of intersection between the straight edge and the ruler in centimeters.
- Normally, the jugular venous pressure is ≤3 cm above the sternal angle.

ABNORMALITIES Elevated jugular venous pressure (>3 cm) occurs with right-sided CHF and is commonly documented as jugular venous distention.

TECHNIQUE

STEP 3

Assess for the Hepatojugular Reflex

Assessment of the **hepatojugular reflex** (Fig. 12-12) is useful in patients exhibiting signs and symptoms of CHF or with elevated jugular venous pressure.

- Place the patient in a supine position. Instruct the patient to breathe quietly through his or her mouth.
- Gently, but firmly, press the palm of your right hand on the right upper quadrant of the patient's abdomen, just below the rib cage.
- Firmly compress the abdomen for 30 to 60 seconds, and observe the rise in the jugular venous pressure.

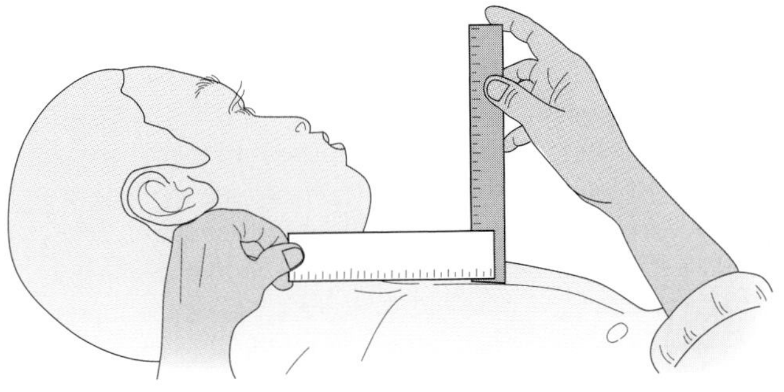

FIGURE 12-11 ■ Estimating the jugular venous pressure.

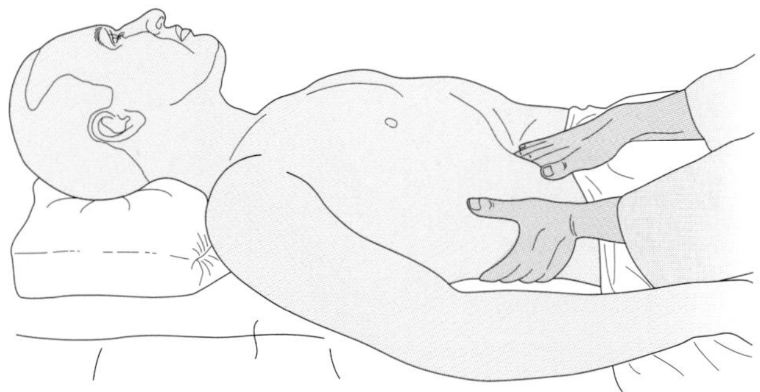

FIGURE 12-12 ■ Palpating the hepatojugular reflex.

- Normally, the jugular venous pressure will drop back to the previous level, after a few beats, while the abdomen is still being compressed. If the jugular venous pressure continues to be elevated during the entire period of abdominal compression, hepatic venous congestion is present. This phenomenon is termed the *hepatojugular reflex.*

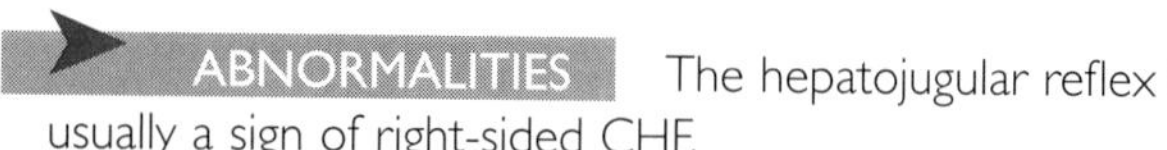

ABNORMALITIES The hepatojugular reflex is usually a sign of right-sided CHF.

Heart

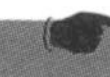

TECHNIQUE

STEP 1

Inspect the Anterior Chest

- Place the patient in a supine position at a 30° angle.
- Carefully inspect the patient's fourth to fifth intercostal space at the midclavicular line of the chest for the apical impulse (i.e., the pulsation of the chest wall created by systole).

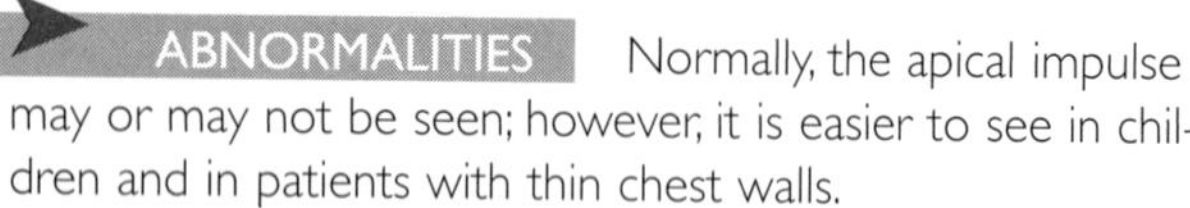

ABNORMALITIES Normally, the apical impulse may or may not be seen; however, it is easier to see in children and in patients with thin chest walls.

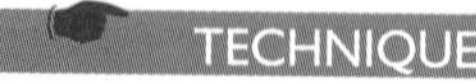

TECHNIQUE

STEP 2

Palpate the Point of Maximal Impulse or Apical Pulse

- Place the pads of your dominant hand's fingers on the patient's chest wall in the region of the apex of the heart (Fig. 12-13). Identify the point of maximal impulse (PMI) or apical pulse with the middle finger.
- To aid in finding the PMI, ask the patient to exhale and then hold the breath. You can also try rolling the patient slightly to the left. Keep in mind that this left lateral position also extends the location of the PMI to the left.
- Note the location of the PMI. Normally, this is the fourth or fifth intercostal space, either at or medial to the midclavicular line, and occupies <3cm in diameter.
- Note the amplitude of the PMI. Normally, it is a short, gentle tapping sensation that occupies the first half of systole.

ABNORMALITIES The PMI may not be palpable in patients with a thick chest wall. The PMI is typically displaced down, to the left, and occupies a larger area in left ventricular dilation (e.g., CHF). The PMI may have increased amplitude and duration with left ventricular hypertrophy, anxiety, fever, hyperthyroidism, and anemia.

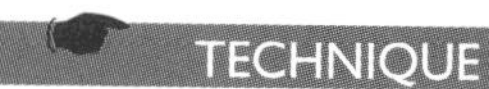

TECHNIQUE

STEP 3

Percussion of the Heart

Percussion provides little additional information for assessment of the cardiovascular system. In the past, it has been used to estimate the size of the heart; however, this information can now be readily obtained from a chest radiograph (X-ray).

STEP 4

Auscultation of the Heart

Auscultate the (1) aortic area, (2) pulmonic area, (3) Erb's point (second pulmonic area), (4) tricuspid area, and (5) mitral area (Fig. 12-14), starting at either the base (the top of the heart) or the apex (the bottom of the heart) and inching your way to each valve area listed. At each area, use the diaphragm of the stethoscope, and listen to the heart's rate and rhythm.

- Count the number of beats for 1 minute. Normally, the rate should be between 60 and 100 bpm.
- Note any irregularities of rhythm. Normally, the rhythm should be regular.

ABNORMALITIES Heart rates <60 bpm are termed bradycardia, and heart rates >100 bpm are termed tachycardia.

- Next, listen for the heart sounds. This is a very difficult technique to master. Most pharmacists do not listen to heart sounds in day-to-day practice; however, interpreting physical examination results from a primary care provider is common for pharmacists in a clinic or a hospital setting.

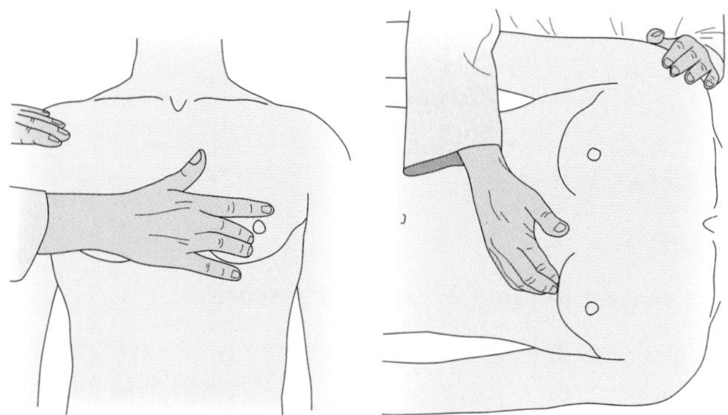

FIGURE 12-13 ■ Position of apical impulse.

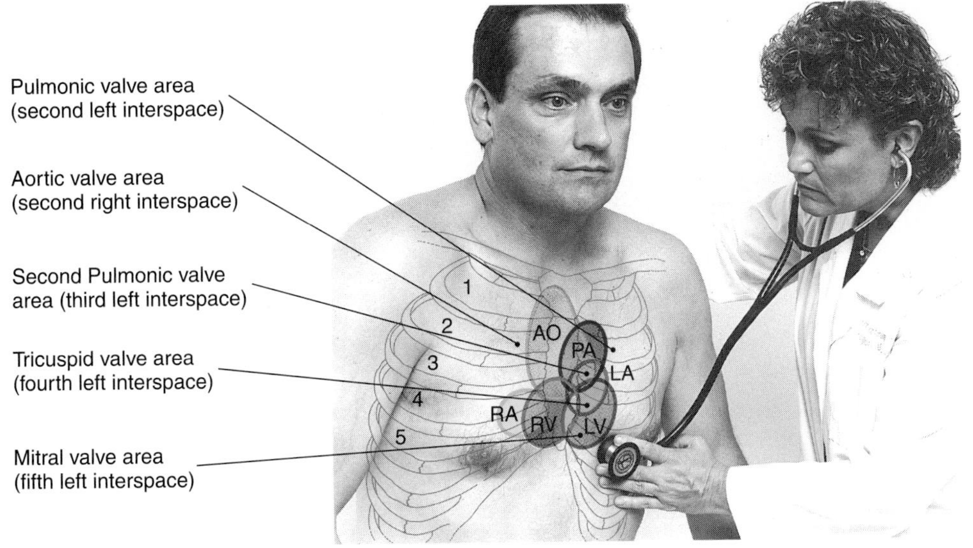

FIGURE 12-14 ■ Cardiac auscultation areas. (*AO*, aorta; *LA*, left atrium; *LV*, left ventricle; *PA*, pulmonary artery; *RA*, right atrium; *RV*, right ventricle.)

- Identify S_1 and S_2 separately. These are usually heard as "lub-dub," and both are normally heard over the entire precordium area. However, S_1 is best heard over the apex, and S_2 is best heard over the base of the heart.
- Using the bell of the stethoscope, listen for extra heart sounds. They will be heard immediately after S_1 and S_2. They are best heard over the apex area of the heart, with the patient lying on his or her left side. Normally, these extra heart sounds should not be heard in patients older than 30 years. If detected, note the timing, and identify as S_3 or S_4.

ABNORMALITIES The S_3 is a ventricular filling sound that occurs in early diastole during the rapid filling phase. In adults, it may be a sign of CHF or volume overload. It typically sounds like "lub-dub-dub." The S_4 is also a ventricular filling sound, but it occurs when the atria contract late in diastole. It is heard immediately before S_1 and typically sounds like "da-lub-dub." It occurs with decreased ventricular compliance (e.g., CHD, cardiomyopathy, aortic stenosis, and hypertension). It may also occur normally in adults older than 40 or 50 years but with no evidence of cardiovascular disease, especially after exercise.

TECHNIQUE

STEP 4 (Continued)

- Listen for murmurs. A murmur will sound like a swooshing or blowing noise. If detected, grade it according to its loudness from I to VI:
  - ***Grade I:*** barely audible
  - ***Grade II:*** audible, but faint
  - ***Grade III:*** moderately loud
  - ***Grade IV:*** loud
  - ***Grade V:*** very loud; heard with stethoscope slightly above the chest wall
  - ***Grade VI:*** loudest; heard without the stethoscope
- Identify the murmur's location by determining where it is best heard.
- Determine the murmur's duration or timing according to the cardiac cycle.

ABNORMALITIES A heart murmur may be normal (e.g., children and adolescents) or abnormal (e.g., valvular defects or congenital heart defects).

Risk Factors for CHD

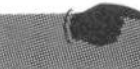
TECHNIQUE

STEP 1

Measure the Blood Pressure

For a detailed discussion of how to measure blood pressure, see Chapter 5.

ABNORMALITIES Elevated blood pressure (>140/90 mm Hg) or use of antihypertensive medications are risk factors for CHD.

Lipid Disorders

In patients suspected of having lipid disorders, a thorough cardiovascular examination should be completed to determine the presence of CHD. (For a detailed discussion of how to complete a cardiovascular examination, see the previous sections of this chapter.) In addition, the eyes and skin should be examined.

TECHNIQUE

STEP 1

Inspect the Eyes

For a detailed discussion of how to inspect the eyes, see Chapter 9.

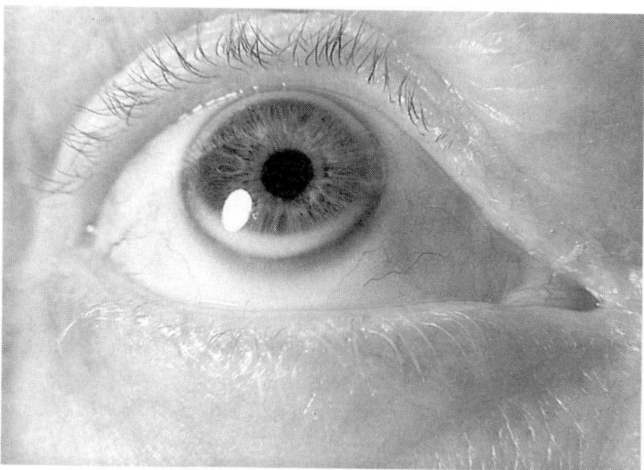

FIGURE 12-15 ■ Corneal arcus. (See Color Plate 34; reprinted with permission from Tasman W, et al. The Wills Eye Hospital atlas of clinical ophthalmology. 2nd ed. Philadelphia: Lippincott Williams & Wilkins, 2001.)

ABNORMALITIES **Corneal arcus** are lipid deposits in the periphery of eye that may be detected when light is directed to the iris (Fig. 12-15). In the area of limbus, where the cornea meets the sclera, a thickened white line represents deposits of fat. These may eventually form a complete circle around the cornea, or a **circus senilis.** In patients younger than 40 years, this may indicate a lipid disorder. It occurs quite commonly in the elderly, however, which may be due to the aging process rather than a lipid disorder.

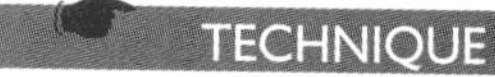

TECHNIQUE

STEP 2

Inspect the Skin Around the Eyes

For a detailed discussion of how to inspect the skin, see Chapter 8.

ABNORMALITIES Xanthelasma of eyelids are lipid-filled lesions of the skin that are commonly located in the periorbital arc of the eye (Fig. 12-16).

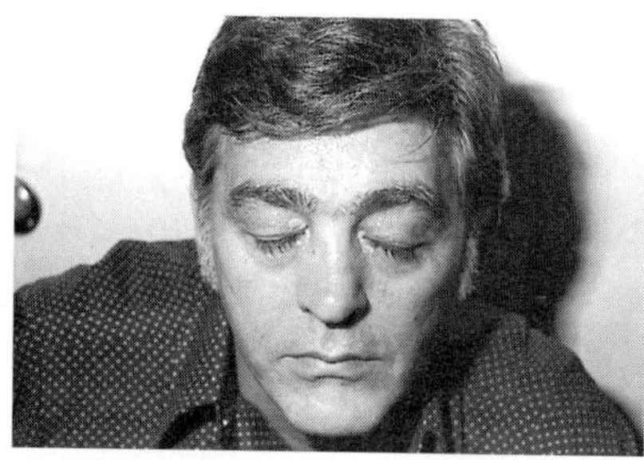

FIGURE 12-16 ■ Xanthelasma. (See Color Plate 35; reprinted with permission from Goodheart HP. A photoguide of common skin disorders: diagnosis and management. Philadelphia: Lippincott Williams & Wilkins, 1999.)

TECHNIQUE

STEP 3

Inspect the Skin Around the Elbows, Knuckles, Buttocks, Soles, Palms, and Achilles Tendon.

ABNORMALITIES Xanthomas in any of these areas may indicate a lipid disorder and are consistent with severe forms of hypercholesterolemia. (Fig. 12-17).

Laboratory and Diagnostic Tests

The following laboratory and diagnostic tests may also be useful in assessing the cardiovascular system:

- Lipid profile, including total cholesterol (TC), HDL, LDL, and triglycerides (TG), evaluates the patient's risk for developing CHD. The LDL is calculated as $LDL = TC - (HDL + TG/5)$. If the triglycerides are higher than 400 mg/dL, then a direct measure of LDL is drawn.
- Glucose determines the presence of diabetes, which is a risk factor for developing CHD.
- Creatinine phosphokinase (CPK) is found predominantly in various muscles within the body. The CPK-MB isoenzyme is specific for myocardial cells and will rise if myocardial damage occurs. Thus, it is used to diagnose and to quantify AMI.
- Lactate dehydrogenase (LDH) is normally found in many body tissues and is comprised of five isoenzymes, LDH_1 to LDH_5. The LDH_1 is found primarily in the heart and blood vessels. Normally, the level of LDH_2 is greater than those of the other four isoenzymes. An LDH_1:LDH_2 ratio that is greater than 1:1 may be a sign of an MI.
- The ECG is a graphic illustration of the electrical impulses that occur during the cardiac cycle. It is useful in identifying abnormal heart rhythms and in diagnosing MI, ventricular hypertrophy, and conduction defects.
- The exercise stress test is a noninvasive procedure during which the patient engages in a physical activity (e.g., walking on a treadmill) while his or her blood pressure, heart rate, and ECG are continuously monitored. The

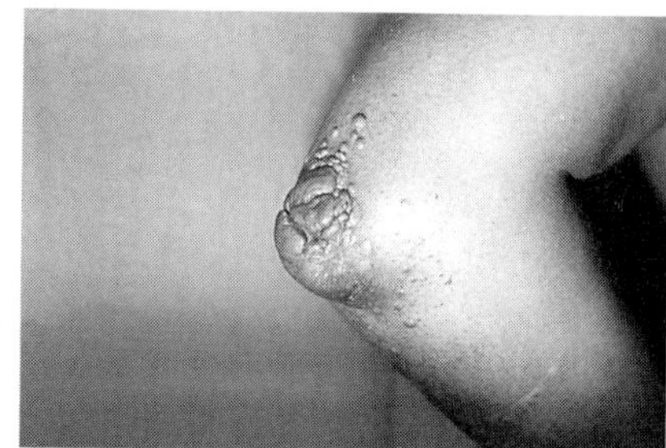

FIGURE 12-17 ■ Xanthomas. (See Color Plate 36; reprinted with permission from Goodheart HP. A photoguide of common skin disorders: diagnosis and management. Philadelphia: Lippincott Williams & Wilkins, 1999.)

speed and grade of incline are slowly increased to raise the heart rate to between 80% and 90% of maximal. This procedure stresses the heart. The test is stopped and considered to be positive if the patient experiences chest pain, dyspnea, fatigue, tachycardia, hypertension, or ECG changes. These signs or symptoms indicate possible coronary disease or occlusion. If the patient reaches his or her target heart rate and does not experience any symptoms or ECG changes, the test is considered to be negative and indicates no coronary insufficiency.
- Coronary angiography is a procedure in which a catheter is passed into the heart through a peripheral vein or artery. Once in place, various cardiac functions are evaluated (e.g., cardiac output). Radiographic dye is also injected into the heart for use with continuous radiographs of the heart, which can be viewed from a computer screen. This procedure is used primarily to evaluate the severity of occlusive CHD.
- The echocardiogram is a noninvasive ultrasound procedure that evaluates the structure and function of the heart.

Special Considerations

Pediatric Patients

Pediatric patients require additional questions to be asked of the parent or guardian.

? INTERVIEW Does the child have any trouble breathing? Any trouble running and playing? Does the child tire easily? Does the child have any history of heart problems? Any siblings with heart problems? Is there a family history of high cholesterol?

➤ ABNORMALITIES When hyperlipidemia occurs in childhood, it usually results from a genetic cause; it is important to determine this for proper evaluation and treatment.

Physical examination of the pediatric patient is very similar to that of the adult. The major differences in children include location of the apical impulse, faster heart rate, heart rhythm of sinus arrhythmia, occurrence of S_3, and heart murmurs. Because the pediatric patient's heart lies more horizontal in the chest wall than it does in adults, the apical impulse is palpated at the fourth intercostal space, just lateral to the midclavicular line. During auscultation, several differences may be found that are considered to be abnormal in adults but normal in pediatric patients. The heart rate typically ranges from 70 to 170 bpm in a newborn and gradually slows as the child ages, ranging from 70 to 110 bpm by 10 years. The heart rhythm of the child is commonly sinus arrhythmia, during which the heart rate speeds up with inspiration and slows down with expiration; this is considered to be normal in children. When listening for heart sounds, an S_3 is occasionally heard, especially at the apex, and again, this is considered to be normal in children. Heart murmurs can also commonly be heard in children. The murmur is considered to be normal (or innocent) if it is grade I or II, of short duration, does not radiate, and is heard at the pulmonic area.

Geriatric Patients

Geriatric patients require additional questions to be asked of either the patient or the caregiver.

? INTERVIEW Do you have a history of heart disease (hypertension, heart failure)? What medications (if any) do you take for your heart? Any problems with dizziness, losing your balance, falls, or ability to climb stairs? Do you take care of your medicine by yourself at home? Does anyone help you with your medicine? What do you do when you forget to take your medicine?

➤ ABNORMALITIES The elderly are more sensitive to certain adverse effects of cardiovascular medications (e.g., dizziness and losing balance), which may increase their risk of falls. If an elderly patient experiences adverse effects from medication, he or she may become noncompliant with that medication, especially antihypertensives and lipid-lowering drugs, because these conditions are asymptomatic.

Aging causes several hemodynamic changes even in the absence of cardiovascular disease. After age 60, peripheral resistance increases and compliance decreases, which causes the systolic blood pressure to rise with no significant change in the diastolic pressure. Thus, the occurrence of isolated systolic hypertension (systolic blood pressure $\geq$ 140 mm Hg, and diastolic blood pressure $<$ 90 mm Hg) also increases after age 60. In addition, elderly patients are more susceptible to orthostatic hypotension (i.e., sudden drop in blood pressure when rising to a sitting or standing position), which is also a common adverse effect of antihypertensive medications. To maintain cardiac output, the stroke volume increases in elderly patients. In addition, left ventricular wall thickness increases, as does the collagen content of the arteries and endocardium.

When auscultating the elderly patient's heart, an S_4 may normally be heard. An S_3 is rarely heard, however, and should be considered abnormal. Occasionally, the elderly patient will have premature atrial beats on the ECG, but this type of arrhythmia does not always indicate cardiovascular disease.

Pregnant Patients

Pregnant patients also require additional questions to be asked.

? INTERVIEW Have you had high blood pressure in the past or during previous pregnancies? How often do you have your blood pressure checked? Have you had any high blood pressure during this pregnancy? Do you have any swelling in your feet, ankles, or lower legs? Has your cholesterol been elevated previously, or is this the first time during this pregnancy? Did you change your diet with this pregnancy?

ABNORMALITIES It is important to determine whether diabetes, thyroid disease, or hyperlipidemia was present before pregnancy or is a result of the condition, because treatment varies depending on the circumstance. If it occurred with previous pregnancies, then the patient has previous experience with the condition, and her history should be examined closely to ensure appropriate monitoring and therapy during the current pregnancy.

During pregnancy, the resting heart rate increases by approximately 10 to 15 bpm, but the blood pressure normally remains stable. As the uterus enlarges, the diaphragm is elevated, and the heart is moved up and to the left. Thus, palpation of the apical impulse is higher and more lateral than in nonpregnant patients. Auscultatory changes that occur with pregnancy include an easily heard and loud S_3 as well as a systolic murmur, which both disappear shortly after delivery. In addition, the ECG shows a slight left-axis deviation because of the heart's altered position.

APPLICATION TO PATIENT SYMPTOMS

Because they are typically in a setting where the patient presents with a specific symptom (or symptoms), pharmacists need to be able to assess the patient's symptom, to identify the most probable cause of the symptom, and to determine the most appropriate action needed to either correct or further evaluate the problem identified. Common symptoms relating to the cardiovascular system include chest pain, dyspnea, and palpitations.

Chest Pain

Severe chest pain that occurs around the heart is termed *angina pectoris.* It is commonly caused by hypoxia of the myocardium, which in turn results from an imbalance of oxygen supply and myocardial demand. Chest pain is not indicative of heart disease, however. It may also result from gastrointestinal, pulmonary, gallbladder, or musculoskeletal disorders. Common causes of the various types of chest pain include:

- *Cardiac:* coronary artery disease, aortic valvular disease, pulmonary hypertension, mitral valve prolapse, and pericarditis.
- *Musculoskeletal:* arthritis, pleuritis, and trauma.
- *Gastrointestinal:* ulcer disease, gastritis, hiatal hernia, pancreatitis, cholecystitis, and gastroesophageal reflux disease.

Table 12-1 lists the differentiating characteristics of cardiac chest pain or angina from other possible causes. Chest pain related to gastrointestinal causes is usually related to food consumption and is relieved with antacids. Musculoskeletal chest pain is related to physical effort or trauma and is often relieved with heat or aspirin. Angina pectoris may be induced by physical exertion or emotional upset and is usually relieved by rest or nitroglycerin administration. Chest pain can also be caused by various medications (Box 12-8).

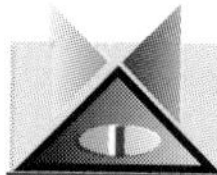

Box 12-8

MEDICATIONS THAT CAN CAUSE CHEST PAIN[a]

CARDIAC

- Amlodipine
- Felodipine
- Isradapine
- Nicardipine
- Nifedipine

GASTROINTESTINAL

- Corticosteroids
- Nonsteroidal anti-inflammatory drugs
- Aspirin
- Alcohol
- Potassium chloride
- Erythromycin
- Ferrous sulfate

[a]Not all inclusive.

CASE STUDY

JH is a 60-year-old white man with a history of CHD and gastritis. He returns to the pharmacy requesting a refill of his sublingual nitroglycerin and complaining that the last bottle didn't work very well. In reviewing his medication profile, the pharmacist notices that it has been nearly a year since his last refill. During counseling, JH states that he has had a few attacks of chest pain during the last couple of months.

ASSESSMENT OF THE PATIENT

Subjective Information

60-year-old white man complaining of chest pain

WHERE IS THE PAIN? In my chest.

DOES IT RADIATE OR SPREAD TO ANY OTHER SPOT? It moves to my jaw and down my left arm.

HOW OFTEN HAVE YOU HAD CHEST PAIN IN THE LAST MONTH? Twice.

HOW LONG DOES THE PAIN LAST? About 5 to 10 minutes, depending on what I am doing.

HOW WOULD YOU DESCRIBE THE PAIN? Like someone is sitting on my chest, or heavy pressure on my chest.

WHAT CAUSES THE PAIN? It usually happens when I am mowing the lawn or get into an argument with my son.

DO YOU HAVE ANY OTHER SYMPTOMS? No.

DOES ANYTHING MAKE THE PAIN WORSE? No.

WHAT MAKES THE PAIN BETTER? If I lie down and rest, it usually goes away. I tried some nitroglycerin this last time, but it didn't help at all.

DO YOU KEEP THE NITROGLYCERIN TABLETS IN THE BOTTLE DISPENSED FROM THE PHARMACY? No, I keep them in my pillbox.

WHERE DO YOU KEEP YOUR NITROGLYCERIN STORED AT HOME? On the window sill by the kitchen sink or in my pocket.

DO YOU FEEL ANY FLUSHING OR HEADACHE AFTER YOU USE THE SUBLINGUAL NITROGLYCERIN? No.

WHAT PRESCRIPTION MEDICATIONS DO YOU TAKE? Isordil and Zantac.

HOW OFTEN DO YOU FORGET TO TAKE YOUR MEDICINE? I forget that middle dose of Isordil almost every day, and sometimes the evening dose, too. I just take the Zantac after I eat a big meal.

HAS YOUR DOCTOR PRESCRIBED ANY NEW MEDICATIONS? No.

HAVE YOU BEEN TAKING ANY NONPRESCRIPTION MEDICATIONS? Yes, antacids for heartburn. When the nitroglycerin didn't help my chest pain, I thought it might be heartburn, so I tried some antacid, but that didn't really help either.

HAVE YOU INCREASED THE AMOUNT OF SPICY FOOD, COFFEE, OR ALCOHOL YOU ARE CONSUMING? No.

Objective Information:

Computerized medication profile:

- Isordil (isosorbide dinitrate): 20 mg, one tablet three times daily; No. 90; Refills: 11; Patient obtains refills every 45 to 60 days.
- Zantac (ranitidine): 150 mg, one tablet every 12 hours; No. 60; Refills: 6; Patient obtains refills every 90 to 120 days.
- Nitrostat (nitroglycerin sublingual): 0.4 mg, put one tablet under the tongue as needed for chest pain; No. 25; Refills: 3; Patient obtained last refill 11 months ago.

Patient in no acute distress
No SOB or light-headedness
Heart rate: 90 bpm
Blood pressure: 130/78 mm Hg
Respiratory rate: 16 rpm
Heart auscultation: regular rate and rhythm, no murmur

DISCUSSION

The concern in this case centers around the occurrence of JH's chest pain. The pharmacist needs to determine whether the increase in chest pain is caused by angina, a flare in JH's gastritis, medications that he is taking, or another type of problem. JH describes the pain like someone is sitting on his chest, and he can feel it in his jaw and down his left arm. It is caused by physical exertion (mowing the lawn) or emotional upset (an argument with his son). During the episodes, stopping his activity and resting relieves the pain. When the pain occurred the last time, however, he tried the sublingual nitroglycerin first, and it did not relieve the pain. He then tried an antacid, but that did not help either. JH is noncompliant with his isosorbide and does not store his nitroglycerin properly or refill it very frequently. On inspection, the pharmacist notices that JH is breathing normally and appears to be at rest and in no current distress or pain. His vital signs and heart sounds are all normal.

After evaluating and synthesizing all the patient's subjective and objective information, the pharmacist concludes that JH's chest pain is most likely angina that is possibly uncontrolled because of noncompliance with the isosorbide. The steps involved in this assessment process are illustrated in the accompanying decision tree (Fig. 12-18). The pharmacist also identifies that the nitroglycerin did not relieve JH's chest pain because of decreased potency, which was probably caused by improper storage and infrequent refilling of the medicine.

Continued

CASE STUDY—continued

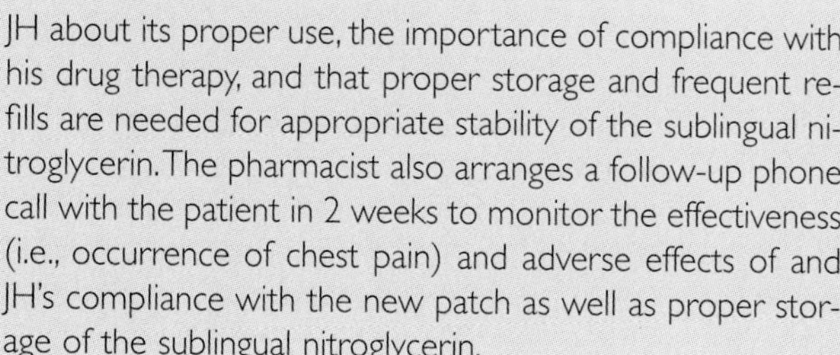

Because JH is in no current distress and his vital signs and heart sounds are all normal, the pharmacist calls JH's physician and discusses JH's complaints and problems of noncompliance with the isosorbide. The pharmacist suggests use of a nitroglycerin patch, because it is applied once daily, to assist JH with medication adherence. The physician agrees and prescribes a nitroglycerin patch. The pharmacist fills the new prescription for the nitroglycerin patch and educates JH about its proper use, the importance of compliance with his drug therapy, and that proper storage and frequent refills are needed for appropriate stability of the sublingual nitroglycerin. The pharmacist also arranges a follow-up phone call with the patient in 2 weeks to monitor the effectiveness (i.e., occurrence of chest pain) and adverse effects of and JH's compliance with the new patch as well as proper storage of the sublingual nitroglycerin.

PHARMACEUTICAL CARE PLAN

Patient Name: JH

Date: 6/18/02

Medical Problems:
- CHD
- Gastritis

Current Medications:
- Isordil (isosorbide dinitrate), 20 mg, one tablet three times daily, No. 90, Refills: 11
- Zantac (ranitidine), 150 mg, one tablet every 12 hours, No. 60, Refills: 6
- Nitrostat (nitroglycerin sublingual), 0.4 mg, put one tablet under the tongue as needed for chest pain, No. 25, Refills: 3

S: 60-year-old white man complaining of chest pain that radiates to his jaw and left arm. Feels like "someone is sitting on my chest." Usually occurs with mowing the lawn or an argument with his son. Is relieved with rest. Is not relieved with nitroglycerin or antacids.

Compliance: Forgets middle dose of isosorbide nearly every day, and occasionally forgets evening dose. Stores nitroglycerin on window sill in plastic pillbox and has not had it refilled for 11 months.

O: Patient in no acute distress. No SOB or lightheadedness.

Heart rate: 90 bpm

Blood pressure: 130/78 mm Hg

Respiratory rate: 16 rpm

Heart auscultation: Regular rate and rhythm

A:
1. Angina pectoris, possibly caused by noncompliance with the isosorbide therapy.
2. Improper storage and refill rate of the nitroglycerin.
3. Noncompliance with Zantac.

P:
1. Call patient's physician, and recommend nitroglycerin patch.
2. New prescription: Nitro-Dur, 0.2 mg/h.
3. Educate JH about the proper use of the patch, the importance of compliance with his drug therapy, and that proper storage and frequent refills are needed for the stability of the sublingual nitroglycerin.
4. Educate JH about how chest pain from gastrointestinal causes would present versus chest pain from cardiac causes.
5. Discuss Zantac use with his physician at next visit, and possibly change to an over-the-counter (OTC) product.
6. F/U phone call in 2 weeks to monitor chest pain, adverse effects of and compliance with Nitro-Dur, and proper storage of sublingual nitroglycerin.

Pharmacist: *Jane Doe, Pharm.D.*

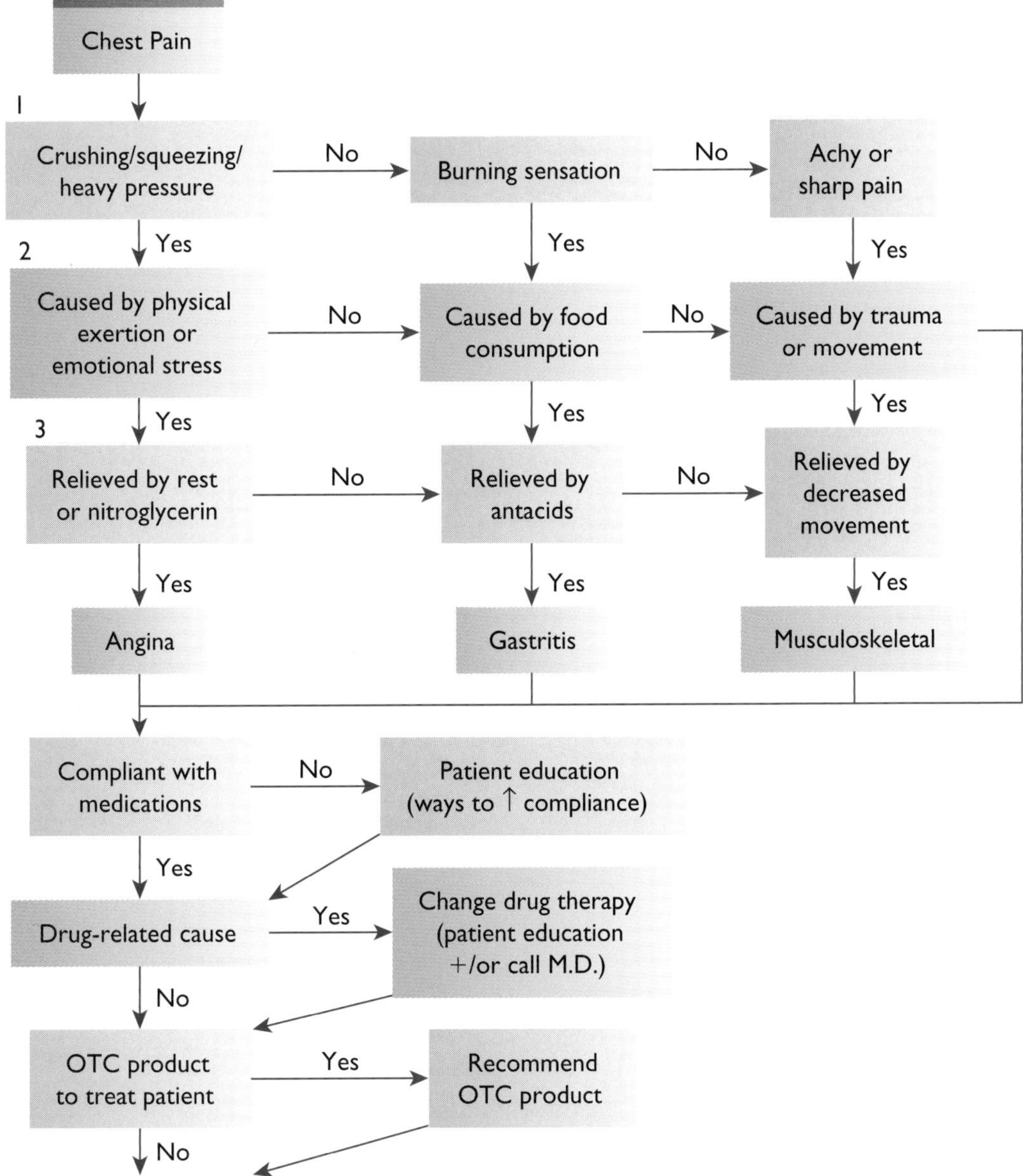

FIGURE 12-18 ■ Decision tree for chest pain. *OTC*, over-the-counter.

Self-Assessment Questions

1. Differentiate the varying characteristics of cardiac, gastrointestinal, and musculoskeletal chest pain.
2. What factors can precipitate stable angina?
3. Compare and contrast the various interview questions that are useful in differentiating the types of chest pain.

Critical Thinking Questions

1. In the case of JH, how would the pharmacist's assessment and plan change if the patient had burning chest pain following a very large meal, which was relieved with antacids?
2. A 54 year-old female complains of severe chest pain that she describes as a heavy pressure on her chest that has been continuing for the past 45 minutes. She is also experiencing SOB, nausea, sweating, and lightheadedness. What would be the assessment and plan for this patient?

Dyspnea

Dyspnea is the subjective feeling of difficult breathing or "shortness of breath." Patients may report that they "can't get enough air." Various causes of dyspnea include:

- *Cardiac:* CHF and MI.
- *Pulmonary:* obstructive lung disease, asthma, restrictive lung disease, and pulmonary embolism.
- *Emotional:* Anxiety.

Patients with dyspnea caused by a cardiac condition usually complain of dyspnea that is brought on by exertion. Dyspnea on exertion can result from CHF, angina, arrhythmias, or chronic pulmonary disease. Paroxysmal nocturnal dyspnea occurs at night or when the patient is supine. The patient falls asleep normally, but he or she awakens two or several hours later gasping for air and coughing. The patient may need to rush to open the window and get some fresh air. PND is relatively specific for CHF. Many times, PND is also associated with orthopnea. Because the dyspnea decreases in the upright position, the patient may need to use two or more pillows to sleep. Box 12-9 lists various medications that may induce or exacerbate dyspnea associated with CHF. (For a discussion of dyspnea caused by respiratory disorders, see Chapter 11.)

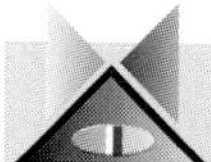

Box 12-9

MEDICATIONS THAT MAY INDUCE CONGESTIVE HEART FAILURE[a]

- β-Blockers[b]
- Calcium-channel blockers[b]
- Antiarrhythmics (disopyramide and quinidine)
- Amphetamines
- Cocaine
- Nonsteroidal anti-inflammatory drugs
- Corticosteroids
- Estrogens
- Hydralazine
- Methyldopa
- Prazosin
- Minoxidil
- Drugs that are high in sodium

[a]Not all inclusive.
[b]β-Blockers and verapamil may be beneficial in diastolic congestive heart failure. β-Blockers may also counteract autonomic hyperactivity in systolic dysfunction.

CASE STUDY

AR is a 67-year-old man who comes into the pharmacy after walking a short distance from his car. As the patient is requesting a refill of his digoxin, the pharmacist notices that AR is having some difficulty breathing. The pharmacist approaches AR and asks him to step into the consultation room to assess his breathing.

ASSESSMENT OF THE PATIENT

Subjective Information

67-year-old man with SOB

MR. R., I NOTICED YOU SEEM SHORT OF BREATH TODAY. IS THIS NORMAL FOR YOU? Not really, but over the past few weeks it seems I have been more short of breath.

WHAT TYPE OF ACTIVITY BRINGS ON YOUR SHORTNESS OF BREATH? Usually if I walk a long way.

HOW MANY BLOCKS CAN YOU WALK NOW BEFORE YOU BECOME SHORT OF BREATH? About one or two blocks.

HOW MANY BLOCKS COULD YOU WALK SIX MONTHS AGO? About six or eight blocks.

HOW OFTEN DO YOU WAKE UP AT NIGHT WITH SHORTNESS OF BREATH? Occasionally, two or three times a week.

HOW MANY PILLOWS DO YOU NEED TO SLEEP AT NIGHT? Sometimes one pillow is okay, and sometimes I need two.

DO YOU EXPERIENCE ANY OTHER SYMPTOMS WITH THE SHORTNESS OF BREATH? CHEST PAIN? NAUSEA? LIGHT-HEADEDNESS OR DIZZINESS? No.

DOES THE SHORTNESS OF BREATH INTERFERE WITH YOUR ACTIVITIES OF DAILY LIVING? No, not really. I just can't work as hard as I used to.

WHAT MEDICAL PROBLEMS DO YOU HAVE? I have heart failure, high blood pressure, and arthritis.

WHAT PRESCRIPTION MEDICATIONS DO YOU TAKE? A tiny white tablet for my heart failure, and another tablet for my blood pressure. I don't know the names of them.

HOW OFTEN DO YOU FORGET TO TAKE YOUR MEDICATION? Probably once or twice a month.

WHAT NONPRESCRIPTION OR OVER-THE-COUNTER MEDICATIONS DO YOU TAKE? I take some antacid for heartburn and ibuprofen for my arthritis when it flares up.

HOW OFTEN DO YOU TAKE THE ANTACID AND THE IBUPROFEN? Over the past month or so, I've needed the antacid four or five times during the day and the ibuprofen, two tablets every 3 or 4 hours throughout the day about five or six times a week.

WHAT TIME DO YOU TAKE THE ANTACID? Right after breakfast, and then about every 3 or 4 hours until bedtime.

Continued

CASE STUDY—continued

WHAT TIME DO YOU TAKE YOUR MEDICINE FOR YOUR HEART FAILURE? I usually take it right after breakfast.

WHAT TIME DO YOU TAKE YOUR OTHER MEDICINE? I take my blood pressure medicine after breakfast, lunch, and dinner.

Objective Information

Computerized medication profile:

- Lanoxin (digoxin): 0.25 mg, one tablet every morning; No. 30; Refills: 11; Patient obtains refills every 25 to 35 days.
- Capoten (captopril): 12.5 mg, one tablet three times a day; No. 90; Refills: 11; Patient obtains refills every 25 to 35 days.

Patient in no acute distress and no use of accessory muscles
Respiratory rate: 18 rpm
Heart rate: 90 bpm
Blood pressure: 136/84 mm Hg
Lung auscultation: bilateral crackles in lower lung fields
Heart auscultation: regular rate and rhythm, a possible S_3 gallop, and no murmur
Extremities: bilateral 2–3+ pitting edema

DISCUSSION

Because dyspnea can be caused by both pulmonary and cardiovascular abnormalities, obtaining a thorough history from patients who complain of SOB is important. In the case of AR, he has had a recent increase of SOB with exertion, and the pharmacist needs to determine the cause. AR also occasionally needs more than one pillow to sleep at night because of possible orthopnea. AR has a history of CHF, which is being treated with digoxin and captopril, and he is taking ibuprofen for his arthritis and an antacid for frequent heartburn. On inspection, AR is in no acute distress and is not using accessory muscles to help with respiration. His respiratory rate and blood pressure are normal, and his heart rate is on the high end of the normal range. Bilateral crackles and a possible S_3 gallop are heard on lung and heart auscultation, respectively. Palpation of AR's extremities shows 2–3+ pitting edema. Because AR has a history of CHF and currently has several of the subjective complaints and objective signs of CHF, the pharmacist concludes that AR has a mild exacerbation of CHF (Fig. 12-19).

Next, the pharmacist must decide the cause of the exacerbation, which includes several possibilities: physiologic worsening of the heart failure, improper drug selection, subtherapeutic drug dosing, patient medication noncompliance, medications, or drug interactions. To determine the most likely cause, the pharmacist must evaluate each possibility.

Physiologic worsening of the heart failure would be illustrated by worsening of the patient's subjective complaints (e.g., SOB, dyspnea on exertion, orthopnea, PND, cough, weakness, fatigue) and objective signs (S_3 gallop, crackles, reflex tachycardia, increased blood urea nitrogen, left ventricular hypertrophy), some of which would need to be determined by tests at the physician's office (e.g., chest radiography, ECG, blood urea nitrogen). Appropriate drug treatment for CHF includes digoxin, ACE inhibitors, diuretics, and vasodilators. Appropriate dosing of these is determined by the appropriate dosage range of the medication, relief of patient signs and symptoms, and serum drug concentrations (e.g., digoxin). Patient noncompliance can be evaluated by asking the patient how he or she takes the medication, asking the patient how often he or she forgets to take the medication, and by checking pharmacy refill records. For medications that can cause drug-induced CHF, see Box 12-9.

Evaluating the causes in AR reveals the following: AR has symptoms of physiologic worsening of the CHF; however, more tests are needed to conclusively determine this. AR's CHF is being treated with appropriate medications; however, a diuretic might be beneficial because of AR's peripheral edema, which is a sign of fluid overload. The dosages of medication are within the normal range. The serum digoxin concentration is unknown. AR is taking ibuprofen frequently, which can cause drug-induced CHF. AR is compliant with his medications; however, he is taking antacids at the same time that he is taking the digoxin, which can decrease the absorption of digoxin and, thus, the digoxin's effectiveness. After evaluating all the possibilities, the pharmacist concludes that AR may be having an exacerbation of CHF, possibly caused by a drug interaction with the digoxin and antacid, frequent use of the ibuprofen, or both.

Because of AR's peripheral edema and need of a serum digoxin concentration, the pharmacist decides to contact AR's physician and recommend a loop diuretic. The physician prescribes furosemide, 20 mg every morning; recommends that AR use acetaminophen for his arthritis; and requests that AR come to her office that afternoon for a digoxin level and then again in 2 weeks to check his electrolytes and to repeat the digoxin level. The pharmacist arranges the appointments for the patient, fills the new prescription, and counsels the patient about the furosemide, using the acetaminophen instead of ibuprofen, and using the antacids 1 to 2 hours before or after the digoxin. The pharmacist also schedules a follow-up assessment with AR in 4 weeks to evaluate his symptoms, medication effectiveness and side effects, respiratory rate, heart rate, blood pressure, lung and heart sounds, and peripheral edema.

Continued

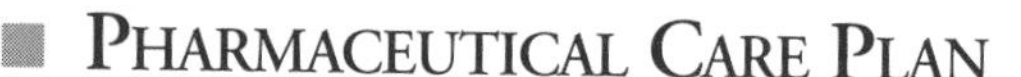

PHARMACEUTICAL CARE PLAN

Patient Name: AR

Date: 3/27/02

Medical Problems:
- CHF
- Hypertension
- Arthritis

Current Medications:
- Lanoxin (digoxin), 0.25 mg, one tablet every morning
- Capoten (captopril), 12.5 mg, one tablet three times a day

S: 67-year-old man with SOB after walking one to two blocks. Worsening over the past few weeks. Occasionally needs two pillows to sleep at night. Compliant with medications. Takes digoxin after breakfast and captopril after meals.

OTC medications: Antacid every morning after breakfast and then every 3 to 4 hours until bedtime. Ibuprofen, 200 mg, two tablets every 3 to 4 hours five or six times per week.

O: Patient in no acute distress and no use of accessory muscles.

Respiratory rate: 18 rpm

Heart rate: 90 bpm

Blood pressure: 136/84 mm Hg

Lung auscultation: Bilateral crackles in lower lung fields.

Heart auscultation: Regular rate and rhythm, possible S_3 gallop, and no murmur.

Extremities: Bilateral 2–3+ pitting edema.

A:
1. Possible exacerbation of CHF caused by a drug interaction between digoxin and the antacid and frequent use of ibuprofen.
2. Gastrointestinal irritation from frequent use of ibuprofen.

P:
1. Call AR's physician to discuss the patient's condition and recommend a loop diuretic.
2. New prescription: furosemide, 20 mg every morning.
3. Follow-up appointment today to check digoxin level.
4. Educate the patient about proper use of furosemide.
5. Recommend using acetaminophen, 500 mg, two tablets every 6 hours as needed for arthritis pain, instead of the ibuprofen to decrease gastrointestinal irritation and need for antacids.
6. Educate patient about separating the use of antacids and medications by 1 to 2 hours and about taking the captopril on an empty stomach.
7. Schedule a follow-up assessment in 4 weeks to assess symptoms, medication efficacy and side effects, respiratory rate, heart rate, blood pressure, lung and heart sounds, and extremities.

Pharmacist: *John James, Pharm.D.*

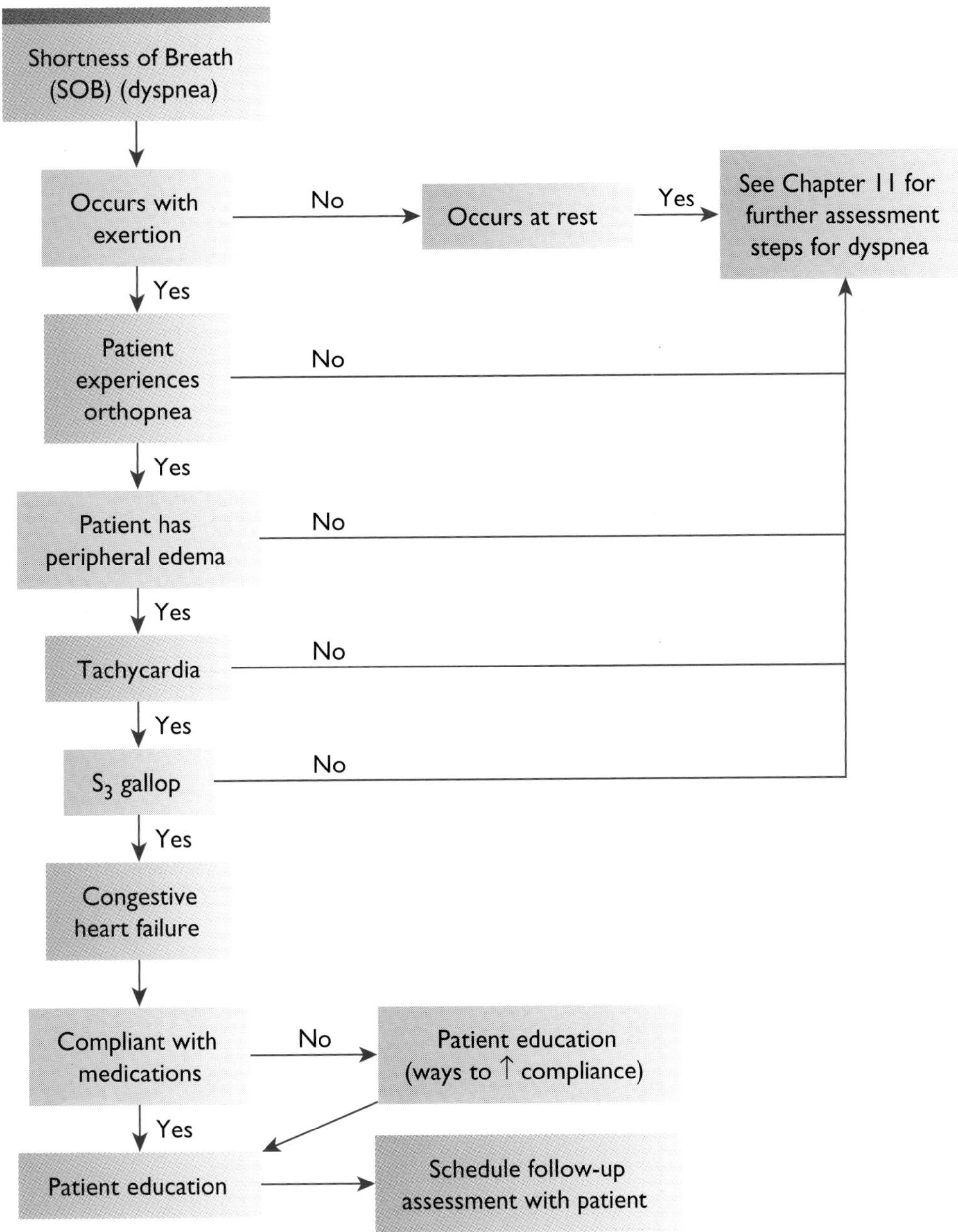

FIGURE 12-19 ■ Decision tree for dyspnea. *OTC*, over-the-counter.

Self-Assessment Questions

1. What signs and symptoms are commonly associated with CHF?
2. What medications may induce or exacerbate CHF?
3. Differentiate the S_3 from the S_1 and S_2 sounds. What is the significance of S_3 in CHF?

Critical Thinking Questions

1. AR comes back to the pharmacy for his follow-up assessment and is still experiencing SOB with exertion. What questions should the pharmacist ask to evaluate AR's SOB?
2. What physical examination procedures would be useful to further evaluate AR? What information will these procedures provide?

Palpitations

A palpitation is an uncomfortable feeling or sensation in the chest that is associated with a wide variety of arrhythmias. Patients may describe palpitations as their heart "beating fast," "fluttering," "beating irregularly," "pounding," "jumping," or "skipping beats." Patients may also complain of SOB or light-headedness with exertion, which results from decreased cardiac output secondary to a possible arrhythmia. Palpitations are common and do not necessarily indicate heart disease. Causes of palpitations include:

- Arrhythmias
- Fever
- Hypoglycemia
- Anxiety
- Aortic stenosis
- Hyperthyroidism
- Heart murmurs
- Tobacco
- Caffeine

Drugs that may induce cardiac arrhythmias are listed in Box 12-10.

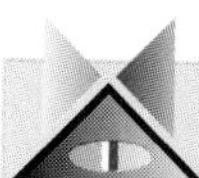

Box 12-10

MEDICATIONS THAT CAN CAUSE PALPITATIONS

- Digoxin
- Sympathomimetic amines
- Antiarrhythmics
- Terfenadine (when used with erythromycin or ketoconazole)
- Caffeine
- Bronchodilators
- Decongestants
- Appetite suppressants
- Amphetamines
- Antidepressants

CASE STUDY

RJ is a 32-year-old woman who presents to the pharmacy asking if one of the new pain killers advertised on television would help the "flutters" that she gets in her chest. Because the pharmacist is concerned that RJ might have an arrhythmia, she asks the patient to step into the consultation room to discuss her symptoms.

ASSESSMENT OF THE PATIENT

Subjective Information

32-year-old woman who complains of fluttering in her chest

HOW LONG HAVE YOU HAD THE FLUTTERING IN YOUR CHEST? For about the last week.

HOW FREQUENTLY DOES IT OCCUR? Usually about once or twice a day.

HOW LONG DOES IT USUALLY LAST? Only a few seconds, but it scares me that it might be my heart.

HAVE YOU NOTICED THE FLUTTERS AFTER YOU WORK HARD OR AFTER STRENUOUS EXERCISE? No.

DURING THESE FLUTTERS, HAVE YOU EVER HAD ANY LIGHT-HEADEDNESS OR FAINTED? No.

HOW MUCH COFFEE, TEA, OR COLA DO YOU CONSUME EACH DAY? I usually have three of four cups of coffee in the morning.

WHAT MEDICAL PROBLEMS DO YOU HAVE? I've had high blood pressure for the last 5 years.

HAVE YOU EVER HAD PROBLEMS WITH YOUR HEART OR THYROID? No.

WHAT PRESCRIPTION MEDICATIONS ARE YOU TAKING? Dyazide every morning.

HOW OFTEN DO YOU FORGET TO TAKE YOUR MEDICATION? Probably once or twice a month.

WHAT NONPRESCRIPTION MEDICATIONS DO YOU TAKE? Usually nothing, but I've been taking a nasal decongestant pill everyday this past week for my allergies and have been taking a pill for weight loss for the last few weeks. It's supposed to help curb my appetite.

DO YOU SMOKE? No, I quit about 5 years ago after smoking for about 10 years.

DO YOU FREQUENTLY CONSUME ALCOHOL? No.

Objective Information

Computerized medication profile:

- Dyazide (hydrochlorothiazide/triamterene): one capsule every morning for blood pressure control; No. 30; Refills: 11; Patient obtains refills every 25–35 days.

Patient in no acute distress
No palpitations, SOB, light-headedness, or dizziness
Heart rate: 110 bpm (regular rhythm)
Blood pressure: 136/78 mm Hg
Respiratory rate: 16 rpm

Continued

CASE STUDY—continued

Heart auscultation: regular rate and rhythm, no murmur
Extremities: no edema present

Discussion

When a patient complains of palpitations, the pharmacist must ask a series of questions to clarify the symptoms and to determine possible causes of the palpitations. In the case of RJ, the pharmacist needs to determine if she is experiencing palpitations because of an arrhythmia or various other causes. RJ states that she has had these palpitations occasionally during the day for the past week. Her only medical problem is hypertension. She denies any history of heart or thyroid problems. She does not smoke; however, she does consume a moderate amount of caffeine and has recently starting taking nasal decongestants and an appetite suppressant for weight loss, any of which could cause palpitations. On physical examination, the pharmacist finds that RJ has tachycardia but a regular heart rhythm.

After evaluating RJ's subjective and objective information, the pharmacist concludes that her palpitations probably result from a combination of excessive caffeine, the nasal decongestant, and the appetite suppressant. To illustrate the steps involved with the assessment process, see the accompanying decision tree (Fig. 12-20). The pharmacist also concludes that a referral to the patient's physician is not warranted at this time, because RJ has a normal heart rhythm and has not experienced any light-headedness or dizziness with the palpitations. The pharmacist educates RJ about slowly decreasing her caffeine consumption, avoiding withdrawal effects, and discontinuing the oral decongestant and the appetite suppressant. The pharmacist also recommends that RJ use a nasal spray decongestant, if needed, to control allergy symptoms and educates RJ about proper diet and exercise for weight loss. In addition, the pharmacist teaches RJ how to monitor her heart rate at home, instructing her about both normal and abnormal findings. The pharmacist schedules a follow-up appointment in 2 weeks to check RJ's heart rate and rhythm, occurrence of palpitations, and weight.

PHARMACEUTICAL CARE PLAN

Patient Name: RJ

Date: 7/21/02

Medical Problems:
Hypertension

Current Medications:
Dyazide (hydrochlorothiazide/triamterene), one capsule every morning

S: 32-year-old woman complaining of a fluttering feeling in her chest for approximately the last week. Occurs approximately once or twice a day but lasts only a few seconds. Denies any dizziness, light-headedness, or fainting. Drinks three or four cups of coffee every morning. Compliant with Dyazide. Takes oral nasal decongestant everyday this past week for allergies and OTC appetite suppressant for weight loss; names and doses unknown. Does not smoke or drink alcohol.

O: Patient in no acute distress.

Heart rate: 110 bpm (regular rhythm)

Blood pressure: 136/78 mm Hg

Respiratory rate: 16 rpm

Heart auscultation: Regular rate and rhythm; no murmur or gallop.

Extremities: No edema present.

A:
1. Palpitations and tachycardia probably caused by excessive caffeine, nasal decongestant, and appetite suppressant.
2. Hypertension: controlled.

P:
1. Patient education: adverse effects of too much caffeine and OTC products that may cause palpitations; slowly decrease coffee to one or two cups per day; appropriate diet and exercise for weight loss.
2. Discontinue oral nasal decongestant and appetite suppressant.
3. Recommend nasal spray decongestant for allergy symptoms, if needed.
4. Follow-up assessment in 2 weeks to monitor heart rate and rhythm, occurrence of palpitations, and weight.

Pharmacist: *Christina Smith, Pharm.D.*

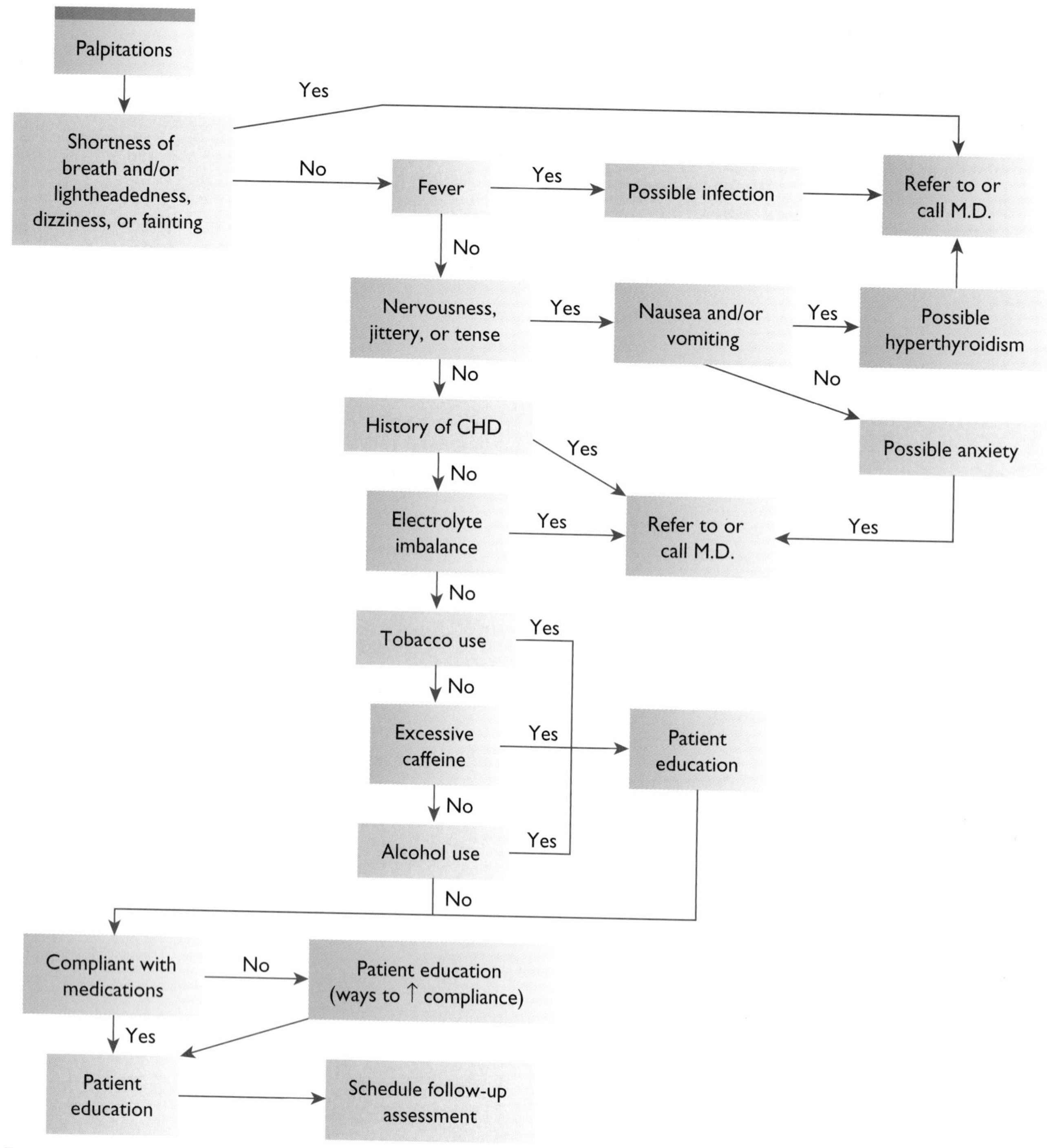

FIGURE 12-20 ■ Decision tree for palpitations. *CHD*, coronary heart disease; *OTC*, over-the-counter.

Self-Assessment Questions

1. What signs and symptoms are associated with arrhythmias?
2. What medications may cause palpitations?
3. Describe the ECG and its use in evaluating arrhythmias.

Critical Thinking Questions

1. In the case of RJ, how would the pharmacist's assessment and plan change if the patient had complained of SOB and dizziness with her palpitations?
2. A 74-year-old man states that his heart feels as if it is skipping beats and is pounding in his chest. What questions should the pharmacist ask to assess his symptoms?

Risk Factors for CHD

The pharmacist is in the perfect position to evaluate risk for CHD, because patients frequently bring in prescriptions for hypertension, diabetes, and high cholesterol, which are CHD risk factors. In addition, customers may request OTC medications or herbal products to treat these diseases. Specific examples of situations in which a pharmacist could assess the patient's overall risk for developing CHD include patients who bring in prescriptions for antihypertensive, antidiabetic, or dyslipidemic medications; patients with high blood pressure, high glucose/blood sugar, or high cholesterol during health screenings in the pharmacy; patients who smoke, are overweight, or are inactive (i.e., do not regularly exercise); and patients who inquire about or purchase smoking cessation products. Patients may also be concerned because of a strong family history of premature CHD. The pharmacist should evaluate all CHD risk factors and educate the patient accordingly. If needed, the pharmacist should also refer the patient to his or her physician for further risk factor evaluation and possible treatment. Aggressive goals and treatment for blood pressure, glucose, and cholesterol significantly decrease the chance of CHD.

CASE STUDY

NR is a 46-year-old man who appears at the pharmacy counter with a prescription for lisinopril. He says that his physician told him his blood pressure was high and could lead to a heart attack. His father died of a heart attack at the age of 42, and NR is scared that it might happen to him as well. He asks that you hurry up and fill the prescription, because he does not want to wait any longer to get started on this new medication.

ASSESSMENT OF THE PATIENT

Subjective Information

46-year-old man with prescription for antihypertensive and frightened of having a heart attack

MR. R., IS THERE A REASON WHY YOU ARE SO ANXIOUS TO START THIS MEDICINE? Yes.

WHAT DID THE DOCTOR TELL YOU WAS THE REASON FOR THIS MEDICINE? To lower my blood pressure.

HAVE YOU EVER HAD ANY OTHER HEART PROBLEMS, SUCH AS HEART ATTACK, STROKE, OR HEART SURGERY BEFORE? No, but it scares me.

WHY DOES IT SCARE YOU? My dad was 42 when he died of a heart attack, and my brother was 49 when he had bypass surgery. I'm scared to death it is going to happen to me.

HOW OLD ARE YOU NOW? 46 years old.

WELL, AGE AND HIGH BLOOD PRESSURE ARE RISKS FOR HEART DISEASE. IF IT IS OKAY WITH YOU, I WOULD LIKE TO ASK YOU ABOUT SOME OF THE OTHER RISK FACTORS. IF YOUR DOCTOR AND I ARE AWARE OF ALL YOUR RISK FACTORS, WE CAN BETTER HELP YOU TO DECREASE YOUR CHANCE FOR HEART DISEASE. Sure, go ahead and ask.

DO YOU HAVE DIABETES? No.

DO YOU SMOKE? No.

HAVE YOU EVER HAD YOUR CHOLESTEROL CHECKED? I don't think I've ever had one taken. I'm sure I'm too young for them to need to check my cholesterol.

WHEN DID YOU EAT YOUR LAST MEAL? Last night at supper. I wasn't hungry at breakfast this morning.

SINCE YOU ARE FASTING, I CAN CHECK YOUR CHOLESTEROL AND GLUCOSE HERE IN THE PHARMACY. WOULD YOU LIKE TO HAVE THAT DONE TODAY? Yes.

OKAY, FIRST LET ME ASK A FEW MORE QUESTIONS. DO YOU TAKE ANY OTHER PRESCRIPTION MEDICATIONS? No.

DO YOU TAKE ANY OTHER MEDICATIONS, SUCH AS NONPRESCRIPTION MEDICATIONS, HERBALS, OR VITAMINS? I have been taking an aspirin a day. Everyone says it will decrease your chance for a heart attack.

WHAT DO YOU TYPICALLY EAT FOR BREAKFAST, LUNCH, AND DINNER? I usually don't eat breakfast. For lunch, I usually eat something quick—it varies quite a bit. Usually fast food, I guess. My wife usually makes dinner, and I eat whatever she fixes. I usually don't pay much attention to what I eat.

WHAT TYPE OF PHYSICAL ACTIVITY DO YOU DO? I mow the lawn once a week, and that's about it, I guess.

Objective Information

Computerized medication profile:

- Aspirin EC: 325 mg, one tablet every morning; No. 100;
- Prinivil (lisinopril): 5 mg, one tablet every morning for blood pressure; No. 30; Refills: 11; new prescription today.

Weight: 185 pounds
Height: approximately 5'10"
Blood pressure: 150/102 mm Hg
Heart rate: 86 bpm
Total cholesterol: 256 mg/dL
Triglycerides: 188 mg/dL
HDL: 24 mg/dL
LDL: 194 mg/dL
Glucose: 82 mg/dL

Continued

CASE STUDY—continued

DISCUSSION

Because NR has been diagnosed with hypertension and his father died from a heart attack at a young age, he is very concerned about also having a heart attack (i.e., CHD). The patient who comes in with prescriptions for medications to treat hypertension, diabetes, or high cholesterol or who may be at risk for these diseases should be evaluated for all CHD risk factors. NR has no history of CHD (i.e., heart attack, stroke, peripheral vascular disease, or bypass surgery). He is 46 years old and is now taking an antihypertensive medication. His father died of a heart attack, and his brother had bypass surgery, both during their forties. NR does not currently smoke or have diabetes and is a normal weight for his height. NR has been fasting for more than 12 hours, so the pharmacist is able to obtain a lipid profile in the pharmacy. His total cholesterol and LDL are high, and his HDL is low. The CHD risk factors that NR has include male age >45 years, family history of premature heart disease, hypertension, high LDL, and low HDL. In addition, he frequently eats potentially high-fat/high-cholesterol foods (i.e., frequently eats fast food for lunch) and is inactive. Because NR has no history of clinical CHD, symptomatic carotid artery disease, peripheral artery disease, abdominal aortic aneurysm, or diabetes, he does not have any CHD risk equivalents.

After evaluating all the risk factors, the next step is to determine the 10-year CHD risk and subsequent LDL goal for the patient (Table 12-4). NR has 2+ risk factors, and his 10-year risk is ≤20% (10%). Based on this, his target LDL is <130 mg/dL (Table 12-4), and his goal blood pressure is <140/90 mm Hg. The first step in attaining his goals includes therapeutic lifestyle changes (i.e., diet and exercise). The pharmacist educates him about a low-fat/low-cholesterol diet and various exercise tips. The pharmacist also encourages him to work with a dietician and physical therapist and schedules a follow-up phone call in 2 weeks and an appointment in 3 months. Figure 12-21 shows the accompanying decision tree for CHD risk assessment.

PHARMACEUTICAL CARE PLAN

Patient Name: NR

Date: 05/09/02

Medical Problems:
Hypertension

Current Medications:
Prinivil (lisinopril), 5 mg, one tablet every morning (new prescription today)
Aspirin EC, 325 mg, one tablet every morning

S: 46-year-old man presenting with prescription for lisinopril and complaining of being frightened about having a heart attack. Risk factors include a positive family history of CHD (brother CABG at age 49; father MI at age 42), age (>45 years) and hypertension (prescription for lisinopril). No personal history of CHD (no previous MI, cerebrovascular accident, transient ischemic attack, PVD, or CABG), diabetes, or cigarette smoking. No regular exercise program. Doesn't limit sodium or fat in diet; eats whatever he wants.

O:

Weight: 185 pounds

Height: 5'10"

Blood pressure: 150/102 mm Hg

Heart rate: 86 bpm

Total cholesterol: 256 mg/dL

Triglycerides: 188 mg/dL

HDL: 24 mg/dL

LDL: 194 mg/dL

Glucose: 82 mg/dL

A:
1. Stage 2 hypertension: uncontrolled.
2. Hyperlipidemia primary prevention with 2+ risk factors uncontrolled. Goal LDL <130 mg/dL

P:
1. Dispense prescription for lisinopril, and educate patient about dosage, adverse effects, monitoring, and follow up.
2. Dispense home blood pressure monitor, and instruct patient about proper procedures and use of machine.
3. Patient needs adequate trial of diet and exercise for hyperlipidemia. Give patient educational handouts along with the names/address/phone number of a local dietician and physical therapist.
4. Educate patient about low-fat/low-cholesterol diet and exercise and about the importance of each.
5. Schedule telephone follow-up appointment for 2 weeks to assess patient's progress, and schedule pharmacy clinic appointment for 3 months to repeat lipid profile.
6. Fax pharmaceutical care plan to patient's primary care physician.

Pharmacist: *Max Monroe, Pharm.D.*

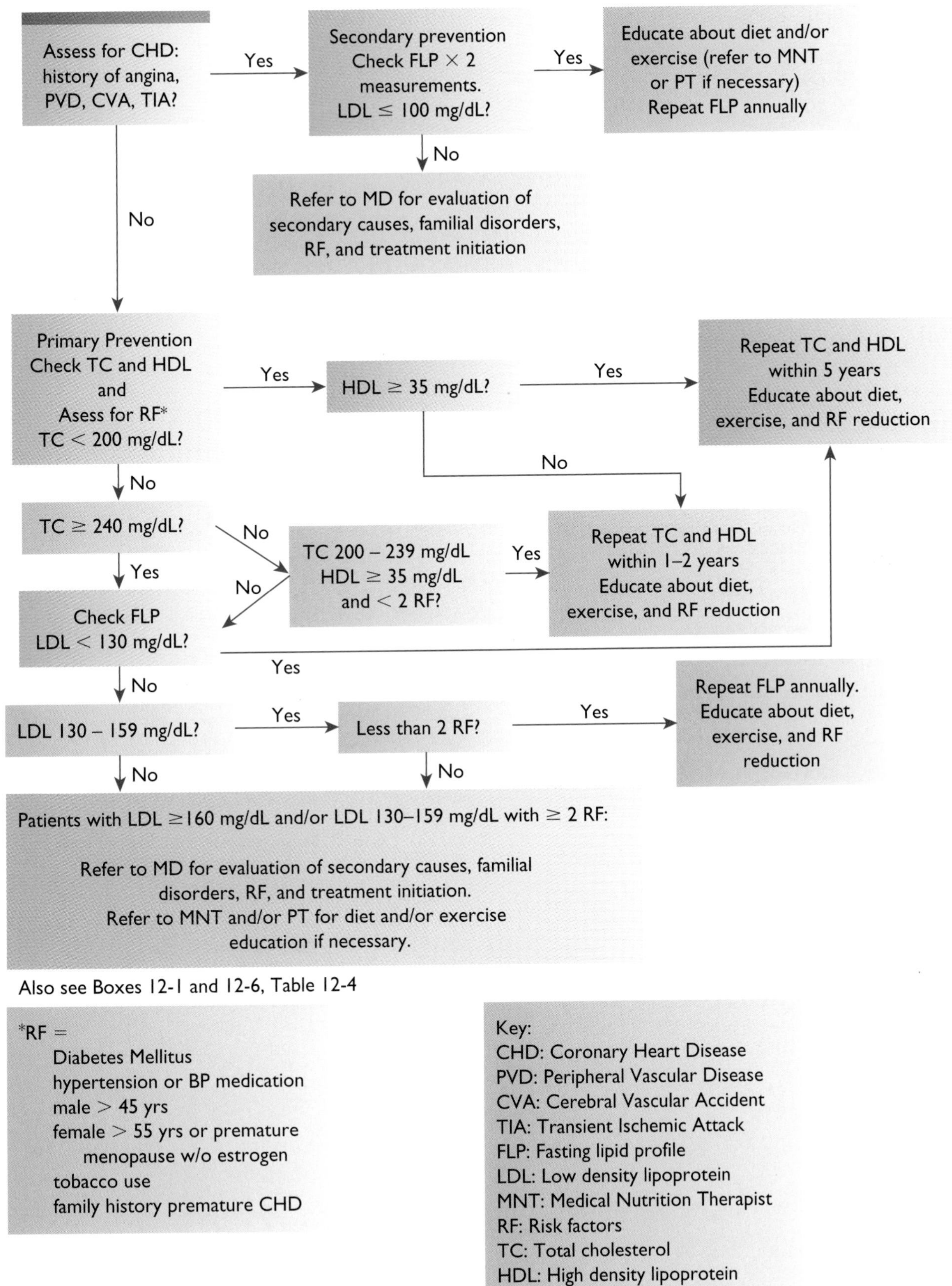

FIGURE 12-21 ■ Decision tree for risk factors of coronary heart disease.

Self-Assessment Questions

1. What are the risk factors for CHD?
2. What are the differences between primary and secondary prevention of CHD? What are the treatment goals of each?
3. What is the difference between HDL and LDL cholesterol?

Critical Thinking Questions

1. KP is a 66-year-old white man who presents to the pharmacy for a lipid profile, which reads as follows: total cholesterol, 240 mg/dL; triglycerides, 620 mg/dL; and HDL, 20 mg/dL. He also has a fasting blood glucose level of 198 mg/dL. What should the pharmacist recommend regarding his lipid profile?
2. PT is a 35-year-old, pregnant black woman who presents to the pharmacy asking what diet-aid the pharmacist would recommend to help her lose weight and decrease her cholesterol. She has just come from her physician, who told her that she was overweight and had dangerously high cholesterol. She wants to fix the problem as soon as possible and asks the pharmacist for advice. Her cholesterol profile today reads as follows: total cholesterol, 280 mg/dL; triglycerides, 290 mg/dL; and HDL, 38. How should the pharmacist educate/counsel this patient?

Bibliography

ACC/AHA guidelines for the management of patients with acute myocardial infarction: 1999 update: a report of the American College of Cardiology/American Heart Association Task Force on Practice Guidelines (Committee on Management of Acute Myocardial Infarction). Available at www.acc.org

ACC/AHA practice guidelines for evaluation and management of chronic heart failure in the Adult. J Am Coll Cardiol 2001;38:2101–2113.

Criscitello MB: Fine-tuning the cardiovascular exam. Patient Care 1990;24(11):51–74.

Cunningham FG, MacDonald PC, Gant NF. Williams obstetrics. 21st ed. New York: McGraw-Hill, 2001.

Davies DM, Ferner RE, de Glanville H. Davies's textbook of adverse drug reactions. 5th ed. New York: Chapman and Hall Medical, 1998.

DeLeon AC: Fine-tuning the examination of the heart. Consultant 1989;29(4):51–61.

DiPiro JT, Talbert RL, Yee GC, et al. Pharmacotherapy: a pathophysiologic approach. 4th ed. Stamford, CT: Appleton & Lange, 1999.

Dorland's illustrated medical dictionary. 29th ed. Philadelphia: WB Saunders, 2000.

Frank MJ, Alvarez-Mena SC, Abdulla AM. Cardiovascular physical diagnosis. 2nd ed. Chicago: Year Book, 1983.

Joint National Committee on Prevention, Detection, Evaluation, and Treatment of High Blood Pressure. The sixth report of the Joint National Committee on Detection, Evaluation, and Treatment of High Blood Pressure (JNC VI). Arch Intern Med 1997;157:2413–2446.

Kradjan WA. Heart failure. In: Applied therapeutics: the clinical use of drugs 7th ed. Baltimore: Lippincott Williams & Wilkins, 2001:1–60.

Kumar V, Cotran RS, Robbins SL. Basic pathology. 6th ed. Philadelphia: WB Saunders, 1997.

Lueckenotte AG. Pocket guide to gerontologic assessment. St. Louis: CV Mosby, 1990.

Mackenna BR, Callander R. Illustrated physiology. 6th ed. New York: Churchill Livingstone, 1997.

Martini FH, Timmons MJ. Human anatomy. 2nd ed. Upper Saddle River, NJ: Prentice-Hall, 1997.

Myers DG. Review of cardiac auscultation (part 1). Hosp Med 1993;29(10):25–52.

Nappi JM. Myocardial infarction. In: Applied therapeutics: the clinical use of drugs 7th ed. Baltimore: Lippincott Williams & Wilkins, 2001:1–24.

National Cholesterol Education Program. Summary of the third report of the national cholesterol education program expert panel on detection, evaluation, and treatment of high blood cholesterol in adults (adult treatment panel III). Bethesda, MD: NIH publication no. 01-3670, 2001.

National Cholesterol Education Program. ATP III guidelines at-a-glance quick desk reference. Bethesda, MD: NIH publication no. 01-3305, 2001.

Pagana KD, Pagana TJ. Mosby's diagnostic and laboratory test reference. 2nd ed. St. Louis: Mosby, 1995.

Perloff JK. Physical examination of the heart and circulation. 2nd ed. Philadelphia: WB Saunders, 1990.

Trujillo TC, Nolan PE. Ischemic heart disease: anginal syndromes. In: Koda-Kimble MA, Young LY, eds. Applied therapeutics: the clinical use of drugs. Baltimore: Lippincott Williams & Wilkins, 2001.

Yacone-Morton LA. Perfecting the art: cardiac assessment. RN 1991;54(12):28–35.

CHAPTER

13

Peripheral Vascular System

Rhonda M. Jones

GLOSSARY TERMS

- Arteriosclerosis
- Atherosclerosis
- Deep venous thrombosis (thrombophlebitis)
- Hypoxia
- Pulmonary embolism

ANATOMY AND PHYSIOLOGY OVERVIEW

Circulation of blood occurs through one continuous loop of arteries and veins that are divided into pulmonary and systemic circuits (Fig. 13-1). The pulmonary circuit transports blood from the heart to the lungs, where it is oxygenated and then returned to the heart. The systemic circulation, or peripheral vascular system, includes arteries, arterioles, veins, venules, and capillaries, which carry blood from the heart to all other organs and tissues and then return the blood back to the heart. In this chapter, only the peripheral vascular system is discussed; see Chapter 12 for a discussion of the pulmonary circulation.

Arteries

The heart pumps newly oxygenated blood through the arteries, arterioles, and capillary beds to all the organs and tissues. The arteries are composed of thick, smooth muscle and elastic fibers. These contractile and elastic fibers help to resist the pressure that is generated when the heart forces blood into the systemic circulation. Major arteries of the systemic circulation include the aorta, carotid, subclavian, and iliac (Fig. 13-2).The aorta arches back behind the heart and descends down the middle of the body. Other arteries branch from the aorta and supply blood to the head, neck, and major organs within the abdomen. The carotid arteries ascend deep within the neck and supply blood to organs within the head and neck, including the brain. The subclavian arteries supply blood to the arms, chest wall, shoulders, back, and central nervous system. The iliac arteries carry blood to the pelvis and the legs.

Arteries in the Arm

After extending through the thoracic cavity, the subclavian artery becomes the axillary artery (Fig. 13-3). The axillary artery then crosses the axilla and becomes the brachial artery, which lies within the biceps-triceps groove in the upper arm. The brachial artery supplies the majority of blood to the arm. At the cubital fossa (i.e., the bend in the elbow), the brachial artery splits into the radial and ulnar arteries, which extend through the lower arm and, in turn, branch into the palmar arches that supply blood to the hand.

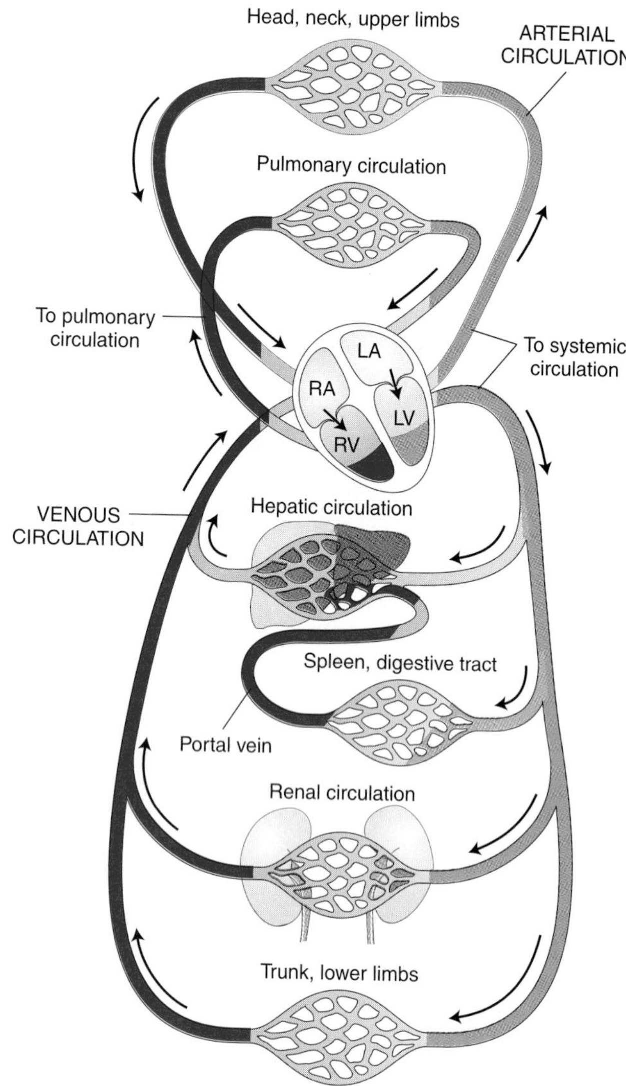

FIGURE 13-1 ■ The circulatory system.

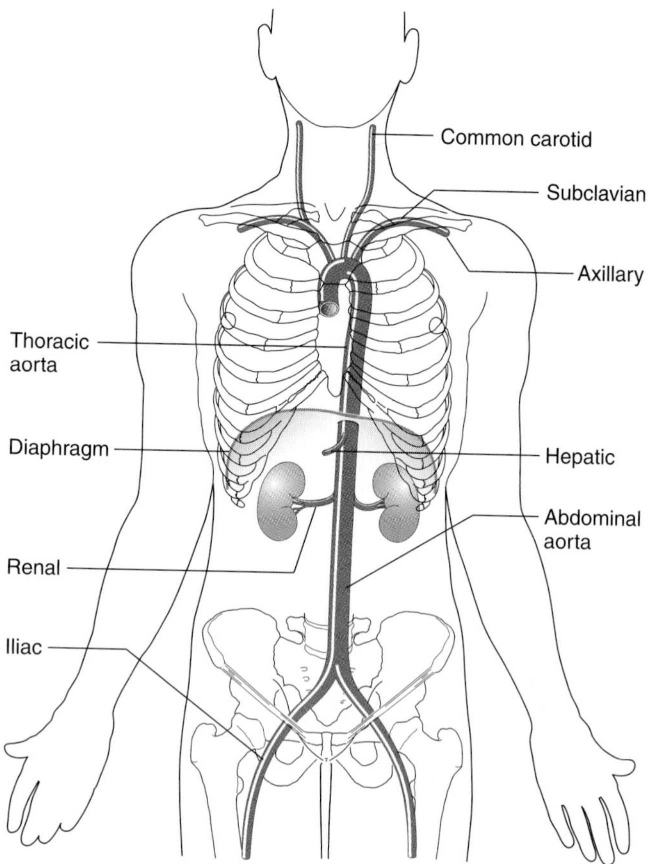

FIGURE 13-2 ■ Major arteries of the systemic circulation.

Arteries in the Leg

After passing through the pelvic region, the iliac artery becomes the femoral artery, which travels down the thigh anteriorly (Fig. 13-4). The femoral artery supplies blood to the skin and deep muscles of the thigh. At the lower thigh, the femoral artery crosses posteriorly and becomes the popliteal artery. Below the knee, the popliteal artery divides into the anterior and posterior tibial arteries. The anterior tibial artery travels down the front of the lower leg onto the dorsa of the foot and becomes the dorsalis pedis. The posterior tibial artery travels down the calf of the lower leg and branches into the plantar arteries within the bottom of the foot.

Veins

After being transported through the arterial vascular system and into the body's tissues and organs, the blood empties into an

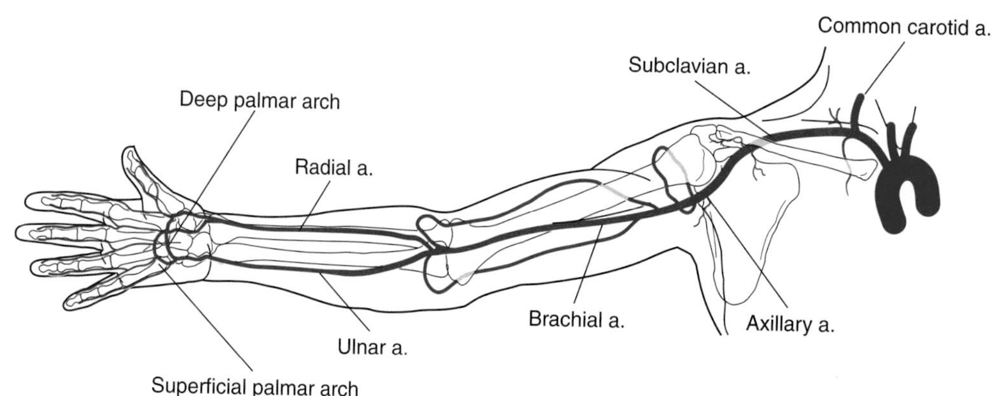

FIGURE 13-3 ■ Arteries in the arm.

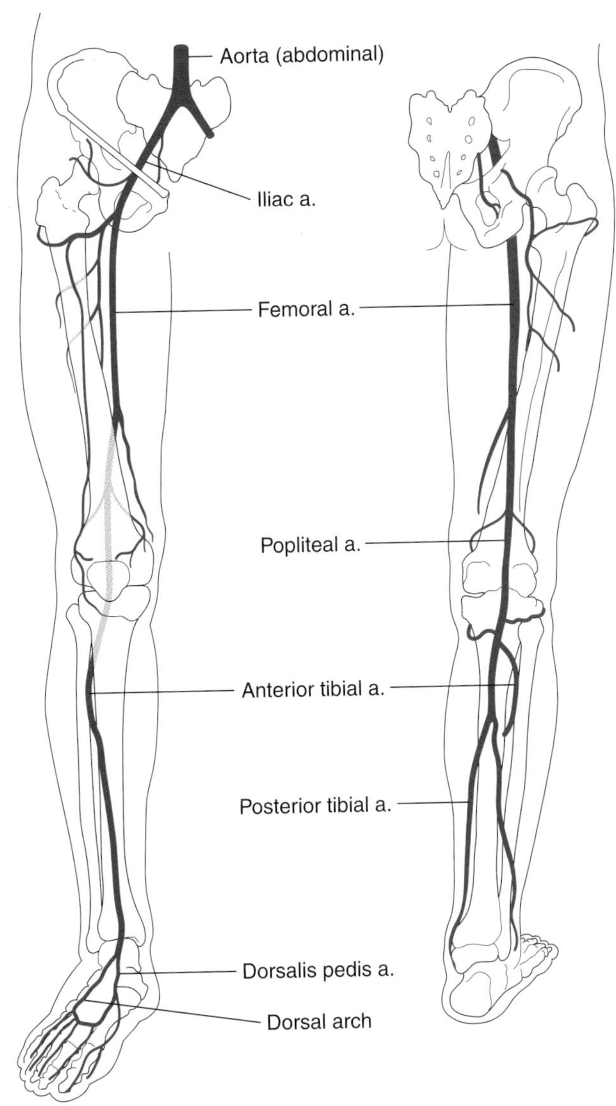

FIGURE 13-4 ■ Arteries in the leg.

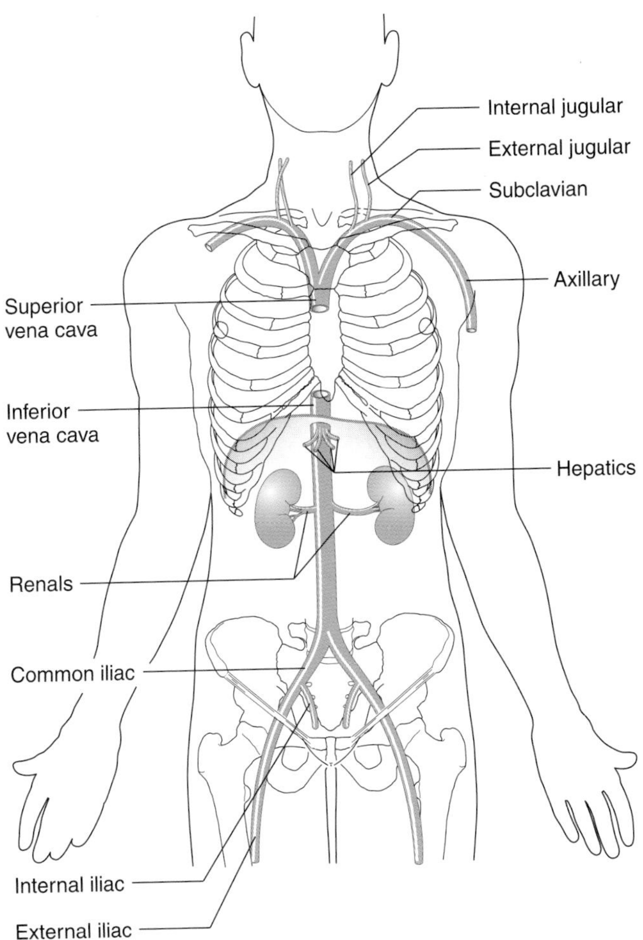

FIGURE 13-5 ■ Major veins of the systemic circulation.

elaborate venous network (Fig. 13-5) that eventually returns it to the right atrium of the heart. The systemic veins run alongside the systemic arteries and have similar names; however, major differences exist between the arterial and venous systems in the neck and extremities. Arteries in these areas are located deep beneath the skin and are protected by bones and soft tissues. In contrast, two sets of peripheral veins usually are found in the neck and extremities: one superficial, and the other deep. Superficial veins are close to the skin surface, can be easily seen, and help to regulate body temperature. When body temperature becomes abnormally low, the arterial blood supply to the skin is reduced, and the superficial veins are bypassed. In turn, when the body becomes overheated, the blood supply to the skin increases, and the superficial veins dilate.

Major veins of the systemic circulation include the superior vena cava, inferior vena cava, and jugular. The superior vena cava receives blood from the tissues and organs of the head, neck, chest, shoulders, and upper extremities. The inferior vena cava collects blood from most of the organs below the diaphragm. Venous blood from the head and face drains into the jugular vein, which is located within the neck.

Veins in the Arm

The palmar venous arches extend from the hand to the lower arm, where they become the ulnar and radial veins (Fig. 13-6). As the ulnar and radial veins reach the cubital fossa (i.e., the bend in the elbow), they combine to form the brachial vein. As the brachial vein extends through the upper arm, it joins the superficial veins of the arm to form the axillary vein, which passes through the axilla and becomes the subclavian vein within the thoracic cavity. The subclavian vein carries blood from the arm and thoracic area into the superior vena cava.

Veins in the Leg

Blood leaving the capillaries in each foot collects into a network of plantar veins (Fig. 13-7). The plantar network drains blood into the deep veins of the leg (i.e., the anterior tibial, posterior tibial, popliteal, and femoral veins). The superficial, great saphenous, and small saphenous veins drain blood in the leg from the dorsal venous arch into the popliteal and femoral veins.

Special Considerations

Pediatric Patients

Physiologic changes in blood pressure and pulse among pediatric patients are discussed in Chapter 5.

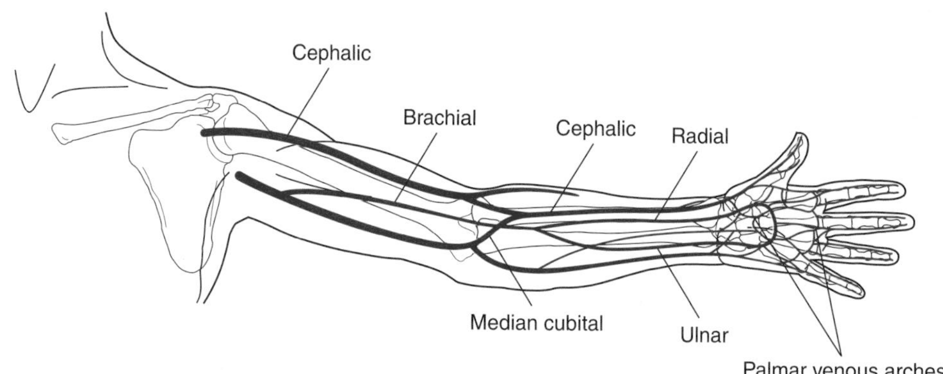

FIGURE 13-6 ■ Veins in the arm

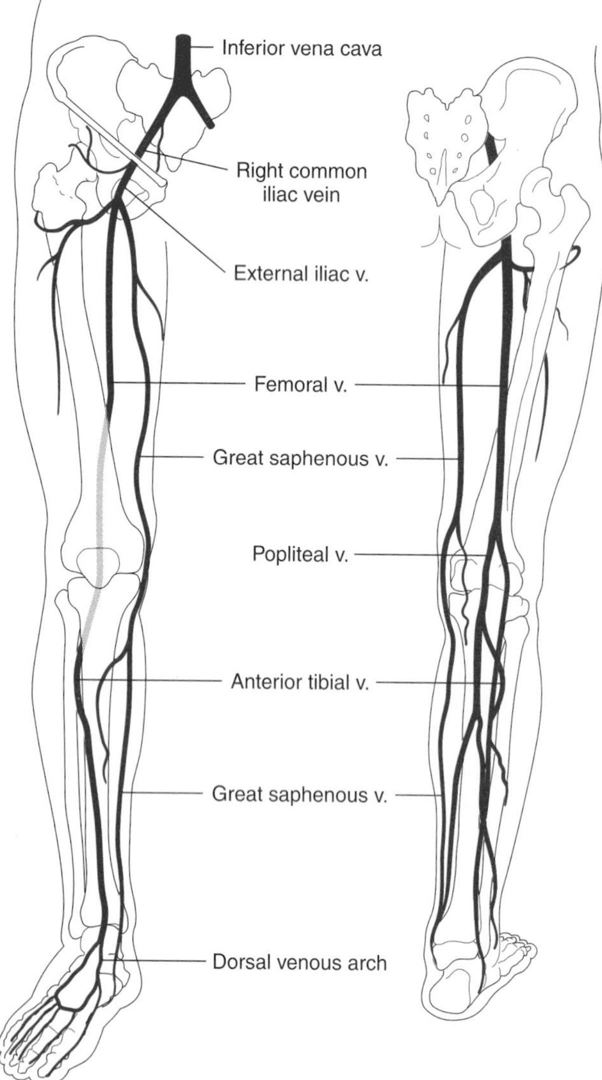

FIGURE 13-7 ■ Veins in the leg.

Geriatric Patients

As the body ages, the blood vessels become more rigid, lose elasticity, and grow thicker, which is commonly termed **arteriosclerosis.** Advancing age also increases the risk of atherosclerotic plaques being deposited in the vascular system, which is termed **atherosclerosis,** and, thus, increases the risk of peripheral vascular disease. Aging progressively enlarges the intramuscular calf veins as well. Deep venous thrombosis and, possibly, subsequent pulmonary embolism may develop as a result of heart failure, prolonged sitting, or prolonged bed rest, which are all common conditions in elderly patients.

Pregnant Patients

An increase in progesterone levels causes a generalized vasodilation. As the fetus grows, the uterus expands and progressively obstructs return of venous blood from the iliac veins and the inferior vena cava. This decrease in venous blood return increases venous pressure in the lower extremities and predisposes the pregnant woman to varicose veins, peripheral edema, varicosities (i.e., hemorrhoids), and venous thrombosis.

PATHOLOGY OVERVIEW

Peripheral Atherosclerosis

Atherosclerosis is a vascular disease that causes the formation of lipid-rich plaques within the vessel wall that protrude into the lumen. As the atherosclerosis progresses, the vessel wall thickens, becomes hard, and loses elasticity, which decreases the flow of blood through the vessel and increases the risk of thrombus formation. Major vessels that are commonly affected include the aorta and the coronary and cerebral arteries. In this chapter, only peripheral atherosclerosis is discussed; for a complete discussion of coronary atherosclerosis, see Chapter 12.

Peripheral atherosclerosis is more commonly called peripheral vascular disease (PVD). It is characterized by the development of atherosclerotic plaques or lesions, primarily in the peripheral arterial vessels. Arteries that are commonly affected include the femoral, popliteal, and tibial arteries of the lower extremities. Risk factors for the development of PVD are very similar to those for coronary artery disease and include:

- Age (males, >45 years; females, >55 years)
- Sex (women are at lower risk than men until after menopause)
- Familial predisposition
- Hyperlipidemia (high low-density lipoprotein or low high-density lipoprotein cholesterol)

- Hypertension
- Diabetes
- Cigarette smoking

The most common symptom associated with PVD is intermittent claudication, which includes pain/aching, cramping, tightness, and weakness/fatigue of the leg muscles (Box 13-1). These symptoms usually occur with exertion and are relieved with rest. Other symptoms may include numbness or continuous pain in the toes or feet, which can lead to ulceration, tissue necrosis, and ultimately, amputation. Medications that may be beneficial in treating PVD include pentoxifylline, aspirin, and possibly, ticlopidine and dipyridamole.

Nonpharmacologic treatment plays a major role in the management of PVD. Any risk factors that the patient may have should be either eliminated (if possible) or appropriately controlled. For example, blood pressure, blood sugar, and cholesterol levels should be within the goal range for the patient. In addition, patients who smoke should be encouraged strongly to quit. Patients also should be educated regarding appropriate foot hygiene, a low-fat/cholesterol diet, and exercise.

Deep Venous Thrombosis

The presence of a *thrombus* (i.e., a blood clot) in a deep vein and the accompanying inflammatory process in the vessel wall is termed a **deep venous thrombosis (DVT),** or **thrombophlebitis.** Blood flow stasis, vascular damage, and hypercoagulability predispose the patient to thrombus formation. Major veins that are commonly affected include the iliac, femoral, and popliteal. Risk factors that are associated with DVT include:

- Orthopedic surgical procedures
- Cancer (pancreas, lung, ovary, testes, urinary tract, breast, and stomach)

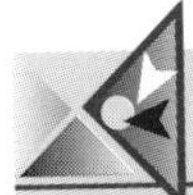

Box 13-1

SIGNS AND SYMPTOMS ASSOCIATED WITH PERIPHERAL VASCULAR DISEASE

- Leg muscle pain and tightness that usually occurs with exertion and is relieved with rest
- Leg muscle weakness or aching that usually occurs with exertion and is relieved with rest
- Numbness or pain in the toes, feet, or lower legs
- Decreased or absent peripheral pulses
- Leg muscle atrophy
- Hair loss on the toes, feet, or lower legs
- Smooth, shiny skin on the feet or lower legs
- Cool skin temperature
- Cyanosis or pallor of the toes, feet, or lower legs
- Thick, hardened toenails
- Ulcers or gangrene of the toes, feet, or lower legs
- Peripheral edema

- Fractures of the spine, pelvis, femur, and tibia
- Immobilization
- Pregnancy
- Estrogen use
- Hypercoagulable diseases (e.g., disseminated intravascular coagulation)

Patients with DVT commonly experience unilateral leg swelling, warmth, erythema, and tenderness (Box 13-2). Occasionally, a cord-like obstruction may be felt on palpation of the affected leg. Skin discoloration may vary between erythema, pallor, or cyanosis. The major, life-threatening concern with DVT is the risk of a thrombus moving to the lung, which is termed **pulmonary embolism.** Therefore, the primary treatment of DVT includes anticoagulation therapy (i.e., heparin and warfarin), which prevents thrombus propagation. Nonpharmacologic therapy, such as elevating the leg above the level of the heart and use of heat, also is common.

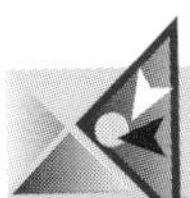

Box 13-2

SIGNS AND SYMPTOMS ASSOCIATED WITH DEEP VENOUS THROMBOSIS

- Unilateral leg swelling
- Pain or tenderness
- Skin discoloration (i.e., erythema, pallor, or cyanosis)
- Palpation of a cork-like obstruction

SYSTEM ASSESSMENT

Subjective Information

Because peripheral vascular problems are primarily diagnosed through subjective complaints, good interviewing skills to obtain information concerning leg pain, peripheral edema, and skin changes are critical. Patients frequently ask their pharmacists about these symptoms; therefore, pharmacists need to be skilled in assessing these symptoms and in determining possible causes, appropriate treatment, and referral to a primary care provider.

Leg Pain

? INTERVIEW Describe the type of pain you are experiencing. Is it burning, aching, cramping? How long have you been experiencing it? Did it come on suddenly or gradually? What brings it on? What makes it better or makes it go away? Does it come on with walking or activity? If so, how many blocks can you walk before the pain begins? Have you recently started a new exercise program?

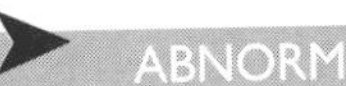

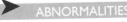

ABNORMALITIES Leg pain associated with PVD usually is an aching/cramping/weak type of pain brought on by walking or exertion and is relieved with rest. As the disease progresses, the distance the patient can walk before experiencing leg pain will decrease. Keep in mind that leg cramping at night is common in elderly patients and pregnant women, so this may not be a sign of PVD.

? INTERVIEW Any history of smoking, high blood pressure, high cholesterol, diabetes, heart problems, recent trauma, bed rest, or surgery?

ABNORMALITIES These are risk factors for PVD and DVT.

Peripheral Skin Changes

? INTERVIEW Any changes in the skin color of your legs (bluish, red, or pale)? Any changes in leg temperature (warm or cool)? Any leg sores or ulcers?

ABNORMALITIES The skin of the lower extremities may appear cyanotic, erythemic, or pale with PVD. The lower extremities may be cool with PVD and warm with DVT. Advanced, chronic PVD may cause leg sores or ulcers.

Edema

? INTERVIEW When does the swelling occur? When is it the worst and best, or is it constant all day? At the end of the day, in the morning, after standing all day? What relieves it? Is it in both legs or only one? Do you have a history of heart failure or kidney problems?

ABNORMALITIES DVT causes swelling in only one leg that will be constant throughout the day. Edema from heart failure or kidney failure usually is bilateral, decreased in the morning, and progressive during the day.

Objective Information

Physical Assessment

Physical assessment of the peripheral vascular system involves inspection, auscultation, and palpation. One basic principle of peripheral vascular assessment is that side-to-side comparison must be made during inspection and palpation of the extremities.

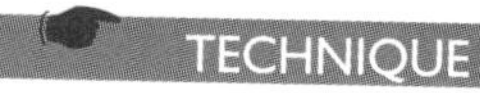

TECHNIQUE

STEP 1

Inspect the Skin of the Arms and Legs

Assess the following:

- Color (note any cyanosis, erythema, or pallor).
- Hair growth (note any areas of decreased hair growth from decreased circulation).
- Muscle atrophy.
- Edema (note any swelling or shiny, taut skin).
- Varicosities.
- Ulcerations (note any open sores).
- Nails (note any thick, hard nails [see Chapter 8]).

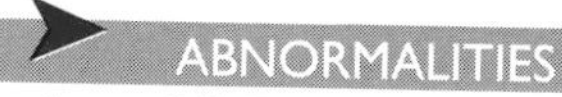

ABNORMALITIES See Boxes 13-1 and 13-2 for signs of PVD and DVT.

TECHNIQUE

STEP 2

Palpate the Arms

- Palpate the radial and brachial pulses (note the rate, rhythm, force, and symmetry of the pulse in both arms) (Figs. 13-8 and 13-9)
- Grade the force (amplitude) of the pulse using a four-point scale:

4+	Bounding
3+	Increased
2+	Normal
1+	Weak/decreased
0	Absent

- The force should be equal bilaterally.

ABNORMALITIES A bounding or increased pulse occurs with hyperkinetic states (e.g., exercise, anxiety, high fever, anemia, and hyperthyroidism). A weak pulse occurs with peripheral arterial disease or shock.

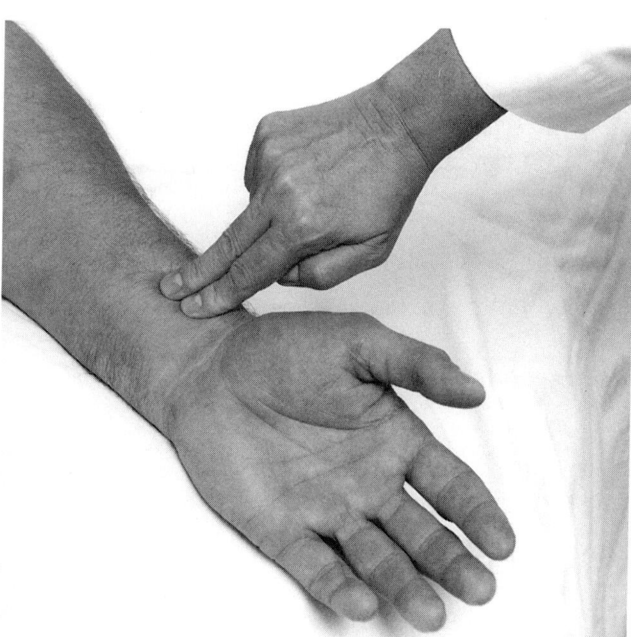

Figure 13-8 ■ Palpation of the radial pulse.

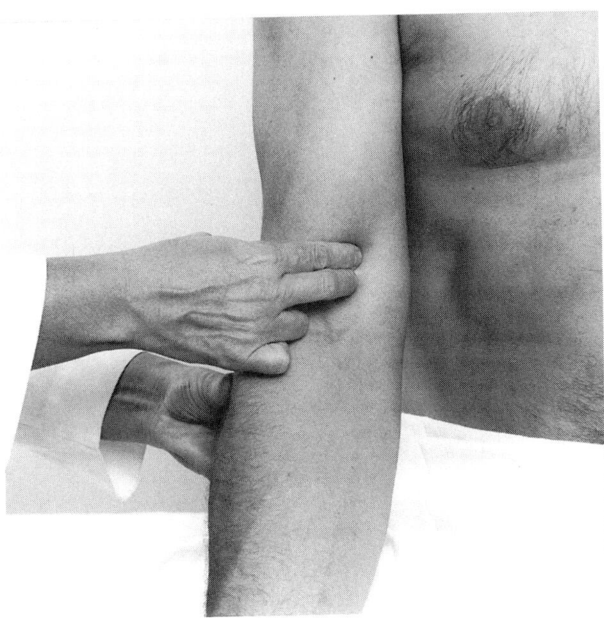

FIGURE 13-9 ■ Palpation of the brachial pulse.

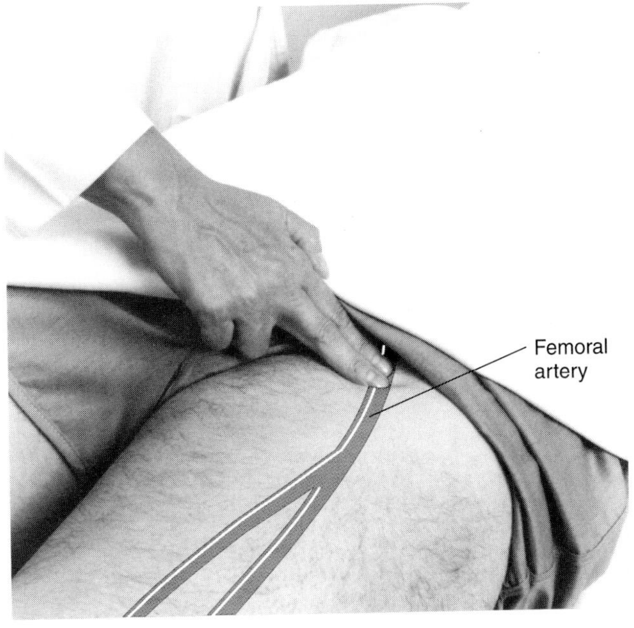

FIGURE 13-10 ■ Palpation of the femoral artery.

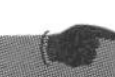 TECHNIQUE

STEP 3

Palpate Capillary Refill

- Extend the person's hands near his or her heart level.
- Depress/squeeze the nail bed of each finger.
- Release, and note the time of color return.
- Color should return to normal within 1 to 2 seconds. Certain conditions (i.e., cool room, decreased body temperature, anemia) may increase this time.

ABNORMALITIES A return time of more than 1 to 2 seconds signifies vasoconstriction, decreased blood flow, or decreased cardiac output (heart failure).

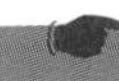 TECHNIQUE

STEP 4

Palpate the Legs

- Check for skin temperature using the back of the fingers along the legs down to the feet, comparing symmetric spots on each leg.
- The skin should be warm and equal bilaterally.
- Using the fingers, palpate pulses in both legs at the femoral, popliteal, dorsalis pedis, and posterior tibial arteries (Figs. 13-10 to 13-13)
- Evaluate the pulse rate, rhythm, force, and symmetry in each leg.
- Grade the force of the pulse using a four-point scale and comparing each leg:

4+ Bounding
3+ Increased
2+ Normal
1+ Weak/decreased
0 Absent

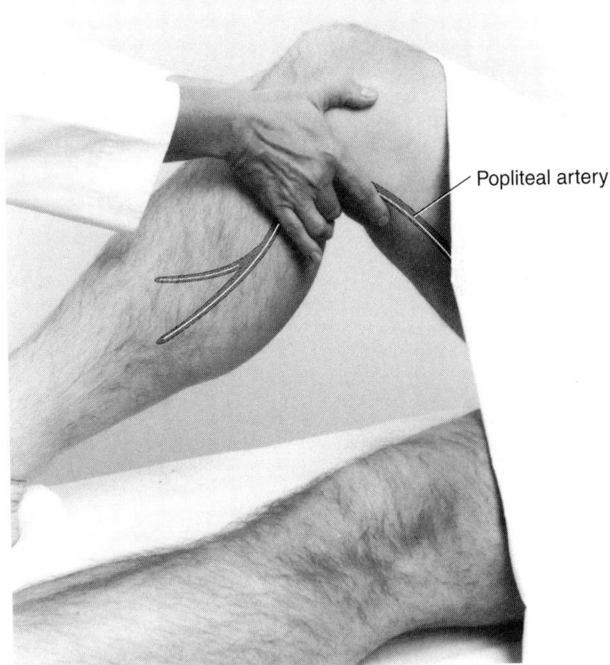

FIGURE 13-11 ■ Palpation of the popliteal artery.

CAUTION The pulse scale is a subjective measurement.

ABNORMALITIES PVD can cause bilateral, diminished, or weak pulses. DVT may cause weak or absent pulses in the affected leg versus the other leg.

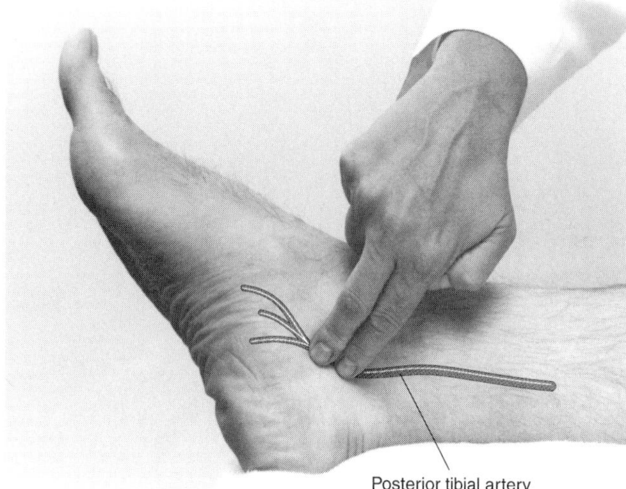

FIGURE 13-12 ■ Palpation of the posterior tibial pulse.

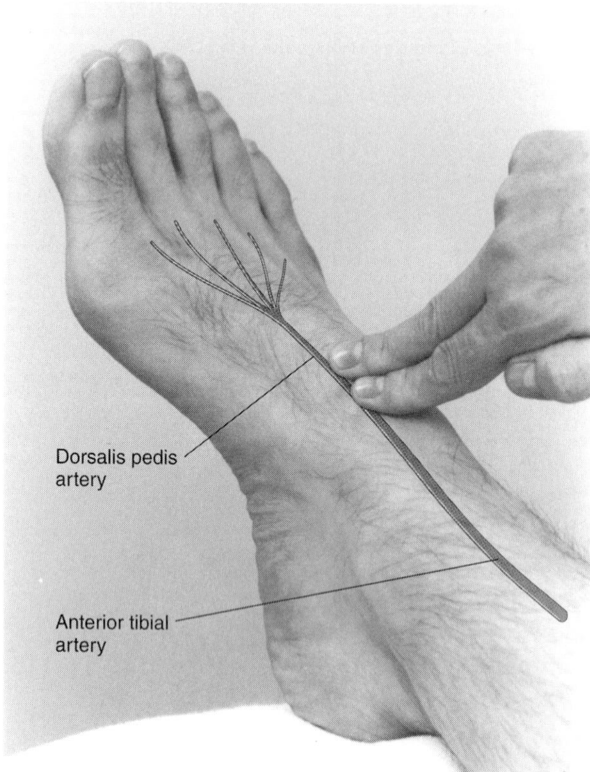

FIGURE 13-13 ■ Palpation of the dorsalis pedis pulse.

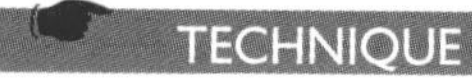
TECHNIQUE

STEP 5

Palpate for Peripheral Edema

- Press down, using your first two fingers, over the tibia (shin) or atop the foot for at least 5 seconds and then release. (Fig. 13-14).
- The skin should pop back and leave no indentation. If pitting edema is present, grade it using a four-point scale:

  4+ Very deep pitting, indentation remains a long time, significant swelling is present.

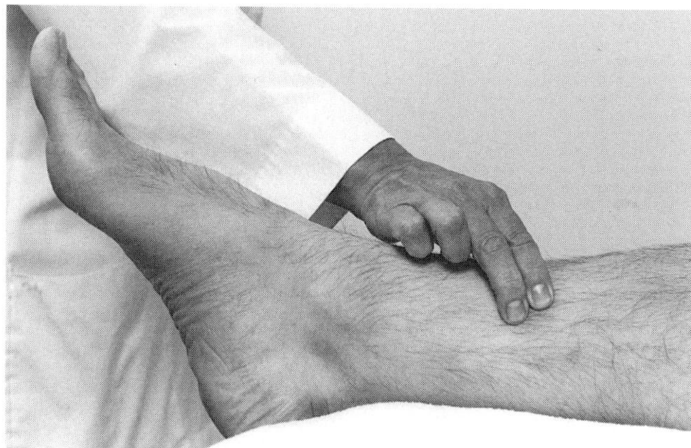

FIGURE 13-14 ■ Palpation for peripheral edema.

  3+ Deep pitting, indentation remains for a short time, visible swelling.

  2+ Moderate pitting, indentation subsides quickly, no visible swelling.

  1+ Mild pitting, slight indentation, no visible swelling.

CAUTION The edema scale is a subjective measurement.

ABNORMALITIES Pitting edema can occur from several different causes (e.g., PVD, DVT, congestive heart failure, trauma, renal failure, etc.). If present, evaluate other signs and symptoms to determine the cause.

Laboratory and Diagnostic Tests

The Doppler ultrasound stethoscope is used to auscultate pulses and to measure blood pressure in the legs. When obtained at the same level in each leg, measurements normally should be equivalent.

Special Considerations

Pediatric Patients

Peripheral assessment is the same in pediatric patients as in adults.

Geriatric Patients

Because of the normal aging process, peripheral pulses may be more difficult to palpate. In addition, skin changes (e.g., loss of hair growth and thick, shiny skin) are normal in elderly patients.

Pregnant Patients

As the pregnancy progresses, varicose veins and pitting edema become common findings on physical examination, especially during the third trimester. If a pregnant patient experiences sudden peripheral edema (especially in the hands and face) accompanied by shortness of breath, increased blood pressure, or both, she should contact her physician.

APPLICATION TO PATIENT SYMPTOMS

Pharmacists frequently are asked questions concerning various health problems. Problems with the extremities, which may relate to the peripheral vascular system, are no exception. A frequent complaint relating to the peripheral vascular system is leg pain.

As discussed, leg pain, cramping, and weakness that occur with walking and are relieved with rest are termed *intermittent claudication,* which is a primary symptom associated with PVD. It is caused by **hypoxia,** or lack of oxygen, in the peripheral vessels and tissues when oxygen demand is increased by activity (e.g., walking). Leg pain, however, also can result from musculoskeletal problems, trauma, and various other causes. For a complete discussion of pain caused by the musculoskeletal system, see Chapter 17. Occasionally, medications also cause muscle weakness and pain (Box 13-3).

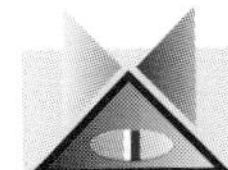

Box 13-3

DRUG-RELATED CAUSES OF MUSCLE PAIN AND WEAKNESS[A]

- 3-Hydroxy-3-methylgluytaryl coenzyme A reductase inhibitors
  - Atorvastatin
  - Fluvastatin
  - Lovastatin
  - Pravastatin
  - Simvastatin
  - Ceravastatin
  - Diuretics

[A]Not an all-inclusive list.

CASE STUDY

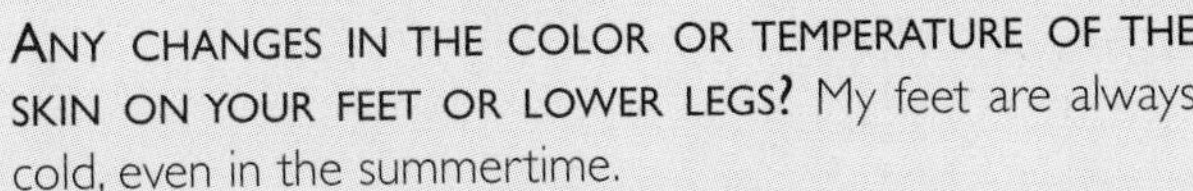

KU is a 68-year-old man who comes to the pharmacy and asks what the best over-the-counter medication would be for his leg pain. Because KU comes to the pharmacy frequently, the pharmacist asks him to step into the patient care room to review his health and medication history before making a recommendation.

ASSESSMENT OF THE PATIENT

Subjective Information

68-year-old man complaining of leg pain

WHERE IS THE PAIN? In both calves of my legs.

HOW LONG HAVE YOU HAD THE PAIN? Oh, I've had it off and on for a long time. It just seems to be getting worse lately.

HAVE YOU RECENTLY STARTED NEW OR DIFFERENT ACTIVITIES INVOLVING YOUR LEGS THAT MAY BE CAUSING THE PAIN, SUCH AS GARDENING, MOWING YOUR LAWN, OR AN EXERCISE PROGRAM? No, not really. Oh, my doctor keeps telling me I should exercise more for my heart and cholesterol, but all I do is walk my dog when he gets restless and I've done that for years.

DESCRIBE THE PAIN. IS IT BURNING, ACHING, CRAMPING? It is a weak, achy feeling.

WHAT DO YOU THINK CAUSES THE PAIN OR BRINGS IT ON? WHAT MAKES IT BETTER OR WORSE? It usually happens when I need to walk long distances, like when I buy groceries or take the dog for a walk. And then when I sit down and rest a while, it goes away.

HOW MANY BLOCKS CAN YOU WALK BEFORE THE PAIN BEGINS? Probably about 8 to 10 blocks.

ANY CHANGES IN THE COLOR OR TEMPERATURE OF THE SKIN ON YOUR FEET OR LOWER LEGS? My feet are always cold, even in the summertime.

ANY PROBLEMS WITH SWELLING IN YOUR FEET OR LOWER LEGS? Sometimes a little at the end of the day, but not really anything bad.

WHAT MEDICAL PROBLEMS DO YOU HAVE? High blood pressure, high cholesterol, and heart problems. And once in a while a little arthritis in my joints.

DO YOU SMOKE? No.

WHAT ARE YOUR USUAL DAILY ACTIVITIES? Mostly, I just putter around the house or work in my garden. I also like to do crossword puzzles. I usually can find something to keep me busy.

WHAT MEDICATIONS ARE YOU TAKING? Atenolol, Mevacor, and a nitroglycerin patch.

HOW DO YOU TAKE THEM? One tablet of each in the morning with breakfast, and I put the patch on then, too.

WHEN DID YOU START TAKING THE MEVACOR? About 2 years ago.

ANY OVER-THE-COUNTER MEDICATIONS? One aspirin every day.

HOW OFTEN DO YOU FORGET TO TAKE YOUR MEDICATION? Oh, I don't forget. I just take them all in the morning with my breakfast.

Objective Information

Computerized medication profile:

- Atenolol: 50 mg, one tablet daily; No. 30; Refills: 11; Patient obtains refills every 25-33 days

Continued

CASE STUDY—continued

- Mevacor (lovastatin): 20 mg, one tablet daily; No. 30; Refills: 11; Patient obtains refills every 28-33 days
- Nitro-Dur (nitroglycerin) patch: 0.4 mg/h, apply one patch once daily; No. 30; Refills: 11; Patient obtains refills every 28–33 days

Patient in no acute distress
Heart rate: 60 bpm
Blood pressure: 128/82 mm Hg
Respiratory rate: 14 rpm
Heart auscultation: regular rate and rhythm, no murmur
Extremities:

- Inspection: mild cyanosis equal bilaterally in feet, no sores or ulcerations, decreased hair growth bilaterally on feet and lower legs
- Palpation: skin cool equal bilaterally in feet, warmer as progress up the lower leg; no edema bilaterally; pulses: femoral, 2+ bilaterally; popliteal. 2+ bilaterally; posterior tibial, 1+ bilaterally; dorsalis pedis, 1+ bilaterally

DISCUSSION

The problem in this case centers around the cause of the patient's leg pain. The pharmacist needs to decide if the leg pain is a symptom of PVD, a musculoskeletal problem, a traumatic incident, a new activity involving the legs, or a side effect of the lovastatin therapy. KU describes the pain as a weak, achy feeling in both calves that is brought on by walking and is relieved with rest. His walking distance is about 8 to 10 blocks, and he has not started any new activities recently. His feet are frequently cold but do not routinely swell. KU has a history of hypertension, hyperlipidemia, and angina. KU is compliant with his medications and started the lovastatin about 2 years ago. All his vital signs are normal; however, on inspection and palpation of his extremities, KU has cyanosis, decreased temperature, and weak pulses in both feet.

After evaluating all the patient information, the pharmacist concludes that KU has three risk factors for PVD (i.e., hypertension, hyperlipidemia, and coronary artery disease) as well as several signs and symptoms that are consistent with PVD. The steps associated with this evaluation process are illustrated in Figure 13-15. Because KU started the lovastatin 2 years ago and does not describe the muscle pain as a "generalized" problem in several different muscles, the pharmacist feels that the muscle pain probably is not caused by the lovastatin. In addition, the pharmacist recalls that myopathy or muscle pain caused by lovastatin has been reported in only 0.1% of patients and occurs most frequently when lovastatin is combined with cyclosporine or gemfibrozil, neither of which KU is taking.

PHARMACEUTICAL CARE PLAN

Patient Name: KU

Date: 9/11/02

Medical Problems:
Hypertension
Hyperlipidemia
Coronary artery disease

Current Medications:
Atenolol, 50 mg, one tablet daily
Mevacor (lovastatin), 20 mg, one tablet daily
Nitro-Dur (nitroglycerin) patch, 0.4 mg/h, apply one patch once daily
Aspirin, 325 mg, one tablet daily

S: 68 year-old man complaining of weak, achy leg pain in both calves. Occurs with walking 8 to 10 blocks and is relieved with rest. Feet are frequently cold. Compliant with medications. Started Mevacor about 2 years ago. No new exercise program. Does not smoke.

O: Patient in no acute distress.

Heart rate: 60 bpm

Blood pressure: 128/82 mm Hg

Respiratory rate: 14 rpm

Heart auscultation: regular rate and rhythm, no murmur

Extremities:

- **Inspection:** mild cyanosis equal bilaterally in feet, no sores or ulcerations, decreased hair growth bilaterally on feet and lower legs
- Palpation: skin cool equal bilaterally in feet, warmer as progress up the lower leg; no edema bilaterally; pulses: femoral, 2+ bilaterally; popliteal, 2+ bilaterally; posterior tibial, 1+ bilaterally; dorsalis pedis, 1+ bilaterally

A: Leg pain possibly caused by PVD.

P:
1. Refer patient to his physician for further evaluation of extremities and possible PVD.
2. Educate patient about proper foot care, low-cholesterol/fat diet, and appropriate exercise.
3. Educate patient about presentation of leg pain as a side effect of lovastatin therapy.
4. Ask patient about physician appointment, foot care, diet, and exercise when he comes in for his next medication refill.

Pharmacist: *Rachel Feinman, Pharm.D.*

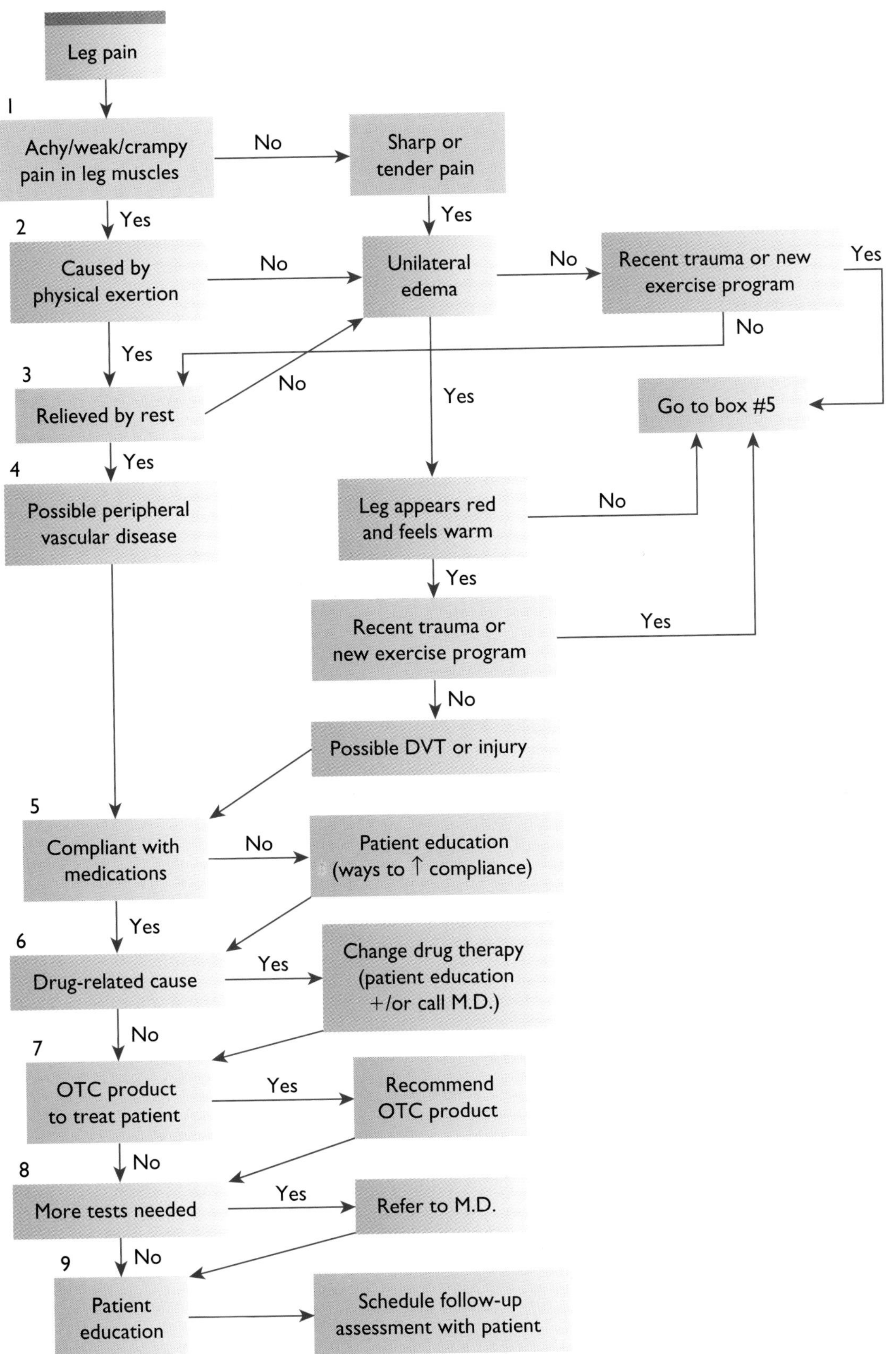

FIGURE 13-15 ■ Decision tree for leg pain.

Self-Assessment Questions

1. What are the risk factors for development of PVD?
2. What signs and symptoms are associated with PVD?
3. Compare and contrast interview questions that are useful in evaluating leg pain.

Critical Thinking Question

1. In the case of KU, what would your assessment be if he had complained of pain and severe swelling in only one leg, which appeared red and felt warm when palpated?
2. In the case of KU, what would you have done if he had complained that all his muscles were weak and achy and had recently started taking lovastatin and gemfibrozil?

Bibliography

Baker JD. Assessment of peripheral arterial occlusive disease. Crit Care Nurs Clin North Am 1991;3:493–498.

Blank CA, Irwin GH. Peripheral vascular disorders: assessment and intervention. Nurs Clin North Am 1990;25:777–794.

Cantwell-Gab K. Identifying chronic peripheral arterial disease. Am J Nurs 1996;96:40–47.

Creager MA, Dzau VJ. Vascular diseases of the extremities In: Harrison's principles of internal medicine. 13th ed. St. Louis: McGraw-Hill, 1994:1135–1151.

Dorland's pocket medical dictionary. 25th ed. Philadelphia: WB Saunders, 1995.

Fellows E, Jocz AM. Getting the upper hand on lower extremity arterial disease. Nursing 1991;21:34–41.

Gehring P. Vascular assessment. RN 1992;55:40–47.

Krenzer ME. Peripheral vascular assessment: finding your way through arteries and veins. AACN Clin Issues 1995;6:631–634.

Kumar V, Cotran RS, Robbins SL. Basic pathology. 6th ed. Philadelphia: WB Saunders, 1997.

Martini FH, Timmons MJ. Human anatomy. 2nd ed. Upper Saddle River, NJ: Prentice-Hall, 1997.

O'Beirne-Woods B. Clinical evaluation of the peripheral vasculature. Cardiol Clin 1991;9:413–427.

Pagana KD, Pagana TJ, Mosby's diagnostic and laboratory test reference. 2nd ed. St. Louis: Mosby, 1995.

Verstraete M. The diagnosis and treatment of deep-vein thrombosis. N Engl J Med 1993;329:1418.

Weitz J, Byrne J. Diagnosis and treatment of chronic arterial insufficiency of the lower extremities: a critical review. Circulation 1996;94:3026–3049.

Wittkowsky AK. Thrombosis. In: Applied therapeutics: the clinical use of drugs. 7th ed. Philadelphia, PA: Lippincott Williams & Wilkins, 2001:1–33.

CHAPTER 14

Gastrointestinal System

Michael S. Monaghan

GLOSSARY TERMS

- Ascites
- Constipation
- Crohn's disease
- Diarrhea
- Gastroesophageal reflux disease
- Peptic ulcer disease
- Peristalsis
- Ulcerative colitis

ANATOMY AND PHYSIOLOGY OVERVIEW

The gastrointestinal (GI) system is composed of the alimentary canal and the digestive organs/glands (Fig. 14-1). This system supplies the body with a continuous source of dietary nutrients, electrolytes, and water. To accomplish this, ingested substances must be moved along the GI tract at an ideal rate for digestion and absorption of nutrients. Hence, **peristalsis** (i.e., the progressive, involuntary, wave-like movements of the alimentary canal) is an essential component of normal function.

The major structures of the alimentary canal are the esophagus, stomach, small intestine, and colon. The digestive glands of the GI system are the liver and pancreas; for a detailed discussion of the liver, see Chapter 15.

Esophagus

The esophagus is a straight, slender tube approximately 20 cm in length in the adult. It functions to deliver the food bolus to the stomach. The upper third of the esophagus is skeletal muscle, the middle third a mixture of skeletal and smooth muscle, and the lower third entirely smooth muscle. Passage of a food bolus into the stomach normally occurs within a few seconds. The esophagus can be affected by motility disorders that disrupt the delivery of food to the stomach (e.g., achalasia and nutcracker esophagus), ulcerations from chronic exposure to acid (e.g., gastroesophageal reflux disease), and carcinomas (e.g., squamous and adenocarcinomas).

Stomach

The stomach is the organ that stores and digests food. The average capacity of the stomach is approximately 1 L. The surface area of the stomach is increased by the presence of folds, called rugae, that contain the gastric pits. The gastric pits are lined with the gastric glands, which are the cells that produce and secrete the functional enzymes of the stomach.

The regions of the stomach are shown in Figure 14-2. The cardia region connects with the esophagus at the esophagogastric junction, the area containing the lower esophageal sphincter (LES). The terminus of the stomach, called the pylorus, connects with the small intestine at the pyloric sphincter.

The stomach contains three major types of secretory cells: 1) the neck mucous cells, which secrete mucus; 2) the chief cells, which secrete pepsin, the proteolytic enzyme; and 3) the parietal cells, which secrete hydrochloric acid. The bulk of the neck mucous cells are in the cardiac and pyloric regions. Both the chief cells and the parietal cells are most numerous in the body and fundus of the stomach.

Like the esophagus, the stomach can be affected by motility disorders (e.g., diabetic gastroparesis), acid-induced ulcerations (e.g., peptic ulcer disease), and carcinomas.

Small Intestine

The small intestine, or small bowel, is approximately 20 feet in length in the average adult and is comprised of the duodenum, jejunum, and ileum. The most superior portion, the duodenum, is approximately 10 inches in length. The jejunum is two-fifths the length of the proximal small intestine, or approximately 8 feet, and the ileum is the distal three-fifths of the small intestine, or approximately 12 feet. The small intestine functions as the major digestive and absorptive organ of the body. All nutrients, amino acids, glucose, and fat are absorbed from the food bolus before it reaches the colon. In addition, most drugs are absorbed in the small intestine.

The small intestine can be affected by motility disorders (e.g., diarrhea and constipation), ulcerations from acid exposure (e.g., duodenal ulcers), inflammatory diseases (e.g., Crohn's disease), and malabsorption syndromes (e.g., caused by celiac disease, sprue, and chronic pancreatitis).

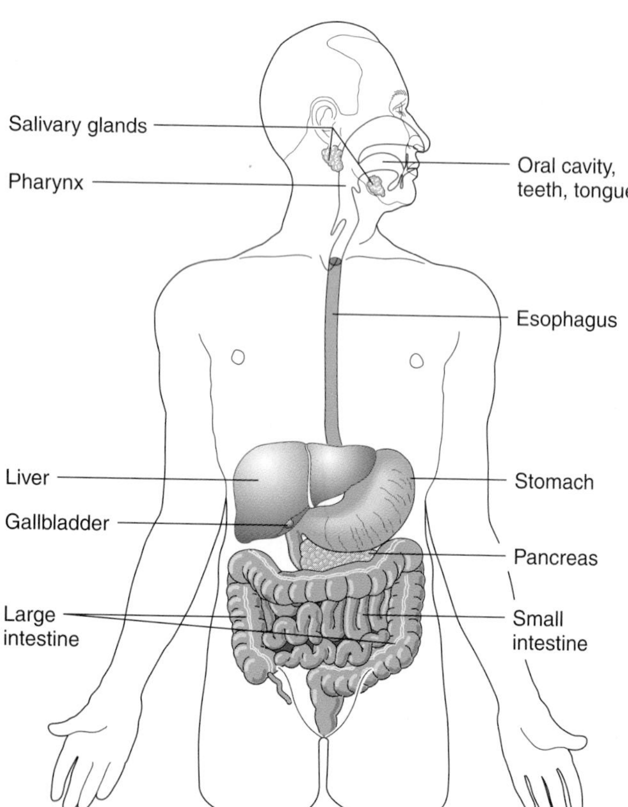

FIGURE 14-1 ■ The gastrointestinal system, including the alimentary canal and digestive organs/glands.

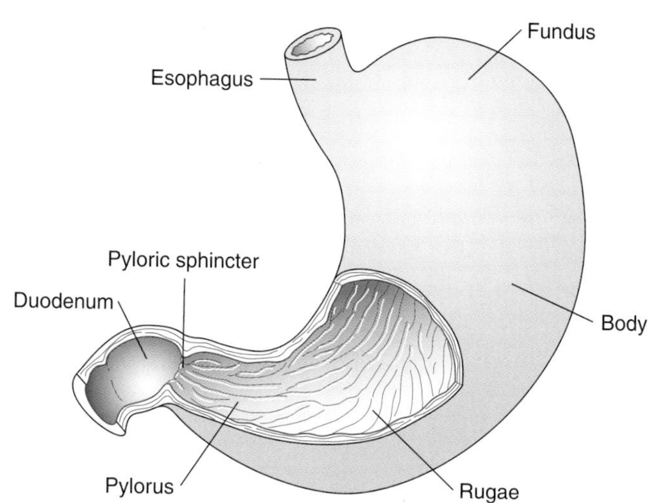

FIGURE 14-2 ■ The stomach, including the anatomic regions.

Colon

The colon, or large bowel, is approximately 5 feet in length in the average adult and is comprised of the cecum, ascending colon, transverse colon, and sigmoid colon. It functions to convert undigested material to feces through dehydration and compaction. The large bowel can be affected by motility disorders (e.g., diarrhea and constipation), inflammatory diseases (e.g., ulcerative colitis and diverticulitis), and cancer.

Pancreas

The pancreas is the largest digestive gland of the body and has both endocrine (i.e., secretion directly into the bloodstream) and exocrine (i.e., secretion through a duct to an epithelial surface) functions. The islets of Langerhans produce insulin and glucagon, fulfilling the endocrine function. The pancreas also secretes bicarbonate and digestive enzymes into the duodenum, fulfilling the exocrine function. The pancreas can be involved in endocrine disease (e.g., diabetes mellitus), ulcerative disease (e.g., duodenal ulcers), motility and malabsorptive diseases (e.g., steatorrhea caused by chronic pancreatitis), and inflammatory diseases (e.g., acute pancreatitis).

Special Considerations

Pediatric Patients

Significant changes occur in the GI tract during the first few days to months of life. These changes include alterations in gastric acidity, GI motility, biliary function, and bacterial flora. During the first 48 hours of life, gastric acidity, which begins at a pH ranging from 6 to 8 at birth, approaches the values of an adult, ranging from a pH of 1 to 3. Gastric emptying is prolonged in neonates and does not reach the adult rate until approximately 6 to 8 months of age. Diarrhea customarily occurs during this phase of life, limiting GI transit time. Bile salt stores and biliary function take months to develop fully. An infant's GI flora depends on diet, and to allow complete colonization, at least a few months of a varied diet are necessary. From a pharmacist's point of view, GI tract maturation affects drug absorption and, hence, the utility of orally administered medications in this age group.

Geriatric Patients

Changes occur in the GI tract with aging, but some debate exists regarding whether these changes are independent of the aging process. For example, motility disorders affecting the esophagus, stomach, and intestine become more frequent with advancing age. These alterations in motility may be caused by the concomitant illnesses (e.g., cerebrovascular disease and diabetes mellitus) or medication use (e.g., anticholinergics and narcotic analgesics) commonly seen in the elderly and not necessarily represent a true deterioration in physiologic function. Alterations in absorption, such as a decrease in the absorption of carbohydrates, vitamin D, and cyanocobalamin, may also occur. Polypharmacy may initiate or exacerbate GI complaints in the elderly; thus, reducing use of medications is a goal for the pharmacist when assessing the GI system in this population.

Pregnant Patients

Pregnancy affects GI function in a variety of ways. Both early and late in pregnancy, nausea and vomiting may occur. As pregnancy progresses, abdominal organs shift to make room for the growing uterus, and this may result in heartburn and regurgitation of gastric contents, constipation, hemorrhoids, or some combination thereof.

PATHOLOGY OVERVIEW

Common GI disorders include diarrhea, constipation, peptic ulcer disease, gastroesophageal reflux disease, and inflammatory bowel disease (ulcerative colitis and Crohn's disease).

Diarrhea

Diarrhea, or an increase in the number and fluid content of bowel movements, is a common complaint from patients seeking medical attention. When diarrhea prompts the patient to seek medical care, the cause is usually infectious, food-related, drug-induced (e.g., antibiotics), or inflammatory bowel disease (discussed later).

Diarrhea is generally classified as acute or chronic, depending on the duration. Acute diarrhea is any diarrhea that continues for less than 3 weeks. Acute diarrhea typically presents with abdominal cramping, nausea, passage of watery stools, weakness, and low-grade fever. Chronic diarrhea has more serious ramifications, because it can lead to skin breakdown, dehydration, weight loss, and malnutrition. It is important to remember, however, that these complications may also occur with severe acute cases of diarrhea.

Acute diarrhea is generally mild and self-limiting, requiring no specific drug therapy. When an infectious cause is present, however, the risk of morbidity is increased, especially in very young and old patients. In these cases, such as dysentery, antibiotic therapy is indicated. The choice of antibiotic is determined by the bacterial cause; for example, dysentery caused by a *Shigella* species can be treated with oral ciprofloxacin.

Chronic diarrhea is generally a symptom of a more serious underlying pathology (e.g., inflammatory bowel disease). Treatment of the underlying cause improves the diarrhea. Stool frequency may also be controlled by use of an antidiarrheal agent such as loperamide, which is indicated for the symptomatic control of both acute and chronic diarrhea. The drug improves stool frequency as well as stool consistency through antiperistaltic action and antisecretory effects. Because loperamide is two- to threefold more potent than diphenoxylate and is not associated with significant respiratory depressant or cardiovascular effects, it is considered to be the antidiarrheal drug of choice.

Because severe diarrhea may cause dehydration, oral rehydration is generally the cornerstone of therapy. This supportive therapy may prevent morbidity in severe acute cases, especially in those patients at the extremes of age (i.e., very young or very old) or with underlying disease states. The first step is to estimate the amount of fluid loss that the patient has experienced. This can be done by calculating the patient's current weight difference (normal weight [kg] − current weight [kg] = weight loss [kg]) and remembering that 1 kg is equivalent to 1 L of fluid. This fluid deficit is then replaced during the next 4 to 6 hours using a commercial product such as Pedialyte. It is important to replace the calculated fluid deficit with an appropriate solution such as Pedialyte, which contains the electrolytes necessary to avoid imbalances. Less-expensive maintenance substitutes, such as Gatorade, decaffeinated soft drinks, and fruit juices, may then be used if desired.

A BRAT (*b*ananas, *r*ice, *a*pplesauce, *t*ea/toast) diet should be recommended to maintain nutritional status during the symptomatic period. In addition, both during and for several days after the diarrhea, adults should avoid dairy products. In most cases, children do not experience lactose intolerance, so dairy products do not have to be restricted.

Good perianal hygiene will help to avoid skin breakdown. The patient should be instructed to rinse the perineum with warm water and to pat the area dry using a cloth towel after each loose stool. If skin irritation is experienced, witch hazel pads may be applied to the area as a soothing agent.

Constipation

The normal bowel habits of people vary widely and depend on factors relating to lifestyle, including diet and exercise. A range of normal bowel habits may be the passage of one stool every 3 days for one individual up to the passage of two or three stools a day for another. This variance must be kept in mind when deciding what is normal for any one person. A change in a person's regular pattern of bowel habits may be a better indicator of a problem than the exact number of bowel movements per day.

Constipation, or the sporadic or arduous passage of stool, is usually caused by lack of exercise, inadequate intake of fluids, and inadequate intake of fiber. These factors, either together or separately, reduce colonic peristaltic movements and delay stool transit and, hence, passage. When children experience constipation, it is usually secondary to ignoring the urge to defecate, which results in infrequent or painful passage of stool.

A variety of agents, ranging from bulk-forming agents to stimulants, may be employed in treatment of constipation. Bulk-forming agents, such as psyllium products, increase the water content of stool, thus making it easier to pass. They are generally best if used on a regular basis. Stool softeners are another "prophylactic" agent, like psyllium products, and generally are more useful for the prevention of constipation rather than its treatment. Mineral oil and stimulants may be used to treat constipation but are associated with more adverse effects, such as GI cramping.

The key to prevention of constipation is nonpharmacologic. Adequate intake of fluids and fiber-containing foods, along with exercise, help a person to maintain normal bowel habits. In general, six to eight glasses of water per day are sufficient to maintain a well-hydrated stool. Bran-containing cereals and breads, along with adequate fruits and vegetables, can function as bulk-forming agents, increasing the fluid content of stool. In addition, exercise (even simple ambulation) stimulates colonic peristalsis and helps to prevent constipation.

Peptic Ulcer Disease

Peptic ulcer disease (PUD) refers to a heterogeneous group of disorders that are characterized by ulceration of the upper GI tract. The cause of the disease is related to ulceration of the mucosa by physiologic action of the acid-pepsin complex, so it can occur wherever acid and pepsin are present.

As recently as 15 years ago, almost all PUD was considered to be idiopathic. Today, specific causes can be identified for virtually every case. The consensus opinion is that infection with *Helicobacter pylori,* a Gram-negative, spiral-shaped, microaerophilic bacterium that inhabits the mucous layer of the stomach, is causally related to most cases (>90% of duodenal ulcers, >70% of gastric ulcers). Infection with *H. pylori* is common (>50% of Americans are infected by 50 years of age), yet most infected individuals do not develop ulcers. The specific risk factors that predispose infected individuals to develop PUD remain to be defined. Many older textbooks, papers, and educational handouts list a number of risk factors (e.g., stressful lifestyle and alcohol use) or findings associated with the occurrence PUD, but their relationship is now questionable in light of the relationship with *H. pylori.* The second most common cause of PUD is the use of nonsteroidal anti-inflammatory drugs (NSAIDs). Before the discovery of *H. pylori,* ulcer treatment was a lifelong commitment for most patients; however, with eradication of this pathogen, ulcer cure should be expected. Box 14-1 lists the most common signs and symptoms associated with PUD.

Medical management of PUD has changed dramatically during the past 20 years. For example, small, frequent meals and drinking of milk were once advocated. Today, however, these modalities are known to increase gastric acid output and, possibly, aggravate the ulcerative condition. With the availability of histamine$_2$-receptor antagonists (H2RAs), PUD therapy was revolutionized, and disease control became possible. Disease cure, however, was rare. Today, because of the recognition of the infectious origin of PUD, antibiotics are now the therapy of choice for most cases, and antiacid therapies (e.g., H2RAs) are combined with antibiotic therapy.

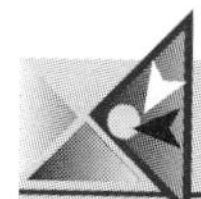

Box 14-1

COMMON SIGNS AND SYMPTOMS ASSOCIATED WITH PEPTIC ULCER DISEASE

SIGNS

- Melena (dark, sticky stools)
- Hematochezia (bright red blood in stools or on toilet paper)
- Anemia

SYMPTOMS

- Epigastric pain (primary complaint in 60%–85% of patients):
- Vague discomfort or cramping
- Burning, gnawing, or hunger-like
- Radiation to the back
- Pain that awakens the patient at night (>50% of patients)
- Pain relief with antacid use or meals
- Anorexia
- Weight loss
- Nausea and vomiting
- Belching/bloating/abdominal distention

Together, these drugs reduce recurrence and are usually curative. Long-term maintenance therapy should be discouraged for all patients except those who fail to heal after eradication of *H. pylori.* In general, triple therapy (i.e., two antibiotics [e.g., tetracycline, amoxicillin, metronidazole, or clarithromycin] combined with either a bismuth compound or omeprazole) can produce a >90% cure rate if patients take the majority of the treatment doses.

The list of possible risk factors for development of PUD is limited, but several may aggravate healing or worsen the symptomatology. Therefore, these factors should be limited to promote healing (and the efficacy of drug therapy) and to lessen the pain associated with PUD. Cigarette smoking, for example, impairs healing, promotes recurrences, and increases the risk of complications. Any limitation in smoking (in terms of the number of cigarettes per day) should be beneficial. Aspirin and NSAIDs can induce erosions and bleeding and are probably responsible for most non–*H. pylori* cases, especially gastric ulcers. Whenever possible, these agents should be discontinued in a patient with suspected PUD. Alcohol, like smoking, may complicate healing; therefore, moderation of alcohol should be stressed as well.

As stated earlier, no bland or small, frequent meals should be recommended for patients with suspected PUD. Avoiding foods that may cause dyspepsia, however, is sound advice in any individual. An increase in dietary fiber may also improve healing rates and, therefore, be appropriate as a dietary recommendation.

Gastroesophageal Reflux Disease

Gastroesophageal reflux disease (GERD) is a disorder in which gastric contents are refluxed into the esophagus. It is the most common disorder of the esophagus, producing pyrosis (i.e., heartburn) in approximately 10% to 20% of the U.S. population. Although this is one of the most common GI problems, few patients experience severe disease that requires medical therapy. The vast majority of patients can be treated periodically through dietary manipulation and over-the-counter (OTC) medications.

The pathogenesis of GERD is probably multifactorial, including one or more of the following three components: (1) patency of LES tone, (2) volume and potency of gastric contents, and (3) effectiveness of esophageal clearance. The major antireflux mechanism in humans is a normal LES pressure, which prevents reflux of gastric contents into the lower esophageal body. In the majority of patients with severe GERD, the tone or pressure of this sphincter is less than that in normal individuals and in patients with mild symptomatic disease. Therefore, most patients with GERD have a lower LES pressure, which allows gastric contents to be refluxed into the esophagus. Gastric volume can also affect reflux episodes: the greater the gastric volume, the greater the number of LES relaxations. This greater number of LES relaxations in turn promotes reflux episodes. The gastric contents also contain acid and pepsin, which are the agents primarily responsible for the epithelial irritation and erosion associated with GERD.

In both persons with GERD and persons without symptomatic disease, esophageal clearance determines the duration of esophageal exposure to any gastric contents that are refluxed. With impaired esophageal motility, the refluxate is in contact with the esophageal mucosa for a greater period of time, increasing the likelihood of esophageal mucosal injury.

Several risk factors are known to predispose one to episodes of reflux; these are listed in Box 14-2. The common signs and symptoms that can be seen when a patient presents with GERD are listed in Box 14-3.

Generally, GERD is a chronic condition that is characterized by recurrent symptoms and, therefore, may require long-term or maintenance therapy to prevent symptomatic recurrences or development of complications. When approaching the symptomatic treatment of GERD, one may visualize a pyramid (Fig. 14-3), in which the vast majority of patients experience minor, intermittent symptoms that may be easily treated with periodic administration of an OTC antacid or H2RA. Those patients with continued symptoms require referral for a prescription medication, but only a small number of all symptomatic patients require long-term maintenance therapy.

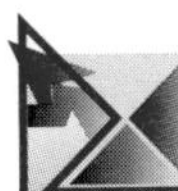

Box 14-2

POTENTIAL FACTORS RELATED TO DEVELOPMENT OR EXACERBATION OF GASTROESOPHAGEAL REFLUX DISEASE

DIETARY

- Large meals and eating before bedtime (increase gastric volume)
- Dietary fat (slows gastric emptying and decreases LES tone)
- Chocolate, alcohol, and caffeine (decrease LES tone)
- Peppermint (decreases LES tone)

MEDICATIONS[a]

- α-Adrenergic antagonists
- Calcium-channel antagonists
- β-adrenergic agonists
- Anticholinergics
- Theophylline
- Morphine and meperidine
- Benzodiazepines
- Barbiturates

MISCELLANEOUS

- Tight clothing (increases intra-abdominal pressure and promotes reflux)
- Pregnancy (increases intra-abdominal pressure and promotes reflux)

LES, lower esophageal sphincter.
[a]All decrease LES tone.

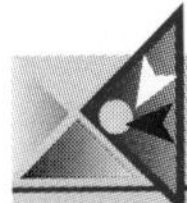

Box 14-3

COMMON SIGNS AND SYMPTOMS ASSOCIATED WITH GASTROESOPHAGEAL REFLUX DISEASE

SIGNS (AND COMPLICATIONS)

- Stricture (10% of severe cases)
- Hemorrhage or perforation (rare)
- Anemia (from insidious blood loss secondary to persistent ulcerations)

SYMPTOMS

- Pyrosis:
  - Heartburn (primary complaint)
  - Retrosternal burning and discomfort
- Intermittent retrosternal chest pain (major cause of noncardiac chest pain)
- Regurgitation
- Dysphagia (swallowing difficulties)
- Respiratory symptoms:
  - Caused by regurgitation and aspiration
  - Morning hoarseness
  - Pneumonitis
  - Asthma-like complaints (wheezing and chest tightness)

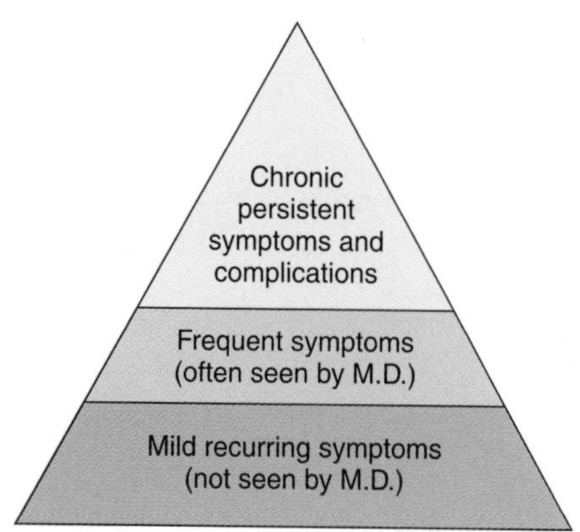

FIGURE 14-3 ■ The gastroesophageal reflux disease pyramid.

One therapeutic approach to GERD is illustrated in Box 14-4. Step one includes nonpharmacologic therapy and may be sufficient to treat some patients with minor, intermittent reflux symptoms. If nonpharmacologic therapy alone is insufficient (i.e., if symptoms recur), OTC therapy should be added to the nonpharmacologic measures. If symptoms are still problematic, the patient should be referred for prescription therapy. A 4- to 8-week trial of a full-strength H2RA may be initiated if the patient is not severely symptomatic and erosive esophagitis is not suspected. If the patient is severely symptomatic or erosive esophagitis is suspected (or confirmed), then the therapy of choice is a proton-pump inhibitor, such as omeprazole, for 4 to 8 weeks of therapy. At the end of the 4- to 8-week trial period, and if the patient is asymptomatic, termination of therapy may be attempted. If symptoms recur or were not controlled during the initial 4- to 8-week trial, then maintenance therapy is indicated. For mild to moderate recurrent disease, a prokinetic agent, such as metoclopramide or cisapride, may be sufficient; for severe recurrent disease, long-term therapy with a proton-pump inhibitor is safe, effective, and the therapy of first choice.

Nonpharmacologic therapy can be useful in the treatment of GERD and should be instituted both before and concurrently with drug therapy to maximize therapeutic efficacy. Box 14-4 delineates these modalities. The first step includes dietary manipulation, such as those risk factors for GERD listed previously (e.g., eating smaller meals, avoiding snacks before sleeping, and avoiding foods that can decrease the LES), as well as increasing the head of the bed using 6-inch wooden blocks to lessen nighttime reflux. Wearing loose clothing decreases intra-abdominal pressure and may decrease episodes of reflux. Chewing gum or sucking on hard candies increases salivation and may also improve esophageal clearance. A pharmacist-specific intervention is adjusting a patient's drug regimen to avoid medications that can decrease the LES (Box 14-2). For example, calcium-channel antagonists may decrease the LES, which promotes reflux. Recommending a change in therapy to a β-adrenergic antagonist, when appropriate, can improve LES tone and decrease episodes of reflux.

Inflammatory Bowel Disease

The two major divisions of inflammatory bowel disease (IBD) are Crohn's disease and ulcerative colitis. **Crohn's disease** is a chronic inflammatory process involving any portion of the GI tract from the mouth to the anus and is transmural in nature, in that the bowel inflammation affects all layers of the GI wall. Crohn's disease most commonly affects the distal ileum and colon. Also, "skip" lesions are common, in that normal or unaffected bowel occurs between areas of disease. Unlike Crohn's disease, the inflammatory process in **ulcerative colitis** is superficial, affecting the mucosa and submucosa of the colon only, and is not transmural in nature. The rectum and descending colon are the areas affected most, but the disease can affect the entire colon. Ulcerative colitis does not affect the GI tract outside the large bowel, however. The lesions are diffuse, with no "skip" areas of normal or unaffected tissue between them. Like Crohn's disease, ulcerative colitis is chronic, being characterized by symptomatic exacerbations.

The exact cause or combination of factors responsible for development of Crohn's disease is unknown. Also, whether Crohn's disease and ulcerative colitis are truly separate disease states or just different manifestations of the same disease is also unknown. Both share similar potential causes.

Box 14-4

ONE THERAPEUTIC APPROACH TO GASTROESOPHAGEAL REFLUX DISEASE

STEP 1: NONPHARMACOLOGIC THERAPY

- Dietary manipulation (avoid fat, chocolate, and caffeine)
- Increase the head of the bed
- Suck on hard candies, or chew gum
- Avoid drugs affecting the lower esophageal sphincter α-adrenergic antagonists)

STEP 2: OVER-THE-COUNTER MEDICATIONS

- Antacids
- Histamine$_2$-receptor antagonists (Zantac 75)
- Alginic acid (Gaviscon)

STEP 3: DECREASING ACID PRODUCTION

- Full-strength histamine$_2$-receptor antagonists (famotidine, 20 mg BID)
- Proton-pump inhibitors (omeprazole, 20 mg QD)

STEP 4: LONG-TERM MAINTENANCE THERAPY

- Prokinetic agents:
  - Metoclopramide, 10 mg QID, AC and HS
  - Cisapride, 10 mg QID, AC and HS
  - More appropriate for recurrent, mild to moderate disease
- Proton-pump inhibitors:
  - Omeprazole, 20 mg QD
  - Lansoprazole may also be used
  - More appropriate for recurrent, severe disease

AC: before meals; HS: at bedtime.

The most likely factors in the development of IBD are an infectious agent or an immunologic cause. An infectious cause for IBD has been sought because some microorganisms produce similar granulomatous diseases in animals. For example, one group of bacteria that has been implicated as a possible cause are the mycobacteria, because *Mycobacterium paratuberculosis* produces a similar disease in goats and several species of mycobacteria have been isolated from patients with Crohn's disease or ulcerative colitis. These findings are not consistent, however, and no causal relationship has been conclusively demonstrated.

Because many inflammatory cells (e.g., lymphocytes, plasma cells, and mast cells) are present in the GI wall when affected by IBD and immunosuppressive therapy (i.e., glucocorticoids) control symptomatic exacerbations, an immunologic cause in the pathogenesis of IBD is likely. Whether IBD is an immunologic response to a microorganism antigen or a genetic or acquired aberration in immunity secondary to an antigen induces the inflammation is not known, but both seem plausible. Emotional, psychologic, or dietary factors may play a role in symptomatic exacerbations, but alone, these factors are probably not responsible for IBD.

Because of both familial and ethnic/racial clustering, an inheritable predisposition to development of IBD may exist. Other risk factors for development remain to be defined. The common signs and symptoms that can be seen when a patient with IBD presents are listed in Box 14-5.

Unlike ulcerative colitis, in which a total colectomy is curative, Crohn's disease is chronic in nature, and remissions in disease activity can occur spontaneously or be induced by drug therapy. During acute exacerbations, pharmacologic intervention remains the therapy of choice. Anti-inflammatory or immunosuppressive therapy to control disease manifestations are most effective. Sulfasalazine and the newer 5-aminosalicylic acid (5-ASA) derivatives are currently the first-line therapy, secondary to the long-term complications associated with glucocorticoids, the second-line therapy. The 5-ASA derivatives are generally most effective for ileocecal involvement and are first-line agents for mild to moderate symptomatic flares. If a patient does not respond to several weeks of therapy with one of these agents, then glucocorticoids are used. During severe exacerbations, glucocorticoids become the agents of choice. In severely ill patients, intravenous administration is used.

If the 5-ASA derivatives and a glucocorticoid (e.g., prednisone) fail to induce a remission, or if steroid requirements cannot be tapered to a desirable dose, then treatment with azathioprine or the active metabolite 6-mercaptopurine may be instituted. These agents are thought to suppress T-cell function and, thereby, to lessen bowel inflammation. Maintenance therapy with either the 5-ASA derivatives or steroids has not been shown to prevent recurrences of disease flares and, therefore, is not indicated in the treatment of Crohn's disease.

Management of Crohn's disease involves maintenance of the patient's nutritional status, supportive therapy (including symptomatic treatment), as well as anti-inflammatory and immunosuppressive therapy (discussed earlier). Nutritional therapy can help to control diarrhea as well as to replete vitamin, calcium, iron, and protein losses. A lactose-free diet may also help to control diarrhea in some progressive cases in which lactose intolerance develops. During acute exacerbations, bowel rest, incorporating parenteral nutrition therapy, may be necessary. Antidiarrheal agents may aid in reducing stool frequency and abdominal cramps and in restoring one's activities of daily living. Currently, loperamide is the therapy of first choice.

The treatment of ulcerative colitis is similar to that of Crohn's disease. The 5-ASA derivatives, glucocorticoids, fluid and electrolyte therapy, nutritional support, and supportive therapy, including antidiarrheals, all play a role in controlling exacerbations. Unlike Crohn's disease, however, maintenance therapy in patients with ulcerative colitis prolongs remissions. Currently, sulfasalazine is the therapy of choice. Other forms of 5-ASA are probably as effective as sulfasalazine for maintenance therapy, but clinical experience is somewhat limited. Therefore, other agents should be used only if the patient is intolerant to sulfasalazine. A total colectomy is curative and repeals the risk of colon cancer, a major concern in ulcerative colitis. Other therapeutic modalities are the same as those for Crohn's disease.

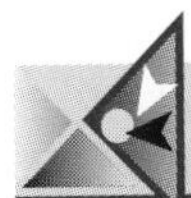

Box 14-5

COMMON SIGNS AND SYMPTOMS ASSOCIATED WITH INFLAMMATORY BOWEL DISEASE

SIGNS

- Fever
- Abdominal mass (focal granuloma)
- Weight loss
- Less common signs:
  - Hypoalbuminemia
  - Vitamin deficiencies
  - Loss of calcium, magnesium, and zinc
  - Anemia
  - Leukocytosis and thrombocytosis
  - Fistula
  - Extraintestinal manifestations:
    - Pyoderma gangrenosum
    - Erythema nodosum and stomatitis
    - Ankylosing spondylitis and sacrolitis
    - Arthritis of large joints

SYMPTOMS

- Diarrhea
- Abdominal pain
- Malaise
- Rectal bleeding

SYSTEM ASSESSMENT

Subjective Information

Gastrointestinal problems account for many of the reasons why patients, especially the elderly, seek health care. With the move to OTC status for H2RAs, the potential for patients to attempt self-treatment for a serious medical problem now exists. Therefore, questioning why patients are seeking medical care or OTC products may be exceedingly important in the pharmacist's evaluation. The following are the most frequently encountered symptoms related to the GI tract, and each should be included in any interview assessing this body system.

Abdominal Pain

Abdominal discomfort is one of the most common GI complaints, because most abdominal diseases manifest with some degree of pain. Questioning the patient about this discomfort can elicit clues regarding the origin of the pain secondary to the relationship between the pain location and the pathology of underlying structures. For example:

- Pain in the epigastrium:
  - Stomach: gastric ulcer
  - Duodenum: duodenal ulcer
  - Gallbladder: cholecystitis
  - Liver: hepatitis
  - Pancreas: pancreatitis
- Pain in the substernal area:
  - Esophagus: gastroesophageal reflux
- Pain near the umbilicus:
  - Small intestine: obstruction or Crohn's disease
- Pain in the hypogastrium:
  - Colon: Crohn's disease, ulcerative colitis, or diverticulitis

? INTERVIEW Tell me more about your pain. When did the pain start? Does the pain come and go, or is it a steady, constant pain? Did the pain have a sudden onset, or did it begin gradually? Describe the pain? Is it knife-like, burning, or cramping? Show me where the pain is. Has this pain moved at all, or has it always been in this spot? Is this the only spot that hurts, or do you have pain anywhere else with it? How often do you have this pain? What makes the pain worse or better? Did you eat any specific foods before the pain began? With this pain, do you experience nausea or vomiting, sweating, bowel changes like diarrhea, or abdominal bloating? Any other symptoms? Are you taking any medications for the pain? Do they help? What other medications are you taking? What over-the-counter medications are you taking? Do you have any allergies?

ABNORMALITIES

Onset	Possible Association
Gradual	Infection
Acute	Perforation
	Torsion of abdominal structure
	Pancreatitis
	Rupture of an ectopic pregnancy

Location	Possible Association
Diffuse	Rupture or perforation of abdominal structure
Localized	Epigastric (PUD or pancreatitis)
Relocation	Umbilical to right lower quadrant

Characteristics	Possible Association
Knife-like	Pancreatitis
Burning	PUD
Cramping	Biliary or renal colic

Concurrent Symptoms	Possible Association
With vomiting	Pancreatitis or rupture/perforation of abdominal structure
With diarrhea	IBD
Rectal bleeding	IBD

Because most pain treated with OTC agents is midepigastric, specific delineation of this complaint is necessary:

? INTERVIEW Do you smoke? Does food affect the pain? Does the pain occur just after meals or hours later? Do you experience pain at night? Does the pain wake you up at night? Is the pain worse when you lie down? Do you drink alcoholic beverages? If so, how often? Do you have dark, sticky stools? What medications, both over-the-counter and prescription, do you take?

ABNORMALITIES

Food	Possible Association
Soon after eating	Gastric ulcer
Hours after eating	Duodenal ulcer

Position	Possible Association
Lying down	GERD

Medications	Possible Association
Ibuprofen/aspirin	PUD

Nausea and Vomiting

Nausea is usually a nonspecific indicator, whereas vomiting is more common with specific abdominal illnesses. If nausea and vomiting are present for approximately 1 week or the vomitus contains blood, the patient should be referred to a diagnostician for further evaluation.

? INTERVIEW How long have you been experiencing the nausea or vomiting? When did it begin? Was it associated with any particular meals or foods? What does the vomited material look like? What does the material smell like? Do you have any abdominal pain with or before the vomiting? Do you have a fever? Are you also experiencing diarrhea?

ABNORMALITIES

Finding	Possible Association
Vomiting	Gastroenteritis, bile duct obstruction, intestinal obstruction, or rupture/perforation of abdominal structure
Nausea	Pregnancy, hepatopancreatic disease, or malignancies

Vomitus	Possible Association
Fecal (smell)	Intestinal obstruction
Blood	PUD
Stomach contents	Gastritis
Greenish fluid	Biliary colic

Pain with Vomiting	Possible Association
Before	Appendicitis or cholecystitis
During	Obstructions

Change in Bowel Habits

Like abdominal pain, changes in bowel habits (e.g., diarrhea or constipation) are frequent complaints for which patients seek OTC products. A thorough history will help the pharmacist to determine if a physician referral is necessary. In general, if the diarrhea/constipation has been present for approximately 1 week or there is evidence of bleeding in the stool or on the toilet paper, the patient should be referred for further evaluation.

? INTERVIEW For those complaining of diarrhea, ask the following questions: How long have you been experiencing the diarrhea? When did it begin? What makes it better or worse? Does it occur after eating? Describe the stools. Are they watery or just loose? Is a copious amount present? Is blood or mucus present? Does the stool float? Do you also experience fever? Chills? Increased thirst? Abdominal pain or cramping? Have you traveled recently? Have you taken any antibiotics recently? Have you lost any weight recently? What prescription medications are you taking? What over-the-counter medications are you taking?

ABNORMALITIES

Acute Onset	Possible Association
After meal	Infection, ingested toxin, or lactose intolerance
Bloody	Shigellosis or amebiasis

Chronic Onset	Possible Association
Bloody	Ulcerative colitis
Mucus	Ulcerative colitis
Watery	Small bowel inflammation (Crohn's disease)
Floating	Malabsorptive states (e.g., chronic pancreatitis)
Weight loss	IBD or carcinoma of the colon
Recent antibiotic use	*Clostridium difficile* toxin

? INTERVIEW For those complaining of constipation, ask the following questions: How long have you been experiencing constipation? When was your last bowel movement? What makes it better or worse? What does the stool look like? What color is the stool? Is any blood present? Any mucus? Do you experience both diarrhea and constipation, back and forth? Any abdominal pain with the passage of the stool? What is the size of the stool? Is the stool thin? Has there been a recent change in its size? Any recent changes in your diet? Have you lost any weight recently? What prescription medications are you taking? What OTC medications are you taking?

 **ABNORMALITIES**

Characteristics	Possible Association
Oscillating with diarrhea	Carcinoma of the colon or diverticular disease
Chalky white stool	Hepatobiliary obstruction
Thin	Carcinoma of the colon
Increase in high-fiber foods	Dietary induced
Blood	Carcinoma of the colon
Weight loss	Carcinoma of the colon

Objective Information

Objective information used during assessment of the GI system includes the physical examination results, laboratory data, and data generated from diagnostic tests.

Physical Assessment

Pharmacists rarely perform physical examination of the abdomen, but while assessing the patient and his or her medications, pharmacists do routinely use data that other health care professionals obtain through the physical examination. The physical examination of the abdomen typically includes, in the following order, inspection, auscultation, percussion, and finally, palpation. After voiding the bladder (a full bladder may alter abdominal findings and make the examination process uncomfortable for the patient), the patient is asked to lie in a supine position that is relaxed and has the arms at the sides (so that flexed abdominal muscles do not interfere with the examination process). The clinician is positioned at the patient's right side.

Physical examination findings are generally recorded in terms of their location on the abdomen as divided into four or nine areas; most clinicians use the four-division approach (Fig. 14-4). By dividing the abdomen into four quadrants, objective findings can be communicated to other health care professionals in a consistent manner.

TECHNIQUE

STEP I

Inspect the Abdomen

Inspect the skin of the abdomen. Look at the color, texture, vascularity, and contour. In most normal patients without disease, the color should be harmonious and nonicteric, or not yellowish (i.e., jaundice), in appearance. The texture should be smooth and usually without striae, the vascularity barely appreciable, and the contour of the belly flat or evenly rounded with

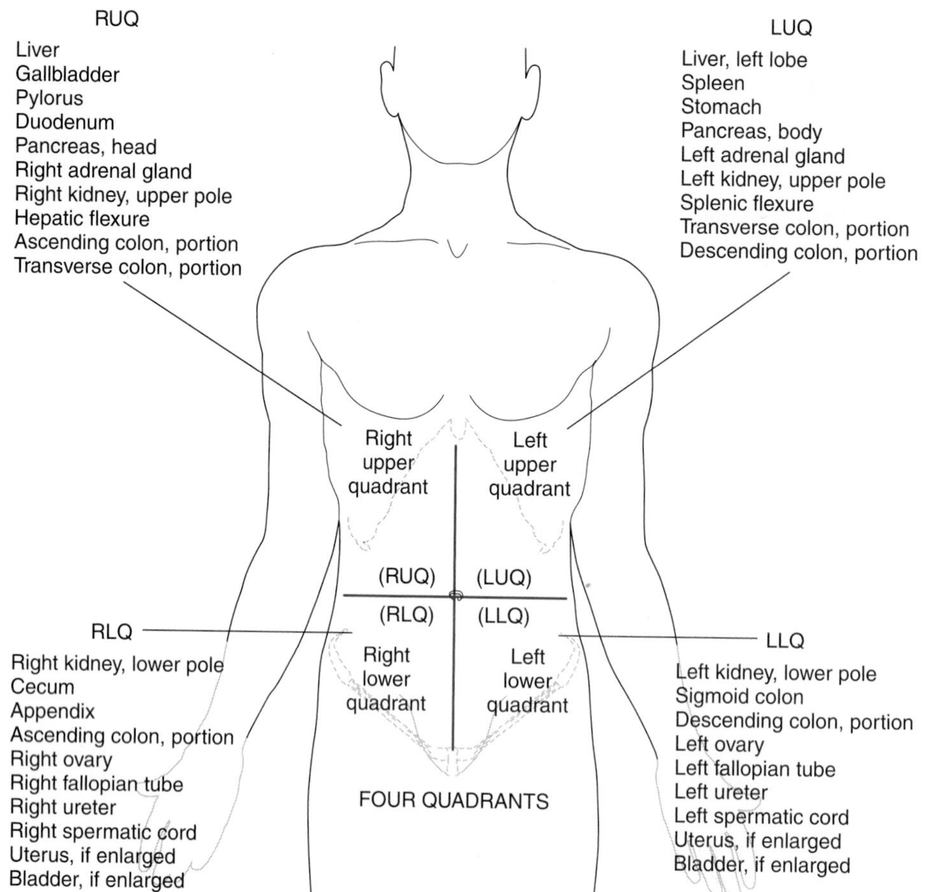

FIGURE 14-4 ■ The four quadrants of the abdomen, including the associated anatomic structures.

the maximum height at the umbilicus. No distention should be present. No masses or nodules should be visible. The umbilicus should be centrally located and without protrusions or swelling.

ABNORMALITIES In a person who is lightly pigmented, yellowing of the skin (i.e., icterus or jaundice) can be noted with hepatic disease; in a person with darker pigmentation, the sclera of the eye will be jaundiced. Spider angiomas, which are small, vascular lesions with a central spot and vascular "legs" extending from this center, are a frequent finding in those with hepatic disease and collagen vascular disease. Ascites, or free fluid in the abdomen, may also be present in patients with significant hepatic disease and some carcinomas. With tense ascites, the skin appears taut and shiny. Other abnormal findings include striae, or "stretch marks," which may result from pregnancy, weight gain, or Cushing's disease. Box 14-6 lists frequent causes of abdominal distention.

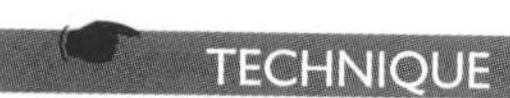

STEP 2

Auscultate the Abdomen

Auscultation is used to assess bowel motility and vascular sounds. It is performed before percussion and palpation when examining the abdomen because of the risk that manipulating the abdomen through percussion and palpation may alter bowel motility (and, hence, bowel sounds) and interfere with auscultatory findings.

- Place the diaphragm of the stethoscope lightly on the midabdomen, near the level of the umbilicus (Fig. 14-5).
- Listen for bowel sounds, noting their frequency and character. Bowel sounds are usually high-pitched (hence the diaphragm) emanations that are heard as clicks and gurgles, occurring randomly, in the range of 5 to 20 per minute.

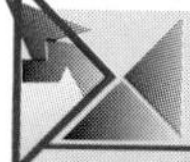

Box 14-6

FREQUENT FINDINGS AS CAUSES OF ABDOMINAL DISTENTION

- Fat (obesity)
- Fluid (ascites)
- Fetus (pregnancy)
- Flatus (gas)
- Feces (stool)
- Fibroid (tumor/mass)

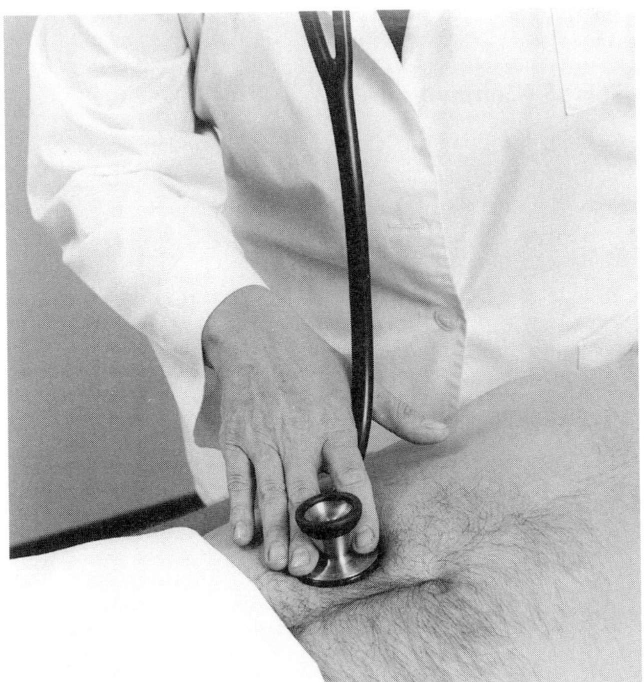

FIGURE 14-5 ■ Auscultation of bowel sounds.

Sounds are produced by the physiologic passage of fluid and gasses through the intestinal tract.

- Place the diaphragm of the stethoscope on all four abdominal quadrants, repeating the previous step.

ABNORMALITIES Abnormal sounds of clinical importance when you listen to the abdomen include those from friction rubs (peritoneal inflammation), arteries (bruits from stenosis of the renal artery or the abdominal aorta), veins (venous hum associated with collateral development in portal hypertension), and peristalsis (hyperactive bowel sounds [GI bleeding] or absence of bowel sounds [ileus]). Increased or hyperactive bowel sounds are common findings in patients with GI bleeding (usually from an upper GI source). Absence of bowel sounds is associated with a paralytic ileus (i.e., cessation of the peristaltic movement through the small bowel), which may result from many causes, ranging from hypokalemia in combination with drugs having anticholinergic effects to a physiologic ileus induced by peritonitis. Friction rubs are best heard over the liver and spleen during inspiration, indicating some inflammatory reaction affecting that organ (e.g., viral hepatitis).

TECHNIQUE

STEP 2 (Continued)

Listen over the renal arteries, iliac arteries, and femoral arteries (Fig. 14-6) for vascular bruits or adventitious (acquired) vascular sounds heard on auscultation as blowing/purring sounds.

ABNORMALITIES Bruits are caused by turbulence in a partially obstructed artery.

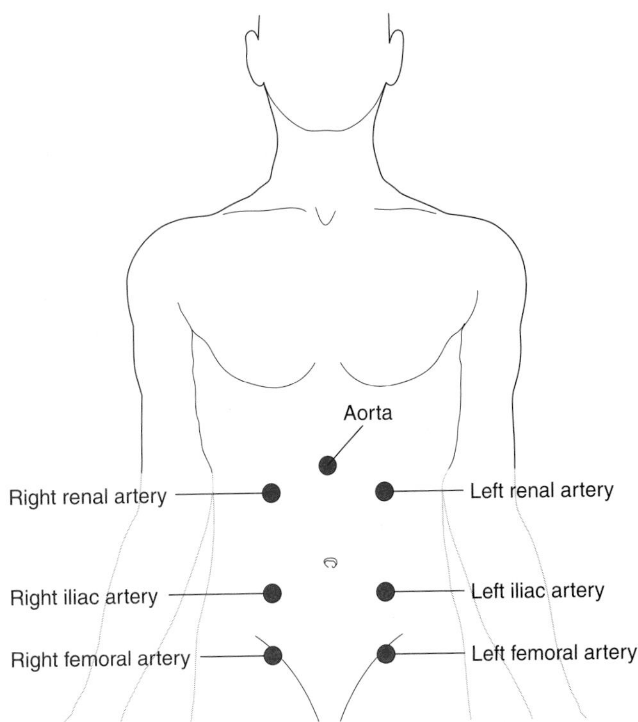

FIGURE 14-6 ■ The abdominal locations for auscultating bruits.

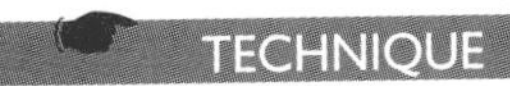

STEP 3

Percuss the Abdomen

The abdomen is percussed to rule out the presence of fluid, gaseous distention, and masses and to evaluate the location and size of the major solid organs.

- Lightly percuss the entire abdomen to obtain an overall assessment of the tympany and dullness (Fig. 14-7). Tympany should predominate secondary to gas present in the stomach, small bowel, and colon. Dullness is usually heard only over organs and, if present, solid masses or a full bladder.

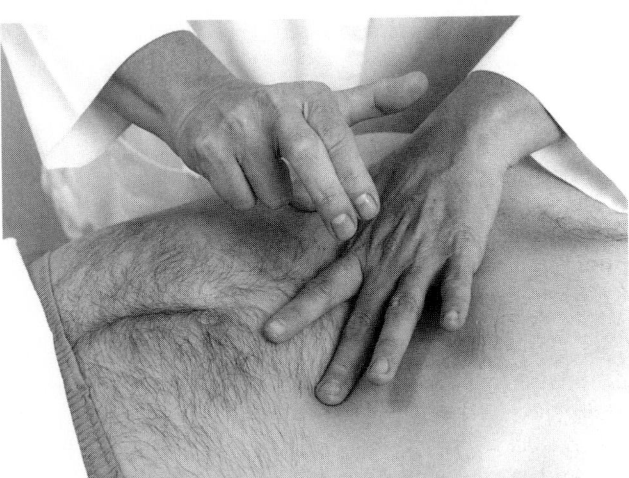

FIGURE 14-7 ■ General percussion of the abdomen.

- Percuss the liver to evaluate the organ size. (For a detailed discussion of percussing the liver, see Chapter 15.)

STEP 4 Test for "Shifting Dullness"

Ascites (i.e., effusion and collection of serous fluid in the abdominal cavity) can be differentiated from simple edema through the test for "shifting dullness."

- Percuss the abdomen laterally to medially while the patient is supine. If ascites is present, a dullness will be heard over the fluid in the flank area, because of gravity, and a tympany will be heard above or medial to this flank area, representing the gas-filled bowel (near the umbilicus).
- Mark the border between the dullness and tympany, which is usually just medial to the costal margins.
- Instruct the patient to lie on one side, and repeat the procedure. If ascites is present, a shifting of dullness will have occurred. Gravity will cause the fluid to flow down toward the dependent side, and the area of dullness will move higher, toward the umbilicus. Thus, a "shifting" occurs in which the area around the umbilicus that was initially tympanic (in the supine position) becomes dull (in the side position) because of the movement of free fluid. This will not occur in patients with simple abdominal wall edema or swelling from another cause (cystic or tumor masses).

STEP 5

Palpate the Abdomen

Palpation may be performed independently of or simultaneously with percussion to authenticate or confirm suspicions identified during the initial portion of the examination. Palpation provides specific organ information (e.g., size, shape, position, consistency, tension, and mobility) and identifies areas of tenderness and muscle spasms or the presence of fluid and masses. The patient must be relaxed as possible, because contraction of the abdominal muscles interferes with this assessment more than with any other technique. All four quadrants are assessed, using both light and deep palpation, but the clinician always begins with light palpation away from any area of known pain to minimize guarding on the part of the patient (see *Abnormal Findings* for this step). Light palpation is used to identify areas of tenderness and muscle resistance.

- Using the palm of the hand with fingers extended and approximated, palpate all four quadrants, depressing the abdominal wall with the finger pads no more than 1 cm. This should be a fluid process, lifting from area to area without short jab motions or digging. The process of light palpation is illustrated in Figure 14-8A.

ABNORMALITIES With light palpation, areas of even mild tenderness can be detected. Abdominal tenderness may cause the patient to "guard" the area, flexing the muscles to protect the underlying tenderness. This guarding can be both voluntary and involuntary; the latter is commonly associated with the presence of peritoneal inflammation.

TECHNIQUE

STEP 5 (Continued)

- Using the same process as described for light palpation, continue to assess all four quadrants, except now press with moderate pressure. With the added pressure, areas not previously perceived as being tender or masses smaller in size may be noted. Some clinicians suggest using the side of the hand when performing this deeper palpation to avoid "finger jabbing."
- Deep palpation is used to further delineate organ structure and consistency and to identify less apparent masses. Using the palmar surface of the fingers, press smoothly and evenly into the abdomen (Fig. 14-8B). One may use just the right hand (for right-handed individuals), or the left hand may be placed over the right, in which case the left hand is used to exert pressure.

ABNORMALITIES During deep palpation in patients with abdominal tenderness, rebound tenderness is usually elicited. Rebound tenderness indicates peritoneal irritation. To elicit this symptom, the clinician palpates deeply and slowly in an area distal to the suspected site of pathology. The hand is then quickly withdrawn; if rebound tenderness is present, the patient will experience a sharp pain on the side where the localized inflammation is present at this time. Although frequently performed, some clinicians have abandoned this practice because, if rebound tenderness is present, significant patient discomfort is produced, which may be accompanied by muscle spasm that interferes with any further examination. If performed, the maneuver should be reserved until the end of the examination process. Abdominal masses may be caused by various carcinomas or cystic diseases.

CAUTION **It is important to visualize the underlying structures when performing deep palpation. This makes it less likely that normal abdominal structures will be mistaken for abnormal findings.**

Laboratory and Diagnostic Tests

Both laboratory data and diagnostic tests are frequently used to evaluate the GI system. Laboratory tests include those to detect *H. pylori* infection and to assess the pancreas.

Helicobacter pylori

The simplest method to determine the presence of *H. pylori* is a serologic test that detects immunoglobulin G antibodies against the organism. The test will be positive in anyone with acute infection, and it will remain positive for months after therapy. Therefore, a repeated antibody titer after eradication therapy is not helpful in assessing the adequacy of therapy. Serology can be repeated at 3 and 6 months after eradication therapy; if titers have dropped by at least 50% and continue to decline between the 3- and 6-month measurements, a cure has probably been attained.

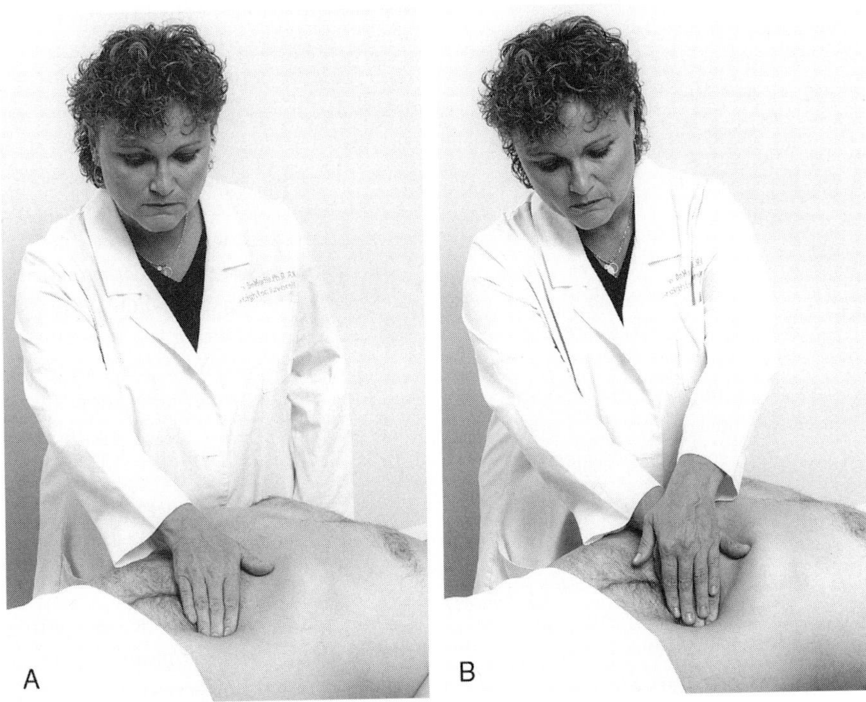

FIGURE 14-8 ■ Palpation of the abdomen. **(A)** Light palpation. **(B)** Deep palpation.

An alternative, less-used method is the breath test, which can be used shortly after drug therapy to assess its effectiveness. *Helicobacter pylori* contains urease. Therefore, radiolabeled urea can be given by mouth, and if the organism is present, the radiolabeled urea will be broken down to radiolabeled carbon dioxide, which can be readily detected in the patient's exhaled air. Currently, office use of this test is limited.

Pancreas

With acute pancreatitis, two laboratory tests can be used to confirm a diagnosis: the serum amylase concentration, and the serum lipase concentration. Both are pancreatic enzymes that are released into the serum with pancreatic inflammation. In acute pancreatitis, the amylase concentration begins to rise 2 to 6 hours after symptoms begin, and the concentration peaks at 12 to 30 hours. Serum lipase elevations roughly parallel serum amylase elevations in acute pancreatitis. Lipase is less sensitive than amylase but is more specific for pancreas inflammation; therefore, it can be used on a confirmatory basis.

Major Diagnostic Tests

Four major diagnostic tests are used in assessing GI diseases: (1) endoscopy, (2) radiography with contrast dye, (3) sonography (ultrasound), and (4) computed tomography. Endoscopy is the use of a fiberoptic instrument to visualize the lumen of the GI tract, both upper and lower (colonoscopy). It can be used to visually establish a diagnosis (e.g., duodenal ulcer or colon cancer) as well as for culturing the GI tract (e.g., *H. pylori*). Endoscopy can also be used for treating GI bleeds through methods such as direct-injection sclerotherapy. Radiography with contrast dye (i.e., barium), which is commonly called a barium swallow, evaluates the esophagus. Ultrasound is used to noninvasively visualize GI structures and to confirm a diagnosis. Common structures visualized include the gallbladder and pancreas. Computed tomography can be used to diagnose numerous ailments affecting the GI tract, including liver disease, pancreatic disease, and colonic disorders (e.g., carcinoma).

Special Considerations

Pediatric Patients

Pediatric patients require additional specific questions to be asked of the parent or guardian.

? INTERVIEW In relation to abdominal pain, does the child attempt to resist abdominal movement? Does the child keep the knees flexed? In relation to constipation, how well is the child toilet-trained? What does the child's typical diet include?

➤ ABNORMALITIES Fear of toilet training and diet (e.g., poor fluid intake) may predispose this age group to constipation.

The physical examination of the pediatric patient is similar to that of the adult patient, except for some minor points. In general, the patient may be more fearful, and placing the pediatric patient at ease and explaining what is or will be happening is even more important. In addition, the kidneys may be identified with deep palpation in children.

Geriatric Patients

Geriatric patients also require additional specific questions to be asked of the patient or caregiver.

? INTERVIEW Have you been experiencing any fecal incontinence? What medications do you take? How much water do you drink per day? How many meals do you eat per day? Do you eat fruit and vegetables? Are you able to ambulate? If so, how much?

ABNORMALITIES Elderly patients frequently take a number of medications that can interfere with normal bowel function; those with anticholinergic effects are most common. Lack of fluid intake and mobility are the two greatest risk factors for constipation in this population. In addition, socioeconomic factors may lead to elderly persons eating smaller, less frequent meals without the proper amount of fruits and vegetables to maintain nutrition and normal GI function.

Elderly patients may have fewer or more mild symptoms on presentation than a younger patient with the same GI problem. Therefore, the clinician must be diligent in his or her interview and physical examination when evaluating older patients. "Silent" GI pathology in elderly persons is associated with significant morbidity, so maintaining a degree of wariness or suspicion may be prudent during the examination.

Pregnant Patients

Interview questions for the pregnant patient should attempt to differentiate common GI complaints during pregnancy (e.g., nausea, vomiting, heartburn, constipation, and hemorrhoids) from those that may be less common.

? INTERVIEW In relation to abdominal pain, where does it hurt? Describe the pain. Is it a burning sensation, or is it a sharp pain? How many weeks along is your pregnancy? Are you experiencing any nausea and vomiting? If so, how much, and how often? Are you experiencing any diarrhea or constipation?

ABNORMALITIES Pain may be experienced in different abdominal regions secondary to pregnancy. Stretching of muscles and ligaments may cause sharp abdominal pain (especially pain that intensifies with movement) or cramping (similar to premenstrual cramping). Severe vomiting may lead to dehydration and, thus, should be monitored by a physician. Frequent constipation may lead to hemorrhoids. High-fiber foods (e.g., whole grains as well as fresh or frozen fruits and vegetables) should be consumed daily to avoid constipation.

Although rarely performed in their practice, pharmacists need to understand the influences of pregnancy on a physical examination. Inspection, percussion, and palpation changes are common in pregnant patients. Women who have given birth may have pinkish to white striae (i.e., stretch marks) associated with the current or previous pregnancies. During percussion, if the uterus is enlarged, a dullness may be appreciated over the suprapubic area. During late pregnancy, the abdominal swelling associated with pregnancy may shift the liver upward, thus interfering with "normal" percussion. Also, during deep palpation, the uterus may be felt as a mass and mistaken for an abnormal finding if the pregnancy is not known or suspected.

APPLICATION TO PATIENT SYMPTOMS

Because they typically practice in a setting where the patient presents with a specific symptom or complaint, pharmacists must be able to assess the severity of the complaint, to identify the most probable cause, and to determine the best course of action. Possible corrective actions include referral to another health care professional for further evaluation, treatment using the current or newly recommended drug regimen, or addition of an OTC agent. Common symptoms of the GI tract include abdominal pain, nausea with or without vomiting, and change in bowel habits, including frequency and presence of blood.

Abdominal Pain

Abdominal pain can be caused by many pathologic processes, as illustrated in Box 14-7, because most abdominal diseases manifest with some degree of pain. In the pharmacist's practice setting, most patients present complaining of midepigastric pain, which is described as a vague discomfort or as cramping, burning, gnawing, or hunger-like. The majority of patients state that the pain awakens them at night, and most also state some relief from antacid use or eating. Nonspecific symptoms may be anorexia, weight loss, related nausea, and feelings of bloating or abdominal distention. Objective signs include indications of GI bleeding (e.g., presence of melena, hematochezia, or mild anemia on laboratory reports), hyperactive bowel sounds heard during auscultation, and mild midepigastric tenderness noted during percussion and palpation. A medication history may identify drugs commonly associated with PUD and GERD (Box 14-8).

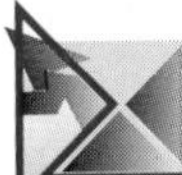

Box 14-7

COMMON PATHOLOGIC CAUSES OF ABDOMINAL PAIN

- Appendicitis
- Ascites
- Cholelithiasis
- Colon cancer
- Crohn's disease
- Diverticulitis
- Gastroesophageal reflux disease
- GI obstruction
- Hepatic cirrhosis
- Hepatitis
- Hepatosplenomegaly
- Kidney infection
- Kidney stones
- Liver cancer
- Ovarian cyst
- Pancreatitis
- Peptic ulcer disease
- Peritonitis
- Pregnancy
- Splenectomy
- Ulcerative colitis
- Urinary tract infection

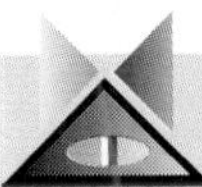

Box 14-8

MEDICATIONS (AND OTHER FACTORS) THAT COMMONLY CAUSE MIDEPIGASTRIC PAIN AND PEPTIC ULCER DISEASE OR SYMPTOMATIC GASTROESOPHAGEAL REFLUX DISEASE

PEPTIC ULCER DISEASE

- Nonsteroidal anti-inflammatory drugs
- Salicylates
- Alcohol
- Cigarette smoking

GASTROESOPHAGEAL REFLUX DISEASE

- α-Alpha-adrenergic antagonists
- Anticholinergics
- Barbiturates
- β-Adrenergic agonists
- Benzodiazepines
- Calcium-channel antagonists
- Morphine and meperidine
- Theophylline

CASE STUDY

A pharmacist approaches a gentleman (MK) standing in front of the GI section of OTC medications and asks if he requires any assistance. MK begins to tell the pharmacist about a 2-week history of midepigastric discomfort characterized by a "burning feeling." The pharmacist asks him to step into the patient counseling area for more privacy. MK agrees and follows the pharmacist.

ASSESSMENT OF THE PATIENT

Subjective Information

32-year-old man with a 2-week history of midepigastric discomfort characterized by a "burning feeling"

WHERE IS THE PAIN? It hurts right about here [MK points to a specific spot in the right upper quadrant, approximately 4 cm off the midline and 8 cm above the umbilicus].

HAS THIS PAIN MOVED AT ALL, OR HAS IT ALWAYS BEEN IN THIS SPOT? It has always been in about this spot.

IS THIS THE ONLY SPOT THAT HURTS, OR DO YOU HAVE PAIN ANYWHERE ELSE WITH IT? That is the only spot.

WHEN DID THE PAIN START? About 2 weeks ago.

DOES THE PAIN COME AND GO, OR IS IT A STEADY, CONSTANT PAIN? It is pretty much constant throughout the day, but it seems worse in the afternoon and evening.

HAS THIS PAIN CHANGED AT ALL LATELY? Yeah. Over the past couple of days, the time of the pain has changed. It hurts more early, like around seven in the morning. And food doesn't seem to help as much anymore.

YOU SAID FOOD HELPS THE PAIN BUT DOESN'T AS MUCH ANYMORE? Yes. At least up to a couple of days ago, the pain would get better after I ate.

WITH THIS PAIN, DO YOU EXPERIENCE NAUSEA OR VOMITING? No.

ANY SWEATING? No.

ANY CHANGES IN BOWEL HABITS, LIKE DIARRHEA? No.

ANY ABDOMINAL BLOATING? No.

DO YOU SMOKE? Yes.

Continued

CASE STUDY—continued

HOW MUCH? About a pack a day.

FOR HOW LONG HAVE YOU SMOKED? About 10 to 15 years.

WHEN DO YOU EXPERIENCE THE PAIN? Usually at night.

DOES THE PAIN WAKE YOU UP AT NIGHT? Once in a while, around two in the morning.

IS THE PAIN WORSE WHEN YOU LIE DOWN? No, not really.

DO YOU DRINK ALCOHOLIC BEVERAGES? No, not really.

ARE YOUR BOWEL MOVEMENTS DARK OR STICKY WHEN YOU WIPE? No, not really.

HAVE YOU EXPERIENCED ANY NEW STRESSES IN YOUR LIFE, LIKE A NEW JOB? No.

HAVE YOU LOST ANY WEIGHT RECENTLY? No.

WHAT PRESCRIPTION MEDICATIONS DO YOU TAKE? None.

WHAT NONPRESCRIPTION MEDICATIONS DO YOU TAKE REGULARLY? None.

DO YOU TAKE ASPIRIN OR IBUPROFEN PRODUCTS OFTEN? Rarely, for an occasional headache.

HAVE YOU TRIED ANY NONPRESCRIPTION MEDICATIONS TO HELP WITH THE PAIN? No, that's why I'm here.

HAVE YOU EVER HAD A PAIN LIKE THIS BEFORE? Yes. I had a similar pain about two times before.

TELL ME ABOUT THIS PREVIOUS PAIN. It happened twice during the past 4 or 5 years and lasted about 2 or 3 weeks each time.

WHAT DID YOU DO FOR THIS PAIN? I took some antacid for a while, and it helped.

HAVE YOU EVER SEEN A PHYSICIAN FOR THIS PAIN? No.

Objective Information

Computerized medication profile:

- No profile on record.

Patient in no acute distress

Vital signs normal

Abdomen: moderate epigastric tenderness to touch and mild upper abdominal distention

DISCUSSION

Severe abdominal pain associated with high-acuity conditions, such as acute pancreatitis or appendicitis, requires a patient to present either to a physician or an emergency department. MK illustrates the more common scenario for pharmacists, in which the patient complains of abdominal discomfort that is not severe enough to seek immediate medical care. Rather, the patient attempts self-treatment with an OTC product. The task for the pharmacist is to assess the severity of the patient's condition to determine if referral to a physician is necessary or if treatment with an OTC agent may be attempted.

MK's complaint of midepigastric burning is consistent with PUD and GERD. Although not pathognomonic, pinpoint tenderness, pain relief with food intake, and worsening of pain toward the evening hours are all indicative of PUD, and specifically of duodenal ulcer. Also, more than 50% of patients with duodenal ulcers state that the pain awakens them at night. Unfortunately, pain at night is also common with GERD. To further differentiate the patient's symptoms from GERD, the pharmacist inquired about pain when supine. Most persons with GERD have more episodes of reflux and, hence, more pain when lying down. This finding is not as common in patients with PUD.

MK has no indications of blood loss or pending dehydration (e.g., melena, complaints of vomiting, orthostasis, or tachycardia) and, therefore, no need for immediate medical attention. His symptoms are consistent with PUD caused by infection with *H. pylori,* because he has no history of NSAID or salicylate use. Because these symptoms are recurrent and a possible cure is available, however, MK should be referred for serologic confirmation of *H. pylori* infection and antibiotic therapy. If MK presented with similar symptoms but for the first time and had no history of similar complaints, the pharmacist could have chosen to treat this episode with an OTC H2RA or antacid, with the understanding that if the symptoms returned, the patient would be referred for further evaluation.

The steps involved in this assessment are illustrated in Figure 14-9.

Continued

CASE STUDY—continued

■ Pharmaceutical Care Plan ■

Patient Name: MK

Date: 5/20/02

Medical Problems:
Epigastric discomfort

Current Medications:
None

S: MK is a 32-year-old man who presents with a 2-week history of midepigastric discomfort characterized by a "burning feeling" alleviated by food. The pain worsens toward evening and has awakened him from sleep. This is the third episode of similar pain in the last 5 years. In the past, he treated the pain with an antacid but has not sought medical care from a physician. No indication of melena, weight loss, or vomiting. No NSAID or salicylate use. Pain is not worse when supine.

O: Patient without any distress.

Blood pressure: 134/78 mm Hg, no orthostasis

Heart rate: 74 bpm

A: Probable PUD, recurrent.

P:
1. Refer to physician for serologic confirmation of PUD.
2. Discuss the role of *H. pylori* as the probable cause of his symptoms and that cure can be expected with proper treatment using antibiotics.
3. Schedule follow-up phone call to ensure that patient sought medical care.

Pharmacist: *Robert Doe, Pharm.D.*

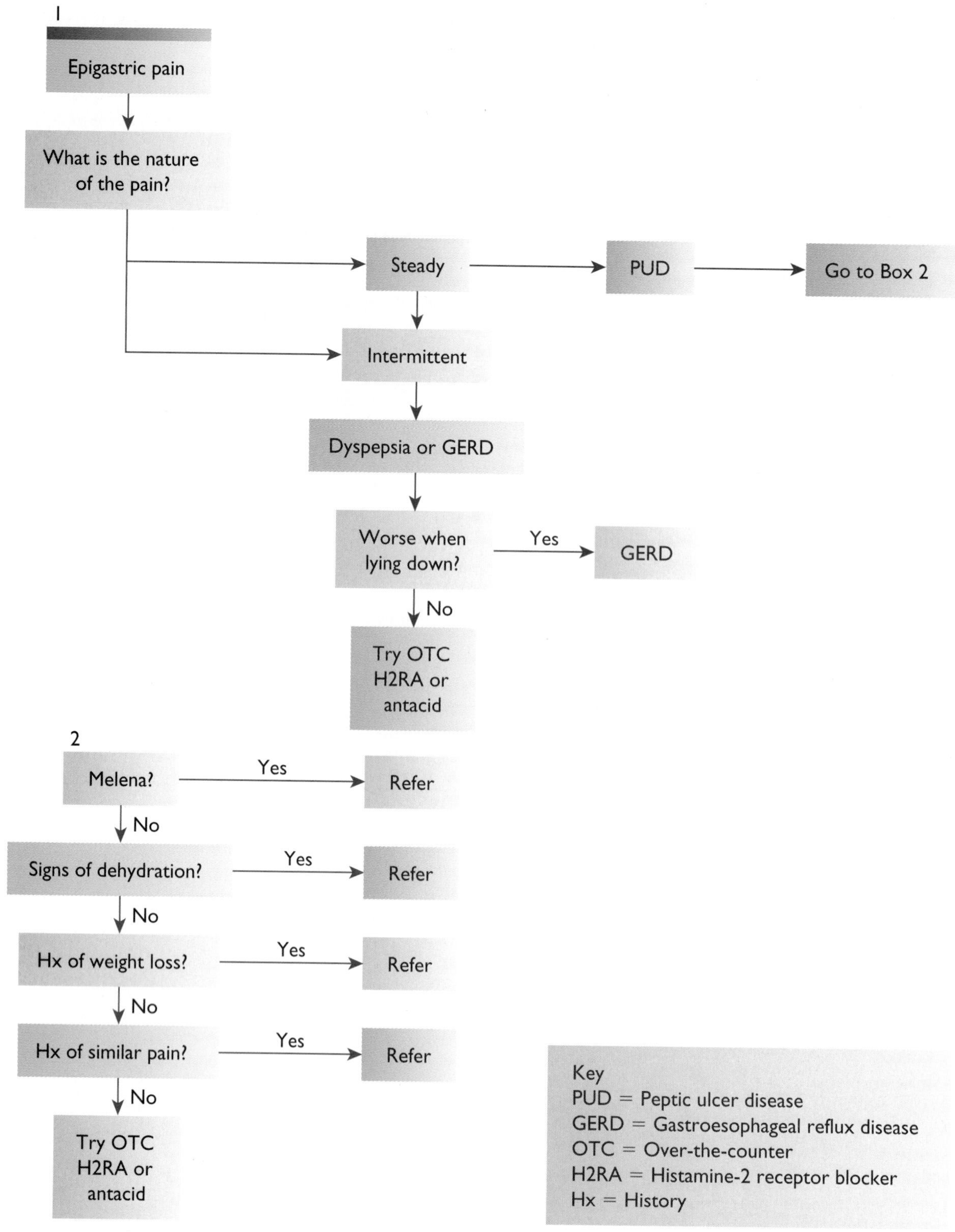

FIGURE 14-9 ■ Decision tree for the assessment of abdominal pain.

Self-Assessment Questions

1. What signs and symptoms are associated with PUD?
2. What signs and symptoms are associated with GERD?
3. When interviewing a patient with complaints of abdominal pain, which questions would help you to differentiate between PUD and GERD?
4. When consulting with a patient, what signs and symptoms would cause you to refer the patient to a health care provider rather than to recommend a self-treatment regimen?

Critical Thinking Questions

1. During the pharmacist's evaluation, MK's vital signs were normal. If MK has extracellular fluid loss, what evidence should be sought when evaluating his vital signs?
2. Pharmacists rarely complete an abdominal examination of a patient, but they are often consulted by patients about abdominal discomfort or pain. Based on what you have learned in previous chapters, what signs in other body systems would you have looked for during the conversation with MK that might indicate a more serious problem?

Nausea and Vomiting

Physiologically, nausea and vomiting are protective measures of the body to evacuate potentially harmful ingestions (e.g., large amounts of alcohol). Medically, nausea and vomiting are important because of the wide range of conditions that can produce them as well as because of the potential complications caused by vomiting.

Nausea and vomiting can be caused by a multitude of conditions, including gastroenteritis, GI obstruction, visceral pain associated with renal or biliary colic, viral and alcoholic hepatitis, pancreatitis, pregnancy, motion sickness, radiation therapy, head trauma, and drug toxicity. Potential complications associated with nausea and vomiting are aspiration pneumonia, Mallory-Weiss tear, esophageal rupture, electrolyte abnormalities, and volume depletion.

Subjective symptoms associated with nausea and vomiting may be described as an "upset stomach," abdominal bloating, increased burping, indigestion, and increased salivation that requires more frequent swallowing. Objective findings will vary based on the cause and severity of the nausea and vomiting, but they can include signs of volume depletion (e.g., tachycardia, deceased skin turgor, and dry mucous membranes), signs of metabolic disturbances (e.g., tachypnea), and mild epigastric tenderness on physical examination. As with abdominal pain, a medication history may indicate drugs that are commonly identified as causing nausea and vomiting (Box 14-9).

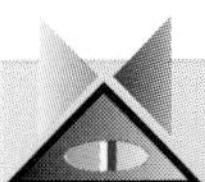

Box 14-9

MEDICATIONS THAT COMMONLY CAUSE NAUSEA AND VOMITING

- Chemotherapeutic agents:
  - Cisplatin
  - Cyclophosphamide
  - Cytarabine
  - Doxorubicin
  - Methotrexate
- Opiate analgesics
- Anticholinergics
- Antibiotics
- Digoxin
- Theophylline

CASE STUDY

The mother of BG, a 20-month-old girl, cannot get through to the pediatrician's office and, therefore, calls the pharmacy instead. The mother sounds somewhat frantic. She states that BG began vomiting this morning and has not stopped and that she, the mother, is worried.

ASSESSMENT OF THE PATIENT

Subjective Information

20-month-old girl with vomiting

HOW MANY TIMES HAS THE CHILD VOMITED? About six times in the last 4 hours.

WHAT DOES THE VOMITED MATERIAL LOOK LIKE? It is mostly a yellowish liquid color now.

WAS IT EVER RED OR BLACK? No.

WHAT DOES THE MATERIAL SMELL LIKE? It smells like vomit.

DOES THE CHILD COMPLAIN OF ABDOMINAL PAIN? No, not really.

DOES THE STOMACH LOOK BLOATED? No.

IS THE CHILD BEHAVING NORMALLY, OTHER THAN FEELING SICK? Yes.

HAS SHE FALLEN RECENTLY OR HIT HER HEAD? No.

IS IT POSSIBLE SHE GOT INTO SOMETHING, LIKE A HOUSEHOLD CLEANER? No, she has been with someone all the time, and we keep everything like that locked up.

DOES THE CHILD HAVE A FEVER? No.

DID YOU TAKE HER TEMPERATURE? Yes. It was normal.

DOES THE CHILD HAVE DIARRHEA? No.

HAS ANYONE ELSE IN THE HOUSEHOLD BEEN SICK? No.

Continued

CASE STUDY—continued

DOES THE CHILD GO TO DAY CARE? Yes.

HAVE ANY CHILDREN THERE BEEN SICK? Yes. There is a virus going around, and some kids have been out for 2 or 3 days.

Objective Information

Computerized medication profile:

- No active prescriptions.

Patient without a fever
Mother in obvious distress

DISCUSSION

This case illustrates the more difficult task of assessing a patient not only over the phone but also through a third party. The first task of the pharmacist is to assess the acuity of the patient. As previously stated, nausea and vomiting can result from numerous causes. Through questioning, however, the pharmacist can determine if specific signs and symptoms are present that would require immediate medical referral. These include (1) color of the vomitus (if the material is red or black, coffee-ground, the child may be experiencing an upper GI bleed and needs immediate medical attention), (2) smell of the vomitus (vomited material with a fecal smell indicates intestinal obstruction and mandates immediate referral), (3) abdominal pain and distention (presence of either may indicate a serious pathologic process, and referral should be considered), (4) abnormal behavior (mental status changes may indicate a metabolic aberration, and immediate referral is necessary), (5) history of head trauma (concussion/head trauma may cause vomiting, and referral is required), and (6) toxic ingestions (vomiting is a protective measure to rid the body of potential toxins). Any chance of a toxic ingestion requires emergency department evaluation and, hence, referral.

Fever is a nonspecific finding, but it may support a diagnosis of viral gastroenteritis. The presence of illness in close contacts (e.g., household members and day care setting) also suggests a communicable pathogen. Concomitant diarrhea is important for two reasons. First, fever and diarrhea commonly accompany gastroenteritis. Second, diarrhea will increase the risk of dehydration, especially in infants and young children. Patients or parents should be educated about the warning signs for dehydration, which include excessive thirst, decreased urine output, dry mucous membranes, fever without sweating, and in infants and children, a sunken fontanelle and crying with little tear production. Severe dehydration may require parenteral hydration and, hence, referral.

Acute gastroenteritis commonly resolves within 48 hours, and most patients can be managed at home with fluid and electrolyte replacement. Oral intake should be held for approximately 2 hours. Then, 5 to 10 mL of an oral electrolyte solution (e.g., Infalyte or Pedialyte) should be given every 15 minutes for 1 hour. If the patient tolerates this amount, the process should be continued, with increasing volumes (5-mL increments) being administered. A clear liquid diet can be initiated in 24 hours, and in most cases, a regular diet can be resumed in 48 hours.

Once it has been concluded that the case is probably caused by simple gastroenteritis, the pharmacist must delineate a treatment regimen, including goals and monitoring parameters. If the patient or parent is unable to meet or does not feel comfortable with the treatment requirements, the patient should be referred for medical care. In this case, the mother believed that she was unable to treat the condition at home, so the pharmacist called the pediatrician's office, and the patient was referred.

The steps involved in this assessment are illustrated in Figure 14-10.

PHARMACEUTICAL CARE PLAN

Patient Name: BG

Date: 4/12/02

Medical Problems:

Probable viral gastroenteritis

Current Medications:

No active medications

S: Received call from a somewhat distraught mother. Her daughter, BG, is a 20-month-old girl who began vomiting this morning. Vomitus is yellowish, with no blood or foul smell. No complaints of abdominal pain. No fever per mother. No diarrhea. No apparent abdominal distention. No history of head trauma or toxic ingestion.

The child behaves appropriately. The child attends day care, which is currently experiencing a "virus" requiring 2 to 3 days at home.

O: Per phone call.

A: Probable viral gastroenteritis.

P:
1. Discussed home treatment with mother, who felt she was unable to meet the treatment regimen.
2. Call pediatrician's office, and arrange an appointment for BG.

Pharmacist: *Jane Doe, Pharm.D.*

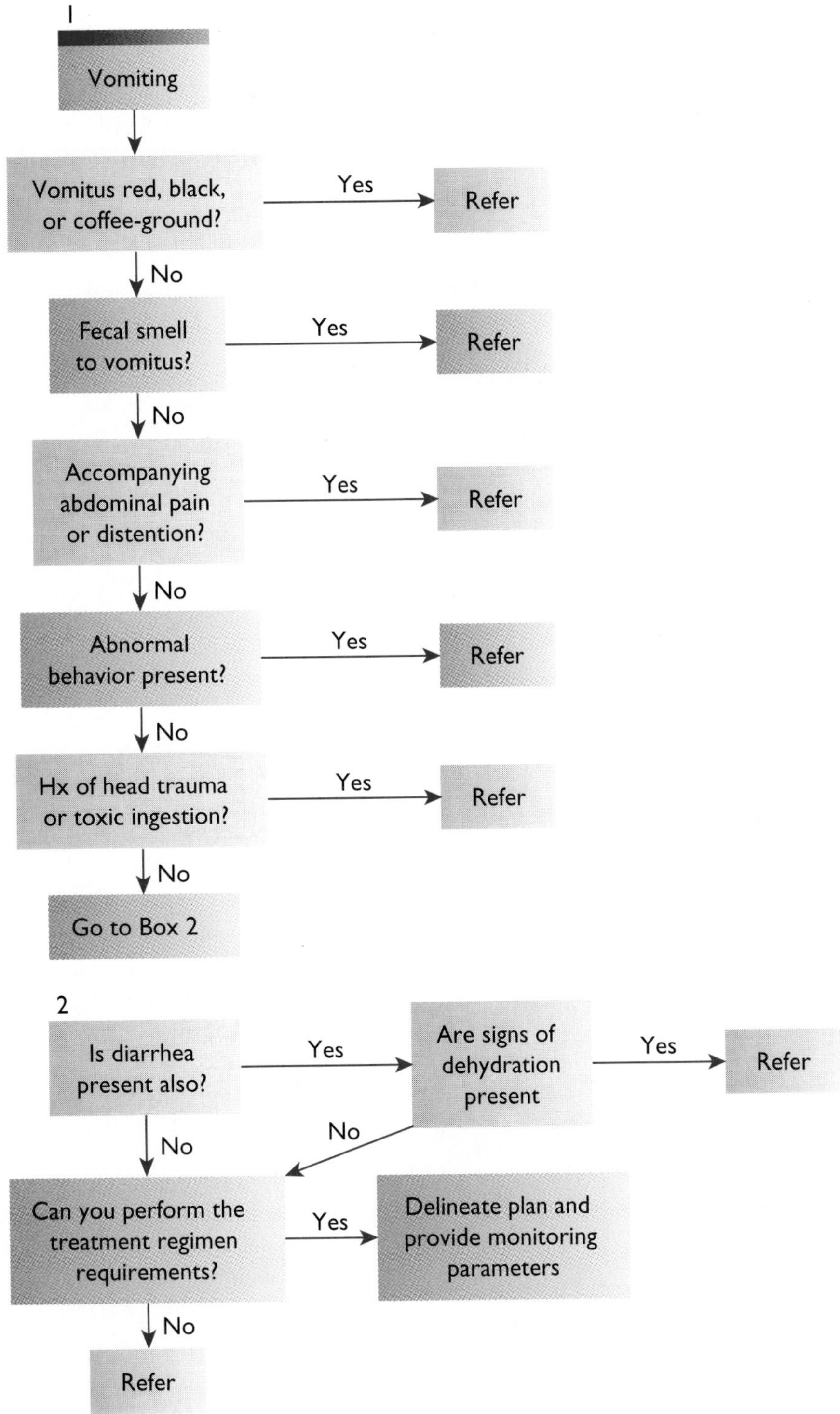

FIGURE 14-10 ■ Decision tree for the assessment of nausea and vomiting.

Self-Assessment Questions

1. What questions would you ask of the geriatric patient experiencing nausea or vomiting?
2. What questions would you ask of the pediatric patient experiencing nausea or vomiting?
3. If BG had been experiencing diarrhea concomitantly, what questions should the pharmacist have asked?
4. What medications commonly cause nausea and vomiting?

Critical Thinking Questions

1. When assessing patients with nausea and vomiting, what signs should you look for to determine whether they need immediate referral to a health care provider?
2. What questions could you ask a mother to obtain more objective information about her child's condition?

3. Compare and contrast the physical findings of nausea and vomiting in an infant, a child, an adult, and an elderly adult.
4. What physical findings would be present in a patient who has suffered from chronic nausea and vomiting?

Change in Bowel Habits

Changes in bowel habits (e.g., diarrhea or constipation) are frequent complaints for which patients seek OTC products and advice from the pharmacist. Diarrhea is the abnormal passage of watery stools. Constipation, by definition, is infrequency of or difficulty in passing stools. Frequent causes of diarrhea and constipation are listed in Box 14-10.

The presentation and findings for patients with diarrhea and constipation may vary depending on the cause. Some common findings that may be present in patients complaining of diarrhea include sudden onset of abnormally frequent stools, which are watery in nature, accompanied by abdominal cramping, weakness, fatigue, abdominal bloating and flatulence, nausea, vomiting, and fever. On physical examination, one may find signs of dehydration (e.g., orthostasis) and electrolyte/metabolic abnormalities (e.g., alkalosis), with mild abdominal discomfort. Some common findings in patients complaining of constipation include low back pain, abdominal distention and vague discomfort, anorexia, and headache. On physical examination, one may find an abdominal mass in the left lower quadrant or over the ileocecal valve and tenderness in the lower abdomen. Medications that commonly cause diarrhea and constipation are listed in Box 14-11, although many more agents have been associated with changes in bowel habits. Again, a guideline to use when assessing changes in bowel habits is that if either diarrhea or constipation has been present for approximately 1 week (or longer) or there is evidence of bleeding in the stool or on the toilet paper, the patient should be referred for further evaluation.

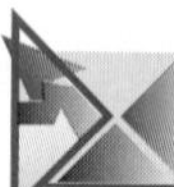

Box 14-10

FREQUENT CAUSES OF DIARRHEA AND CONSTIPATION

DIARRHEA

- Intestinal disease (ulcerative colitis or Crohn's disease)
- Medication (overuse of magnesium-containing antacids)
- Dietary (lactase deficiency)
- Infectious (*Escherichia coli* food poisoning)

CONSTIPATION

- Intestinal disease (diverticular disease)
- Medication (overuse of aluminum-containing antacids)
- Dietary (inadequate fluid intake and low-fiber diet)
- Metabolic (hypokalemia)
- Endocrine (hypothyroidism)

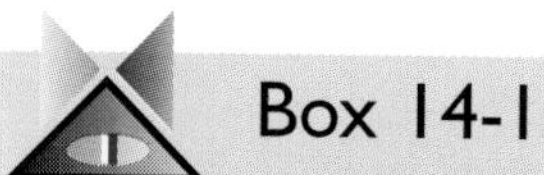

Box 14-11

MEDICATIONS THAT COMMONLY CAUSE DIARRHEA AND CONSTIPATION

DIARRHEA

- Antibiotics
- Antacids (containing magnesium)
- Acarbose
- Bethanecol
- Colchicine
- Metformin
- Metoclopramide
- Quinidine

CONSTIPATION

- Opiate analgesics
- Antacids (containing aluminum or calcium)
- Anticholinergics
- Antihypertensives
- Diuretics
- Iron supplements
- Neuroleptics
- Vincristine

CASE STUDY

AS is a 22-year-old woman who asks the pharmacist to recommend a product for diarrhea. She is somewhat tearful and anxious. She states that she is a college student and sometimes has trouble sitting through class because of the urge to defecate and that the diarrhea is "messing up her life." The pharmacist asks her to step into the patient counseling area for more privacy. She agrees and follows the pharmacist.

ASSESSMENT OF THE PATIENT

Subjective Information

22-year-old woman complaining of diarrhea

How long have you been experiencing the diarrhea? Almost 8 months now.

How often do you have to go to the bathroom? Probably five times a day, on average.

Does it occur after eating or drinking? No, not just after eating or drinking. It happens throughout the day.

Are the stools watery or just loose? They are just loose.

Is there a copious amount present? No. Sometimes it is as little as one-half cupful.

Is there blood or mucus present? No, not that I can see.

Does the stool float? No.

Do you also experience fever? Well, maybe. I'm not sure.

Chills? No.

Increased thirst? No.

Abdominal pain or cramping? Yes. I get a colicky pain that goes away after I have the diarrhea.

Have you traveled recently? No.

Have you taken any antibiotics recently? No.

Have you lost any weight recently? Yes, about a 10-pound weight loss over the last 6 months.

Do you use any medications, either prescription or nonprescription? I don't take any prescription medications, but I have been using Imodium AD for the diarrhea. It isn't helping much, though.

Does anyone in your family have inflammatory bowel disease? Yes, I think my aunt does.

Objective Information

Computerized medication profile:

- No active prescriptions.

Patient mildly anxious
Blood pressure: 122/78 mm Hg
Heart rate: 96 bpm
Respiratory rate: 16 rpm
Temperature (tympanic): 100°F

Discussion

Changes in bowel habits are a frequent reason for use of OTC medications. In many cases, OTC agents may be appropriate adjuvant therapies. Without careful clarification of the history, however, a pharmacist may not be able to determine if an OTC agent is beneficial or even harmful. For example, in some cases of infectious diarrhea, antidiarrheal agents may interfere with the natural course of the infection and prolong the symptomatic phase.

When a patient presents with a complaint of diarrhea, the first questions should address the symptomatic onset to determine if it was acute or chronic. Most acute cases relate to infectious causes or lactose intolerance. The stool consistency can aid in identifying the GI source of the disturbance. In most cases, small bowel pathology produces loose stools, whereas colonic pathology produces watery stools. Blood and mucus are also more common with colonic involvement. Floating stools sometimes indicate a malabsorptive process, such as steatorrhea associated with pancreatitis. Systemic symptoms (e.g., fever) with an acute onset indicate an infectious cause, whereas fever and chronic onset indicate IBD. Similarly, a sudden onset with abdominal pain or cramping is more indicative of a toxin, whereas a chronic onset with abdominal pain is common with IBD. Travel history and recent antibiotic use suggest an infectious cause, whereas weight loss indicates a systemic disease (e.g., IBD or cancer). Familial clustering also is seen with IBD.

The objective data (e.g., low-grade fever and tachycardia) support IBD as the probable cause of AS's diarrhea. Because of the need for a diagnostic workup, the patient was instructed to see a physician. The pharmacist took some time to explain that medical therapy is effective in controlling diarrhea once a cause is firmly established. The patient was reassured, and diet therapy was discussed.

Figure 14-11 illustrates the steps used in evaluating a patient presenting with diarrhea.

Continued

CASE STUDY—continued

PHARMACEUTICAL CARE PLAN

Patient Name: AS

Date: 10/1/02

Medical Problems:
Diarrhea, chronic

Current Medications:
Imodium AD: 1-2 PO PRN

S: 22-year-old female college student seeking an OTC to treat diarrhea. Patient relates a 7- to 8-month history of approximately five loose stools per day unrelated to food ingestion. Diarrhea is accompanied by colicky abdominal pain; defecation relieves the pain. Questionable history of low-grade fever. History of a 10-pound weight loss. No history of recent antibiotic use or foreign travel. Family history of IBD.

O: No active prescriptions. Patient mildly anxious.

Temperature: 100°F

Heart rate: 96 bpm

A: Probable IBD.

P:
1. Refer to a physician for further evaluation.
2. Reassure patient about symptomatic control once the cause is identified.
3. Provide some dietary interventions that may help to control stool output.

Pharmacist: *John Smith, Pharm.D.*

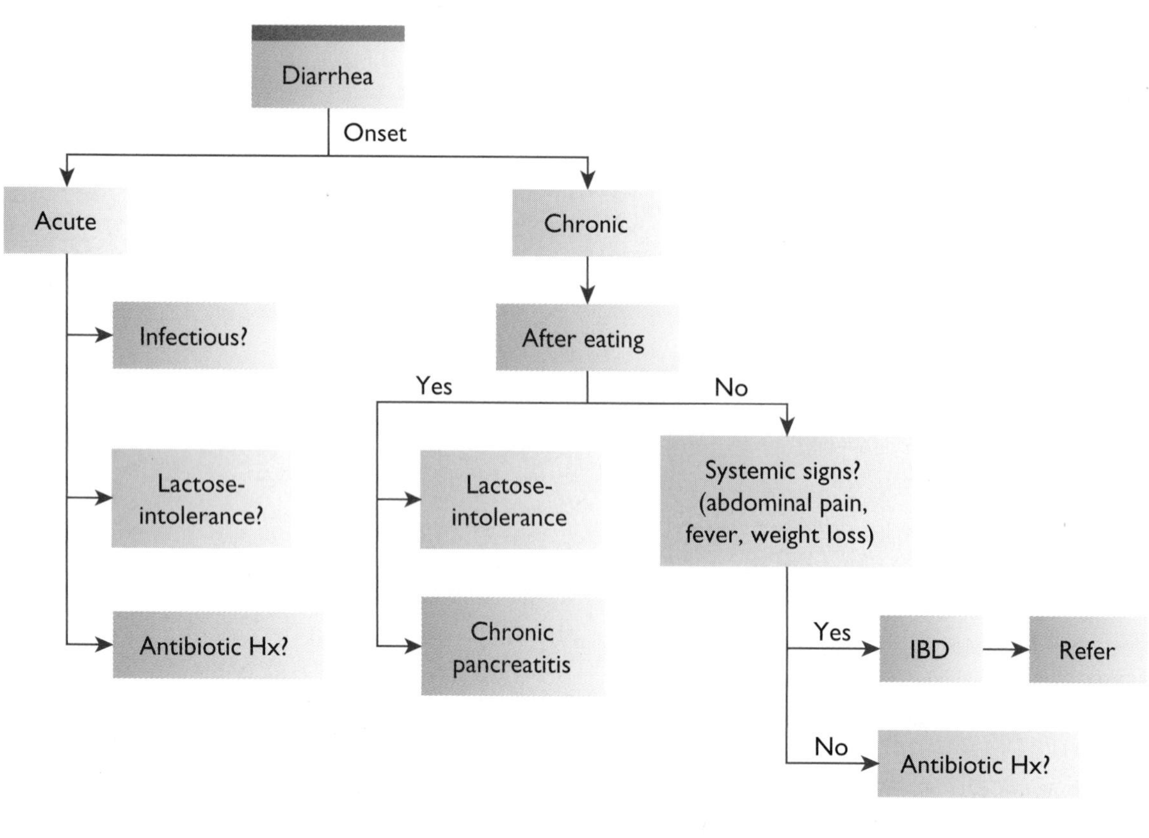

FIGURE 14-11 ■ Decision tree for the assessment of diarrhea.

Self-Assessment Questions

1. What signs and symptoms are associated with IBD? What signs and symptoms did AS have?
2. What questions would you ask someone suffering from diarrhea that would help to differentiate whether the patient could safely self-treat with an OTC product or should be referred to a physician?
3. What medications are commonly associated with constipation?
4. What medications are commonly associated with diarrhea?

Critical Thinking Questions

1. Inspection is the pharmacist's primary mode of physical assessment. As you review the signs associated with IBD, what physical findings would indicate that those signs were present in your patient?
2. In monitoring a patient with IBD, what physical findings would you monitor to determine if the treatment was efficacious?

Bibliography

Farkas P, Hyde D. Liver and gastroenterology tests. In: Taub SL, ed. Basic skills in interpreting laboratory data. 2nd ed. Bethesda, MD: American Society of Health-Systems Pharmacists, 1996:213–244.

Hanauer SB, Meyers S. Management of Crohn's disease in adults. Am J Gastroenterol 1997;92:559–566.

Kornbluth A, Sachar DB. Ulcerative colitis: practice guidelines in adults. American College of Gastroenterology, Practice Parameters Committee. Am J Gastroenterol 1997;92:204–211.

Levitan R. GI problems in the elderly. Part I: aging-related considerations. Geriatrics 1989;44:53–56.

Skoutakis VA, Joe RH, Hara DS. Comparative role of omeprazole in the treatment of gastroesophageal reflux disease. Ann Pharmacother 1995;29:1252–1262.

Soll AH, et al. Medical treatment of peptic ulcer disease. Practice guidelines. JAMA 1996;275:622–629.

Steingart R. Management of patients with sickle cell disease. Med Clin North Am 1992;76:669–681.

CHAPTER

15

Hepatic System

Wendy Mills

Glossary Terms

- Hepatitis
- Cholecystitis
- Cirrhosis
- Pancreatitis

ANATOMY AND PHYSIOLOGY OVERVIEW

The organs of the hepatic system, including the liver, pancreas, and gallbladder, are sometimes classified as accessory digestive organs. Though part of the gastrointestinal system, these organs do more than simply help to digest our food. In fact, the liver alone performs more than 500 functions. Because of their versatility, these organs, when not functioning properly, can cause significant morbidity and mortality.

Drug-related morbidity and mortality is of special importance to pharmacists. The liver plays a major role in metabolism of medications. Thus, liver damage or dysfunction can either enhance or delay metabolism of medications, resulting in a lack of treatment efficacy or an enhancement of the medication's adverse effects. Therefore, pharmacists must develop skills for assessment of the liver and its functioning.

The Liver

The liver is the largest visceral organ in the body, weighing approximately 1.5 kg, or approximately 3 pounds (Fig. 15-1). It is located under the diaphragm, and it occupies most of the right hypochondriac and part of the epigastric regions of the abdomen (see Fig. 14-4). The anterior surface of the liver follows the smooth curve of the body wall, but the posterior surface bears the impression of the stomach, small and large intestines, and right kidney. The falciform ligament marks the division between the right and left lobes.

Two blood vessels, the hepatic artery and the portal vein, provide the blood supply to the liver. The hepatic artery supplies oxygenated blood, whereas the hepatic portal vein supplies deoxygenated blood, containing nutrients, and accounts for approximately two-thirds of the blood supply that is provided to the liver. Blood from the stomach, small intestine, spleen, and pancreas passes through the liver via the portal vein before entering the systemic circulation. This allows the liver to remove bacteria and other particulate matter that might enter the blood from the gastrointestinal tract, and it helps to prevent direct access of potentially harmful agents to the rest of the body.

The basic functional unit of the liver is the liver lobule. The lobule consists of hepatocytes that are primarily responsible for the liver's three major categories of function: (1) metabolism, (2) synthesis, and (3) storage. The major functions of the liver in each category are listed in Table 15-1.

The Gallbladder

The gallbladder is a hollow, pear-shaped organ near the posterior surface of the liver (Fig. 15-1). It stores and concentrates bile as much as 10-fold, by absorbing water and some ions, until bile is needed in the small intestine.

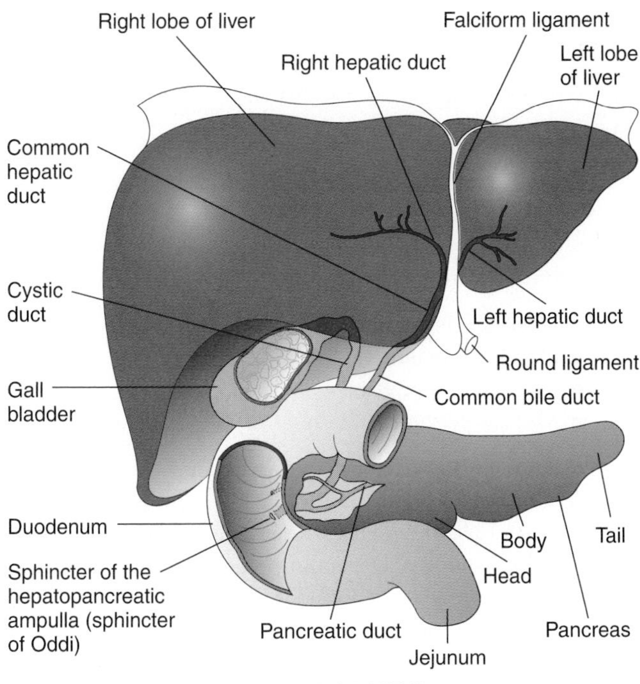

FIGURE 15-1 ■ Anatomy of the liver, gallbladder, and pancreas.

Bile is formed in the liver and contains mostly water, bile salts, cholesterol, lecithin, bile pigments (primarily bilirubin), and several ions. Bile salts play a role in the emulsification and absorption of fats and, along with lecithin, make cholesterol soluble. Bilirubin, a breakdown product from red blood cells, is excreted through the bile and is metabolized in the intestine.

Bile enters the small intestine through the common bile duct. When the small intestine is empty, the sphincter of Oddi (or pancreaticohepatic sphincter) contracts, sealing off the passageway and preventing bile from entering the small intestine. Bile then backs up and enters the expandable gallbladder (via the cystic duct) for storage.

Bile ejection occurs under stimulation by cholecystokinin. When chyme (the semiliquid, acidic mass in which food passes from the stomach and into the small intestine) arrives at the duodenum, cholecystokinin is released. The cholecystokinin relaxes the sphincter of Oddi, and the gallbladder contracts, sending bile into the small intestine.

The Pancreas

The pancreas is oblong, pinkish-gray, and lies posterior to the greater curvature of the stomach, extending laterally toward the spleen (Fig. 15-1). It has functions of both exocrine, digestive secretion as well as endocrine, hormonal secretion. Ninety-nine percent of the pancreatic cell clusters, called acini, are exocrine. They secrete pancreatic juice and isotonic fluid that contains sodium, potassium, chloride, calcium, bicarbonate, water, and protein. Most of the protein in the pancreatic juice consists of pancreatic digestive enzymes, which must be secreted into the intestinal tract before they can become active. Secretion occurs primarily in response to hormonal stimulation from the duodenum via secretin and cholecystokinin. Once secreted, pancreatic juice stops the action of pepsin from the stomach, thus creating the proper environment for the small intestine.

The other 1% of the small, glandular clusters includes the islets of Langerhans and forms the endocrine portion of the organ. The islets of Langerhans consist of four different cell types, alpha, beta, delta, and F cells, that secrete the hormones glucagon, insulin, somatostatin, and pancreatic polypeptide, respectively.

Special Considerations

Pediatric Patients

In the embryo, the hepatic system begins to develop within the first month of gestation, and most of the enzymatic microsomal systems for metabolism are present at birth. At delivery, the infant possesses full capacity for reduction and increased capacity for methylation reactions in the liver as well as a well-developed ability for sulfate conjugation. Other metabolic pathways generally have decreased activity compared to those in the adult, including decreased hydroxylation, *N*-demethylation, conjugation of bilirubin, and activity of the major components of the mixed-function oxidase system, including the cytochrome P-450 system. Also present are decreased hepatic uptake, low concentration of intracellular carrier proteins, and decreased bile production, which can further influence possible problems in metabolism of substances by the liver. Maturation of hepatic enzymes varies based on the specific enzyme and can be influenced by exposure to enzyme-inducing agents. In fact, infants may have a faster (and greater) response than adults to enzyme-inducing agents. These differences in enzymatic maturation are important when considering variations in drug metabolism that occur between infants, children, and adults.

Premature infants and newborns have a diminished bile acid pool, biliary function, and pancreatic enzymes, specifically pancreatic amylase, which leads to decreased absorption of fat and fat-soluble vitamins as well as decreased utilization of starches. Because of this immaturity, neonatal jaundice (unconjugated hyperbilirubinemia) is common, occurring in 60% of

TABLE 15-1 ➤ FUNCTIONS OF THE LIVER

FUNCTION	
Metabolism	Carbohydrate
	Lipids and lipoproteins
	Amino acids
	Drugs and hormones
	Bilirubin
	Phagocytosis of red blood cells and bacteria
Synthesis	Lipids and lipoproteins
	Proteins
	Coagulation factors
	Activation of vitamin D
	Glucose
	Bile salts
Storage	Glycogen
	Vitamins A, B_{12}, C, D, E, and K
	Minerals

normal, full-term infants and in 80% of preterm infants. Protein, especially albumin, is decreased in the neonate but increases to adult concentrations by the end of the first year of life.

Liver functions in general are imperfect during at least the first week of life, leading to unstable and often low blood glucose concentrations. Most liver functions begin to mature within the first 1 to 3 years. In fact, drug metabolism in children may occur at a more rapid rate, especially for drugs metabolized by the liver, than in adults.

Geriatric Patients

As a person ages, the likelihood of hepatic system dysfunction secondary to chemical and infectious causes increases. During normal aging, both oxidative metabolism and general enzyme activity appear to decrease. Unlike younger adults and children, older adults may be less prone to the effects of enzyme-inducing agents. A decrease in portal blood flow and in liver mass may account for this decreased enzyme activity as well; however, this is not specifically known.

The production and secretion of digestive enzymes also may decrease with age, but they still appear to be sufficient for digestive purposes. In general, little information is available regarding the changes in hepatic function that occur with age, and direct determinants of hepatic function can be difficult to assess.

Pregnant Patients

During pregnancy, an overall increase in cardiac output and total body water occurs; however, a corresponding increase in hepatic blood flow does not. There may be an increase or decrease in the metabolism of specific medications, depending on the stage of pregnancy and the specific enzymatic pathway that is involved. Protein binding is decreased, as are total albumin concentrations, especially during the third trimester. Insulin production may increase or remain the same, and glucagon suppression is enhanced in normal women. Insulin sensitivity may decrease throughout pregnancy, which can lead to an increase in hyperglycemia and in vulnerability to ketosis after food deprivation, especially in women who are predisposed to gestational diabetes. The gallbladder will experience the same general motor sluggishness as the rest of the gastrointestinal tract does throughout pregnancy, predisposing pregnant women to gallstones.

PATHOLOGY OVERVIEW

Diseases of the hepatic system can account for significant morbidity and mortality. Major diseases of this system include hepatitis, cirrhosis, chemical- or drug-induced liver dysfunction, pancreatitis, and cholecystitis.

Hepatitis

Hepatitis is an inflammation of the liver that results primarily from viral and chemical or drug-related causes. (For further information regarding chemical or drug-related causes, see the section on chemical or drug-induced liver dysfunction later in this chapter.) Multiple different viruses, including hepatitis A (HAV), hepatitis B (HBV), and hepatitis C (HCV), can cause viral hepatitis.

Hepatitis A

An RNA virus causes hepatitis A, which is also known as infectious hepatitis. It is primarily spread by the fecal-oral route and has an incubation period of approximately 3 to 5 weeks. People at risk for contracting HAV include:

- People having contact with infected persons
- Day care workers and attendees
- Institutional travelers
- Military personnel

Unlike hepatitis B or C, hepatitis A does not cause chronic disease. Most patients with hepatitis A (≈90%) are asymptomatic. Of the other 10% of patients who become symptomatic, only 10% develop jaundice. Depending on the age of the patient, symptoms can range from a mild, influenza-like illness to elevated hepatic transaminase levels and jaundice. In general, symptoms worsen as the patient age increases. Treatment focuses on prevention with the hepatitis A vaccine. Once a patient experiences acute illness, however, treatment is primarily supportive, including general measures such as a healthy diet, rest, maintaining fluid balance, and avoiding hepatotoxic substances.

Hepatitis B

Unlike HAV, HBV is a DNA virus that undergoes primary replication in the liver. It is spread through body fluids; therefore, sexual activity, blood products, and contaminated needles are the most common routes of transmission. Infection with HBV infection is a worldwide concern because of the chronic liver disease and primary hepatocellular carcinoma that infection can induce. Chronic HBV infection itself is a tremendous health problem, with more than 1 million carriers in the United States alone. People at risk for contracting HBV include:

- Family of infected persons
- Health care professionals
- Hemodialysis patients
- Homosexual men
- Intravenous (IV) drug users
- Morticians
- Multipartner heterosexuals
- Newborns of HBV-carrier mothers
- Sexual partners of HBV carriers
- Tattooed or body-pierced persons
- People living in highly endemic areas

The course of hepatitis B is best considered in four stages. The first is the incubation period, which generally lasts longer than in hepatitis A (anywhere from 1-6 months). In neonatal infections, the incubation period may last for years or decades. The second stage is characterized by an immune response, direct hepatocyte lysis, and the inflammatory process. This is the period of symptomatic hepatitis and typically lasts from 3 to 4 weeks; signs and symptoms are listed in Box 15-1. The greater

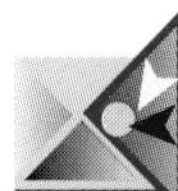

Box 15-1

SYMPTOMS AND SIGNS OF HEPATITIS B

SYMPTOMS

- Malaise
- Fatigue
- Weakness
- Anorexia
- Myalgias
- Arthralgias
- Jaundice

SIGNS

- Increase in ALT and AST
- Increase in bilirubin (especially unconjugated)
- Increase in GGTP
- Increase in LDH
- Positive antibody studies
- Decrease in total protein

an immune response the patient has, the more severe the signs and symptoms. Patients who do not have a large immune response to HBV infection are more likely to develop chronic hepatitis. In the third stage, active replication of HBV ends, and aminotransferase levels become normal. The fourth and final stage is immunity to HBV, at which point the patient is unlikely to become reinfected or to experience reactivation of the infection.

Prevention of HBV infection is important. Vaccination against HBV provides the same immunity to HBV as gained from a previous active infection. Immunoglobulin can be given to patients exposed to HBV to prevent infection; however, once infection occurs, treatment is primarily supportive, especially during the acute phase of the illness. Interferon-α and -β have been investigated for treatment options during the acute phase, but their role in such treatment is undefined. In chronic HBV infection, interferon-α_{2a} has been effective in one-third to one-half of cases. Patients also may relapse after therapy is discontinued. Combinations of interferon and prednisone as well as antiviral agents have also been used with varying success.

Hepatitis C

Before its discovery in 1989, hepatitis C was referred to as non-A, non-B hepatitis. Like HAV, HCV is a single-strand RNA virus; however, it is quite different from other hepatitis viruses. Though it is transmitted primarily parenterally, HCV also may be transmitted sexually. Unlike HBV, however, hepatitis C has a higher chronic carrier rate (20% vs. 80%, respectively). It also evades the immune system more readily and mutates more rapidly than HBV. In fact, a patient may be infected with more than one subtype of HCV at any given time. The multiple subtypes and rapid mutation of HCV lessen the likelihood of developing an effective vaccine in the near future. Patients at risk for developing HCV infection include:

- Those undergoing dialysis and transplant
- Health care professionals
- IV drug users
- Multipartner heterosexuals
- Multiply transfused patients
- Tattooed or body-pierced persons

The incubation period of HCV is generally 6 to 12 weeks, or in between those of HAV and HBV. Most patients with acute and chronic HCV infection are asymptomatic. Some may complain of fatigue, vague discomfort in the right upper quadrant (particularly at night), and flu-like symptoms, but many will initially present with cirrhosis or chronic elevation in transaminase levels. The only currently approved treatment for chronic hepatitis C is interferon-α_{2b}. Treatment generally does not provide a cure, but it may decrease the risk of progression to hepatocellular carcinoma. Another treatment option includes combination therapy with interferon and ribavirin. Further research into diagnostic and therapeutic options continues.

Cirrhosis

Cirrhosis is a chronic disease of the liver in which widespread hepatic cell destruction causes formation of connective tissue and nodular regeneration, with consequent disorganization of the normal architecture. Cirrhosis can be idiopathic or result from alcohol, viral hepatitis, bile duct obstruction, or chronic congestive heart failure (CHF). Alcohol is the most common cause of cirrhosis in the United States. Clinical manifestations may be absent or may include the signs and symptoms listed in Box 15-2. Cirrhosis can lead to the development of portal hypertension, encephalopathy, and hemorrhagic complications. Treatment generally includes therapy for the underlying cause, avoidance of hepatotoxic substances, and symptomatic relief.

Drug-Induced Liver Dysfunction

Drug-induced liver dysfunction can be predictable or idiosyncratic in nature. Predictable reactions are caused by toxic response to a drug. Patients with acquired or genetic metabolic abnormality may be at increased risk for such reactions. Idiosyncratic reactions generally have no association with concentration or with a specifically identified metabolic abnormality. Signs and symptoms of drug-induced liver dysfunction are primarily nonspecific and can include fatigue, jaundice, anorexia, nausea, vomiting, and diarrhea. More than 600 medications have been incriminated in causing liver dysfunction, but a few are more relevant clinically (Box 15-3). Drug-induced liver dysfunction may cause direct hepatocyte injury, cholestatic injury (manifested by decreased bile flow), or both. Direct hepatocyte injury is more serious and can lead to death. Treatment includes removal of the offending agent, supportive therapy, and specific treatment based on the agent causing the liver dysfunction (e.g., acetylcysteine for acetaminophen toxicity).

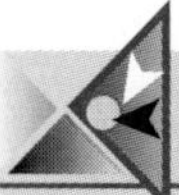

Box 15-2

SIGNS AND SYMPTOMS OF CIRRHOSIS

SIGNS

- Ascites
- Gastrointestinal bleeding
- Anemia
- Prolonged PT
- Hypoalbuminemia
- Hyponatremia
- Increased or decreased liver function tests (AST, ALT, GGTP, Bilirubin)

SYMPTOMS

- Anorexia
- Nausea
- Vomiting
- Diarrhea
- Fatigue
- Weakness
- Fever
- Pruritis
- Jaundice

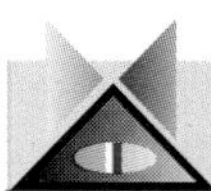

Box 15-3

DRUGS THAT MAY CAUSE DRUG-INDUCED LIVER DYSFUNCTION AND JAUNDICE

- Acetaminophen
- Alcohol
- Amiodarone
- Anabolic steroids
- Anesthetic agents (halothane)
- Anticonvulsants (phenytoin, carbamazepine, valproic acid)
- Aspirin (toxicity or development of Reye's syndrome)
- Carbon tetrachloride
- Chlorpromazine
- Estrogens
- Halothane
- 3-Hydroxy-3-methylglutaric acid coenzyme A reductase inhibitors
- Isoniazid
- Nonsteroidal anti-inflammatory drugs
- Nicotinic acid
- Tetracycline
- Troglitazone
- Vitamin A

Pancreatitis

Pancreatitis, or inflammation of the pancreas, can be acute or chronic. Acute pancreatitis results from premature activation of the proteolytic enzymes within the pancreas; alcohol abuse or gallstones cause 60% to 80% of cases. Other causes include abdominal trauma, postoperative complications, hypertriglyceridemia, hypercalcemia, infection, and medications. Medications that may cause pancreatitis are listed in Box 15-4. Box 15-5 lists the signs and symptoms of acute pancreatitis. The risk of mortality is higher during the first episode of pancreatitis than during subsequent episodes. Complications can be severe and may include pseudocyst, phlegmon (mass of inflamed pancreas containing patchy areas of necrosis), hemorrhage, abscess, ascites, and chronic pancreatitis.

Treatment aims to minimize pain and complications to prevent subsequent episodes. The goal is to decrease pancreatic activation. Most patients respond to discontinuing food and fluid intake and medications until symptoms resolve. Most patients with mild to moderate pancreatitis can be restarted on a clear liquid diet after 3 to 6 days. Intravenous fluid and electrolyte replacement is necessary in those patients with pancre-

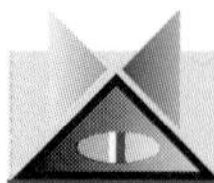

Box 15-4

MEDICATIONS THAT MAY CAUSE DRUG-INDUCED PANCREATITIS[a]

DEFINITE ASSOCIATION

- 5-Aminosalicylic acid
- Asparaginase
- Azathioprine
- Dideoxyinosine
- Estrogens (oral contraceptives)
- Furosemide
- 6-Mercaptopurine
- Methyldopa
- Metronidazole
- Pentamidine
- Sulfonamides
- Sulindac
- Thiazide diuretics
- Tetracycline
- Valproic acid

PROBABLE ASSOCIATION

- Ampicillin
- Angiotensin-converting enzyme inhibitors
- Bumetanide
- Calcium
- Cimetidine
- Nonsteroidal anti-inflammatory drugs
- Salicylates

[a]Not all inclusive.

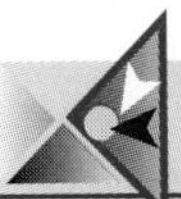

Box 15-5

SIGNS AND SYMPTOMS OF PANCREATITIS

SIGNS

- Low-grade fever
- Hypotension
- Elevation in serum alkaline phosphatase
- Elevation in liver transaminases
- Hypoalbuminemia
- Hypocalcemia

SYMPTOMS

- Severe midepigastric pain
- Radiation of pain to the back
- Abdominal distention
- Nausea
- Vomiting
- Jaundice

atitis caused by loss of fluid from nausea, vomiting, and restriction of fluids by mouth. The drug of choice for analgesia in acute pancreatitis is meperidine. Discontinuance of any known causes of the pancreatitis, including possible medications, is prudent. Other measures may be needed depending on the severity of the pancreatitis and any other concomitant disease states or additional signs and symptoms.

Chronic pancreatitis is progressive, irreversible, and results from functional and structural damage to the pancreas. The most common cause of chronic pancreatitis in the United States is alcohol. Signs and symptoms may be similar to those of acute pancreatitis and include abdominal pain, malabsorption, weight loss, and diabetes; however, the abdominal pain is duller than during acute exacerbations. Though a patient may have chronic pancreatitis, the possibility of acute exacerbations remains, and these should be treated as any other episode of acute pancreatitis. Treatment for chronic pancreatitis aims to control pain and malabsorption. Alcohol and large fatty meals should be avoided. A stepwise approach to pain management should be used, and if necessary, surgery should be considered. Pain may be exacerbated by food; therefore, pain medication should be given regularly with each meal. Pancreatic enzyme replacement may be needed to control malabsorption and may decrease pain. Glucose intolerance is treated with insulin.

Cholecystitis

Acute **cholecystitis,** or inflammation of the gallbladder, is usually caused by cystic duct obstruction from an impacted stone. Gallstones may be caused by too much cholesterol in bile, inflammation of the epithelium, or both. Patients who are on oral contraceptives and those with a high-fat diet have an increased risk of gallstones. Signs and symptoms may range from mild to severe (Box 15-6). Treatment includes bowel rest, IV fluid and electrolytes, analgesia, and ultimately, surgery.

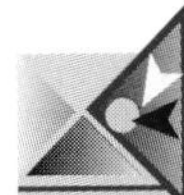

Box 15-6

SIGNS AND SYMPTOMS OF CHOLECYSTITIS

SIGNS

- Fever
- Mildly elevated serum bilirubin
- Mildly elevated serum alkaline phosphatase

SYMPTOMS

- Abdominal pain
- Nausea
- Vomiting
- Anorexia

SYSTEM ASSESSMENT

Subjective Information

When assessing the hepatic system, subjective information may be somewhat vague. Many times, symptoms relating to the hepatic system will overlap with those relating to the gastrointestinal system (see the previous chapter for additional information). Thus, the pharmacist must ask the patient appropriate questions to elicit specific data.

Abdominal Pain

? INTERVIEW Do you ever have any abdominal pain or discomfort? If yes,

Onset and duration: When did it start? Did the pain start suddenly? How long does it last? How does it change throughout the day? Have you had this type of abdominal pain before? How often do you experience abdominal pain?

Characteristics: Describe the pain. Is it severe and stabbing, or is it dull and constant? Aching? Cramping? Burning? Gnawing? Have you ever had this type of pain before? Is it the same or different? How severe is it?

➤ ABNORMALITIES Abdominal pain from acute pancreatitis typically is described as a severe, stabbing pain. Patients sometimes describe abdominal pain as chest pain (see Table 12-1 to differentiate among types of chest pain and Box 14-7 to differentiate among potential causes of abdominal pain). If a patient has had the same type of pain previously, this may give you information regarding the possible cause and any changes in condition.

? INTERVIEW Where is the pain located? Does the pain radiate to any other areas?

ABNORMALITIES Pain described in the epigastric area or in the right upper quadrant may result from hepatic system disorders. Pain secondary to pancreatitis may be described as radiating to the back. Pain secondary to cholecystitis occasionally may radiate to the right scapula and back.

INTERVIEW What brings on the pain? What makes it worse? Does the pain get worse with food intake? Does it get worse with changes in position?

ABNORMALITIES Pain can be increased by food in patients with pancreatitis or cholecystitis; it generally is not increased by food in patients with hepatitis. Pain generally comes on suddenly with acute pancreatitis and cholecystitis. In acute pancreatitis, the pain is frequently increased in the supine position. In cholecystitis, patients may have a constant, dull pain that increases approximately 60 to 90 minutes after meals, especially those containing fatty foods, and can last for several hours. Chronic pancreatitis may have a constant pain, but the patient may not be able to specifically identify when it started.

INTERVIEW

Relief: What relieves the pain? Food? Lying down?

Symptoms: Do you experience any other symptoms with the pain? Nausea? Vomiting? Diarrhea? Itching? Yellow skin?

ABNORMALITIES Pruritis can be a symptom of cirrhosis or cholecystitis. Yellow discoloration of the skin and eyes can indicate jaundice, which will help to differentiate the pain from that of other gastrointestinal disorders.

Ascites

INTERVIEW Do you ever experience a feeling of tightness and extra fluid being around your stomach? If yes,

Onset and duration: When did this begin? How long does it last? Is it constant, or does it come and go?

Cause: What brings it on?

Relief: What makes it better or makes it go away?

ABNORMALITIES Typically, ascites secondary to hepatic disease is not salt sensitive compared to CHF.

INTERVIEW Do you experience any other symptoms with it? Shortness of breath? Abdominal pain? Edema?

ABNORMALITIES Ascites from hepatic causes may be associated with abdominal discomfort or pain and shortness of breath. Typically, if associated with edema in the ankles, feet, and lower legs, ascites is more suggestive of CHF.

Jaundice

INTERVIEW Have you ever had yellow discoloration of your skin or the whites of your eyes? If yes,

Onset and duration: When did it occur? How long has it lasted?

Cause: What brought on this change in color?

Relief: What made it go away?

Symptoms: What other symptoms do you experience? What color are your stools? What color is your urine? Do you have itching for unknown reason?

ABNORMALITIES Yellow discoloration of the skin or sclera indicates jaundice from some type of hepatic disease. When bile excretion becomes completely obstructed, stools become light-colored and gray. Urine, however, may turn yellowish-brown or like the color of tea. Itching for an unknown reason favors cholestasis or obstructive jaundice.

INTERVIEW

Past history: Do you have any history of liver problems? Have you had hepatitis in the past? If so, what kind? Do you have any history of problems with your gallbladder or pancreas? Do you have any history of problems with your stomach or intestines?

Family history: Do you have any immediate family members with liver problems?

Medication history: What prescription and nonprescription medications are you currently taking?

Social history: Do you smoke or chew tobacco? If yes, how much each day? For how many years? Do you drink any alcohol (beer, wine, liquor)? If yes, how much each day or week? For how many years? Have you ever used injectable drugs? Have you recently traveled outside the United States? Have you been around someone with hepatitis or another liver disease? Have you had any abdominal surgery lately? What do you do for a living?

ABNORMALITIES Some patients may be more at risk for developing hepatitis because of job exposure. People at increased risk for HAV infection include day care workers, international travelers, and military personnel. People at increased risk of HBV infection include health care workers and morticians.

INTERVIEW Have you ever received a blood transfusion? If so, was it before 1991?

ABNORMALITIES Patient may be at greater risk for HCV infection if they received transfused blood products before 1991. Blood products have been tested for HCV since that time.

Objective Information

Physical Assessment

For good assessment of the abdomen in general and of the hepatic system in particular, you need (1) good light, (2) full exposure of the abdomen, (3) warm hands and short fingernails, and (4) a comfortable, relaxed patient. Physical examination of the hepatic system involves inspection, palpation, and percussion of the abdomen and liver. Routine practice by the pharmacist does not include this type of physical examination, but a clear understanding of it allows the pharmacist to ask patients more pertinent and relevant questions.

The Abdomen

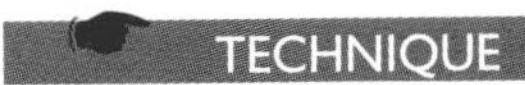
TECHNIQUE

STEP 1

Encourage Relaxation

The patient must be comfortable and relaxed. To encourage relaxation:

- Have the patient void his or her bladder before the examination.

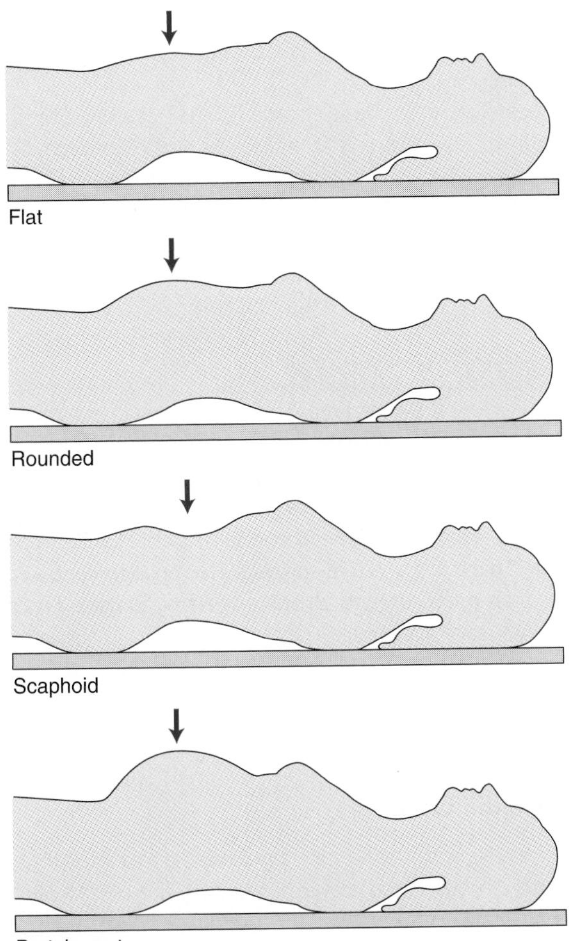

FIGURE 15-2 ■ Contours of the abdomen.

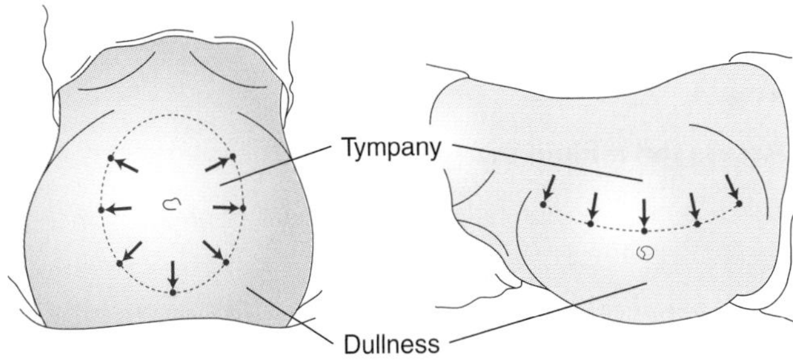

FIGURE 15-3 ■ Shifting dullness.

- Lie the patient in a supine position, with a pillow beneath the head and the knees slightly flexed. The patient's arms should be at the sides.
- Stand on the patient's right side.
- Watch the patient's face for signs of discomfort or pain.
- Distract the patient, if necessary, with conversation or questions.
- Avoid unexpected and abrupt movements.

STEP 2

Inspect the Abdomen

- Inspect the abdomen's skin, noting the color and surface characteristics.
- Inspect and note the abdomen's contour (profile from the rib margin to the pubis, viewed on a horizontal plane) (Fig. 15-2).
- Inspect the abdomen for bulges, symmetry, or an enlarged organ or mass.

ABNORMALITIES Yellow skin suggests jaundice; a glistening, taut appearance suggests ascites. A protuberant abdomen can be a sign for many conditions, including obesity, gaseous distention, tumor, pregnancy, and ascites. An enlarged liver may be seen. Ascites may be seen as flanks that bulge in the supine position. (See Chapter 14 for auscultation and general palpation and percussion of the abdomen.)

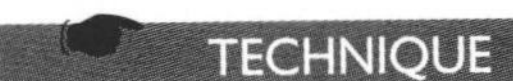
TECHNIQUE

Step 3

Percuss for Shifting Dullness

In patients with a protuberant abdomen or flanks that bulge in the supine position, ascites may be suspected.

- Percuss for areas of dullness and resonance with the patient in the supine position (Fig. 15-3). If found, mark the area.
- Have the patient lie on one side, and again percuss for tympany and dullness. If found, mark the area.

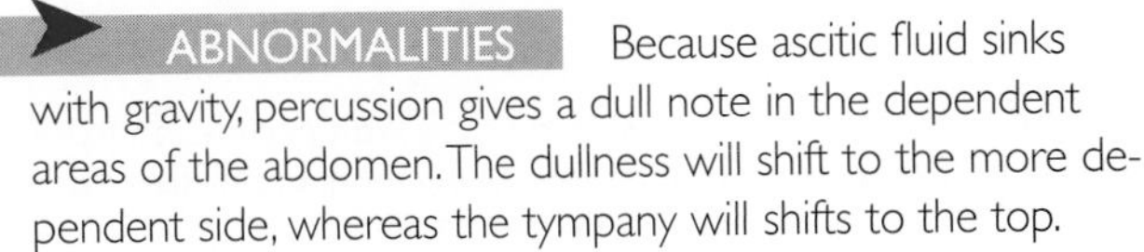
ABNORMALITIES Because ascitic fluid sinks with gravity, percussion gives a dull note in the dependent areas of the abdomen. The dullness will shift to the more dependent side, whereas the tympany will shifts to the top.

TECHNIQUE

Step 4

Assess for a Fluid Wave

This test requires assistance of the patient or an additional person (Fig. 15-4).

- Have the other person press the edge of his of her hand and forearm firmly along the vertical midline of the abdomen.
- Place your hands on each side of the abdomen, and strike one side sharply with your fingertips.
- Feel for the impulse of a fluid wave with the fingertips of your other hand.

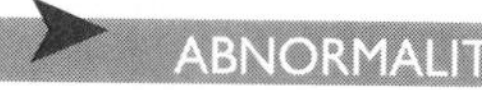

ABNORMALITIES An easily detected fluid wave suggests ascites.

CAUTION A fluid wave can sometimes be felt in patients without ascites and, conversely, may not occur in those with early ascites.

The Liver

TECHNIQUE

Step 1

Percuss the Liver

For ease of examination and patient comfort, you may wish to complete percussion of the liver during percussion of the rest of the abdomen (see Chapter 14).

- Lie the patient in a supine position with the knees bent.
- Percuss the abdomen starting at the right midclavicular line over an area of tympany.

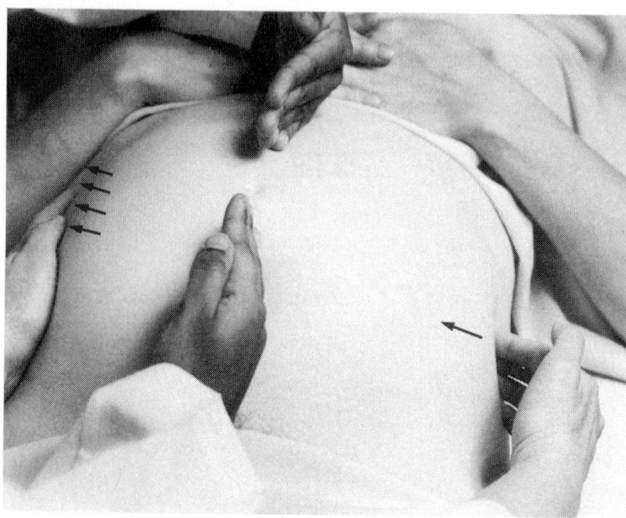

FIGURE 15-4 ■ A fluid wave. (Reprinted with permission from Bickley LS. Bates' guide to physical examination and history taking. 7th ed. Philadelphia: Lippincott Williams & Wilkins, 1999.)

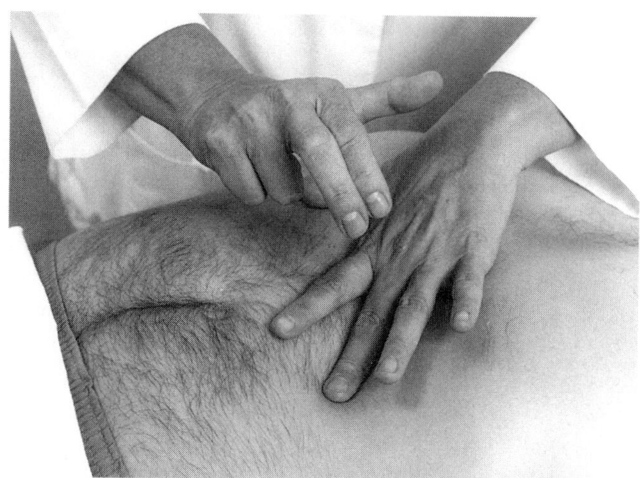

FIGURE 15-5 ■ Percussing the liver span.

CAUTION Always begin percussion over an area of tympany and proceed to an area of dullness, because that sound change is easier to detect than vice versa.

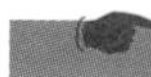

TECHNIQUE

Step 1 (Continued)

- Percuss upward along the midclavicular line (Fig. 15-5) to determine the lower border of the liver. Mark the lower border.
- To determine the upper border, begin percussion on the right midclavicular line at an area of lung resonance. Percuss downward until the tone changes to dullness. The upper border usually begins at the fifth to seventh intercostal space. Mark the upper border.
- Measure the distance between the borders to estimate the vertical span. (Normal is approximately 6-12 cm.)

ABNORMALITIES A lower liver border 2 or 3 cm below the costal margin indicates organ enlargement or a downward displacement of the diaphragm that may be from disease. A border below normal indicates downward displacement from pulmonary causes; a higher border indicates upward displacement from a mass or fluid. A liver span greater than 12 cm suggests liver enlargement; a span less than 6 cm suggests atrophy. Age, sex, and size of a person influence liver span.

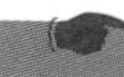

TECHNIQUE

Step 2

Palpate the Liver

- Place your left hand under the patient parallel to the 11th and 12th ribs. Press upward to elevate the liver toward the abdominal wall.
- Place your right hand on the abdomen with your fingers pointing toward the head and extended so your fingertips

rest at the right midclavicular line below the lower liver border previously percussed (Fig. 15-6).

- Press your right hand gently, but deeply, in and up.
- As the patient breathes deeply, try to feel the liver edge.
- When felt, the liver should be firm, smooth, even, and not tender.

ABNORMALITIES Hardness of the liver, bluntness or rounding of its edges, and irregularity of its contour suggest abnormalities.

TECHNIQUE

Step 2 (Continued)

An alternative method of palpating the liver (Fig. 15-7) is:

- Stand at the patient's shoulder, facing the feet.
- Hook your fingers over the costal margin from above.
- Have the person take a deep breath, and then feel for the lower edge of the liver.

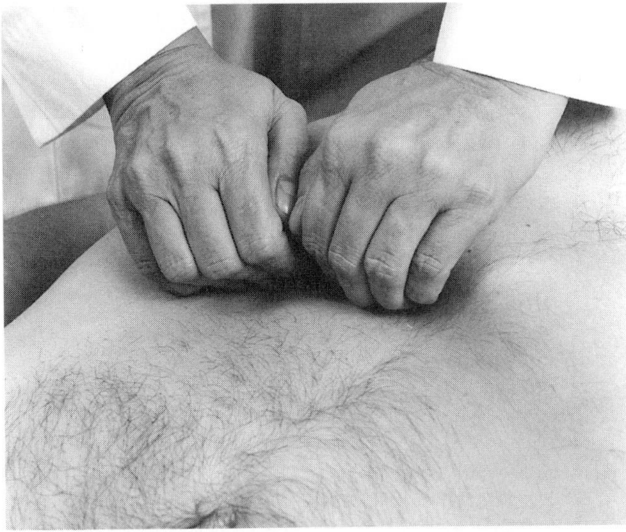

FIGURE 15-7 ■ Palpating the liver (hook technique).

Laboratory and Diagnostic Tests

Laboratory and diagnostic tests that may be useful in assessing the hepatic system include:

- Total cholesterol, high-density lipoprotein cholesterol, low-density lipoprotein cholesterol, and triglycerides to determine functioning of the pancreas and liver.
- Albumin, which is synthesized by the liver and can be measured to assess the liver's ability to synthesize proteins. It has a long life span (half-life, 20 days) and is slow to fall after the onset of hepatic dysfunction. Complete cessation of albumin production results in a 25% decrease in the serum albumin level after 8 days. Therefore, low concentrations (<2.5 g/dL) are associated with a poor prognosis in patients with liver disease. Because of the long half-life, albumin may be slow to increase after remission of hepatic disease.
- Prealbumin, which is also synthesized by the liver and is generally used to assess the patient's nutritional status rather than the liver's synthetic capability. Its half-life is shorter than that of albumin (2 vs. 20 days, respectively); therefore, it is a sensitive marker for acute liver and nutritional status changes.
- Total protein, which is the sum of albumin and globulin and follows the same trend as albumin.
- Prothrombin time (PT), which can be elevated significantly in patients with advanced liver disease. The liver synthesizes coagulation factors I, II (prothrombin), V, VII, IX, and X. It has tremendous synthetic reserves, and more coagulation factors are produced than are needed. Only severe hepatic dysfunction decreases synthesis and impairs clotting. A PT that remains prolonged after the administration of vitamin K is caused by hepatic impairment.
- Alkaline phosphatase, which refers to a group of enzymes present in a variety of body tissues, including liver, bone, and intestine. This is not a specific test for liver dysfunction. Serum levels may be increased in biliary diseases, tumors, or cirrhosis.
- Gamma-glutamyl transpeptidase (GGTP), which is a biliary excretory enzyme that participates in the transfer of amino acids and peptides across cellular membranes. It may be found in the liver, kidney, spleen, and prostate gland. Because it is not found in bone, it can help to explain elevated alkaline phosphatase levels. The GGTP increases with alcohol ingestion, hepatitis, cirrhosis, hepatic necrosis, and ischemia.
- The aminotransferases, alanine aminotransferase (ALT) and aspartate aminotransferase (AST), which indicate hepatic inflammation and necrosis. Markedly elevated concentrations are associated with acute viral hepatitis, severe drug or toxic reactions, and hepatic necrosis. Infants and elderly patients may normally have higher levels than the average adult.
- Lactate dehydrogenase (LDH), which is found in most human tissues, especially the liver, myocardium, skeletal muscle, brain, kidneys, and red blood cells. It is

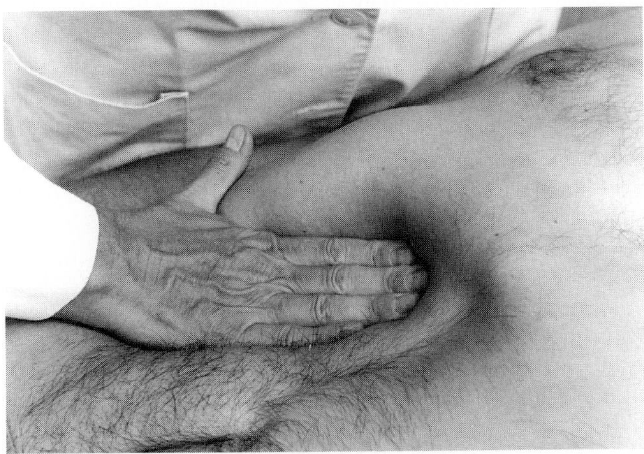

FIGURE 15-6 ■ Palpating the liver.

composed of five isoenzymes; elevation in LDH5 corresponds with liver disease.

- Bilirubin, which is a degradation product of heme and the levels of which represent a balance between production and excretion. Total bilirubin is the sum of conjugated (direct) and unconjugated (indirect) bilirubin. An elevated total bilirubin is not a sensitive indicator of hepatic disease. Jaundice usually becomes visible when the total bilirubin concentration is 2-4 mg/dL. Other hepatic tests should be used in combination with an elevated bilirubin level. Predominantly indirect bilirubin is elevated by excessive bilirubin production, impaired bilirubin conjugation, or reduced hepatic bilirubin uptake. Conjugated bilirubin becomes elevated in response to biliary obstruction or hepatocellular dysfunction.
- Ammonia, which is a byproduct of protein breakdown and is metabolized by the liver into urea and then excreted by the kidneys. In liver dysfunction, or when blood flow to the liver changes (e.g., portal hypertension), ammonia cannot be catabolized, and the levels rise.
- Amylase and lipase, which are enzymes produced by the pancreas to promote the breakdown of starches and fats, respectively. Both concentrations are elevated during acute pancreatitis; other causes of elevated concentrations include alcoholism and gallstones. Serum lipase is generally less sensitive but more specific than amylase in pancreatitis.
- Antigens of hepatitis viruses and antibodies, which can be measured to determine if a patient has an acute, chronic, or resolving viral hepatitis infection.
- Ultrasound, which is primarily used to depict biliary dilation and gallstones.
- Computed tomography with IV contrast material, which is generally used to evaluate for abscesses, tumors, pancreatitis, and other parenchymal diseases.
- Magnetic resonance imaging, which is used to assess for tumors and other growths (contrast material is not needed).

Special Considerations

Pediatric Patients

Additional questions to ask the pediatric patient's parent or guardian include:

? INTERVIEW Has your child received hepatitis B vaccinations? Does your child go to day care? Does your child tire easily? Does the child have any history of liver problems?

ABNORMALITIES Children in day care or public or private school have additional risk for hepatitis A because of inappropriate food preparation or sharing of food from home.

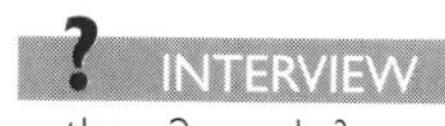
Has your baby had jaundice for more than 2 weeks?

ABNORMALITIES Persistence of neonatal jaundice beyond 2 weeks should be evaluated for an organic cause. The three most common include hepatitis, biliary atresia, and choledochal cyst (inflammation and dilation of the common bile duct from reflex on pancreatic enzymes into the pancreatic duct).

Physical examination of pediatric patients is similar to that of adults. Major differences include the liver being more easily palpated, especially in infants and young children. The size of the liver is better determined by percussion than by palpation. If the liver extends 3 cm or more below the costal margin, this suggests infection, cardiac failure, or liver disease. The contours of young children's abdomens are normally protuberant when standing and supine because of immature abdominal musculature; as the child ages, the protuberant nature of the abdomen decreases, first in the supine position and then when standing.

Geriatric Patients

Additional questions to ask geriatric patients or their caregivers include:

? INTERVIEW Do you take care of your medicine by yourself at home? Does anyone help you with your medicine? What do you do when you forget to take your medicine?

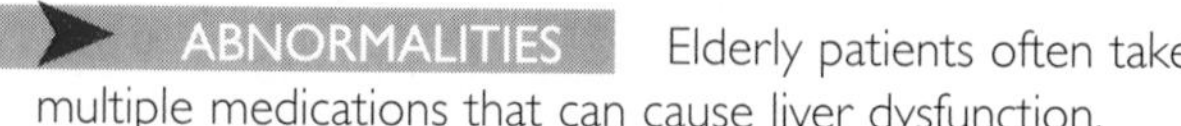
multiple medications that can cause liver dysfunction.

Physical examination of older adults is the same as that of younger adults. In geriatric patients, however, the abdominal wall is thinner and softer, allowing easier palpation of the liver in the absence of obesity. Palpation may be relatively easier than percussion and provide more accurate findings. The liver may be palpated lower than in younger adults because of distended lungs and a depressed diaphragm, especially in patients with chronic obstructive pulmonary disease. The liver may be enlarged or atrophy slightly with increasing age. Use judgment to determine whether patients can comfortably assume a particular position for assessment, and change your examination techniques as needed.

Pregnant Patients

Additional questions to ask pregnant patients include:

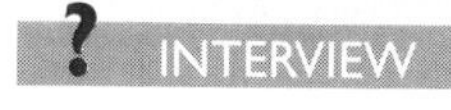
How many weeks pregnant are you?

ABNORMALITIES Pregnancy may alter the usual location of abdominal pain.

? INTERVIEW Have you had difficulties with swelling of your hands and feet? Any unusual or new problems with nausea, vomiting, headache, itching, or abdominal pain? Do you know what your blood pressure has been?

ABNORMALITIES Pregnant women, especially those with preeclampsia, are at risk for acute fatty liver of pregnancy, cholestasis of pregnancy, eclampsia, and the HELLP syndrome (hemolysis, elevated liver tests, and low platelets). Though rare, these syndromes occur primarily during the third trimester. These women are at great risk of morbidity and mortality for both themselves and the fetus and should immediately seek care from a physician.

The liver is more difficult to assess in pregnant patients because of the increasing size of the uterus. Gastrointestinal complaints of nausea and vomiting are common during the first trimester, and heartburn may be more frequent as the pregnancy progresses. (See Chapter 14 for a more detailed discussion on the gastrointestinal system in pregnancy.)

APPLICATION TO PATIENT SYMPTOMS

Because they typically practice in a setting where patients present with specific symptoms, pharmacists should be able to assess these symptoms, identify their most probable cause, and determine the most appropriate action to either correct or further evaluate the problem. Common symptoms relating to the hepatic system include abdominal pain, ascites, and jaundice.

Abdominal Pain

Abdominal pain can result from many different causes and does not necessarily indicate hepatic disease. It may also result from cardiac, gastrointestinal, musculoskeletal, and genitourinary disorders. Common causes for the various types of abdominal pain include:

- *Cardiac:* coronary artery disease, pericarditis, and angina pectoris.
- *Musculoskeletal:* arthritis and trauma.
- *Gastrointestinal:* ulcer disease, gastritis, hiatal hernia, gastroesophageal reflux disease, constipation, and inflammatory bowel disease.
- *Genitourinary:* sexually transmitted diseases, cystitis, pyelonephritis, ectopic pregnancy, labor, and menstrual cramps.

Aspirin or heat generally relieves musculoskeletal pain. Angina can be induced by physical exertion or emotional stress and usually is relieved by rest or nitroglycerin. Genitourinary problems generally occur lower in the abdomen, whereas hepatic illnesses generally occur in the upper quadrants. (See Chapter 14 for specific gastrointestinal causes of abdominal pain.) Hepatic abdominal pain might relate to nausea and vomiting of bile, tenderness in the epigastric area, and increased liver enzymes. Many medications can cause abdominal pain; some of the more common are listed in Box 15-7.

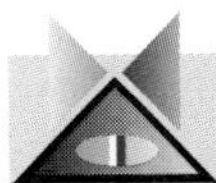

Box 15-7

DRUGS THAT MAY CAUSE ABDOMINAL PAIN

- Acyclovir
- Nonsteroidal anti-inflammatory drugs
- Antibiotics
- 3-Hydroxy-3-methylglutaric acid coenzyme A reductase inhibitors
- Steroids
- Hormones
- Antihypertensives

CASE STUDY

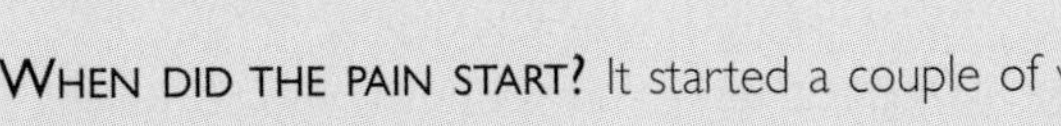

FV is a 46-year-old, obese woman with a history of s/p (status post) hysterectomy and bilateral oophorectomy, hyperlipidemia, and hypothyroidism who comes into the pharmacy for refills of her medications. During counseling, she states she has been having a lot of abdominal pain over the last couple of weeks and would like to purchase some Pepcid.

ASSESSMENT OF THE PATIENT

Subjective Information

46-year-old woman complaining of abdominal pain

WHEN DID THE PAIN START? It started a couple of weeks ago.

WHERE IS THE PAIN? In the upper part of my stomach, kind of near my ribs, more to the right of center.

DESCRIBE THE PAIN. It is mostly dull and feels really tender.

DOES IT GO ANYWHERE? No. It pretty much stays in the same spot.

HOW LONG DOES THE PAIN LAST? It lasts off and on throughout the day, but it gets worse after I eat.

Continued

CASE STUDY—continued

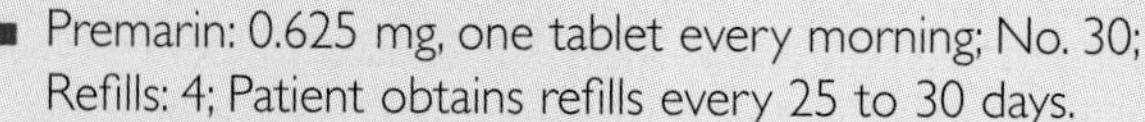

HAVE YOU EVER HAD THIS TYPE OF ABDOMINAL PAIN BEFORE? No.

HOW OFTEN DO YOU EXPERIENCE THIS PAIN? Pretty much every day.

WHAT MAKES THE PAIN WORSE? Eating, especially anything greasy.

WHAT MAKES THE PAIN BETTER? It normally goes away about 3 or 4 hours after I eat.

DOES IT FEEL LIKE IT IS BURNING? Every now and then, but most of the time no.

CAN YOU EVER TASTE ACID IN YOUR MOUTH? No.

DOES IT EVER WAKEN YOU FROM SLEEP? No.

DOES LYING DOWN CAUSE THE PAIN TO INCREASE? No, not really.

DO YOU FEEL LIKE YOU WANT TO VOMIT? No, not really, except yesterday.

DID YOU VOMIT? Yes, after I ate fast food yesterday.

WHAT DID IT LOOK LIKE? It kind of had a yellowish-greenish hue to it.

WAS THERE ANY BLOOD IN THE VOMIT, EITHER BRIGHT RED OR ANYTHING THAT LOOKED LIKE COFFEE GROUNDS? No, not that I've seen.

HAVE YOU HAD ANY DIARRHEA? No.

WHAT DOES YOUR STOOL LOOK LIKE? Like normal, I guess.

HAVE YOU LOST ANY WEIGHT LATELY? I've lost about 40 pounds over the last 5 months on Weight Watchers.

DO YOU DRINK ALCOHOL? Very rarely. Maybe a glass of wine with dinner every couple of months.

WHAT MEDICATIONS ARE YOU CURRENTLY TAKING? Only the ones I get here.

Objective Information

Computerized medication profile:

- Synthroid: 0.112 mg, one tablet every morning; No. 30; Refills: 5; Patient obtains refills every 25 to 30 days.
- Zocor: 40 mg, one tablet every morning; No. 30; Refills: 5; Patient obtains refills every 25 to 30 days.
- Premarin: 0.625 mg, one tablet every morning; No. 30; Refills: 4; Patient obtains refills every 25 to 30 days.

Patient is in no acute distress; no shortness of breath or light-headedness
Heart rate: 86 bpm
Blood pressure: 124/76 mm Hg
Respiratory rate: 18 rpm
Temperature: 98.4°F
Abdomen: No lesions or discolorations; protuberant abdomen from obesity; bowel sounds normal; tender to palpation in right upper quadrant (RUQ); liver within normal limits (WNL)

DISCUSSION

The concern centers around the occurrence of FV's chest pain. The pharmacist needs to determine what type of abdominal pain the patient most likely is experiencing and if Pepcid is an appropriate choice. FV has been having abdominal pain that is worsened by eating high-fat foods. She rarely has a burning sensation, does not taste acid in her mouth, and the pain does not increase on lying down. She did say that she vomited a greenish-yellow liquid.

After evaluating and synthesizing all the patient's subjective and objective information, the pharmacist concludes that Pepcid is not an appropriate option. The pain may be caused by cholestasis or cholelithiasis, and the patient should be referred to her physician for further evaluation. The steps involved in this assessment process are illustrated in Figure 15-8. The pharmacist also recognizes that the estrogen replacement therapy may be a potential cause or aggravating factor. Because FV is not in any current severe distress and her temperature is not elevated, she should be referred to her physician within the next few days. The pharmacist calls the physician and discusses FV's complaints as well as the potential aggravation of FV's condition by the estrogen replacement therapy. The physician agrees to hold the Premarin until evaluation can be completed. The patient is scheduled for an appointment in 2 days, and the pharmacist arranges for a follow-up phone call in 3 days to see how her abdominal pain is doing.

Continued

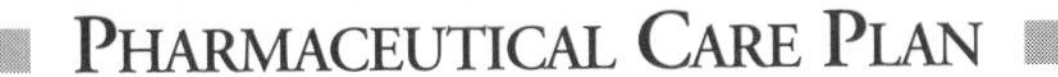

CASE STUDY—continued

PHARMACEUTICAL CARE PLAN

Patient Name: FV

Date: 8/26/02

Medical Problems:
- Hyperlipidemia
- Hypothyroidism
- Postmenopausal secondary to hysterectomy with bilateral oophorectomy

Current Medications:
- Synthroid, 0.112 mg, one tablet every morning, No. 30, Refills: 5
- Zocor, 40 mg, one tablet every morning, No.30, Refills: 5
- Premarin, 0.625 mg, one tablet every morning, No. 30, Refills: 4

S: 46-year-old obese white woman complains of RUQ abdominal pain worsened by fatty meals and requests Pepcid. Pain occurs after eating and lasts for a couple of hours. Vomited once, greenish-yellow liquid. Denies vomiting blood. Is currently on a diet and has lost 40 pounds in the last 5 months.

O: Patient in no acute distress. No shortness of breath or light-headedness.

Heart rate: 86 bpm

Blood pressure: 124/76 mm Hg

Respiratory rate: 18 rpm

Temperature: 98.4°F

Abdomen: No lesions or discolorations. Protuberant abdomen from obesity. Bowel sounds normal. Tender to palpation in RUQ. Liver WNL.

A: Possible cholestasis or cholelithiasis

P:
1. Call physician to discuss patient's complaints.
2. Set up an appointment with physician in 2 days.
3. Hold Premarin therapy.
4. Educate patient about avoiding high-fat foods and eating small portions.
5. Inform patient to go to the emergency room if she develops a fever or begins to vomit more bile.
6. Follow-up phone call in 3 days to assess patient's abdominal pain and further evaluation.

Pharmacist: *Jacob Reitman, Pharm.D.*

Self-Assessment Questions

1. Compare and contrast the various interview questions that are useful in differentiating the types of abdominal pain.
2. What are the signs and symptoms of cholelithiasis and cholestasis?
3. What medications can cause liver dysfunction?

Critical Thinking Questions

1. How would your assessment and care plan change if FV had a long history of alcohol abuse?
2. What other objective measures would be useful in further evaluating FV? What information will these measures provide?

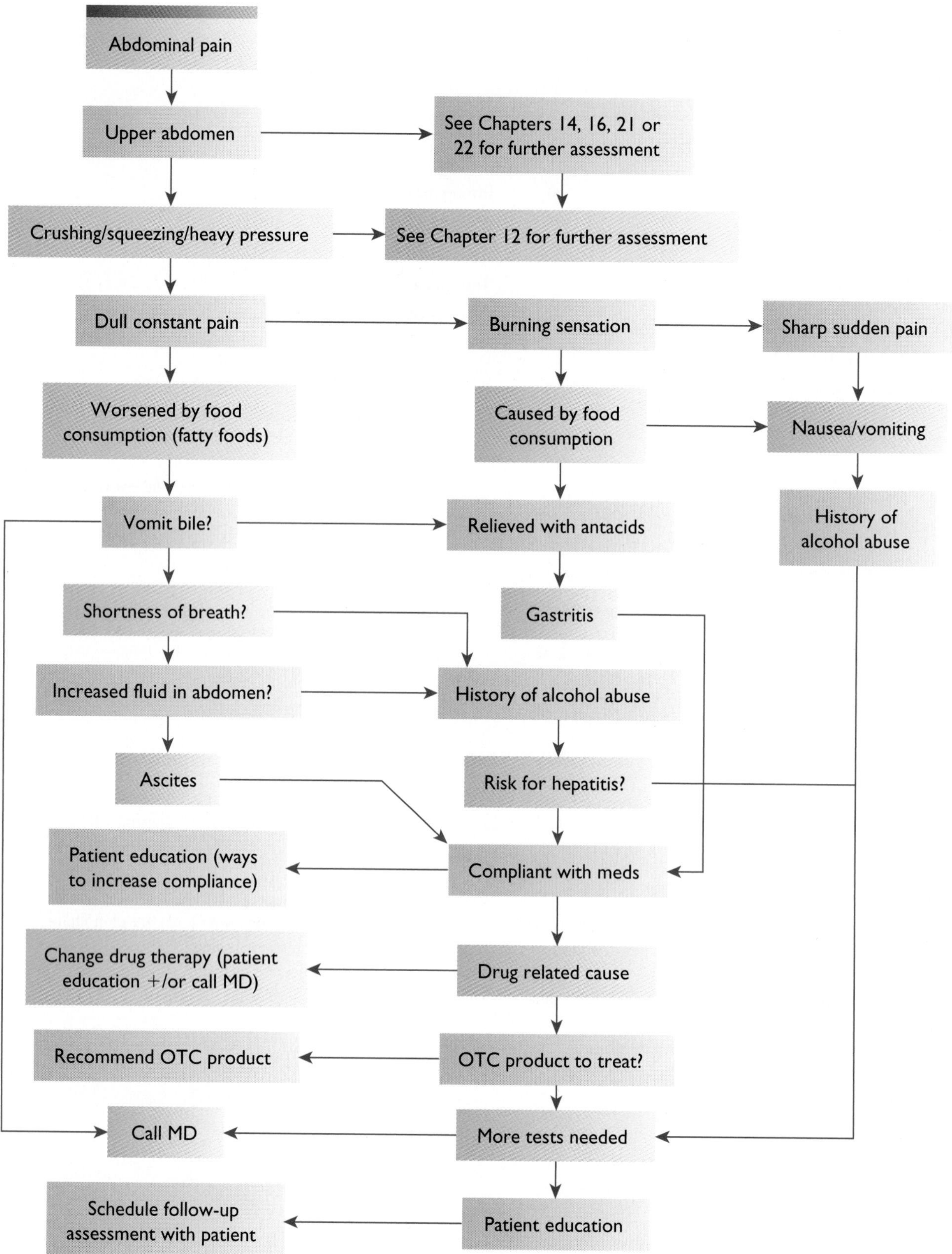

FIGURE 15-8 ■ Decision tree for abdominal pain.

Ascites

Ascites is the accumulation of fluid in the peritoneal cavity. This accumulation leads to abdominal swelling. Causes of ascites include:

- Infections
- Heart failure
- Portal hypertension
- Cirrhosis
- Various cancers (especially of the ovary and liver)
- Medications (Box 15-8)

Different diseases of the peritoneum should be ruled out; these include infections, neoplasms, vasculitis, and other possible causes of peritoneal inflammation. Ascites can be classified as low-gradient ascites, in which the serum ascites albumin gradient is less than 1.1, or as high-gradient ascites, in which this gradient is more than 1.1. The ascitic fluid may contain red blood cells, white blood cells, protein, organisms, amylase, or some combination thereof, which can help in determining the cause.

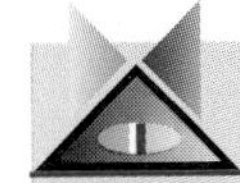

Box 15-8

DRUGS THAT MAY CAUSE ASCITES

- Tricyclic antidepressants
- Lithium
- Vitamin A and derivatives
- Leuprolide
- Dextran

CASE STUDY

JP is a 52-year-old black man with a history of alcohol abuse, atrial fibrillation, and cirrhosis who comes into the pharmacy for a refill of his medications. During counseling, he states that his abdomen feels full and his clothes are fitting more tightly.

ASSESSMENT OF THE PATIENT

Subjective Information

52-year-old male patient who complains of fullness in the abdomen and "tighter fitting clothes"

WHEN DID THIS BEGIN? It has seemed worse for the past month or so. It was better about 3 months ago, and then it just seems to have gotten worse.

WHAT BRINGS IT ON? I don't really know.

WHAT MAKES IT BETTER OR GO AWAY? Sometimes the doctor gives me medicine and that seems to help; that's why I came into the pharmacy today.

DO YOU EXPERIENCE ANY OTHER SYMPTOMS WITH IT? SHORTNESS OF BREATH? It does seem like my breath had been harder to catch if I walk around a lot or if I lay flat on my back. It is like there is too much pressure to breathe.

ABDOMINAL PAIN? Just a lot of pressure. It feels tight.

SWELLING IN YOUR LEGS OR FEET? No, those normally do real well.

DO YOU HAVE ANY IMMEDIATE FAMILY MEMBERS WHO HAVE HAD PROBLEMS WITH THEIR LIVER? Not that I know of.

WHAT PRESCRIPTIONS AND NONPRESCRIPTION MEDICATIONS ARE YOU CURRENTLY TAKING? Just the ones I get here. I do take some acetaminophen every now and then.

DO YOU SMOKE OR CHEW TOBACCO? Nope, never have.

HOW MUCH DO YOU DRINK (BEER, WINE, LIQUOR)? I have a wine cooler or two just about every day.

Objective Information

Computerized medication profile:

- Furosemide: 80 mg, one tablet twice daily; No. 60; Refills: 3; Patient obtains refills every 35 to 40 days
- Spironolactone: 25 mg, one tablet twice daily; No. 60; Refills: 5; Patient obtains refills every 40 to 45 days
- Lisinopril: 10 mg, one tablet daily; No. 30; Refills: 3; Patient obtains refills every 35 to 40 days
- Digoxin: 0.125 mg, one table daily; No. 30; Refills: 3; Patient obtains refills every 35 to 40 days
- Thiamine: 100 mg, one tablet daily; No. 100; Refills: 2; Patient obtains refills every 100 to 110 days

Patient in no acute distress
No palpitations, light-headedness, or dizziness
Positive dyspnea on exertion and shortness of breath lying down
Height: 5'9"
Weight: 158 pounds
Heart rate: 104 bpm (irregular rhythm)
Blood pressure: 110/86 mm Hg
Respiratory rate: 16 rpm
Heart auscultation: irregular rate; irregular rhythm; no murmurs, rubs, or gallops
Pulmonary: clear throughout bilaterally
Abdomen: protuberant abdomen, slightly tender on palpation, lower liver border 7 cm below costal margin, positive shifting dullness, negative fluid wave
Extremities: no edema present

Continued

CASE STUDY—continued

DISCUSSION

When a patient complains of fullness in the abdomen, the pharmacist must clarify the symptoms and determine the possible causes. With JP, the pharmacist needs to determine if the patient is experiencing fullness in his abdomen because of liver failure, worsening of cirrhosis, or development of CHF. JP states that he is drinking every day. His abdominal fullness has responded previously to pharmacologic treatment. He currently does not have an S_3 gallop, so overt heart failure may not be a possibility.

After evaluating JP's subjective and objective information, the pharmacist concludes that the abdominal fullness is caused by ascites from his liver disease, secondary to noncompliance. To illustrate the steps involved with the assessment process, see Figure 15-9. The pharmacist also concludes that a referral to the physician is not warranted at this time because of JP's noncompliance and lack of distress. The pharmacist educates the patient about improving compliance with his medications to help with the abdominal fullness, advises him to decrease or completely stop his alcohol intake, and says that if JP starts having difficulty breathing or feels worse, he should see his physician. The pharmacist schedules a follow-up appointment in 1 week to check JP's signs and symptoms, compliance with his medications, and weight.

PHARMACEUTICAL CARE PLAN

Patient Name: JP

Date: 10/28/02

Medical Problems:
- Alcohol abuse
- Atrial fibrillation
- Cirrhosis

Current Medications:
- Furosemide, 80 mg, one tablet twice daily
- Spironolactone, 25 mg, one tablet twice daily
- Lisinopril, 10 mg, one tablet daily
- Digoxin, 0.125 mg, one tablet daily
- Thiamine, 100 mg, one tablet daily

S: 52-year-old male patient who complains of fullness and tightness in the abdomen and "tighter fitting clothes," worsening over the last month. States shortness of breath when lying down and on exertion. States he has previously had the same symptoms, but they were relieved by medications. Still states ingestion of one to two wine coolers per day.

O: Patient in no acute distress. No palpitations, lightheadedness, or dizziness. Positive dyspnea on exertion and shortness of breath lying down.

Height: 5'9"

Weight: 158 pounds

Heart rate: 104 bpm (irregular rhythm)

Blood pressure: 110/86 mm Hg

Respiratory rate: 16 rpm

Heart auscultation: irregular rate, irregular rhythm, no murmurs, rubs, or gallops

Pulmonary: clear throughout bilaterally

Abdomen: protuberant abdomen, slightly tender on palpation, lower liver border 7 cm below costal margin, positive shifting dullness, negative fluid wave

Extremities: no edema present

A:
1. Ascites caused by liver disease and noncompliance with current regimen.
2. Alcoholism.

P:
1. Patient education: increase compliance with medications, and stress importance of medications.
2. Counsel on alcohol abstinence or decrease and possibility of rehabilitation programs.
3. Follow-up in 1 week to evaluate signs and symptoms, weight, compliance with medications, and side effects.

Pharmacist: *Rita Buk, Pharm.D.*

Self-Assessment Questions

1. Why might JP not have had a fluid wave on physical examination even though he has ascites?
2. What medications may cause ascites?
3. Describe the shifting dullness test and its use in evaluating ascites.

Critical Thinking Questions

1. How would your assessment and care plan change if JP also had CHF? What other physical assessment techniques would be useful?
2. How would medications be affected by ascites, and what would you need to consider?

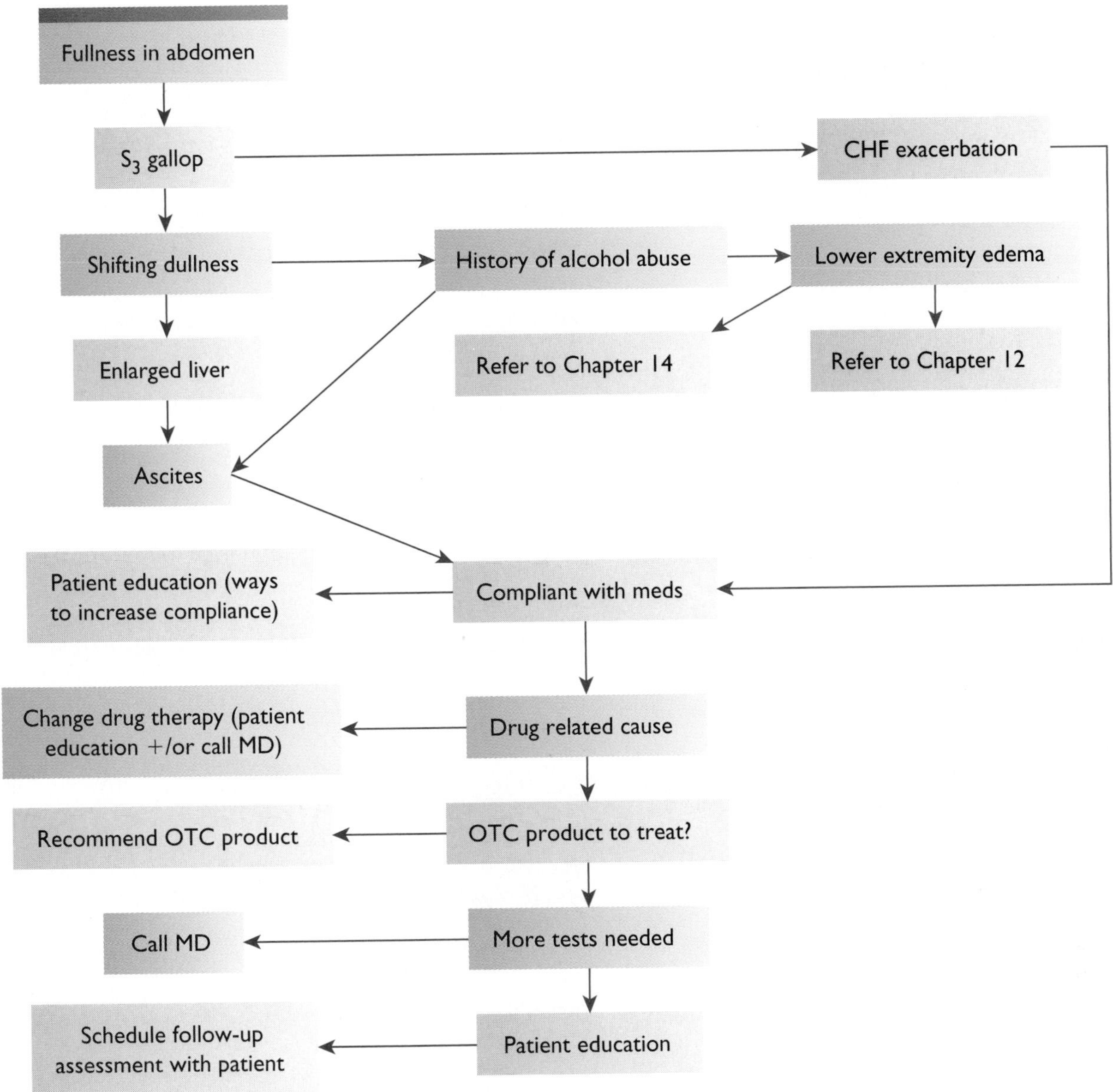

FIGURE 15-9 ■ Decision tree for ascites.

Jaundice

Jaundice, a yellowing of the skin and whites of the eyes, is a sign of increased bilirubin. Causes of jaundice include:

- Obstruction
- Liver dysfunction
- Hemolysis
- Medications (Box 15-3)

Table 15-2 differentiates causes of jaundice. Color changes in the urine and feces can give good information regarding the possible cause, but jaundice itself always indicates a problem.

TABLE 15-2 ➤ DIFFERENTIATING CHARACTERISTICS OF TYPES OF JAUNDICE

TYPE	CAUSE	URINE	FECES	OTHER
Obstructive	Bile fails to reach the intestine because of obstruction in the bile ducts or cholestasis	Dark	Pale	Patient may itch
Hepatocellular	Liver is unable to use the bilirubin that accumulates in the blood	Dark	Normal	Increased liver function tests
Hemolytic	Excessive destruction of red cells in the blood	Normal	Normal	Low hemoglobin and hematocrit

CASE STUDY

MW is a 23-year-old woman with a history of allergies who calls the pharmacy wanting to pick up her nasal spray. While talking to you, she asks if the medication can make her skin or eyes turn yellow.

ASSESSMENT OF THE PATIENT

Subjective Information

23-year-old woman complaining of yellow skin and eyes

When did your eyes and skin turn yellow? About 3 or 4 days ago.

What other symptoms are you experiencing? I have just been kind of tired and achy lately, but I have attributed that to school.

Have you experienced nausea or vomiting? No.

What color are your stools? Normal.

What color is your urine? It kind of looks like really diluted tea.

Itching for unknown reason? No.

Do you have any history of liver problems? No.

Do you have any history of problems with your gallbladder or pancreas? No.

What prescription and nonprescription medications are you currently taking? I take the Flonase for my allergies and then some Naproxen when I need something for a headache, but that isn't very often.

Do you smoke or chew tobacco? Yes. I smoke about half a pack a day.

How often do you drink alcohol (beer, wine liquor)? A couple of times a week.

Have you ever used injectable drugs? No.

Have you recently traveled outside of the United States? I just got back about a month ago from a trip to Africa.

Have you been around someone with hepatitis or other liver disease? Not that I know of.

Have you had any abdominal surgery lately? No.

What do you do for a living? I am a student and live in the sorority house.

Have you ever received a blood transfusion? No.

Objective Information

Computerized medication profile:

- Flonase Nasal Spray: 50 g, two sprays per nostril once daily; No. 9; Refills: 1; Patient refills medication every 25 to 35 days

Patient in no acute distress
Heart rate: 68 bpm
Blood pressure: 106/72 mm Hg
Abdomen: No lesions, skin yellow, no tenderness to palpation, liver within normal limits
Head, eyes, ears, nose, and throat (HEENT): White of eyes yellow

DISCUSSION

The concern centers around the possible causes of jaundice; the pharmacist needs to determine the most likely one. MW just returned from a trip to Africa, in which HAV in endemic. She also has had very vague complaints of fatigue and feeling achy. Her stools are normal in color, but her urine is dark. She does not have any tenderness on palpation, which you might expect if her jaundice was related to gallbladder disease.

After evaluating and synthesizing all the patient's subjective and objective information, the pharmacist concludes that MW's jaundice could be caused by HAV infection. The steps involved in this assessment process are illustrated in Figure 15-10. The pharmacist calls MW's physician, notifies him of MW's symptoms, and sets up an appointment. MW is counseled on avoiding any medications and alcohol and on eating a healthy diet, resting well, and maintaining a good fluid balance.

Continued

Self-Assessment Questions

1. How do you differentiate between the types of jaundice?
2. What medications can worsen jaundice?
3. Do HBV and HCV have different rates of chronic infection? Why?

Critical Thinking Questions

1. What laboratory tests would you order when assessing a patient with potential viral hepatitis, and what would these results tell you?
2. A 30-year-old man comes into the pharmacy asking about the hepatitis B vaccine, because his roommate has just been diagnosed with HBV infection. What do you tell him?

CASE STUDY—continued

Pharmaceutical Care Plan

Patient Name: MW

Date: 9/10/02

Medical Problems:

Seasonal allergies

Current Medications:

Flonase Nasal Spray, 50 g, two sprays per nostril once daily

Naproxen, 220 mg, one or two tablets daily as needed

S: 23-year-old woman who lives in a local sorority house complaining of yellow skin and eyes for the last 3 or 4 days. States that she returned from a trip to Africa about a month ago. Has recently been more fatigued and achy than normal. Smokes half a pack of cigarettes daily and drinks two or three times per week.

O: Patient is in no acute distress.

Heart rate: 68 bpm

Blood pressure: 106/72 mm Hg

Abdomen: no lesions, skin yellow, no tenderness to palpation, liver within normal limits

HEENT: white of eyes yellow

A: Jaundice.

P: 1. Talk to physician concerning signs and symptoms.

2. Refer to physician for further tests to evaluate for HAV infection.
3. Counseled on avoiding medications and alcohol, eating a healthy diet, resting well, and maintaining a good fluid balance.
4. Call in 1 week to evaluate signs and symptoms.

Pharmacist: *Richard Silverstein, Pharm.D.*

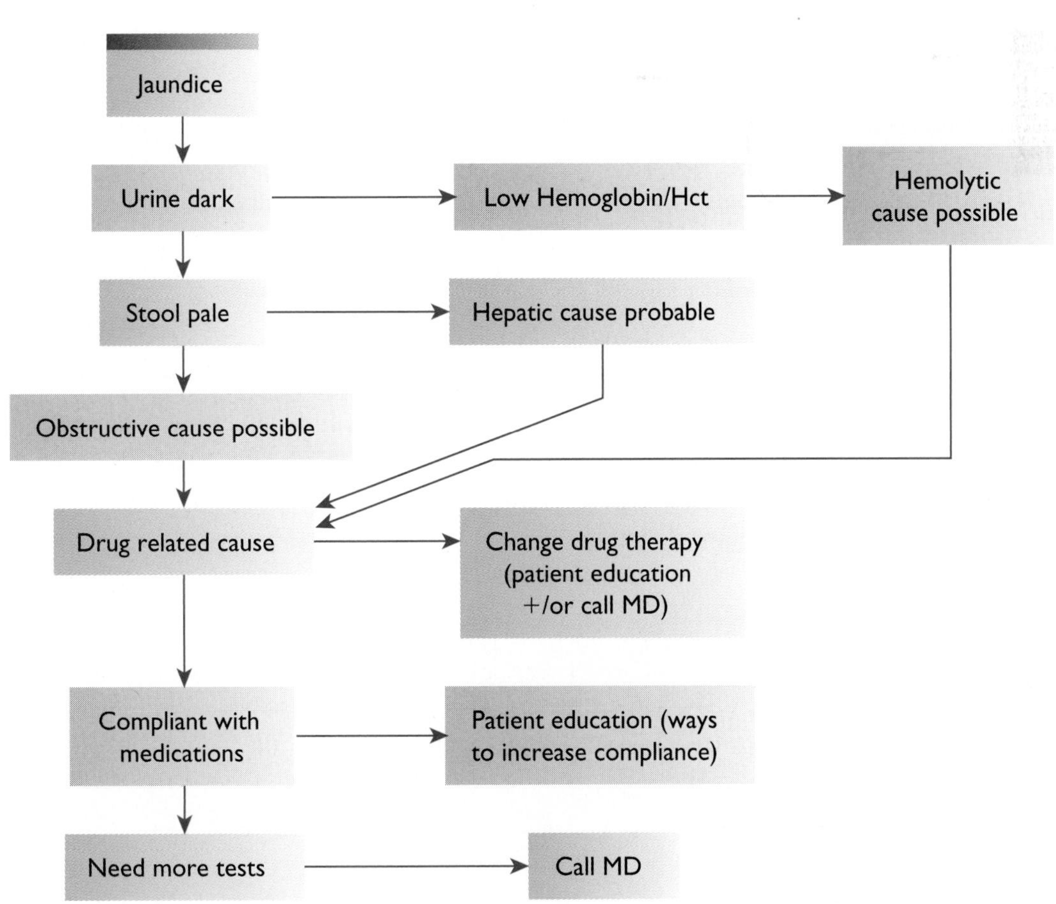

Figure 15-10 ■ Decision tree for jaundice.

Bibliography

Albrecht JH, Jensen DM, Peine CJ, Schieff ER. Transfusions to tattoos: the danger of hepatitis C. Patient Care 1996;13:113–139.

Amann ST, Di Magno E, Rubin W. Pancreatitis: diagnostic and therapeutic interventions. Patient Care 1997;18:200–215.

Bataller R, Gines P, Arroyo V. Practical recommendations for the treatment of ascites and its complications. Drugs 1997;54:571–580.

Berger A. Behavior of hepatitis C virus. BMJ 1998;317:437.

Braunwald E, Fauncias Kasper DL, Hauser SL, Longo DL, Jameson JL. Harrison's principles of internal medicine. 15th ed. New York: McGraw-Hill, 2001.

Ciba Foundation Symposium 63. Pregnancy metabolism, diabetes and the fetus. Amsterdam: Excerpta Medica, 1979.

Evans WE, Schentag JJ, Jusko WJ. Applied pharmacokinetics: principles of therapeutic drug monitoring. 3rd ed. Vancouver, Washington: Applied Therapeutics, 1992.

Gartner LM, Herschel M. Jaundice and breastfeeding. Pediatr Clin North Am 2001;48;389–399.

Gill MA, Kirchain WR. Portal hypertension and cirrhosis. In: Dipiro JT, Talbert RL, Yee GC, et al., eds. Pharmacotherapy: a pathophysiologic approach. 4th ed. Stamford, CT: Appleton & Lange, 1999:614–627.

Gubernick JA, Rosenberg HK, Ilaslan H, Kessler A. US approach to jaundice in infants and children. Radiographics 2000;20:173–195.

Guyton AC, Hall JE. Human physiology and mechanisms of disease. 6th ed. Philadelphia: WB Saunders, 1997.

Hart MN, Kent TH. Introduction to human disease. 4th ed. Upper Saddle River, NJ: Prentice-Hall, 1998.

Herfindal ET, Gourley DR. Textbook of therapeutics: drug and disease management. 7th ed. Baltimore: Lippincott Williams & Wilkins, 2000.

Houston R, Hayes J. Wildman K, Allerheiligen D. Jaundice and disseminated intravascular coagulopathy in pregnancy. J Am Board Fam Pract 2000;13:70–72.

Hunt CM, Sharara AI. Liver disease in pregnancy. Am Fam Physician 1999;59:1–10.

Kirchain WR, Gill MA. Drug-induced liver disease. In: Dipiro JT, Talbert RL, Yee GC, et al., eds. Pharmacotherapy: a pathophysiologic approach. 4th ed. Stamford, CT: Appleton & Lange, 1999:614–627.

Koda-Kimble MA, Young LY. Applied therapeutics: the clinical use of drugs. Baltimore: Lippincott Williams & Wilkins, 2001.

Krige JE, Beckinham IJ. ABC of diseases of liver, pancreas, and biliary system: Portal hypertension-2. Ascites, encephalopathy, and other conditions. BMJ 2001;322:416–418.

Kumar RK. Neonatal jaundice. An update for family physicians. Aust Fam Physician 1999;28:679–682.

Lafferty K. Understanding abdominal pain. Practitioner 2001;245:156,159–161.

Lee WM. Hepatitis B virus infection. N Engl J Med 1997;337:1733–1745.

Mackenna BR, Callander R. Illustrated physiology. 6th ed. New York: Churchill Livingstone, 1997.

Martini FH, Timmon MJ. Human anatomy. 2nd ed. Upper Saddle River, NJ: Prentice-Hall, 1997.

Pagana KD, Pagana TJ. Mosby's diagnostic and laboratory test reference. 5th ed. St. Louis: Mosby-Year Book, 2001.

Raebel MA, Palmer SM. Viral hepatitis. In: Dipiro JT, Talbert RL, Yee GC, et al., eds. Pharmacotherapy: a pathophysiologic approach. 4th ed. Stamford, CT: Appleton & Lange, 1999:614–627.

Reynolds TB. Ascites. Clin Liver Dis 2000;4:151–168.

Riddel A, Carr SB. Recurrent abdominal pain in childhood. Practitioner 2000;244:346–350.

Sanson TG, O'Keefe KP. Evaluation of abdominal pain in the elderly. Emerg Med Clin North Am 1996;14:615–627.

Traub SL. Basic skills in interpreting laboratory data. 2nd ed. Bethesda, MD: America Society of Health-System Pharmacists, 1996.

Tortora GJ. Principles of human anatomy. 8th ed. New York: John Wiley & Sons, 2000.

Uriz J, Cardenas A, Arroyo V. Pathophysiology, diagnosis and treatment of ascites in cirrhosis. Baillieres Best Pract Res Clin Gastroenterol 2000;14:927–943.

Waterston T. A strategy for abdominal pain. Practitioner 1997;241:316–318,320.

CHAPTER

16

Renal System

Rhonda M. Jones

GLOSSARY TERMS

- Acute renal failure
- Anuria
- Azotemia
- Blood urea nitrogen
- Chronic renal failure
- Creatinine clearance
- Hematuria
- Incontinence
- Oliguria
- Proteinuria
- Pyelonephritis
- Pyuria
- Renal insufficiency
- Serum creatinine
- Uremia
- Urinalysis

ANATOMY AND PHYSIOLOGY OVERVIEW

The renal system includes the kidneys, ureters, bladder, and urethra (Fig. 16-1). It performs vital processes of excretion (i.e., filtration, secretion, and reabsorption) as well as endocrine and metabolic functions. More specifically, functions of the renal system include:

- Regulating sodium, potassium, chloride, calcium, and other ion concentrations in the plasma.
- Regulating blood volume and blood pressure (by controlling the volume of water excreted in urine and releasing erythropoietin and renin).
- Excreting urea and uric acid, toxic substances, and drugs.
- Stabilizing the blood pH.
- Synthesizing calcitriol, a vitamin D_3 derivative that stimulates calcium ion absorption by the intestines.

Kidneys

The kidneys are two bean-shaped organs approximately 12 cm in length and 6 cm in width. They are located lateral to the vertebral column between T12 and L3. Usually, the right kidney is slightly lower than the left kidney. Blood vessels and nerves enter and leave the kidney at the vertical cleft, which is called the renal hilus. Superior to each kidney rests an adrenal gland, which is so named for its position even though it is functionally unrelated.

Each kidney contains approximately 1.25 million structural units called nephrons, which are the primary functional units of the kidney (Fig. 16-2). Filtration, reabsorption, and secretion of fluids occurs throughout each nephron's various components. Filtration begins in the Bowman's capsule, which contains several intertwining capillaries that collectively are called a glomerulus. Filtration across the glomerulus walls produces a protein-free solution, which is called the filtrate. The filtrate then passes through the various tubular components, including the proximal convoluted tubule, descending and ascending loop of Henle, distal convoluted tubule, and collecting duct. Selective reabsorption and filtration of substances occur throughout the tubular segments according to the body's needs and the presence of medications and hormones. Vital substances and fluids are reabsorbed into the interstitium of the kidney. Waste products unneeded by the body remain in the tubules and are excreted as urine.

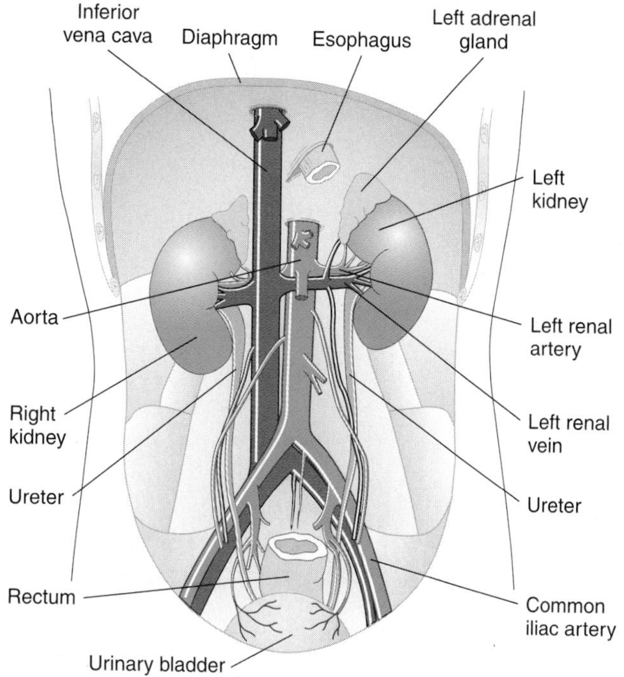

FIGURE 16-1 ■ Components of the renal system.

Ureters

The ureters are a pair of tubules that extend from the kidneys to the bladder (Fig. 16-1). Smooth muscles within the ureters contract rhythmically, thus propelling urine from the kidneys to the bladder.

Bladder

The bladder is a hollow, muscular organ that functions as a storage reservoir for urine (Fig. 16-1). It lies just posterior to the pubic symphysis and has the capacity to hold approximately 1000 mL of urine. When the bladder contains 200 to 300 mL, however, the autonomic nervous system signals the brain, which in turn causes the urge to urinate.

Urethra

The urethra is a small tube that extends from the bladder to the exterior surface of the body and through which urine is emptied from the bladder. In females, the urethra is approximately 3 to 4 cm in length, whereas in males, it is approximately 20 cm in length. Approximately 2.5 cm of the male urethra runs within the prostate gland, which sits just below the bladder.

The urinary sphincter, a band of skeletal muscles, encircles the urethra and controls the initiation of urination through the external opening, which is called the urinary meatus. In males, the urethra carries semen as well as urine, though never at the same time.

Special Considerations

Pediatric Patients

In children, the bladder is located higher than it is in adults, lying between the pubic symphysis and the umbilicus. The bladder and kidneys also may be easier to palpate in children, be-

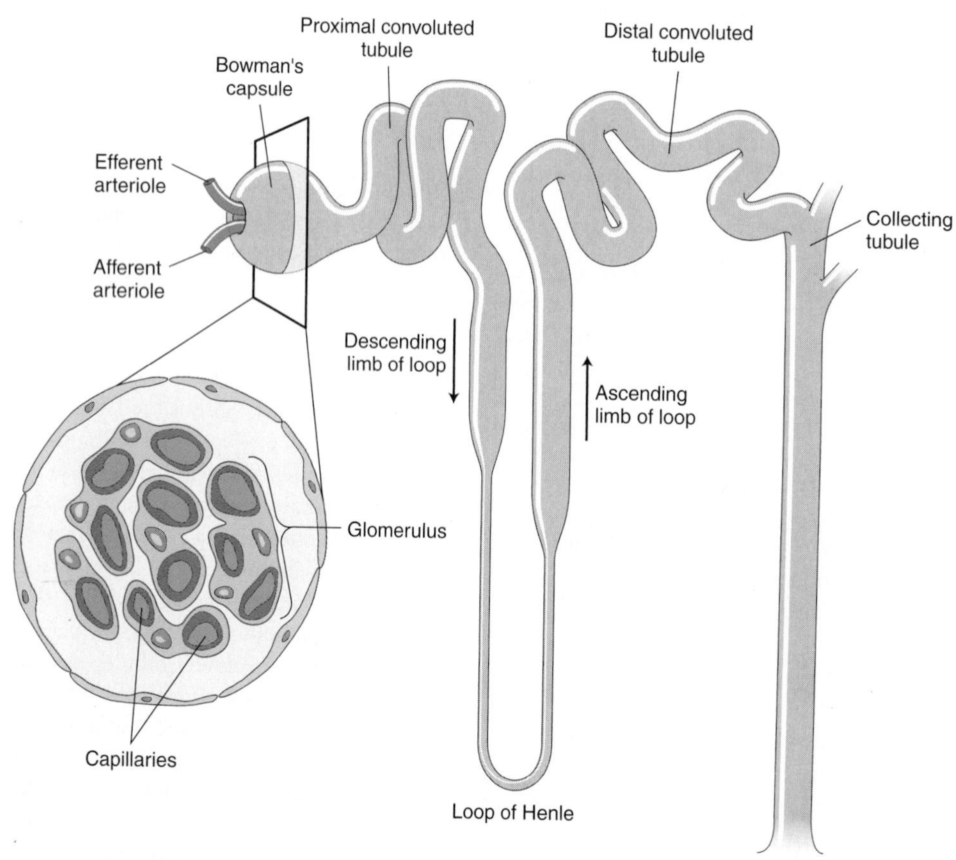

FIGURE 16-2 ■ The nephron.

cause their abdominal walls are less muscular than those of adults.

Geriatric Patients

Physiologic renal changes that occur with the aging process include decreased renal blood flow, decreased tubular function, decreased ability to concentrate urine, and decreased number of functional nephrons and glomeruli in the kidney. These changes cause a significant decline in creatinine clearance and renal function. The serum creatinine level may not increase, however, because the normal aging process also causes a decrease in muscle mass.

In addition, the sphincter muscles lose tone and, thus, become less effective at retaining urine. This loss in muscle tone predisposes elderly patients to **incontinence,** which is an involuntary loss of urine. Stress incontinence is an especially common problem in elderly women. In this condition, when abdominal pressure increases, such as when a woman coughs or laughs, an involuntary loss of urine occurs. The amount of urine that is expelled with stress incontinence may vary, however, from a few drops to a significant amount.

Elderly male patients may experience benign prostatic hypertrophy. Because the prostate surrounds the urethra, an enlarged prostate obstructs the flow of urine. Thus, patients with benign prostatic hypertrophy may complain of frequency, urgency, hesitancy, dribbling, nocturia, and dysuria. (See Chapter 21 for more details.)

Pregnant Patients

Pregnancy causes an increase in renal blood flow and glomerular filtration rate (GFR). In addition, the growing uterus displaces the kidneys and the ureters as well as increases pressure on the bladder, especially during the first and third trimesters. Therefore, urinary frequency is a common consequence of pregnancy.

PATHOLOGY OVERVIEW

Renal Failure

Renal failure is a major cause of morbidity and mortality. It usually is classified as either acute or chronic, according to the rate of decline in renal function.

Acute Renal Failure

Acute renal failure (ARF) is a decline in renal function that occurs rapidly and results in **azotemia,** an accumulation in the blood of nitrogenous waste products (i.e., blood urea nitrogen [BUN] and creatinine) that normally are excreted in the urine. It can be caused by various factors.

For normally functioning kidneys to produce urine, several conditions are required. First, a minimum volume of blood must be delivered to the kidneys. Second, the glomeruli must form a filtrate, which then must be processed through the nephron's tubular system to form urine. Finally, the urine must be excreted through the ureters. Any reduction in blood delivery, damage to the renal parenchymal tissue, or obstruction to the flow of urine can increase the risk of ARF. Common causes of ARF include:

- Volume depletion (e.g., diarrhea, vomiting, diuretics)
- Acute hemorrhage
- Hypotension
- Ischemia
- Glomerulonephritis
- Pyelonephritis
- Calculi

Certain drugs can also cause ARF (Box 16-1). Signs and symptoms associated with ARF are listed in Box 16-2.

The clinical course of ARF usually evolves through three phases. The oliguric phase begins with the onset of decreased urine output, usually with increased serum concentrations of BUN and serum creatinine; this phase may last from several days to weeks. The diuretic phase typically begins with an increase in urine output; the BUN and serum creatinine concentrations remain high. This phase usually lasts for several days. The recovery phase begins with a gradual decline in the BUN and serum creatinine concentrations. Urine production continues, and the kidney's ability to concentrate and dilute urine returns to normal. Depending on damage to the kidneys, the recovery phase continues over weeks to months, with the time for complete recovery to baseline functions varying in each patient.

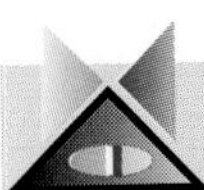

Box 16-1

DRUGS THAT CAN CAUSE ACUTE RENAL FAILURE

- Angiotensin-converting enzyme inhibitors
- Nonsteroidal anti-inflammatory drugs
- Diuretics
- Aminoglycosides
- Amphotericin
- Ciprofloxacin

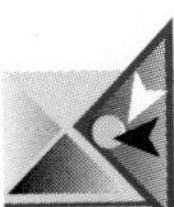

Box 16-2

SIGNS AND SYMPTOMS ASSOCIATED WITH ACUTE RENAL FAILURE

- Proteinuria
- Increased BUN
- Increased serum creatinine
- Decreased urine output (oliguria)
- Peripheral edema
- Increased blood pressure

Treatment of ARF depends on the cause. For example, if a drug is causing the ARF, treatment includes discontinuation of the causative agent. Other treatments include hydration, supportive treatment, and immunosuppressive drug therapy.

Chronic Renal Failure

Chronic renal failure (CRF) involves extensively diminished renal function that has occurred for an extended period of time and that is unlikely to improve. It develops gradually, and it typically is characterized by four stages of progressing dysfunction: renal insufficiency, azotemia, uremia, and end-stage renal disease. **Renal insufficiency** is a mild reduction in the GFR with no occurrence of signs or symptoms. As the GFR continues to decline, nitrogenous waste products (e.g., BUN and creatinine) accumulate. This stage is termed azotemia. As the renal function declines to approximately 10% of normal, nitrogenous waste products accumulate in the bloodstream, and the patient begins to experience a cluster of signs and symptoms (Box 16-3). These signs and symptoms result from the kidney's inability to excrete sodium, water, potassium, magnesium, phosphate, BUN, creatinine, and uric acid. In turn, this leads to fluid retention, weight gain, and increased blood pressure. Lack of erythropoietin production by the kidney causes a decrease in hemoglobin and hematocrit; this stage is called **uremia.** The stage at which renal function has so declined that dialysis is necessary to sustain life is termed end-stage renal disease.

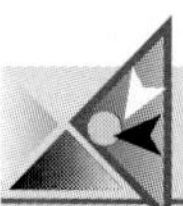

Box 16-3

SIGNS AND SYMPTOMS ASSOCIATED WITH UREMIC SYNDROME IN CHRONIC RENAL FAILURE

- Edema
- Hyperkalemia
- Hypermagnesemia
- Hyperphosphatemia
- Hypocalcemia
- Metabolic acidosis
- Decreased hemoglobin and hematocrit
- Increased BUN and serum creatinine
- Increased blood pressure
- Anorexia
- Flank pain
- Nausea/vomiting
- Lethargy
- Muscular cramps and weakness
- Altered skin pigmentation
- Pruritus
- Depression
- Anxiety
- Shortness of breath

Chronic renal failure may result from long-standing diseases (Box 16-4) or simply be part of the normal aging process. Risk factors for CRF include:

- Diabetes
- Hypertension
- Polycystic kidney disease
- Glomerulonephritis
- Interstitial nephritis
- Advancing age

Because CRF presently has no cure, treatment involves medical management of the various signs and symptoms, dialysis, and ultimately, transplantation.

Urinary Tract Infections

A urinary tract infection (UTI) is the presence of microorganisms (e.g., bacteria) in the urinary tract, which includes the bladder, prostate, kidney, and collecting duct. Urinary tract infections include a wide variety of clinical entities, ranging from asymptomatic infection to acute **pyelonephritis,** which is an inflammation of the kidney caused by severe bacterial infection.

The most common cause of uncomplicated UTIs is *Escherichia coli,* which accounts for approximately 85% of community-acquired UTIs. Other organisms that cause uncomplicated UTIs include *Staphylococcus saprophyticus* (5%–15%), *Klebsiella pneumoniae, Proteus mirabilis,* and *Pseudomonas aeruginosa* (5%–10%). Various and more resistant organisms cause complicated infections. *Escherichia coli* is still a frequently found pathogen, but it accounts for less than 50% of complicated infections. Other frequently isolated organisms include *Proteus* sp., *K. pneumoniae, Enterobacter* sp., *Pseudomonas aeruginosa,* staphylococci, and enterococci. Most UTIs are caused by one organism; however, multiple organisms may be found in patients with indwelling catheters, kidney stones, or chronic renal abscess.

Bacteria most commonly gain entrance into the urinary tract from an ascending pathway. The female urethra frequently is colonized with bacteria that originate from fecal flora in the gastrointestinal tract. This colonization results from the proximity of the female urethra to the perirectal area and from its short length as compared to that in men. The anatomic differences cause UTIs to occur more frequently in

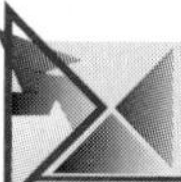

Box 16-4

DISEASES ASSOCIATED WITH CHRONIC RENAL FAILURE

- Diabetes
- Hypertension
- Glomerulonephritis
- Polycystic kidney disease
- Interstitial nephritis

women than in men. The exact mode of bacterial ascent into the bladder is not completely understood; however, massage of the female urethra and sexual intercourse are believed to be two possible mechanisms.

Risk factors for development of UTIs include:

- Extremes of age
- Female gender
- Pregnancy
- Catheterization
- Neurologic dysfunction
- Renal disease
- Urinary tract obstruction

Signs and symptoms that are commonly associated with UTIs are listed in Box 16-5. Patients with pyelonephritis typically present with high-grade fever, severe flank pain, and possibly, nausea, vomiting, and dehydration. The actual presence of an infection as well as the severity and location of the UTI (i.e., lower urinary tract vs. pyelonephritis), however, do not correlate well with these signs and symptoms.

Treatment of uncomplicated UTIs includes antibiotic therapy, which commonly involves oral trimethoprim-sulfamethoxazole, cephalosporins, ampicillin, or fluoroquinolones for lower tract infections. Mild cases of pyelonephritis are treated on an outpatient basis with these oral antibiotics as well. Severely ill patients, however, are hospitalized and treated with intravenous antibiotics, such as third-generation cephalosporins, aminoglycosides (gentamicin) and ampicillin, fluoroquinolones, β-lactamase inhibitor combinations (ampicillin/sulbactam, ticarcillin/clavulanate, and piperacillin/tazobactam), or imipenem. A significant reduction in urine bacteria should occur within 48 hours. Once the patient is afrebrile for 24 hours, parenteral therapy is discontinued and oral antibiotic therapy is started to complete a 2-week course of therapy.

Renal Stones

Renal stones usually result from a breakdown in the delicate balance in the kidneys between conserving water and excreting materials with a low solubility. When urine becomes supersaturated with insoluble products (because of excessive excretion rates, extreme water conservation, or both), crystals form that eventually may develop into a stone. Most kidney stones are caused by accumulation of calcium salts, uric acid, or struvite on the surface of the renal papillae or within the collecting system. Calcium stones are the most common type, appearing in 75% to 85% of all kidney stones. Calcium stones occur more commonly in men, with an average age of onset during the third decade of life. Patients with uric acid stones also frequently have gout, and uric acid stones are more common in men. Struvite stones occur more frequently in women and commonly result from UTI with a urease-producing bacteria (e.g., *Proteus* sp.).

Stones may accumulate within the kidney asymptomatically. When a stone breaks loose, however, and enters the ureter or occludes the ureteropelvic junction, it causes severe pain and hematuria. The pain typically begins gradually, usually in the flank area, and steadily increases to a severe level during the next 20 to 60 minutes. The pain may remain in the flank or spread downward toward the loin, testis, or vulva. If the stone is in the portion of the ureter within the bladder, the patient also may experience frequency, urgency, dysuria, and hematuria (particularly when the stone is passed).

Risk factors for development of kidney stones include:

- Idiopathic hypercalciuria
- Hyperuricosuria
- Gout
- Primary hyperparathyroidism
- Dehydration

In addition, most patients with kidney stones have metabolic disorders that cause the stones and that can be detected by chemical analysis of serum and urine (calcium, uric acid, creatinine, and serum electrolytes typically are measured). Treatment of stones in the kidneys or urinary tract requires a combination of medical and surgical procedures, with the specific approach depending on the stone location, amount of obstruction, presence or absence of UTI, progress of stone passage, and the risk versus benefit of surgery.

Three procedural alternatives include extracorporeal lithotripsy, percutaneous lithotripsy, and cystoscopy. Extracorporeal lithotripsy fragments stones by exposing them to shock waves. The patient is submerged in a water tank, the kidney stones are centered at the focal point of parabolic reflectors, and high-intensity shock waves are then produced with a high-voltage discharge. The waves pass through the patient and fracture the stone. After multiple discharges, most stones are reduced to a powder, which passes through the ureter and into the bladder. Percutaneous ultrasonic lithotripsy requires passage of a cystoscope-like instrument into the renal pelvis through a small incision in the flank. Stones are disrupted by an ultrasonic transducer, and fragments are directly removed. Ureteral stones that are inaccessible to extracorporeal or percutaneous lithotripsy are fragmented and then removed using an ultrasonic transducer that is endoscopically inserted into the ureter via a cystoscope.

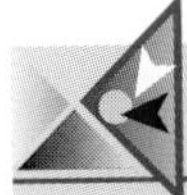

Box 16-5

SIGNS AND SYMPTOMS ASSOCIATED WITH URINARY TRACT INFECTIONS

- Dysuria (painful, burning sensation while urinating)
- Frequent urination
- Suprapubic pain
- Urgency
- Fever
- Chills
- Nausea/vomiting
- Hematuria
- Bacteriuria

SYSTEM ASSESSMENT

Subjective Information

When assessing the renal system, subjective patient symptoms or complaints can be vague and nonspecific. Some symptoms, however, may lead pharmacists to consider problems with the renal system. To determine if a patient is experiencing these symptoms, ask the following questions.

Urinary Symptoms

? INTERVIEW Are you experiencing any problems with urination? Any problems with frequency in urination or having the urge to urinate but only producing a small amount? How often do you get up at night to urinate? Any pain or burning sensation when you urinate? What typically is the color of your urine? Any changes in the amount or frequency of urination?

ABNORMALITIES UTIs may cause burning/pain, frequency, and urgency with urination. Red or pink urine may be a sign of blood in the urine (i.e., **hematuria**); cloudy urine may be a sign of white blood cells (WBCs) and infection. Renal dysfunction may cause various changes in the urine depending on the severity of renal dysfunction (i.e., decreased urine output [**oliguria**] or change in urine color and appearance to clear/colorless, cloudy, foamy, pink, or red).

Renal Dysfunction

? INTERVIEW Do you experience pain in the flank area (side pain between the ribs and ilium)? Is the pain relieved by changing positions?

ABNORMALITIES Flank pain unrelieved by changing position may suggest renal stones or colic; flank pain relieved by lying down may suggest infection.

? INTERVIEW Any problems with swelling in your feet and ankles? Any mental changes (e.g., decreased attention span, anxiety, or depression)? Any muscle cramps or "restless leg" sensation? Any changes in skin color or problems with itching? Any changes in appetite? Nausea or vomiting? Any problems with breathing?

ABNORMALITIES See Box 16-3 for symptoms associated with CRF.

Objective Information

Because renal system function affects the entire body, assessing the renal system involves physical examination of the kidneys, laboratory and diagnostic tests, and evaluation of the skin, neuromuscular, cardiovascular, respiratory, and gastrointestinal systems. Assessment findings depend on the severity of renal dysfunction and the length of time that the renal system has been impaired.

Many medications are renally excreted and, thus, are affected by renal dysfunction, so pharmacists routinely assesses renal function in their patients. Pharmacists usually assess kidney function by reviewing laboratory data (described later), and they recommend medication and dosing changes accordingly. Because pharmacists have easy access to laboratory data in the hospital, long-term care, and home health care settings, they assess kidney function most commonly in these environments.

Physical Assessment

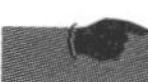
TECHNIQUE

Step 1

Check the Patient's Weight to Determine Changes in Fluid Status

See Chapter 5 for detailed discussion of how to determine weight.

ABNORMALITIES Patients may develop hypervolemia or hypovolemia depending on the disease causing the renal dysfunction. Patients who gain more than 1.1 pounds per day are retaining fluid; patients who lose 0.5 pounds or more over 2 days may be losing fluid.

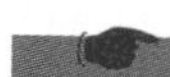
TECHNIQUE

Step 2

Measure the Patient's Vital Signs

Vital signs include heart rate, respiratory rate, and blood pressure. See Chapter 5 for detailed discussion of how to measure vital signs.

ABNORMALITIES Patients with fluid and electrolyte imbalances caused by renal dysfunction may have a bounding pulse (volume overload); a rapid, weak, thready pulse (dehydration); or dysrhythmias (excess sodium and potassium, or deficient magnesium or potassium). Patients with severe metabolic acidosis caused by renal failure may exhibit rapid deep breaths (Kussmaul respirations) in an attempt to normalize blood pH by excreting increased amounts of carbon dioxide. Patients with severe metabolic alkalosis hypoventilate to normalize blood pH by retaining carbon dioxide. Blood pressure may be high (volume overload) or low (dehydration).

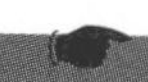
TECHNIQUE

Step 3

Inspect the Patient's Affect, Mouth, and Skin

Affect refers to the patient's facial expression. For detailed discussions of how to inspect the patient's affect, mouth, and skin, see Chapters 19, 14, and 8, respectively.

ABNORMALITIES As uremic toxins increase, patients may display a flat affect or depressed appearance. Other possible mental changes include shortened attention span, poor memory, and confusion. Uremic toxins also may cause ulcerations in the mouth and ammonia breath. A dry mouth and thick, pasty sputum are typical in dehydrated patients. Patients with renal failure may exhibit various skin color changes, ranging from grayish/bronze to yellowish. If anemic, patients have an underlying pallor. Ecchymosis or petechiae also may be present because of abnormal platelet adhesion, which occurs when the kidneys cannot maintain a normal acid-base balance.

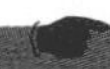
TECHNIQUE

Step 4

Palpate the Patient's Lower Legs and Feet for Peripheral Edema

See Chapter 13 for a detailed discussion on how to palpate for edema.

ABNORMALITIES If patients are retaining fluid, edema will be present. Remember, however, that several causes of edema are possible besides renal failure (e.g., congestive heart failure, inflammation from heat or trauma, cirrhosis, peripheral vascular disease, and excessive salt intake).

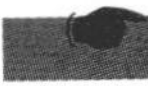
TECHNIQUE

Step 5

Auscultate the Patient's Breath Sounds

See Chapter 11 for a detailed discussion of how to auscultate breath sounds.

ABNORMALITIES Crackles or rales indicate fluid accumulation.

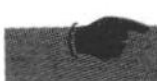
TECHNIQUE

Step 6

Auscultate the Patient's Heart Sounds

See Chapter 12 for a detailed discussion of how to auscultate heart sounds.

ABNORMALITIES An S_3 sound may indicate fluid overload. An S_4 sound may indicate prolonged systemic hypertension caused by renal failure.

Pharmacists rarely palpate the kidneys; however, the skill is described here for completeness.

TECHNIQUE

Step 7

Palpate the Kidneys

- Instruct the patient to lie flat on the examination table.
- To palpate the right kidney, place your hands together over the patient's right flank area (Fig. 16-3). Press your hands together firmly, and have the patient take a deep breath. Normally, you should feel no change or, possibly, a round, smooth mass slide between your hands.
- To palpate the left kidney, reach with your left hand across the abdomen and behind the left flank (Fig. 16.3). Remember that the left kidney is positioned approximately 1 cm higher than the right kidney. Press your right hand deep into the abdomen, and have the patient take a deep breath. Normally, no change should be felt.

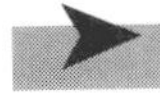
ABNORMALITIES An enlarged kidney may be caused by cysts or a neoplasm.

Laboratory and Diagnostic Tests

Physical examination of the kidneys provides imprecise and limited information. Therefore, laboratory tests frequently are used to specifically evaluate kidney function. Common laboratory tests include urinalysis, serum creatinine, BUN, and electrolytes. In addition, pharmacists routinely use the patient's creatinine clearance (see detailed discussion later) to evaluate medication doses and to make recommendations for dosing changes.

A common way to assess the kidney's ability to maintain normal fluid levels is to monitor the patient's fluid intake and urinary output. Normal urinary output is 1000 to 1500 mL in 24 hours. Urine output of 100 to 400 mL in 24 hours is considered to be oliguria. Monitoring of fluid intake and urine out-

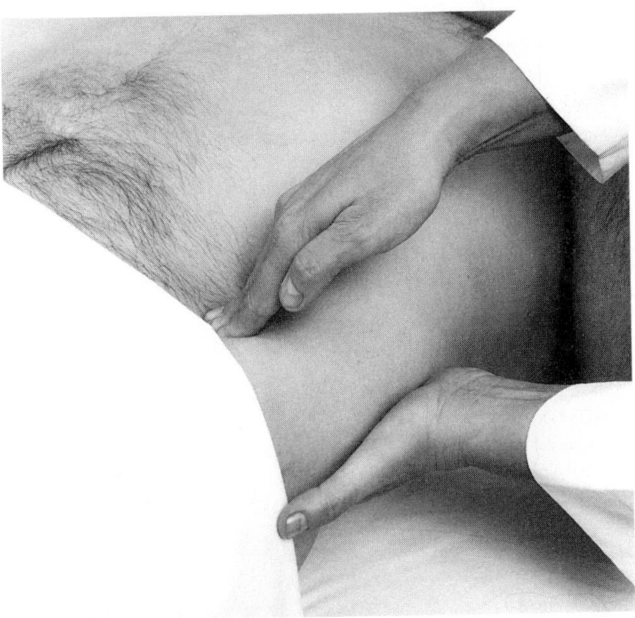

FIGURE 16-3 ■ Palpation of the kidneys.

put (commonly referred to as the patient's "in's and out's") usually is done in the hospital setting, because accurate measurements are difficult to obtain in the ambulatory setting.

A clean-catch or midstream urine specimen provides useful information concerning kidney function. The urine's color and clarity indicate which substances are being filtered and retained. Normally, the urine should be clear, with an amber-yellow color. Abnormal urine appearances and their possible causes are listed in Table 16-1. Various medications also may affect the urine color (Table 16-2).

Urinalysis, which is a dipstick examination of the urine specimen, provides information concerning the presence of blood, protein, glucose, and bile in the urine. In addition, the pH and specific gravity of the urine can be determined. Protein in the urine, (i.e., **proteinuria**) reflects loss of the normal glomerular impermeability to filtration of plasma proteins. Proteinuria is an early sign of kidney dysfunction, and it is a hallmark sign of kidney disease (i.e., most kidney diseases are discovered through detection of proteinuria). Further quantification of proteinuria may be useful in determining the cause of the kidney disease and in monitoring its progression and treatment.

Microscopic examination of the urine specimen is a simple procedure to determine the presence of bacteria and leukocytes in patients with suspected UTI. Because urine in the bladder normally is sterile, a significant number of bacteria in the urine indicates UTI. **Pyuria,** which is the presence of pus/WBCs in the urine, is specifically defined as a WBC count in the urine of more than 10 WBCs/mL. Pyuria is nonspecific; it only reflects the presence of inflammation rather than of infection. Pyuria in symptomatic patients, however, typically correlates with bacturia.

A urine culture is the most reliable method to identify UTI. Patients with infection usually have more than 100,000 bacteria/mL, but a significant portion of both symptomatic and asymptomatic patients have less than this. Once the presence of bacteria has been determined, the bacteria are specifically identified using a calibrated loop technique to streak a fixed amount of urine on an agar plate. The specific bacteria are then further tested for susceptibility to various antibiotics.

Serum creatinine is a normal metabolic product of skeletal muscle breakdown in the body. Thus, its production is determined by muscle mass, which is constant in most individuals. Creatinine normally is excreted by the kidneys on a daily basis, and the amount excreted is directly proportional to the renal excretory function. Therefore, the serum creatinine concentration will remain at a relative steady state in healthy individuals and rise abnormally in those with renal dysfunction.

Creatinine clearance is a measure of the GFR and an evaluative measure of renal function. A 24-hour urine collection is obtained from the patient, and the creatinine clearance (mL/min) is then calculated using the following equation:

$$\text{CrCl mL/min} = \frac{(U_v)(Cr_{urine})}{(Cr_s)(1440)}$$

in which CrCl is the creatinine clearance (mL/min), U_v is the 24-hour volume of urine (mL), Cr_{urine} is the creatinine concentration in the 24-hour urine (mg/dL), Cr_s is the serum creatinine concentration, and 1440 is the number of minutes in 24 hours. Because obtaining a 24-hour urine sample is inconvenient, the creatinine clearance is commonly calculated using the Cockcroft-Gault formula:

$$\text{CrCl mL/min} = \frac{(140 - \text{age})(\text{LBW})}{(72)(Cr_s)}$$

in which LBW is the person's lean body weight (kg). Because women have less muscle mass than men, this equation must be multiplied by 0.85 with female patients. For example,

34-year-old woman

$Cr_s = 0.8$

Weight = 160 pounds (72.7 kg)

Height = 5'9"

$$\text{CrCl} = \frac{(140 - 34)(72.7)}{(72)(0.8)}$$

$$\text{CrCl} = 133.8(0.85)$$

$$\text{CrCl} = 113.7 \text{ mL/min}$$

In healthy individuals, the creatinine clearance remains constant. As renal function declines, however, the creatinine clearance also declines.

TABLE 16-1 ABNORMAL URINE APPEARANCES AND POSSIBLE CAUSES

COLOR	CLARITY	POSSIBLE CAUSE
Colorless	Clear	Tubules are unable to effectively concentrate urine (beginning or resolution of acute renal failure, stress)
Pink or red	Foamy	Presence of red blood cells Presence of albumin
Dark amber	Cloudy	Dehydration Presence of white blood cells (e.g., infection)

TABLE 16-2 MEDICATIONS THAT MAY AFFECT URINE COLOR[a]

MEDICATION	URINE COLOR
Dioctyl calcium sulfosuccinate (Surfak)	Pink, red, or red-brown
Iron preparations	Dark brown
Levodopa	Dark brown on standing
Nitrofurantoin (Macrodantin)	Brown
Phenazopyridine (Pyridium)	Orange to red
Phenolphthalein (Ex-Lax)	Red or purplish-pink in alkaline urine
Phenothiazines	Red-brown
Phenytoin (Dilantin)	Pink, red, or red-brown
Riboflavin	Intense yellow
Rifampin	Red-orange
Sulfasalazine (Azulfidine)	Orange-yellow in alkaline urine

[a]Not an all-inclusive list.

Blood urea nitrogen measures the amount of urea nitrogen in the blood. As protein is metabolized in the liver, it is broken down into amino acids, which are then catabolized and used to make free ammonia and urea. The urea is deposited into the blood and excreted by the kidneys. Thus, the BUN directly relates to the excretory function of the kidneys. As renal function declines, the BUN increases.

The kidneys help to maintain narrow ranges of electrolyte plasma concentrations by regulating the excretion and reabsorption of water and electrolytes (i.e., sodium, potassium, calcium, and magnesium) within the nephron. In patients with renal dysfunction, electrolyte values may be abnormal (i.e., hyperkalemia, hypermagnesemia, hyperphosphatemia, and hypocalcemia).

Normally, the kidneys produce and release erythropoietin, which stimulates the bone marrow to produce red blood cells. In chronic renal dysfunction, the complete blood count is commonly used to determine the presence of anemia.

SPECIAL CONSIDERATIONS

Pediatric Patients

? INTERVIEW If the child is of "potty-training" age (18–36 months), any problems with "accidents"? Any problems with bed-wetting? Any pain or burning sensation when urinating?

➤ ABNORMALITIES When potty-training a child, accidents are common and normal. Frequent accidents are considered to be abnormal, however, in children who have been potty-trained for several months. Accidents may result from a stressful situation or a change in the child's routine or surroundings (e.g., taking the child to a new baby-sitter or day care center). Urinary tract infections are uncommon in children overall. In preschool females, however, they typically result from poor self-hygiene and the close anatomic proximity of the urethra to the perirectal area. In preschool males, they usually result from structural or functional abnormalities of the urinary tract.

Geriatric Patients

? INTERVIEW As people age, many notice they no longer have full control of their bladder. Have you noticed this? Under what circumstances do you find it difficult to control your bladder? Do you have any problems with frequency, urgency, dribbling, or hesitancy?

➤ ABNORMALITIES Incontinence with laughing, coughing, or sneezing is a common problem in elderly women. Benign prostatic hypertrophy is common in elderly men and may cause frequency, urgency, dribbling, and hesitancy; it also increases the risk of UTI and is a significant factor in why the occurrence of UTI in men and women changes significantly in the elderly. In patients older than 65 years, the occurrence of UTIs is approximately equal in men and women. The rate of infection increases further for elderly patients in hospitals and nursing homes; however, these patients may be asymptomatic or have atypical symptoms (e.g., increased agitation or confusion). This increased incidence results from several factors, including poor bladder emptying (possibly from prolapse in females or anticholinergic medications), fecal incontinence, neuromuscular disease, and use of urinary catheters.

Kidney function normally declines as a result of the aging process. Interpretation of the serum creatinine concentration alone, however, is difficult in elderly patients because of their decreased muscle mass and lower production of creatinine. Therefore, use of the Cockcroft-Gault formula (as described earlier) is recommended to estimate the elderly patient's creatinine clearance.

Pregnant Patients

? INTERVIEW How frequently do you go to the bathroom? How frequently do you go to the bathroom at night? Any problems with pain or a burning sensation when urinating?

➤ ABNORMALITIES Urinary frequency is a common finding during pregnancy, especially in the first and third trimesters. Kidney function, however, should remain the same. Pregnant patients are at a higher risk of developing UTI.

APPLICATION TO PATIENT SYMPTOMS

Renal dysfunction typically is asymptomatic until significant changes have occurred, but pharmacists need to be aware of possible symptoms (see Boxes 16-2 and 16-3). One possible symptom during the early stages of ARF is oliguria.

Oliguria

Oliguria is a decrease in urine output to between 50 and 400 mL/day. If the urine output is less than 50 mL/day, it is termed **anuria.** Oliguria and anuria can be caused by various renal problems.

CASE STUDY

MR is a 72-year-old white woman with a history of diabetes, hypertension, and arthritis. She approaches you at your pharmacy with a new prescription for Celebrex, a pain medication for her arthritis. The doctor gave her some samples of this medication a few weeks ago. It seems to be helping a little, but her arthritis is still bothering her quite a bit. As you are filling this prescription, you ask MR if she needs any of her other medications refilled. She states that she needs her furosemide filled but complains that she doesn't think it does any good. You ask her about this, and she says that she hardly goes to the bathroom anymore and her legs are always swollen.

ASSESSMENT OF THE PATIENT

Subjective Information

72-year-old woman complaining of decreased urine output and fluid retention

HOW OFTEN DID YOU USED TO GO THE BATHROOM? I used to go several times a day, especially when I started taking the furosemide. But now I only go a couple of times a day.

WHEN DID YOU NOTICE THIS CHANGE IN HOW OFTEN YOU URINATE? It's probably been slowly decreasing for the past few months, but the last two weeks have been really bad.

DO YOU HAVE ANY PAIN OR BURNING WHEN YOU URINATE? No.

HOW LONG HAVE YOU NOTICED THE SWELLING IN YOUR LEGS? Over the last few months, but the furosemide usually helped quite a bit until the last couple of weeks.

IS THE SWELLING DOWN WHEN YOU WAKE UP IN THE MORNING? A little, but not a whole lot.

ARE YOU HAVING ANY PROBLEMS WITH SHORTNESS OF BREATH OR CHEST PAIN? No.

WHAT MEDICATIONS ARE YOU TAKING? Furosemide, one tablet every morning, Zestril once a day, Glucotrol XL once a day, and this new Celebrex once a day.

HOW OFTEN DO YOU FORGET TO TAKE YOUR MEDICATION? Oh, I don't forget. In fact, I frequently take an extra water pill at noon to get rid of the fluid in my legs.

HOW MANY TIMES A WEEK DO YOU DO THIS? Three or four times per week.

HAVE YOU BEEN TAKING ANY NONPRESCRIPTION OR OVER-THE-COUNTER MEDICATIONS? Yes, I take ibuprofen every day for my arthritis.

HOW MUCH DO YOU TAKE EVERY DAY? Two tablets, four to five times a day.

HOW LONG HAVE YOU BEEN TAKING THE IBUPROFEN? Oh, I've been taking it for years to help my arthritis.

Objective Information

Computerized medication profile:

- Furosemide: 40 mg, one tablet every morning; No. 30; Refills: 6; Patient obtains refills every 25 to 30 days; Last refill 2 weeks ago
- Zestril (lisinopril): 40 mg, one tablet every day; No. 30; Refills 3; Patient obtains refills every 25 to 30 days
- Glucotrol XL (glipizide): 10 mg, one tablet every morning; No. 30; Refills 5; Patient obtains refills every 25 to 30 days

Patient in no acute distress.
Heart rate: 78 bpm
Blood pressure: 158/90 mm Hg
Heart auscultation: regular rate and rhythm, no murmur
Extremities: 3+ pitting edema in lower extremities

DISCUSSION

The concern centers on MR's decreased urine output and worsening peripheral edema. The pharmacist needs to determine whether the oliguria results from a possible UTI or possible renal dysfunction caused by diabetes or one of the medications. MR states the oliguria and edema have been worsening gradually, but that they have significantly worsened over the last 2 weeks. She denies any pain or burning with urination. In reviewing MR's medications, the pharmacist notes that she started taking a new nonsteroidal anti-inflammatory drug (NSAID) approximately 2 weeks ago, and that she frequently takes a second dose of furosemide. In addition, she takes an angiotensin-converting enzyme inhibitor and also takes ibuprofen, an NSAID, routinely throughout the day each day. MR is hypertensive and, on palpation, has significant peripheral edema.

After evaluating MR's situation, the pharmacist concludes she could be in ARF, because she has several factors that increase her risk (Fig. 16-4). These factors include diabetes, chronic use of two NSAIDs, and volume depletion from the diuretic. The pharmacist calls MR's physician, who requests that she come in to be seen that day.

Continued

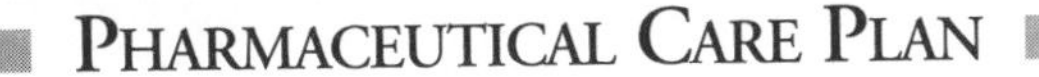

CASE STUDY—continued

Pharmaceutical Care Plan

Patient Name: MR

Date: 6/15/02

Medical Problems:
- Diabetes
- Hypertension
- Arthritis

Current Medications:
- Furosemide, 40 mg, one tablet daily
- Zestril (lisinopril), 40 mg, one tablet daily
- Glucotrol XL (glipizide), 10 mg, one tablet every morning

S: 72-year-old woman complaining of worsening fluid retention and decreasing urination; only goes to the bathroom a couple of times a day. Also has severe arthritis pain.

Compliance: Takes an extra dose of furosemide three or four times per week. Also takes over-the-counter ibuprofen, 400 mg, four to five times per day.

O: Patient in no acute distress.

Heart rate: 78 bpm

Blood pressure: 158/90 mm Hg

Heart auscultation: regular rate and rhythm, no murmur

Extremities: 3+ pitting edema in lower extremities

A: Possible ARF caused by volume depletion, chronic use of two NSAIDs, and diabetes.

P:
1. Call MR's physician, and describe findings.
2. Instruct MR to see her physician immediately.
3. Educate NR about not using over-the-counter ibuprofen with Celebrex.

Pharmacist: *Joe Ulrich, Pharm. D.*

Self-Assessment Questions

1. What are the major functions of the renal system?
2. What signs and symptoms are associated with ARF?
3. Calculate the creatinine clearance for an 82-year-old woman who weighs 145 pounds, is 5'9" tall, and has a serum creatinine of 1.4 mg/dL.

Critical Thinking Question

1. A 23-year-old woman calls your pharmacy and requests a refill of Bactrim DS, one tablet twice a day for 3 days, because she thinks she has another UTI. She states that it really hurts and itches when she goes to the bathroom. You notice that she just got the original prescription filled 5 days ago, and that there is one refill on the prescription. What would you do? What would you ask her to determine if she was experiencing a UTI? Would you fill the prescription? Why, or why not?

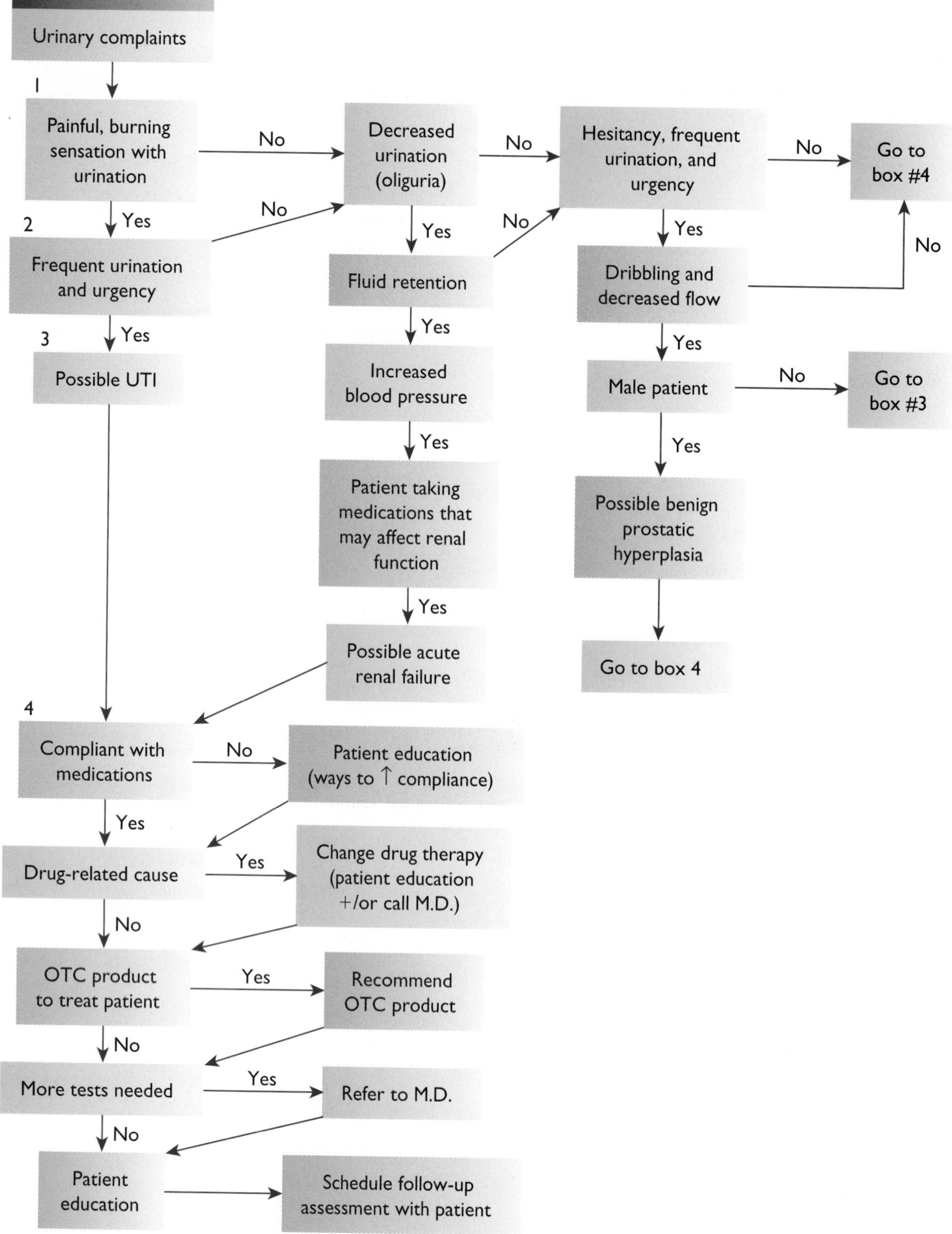

FIGURE 16-4 ■ Decision tree for urinary problems. *OTC*, over-the-counter.

Bibliography

Bolton WK, Kliger AS. Chronic renal insufficiency: current understandings and their implications. Am J Kidney Dis 2000;36(suppl 3):S4–S12.

Brophy DF. Acute renal failure. In: Applied therapeutics: the clinical use of drugs. 7th ed. Baltimore: Lippincott Williams & Wilkins, 2001:29.1–29.23.

Cohen EP, Lemann JJ. The role of the laboratory in evaluation of kidney function. Clin Chem 1991;37:785–796.

Comstock TJ. Assessment of renal function. In: Pharmacotherapy: a pathophysiologic approach. 4th ed. Stamford, CT: Appleton and Lange, 1999: 686–705.

Chronic renal failure. In: Applied therapeutics: the clinical use of drugs. 7th ed. Baltimore: Lippincott Williams & Wilkins, 2001.

Dorland's pocket medical dictionary. 29th ed. Philadelphia: WB Saunders, 2000:30.1–30.38.

Driver DS. Renal assessment: back to basics. ANNA J, 1996;23:361–366.

Goldberg EA. Physical assessment of children ages 1 to 10 years. ANNA J, 1997;24:209–217.

Goldberg EA. Physical assessment of children ages 1 to 10 years with renal disease. ANNA J, 1997;24:222–228.

Kumar V, Cotran RS, Robbins SL. Basic pathology. 6th ed. Philadelphia: WB Saunders, 1997.

Martini FH, Timmons MJ. Human anatomy. 2nd ed. Upper Saddle River, NJ: Prentice-Hall, 1997.

Mullenix TA, Prince RA. Urinary tract infections and prostatitis. In: Pharmacotherapy: a pathophysiologic approach. 4th ed. Stamford, CT: Appleton and Lange, 1999:1779–1794.

Pagana KD, Pagana TJ. Mosby's diagnostic and laboratory test reference. 5th ed. St. Louis: Mosby–Yearbook, 2001.

Powell AA, Armstrong MA. Peripheral edema. Am Fam Physician 1997;55:1721–1726.

Yucha CB, Shapiro JI. Acute renal failure: recognition and prevention. Primary Care Practice 1997;1:388–398.

17

Musculoskeletal System

Amy F. Wilson

GLOSSARY TERMS

- Ataxia
- Antalgic gait
- Ballottement
- Boutonniere deformities
- Bulge sign
- Bursitis
- Carpal tunnel syndrome
- Crepitus
- Degenerative joint disease
- Dermatomyositis
- Diplopia
- Dislocation
- Fibromyalgia
- Fracture
- Goniometer
- Gout
- Heberden's or Bouchard's nodules
- Kyphosis
- Lordosis
- McMurray's test
- Myasthenia gravis
- Myopathy
- Neuropathy
- Osteoarthritis
- Osteomyelitis
- Osteoporosis
- Polymyositis
- Rheumatoid arthritis
- Sciatica
- Scoliosis
- Sprain
- Strain
- Swan-neck deformities
- Temporomandibular joint syndrome
- Tendinitis
- Tenosynovitis

ANATOMY AND PHYSIOLOGY OVERVIEW

The musculoskeletal system forms the framework of the body. It is composed of 206 bones, more than 600 striated (or voluntary) muscles, and several types of articulations that form unions between two or more bones. The entire skeletal framework is held together by a system of tendons and ligaments that attach muscle to bone and bone to bone, respectively. In addition to providing support for and enabling movement of the human body, the musculoskeletal system also protects vital organs from damage, produces blood cells via the process of hematopoiesis in certain bones, and stores minerals (principally calcium and phosphorus) for distribution to other areas of the body.

To assess the musculoskeletal system, it is important to have a general understanding of the various components and the role that each component plays within the system.

Bone

Within the skeletal system are two types of connective tissue: cartilage, and bone.

Cartilage is a specialized type of dense connective tissue that is embedded in chondroitin sulfate, a jelly-like substance. Cartilage forms part of the skeleton and is found throughout the body, including the costal cartilages of the ribs, at joints over the ends of long bones, nasal septum, external ear, wall of the larynx, intervertebral discs between vertebrae, and in the trachea and bronchi. Cartilage offers both strength (from collagenous fibers of connective tissue) and resilience (from the chondroitin sulfate) to the human skeleton.

Bone, which is also known as osseous tissue, is a specialized form of dense connective tissue consisting of osteocytes, or bone cells, embedded in a matrix of calcified intercellular substance. Bones are considered to be the individual units of the skeleton. Bone can generally be classified into four types on the basis of shape:

- Long (legs and arms)
- Short (wrists and ankles)
- Flat (sternum and scapulae)
- Irregular (vertebrae and facial bones)

The bones of the human skeleton are shown in Figure 17-1.

Long bones consist of three regions. The diaphysis is the shaft, or main portion, of a long bone. The ends of the bone are known as the epiphyses. The metaphysis forms the junction of the diaphysis and the epiphyses (Fig. 17-2).

Joints

A joint is the basic functional unit of the musculoskeletal system and forms the union of two or more bones. The degree of mobility within the joints can vary from no movement to freely movable. Movable joints, also known as synovial joints, are classified according to the type of movement that their structure permits. Table 17-1 lists the common synovial joints and the movements allowed.

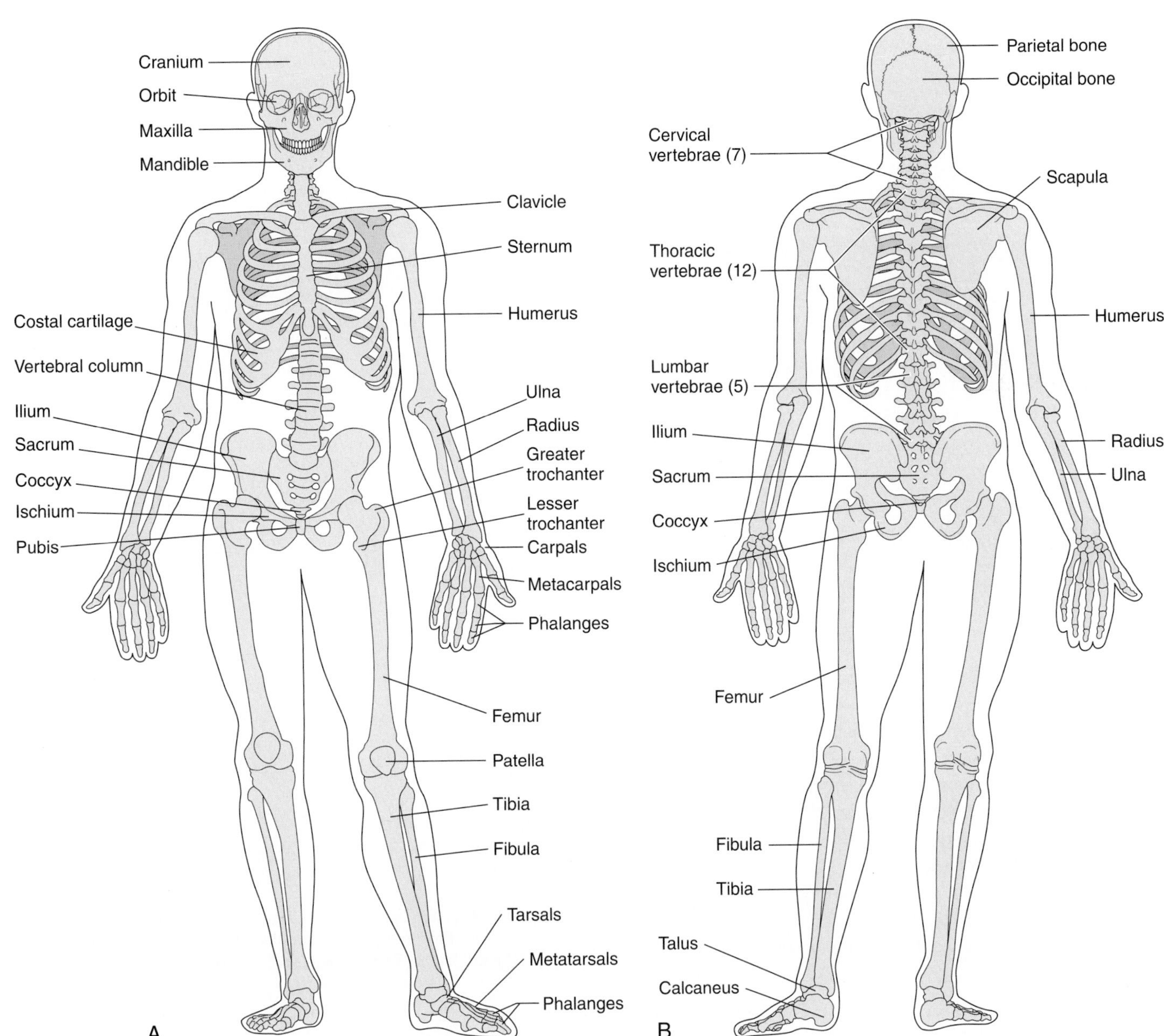

Figure 17-1 ■ The human skeleton. **(A)** Anterior view. **(B)** Posterior view.

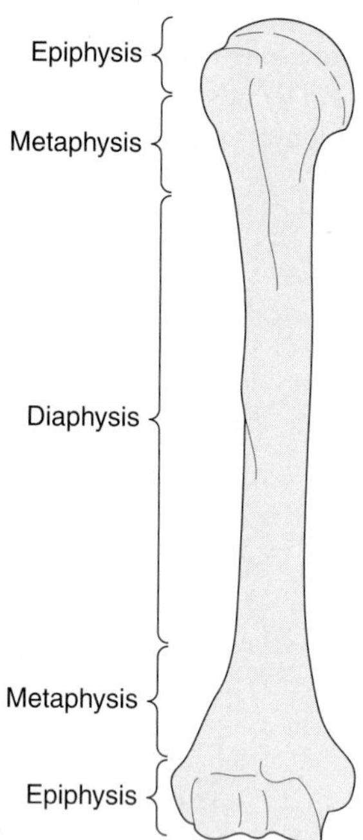

FIGURE 17-2 ■ Regions of a long bone.

TABLE 17-1 ➤ SYNOVIAL JOINTS

TYPE OF JOINT	EXAMPLE	MOVEMENTS ALLOWED
Hinge (ginglymus)	Elbow, ankle	Flexion-extension
Pivot	Proximal radioulnar	Rotation
Condyloid (ellipsoidal)	Wrist	Flexion-extension, abduction-adduction
Saddle	Carpometacarpal joint of thumb	Flexion-extension, abduction-adduction
Ball-and-socket	Shoulder, hip	Flexion-extension, abduction-adduction, rotation
Gliding (arthrodia)	Between sternum and clavicle, scapulae and clavice	Side-to-side, back-and-forth

Seven types of joint motion exist:

- *Flexion:* decrease in angle between the surfaces of articulating bones.
- *Extension:* increase in angle between the surfaces of articulating bones.
- *Abduction:* movement away from the midline of the body.
- *Adduction:* movement toward the midline of the body.
- *Internal (medial) rotation:* turning inward of the anterior surface of a limb.
- *External (lateral) rotation:* turning outward of the anterior surface of a limb.
- *Circumduction:* 360° rotation or combination of other motions.

Joints are often a source of injury. The most commonly injured joints include the shoulder, elbow, hip, knee, ankle, and spine. Figure 17-3 illustrates these clinically significant joints.

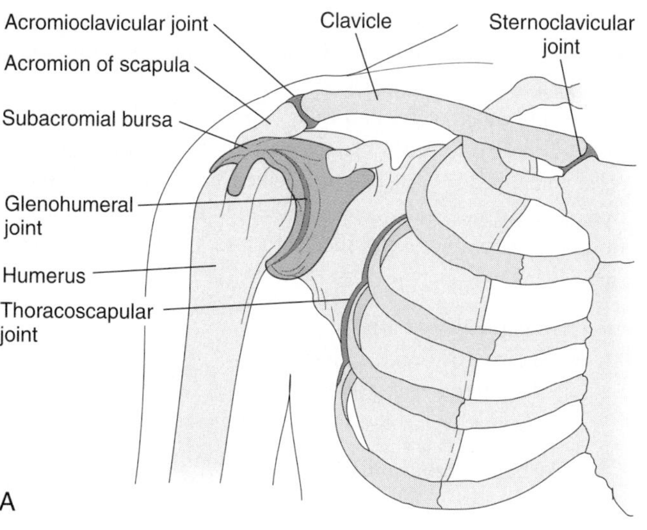

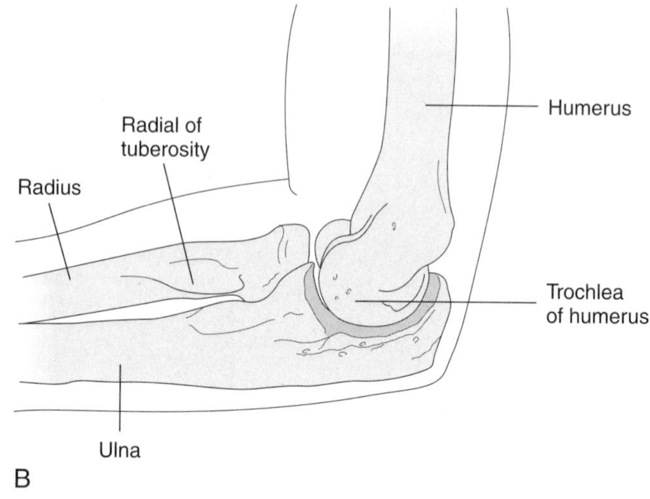

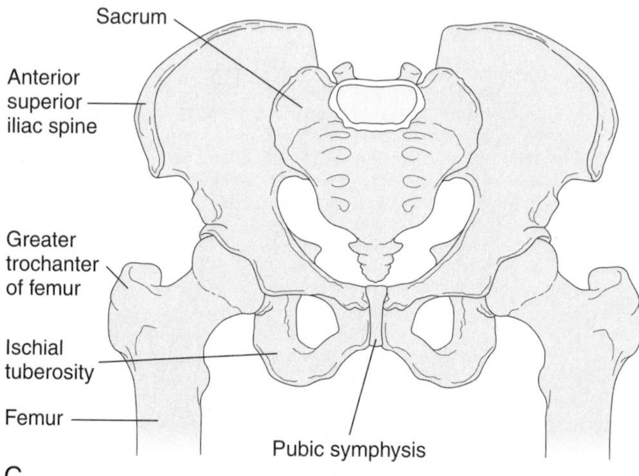

FIGURE 17-3 ■ Clinically significant joints. The joints most commonly injured include **(A)** the shoulder, **(B)** the elbow, **(C)** the hip, **(D)** the knee, **(E)** the ankle/foot, and **(F)** the spine.

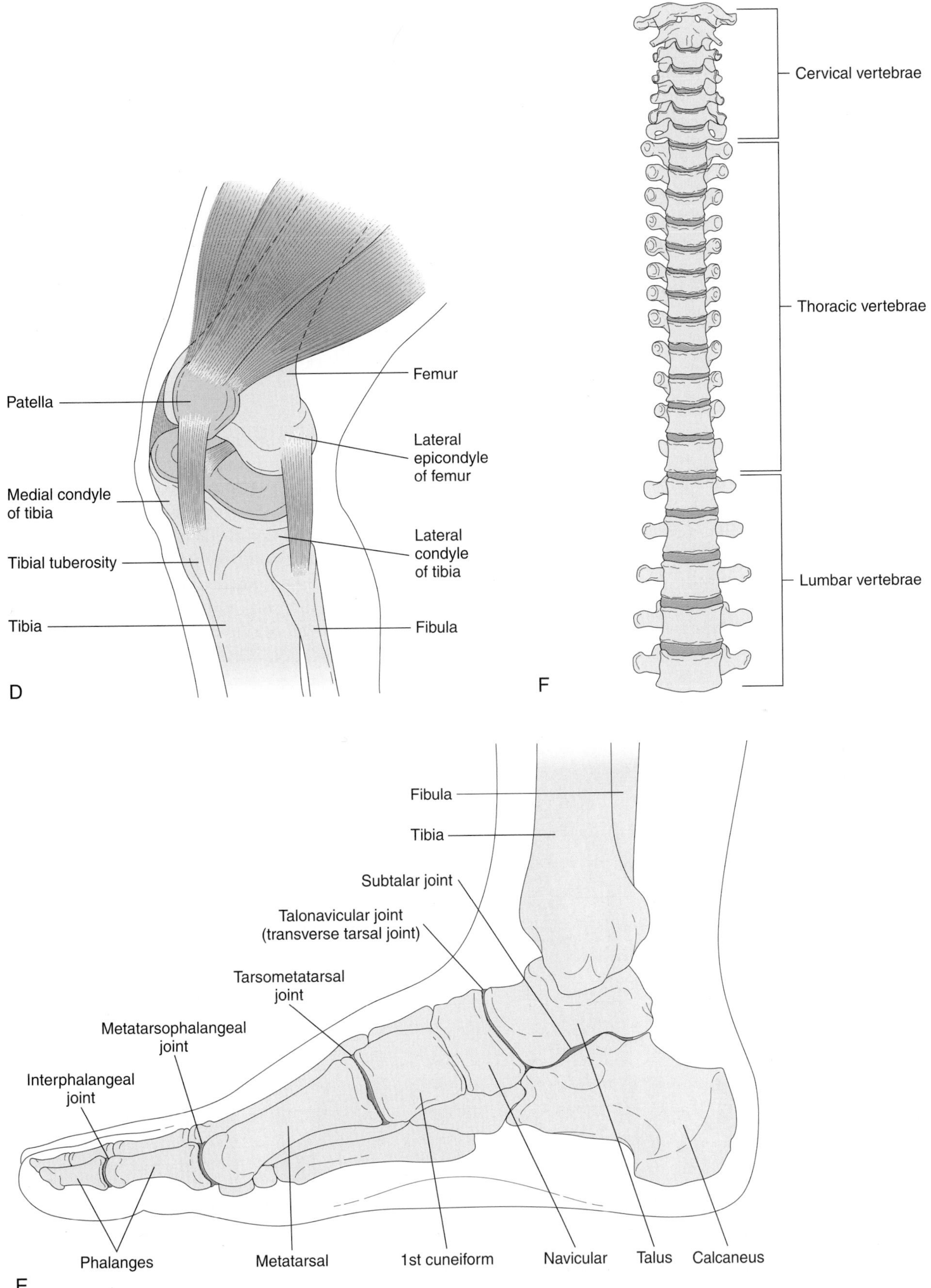
Patella
Femur
Lateral epicondyle of femur
Medial condyle of tibia
Tibial tuberosity
Lateral condyle of tibia
Tibia
Fibula
D
Cervical vertebrae
Thoracic vertebrae
Lumbar vertebrae
F
Fibula
Tibia
Subtalar joint
Talonavicular joint (transverse tarsal joint)
Tarsometatarsal joint
Metatarsophalangeal joint
Interphalangeal joint
Phalanges
Metatarsal
1st cuneiform
Navicular
Talus
Calcaneus
E

Figure 17-3 ■ Cont'd

Muscle

Muscle makes up almost half the body's mass, and within the framework of the musculoskeletal system, muscle contributes to motion through the mechanisms of contraction and relaxation. In addition to motion, muscle also maintains posture, stabilizes joints, and is responsible for the production of body heat.

Three types of muscle tissue exist: (1) skeletal, (2) cardiac, and (3) smooth. Skeletal muscle tissue is the only type to be classified as "voluntary." That is, conscious control allows skeletal muscle to contract. Cardiac muscle, which makes up the wall of the heart, and smooth muscle, which is found in the walls of the bronchioles, in blood vessels, and in some internal organs, are considered to be involuntary, because no conscious control is necessary to enact movement. During physical assessment of patients, pharmacists concentrate on the skeletal muscle tissue.

The act of muscle contraction is a very complex process. For skeletal muscle to contract, it must have a stimulus applied to it. This stimulus is delivered by a nerve cell, or neuron. Neurons have a fiber, or axon, that runs to the muscle. A neuron that stimulates skeletal muscle is a motor neuron. When a motor neuron enters skeletal muscle, the axon branches into axon terminals. The distal ends of these terminals contain chemicals called neurotransmitters, which determine whether a nerve impulse is passed along to a muscle. When a nerve impulse reaches an axon terminal, it initiates the release of acetylcholine, which is the neurotransmitter at neuromuscular junctions. This release of acetylcholine ultimately results in development of a muscle action potential, which initiates the events leading to contraction.

Skeletal muscle is classified according to the joint movement that produces the contraction. So, referring back to the discussion of joint movement, muscles are categorized as flexors, extensors, abductors, adductors, internal or medial rotators, external or lateral rotators, or circumflexors. The main muscles of the human body are shown in Figure 17-4.

To fully understand the musculoskeletal system and easily discuss patient information with other health care professionals, pharmacists need to be familiar with the nomenclature used to describe the location and relative position of various anatomic structures. Table 17-2 lists and defines these anatomic directional terms.

Special Considerations

Pediatric Patients

The musculoskeletal system of pediatric patients develops throughout childhood. Bone growth continues in many children through adolescence, until the epiphyseal plate is firmly fused. At this time, bone growth is complete. Ligaments are stronger than bone during childhood; thus, injuries in pediatric patients more commonly result in fractures rather than in sprains. At adolescence, rapid growth results in decreased epiphyseal strength, decreased general strength, and decreased flexibility. This can result in a greater potential for injury in the adolescent patient.

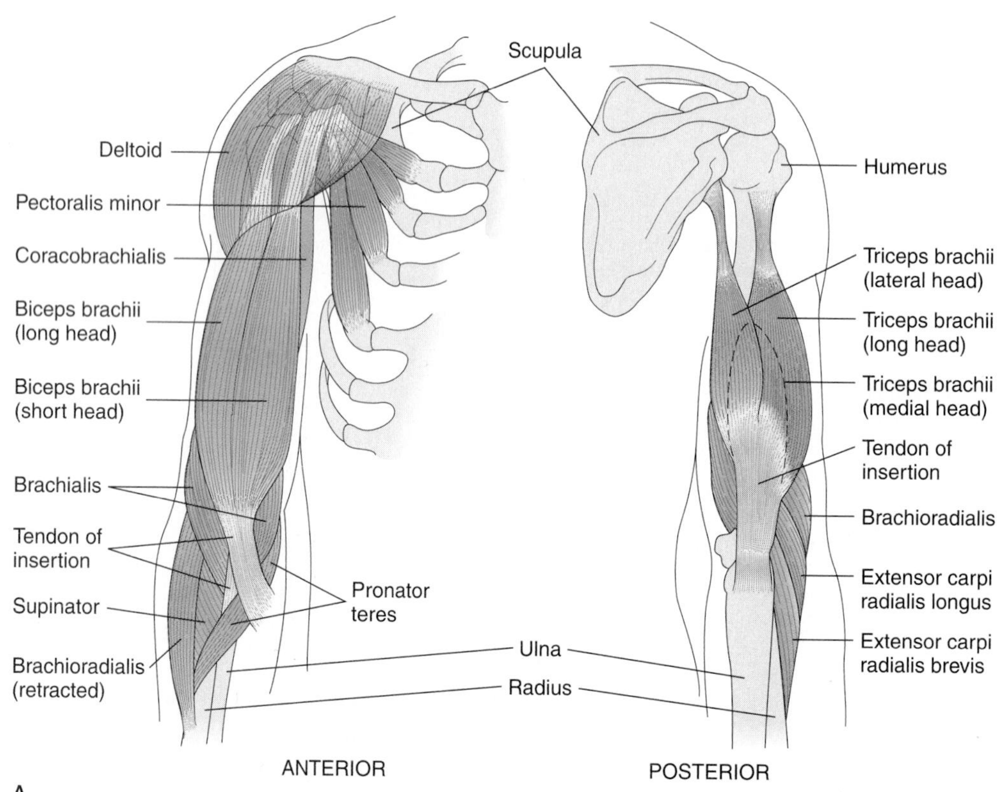

FIGURE 17-4 ■ Muscles of the human body. **(A)** Upper extremities. **(B)** Lower extremities. **(C)** Abdominal wall.

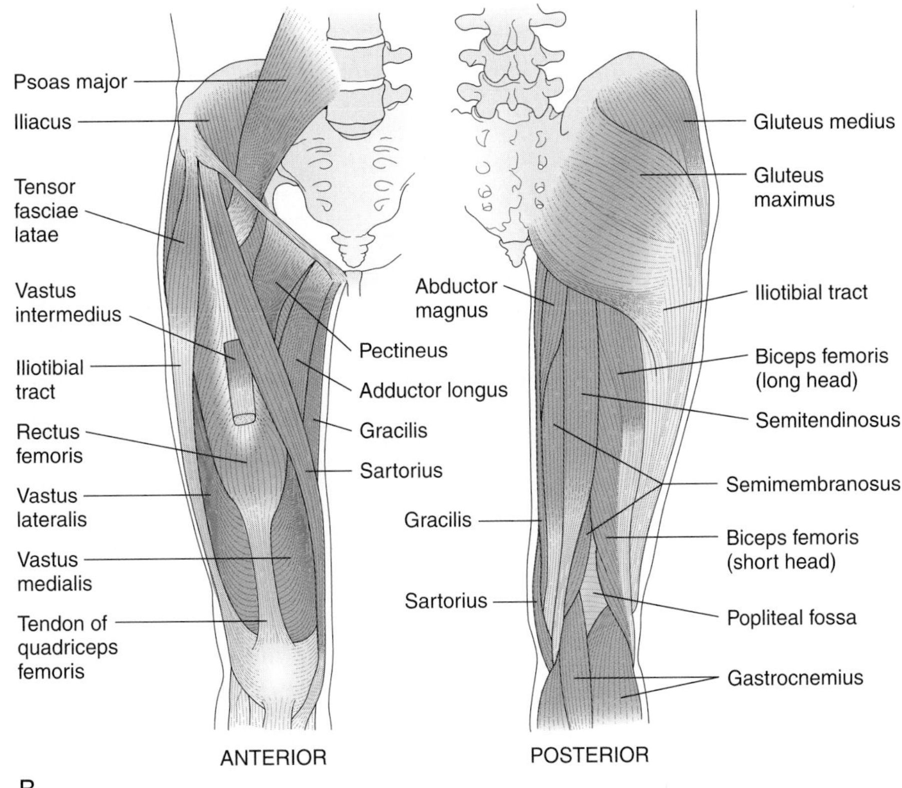
Psoas major
Iliacus
Tensor fasciae latae
Vastus intermedius
Iliotibial tract
Rectus femoris
Vastus lateralis
Vastus medialis
Tendon of quadriceps femoris
Pectineus
Adductor longus
Gracilis
Sartorius
ANTERIOR
Gluteus medius
Gluteus maximus
Abductor magnus
Iliotibial tract
Biceps femoris (long head)
Semitendinosus
Semimembranosus
Gracilis
Biceps femoris (short head)
Sartorius
Popliteal fossa
Gastrocnemius
POSTERIOR
B

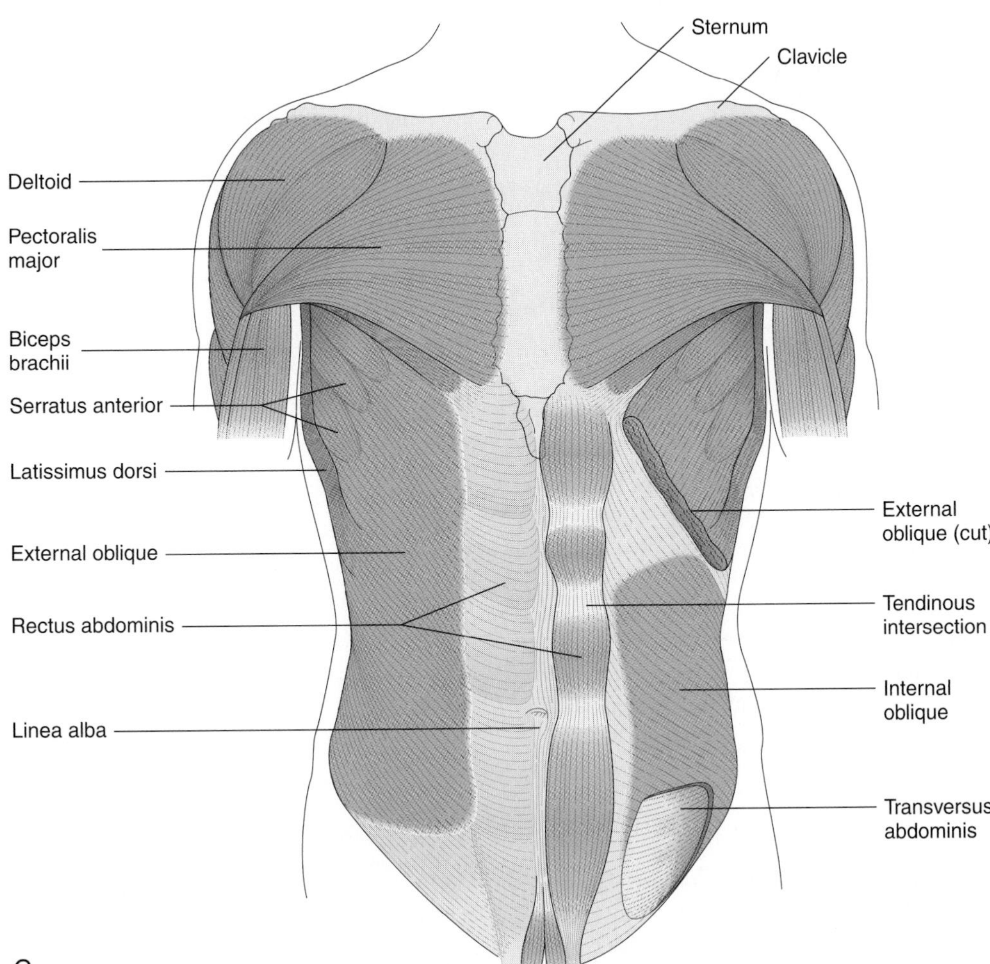
Sternum
Clavicle
Deltoid
Pectoralis major
Biceps brachii
Serratus anterior
Latissimus dorsi
External oblique
Rectus abdominis
Linea alba
External oblique (cut)
Tendinous intersection
Internal oblique
Transversus abdominis
C

FIGURE 17-4 ■ Cont'd

TABLE 17-2 ➤ ANATOMIC DIRECTIONAL TERMS

TERM	DEFINITION	EXAMPLES
Superior (cephalic, cranial)	Toward the head	The heart is superior to the stomach.
Inferior (caudad)	Away from the head, toward lower part of a structure	The liver is inferior to the lungs.
Anterior (ventral)	At or nearer the front of the body	The sternum is anterior to the heart.
Posterior (dorsal)	At or nearer the back of the body	The esophagus is posterior to the trachea.
Prone position	Body lies anterior-side down	
Supine position	Body lies anterior-side up	
Medial	Nearer the midline of the body	The ulna is on the medial side of the forearm.
Lateral	Farther from the midline of the body	The lungs are lateral to the heart.
Ipsilateral	On the same side of the body	The gallbladder and ascending colon of the large intestine are ipsilateral.
Contralateral	On the opposite side of the body	The ascending and descending colons of the large intestine are contralateral.
Proximal	Nearer to the point of origin	The humerus is proximal to the ulna.
Distal	Farther from the point of origin	The metacarpals are distal to the carpals.

Geriatric Patients

The musculoskeletal system normally maintains an equilibrium between bone deposition and bone resorption (i.e., breakdown) throughout adulthood. As the body ages, however, this equilibrium shifts toward a higher rate of bone resorption. Consequently, bone mass decreases throughout the entire skeletal system, particularly in the long bones and vertebrae, in elderly patients. This loss of bone mass predisposes these patients to increased risk of fracture. This mechanism is the basis of osteoporosis (discussed in detail later).

Alterations in muscle mass are also experienced with aging. Collagen begins to accumulate in the tissue, followed by fibrosis of connective tissue and loss of tendon elasticity. Total muscle mass, strength, and tone are reduced. This accounts for decreases in agility, speed, and endurance in elderly patients.

Pregnant Patients

During pregnancy, musculoskeletal changes take place to assist with carrying and delivering the child. Examples of these changes include loosening of the pelvic joints and widening of the hips. As the pregnancy progresses, women may experience lordosis, or a pronounced lumbar curve, as the body attempts to shift the center of gravity back over the lower extremities. Low back pain is often experienced during pregnancy because of stressed ligaments and muscles. A significant number of pregnant women experience nocturnal or activity-induced cramps in the gluteal or thigh muscles, but the cause of these cramps is unknown.

PATHOLOGY OVERVIEW

Diseases of the musculoskeletal system may be localized (i.e., affecting only one or a limited number of areas) or systemic (i.e., affecting much of the musculoskeletal system). Typically, patients with systemic musculoskeletal diseases, particularly those that are immune modulated, present with the signs and symptoms of a chronic illness. These patients may experience generalized pain, weakness, and stiffness on a regular basis. It is important to remember that some localized diseases, such as osteoarthritis or osteomyelitis, may be categorized as systemic, depending on the location, severity, and progression of the disease. Table 17-3 lists examples of typical local and systemic musculoskeletal diseases. The most common diseases and disorders of the musculoskeletal system include: (1) rheumatoid arthritis, (2) osteoarthritis, (3) osteoporosis, (4) osteomyelitis, (5) gout, (6) bursitis, (7) temporomandibular joint syndrome. Trauma can also be a factor.

Rheumatoid Arthritis

Rheumatoid arthritis (RA) is a systemic musculoskeletal disease that is characterized by symmetric inflammation of synovial tissues. The cause of RA is unknown, but one theory identifies infectious agents as a possible cause. Because the cause is unknown, no specific risk factors for development of RA have been identified. It has been shown, however, that RA is two to three times more common in women than in men, and that the prevalence of the disease increases with advancing age. The signs and symptoms of RA are listed in Box 17-1.

The initial choice of drug therapy for RA is either salicylates or nonsteroidal anti-inflammatory drugs (NSAIDs). Because RA

TABLE 17-3 ➤ GENERAL CLASSIFICATION OF MUSCULOSKELETAL DISEASES

LOCALIZED	SYSTEMIC
Osteoarthritis	Rheumatoid arthritis
Osteomyelitis	Osteoporosis
Carpal tunnel syndrome	Ankylosing spondylitis
Gout	Fibromyalgia
Temporomandibular joint syndrome	Systemic lupus erythematosus
Bursitis	Muscular dystrophy
Back pain	Amyotrophic lateral sclerosis

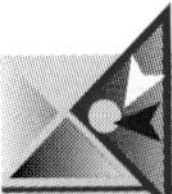

Box 17-1

SIGNS AND SYMPTOMS OF RHEUMATOID ARTHRITIS[a]

SIGNS

- Presence of serum rheumatoid factor
- Radiographic changes typical of rheumatoid arthritis (erosions or unequivocal bony decalcification)
- Swan-neck or boutonniere deformities
- Subcutaneous nodules

SYMPTOMS[b]

- Morning stiffness (lasting at least 1 hour before maximal improvement)
- Arthritis of three or more joint areas simultaneously
- Arthritis of hand joints
- Symmetric arthritis

[a]According to the American Rheumatism Association, a patient must satisfy at least four of the criteria.
[b]Must be present for at least 6 weeks.

is an inflammatory disease, higher doses of these agents are required than are necessary for analgesic purposes. If an adequate trial (2 weeks) of anti-inflammatory–dose salicylates or NSAIDs does not elicit an acceptable patient response, another NSAID is usually prescribed. Concurrent use of more than one NSAID is not recommended: There is no evidence of increased efficacy, but the risk of potential adverse effects is increased. Because of gastrointestinal, hematologic, and renal effects associated with these agents, patients should be carefully monitored after initiation of therapy. A new category of NSAIDs, the COX-2 Inhibitors, may be of value in patients who cannot tolerate the gastrointestinal side effects of traditional NSAIDs.

Some patients will not respond to NSAID therapy and, thus, will need to use second-line agents. Glucocorticoids, methotrexate, gold, hydroxychloroquine, sulfasalazine, azathioprine, and cyclophosphamide, among others, have shown benefit in maintenance treatment of RA. These agents also, however, have the potential to cause adverse effects and require close monitoring. Two biotechnology products, etanercept and infliximab, have recently been approved and have shown promise in treating refractory cases of RA.

Nondrug therapy, including rest, exercise, and heat, are also part of the regimen for treating RA. Both physical and occupational therapy, as well as ongoing emotional support, may be of benefit to the patient. In those with disease that is difficult to manage, surgical removal of the synovium may be an option.

Osteoarthritis

Osteoarthritis (OA), or **degenerative joint disease,** is characterized by deterioration of articular cartilage that results in formation of new bone at the surfaces of the joint. It differs from RA in that it is a noninflammatory disorder with symptoms typically limited to the joints where cartilage degeneration is occurring, which are most commonly the weight-bearing joints.

Osteoarthritis can be categorized as either primary or secondary. Primary OA is idiopathic in nature (i.e., no predisposing factor is known for the cartilage failure). Secondary OA results from underlying trauma, another joint disorder, or a systemic metabolic or endocrine disorder.

Risk factors for OA include:

- Age
- History of trauma to the joints
- History of fracture or infection

Obesity and stress from the patient's occupation or sports are controversial; the relationship of these risk factors with OA has not been clearly defined.

The signs and symptoms of OA are listed in Box 17-2. Table 17-4 lists the differential diagnosis of OA and RA.

Analgesics and anti-inflammatories are the cornerstones of therapy for OA; however, this treatment is only symptomatic. As in RA, analgesics and anti-inflammatories do not alter the progression of OA. Acetaminophen, 1000 mg four times daily, has benefit in patients who do not require anti-inflammatory effects. Caution against excessive use or use in patients with liver disease is necessary, however, because of the risk of hepatoxicity associated with acetaminophen. If simple analgesics fail or toxic effects or inflammation is present, NSAID therapy should be initiated. Again, cautionary use is advised because of possible adverse effects associated with this class of drugs. The COX-2 inhibitors may offer benefit to patients who cannot tolerate the gastrointestinal side effects of traditional NSAIDs.

New agents, which are derivatives of hyaluronic acid, have been introduced to the market. These agents, which are injected directly into the joint, have shown benefit in some patients with OA. Currently, however, these products are only approved for use in the knee.

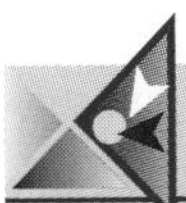

Box 17-2

SIGNS AND SYMPTOMS OF OSTEOARTHRITIS

SIGNS

- Radiographic evidence of joint degeneration
- Visible deformities of fingers

SYMPTOMS

- Pain (with or without motion)
- Morning stiffness (typically ≤15 min)
- Limited range of motion
- Crepitus (crackling or grating sound/feeling caused by bone rubbing on bone or cartilage)
- Instability
- Joint tenderness
- Muscle atrophy

TABLE 17-4 DIFFERENTIAL DIAGNOSIS OF RHEUMATOID ARTHRITIS AND OSTEOARTHRITIS

SYMPTOM	RHEUMATOID ARTHRITIS	OSTEOARTHRITIS
Morning stiffness	>1 hour	≤15 minutes
Inflammation	Present	Absent or mild
Disease distribution	Systemic	Local
Serum rheumatoid factor	Frequently positive	Negative
Erythrocyte sedimentation rate	Increased	Normal
Swelling	Symmetrical	Irregular
Subcutaneous nodules	Frequently present	Absent
Joint involvement	Bilateral, symmetrical	Unilateral or bilateral, symmetric or asymmetric

As in RA, nondrug therapies are also important in OA. Overweight patients should be counseled regarding weight loss to decrease stress on the weight-bearing joints. Physical therapy, including exercise and appropriate use of heat and cold, may help to maintain joint function and to relieve pain. Patients with severe, debilitating disease may be candidates for surgical intervention.

Osteoporosis

Osteoporosis is a disease that is characterized by low bone mass and microarchitectural deterioration of bone tissue, leading to increased bone fragility and susceptibility to fracture. Mainly seen in postmenopausal women, the cause of osteoporosis is multifactorial. These factors include age-related changes in bone resulting from decreased bone formation, decreased calcium absorption, biochemical imbalances, and in women, menopause.

Generally speaking, two types of osteoporosis exist: type I, or postmenopausal, which typically manifests approximately 10 years after menopause in women; and type II, or senile, which presents around age 70 in both sexes. Two types of bone can be affected by osteoporosis: trabecular, and cortical. Trabecular bone, also known as spongy bone, is a series of thin plates forming the interior latticework of bone. It constitutes approximately 20% of the human skeleton. Cortical bone is the compact layer that forms the outer shell of the bone and constitutes approximately 80% of the human skeleton. Type I osteoporosis is characterized mainly by trabecular bone loss, whereas type 2 osteoporosis is characterized by both trabecular and cortical bone loss. Osteoporosis can also occur secondary to conditions and medications. The most common type of secondary osteoporosis is glucocorticoid-induced osteoporosis, which is associated with chronic administration of glucocorticoids.

Risk factors for osteoporosis include:

- Advanced age
- Female sex
- Caucasian/Asian descent
- Small build
- Estrogen deficiency
- Chronic use of steroids
- Family history of osteoporosis
- Low calcium intake

The signs and symptoms of osteoporosis are listed in Box 17-3.

The treatment of choice for postmenopausal osteoporosis is estrogen replacement therapy. With hormone therapy, a risk of breast or endometrial cancer (or both) does exist, particularly in patients with a personal or family history of these diseases. Although the literature supporting these risks is somewhat controversial, many women are uncomfortable using hormone replacement therapy for osteoporosis. Alendronate, a bisphosphonate, and calcitonin, a naturally occurring hormone, both inhibit bone resorption. The National Osteoporosis Foundation Consensus Statement recommends the use of one of these agents when estrogen replacement therapy is contraindicated or not accepted by patients. Results of clinical trials also suggest that these agents have benefit in preventing bone loss in patients with glucocorticoid-induced osteoporosis.

Alendronate and raloxifene, a selective estrogen-receptor modulator, are both indicated for prevention of osteoporosis in postmenopausal women. Postmenopausal women who are at increased risk of developing osteoporosis and in whom estrogen therapy is contraindicated may benefit from one of these agents. Early literature suggests a lesser association with the development of breast and endometrial carcinoma with use of raloxifene than with use of traditional estrogen replacement.

Adequate vitamin D and calcium intake is also fundamental to both prevention and treatment of postmenopausal osteoporosis. Postmenopausal women older than 65 years and who are receiving estrogen replacement therapy should take 1000 mg of calcium daily; those not receiving estrogen should take 1500 mg daily. All women with osteoporosis and who are younger

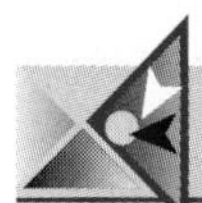

Box 17-3

SIGNS AND SYMPTOMS OF OSTEOPOROSIS

SIGNS

- Decreased bone mineral density

SYMPTOMS

- Fracture (usually after minor trauma)
- Pain
- Dorsal kyphosis
- Cervical lordosis (dowager's hump)

than 65 years, regardless of hormonal supplementation, should take 1500 mg of calcium daily. Vitamin D supplementation is also imperative in women who do not receive enough through their diet. Thus, it may be best for those who need to take calcium supplementation to take calcium with vitamin D.

In addition to pharmacotherapy, weight-bearing (e.g., walking, jogging, stair-climbing, or dancing) and resistance (e.g., weight-lifting) exercise may also slow bone loss. Prevention of injury is also important, because fractures present additional problems for older patients. Approximately 20% of elderly women who experience a hip fracture do not survive the first year after the incident, and an additional 20% do not regain the ability to walk without some type of assistance.

Osteomyelitis

Osteomyelitis is an inflammation of the bone marrow and surrounding bone caused by an infecting organism. It can occur in any bone, and it often leads to serious morbidity.

Bone can be infected by three main routes:

- Hematogenous spread from a distal infection site
- Direct infection from an adjacent infection
- Infection secondary to vascular insufficiency

Staphylococcus aureus is the most common infecting organism; however, Gram-negative and anaerobic bacteria may also cause osteomyelitis.

Risk factors for osteomyelitis include:

- Bacteremia
- Trauma
- Surgery
- Cellulitis
- Diabetes
- Peripheral vascular disease

Signs and symptoms of osteomyelitis are listed in Box 17-4.

Treatment of osteomyelitis requires antibiotic therapy with an agent that covers the results of culture and sensitivity testing. Typically, at least 6 weeks of antibiotic therapy are necessary, with at least the first 2 to 3 weeks being parenteral therapy. Depending on the individual situation, oral therapy may be acceptable for the latter course of treatment.

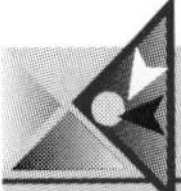

Box 17-4

SIGNS AND SYMPTOMS OF OSTEOMYELITIS

SIGNS

- Bone changes on radiograph
- Elevated erythrocyte sedimentation rate
- Elevated white-blood-cell count

SYMPTOMS

- Fever
- Tenderness
- Swelling
- Warmth
- Limited motion
- Drainage

Gout

Gout is a disorder of uric acid metabolism. The resultant hyperuricemia is either a result of overproduction or underexcretion of uric acid (or some combination of the two). When uric acid accumulates, a crystal-induced inflammation occurs. Acute attacks are characterized by the rapid onset of excruciating pain, swelling, and inflammation. When an acute attack occurs, it is typically localized to a single joint in the foot or ankle, most commonly the first metatarsophalangeal joint (i.e., the great toe). Attacks of gout, however, may occur in other joints as well. Attacks are often sporadic, with pain-free intervals lasting from months to years. Attacks can be precipitated by dehydration, fasting, binge eating, or excessive alcohol ingestion.

Risk factors for gout include:

- Myeloproliferative disorders
- Lymphoproliferative disorders
- Renal dysfunction
- Psoriasis
- Acute alcoholism
- Diabetic ketoacidosis
- Obesity
- Congestive heart failure
- Hypothyroidism
- Hyperparathyroidism
- Hypoparathyroidism
- Uric acid–modifying agents (e.g., diuretics, niacin, and others)
- Stress
- Trauma
- Surgery

Signs and symptoms of gout are listed in Box 17-5.

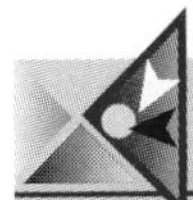

Box 17-5

SIGNS AND SYMPTOMS OF GOUT

SIGNS

- Increased serum uric acid level
- Erythema of affected joint

SYMPTOMS

- Rapid onset of excruciating pain (most commonly in a single joint)
- Swelling
- Inflammation

Commonly, NSAIDs are used for treatment of acute gout attacks. Initial doses should be high, followed by rapid tapering over the course of a week. Indomethacin has been used extensively in the treatment of acute gout attacks. Long-acting NSAIDs are generally not recommended for gout. Colchicine is an option in the treatment of acute attacks that do not respond to NSAID therapy. Prophylactic treatment of gout can be managed by either allopurinol, which decreases serum uric acid synthesis, or uricosuric drugs such probenecid and sulfinpyrazone, which increase renal excretion of uric acid.

Nondrug therapy does not have a large role in the treatment of gout. Patients should be counseled to avoid any dietary triggers, such as anchovies, sardines, liver, or other foods that are high in purines, because these may precipitate an attack.

Bursitis, Tendinitis, and Tenosynovitis

Inflammation of periarticular soft tissue structures can result in painful attacks of bursitis, tendinitis, and tenosynovitis. **Bursitis** is an inflammation of the bursa, a sac or cavity filled with synovial fluid that is usually located near joints. Bursae function to reduce friction between structures. **Tendinitis** is an inflammation of the tendon; tendons are connective tissue that attach muscle to bone. **Tenosynovitis** is an inflammation of the tendon and the synovial membrane at the joint. These inflammatory processes may be the result of trauma, rheumatic processes, or infection.

Risk factors for these conditions include:

- Trauma:
  - Strain
  - Direct injury
- RA
- Reiter's syndrome
- Gout
- Infection (especially gonorrhea)

Signs and symptoms of bursitis, tendinitis, and tenosynovitis are listed in Box 17-6.

Often, NSAIDs are useful for the acute pain associated with these types of inflammation. Steroid injections (e.g., triamcinolone) may also provide relief. In addition, joint rest and immobilization are important components of therapy.

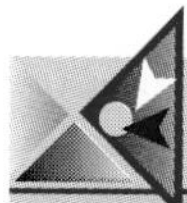

Box 17-6

SIGNS AND SYMPTOMS OF BURSITIS, TENDONITIS, AND TENOSYNOVITIS

SIGNS

- Fluid on the affected joint

SYMPTOMS

- Inflammation
- Pain
- Common sites:
  - Shoulder
  - Elbow (tennis elbow)
  - Hip
  - Thumb
  - Knee
  - Heel

Temporomandibular Joint Syndrome

Temporomandibular joint (TMJ) syndrome is a painful jaw movement that is characterized by dull pain and tenderness in the joint area. It has several potential causes, including congenital abnormalities, trauma, or arthritis.

Risk factors for TMJ syndrome include:

- Congenital abnormalities
- Trauma
- Arthritis
- Improperly aligned teeth
- Grinding/clenching of teeth

Signs and symptoms of TMJ syndrome are listed in Box 17-7.

Symptomatic treatment with NSAIDs decreases the pain in most patients. In addition, nondrug therapies play an important role. Heat or cold applications, limited movement, and a soft diet seem to improve symptoms. Elimination of caffeine and stress-reduction therapies are also effective in some patients. In more severe cases, splinting, adjustment, or reshaping of the teeth—or surgical intervention—may be necessary.

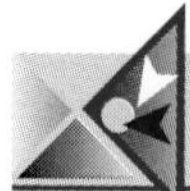

Box 17-7

SIGNS AND SYMPTOMS OF TEMPOROMANDIBULAR JOINT SYNDROME

SIGNS

- Abnormal wearing of the teeth (on visual or radiographic examination)
- Tenderness and crepitus on palpation
- Decreased range of motion

SYMPTOMS

- Dull pain around the ear
- Unilateral face pain (may refer to the neck)
- Jaw tenderness
- Clicking or popping noise when opening or closing the mouth
- Abnormal opening of the mouth
- Headache
- Tooth sensitivity

Trauma

In addition to the diseases that can affect the musculoskeletal system, patients can also exhibit skeletal signs and symptoms secondary to injury or trauma. These conditions include strains, sprains, dislocations, or fractures.

A **strain** is the overstretching of a muscle. While strains may be painful, they are not as serious as sprains and are commonly treated only with joint rest.

A **sprain** is trauma to a joint that includes damage to the ligaments. In severe sprains, ligaments may be completely torn. Sprains are commonly treated by cold therapy for 24 to 48 hours, which is then followed by heat therapy, if necessary, and joint elevation. In severe cases, joint immobilization may be necessary.

A **dislocation** occurs when a bone is displaced from a joint, with tearing of ligaments, tendons, and articular capsules. A dislocation usually results from a blow or a fall. Dislocations may also be referred to as luxations. A partial or incomplete dislocation is referred to as a subluxation. Joint dislocations are treated by manipulation of the bone back into the appropriate position.

A **fracture** is any break in a bone. Depending on the degree of the break, the severity of the fracture will vary. Typically, the broken bone must be manipulated into the proper position and then cast to prevent movement until union has taken place.

SYSTEM ASSESSMENT

Because musculoskeletal problems are commonly treated with over-the-counter medications and nonpharmacologic products, the pharmacist is frequently consulted about signs and symptoms associated with the musculoskeletal system. To thoroughly evaluate these complaints, the pharmacist should use the following interview questions.

Subjective Information

Pain

Pain is the most frequent symptom of disease or disorder within the musculoskeletal system; however, it can also be a very elusive symptom. Careful questioning of the patient by the pharmacist and a thorough objective assessment of the patient's skeletal system are necessary to establish an accurate assessment and to form recommendations for managing the care of the patient. The following questions should be included in the assessment of patients complaining of musculoskeletal pain.

? INTERVIEW Do you ever experience any pain in your joints, muscles, or bones? If so, how would you classify the pain? Is it dull, sharp, aching?

➤ ABNORMALITIES Dull or aching pain is characteristic of arthritic conditions. Sharp pain may indicate acute trauma, injury, or gout.

? INTERVIEW Where is the pain located? Is it localized or diffuse in nature? Do you notice it on one side or on both sides?

➤ ABNORMALITIES Knowing if the pain is localized or diffuse and symmetric will help to determine the type of disorder. RA is characterized by diffuse pain that is symmetric in nature; OA and gout manifest as localized pain at a single or limited number of joints.

? INTERVIEW How long has the pain been occurring? Is it continual or sporadic in nature? Does it occur frequently?

➤ ABNORMALITIES If the pain is new in onset, determine if a relationship with any trauma or stress in the recent past can be established. Continual pain suggests a chronic musculoskeletal disease.

? INTERVIEW Is the pain worse at any certain time of the day?

➤ ABNORMALITIES Pain from rheumatic disorders tends to be worse in the morning. Tendinitis pain is severe in the morning but often tapers off by midday. Osteoarthritic pain worsens throughout the day.

? INTERVIEW Does anything make the pain better or worse? Movement? Rest? Weather?

➤ ABNORMALITIES In most musculoskeletal conditions, movement worsens the pain. In RA, however, movement often decreases pain, and rest increases pain. Although controversial, many patients state that their arthritis is worse during rainy weather.

? INTERVIEW Does the pain involve muscle cramping? If so, is it accompanied by weakness? Which muscles experience this pain? Does it occur in the calf muscle? Does walking aggravate the pain?

➤ ABNORMALITIES Muscle pain often may result from overexertion. Question the patient regarding recent behavior. Muscle pain in conjunction with weakness may indicate a primary muscle disorder. Calf muscle pain may indicate intermittent claudication, especially if it is experienced with walking.

? INTERVIEW Have you tried anything to relieve the pain? If so, what have you tried? Was it helpful?

➤ ABNORMALITIES Noninflammatory disorders often respond to simple analgesics (e.g., acetaminophen).

Inflammatory disorders, including RA, bursitis, or gout, require therapy with NSAIDs for relief. Rest will relieve pain for most musculoskeletal conditions, with the exception of RA. Cold often relieves the pain of local trauma; arthritic conditions may respond better to heat.

INTERVIEW Is the pain associated with chills, fever, nausea, or sore throat? Have you had a recent illness?

ABNORMALITIES Viral illnesses are frequently associated with myalgia. If osteomyelitis is suspected, recent infection could assist in determining the cause of the infection. A recent history of sore throat followed by joint pain 1 to 2 weeks later may be associated with rheumatic fever.

INTERVIEW Is the pain severe enough to cause difficulty in your daily routines? Rate the pain on a scale from 0 (no pain) to 10 (worst pain you've ever experienced).

ABNORMALITIES If pain keeps patients from daily activities, it often is quite severe. Assessment of physical mobility during the objective examination will be important.

INTERVIEW Does the pain wake you up at night? Does the pain make it difficult for you to get to sleep?

ABNORMALITIES Severe pain makes it difficult to sleep, particularly if the patient is lying on the affected area. RA and tendinitis often wake people in the early morning because of pain caused by lack of movement.

Swelling

Swelling within the musculoskeletal system is often a sign of inflammation. When a muscle or joint is noted to have edema, it may be accompanied by local signs of erythema and limitation of movement. Swelling can also indicate fluid on a joint and be the result of an acute traumatic event or the manifestation of an ongoing, systemic inflammatory condition. Although establishing a diagnosis may not be possible through identification of this one symptom, swelling, erythema, and tenderness can be important clues when integrated with other subjective and objective data. The following questions should be asked when assessing musculoskeletal swelling in a patient.

INTERVIEW Have you experienced any swelling? If so, is the swelling present continuously, or does it occur sporadically? Is the swelling an isolated incident?

ABNORMALITIES Swelling may indicate inflammation and may involve accumulation of fluid on a joint. Chronic conditions (e.g., RA) may have continuous swelling. Acute trauma, inflammation, or infection may present suddenly with swelling. Swelling may occur with stress or trauma to a joint and, therefore, be seen sporadically.

INTERVIEW Have you recently experienced any trauma to the affected area? If so, what happened?

ABNORMALITIES Localized trauma to a joint (e.g., sprains) causes swelling and pain at the point of injury. Often, ice applied to the spot decreases the swelling.

INTERVIEW Do you ever experience swelling and erythema in other joints?

ABNORMALITIES Diffuse swelling and erythema are characteristic of a systemic inflammatory condition. Given other objective and subjective information, consider a systemic disease.

INTERVIEW What seems to trigger the swelling?

ABNORMALITIES Previously injured joints may swell only on subsequent trauma to the area. Joints that swell on stress or exertion should be carefully examined for previous trauma to the area.

INTERVIEW Does anything cause relief of the swelling?

ABNORMALITIES Ice applied to a traumatized joint may decrease swelling. Swelling from a chronic disease may not respond to cold therapy.

INTERVIEW Do you have any medical history of cardiac disease? If so, of what type?

ABNORMALITIES Pitting edema can be a sign of cardiac disease, particularly heart failure. This edema is quite prevalent in the ankles.

INTERVIEW What medications do you currently take?

ABNORMALITIES Some medications can cause fluid retention, leading to edema. Box 17-8 lists drugs that may cause swelling.

Stiffness/Range of Motion

Stiffness is a very common symptom of musculoskeletal disease and can be associated with situations ranging from overexertion to RA. Because stiffness can be a very nonspecific symptom, it is important to gather as much specific information as possible to

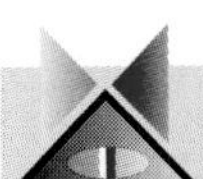

Box 17-8

DRUGS THAT MAY CAUSE SWELLING

- Calcium-channel blockers
- Nonsteroidal anti-inflammatory drugs
- Glucocorticoids
- Oral contraceptives
- Estrogen

assist in identifying the cause. Stiffness may be associated with difficulties in range of motion (ROM). Limitation of movement can be caused by several factors. For example, intrinsic joint disease, thickening of extra-articular structures (i.e., joint capsules or ligaments), fibrosis, or muscle contractures can limit motion in a patient. When patients begin to suffer a decrease in motion, it can interfere with daily activity. To assess the severity of stiffness and movement limitation, the following questions should be asked.

? INTERVIEW Do you frequently experience stiffness?

➤ ABNORMALITIES Patients with chronic musculoskeletal diseases such as arthritis or **fibromyalgia,** a systemic condition resulting in chronic muscle and soft tissue pain, frequently have daily stiffness associated with the disorder.

? INTERVIEW Is it a generalized condition, or is it localized to a single joint or to limited joints or muscles?

➤ ABNORMALITIES Again, this refers to the distribution of the disease. Systemic diseases manifest as a chronic disease affecting much of the body.

? INTERVIEW Have you had any overexertion recently?

➤ ABNORMALITIES Overexertion, particularly in patients who are not frequently active, can cause muscle stiffness. Chronic stiffness should be evaluated further for underlying causes. Stiffness and limited ROM caused by overexertion should not be a chronic condition.

? INTERVIEW Do you experience stiffness at any particular time of the day? Is morning stiffness present? If so, how long does it typically take to resolve?

➤ ABNORMALITIES Morning stiffness is associated with rheumatic diseases. Patients with OA tend to experience stiffness for only a short period of time (usually ≤15 min), whereas patients with RA may have stiffness for an hour or longer. Stiffness caused by overexertion is typically worse in the morning and improves as the day goes on and the joint "loosens up."

? INTERVIEW Can you do anything to help relieve the stiffness? Does heat help?

➤ ABNORMALITIES Heat typically helps to improve muscle-related stiffness. Stiffness associated with injury may or may not respond to heat.

? INTERVIEW Are you having difficulty moving any parts of your body? If so, which ones? Have you overexerted yourself recently?

➤ ABNORMALITIES A generalized limitation in movement would be caused by a systemic musculoskeletal disorder or by recent overexertion.

Weakness

Weakness can be a very important symptom of musculoskeletal disease. It is important to differentiate between muscle weakness and generalized fatigue when assessing a patient. When weakness exists, identifying which muscle groups are affected assists in assessing the problem. Typically, proximal weakness is associated with **myopathy** (i.e., disease of the muscle), whereas distal weakness is associated more commonly with **neuropathy** (i.e., disease of the nervous system). Weakness can indicate serious neurologic disorders and should be taken seriously. To help identify the cause of muscle weakness, the following questions should be asked.

? INTERVIEW Have you noticed any weakness in your muscles? Is this something new?

➤ ABNORMALITIES Muscle weakness may result from overexertion or systemic musculoskeletal disorders, such as myasthenia gravis, polymyositis, and dermatomyositis. **Myasthenia gravis** is an autoimmune disease marked by skeletal muscle fatigue in which antibodies are directed against acetylcholine receptors, causing the inhibition of muscle contraction. **Polymyositis** is an inflammatory disease of the skeletal muscle tissue characterized by symmetric weakness of proximal muscles of the limbs, neck, and pharynx. **Dermatomyositis** is an inflammatory disease of the connective tissue that causes muscle inflammation, edema, and dermatitis.

? INTERVIEW If the weakness in your muscles is not something new, does it occur continuously or sporadically?

➤ ABNORMALITIES Myasthenia gravis may have a variable clinical course; spontaneous remissions and exacerbations frequently occur. Polymyositis and dermatomyositis typically are rapidly progressive diseases without remissions.

? INTERVIEW Does the weakness change depending on the time of day?

ABNORMALITIES It is important to differentiate weakness from fatigue. Patients who complain of progressive weakness throughout the day may be describing fatigue or have a systemic disorder (e.g., myasthenia gravis).

? INTERVIEW Is the weakness limited to a certain muscle, or have you noticed generalized weakness?

ABNORMALITIES Generalized weakness is a sign of a systemic disorder (e.g., myasthenia gravis). Weakness limited to a certain muscle may indicate overexertion or injury or be neurologic in nature. A neurologic examination may be necessary.

? INTERVIEW Do you have pain or stiffness associated with the weakness?

ABNORMALITIES Pain and stiffness may be associated with a systemic muscular disorder (e.g., myasthenia gravis) or with overexertion. Less than half the cases of polymyositis have associated muscle pain.

? INTERVIEW Do you have difficulty combing your hair? Do you have difficulty lifting objects?

ABNORMALITIES A proximal weakness of the upper extremities will cause difficulties with these tasks.

? INTERVIEW Have you noticed problems with writing or turning a doorknob?

ABNORMALITIES A distal weakness of the upper extremities will cause difficulties with these tasks. It may also cause difficulties with fine motor skills (e.g., buttoning a shirt).

? INTERVIEW Have you noticed the muscle(s) to be smaller than usual, or to be stiff?

ABNORMALITIES This could signal atrophy of the muscles. Atrophy is typically associated with lack of use of the muscles. Patients who have suffered a stroke or other neurologic disorder that could impair muscle function may experience atrophic changes.

? INTERVIEW Has anything helped this weakness? Does rest help?

ABNORMALITIES The weakness associated with myasthenia gravis is typically worse after exercise and better after rest, but a general weakness remains constant.

? INTERVIEW Have you noticed any double vision? Any difficulty swallowing or chewing?

ABNORMALITIES Patients with myasthenia gravis often experience **diplopia,** or double vision. These patients also experience difficulties with swallowing or chewing.

Objective Information

Physical Assessment

Physical assessment of the musculoskeletal system consists of four basic components: (1) inspection, (2) palpation, (3) ROM evaluation, and (4) muscle strength testing. Each is important, because each reveals individual clues regarding the patient's condition. When performing these components of the musculoskeletal assessment, it is best to use the cephalocaudal (i.e., head-to-toe) approach. Using this system decreases the possibility of omissions. In addition, when specifically examining muscles and joints, they should be examined as symmetric pairs to allow for comparison in appearance, size, and strength. Keep in mind that unequal muscles or joints can indicate possible disorders.

All joints, bones, and surrounding muscles should be palpated for abnormalities. Heat, swelling, tenderness, or masses should be closely examined. Joints should be nontender. Palpable fluid is abnormal. Hard or doughy muscle tone may represent atrophy. Any hard masses that are found on examination should be referred for evaluation of possible malignancy.

Testing ROM compares the patient's ability to move a particular joint against the expected normal motion of that joint. The ROM may be measured with a **goniometer,** which is a protractor with moveable arms that is used to measure the range of joint motion in degrees. This assessment is also performed through a series of movements (discussed in detail later). A decreased ROM can be the result of trauma, stiffness, swelling (with or without fluid accumulation), or neurologic problems. Limited ROM must be further investigated to diagnose the underlying disorder. Patients with limited ROM may suffer from pain on movement, so go slowly when evaluating mobility to minimize patient discomfort.

Evaluation of muscle strength is generally incorporated in the ROM assessment. Muscle strength should be bilaterally symmetric, with full resistance to opposition. Weakness can be a sign of atrophy, fatigue, pain, or neurologic disorder. Significant muscle weakness must be further investigated.

The pharmacist rarely completes a full musculoskeletal examination; however, it is described here for completeness.

Gait

The initial step in a full musculoskeletal assessment is inspection of the gait and posture of a patient. Normal posture is illustrated in Figure 17-5.

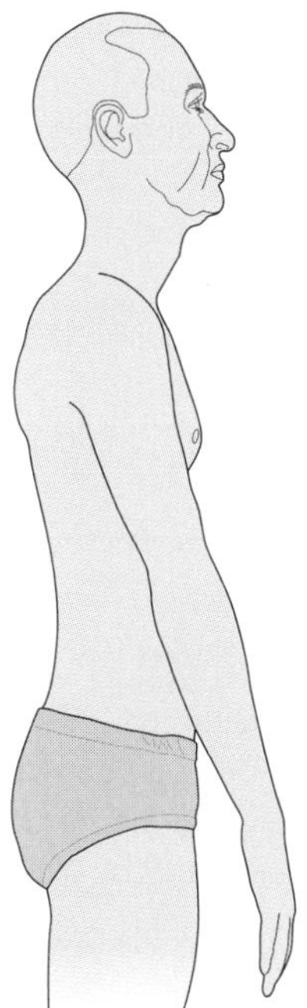

FIGURE 17-5 ■ Normal posture. Note the curvature of the spine and the even contour of the shoulders.

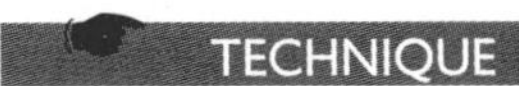

TECHNIQUE

STEP 1

Evaluate the Patient's Gait

Observe the rate, rhythm, and arm motion of the patient while walking:

- Ask the patient to walk away from you normally.
- Ask the patient to walk toward you on tiptoe.
- Ask the patient to walk away from you on the heels.
- Ask the patient to walk back to you in a normal gait.

ABNORMALITIES A short, shuffling gait could indicate Parkinson's disease or other neurologic disorders. **Ataxia** (i.e., the inability to coordinate muscular movements) is typically associated with cerebellar dysfunction or adverse effects of drugs (e.g., alcohol intoxication or benzodiazepines). An **antalgic gait** occurs when a patient experiences pain during the stance phase and, therefore, remains on the painful leg for as short a time as possible. This may indicate a painful hip.

Inspection of Muscles and Joints

TECHNIQUE

STEP 1

Inspection of the Muscles and Joints

- Complete a visual scan of the muscles and joints, including the following:
- Size (muscles and joints should generally be similar in size).
- Symmetry (joints and muscles should be symmetrical bilaterally).
- Skin (look for any redness, swelling, masses, or deformities).
- Note any obvious abnormalities.

ABNORMALITIES Atrophy or hypertrophy may indicate disease, including malnutrition or lipodystrophy. Asymmetric joint swelling may be associated with trauma or systemic disease. Redness and swelling can indicate inflammation and most often is associated with warmth and tenderness. Ecchymosis may indicate recent acute trauma.

Temporomandibular Joint Syndrome

Assessment of TMJ is illustrated in Figure 17-6.

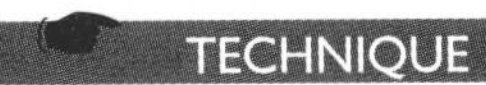

TECHNIQUE

STEP 1

Inspect the TMJ Area

- Position the patient standing facing you.
- Observe any swelling or discoloration in the TMJ area.

STEP 2

Palpate the TMJs

- Locate the TMJs with your fingertips placed anterior to the tragus of each ear.
- Instruct the patient to open and close the mouth slowly.
- Confirm that the jaw opens and closes smoothly.
- Note any swelling, tenderness, or crepitus.

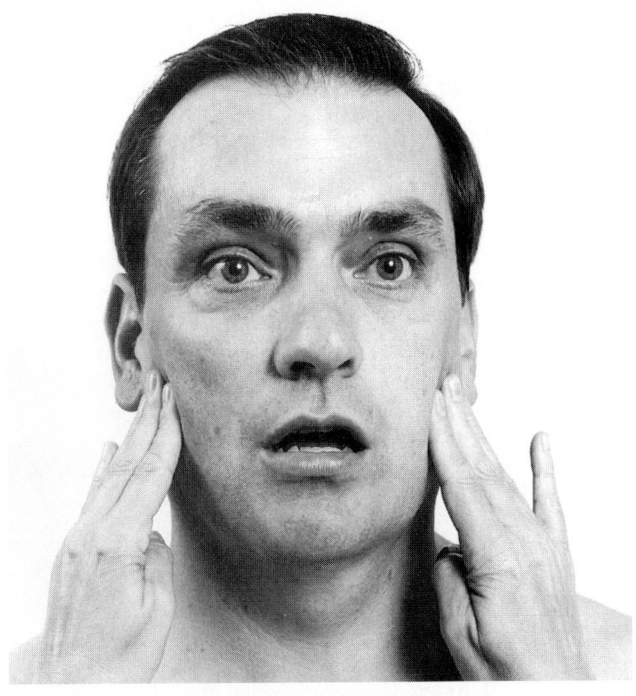

FIGURE 17-6 ■ Assessing the temporomandibular joint.

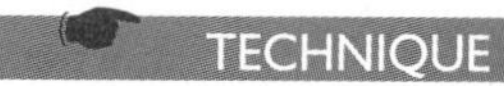

ABNORMALITIES **Crepitus,** a crackling sound heard during movement of the joints because of irregularities in the articulating surfaces, can be a normal finding. Pain, locking of the jaw, or a "popping" or "clicking" sound may indicate TMJ syndrome.

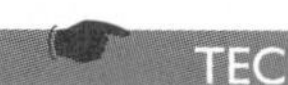

TECHNIQUE

STEP 3

Evaluate the ROM of the TMJs

- Ask the patient to move the jaw from side to side.
- Ask the patient to move the jaw forward and backward.
- Note any decreased ROM.

Cervical Spine

TECHNIQUE

STEP 1

Inspect the Alignment of the Head and Neck

- Position the patient standing facing you.
- Confirm that the alignment is appropriate, the head erect, and the cervical spine concave.

STEP 2

Inspect and Palpate the Neck and Surrounding Muscles

- Inspect the neck and surrounding muscles.
- Confirm that the muscles are symmetric in size.
- Palpate the neck and surrounding muscles.
- Note any heat, tenderness, swelling, and masses. Confirm there is firm tone without tenderness.

STEP 3

Assess the ROM of the Cervical Spine

Do not ask patient to perform these movements if neck trauma is suspected.

- Position the patient standing facing you.
- Instruct the patient to bend the head forward, chin to chest (Fig. 17-7A).
- Measure motion with a goniometer. Expect flexion of 45°.
- Instruct the patient to bend the head back, chin to ceiling.
- Measure motion with a goniometer. Expect hyperextension of 55°.
- Instruct the patient to bend the head to each side, ear to each shoulder (Fig. 17-7B).
- Measure motion with a goniometer. Expect lateral bending of 40°.
- Instruct the patient to turn the chin to each shoulder (Fig. 17-7C).
- Measure motion with a goniometer. Expect rotation of 70°.

ABNORMALITIES Pain, limited ROM, or both could indicate strain, arthritis, or a neurologic condition. Hard or doughy muscle may represent atrophy. Any hard masses should be referred for evaluation of possible malignancy. Muscle weakness may be a sign of atrophy, fatigue, pain, or a neurologic disorder.

STEP 4

Inspect the Spine for Alignment

- Position the patient standing in front of you.
- Inspect the spine from side and back for alignment.
- Confirm that the curves of the lumbar spine are concave and that the curve of the thoracic spine is convex (Fig. 17-8).
- Note the presence or absence of symmetry of the shoulders, scapula, iliac crests, and gluteal folds.

ABNORMALITIES A difference in shoulder elevation could indicate **scoliosis,** a lateral thoracic curvature. **Kyphosis,** an enhanced thoracic curve, is commonly seen in elderly patients. **Lordosis,** a pronounced lumbar curve, is common in obese or pregnant patients.

TECHNIQUE

STEP 5

Palpate the Spinal Processes

- Position yourself standing behind the patient.
- Palpate the spinal processes.

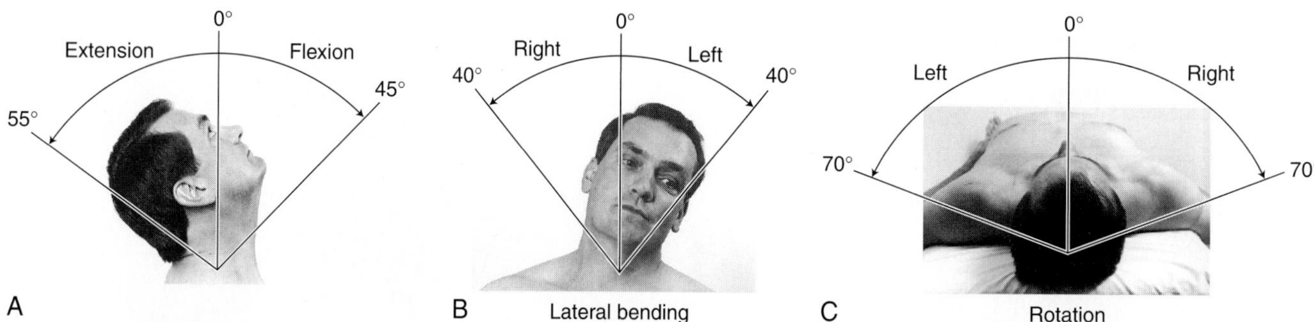

FIGURE 17-7 ■ Assessing range of motion of the cervical spine. **(A)** Proximal bending, **(B)** Lateral bending, **(C)** Rotation.

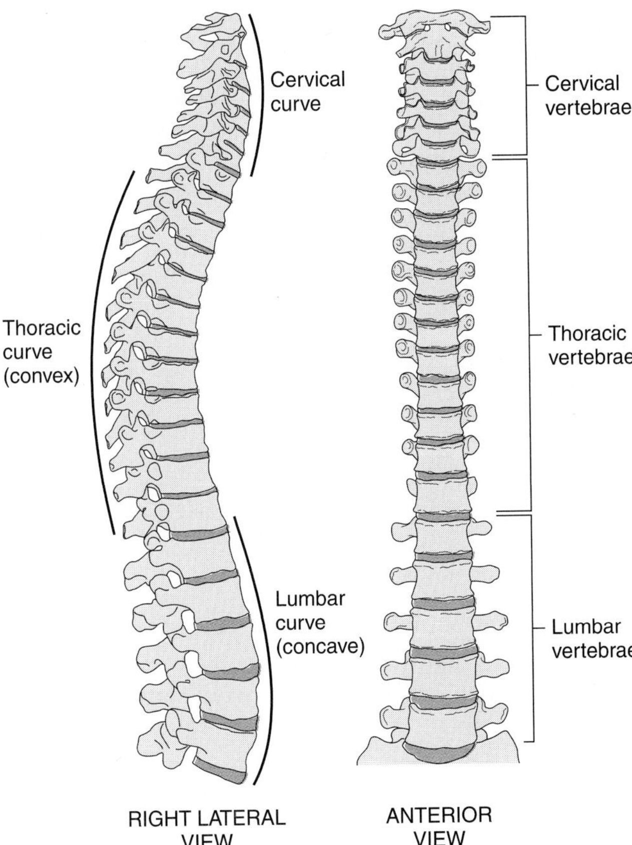

FIGURE 17-8 ■ The normal spine has a concave lumbar curve and a convex thoracic curve.

- Confirm that the spinal processes are straight and nontender.
- Palpate the paravertebral muscles.
- Confirm that the paravertebral muscles are firm and nontender.

ABNORMALITIES Spinal pain is a common complaint and can indicate a number of conditions. Pain associated with coughing may be associated with a herniated disc. Pain associated with numbness or tingling in the lower extremities can signal a nerve root disorder and warrants further neurologic testing. If patients complain of a burning or aching pain that radiates to the leg, foot, or toe, assess for **sciatica** (i.e., severe pain in the leg felt at the back of the thigh and running down along the sciatic nerve) via the straight leg-raising test, which will stretch the sciatic nerve.

TECHNIQUE

STEP 6

Perform the Straight Leg-Raising Test

- Position the patient lying supine.
- Direct patient to extend the affected leg, flexed at the hip.
- Ask the patient to plantar flex (i.e., point toes toward the floor) and dorsiflex (i.e., point toes toward his or her nose) the foot.
- Repeat with the opposite leg.

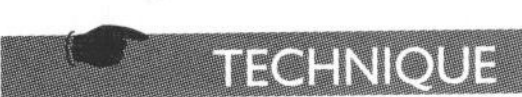

ABNORMALITIES Pain associated with this test indicates sciatica.

Shoulder

The shoulder joint is a ball-and-socket joint that is the articulation of the glenoid fossa of the scapula and the humerus. Bursae are situated around the shoulder joint to decrease friction between the moving parts. The muscles and tendons around the socket form the rotator cuff of the shoulder.

TECHNIQUE

STEP 1

Inspect the Shoulder

- Position the standing patient facing you.
- Inspect the shoulder for symmetry, deformity, and size.

ABNORMALITIES If the contour of the shoulders is asymmetric and appears "hollow," a shoulder dislocation may be present (Fig. 17-9).

STEP 2

Palpate the Shoulder

- Palpate the right shoulder for areas of pain, warmth, or tenderness.
- Repeat with the opposite shoulder.

ABNORMALITIES Tenderness and warmth of the bursae could indicate bursitis. Pain and tenderness of the bursa and the biceps or triceps tendons could indicate impingement syndrome or rotator cuff tendinitis. Continued

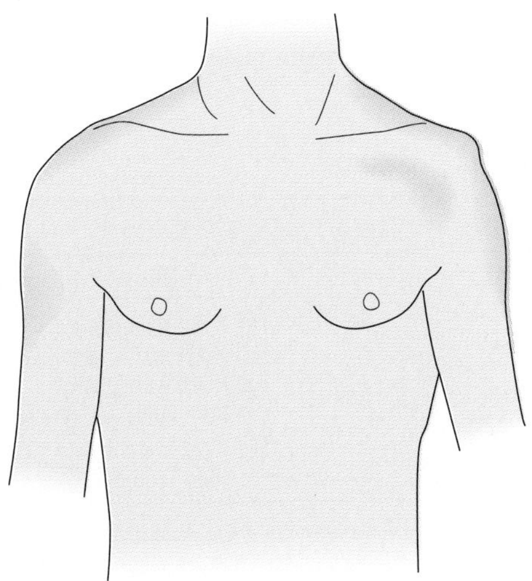

FIGURE 17-9 ■ Dislocation of the shoulder.

trauma of this condition could lead to a rotator cuff tear. Pain and extreme tenderness at the greater tuberosity of the humerus could indicate a rotator cuff tear; perform ROM examination to obtain further diagnostic information.

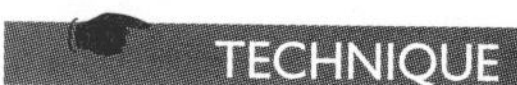

TECHNIQUE

STEP 3

Assess the ROM of the Shoulder

- Position the standing patient facing you.
- Cup a hand over the patient's shoulder to assess for any crepitus.
- Ask the patient to place the arms at sides with the elbows extended (Fig. 17-10*A*).
- Instruct the patient to move the arms forward, up, and back.
- Expect forward flexion of 180° and hyperextension of approximately 50°.
- Instruct the patient to rotate the arms internally and place the back of the hands toward the scapulae (Fig. 17-10*B*.)
- Expect internal (medial) rotation of 90°.
- Instruct the patient to raise both arms and touch the palms above the head, with arms at the sides and elbows extended (Fig. 17-10*C*).
- Expect abduction of 180° and adduction of 50°.
- Ask patient to touch both hands behind the head, with the elbows flexed and rotated posteriorly (Fig. 17-10*D*).
- Expect external (lateral) rotation of 90°.

STEP 4

Assess Muscle Strength of Shoulder

- The examiner should apply his or her hands, with light pressure, to the patient's shoulder.
- Instruct the patient to flex the shoulders forward and up, against the resistance of the examiner.
- Grade the muscle strength (Table 17-5).

ABNORMALITIES Limited ROM could indicate several things. Limited ROM, pain, and muscle spasms on abduction could indicate rotator cuff lesions. If the arm drops suddenly during the drop-arm test (described later), suspect a rotator cuff tear. Crepitus noted on movement may indicate OA. Difficulty in shrugging the shoulder against resistance may indicate cranial nerve XII dysfunction.

TECHNIQUE

STEP 5

Assess the Rotator Cuff

- Instruct the patient to abduct and slowly lower the arm.
- Confirm that the arm abducts and lowers smoothly.

ABNORMALITIES Patients with rotator cuff disorders may have normal forward flexion. If the arm drops suddenly during the drop-arm test, suspect a rotator cuff tear.

Elbow

The elbow joint is a hinge joint that is the articulation of the humerus, radius, and ulna. Several bursae are located around the joint to reduce friction.

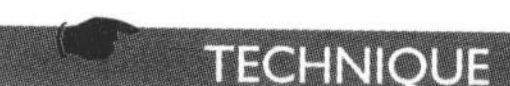

TECHNIQUE

STEP 1

Inspect the Size and Contour of the Elbow

- Position the patient sitting on the examination table.
- Instruct the patient to flex the elbow.
- Inspect the size and contour of the elbow.
- Instruct the patient to extend the elbow.
- Again inspect the size and contour of the elbow.
- Note any redness, asymmetry, and masses.

TABLE 17-5 ➤ GRADING MUSCLE STRENGTH

GRADE	LEVEL OF MUSCLE FUNCTION	% NORMAL	ASSESSMENT
5	Full ROM against gravity, full resistance	100	Normal
4	Full ROM against gravity, some resistance	75	Good
3	Full ROM with gravity	50	Fair
2	Full ROM with gravity eliminated (passive movement)	25	Poor
1	Slight contraction	10	Trace
0	No contraction	0	Zero

ROM, Range of motion.
Adapted from Musculoskeletal system. In: Mosby's Guide to Physical Examination. Seidel HM, Ball JW, Dains JE, et al (eds.), 4th ed. St. Louis: Mosby, 1999:707.

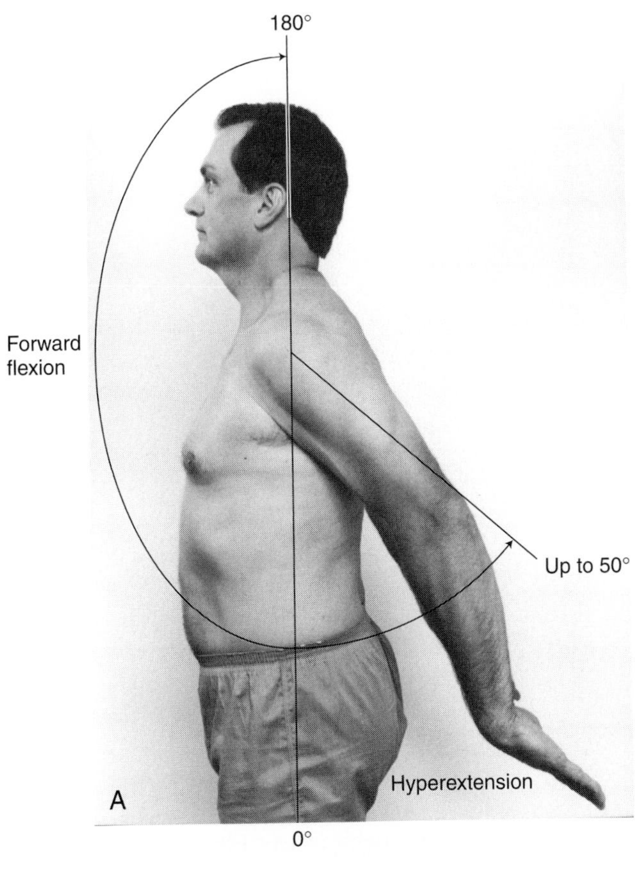

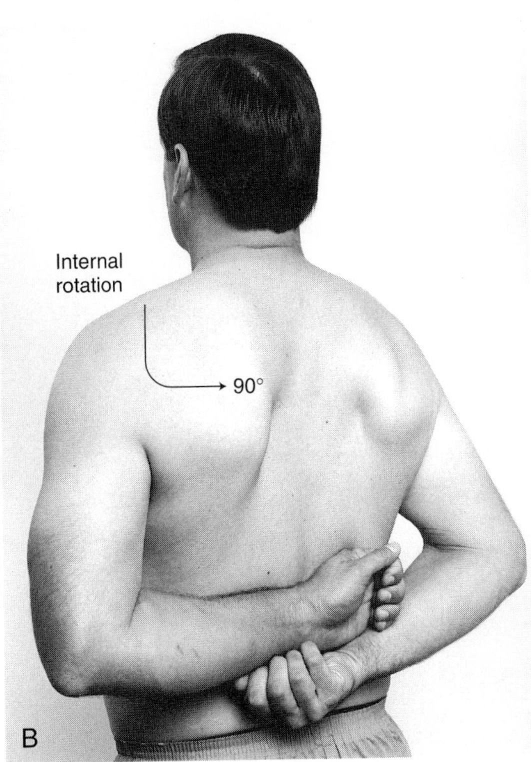

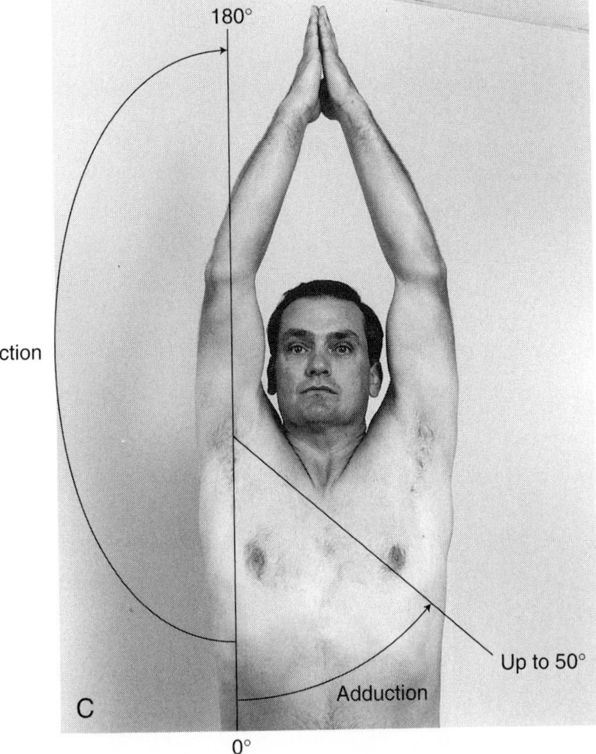

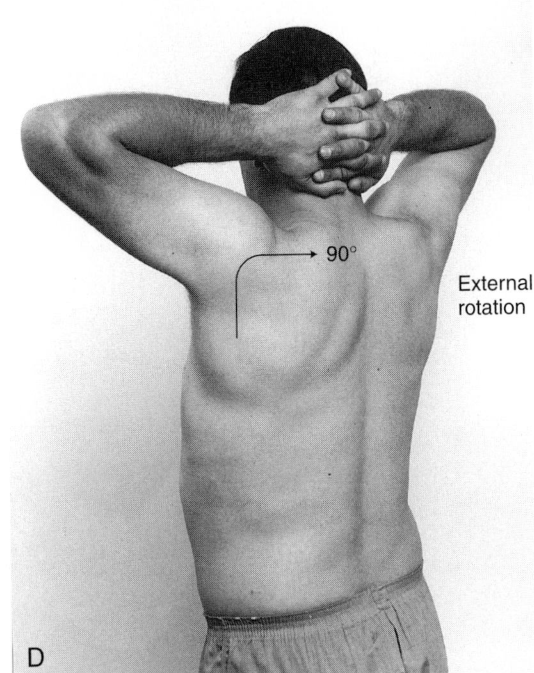

FIGURE 17-10 ■ Range of motion of the shoulders.

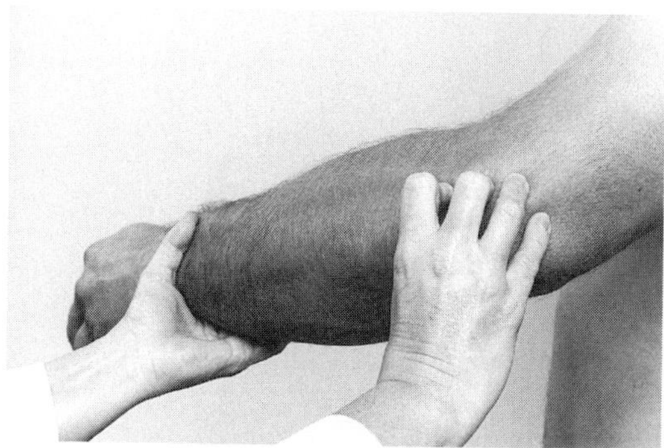

FIGURE 17-11 ■ Palpation of the elbow.

STEP 2

Palpate for Deformity, Redness, Warmth, or Swelling

- Position the examiner's hand on the patient's forearm for support.
- Palpate the extensor surface of the elbow with the thumb and forefingers of the other hand (Fig. 17-11).
- Identify any areas of deformity, redness, warmth, or swelling.

ABNORMALITIES Swelling and erythema can signify bursitis. Swelling related to effusion or synovial thickening could be associated with gouty arthritis. Subcutaneous nodules along the extensor surface of the ulna or the bursa may indicate RA. Inflammation and local tenderness at the tendons, head of the radius, or the epicondyles can also be associated with lateral epicondylitis or "tennis elbow."

TECHNIQUE

STEP 3

Assess the ROM of the Elbow

Assessment of the elbow's ROM is illustrated in Figure 17-12*A*.

- Position the patient seated on the examination table.
- Instruct the patient to bend and straighten the elbow.
- Expect flexion of 160° and full extension of 180°.
- Instruct the patient to flex the elbow to a right angle and to rotate the hand from palm down to palm up (Fig. 17-12*B*).
- Expect both pronation (palm faces downward) and supination (palm faces upward) of 90° each.

ABNORMALITIES Limited ROM without other signs of inflammation could be associated with OA or acute strain or trauma to the joint.

TECHNIQUE

STEP 4

Assess Muscle Strength of the Elbow

- Position the patient seated on the examination table.
- Stabilize the patient's arm with one hand under the elbow and one hand holding onto the wrist (proximal).

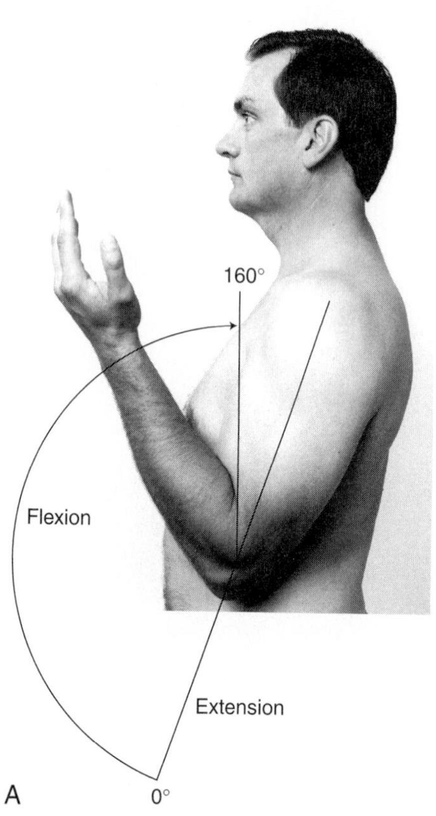

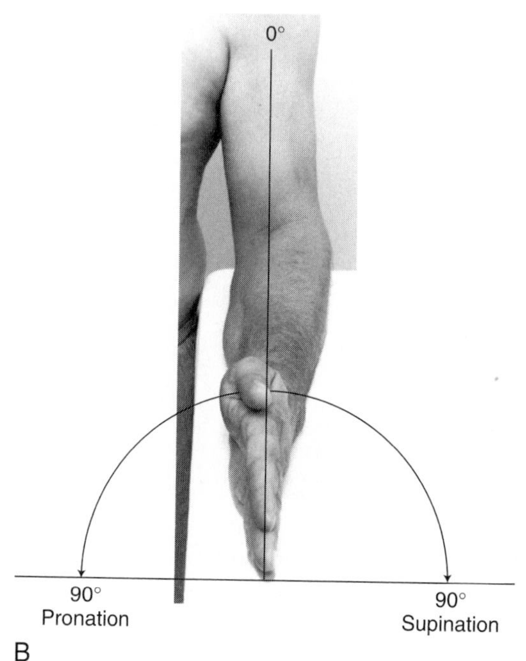

FIGURE 17-12 ■ Range of motion of the elbow.

- Instruct the patient to flex the elbow against your resistance.
- Instruct the patient to extend the elbow against your resistance.
- Grade muscle strength (Table 17-5).

Wrist and Hand

The wrist is the articulation of the radius and proximal row of the carpal bones of the hand. The carpal ligament connects the carpal bones, and the median nerve and all flexors of the wrist pass under this ligament through the carpal tunnel. Entrapment of the median nerve is known as **carpal tunnel syndrome** (CTS).

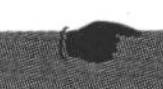 TECHNIQUE

STEP 1

Inspect the Wrist and Hand

- Position the patient seated on the examination table.
- Inspect on the dorsal and palmar sides of the hands for position, contour, and shape.
- Confirm the fingers lie straight in the same axis as the forearm.

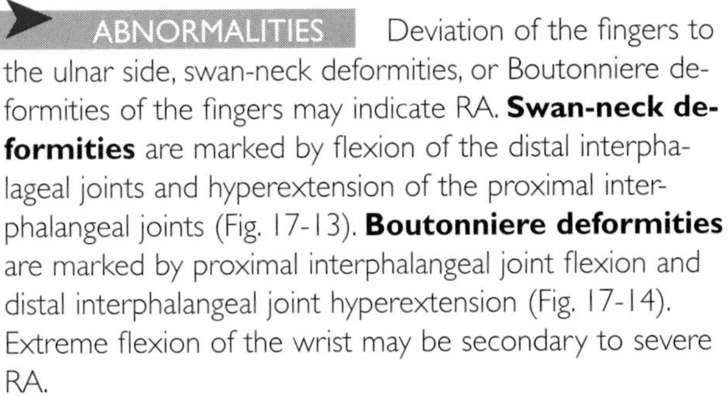

ABNORMALITIES Deviation of the fingers to the ulnar side, swan-neck deformities, or Boutonniere deformities of the fingers may indicate RA. **Swan-neck deformities** are marked by flexion of the distal interphalageal joints and hyperextension of the proximal interphalangeal joints (Fig. 17-13). **Boutonniere deformities** are marked by proximal interphalangeal joint flexion and distal interphalangeal joint hyperextension (Fig. 17-14). Extreme flexion of the wrist may be secondary to severe RA.

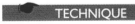

 TECHNIQUE

STEP 2

Palpate the Wrist and Hand

Palpation of the wrist is illustrated in Figure 17-15.

- Using the thumb and index fingers, palpate the patient's wrist.
- Identify any swelling, tenderness, bogginess, or deformities.
- Palpate the proximal and distal interphalangeal joints using the thumb and index fingers.
- Note any swelling, redness, or tenderness.

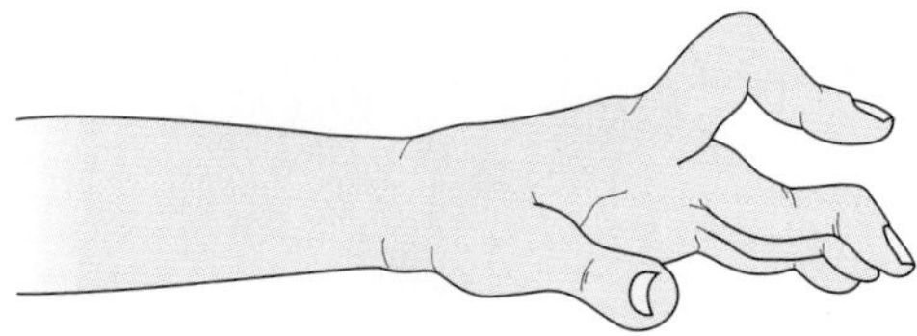

FIGURE 17-13 ■ Swan-neck deformity of the fingers.

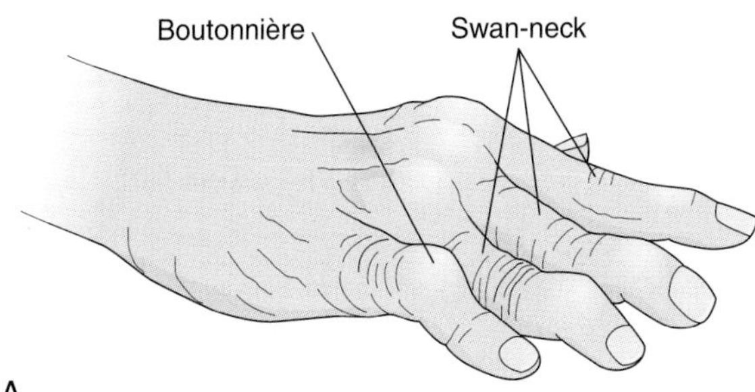

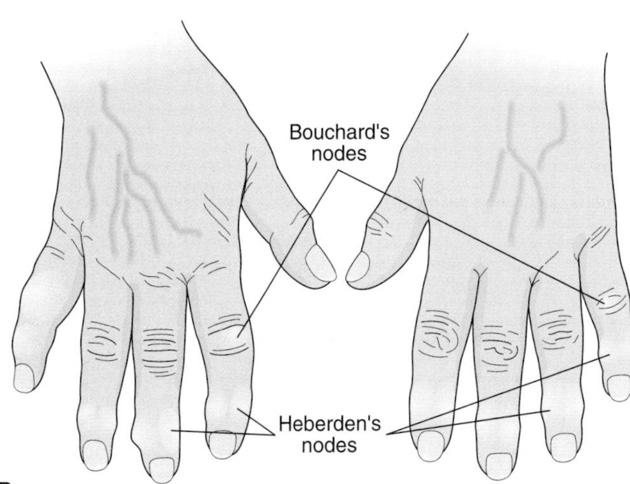

FIGURE 17-14 ■ Deformities of the fingers.

ABNORMALITIES Hard, nontender nodules on the distal interphalangeal joints are referred to as **Heberden's or Bouchard's nodules** and are frequently associated with OA. Generalized swelling and tenderness of the joints may be associated with RA.

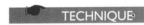

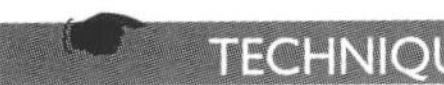

STEP 3

Assess the ROM of the Wrist and Hand

- Ask the patient to bend the fingers forward at the metacarpophalangeal joint (Fig. 17-16A).
- Expect flexion of 90°.

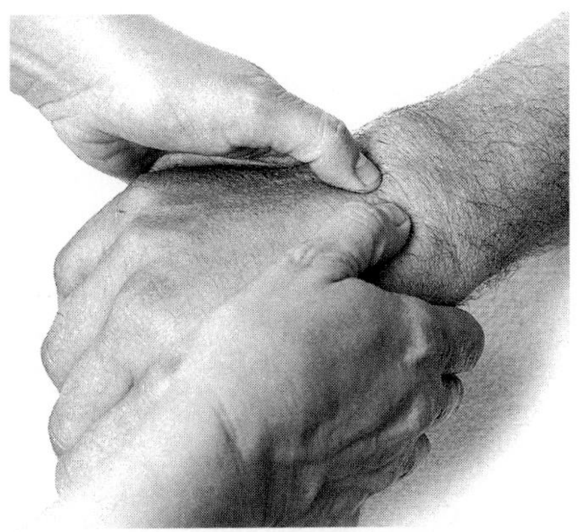

FIGURE 17-15 ■ Palpation of the wrist.

FIGURE 17-16 ■ Range of motion of the wrist and fingers.

- Instruct the patient to touch the thumb to each fingertip and make a fist (Fig. 17-16*B*.)
- Instruct the patient to spread the fingers apart and then touch them together (Fig. 17-16*C* and *D*).
- Confirm that all movements can be done without pain.
- Ask the patient to bend the hand up and down at the wrist (Fig. 17-16*E*).
- Expect flexion of 90° and hyperextension of approximately 70°.

STEP 4

Assess Muscle Strength of the Wrist and Hand

- Evaluate hand strength by having the patient grip two of the examiner's fingers.
- The patient should flex the thumb and close the fingers over it, then attempt to move the hand into ulnar deviation.
- Grade muscle strength (Table 17-5).

ABNORMALITIES Excruciating pain signifies tenosynovitis of the thumb abductors and extensors.

Carpal Tunnel Syndrome

Carpal tunnel syndrome is associated with pain, numbness, and paresthesia in the hands. Two specific tests for CTS may be of benefit in evaluating patients with these symptoms.

TECHNIQUE

STEP 1

Phalen's Test

- Instruct patient to maintain palmar flexion for 1 minute (Fig. 17-17).

ABNORMALITIES If numbness and paresthesia are experienced over the palmar surface of the hand and

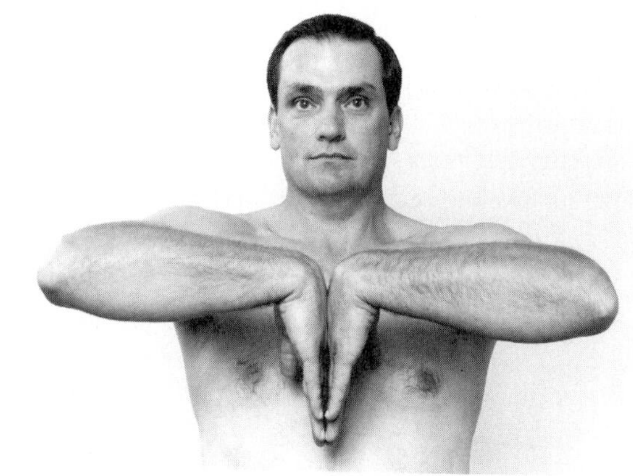

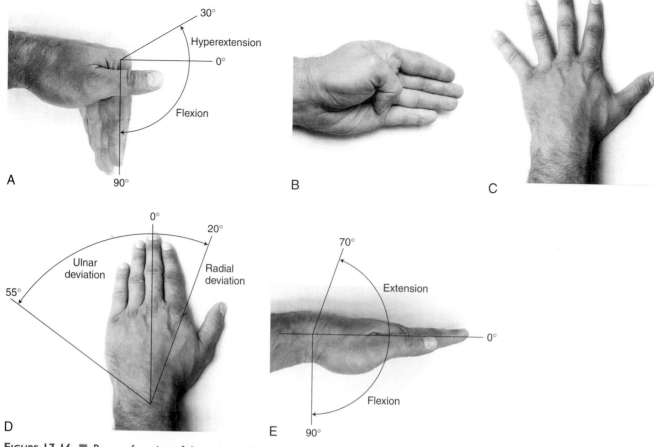

FIGURE 17-17 ■ Phalen's test.

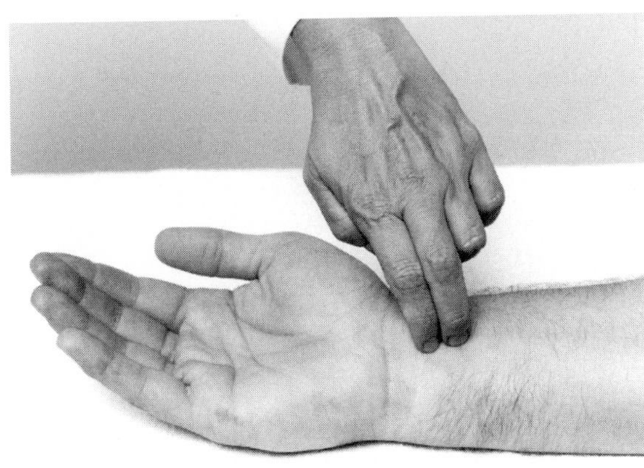

Figure 17-18 ■ Tinel's sign.

the first three fingers, the sign is positive for CTS. The symptoms should resolve with the return of the hand to the resting position.

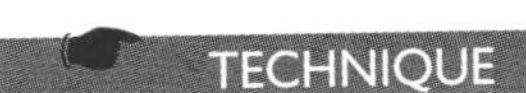

STEP 2

Tinel's Sign

Lightly tap over the median nerve of the patient (Fig. 17-18).

ABNORMALITIES If tingling or prickling occurs, the sign is positive for CTS. Limited ROM in the hand and wrist can be associated with OA or RA. Detection of crepitus also indicates OA. Sprains or strains secondary to acute trauma may limit the ROM of the wrist.

Hip

The hip is a ball-and-socket joint that is the articulation of the femur and the acetabulum. The acetabulum is a depression on the lateral surface of the hip bone that provides the socket into which the head of the femur fits. Three bursae are present to reduce friction.

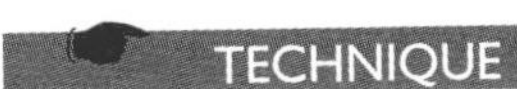

STEP 1

Inspection of the Gait

Inspection of the gait was described earlier in the exam process. This assists in assessing function of the hip. A smooth, even gait reflects appropriate hip motion.

STEP 2

Palpate the Hip Joints

- Ask the patient to assume a supine position.
- Palpate the hip joints.
- Confirm that the joints feel stable and symmetric.
- Note any tenderness or crepitus.

ABNORMALITIES Pain, tenderness, or inflammation could indicate bursitis of the hip joint. Crepitus of the joint may be associated with OA.

TECHNIQUE

STEP 3

Evaluation of Leg Length

- Have patient remain in the supine position.
- Measure the leg length from the anterior superior iliac spine to the tip of the medial malleolus (the protuberance at the ankle joint that is at the lower end of the tibia).
- Repeat for other side of the body, and compare the results.

ABNORMALITIES Differences in leg lengths can be associated with hip joint disorders.

TECHNIQUE

STEP 4

Assess the ROM of the Hip Joint

- Instruct the patient to remain in the supine position.
- Instruct the patient to raise each leg, with the knee extended (Fig. 17-19*A*).
- Expect hip flexion of 90°.
- Repeat with the opposite leg.
- With the patient on his or her back, flex the knee and hip to 90° (Fig. 17-19*B*). Stabilize by placing one hand on the thigh and one hand on the ankle.
- Rotate the patient's foot inward and outward.

ABNORMALITIES Restriction of rotation is a reliable sign of degenerative hip disease.

- With knees straight, have patients swing the leg laterally and medially (Fig. 17-19*C*).
- Expect abduction of approximately 45° and adduction of approximately 30°.

ABNORMALITIES Limitation of hip abduction is the most common functional disability of the hip joint.

TECHNIQUE

STEP 5

Assess for any Hip Deformity

- Instruct the patient to bend each knee to the chest while keeping the other leg straight (Fig. 17-19*D*).
- Confirm that the opposite thigh remains on the table.
- Expect hip flexion of 120°.

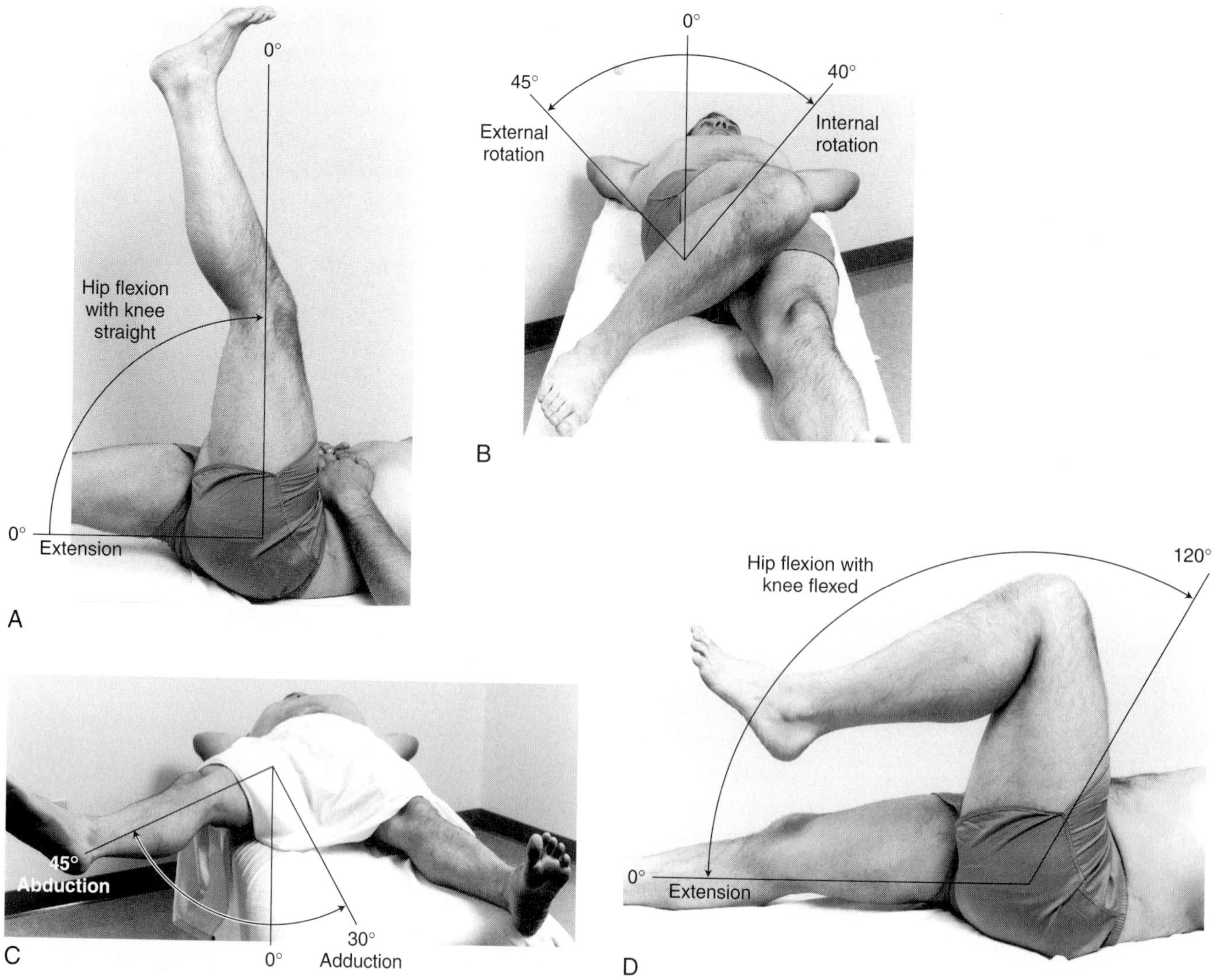

FIGURE 17-19 ■ Range of motion of the hip.

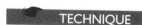

ABNORMALITIES If the opposite thigh is flexed, it represents a flexion deformity in that hip.

Knee

The knee, the largest joint in the body, is a hinge joint that is the articulation of the femur and the tibia. Muscles and ligaments around the joint provide stability, and bursae are present to decrease friction.

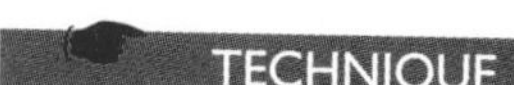

STEP 1

Inspect the Knee Joint

- Position the standing patient facing you.
- Inspect the knee for any deformity, swelling, or discoloration.

STEP 2

Palpate the Knee Joint

- Position the patient lying supine.
- Starting approximately 10 cm above the patella, palpate with the left thumb and fingers in a grasping fashion, proceeding down to the knee (Fig. 17-20).
- Confirm that the joint margins feel smooth, and that the muscles and surrounding tissue are firm without thickening, warmth, or tenderness.

ABNORMALITIES If swelling is present, the cause must be determined and differentiated between soft-tissue swelling and increased fluid in the joint. The **bulge sign** confirms the presence of fluid in the suprapatellar pouch.

- Firmly stroke up the medial aspect of the knee three times. This will displace any accumulated fluid.

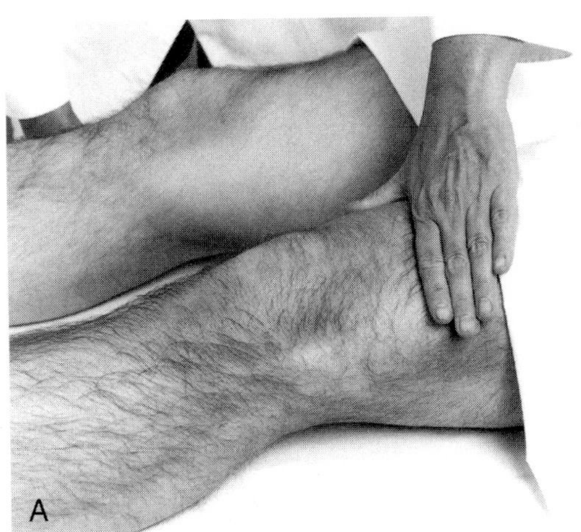

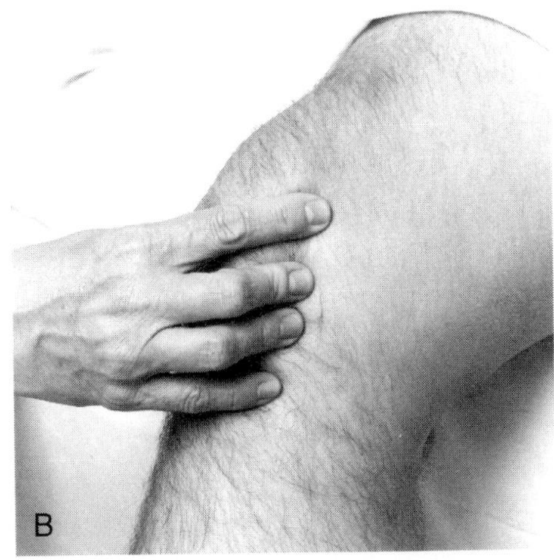

FIGURE 17-20 ■ Palpation of the knee joint.

- Tap the lateral aspect of the knee, and watch the medial side in the hollow for a bulge from a fluid wave.

ABNORMALITIES A positive bulge sign can detect small amounts (10 mL) of fluid on the joint. **Ballottement,** a palpatory technique to examine for excess fluid on the patella, may be useful when larger amounts of fluid are present on the knee.

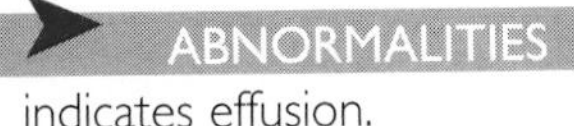

TECHNIQUE

STEP 2 (Continued)

- Compress the suprapatellar pouch with the left hand while pushing the patella sharply against the femur with the right hand. (If the patella is snug against the femur, no fluid is present.)
- Tap on the patella.
- Listen for an auditory tap as the patella bumps the femur.

ABNORMALITIES Presence of this auditory tap indicates effusion.

TECHNIQUE

STEP 2 (Continued)

- Hold a hand on the patella as the knee is flexed and extended.
- Identify any signs of crepitus.

ABNORMALITIES Irregular joint margins are characteristic of OA. Pain, tenderness, and swelling can be associated with OA, RA, or acute trauma. Shiny skin, which is characteristic of psoriasis, should be noted, because psoriatic arthritis is possible. Fluid can result from chronic inflammatory conditions, infectious processes, or trauma. Excessive amounts of fluid should be aspirated by the physician and sent to a laboratory for evaluation.

TECHNIQUE

STEP 3

Assess the ROM of the Knee

- Position the patient to stand on one leg (have the patient hold onto a countertop or the examination table for balance).
- Instruct the patient to bend and extend each knee (Fig. 17-21).
- Expect flexion of 130° to 150° and extension to a straight line (0°).

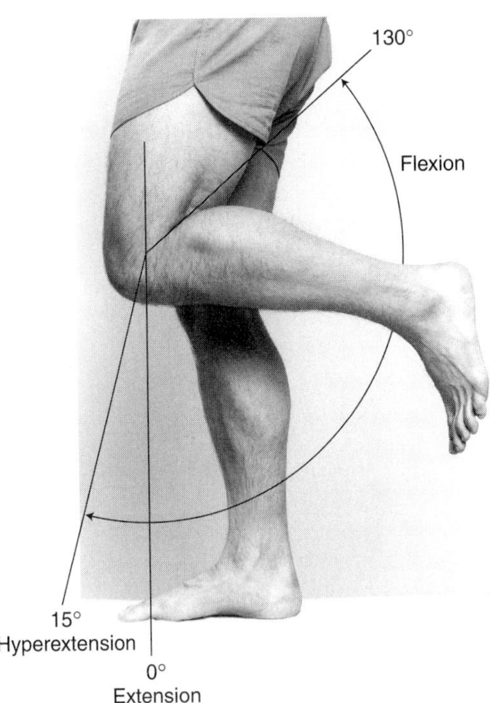

FIGURE 17-21 ■ Range of motion of the knee.

STEP 4

Assess Muscle Strength of the Knee

- Instruct the patient to maintain knee flexion (bend the knee).
- The examiner opposes by trying to pull the patient's leg forward.
- Grade muscle strength (Table 17-5).

ABNORMALITIES Patients with repeated history of trauma, particularly those who have experienced a knee "giving out," should be checked for a torn meniscus. The **McMurray's test** will assess patency of the meniscus. When a torn meniscus is suspected, use caution when rotating the leg. This rotation can be extremely painful for the patient and cause additional damage if done incorrectly.

TECHNIQUE

STEP 5

Assess the Meniscus

- Instruct the patient to lie supine.
- Hold the patient's heel, and flex the patient's knee and hip (Fig. 17-22).
- Place the other hand on the patient's knee, with fingers on the medial side.
- Initially rotate the leg in and out to loosen joint; then externally rotate the leg and place inward stress on the knee.
- Slowly extend the knee (the leg should extend without pain).

ABNORMALITIES Limited ROM in the knee joint can be caused by joint inflammation, degeneration, or acute injury. Significant crepitus indicates OA; however, some crepitus in an otherwise asymptomatic knee is normal. A "click" or "pop" elicited from a McMurray's test is positive for a torn meniscus. Sudden locking of the knee, characterized as "buckling" or "giving out," occurs with ligament injury.

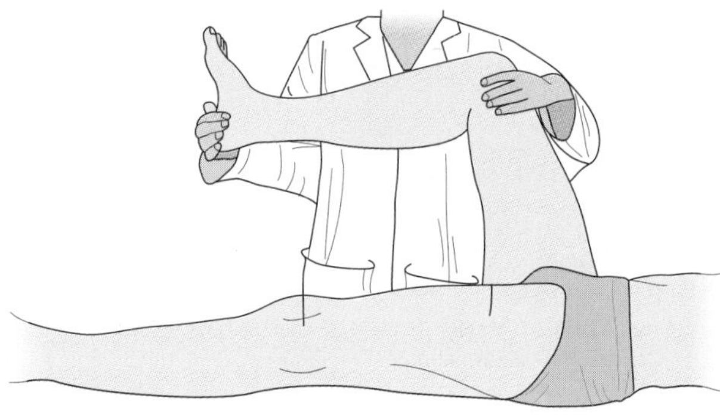

Figure 17-22 ■ McMurray's test.

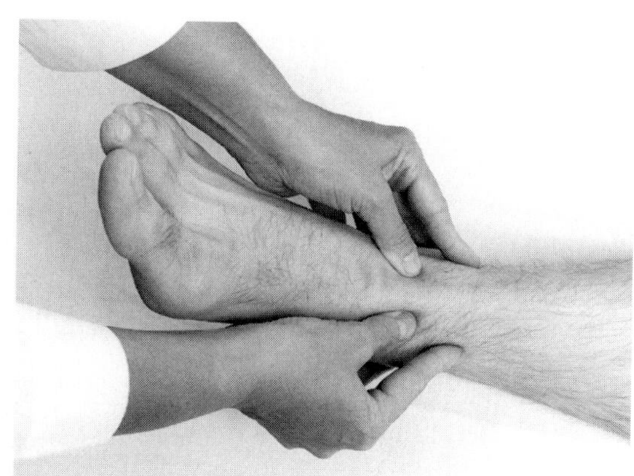

Figure 17-23 ■ Palpation of the ankle.

Ankle and Foot

The ankle (tibiotalar) joint is a hinge joint that is the articulation of the tibia, fibula, and talus. It is protected by ligaments on the medial and lateral surfaces. Ankle and foot symptoms typically have a local cause.

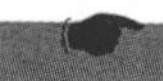

TECHNIQUE

STEP 1

Inspect the Ankle and Foot

- Position the standing patient facing you.
- Inspect the ankle and foot for any swelling, deformities, calluses, or lesions.
- Confirm that the toes point straight and lie flat.
- Inspect the height of the arches.

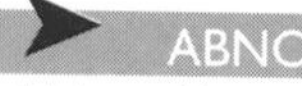

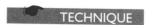

ABNORMALITIES A cavus foot (i.e., abnormally high arch) or flat foot may cause pain.

TECHNIQUE

STEP 2

Palpate the Joint Spaces of the Ankle

- Position the patient seated on the examination table.
- Palpate the joint spaces of the ankle for tenderness, swelling, and deformity (Fig. 17-23).
- Confirm that the joint spaces feel smooth and depressed.
- Palpate the metatarsophalangeal and interphalangeal joints by grasping the metatarsophalangeal joints between the thumb and index fingers and then compressing the forefoot.
- Confirm that this does not cause pain.

ABNORMALITIES Tenderness and swelling within the ankle joint are often associated with local trauma. Crepitus may be associated with degeneration of the joints. Extreme tenderness of the metatarsophalangeal joints may be associated with gout. Pain on attempting to compress the forefoot may be an early sign of RA.

TECHNIQUE

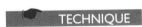

STEP 3

Assess the ROM of the Ankle and Foot

- Ask the patient to dorsiflex and plantar flex and to evert and invert the ankle and foot (Fig. 17-24*A* and *B*).

ABNORMALITIES Pain or limited motion may signify trauma, an arthritic condition, or other localized condition (e.g., gout). It can also signify strain on the ligaments of the foot, ankle, or both.

TECHNIQUE

STEP 4

Assess Muscle Strength of Ankle and Foot

- Instruct the patient to maintain dorsiflexion and plantar flexion against your resistance.
- Grade muscle strength (Table 17-5).

Laboratory and Diagnostic Tests

Unlike that for other body systems, evaluation of the musculoskeletal system focuses more on the physical examination and less on laboratory or diagnostic tests. In certain diseases of the musculoskeletal system, however, laboratory or diagnostic results can offer beneficial information. Some of the laboratory tests that are helpful in musculoskeletal problems include:

- A complete blood count (CBC) may provide useful information for establishing the diagnosis of certain musculoskeletal disorders. High white-blood-cell (WBC) counts are associated with infectious processes. Osteomyelitis and infectious arthritis may present with increased WBC counts. Patients with RA often experience a mild to moderate normocytic, normochromic anemia; RA arthritis is also associated with thrombocytosis. Platelet counts often rise and fall in direct correlation to disease activity.
- The erythrocyte sedimentation rate (ESR) is a nonspecific indicator of inflammation. It is elevated in patients with acute and chronic inflammatory processes, infections, and rheumatic diseases, among other conditions. Although patients with localized or systemic inflammatory disorders may have elevated ESR levels, the lack of specificity of this test results in it providing more assistance in confirming a diagnosis than in establishing one.
- Serum rheumatoid factor is an antibody-specific laboratory test that is positive in approximately two-thirds of patients with RA. Like the ESR, this test also lacks specificity, because patients may have a diagnosis of RA without a positive test for rheumatoid factor. The presence of rheumatoid factor should be used as a tool to aid in establishing a diagnosis.
- Synovial fluid from a joint should be aspirated and evaluated in patients with an effusion of unknown cause. Normal synovial fluid is transparent. Inflammatory fluid is turbid because of the large numbers of leukocytes present. WBC counts of 5000 to 50,000 cells/mm^3 are not uncommon in inflamed joints. Septic joints may have even higher numbers of leukocytes (>75,000 cells/mm^3). The synovial fluid of septic joints are often culture positive.
- Screening for bone mineral density (BMD) is the most accurate predictor of lifetime fracture risk. However, the National Osteoporosis Foundation recommends

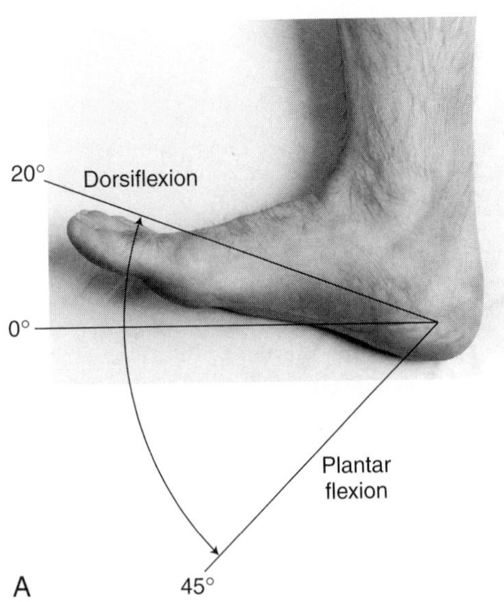

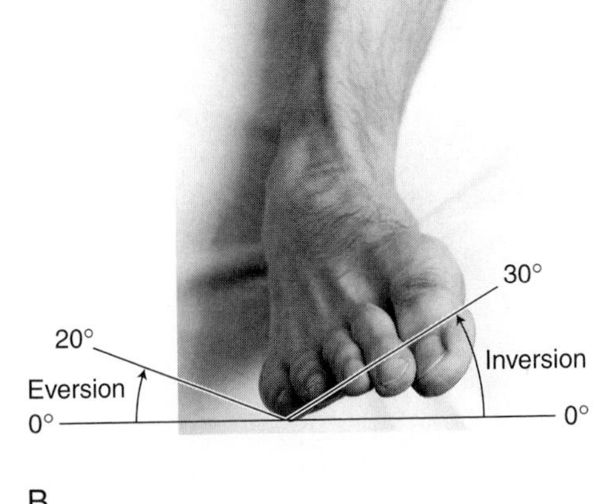

FIGURE 17-24 ■ Range of motion of the ankle and foot.

BMD screening only when osteoporosis is suspected. One of the most common radiographic scanning techniques used for such screening is the dual-energy x-ray absorptiometry.

Special Considerations

Pediatric Patients

Pediatric patients require that additional questions be asked of the patient or parent.

? INTERVIEW Was there any trauma to the infant during labor and delivery? Has the baby reached motor-skill milestones at appropriate ages (e.g., sitting up alone, rolling over, crawling, and walking)?

ABNORMALITIES Traumatic delivery increases the risk of fractures, especially of the clavicle and humerus.

? INTERVIEW What activities/sports does your child like to play? Does the child use protective safety equipment?

ABNORMALITIES Sports activities increase the child's risk of musculoskeletal injury. Use of safety equipment decreases the risk of injury.

Musculoskeletal anomalies may result from genetic or fetal insults. Because of various pressures placed on the fetus in utero, manifestations may be seen in infants. Complete assessment of the infant is an extensive undertaking, but the following practical points will assist the pharmacist in performing a general musculoskeletal examination:

- Inspect all extremities for symmetry in flexion, position, and shape.
- Movements should be symmetrical.
- Check the hips routinely for congenital dislocation during the first year of life.
- An inspection of the leg lengths of the infant can be of assistance. Place the infant's feet flat on the table, and flex the knees up. One knee significantly lower than the other may signify a dislocated hip.

Geriatric Patients

Because the aging process causes musculoskeletal changes, elderly patients also require that additional questions be asked of the patient or caregiver to assess the risk of injury.

? INTERVIEW Have you noticed any changes in your muscle strength recently? Have you had any problems with weakness lately? Have you had any problems with falls or stumbling? If so, do you use mobility aids such as a cane or a walker to help you get around?

ABNORMALITIES Elderly patients are at increased risk of falls, especially if they have musculoskeletal problems (e.g., OA). Use of mobility aids decreases this risk.

Physical assessment of an elderly patient follows that of a normal adult, although the patient's response may be slowed. Decreased joint and muscle agility may cause difficulties with motor function. Fine and gross motor function associated with activities of daily living may be affected because of this decrease in agility. Muscle atrophy may be apparent, leading to decreased total muscle mass. This can result from disuse, such as seen in patients with arthritis, or from a loss of nervous innervation, such as seen in patients with diabetic neuropathy. During inspection, a broad base with feet widely spaced may be apparent. In addition, arms may be held away from the body to maintain balance.

Pregnant Patients

Assessment of the pregnant patient should be similar to that of a typical adult, with caution being used to avoid stress. Postural changes occur as pregnancy progresses because of the shifting forward of the center of gravity, including lordosis, anterior cervical flexion, kyphosis, and slumped shoulders. Joints experience increased mobility and instability, contributing to the "waddling" gait. Women may experience CTS secondary to fluid retention. Symptoms should resolve after delivery.

APPLICATION TO PATIENT SYMPTOMS

The pharmacist's accessibility provides a unique advantage to assess patient symptoms, identify potential causes, evaluate current disease status, and guide patients toward appropriate treatment. Common symptoms of musculoskeletal disorders include pain, swelling, and stiffness or limitation of movement.

Musculoskeletal Pain

Pain is one of the most common—and least specific—symptoms of the musculoskeletal system. The extent of pain can be localized to a single joint or the result of a systemic disease causing generalized discomfort. It may be associated with a traumatic event, a systemic illness, or other musculoskeletal disorders. Because musculoskeletal pain is highly nonspecific, the pharmacist must be able to assess and identify the actual cause.

Pain itself is a very subjective symptom. In addition to having the patient rate his or her pain, the pharmacist must also observe for nonverbal signs to judge the severity of pain. Nonverbal signs such as affected gait, wincing, and a haggard appearance also form a basis for evaluating the patient, because many patients will not admit fully to having intolerance to pain.

CASE STUDY

GJ is a 52-year-old man who comes into the pharmacy wanting an over-the-counter pain reliever and asks the pharmacist what she recommends.

ASSESSMENT OF THE PATIENT

Subjective Information

52-year-old male wanting an over-the-counter (OTC) pain reliever

Tell me about the pain that you are having. Where exactly is the pain? In my right big toe.

When did it start? I just noticed it yesterday for the first time.

How would you characterize the pain? It is terrible, almost like my big toe is on fire. I can barely wear my shoe.

With 10 being the worst pain you have ever experienced, rate your pain on a scale of 1 to 10. Oh, it's at least an eight or a nine.

Do you have pain anywhere else? No, just my big toe.

What makes the pain better and worse? Well, wearing my shoe and walking on it seems to make it worse, and I haven't tried anything for it yet—that's why I'm here.

Any other symptoms? No.

Did you injure your toe recently? No, not that I can recall. I played some golf with my buddies the night before last, but don't recall hurting it.

Have you been taking any over the counter medications or any new medications? No, I've just been taking my water pill and my sugar pill like I always do. Oh, and my blood pressure pill, too.

So, you have high blood pressure and diabetes? Yes.

What other medical problems do you have? None.

Have you been eating or drinking any differently than usual? Not really. The other night though, I probably had five of six beers after the golf game. And a great dinner, the best steak I've had in a long time. I'm still full!

Objective Information

Computerized medication profile:

- Hydrochlorothiazide: 50 mg every day.
- Glucotrol XL (glipizide): 10 mg PO BID.
- Vasotec (enalapril): 20 mg PO every day.
- Aspirin: 325 mg PO every day.

Heart rate: 72 bpm
Blood pressure: 130/78 mm Hg
Blood sugar (random): 114 mg/dL
Monoarticular swelling and erythema of the right great metatarsophalangeal (MTP) joint.

DISCUSSION

This case centers around GJ's recent onset of pain in his right big toe. The pharmacist must determine if this pain is secondary to injury, a degeneration within the joint, or an inflammatory disorder. The patient has a history of diabetes and hypertension, for which he is taking hydrochlorothiazide, Glucotrol XL, and Vasotec. In addition, he takes an aspirin daily for prevention of coronary heart disease. GJ describes the pain as being sudden in onset, with a fire/burning sensation. The pain is localized to his great toe and cannot be associated with any recent injury. He has no other symptoms. Wearing his shoe has made the pain worse, and he hasn't tried anything yet to help with the pain. He does state that he played golf the night before last, but he does not recall any trauma to his foot. He also admits to having a large amount of beer and a large meal after golfing. His heart rate, blood pressure, and blood glucose are all normal, however. Physical examination of the patient's foot revealed a tender, swollen, erythematous great right MTP joint.

After evaluating all the subjective and objective information, the pharmacist suspects that GJ is suffering from an acute gout attack. The steps involved in the assessment of this patient are illustrated in the accompanying decision tree (Fig. 17-25). The patient has a history of diabetes and hypertension and is on a thiazide diuretic, an angiotensin-converting enzyme inhibitor, an oral sulfonylurea, and a daily aspirin. Diuretics and high-dose salicylates have been implicated in the induction of hyperuricemia. Although the patient was on a lower dose of aspirin, an additive effect may be seen. In addition, GJ has a history of hypertension and diabetes, which can increase his risk of renal dysfunction. If GJ does have renal dysfunction, it can cause a decrease in uric acid excretion. Overeating, especially with a high protein intake, and alcohol use may precipitate acute episodes of gout; GJ admits to these activities 2 days previously.

Because GJ is probably suffering from an acute gout attack, the pharmacist recommends that he make an appointment with his physician. The pharmacist educates GJ that his physician will likely prescribe a short-term NSAID to treat this acute attack. Any NSAID will work; however, indomethacin is often used with excellent results, starting with a high dose and then rapidly tapering off during the course of a week. Sulindac, another NSAID, is thought to be somewhat "renal sparing." If the patient should need frequent abortive therapy, this may be a reasonable option, particularly if renal function declines.

GJ later returns with a prescription for indomethacin, 75 mg (immediate release) for one dose followed by 50 mg every 6 hours for 48 hours and then 50 mg every 8 hours for 24 to 72 hours. The patient is counseled to take the medication with food and to consult the pharmacist if any side effects occur. The patient is also counseled to avoid overeating

Continued

CASE STUDY—continued

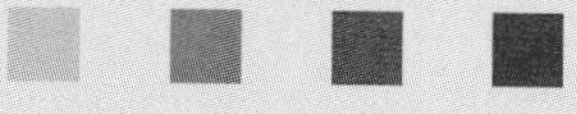

and alcohol, because these may precipitate another attack. Depending on patient response and attack frequency, prophylactic therapy may be warranted in the future. The pharmacist plans a follow-up call within the next 2 days to assess treatment of the acute attack and any potential adverse effects that may have occurred.

PHARMACEUTICAL CARE PLAN

Patient Name: GJ

Date: 08/31/02

Medical Problems:

- Type 2 diabetes
- Hypertension
- Gout

Current Medications:

- Hydrochlorothiazide, 50 mg every day
- Glucotrol XL (glipizide), 10 mg PO BID
- Vasotec (enalapril), 20 mg PO every day
- Aspirin, 325 mg PO every day

S: 52-year-old man complaining of severe, burning pain of the right great toe, which started yesterday. Rates pain an 8 or a 9 on 1–10 scale. No other pain or symptoms. No recent trauma.

O: Monoarticular swelling and erythema of the right great MTP joint.

Heart rate: 72 bpm

Blood pressure: 130/78 mm Hg

Blood sugar (random): 114 mg/dL

A: Probable acute gout attack.

P:
1. Refer patient to physician for prescription NSAID.
2. New prescription: indomethacin, 75 mg (immediate release) for one dose, followed by 50 mg every 6 hours for 48 hours and then 50 mg every 8 hours for 24 to 72 hours.
3. Educate GJ regarding administration and possible adverse reactions of the drug.
4. Educate GJ regarding lifestyle modifications.
5. Schedule follow-up phone call in 1 to 2 days to assess treatment.

Pharmacist: *Jane Kennedy, Pharm.D.*

Self-Assessment Questions

1. Differentiate the signs and symptoms of gout versus acute musculoskeletal trauma.
2. What interview questions would elicit subjective symptoms of gout versus acute trauma?
3. Discuss nonpharmacologic therapies that may be of benefit to the patient.

Critical Thinking Questions

1. Would you recommend prophylactic treatment for GJ? Why, or why not?
2. Synthesize a long-term approach to the pharmaceutical management of GJ's case. What factors could be important as this patient grows older?

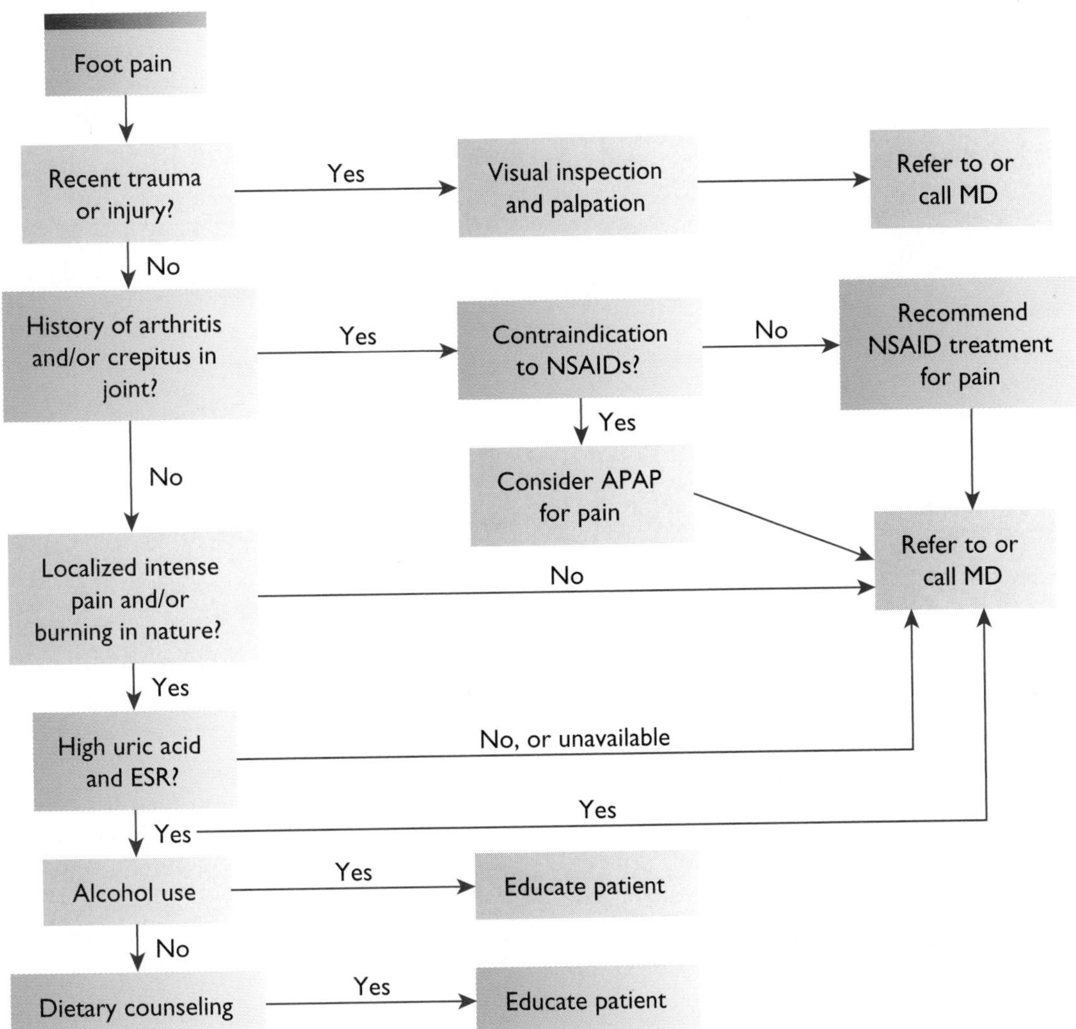

FIGURE 17-25 ■ Decision tree for musculoskeletal pain.

Musculoskeletal Swelling or Edema

Swelling within the musculoskeletal system is often a sign of inflammation. When a muscle or joint is edematous, it may also have local signs of erythema and limitation of movement. Swelling may indicate presence of fluid on a joint as well and can be the result of an acute traumatic event or the manifestation of an ongoing, systemic inflammatory condition. Swelling can play an important role when determining the overall diagnosis of a musculoskeletal complaint.

CASE STUDY

SN, a 64-year-old woman and a regular customer of a retail pharmacy, comes in to pick up her monthly prescriptions. She comes to the counter with a large bottle of ibuprofen and an electric heating pad. While fumbling to sign for her prescriptions, she asks if that new "twice-daily" OTC pain medication she heard about on television will help her rheumatism. Assuming that she is experiencing trouble with increased pain, the pharmacist asks the patient to step into the counseling room to discuss her symptoms.

ASSESSMENT OF THE PATIENT

Subjective Information

64-year-old woman complaining of increased pain

HOW LONG HAVE YOU HAD THIS PAIN? I've always had some pain, but over the last few months, it seems to have been getting worse. It must be part of getting old.

WHERE EXACTLY DOES IT HURT? Pretty much all over. My joints just ache. Some days my hands hurt so bad I can't even write my own name.

DO YOU HAVE PAIN ALL THE TIME, OR DOES IT COME AND GO? Some days are worse than others, but I always have some pain. If I move around quite a bit, it seems to help.

DO YOU HAVE PAIN AT NIGHT? Not so much when I go to bed, but I often wake up from the pain.

ARE YOU ALSO STIFF? Yes, very stiff. Sometimes I can barely move in the morning. I was hoping the heating pad would help.

HAVE YOU BEEN SICK WITH A SORE THROAT OR COLD LATELY? No.

HOW LONG WOULD YOU SAY YOUR STIFFNESS LASTS IN THE MORNING? Usually it takes me until midmorning to get going. Once I do start moving, though, I feel a little better.

HAVE YOU NOTICED ANY SWELLING? Well, my hands are swollen all of the time. Makes it hard to do anything! Also, my knees and ankles are usually swollen also.

HAVE YOU TAKEN ANYTHING FOR THE PAIN? Yes, I take one of these ibuprofen three to four times a day, but they don't seem to do much. That's why I'm thinking about that new one I saw on television.

DID YOU MENTION THIS THE LAST TIME YOU WERE IN TO SEE THE DOCTOR? No, I haven't seen him for about 6 months. I probably should. I've never been sick a day in my life, but lately, I've been so tired and sore. I don't know what is wrong. I went to a health fair at the clinic and had my blood drawn to see if I was okay. I think I have the results in my purse. Here they are. [*SN produces a computerized lab report of a CBC and Chem-7. The labs were drawn about 6 weeks ago.*]

Objective Information

Computerized medication profile:

- Premarin (conjugated estrogens): 0.625 mg PO every day.
- Provera (medroxyprogesterone): 5 mg PO every day on days 10–25.

Physical Examination of Extremities

Hands: Appear erythematous and swollen; inspection and palpation of the hands reveals slight swan-neck deformities and nodules on the metacarpal joints

Ankles: Appear bilaterally swollen, tender, and red; palpation reveals no significant fluid, but thickening of the soft tissue

Knees: Not examined

Significant Laboratory Results

Obtained 6 weeks ago

Hematocrit: 32%

Platelets: 600,000/mm^3

DISCUSSION

This case centers around SN's complaints of recurrent joint pain and swelling. The pharmacist needs to determine the cause of the symptoms. When a patient complains of chronic musculoskeletal pain, a systemic disorder must be considered. SN is a patient with no significant medical history other than her current complaints. Her only medications are hormone replacement therapy and ibuprofen as required for her musculoskeletal symptoms. The patient related that she is bothered by chronic pain and swelling, which is present most of the time. She does relate that the pain and associated stiffness are better after she moves around, cause her to wake at night, and limits her movement until midmorning. SN has been taking OTC ibuprofen in an attempt to control her symptoms with little success.

SN exhibits swelling and erythema in her hands and symmetric swelling in her knees and ankles. Laboratory tests that were performed approximately 6 weeks earlier revealed a

Continued

CASE STUDY—continued

mild anemia and thrombocytosis. Palpation of her hands was positive for nodules and showed early swan-neck deformities. Palpation of the ankles revealed swelling of the soft tissue without fluid.

After evaluating the subjective and objective information, the pharmacist suspects that the patient may have RA. The steps involved in the assessment of this patient are illustrated in the accompanying decision tree (Fig. 17-26). RA is a systemic inflammatory disorder that manifests with diffuse pain and swelling throughout the musculoskeletal system. Patients with RA often experience arthritis in three or more joints, including the hands, and morning stiffness, which is not quick to resolve. Joint swelling is a hallmark of the disease. The presence of rheumatoid nodules, anemia, and thrombocytosis also correlate with the suspected diagnosis.

Although NSAID therapy is the initial treatment of choice, SN currently is only taking analgesic doses of ibuprofen. Anti-inflammatory processes, such as RA, require higher doses of NSAIDs. Because of the findings, the pharmacist calls the physician to discuss SN. The physician agrees with the pharmacist and advises the patient to make an appointment for an examination and full workup. SN is advised to increase the dose of her ibuprofen to 600 mg PO QID and to apply the heating pad as necessary to assist in relieving pain. The patient is counseled regarding administration of ibuprofen with food and is again reminded to contact the physician's office for an appointment. The pharmacist also schedules a follow-up call with SN in 1 week to assess the impact of increasing the anti-inflammatory dosing on her symptoms.

PHARMACEUTICAL CARE PLAN

Patient Name: SN

Date: 08/31/02

Medical Problems:
Postmenopausal

Current Medications:
Conjugated estrogens, 0.625 mg PO every day
Medroxyprogesterone, 5 mg PO every day on days 10–25

S: 64-year-old woman with complaints of diffuse pain and swelling of the musculoskeletal system. Pain and stiffness are chronic but seem to decrease with motion. Pain causes patient to awaken from sleep, and morning stiffness is present until midmorning. Pain and stiffness are causing some difficulty in activities of daily living. Patient has been self-medicating with ibuprofen, 200 mg TID to QID as needed, but with little symptom relief.

O: Erythematous, swollen joints of the hands, ankles, and knees. Joint swelling appears symmetric. Rheumatoid nodules and early swan-neck deformities are noted in the hands.

Hematocrit: 32% (6 weeks ago)

Platelets: 600,000/mm^3 (6 weeks ago)

A: Systemic inflammatory musculoskeletal disorder, most likely RA.

P:
1. Call physician to discuss case and recommend increased anti-inflammatory therapy. Patient will likely need a full examination and workup by her physician.
2. Advise patient to increase ibuprofen to 600 mg QID.
3. Educate patient regarding adverse effects of ibuprofen therapy, and instruct on nondrug therapy of rest and use of heat.
4. Patient to see physician for thorough examination and workup.
5. Schedule follow-up call in 1 week to assess impact of ibuprofen therapy and any potential adverse effects.

Pharmacist: *Richard Feldstein, Pharm.D.*

Self-Assessment Questions:

1. Compare and contrast the signs and symptoms associated with RA and with OA.
2. What interview questions are useful in eliciting subjective information concerning RA and OA?
3. Discuss nonpharmacologic therapies that may be of benefit to SN based on the current symptoms she is experiencing.

Critical Thinking Questions

1. Assuming that the pharmacist's assessment of SN is correct, what course of therapy should be considered if anti-inflammatory treatment fails to relieve SN's symptoms?
2. If SN had complained of severe weakness in addition to her other symptoms, how might you have approached the case differently? What additional questions and objective tests would you have included in your assessment?

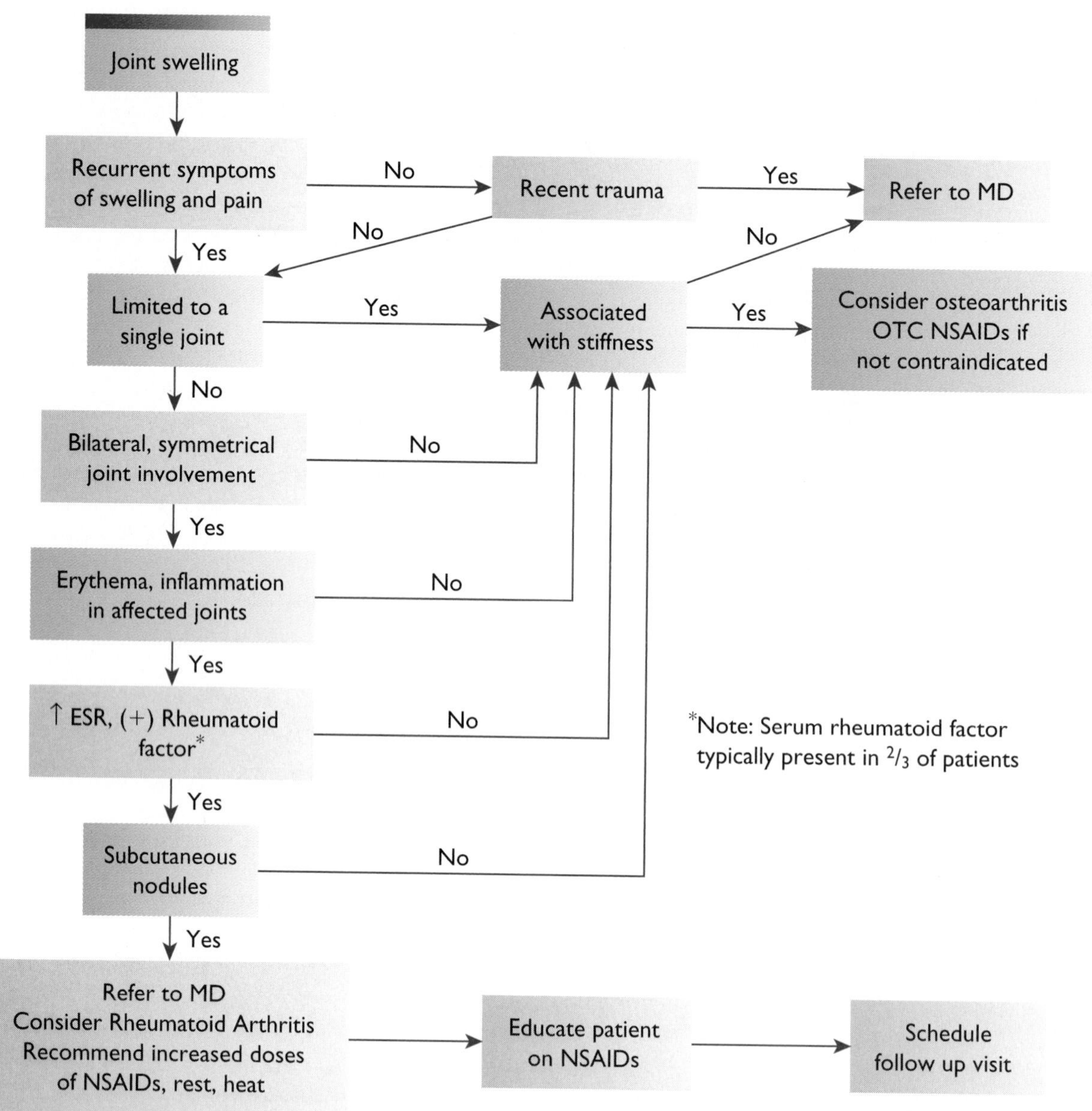

FIGURE 17-26 ■ Decision tree for musculoskeletal swelling or edema.

Stiffness and Decreased ROM

Stiffness and decreased ROM are common complaints in patients with musculoskeletal disorders. They can occur independently but are often associated. Unfortunately, like other musculoskeletal symptoms, they are also very nonspecific. Stiffness and decreased ROM can result from many things, including acute trauma, overexertion, localized joint inflammation, deformity, or systemic disease. Because of this variability in causes, the pharmacist must elicit thorough subjective information and objective data to clearly assess the patient's condition.

CASE STUDY

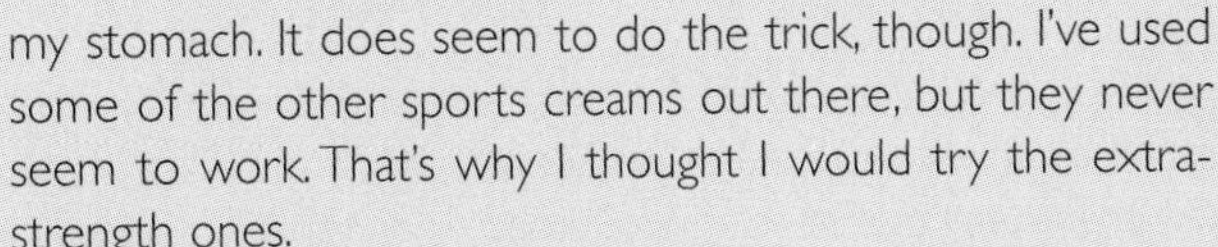

EC, a 37-year-old man, comes to the pharmacy with two tubes of OTC sports cream in his hand. He appears to be in a hurry as he asks for the pharmacist's opinion regarding which cream is stronger. "They both say extra-strength," he asks. "Which one would you use?" To help this patient get the relief he needs, the pharmacist must first determine why EC needs the product. As the pharmacist takes the two tubes from EC to examine the ingredients, the following questions are asked to assist the patient in obtaining the appropriate treatment.

ASSESSMENT OF THE PATIENT

Subjective Information

37-year-old man asking which sports cream is stronger

ARE THESE FOR YOU OR FOR SOMEONE ELSE? For me.

ARE YOU HAVING SOME KIND OF PAIN? Yeah, I've had a sore knee for a while now. I'm on my way to a family reunion, and I want to be able to play softball. I wanted to put something on to loosen it up a little.

WHERE ARE YOU EXPERIENCING THE PAIN? My knee has been a little painful and tight. Like I said, I wanted to loosen it up a little bit. It just isn't moving like it should.

ARE YOU EXPERIENCING STIFFNESS AS WELL? Yes, I have a hard time moving my leg like I used to. Especially when I roll out of bed in the morning. Some days it takes 15 minutes for me to be able to walk very well.

HAVE YOU HURT YOUR KNEE RECENTLY OR IN THE PAST? No, I've just had some pain. I think I may have twisted it running last week. So which one of these is better?

ACTUALLY, THE TWO ARE QUITE SIMILAR, BUT I'M NOT SURE EITHER ONE IS GOING TO OFFER YOU THE RELIEF THAT YOU WANT. ARE YOU HAVING PAIN IN ANY OF YOUR OTHER JOINTS? No, just my knee. Otherwise I feel great. I've been out running 5 miles every day, just like when I was in college training. My old football coach would be proud. I've only gained five pounds since I graduated!

HAVE YOU TRIED ANYTHING ELSE FOR THE PAIN AND STIFFNESS? Once in a while I'll take some ibuprofen, but it upsets my stomach. It does seem to do the trick, though. I've used some of the other sports creams out there, but they never seem to work. That's why I thought I would try the extra-strength ones.

DO YOU HAVE A HISTORY OF ULCERS? I do. I've been taking Zantac on and off for the last year or so. My stomach is pretty good now, but I hate to mess it up. My doctor told me to stay away from the ibuprofen, so I've been avoiding it. But it seems like my knee has been getting worse. I wonder if it's a sprain.

DO YOU HAVE ANY MEDICAL PROBLEMS OTHER THAN YOUR STOMACH? No, that's it.

HOW OFTEN DO YOU DRINK ALCOHOL? Rarely. Once in a while my wife and I will have a drink with dinner, but that isn't very often.

Objective Information

Medication profile (per patient report):

- Zantac (ranitidine): 150 mg PO QHS as needed.
- Multivitamin: one tablet PO every day.

Left knee: swollen, without signs of erythema; palpation reveals swelling of the soft tissue, without any apparent fluid; ROM appears limited; crepitus detected during movement
Right knee: nontender, with no crepitus or swelling noted
Other joints: no signs of swelling; other weight-bearing joints show no signs of distress
Hands: appear normal, without any redness or tenderness

DISCUSSION

This case centers around EC's stiffness and restricted motion in his left knee. The pharmacist must determine if the stiffness is the result of acute injury or trauma, degeneration of the joint, or systemic disease. Physical assessment of the knee reveals a swollen joint that does not appear inflamed. Crepitus is noted as well. The patient describes the joint as being "tight" and denies any recent significant injury, other than the possibility of a recent twist while running.

The subjective information in this case proves to be important. The patient is a former football player who now is a routine runner. Per the patient conversation, it appears that

Continued

CASE STUDY—continued

the intensity of the stiffness is variable, and that he has attempted to manage it symptomatically in the past with topical analgesic products. He also indicated that the stiffness was increased in the morning but quickly resolved. This stiffness could relate to a past history of injury, and the daily running may aggravate this weight-bearing joint. Another important fact is that EC has a history of peptic ulcer disease. The patient avoids NSAIDs but, unfortunately is not getting the relief that is necessary from the topical products he has been using.

After gathering the subjective and objective information from the patient, the pharmacist concludes that EC is most likely experiencing OA in the left knee. The steps involved in the assessment of this patient are illustrated in the accompanying decision tree (Fig. 17-27). Factors that lead to this conclusion include localization of stiffness, decreased motion, pain in the joint, lack of inflammatory response, positive joint crepitus on examination, morning stiffness that resolves quickly, and the history of sports, which included college football and continuous weight-bearing exercise.

Although the usual treatment of choice in patients with OA is NSAID therapy, EC's history of peptic ulcer disease is a consideration. The patient indicates that ibuprofen has caused stomach upset in the past; however, topical therapy has not shown a benefit at this point. Because the patient is not suffering from an inflammatory arthritis, analgesic therapy with acetaminophen may be a good option. In addition, the patient may get relief from topical capsaicin, because capsaicin induces the release of substance P, the principal chemomediator of pain impulses from the periphery to the central nervous system. This topical product has shown benefit in some patients with OA, RA arthritis, diabetic neuropathies, and postherpetic neuralgias. It is important to emphasize to EC that this medication must be applied on a regular basis for at least 2 weeks to see results, and that maximal benefits may not be seen for 4 to 6 weeks.

The pharmacist feels comfortable making these recommendations for short-term management of EC's pain and stiffness. The pharmacist also recommends, however, that EC see his physician in the near future for a complete examination and workup of his knee. The pharmacist instructs EC to take acetaminophen, 650 mg every 4 to 6 hours, and see how the joint feels. If needed, EC may increase the dose to 1000 mg every 6 hours, but he should not exceed 4000 mg/day. The capsaicin is also discussed as an option if the arthritis continues to progress and the pain is not manageable. The pharmacist recommends waiting to see how the acetaminophen affects the joint initially, however. In addition, application of heat to the area and rest are also recommended.

PHARMACEUTICAL CARE PLAN

Patient Name: EC

Date: 10/31/02

Medical Problems: History of peptic ulcer disease

Current Medications:

Zantac (ranitidine), 150 mg PO every day as needed for stomach pain

Multivitamin, one tablet every day

S: 37-year-old male complaining of stiffness, limited motion, and pain in the left knee joint that subsides quickly in the morning after rising. Has tried topical analgesics in the past without success. Cannot take NSAIDs because of history of peptic ulcer disease. No recent trauma. Football player in college. Currently runs 5 miles/day.

O: Joint inspection reveals a swollen knee, without signs of erythema. Palpation reveals swelling of the soft tissue, without any apparent fluid. ROM appears limited, and crepitus is detected during movement. Inspection of other joints does not show any swelling. The right knee is nontender, with no crepitus or swelling noted. Involvement appears limited to the left knee.

A: Possible OA of the left knee joint.

P:

1. Recommend acetaminophen, 650 mg every 4 to 6 hours. If pain and stiffness do not improve, increase to 1000 mg every 6 hours, not to exceed 4000 mg/day.
2. Educate EC regarding nonpharmacologic therapies that may be of benefit, including rest and application of heat.
3. Recommend referral to physician for complete examination and workup in the near future.

Pharmacist: *Helen Gabriel, Pharm.D.*

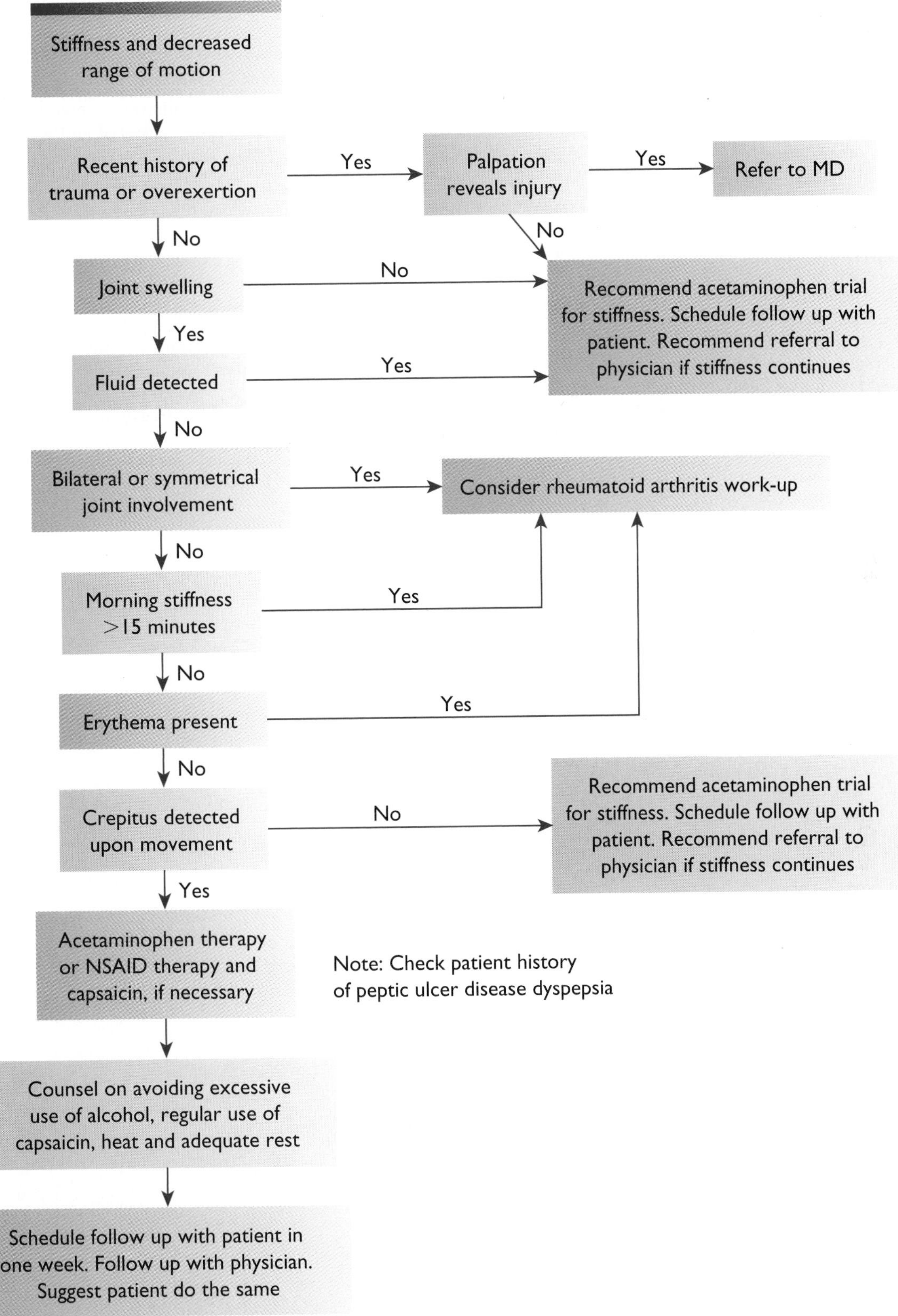

FIGURE 17-27 ■ Decision tree for stiffness and decreased range of motion.

Self-Assessment Questions

1. What specific findings support OA versus RA or acute injury in EC?
2. What potential complications can occur with chronic, high-dose acetaminophen therapy?
3. What other options are available for EC if acetaminophen does not help?

Critical Thinking Questions

1. What role, if any, would topical analgesics play in the treatment of OA?
2. If EC's symptoms progress to an erythematous joint in addition to the pain, stiffness, and swelling, what are the possible causes?

Bibliography

Amarshi N, Scoggin JA, Ensworth S. Osteoporosis: review of guidelines and consensus statements. Am J Manage Care 1997;3:1077–1084.

American Association of Clinical Endocrinologists. AACE Clinical Practice Guidelines for the Prevention and Treatment of Postmenopausal Osteoporosis. Endocr Pract 1996;2:157–171.

Cary C, Lee H, Woeltje K. The Washington manual of medical therapeutics. 29th ed. St. Louis: Little, Brown, 1998.

DiPiro JT, Talbert RL, Yee GC, et al. Pharmacotherapy: a pathophysiological approach. 4th ed. Stamford, CT: Appleton and Lange, 1999.

Fauci AS, Braunwald E, Isselbacher KJ, et al. Harrison's principles of internal medicine. 14th ed. New York: McGraw-Hill, 1998.

Kelley WN. Textbook of internal medicine. 3rd ed. Philadelphia: JB Lippincott, 1997.

Koda-Kimble MA, Young LY. Applied therapeutics: the clinical use of drugs. Baltimore: Lippincott Williams & Wilkins, 2001.

Mangini M. Physical assessment of the musculoskeletal system. Nurs Clin North Am 1998;33:643–652.

Musculoskeletal system. In: Seidel HM, Ball JW, Dains JE, et al., eds. Mosby's guide to physical examination. 4th ed. St. Louis: Mosby, 1999.

Swartz MH. Textbook of physical diagnosis. 3rd ed. Philadelphia: WB Saunders, 1998.

Thomas CL. Taber's cyclopedic medical dictionary. 18th ed. Philadelphia: FA Davis, 1997.

Tortora GJ. Principles of human anatomy. 5th ed. New York: HarperCollins, 1989.

Tortora GJ. Principles of human anatomy. 6th ed. New York: HarperCollins, 1992.

CHAPTER

18

Nervous System

Wendy Mills

GLOSSARY TERMS

- Absence seizures
- Atonic seizures
- Cerebrovascular accidents
- Cerebrovascular disease
- Cluster headache
- Epilepsy
- Generalized seizures
- Graphesthesia
- Hyperreflexia
- Ischemia
- Migraine headaches
- Myoclonic seizures
- Neuropathy
- Paresthesia
- Parkinson's disease
- Partial seizures
- Retropulsion
- Seizure
- Status epilepticus
- Stereognosis
- Tension headaches
- Tonic-clonic seizures
- Transient ischemic attacks

ANATOMY AND PHYSIOLOGY OVERVIEW

The function of the nervous system is to receive, interpret, and respond to stimuli and, thus, to maintain a network of coordination and control for the body. The two components of the nervous system include the central nervous system and the peripheral nervous system (Fig. 18-1).

Central Nervous System

The central nervous system (CNS) consists of the brain and the spinal cord, and it is the control center for the entire nervous system. Within the CNS, sensory information is correlated and interpreted, emotions and thoughts are formed, and muscles and glands are stimulated via outgoing nerve impulses.

Brain

The brain in the average adult consists of approximately 1000 billion neurons and is one of the largest organs in the body. Brain tissue may be gray or white. Gray matter consists primarily of neuronal cell bodies. It covers the surfaces of the cerebral hemispheres, and it forms additional structures within the brain, such as the basal ganglia, the thalamus, and the hypothalamus. White matter consists primarily of myelinated neuronal axons, which connect and transmit nerve impulses between different parts of the CNS.

Two internal carotid arteries, two vertebral arteries, and the basilar artery form the cerebral arterial circle (i.e., circle of Willis), which supplies the brain with oxygen and nutrients (Fig. 18-2). Even though the brain weighs approximately 2% of total body weight, it consumes approximately 20% of the body's oxygen requirement at rest. If the brain's oxygen supply is inter-

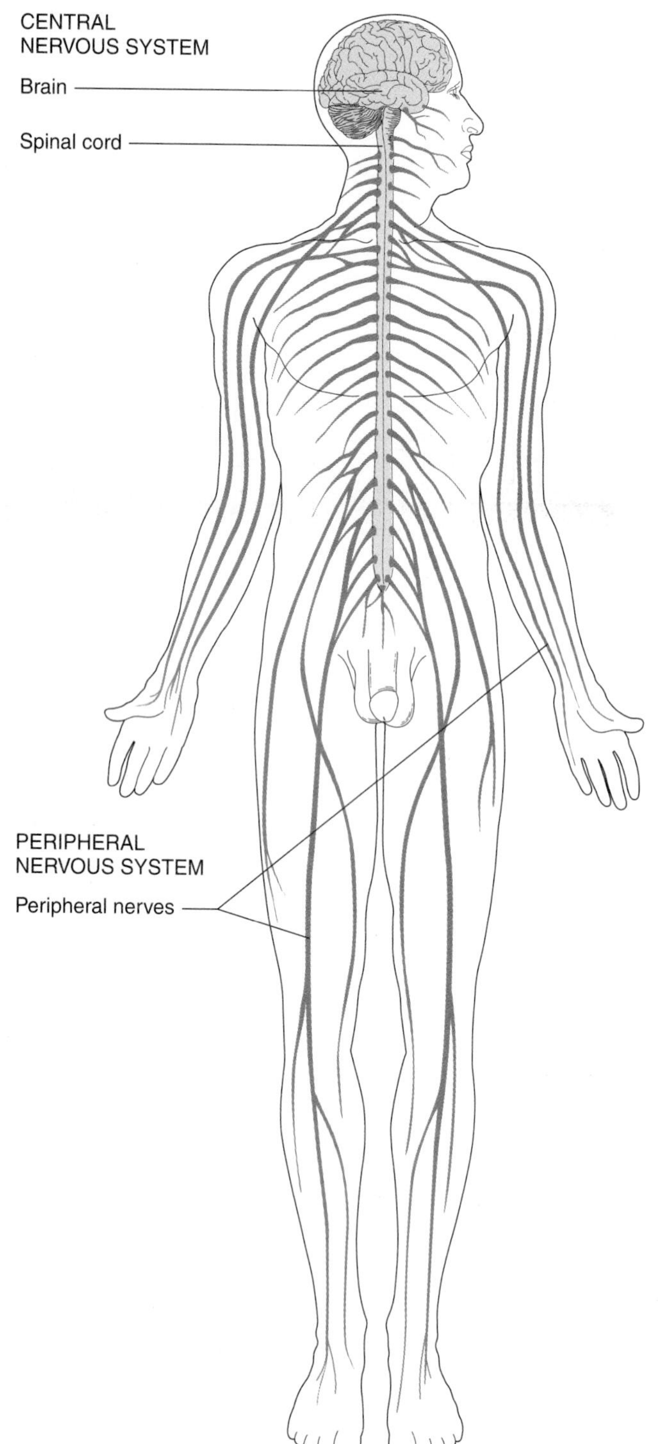

FIGURE 18-1 ■ The nervous system.

rupted for as little as 4 minutes, permanent brain damage can result.

The endothelial cells that line the capillaries supplying the brain are densely packed, forming a blood-brain barrier. This allows the passage of different substances from the blood into the brain cells to be regulated and, thus, protects the brain from harmful substances. Most lipid-soluble substances, glucose, oxygen, carbon dioxide, and water pass directly from the circulating

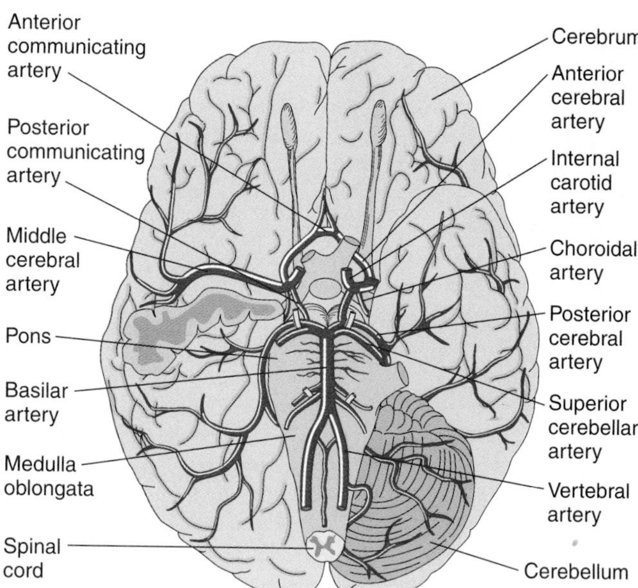

FIGURE 18-2 ■ Posterior view of the arterial supply to the brain.

blood into the brain cells. Other substances, such as sodium and potassium, enter slowly, and some antibiotics and proteins do not pass into the brain cells at all.

The brain is further protected by the cranial bones, the cerebrospinal fluid (CSF), and the cranial meninges. The cranial meninges are connective tissue membranes that cushion the brain within the skull. They are continuous with the spinal meninges, and they are composed of the dura mater, arachnoid mater, and pia mater. The CSF is continuously circulating around the brain and the spinal cord, providing protection and nourishment.

The brain has four principal divisions: (1) the cerebrum, (2) the diencephalon, (3) the cerebellum, and (4) the brainstem (Fig. 18-3). The cerebrum is situated on top of the brainstem and diencephalon, and it forms the bulk of the brain. The gray outer layer (i.e., the cerebral cortex) contains sensory, motor, and association areas, which are responsible for sensory infor-

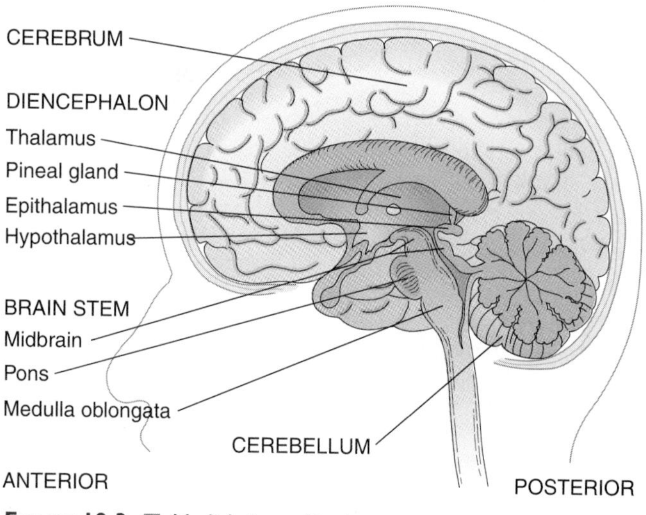

FIGURE 18-3 ■ Medial view of brain.

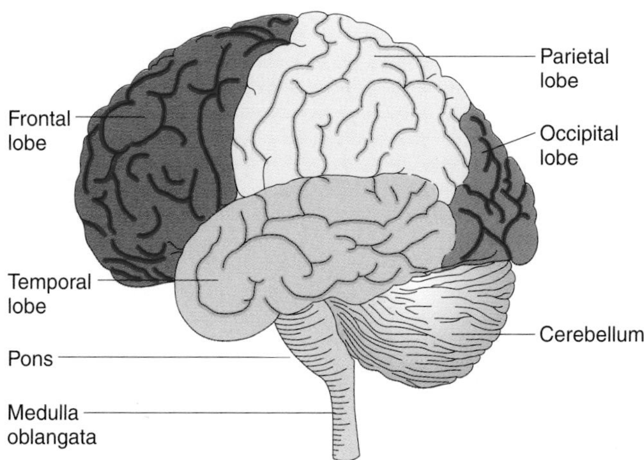

FIGURE 18-4 ■ Left lateral view of the brain.

mation, muscular movement, and emotional and intellectual processes. The white matter underlying the cortex contains myelinated axons, which connect and transmit nerve impulses between different parts of the brain. The cerebrum is composed of two hemispheres, which are subdivided into the frontal, parietal, occipital, and temporal lobes (Fig. 18-4).

The frontal lobes control voluntary skeletal muscle movements, speech formation, emotions, affect, and awareness of self. Processing of sensory data as it is received as well as more complex functions, such as comprehension, reasoning, and awareness of body position (i.e., proprioception), occur in the parietal lobes. The occipital lobes are primarily responsible for vision and interpretation of visual data. The temporal lobes are involved in the perception and interpretation of sound, taste, smell, and balance.

The diencephalon consists of the thalamus, the hypothalamus, and the pineal gland, and it provides the relay centers for both the sensory and motor pathways (Fig. 18-3). The thalamus functions as an interpreter and messenger of sensory information to the cerebral cortex. Maintenance of homeostasis and the endocrine system is provided by the hypothalamus. The circadian rhythms are regulated by melatonin, a hormone secreted by the pineal gland.

The cerebellum is the second-largest portion of the brain and is located under the occipital lobe of the cerebrum. It is concerned with balance, sensory information, and subconscious skeletal motor commands.

The medulla, pons, and midbrain form the brainstem, which is the pathway between the cerebral cortex and the spinal cord. The medulla physically connects the brain and the spinal cord. It contains all ascending (i.e., sensory) and descending (i.e., motor) tracks, and it controls many of the involuntary functions. The pons links the cerebellar hemispheres with the rest of the brain. Reticular formation as well as processing of visual and auditory information are located in the midbrain.

Spinal Cord

The vertebral column, ligaments, spinal meninges, and CSF protect the spinal cord. In young children, the vertebral column and the spinal cord grow longer with body growth. As children approach 5 years of age, however, the spinal cord no longer grows. Therefore, the spinal cord occupies only the upper two-thirds of the vertebral canal, and it consists of both gray and white matter. The gray matter is organized into an "H" shape, with anterior and posterior horns, and it is surrounded by white tracts of nerves that serve as the highway for information between the brain and the peripheral nervous system. Ascending tracts provide sensory information from the peripheral nervous system to the brain; descending tracts provide motor information from the brain to the peripheral nervous system.

Spinal tracts also provide a means of integrating reflexes, or fast responses to stimuli in the internal or external environment to maintain homeostasis. Reflexes may be classified as cranial, somatic, or autonomic (visceral). Cranial reflexes involve cranial nerves and occur through the brainstem. Somatic reflexes occur through the spinal cord and involve skeletal muscle contraction. Autonomic, or visceral, reflexes involve cardiac muscle, glands, and smooth muscle; one is not usually aware of autonomic reflexes when they occur.

Reflexes occur when nerve impulses flow through a pathway known as a reflex arc (Fig. 18-5). For a reflex arc to be complete and to elicit the desired reflex, five components are neces-

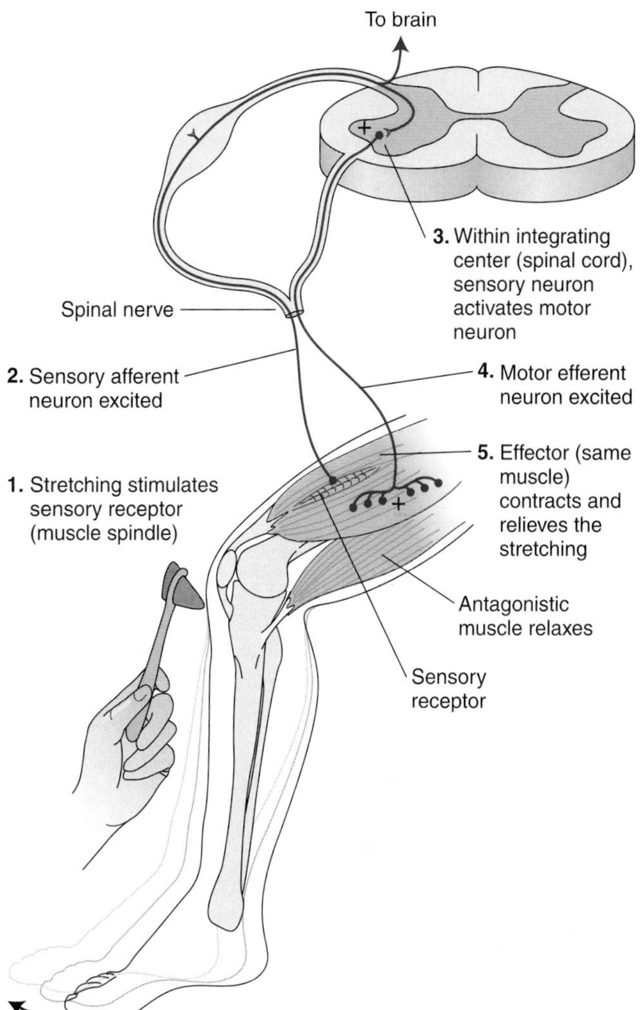

FIGURE 18-5 ■ Reflex arc.

sary: (1) sensory receptor, (2) sensory (i.e., afferent) neuron, (3) integrating center, (4) motor (i.e., efferent) neuron, and (5) effector. Simply stated, the sensory receptor responds to a stimulus and triggers nerve impulses in the sensory neuron. The nerve impulses then travel along the axon to the integrating center, where they are relayed to a motor neuron. The motor neuron then conducts these impulses to the effector, which is the muscle or gland that will respond. The response the effector makes is a reflex. A reflex may involve as few as two neurons (one sensory and one motor) across a single synapse. Reflexes depend on intact sensory and motor fibers, functional synapses, and competent neuromuscular junctions and muscle fibers. Deep tendon reflexes are examples of such monosynaptic reflexes and involve specific spinal segments.

Peripheral Nervous System

The peripheral nervous system contains 12 cranial nerves, which enter and exit the brain, and 31 pairs of spinal nerves. Ten of the 12 cranial nerves arise from the diencephalon. Cranial nerves are either sensory in function or mixed, including both sensory and motor functions. Cell bodies of sensory nerves lie outside the CNS; cell bodies of motor fibers lie within the CNS. Sensations that occur include sense of position (i.e., proprioception), temperature, light touch, vibration, and pain. These stimuli travel to the brain through different pathways, three of which are clinically significant. The posterior column pathway is the sensory pathway for light touch, proprioception, and vibration. The lateral spinothalamic pathway conveys sensory impulses for temperature and pain. The anterior spinothalamic pathway communicates sensory impulses for crude touch and pressure. Identifying deficits in any of these sensory impulses assists in directing further clinical investigation. The motor pathway from the motor cortex in the frontal lobe to the skeletal muscles consists of pyramidal and peripheral nerve fibers. Pyramidal nerve fibers are associated with upper motor neurons, and peripheral nerve fibers are associated with lower motor neurons. Lesions or damage to the upper motor neurons are typically associated with more generalized disorders, whereas damage to the lower motor neurons may affect a more localized muscle group. The 12 cranial nerves primarily supply the head and neck, except for the vagus nerve, which also supplies organs such as the heart and stomach (Table 18-1).

Table 18-1 ➤ CRANIAL NERVES

Cranial Nerve	Function
I: Olfactory	Sensory: smell
II: Optic	Sensory: vision
III: Oculomotor	Motor: extraocular movement, upper eyelid
	Parasympathetic: adjust lens and pupil constriction
IV: Trochlear	Motor: downward and inward movement of the eye
	Sensory: muscle sense
V: Trigeminal	Motor: muscles of mastication
	Sensory: touch, pain, and temperature in the eye, mucous membranes of the mouth and nose, scalp
VI: Abducens	Motor: lateral movement of eye
	Sensory: muscle sense
VII: Facial	Motor: facial movements, close eye and mouth
	Sensory: anterior two-thirds of tongue, taste
VIII: Vestibulocochlear	Sensory: hearing and balance
IX: Glossopharyngeal	Motor: swallowing, salivary glands
	Sensory: pharynx and posterior third of tongue, taste, carotid reflex
X: Vagus	Motor: palate, pharynx, larynx
	Sensory: general sensation from pharynx, viscera, external auditory canal
	Autonomic: gastrointestinal, cardiac
XI: Accessory	Motor: voluntary swallowing, sternocleidomastoid and trapezius muscles
XII: Hypoglossal	Motor: movements of the tongue

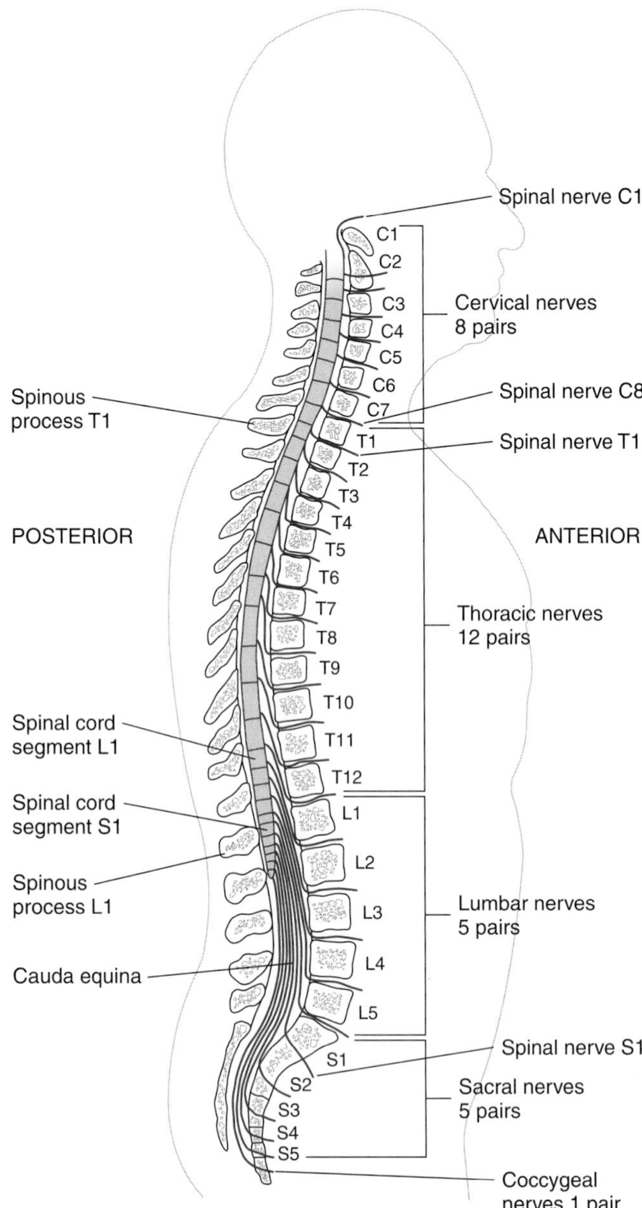

Figure 18-6 ■ Lateral view of the spinal cord and nerves.

Thirty-one pairs of nerves emerge from the spinal cord: 8 cervical, 12 thoracic, 5 lumbar, 5 sacral, and 1 coccygeal (Fig.

18-6). All the spinal nerves are mixed nerves, because they contain both sensory and motor fibers. Within the spinal column, each spinal nerve separates out into the ventral and dorsal root. The sensory fibers of the dorsal root and the motor fibers of the ventral root carry information to and from the CNS, respectively.

Knowledge of dermatomes (i.e., the bands of skin that are innervated by the sensory nerve root of a single spinal segment) can aid in localizing neurologic lesions (Fig. 18-7). Their levels are considerably more variable than those that have been mapped, however, and tend to overlap at the midline.

The peripheral nervous system is further divided into the somatic nervous system (SNS) and the autonomic nervous system (ANS). The SNS contains sensory neurons that convey information from receptors in the head, body wall, and extremities to the CNS and that innervate skeletal muscle only. The motor responses of the SNS are voluntary. In contrast, the ANS consists of sensory neurons that convey homeostatic information and that innervate smooth muscle, cardiac muscle, and glands. The motor responses of the ANS are involuntary. The ANS is further subdivided into the sympathetic system, which stimulates organs during stress, and the parasympathetic system, which stimulates organs for normal functioning.

Special Considerations

Pediatric Patients

In the embryo, the CNS starts to appear during the third week of gestation. The backbone and vertebral canal have formed at the end of the first month. At the end of 7 months of gestation, the CNS is able to control respiration and body temperature, and if born prematurely, the newborn is now capable of survival.

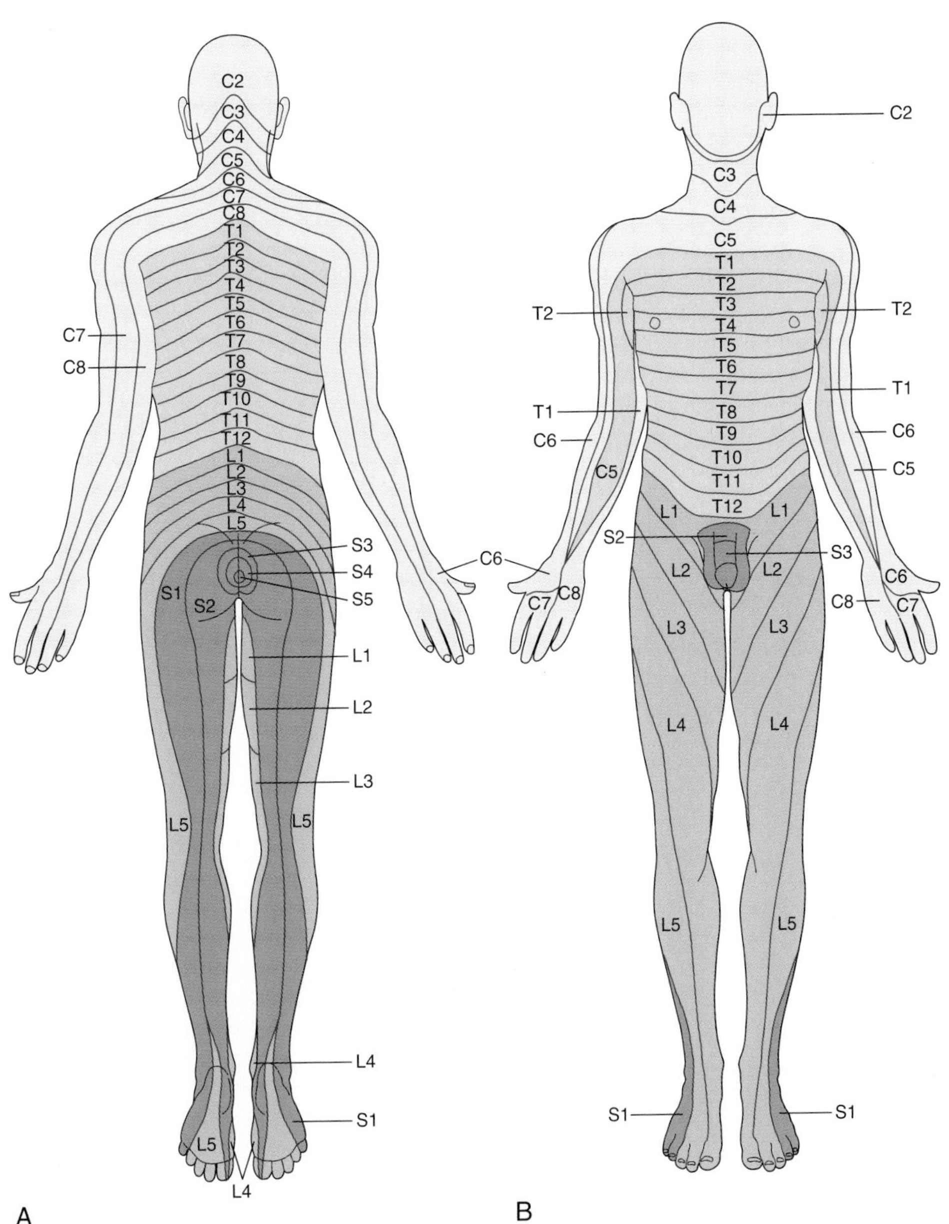

FIGURE 18-7 ■ Dermatomes. **(A)** Posterior view. **(B)** Anterior view.

Even in full-term infants, the nervous system is not completely developed; however, primitive reflexes, such as yawning, sneezing, and blinking at a bright light, do exist. The major portion of brain growth, myelinization of the nerves and neuronal axons, and further development of the blood-brain barrier occurs during the first year of life. The infant's sensory and motor development proceeds along with the acquisition of myelin (in the same order that the child is observed to gain motor control).

Geriatric Patients

As an individual ages, the number of neurons in the brain and the spinal cord decreases, which can produce changes that would be considered abnormal in a patient younger than 65 years. Alterations in hearing, vision, extraocular movements, and pupillary reactivity may occur, as may decreases in muscle mass and vibration sensation. The nerve impulse velocity decreases by as much as 10% with aging. Therefore, various responses take longer, and reflexes may decrease. There is also a decrease in the synthesis and metabolism of neurotransmitters, such as norepinephrine, serotonin, and dopamine, which may decrease a person's ability to respond in times of stress and increase the risk of delirium. Long-term memory may decrease with age as well; however, no decline in general intelligence should be seen unless a systemic or neurologic disorder develops.

Pregnant Patients

Specific alterations in pregnant patients are generally not well-defined; however, neurohormonal changes in the hypothalamic-pituitary system are seen throughout pregnancy. These patients may experience tension headaches, numbness or tingling in the hands, and changes in sleep patterns throughout their pregnancy.

PATHOLOGY OVERVIEW

Neurologic diseases can account for significant morbidity and mortality throughout a patient's life. Major neurologic disorders include headache disorders, epilepsy, Parkinson's disease, cerebrovascular disease, and peripheral neuropathies.

Headache Disorders

Headache disorders can be classified as either primary or secondary. If the headache is a symptom of another disease, it is considered to be secondary. Causes of secondary headaches include:

- Trauma
- Tumors
- Infection
- Menstruation
- Pregnancy
- Stroke

Primary headaches consist of tension headaches, migraine headaches (with and without aura), and cluster headaches.

Tension Headaches

Tension headaches are the most common type of headache complaint. They are generally a pressing/tightening, nonpulsating, bilateral pain. Physical activity does not usually aggravate tension headaches. Initial treatment consists of over-the-counter analgesics (e.g., aspirin, acetaminophen, or ibuprofen). If these agents are not effective, then prescription analgesics, including nonsteroidal anti-inflammatory drugs (NSAIDs) and combination analgesics, are used. Prophylaxis is rarely needed.

Migraine Headaches

Migraine headaches are thought to result from a combination of vascular and neurohormonal mechanisms. Signs and symptoms are listed in Box 18-1. Women generally experience migraine headaches more often than men, as do individuals with a family history of migraine headaches. Many patients with migraine headaches also experience tension headaches. Factors that may precipitate migraine headaches include:

- Medications
- Emotional stress
- Depression
- Tobacco smoke
- Sensory stimulation (e.g., light, sound, and odors)
- Diet
- Hormonal changes
- Hypoglycemia
- Changes in sleep or exercise patterns

Nonpharmacologic treatment of migraine headache pain consists of resting in a dark, quiet room free from external stimulus. Medications used to abort migraine headaches include NSAIDs, combination analgesics, serotonin agonists, and ergot-

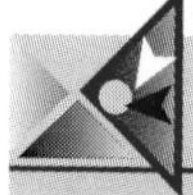

Box 18-1

SIGNS AND SYMPTOMS OF MIGRAINE HEADACHES

SIGNS

- Aura
- Visual disturbances
- Sensory disturbances
- Local weakness

SYMPTOMS

- Unilateral
- Pulsating pain
- Nausea
- Vomiting
- Photophobia
- Phonophobia
- Pain aggravated by physical activity

amine and its derivatives. Prophylactic therapy is used in patients with contraindications to abortive therapies, debilitating headaches, and more than two headaches per month. Medications, including β-blockers, tricyclic antidepressants, calcium-channel blockers, and selective serotonin-reuptake inhibitors have been useful for prophylaxis.

Cluster Headaches

Cluster headaches generally occur during the early morning hours and more often in men than in women. The pain is described as an excruciating, stabbing pain that is unilateral and clusters over an eye. Cluster headaches generally last for only 30 to 90 minutes, but they may "cluster" in occurrence during certain times of the year. Patients may experience headaches ranging from several daily to several weekly for a period of time, then complete remission for weeks or months. Oxygen therapy, injectable sumatriptan, or dihydroergotamine have been useful in the abortive treatment of cluster headaches. Agents such as lithium, ergotamine, and methysergide have been used for prophylaxis.

Epilepsy

At some point during their lifetimes, approximately 8% of the general population will experience a **seizure,** which is a focal and/or generalized disturbance of neuronal electrical activity that may manifest by abnormal movements or sensations and a loss of reflexes, memory, or consciousness. Incidence is highest until 10 years of age, at which point it decreases until 50 years of age and then increases throughout the rest of life. **Epilepsy** is generally defined as two or more unprovoked seizures without an identifiable cause. If a seizure has an identifiable cause, then a person does not have epilepsy; however, treatment may still be required. Seizures can have many causes, including mechanical causes (e.g., trauma and neoplasms), metabolic abnormalities, medications and withdrawal, infection, and fever. Patients can have partial seizures, generalized seizures, status epilepticus, or some combination thereof. Table 18-2 differentiates among the various seizure types.

Partial Seizures

Partial seizures begin in an area of the brain that is limited to one hemisphere, and they are often suggestive of an underlying focal brain lesion. Partial seizures can be classified as simple partial, in which consciousness is preserved, or as complex partial, in which consciousness is impaired. Both simple and complex partial seizures may secondarily generalize, causing a loss of consciousness. Medications that are useful during the initial treatment of partial seizures include phenytoin, carbamazepine, and valproic acid. Lamotrigine, topiramate, gabapentin, tiagabine, and phenobarbital have all been successfully used as second-line agents in the treatment of partial seizures.

Generalized Seizures

Generalized seizures usually cause a patient to lose consciousness and are primarily differentiated on symptomatology (Table 18-2). **Tonic-clonic seizures** are the most recognized seizure type, and they have a prolonged postseizure, or postictal, stage during which the person can experience symptoms such as fatigue, muscle pain, and confusion. Phenytoin, valproic acid, lamotrigine, topiramate, and phenobarbital are the medications generally used in treatment of tonic-clonic seizures. **Absence seizures** are more common in children and may be initially confused with daydreaming. The loss of consciousness as well as the return to consciousness occurs very rapidly. Generally, absence seizures do not continue into adulthood. Valproic acid, ethosuximide, lamotrigine, and topiramate are all effective treatments. **Myoclonic seizures** are characterized by sudden and brief muscle contractions, either in a single part of the body or the entire body. **Atonic seizures** present with a sudden loss of postural muscle tone, usually lasting only for 1 or 2 seconds. Both myoclonic and atonic seizures are not as common as the other types and may be treated with valproic acid, lamotrigine, and topiramate.

TABLE 18-2 ➤ TYPES OF SEIZURES

PARTIAL SEIZURES	
Simple partial	Repetitive, purposeless movements such as chewing, rubbing, patting, and picking movements that generally last for as long as 5 minutes. Patient maintains consciousness.
Complex partial	Repetitive, purposeless movements. Patient loses consciousness.
Secondarily generalized	Begins as a partial seizure but progresses to a generalized seizure. Patients with an aura before a generalized seizure have secondarily generalized seizures.
GENERALIZED SEIZURES	
Tonic-clonic	Major muscle groups undergo toxic extension followed by rhythmic contraction. Patient loses consciousness and may be incontinent of bowel or bladder. A postictal state, including dizziness, drowsiness, and confusion, generally follows.
Absence	Loss of consciousness for a few seconds, and then normal activities are resumed.
Atonic	Sudden loss of muscle tone. May cause head to drop suddenly (or entire body to drop to the floor).
Myoclonic	Muscles jerk (single or cluster).

Adapted from Welty T. Managing the patient with epilepsy. Clinical Pharmacy Newswatch 1997;4:1–6.

Status Epilepticus

Status epilepticus is defined as repetitive seizure activity, with or without convulsions, and without recovery of consciousness between attacks lasting 30 minutes or more. It is considered to be a medical emergency. If untreated, status epilepticus can cause permanent neurologic damage and even death. Patients at increased risk for developing status epilepticus include those with:

- Focal background abnormalities at electroencephalography.
- A history of partial seizures with secondary generalization.
- Generalized abnormalities at neuroimaging.
- A history of first seizure as status epilepticus.

TABLE 18-3 ➤ STAGING OF DISABILITY IN PATIENTS WITH PARKINSON'S DISEASE

Stage I	Unilateral involvement only. Minimal or no functional impairment.
Stage II	Bilateral involvement. No impairment of balance.
Stage III	Evidence of postural imbalance. Some restriction of activities. Mild to moderate disability. Capable of leading an independent life.
Stage IV	Severely disabled. Unable to walk or stand unassisted. Markedly incapacitated.
Stage V	Restricted to bed or a wheelchair unless assisted.

Status epilepticus can be secondary to withdrawal of antiepileptic medication, alcohol withdrawal, drug toxicity, CNS infection, metabolic disorders, and cerebrovascular disease. Treatment is generally initiated with either diazepam or lorazepam, but it may also include phenytoin, valproic acid, phenobarbital, and pentobarbital.

Parkinson's Disease

Doctor James Parkinson first described **Parkinson's disease** in 1817. It is a chronic, progressive disease that occurs in 1% to 3% of the population. The staging of Parkinson's disease is provided in Table 18-3. In the advanced stages, Parkinson's disease produces very dramatic symptoms. In the early stages, initial symptoms may include aching pains, numbness, paresthesias, and coldness (Box 18-2). Most cases of Parkinson's disease occur in individuals who are older than 50 years and are idiopathic. Secondary causes include trauma, tumors, infections, chemicals, and medications. Tremors, a symptom of Parkinson's disease, can also be caused by the medications listed in Box 18-3.

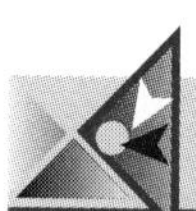

Box 18-2

SIGNS AND SYMPTOMS OF PARKINSON'S DISEASE

SIGNS

- Lewy bodies in the substantia nigra
- Cogwheel rigidity
- Festinating gait
- Frozen, mask-like face
- Postural instability
- Micrographia
- Retropulsion

SYMPTOMS

- Pill-rolling tremor at rest
- Weakness
- Drooling
- Paresthesias
- Numbness
- Aching pains
- Difficulty swallowing

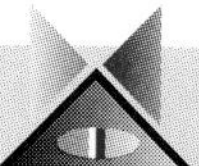

Box 18-3

MEDICATIONS THAT CAN CAUSE TREMORS

- Antipsychotics
- Metoclopramide
- Prochlorperazine
- Reserpine
- Methyldopa
- MPTP
- Tricyclic antidepressants
- Sympathomimetics
- Theophylline
- β-Agonists

Parkinson's is a disease of the extrapyramidal system of the brain—specifically, of the basal ganglia, which is responsible for the maintenance of posture and muscle tone as well as for the regulation of voluntary smooth motor activity. Dopamine is synthesized in the cell bodies of the neurons in the substantia nigra within the basal ganglia, and the loss of these neurons causes the symptoms of Parkinson's disease. Because dopamine, an inhibitory neurotransmitter, is progressively lost within the nigrostriatal tracts, there is a relative increase in the excitatory neurotransmitter, acetylcholine, as well as an onset and increase in severity of Parkinson's symptoms. As a threshold, approximately 80% of the melanin-containing neurons in the substantia nigra are lost before the onset of symptoms.

Traditional treatment has relied on anticholinergics, carbidopa and levodopa combinations, dopamine agonists, and monoamine oxidase B inhibitors. Supportive care, including exercise, physical therapy, speech therapy, and psychologic support, are important components in treatment. New treatments include catechol-*O*-methyltransferase inhibitors and, investigationally, fetal substantia nigra implants.

Cerebrovascular Disease

Cerebrovascular disease is a broad term encompassing disease relating to the blood vessels of the CNS, which is one of the leading causes of morbidity and mortality in the United States. It results from decreased blood flow to the brain (i.e., **ischemia**) or hemorrhage into the CNS with subsequent neurologic dysfunction. Risk factors for developing cerebrovascular disease include:

- Hypertension
- Hyperlipidemia
- Diabetes mellitus
- Cardiac disease

- Increased age
- Carotid bruit
- Increased hematocrit
- Sickle cell disease
- Cigarette smoking
- Male sex
- Alcohol abuse
- Family history
- Previous history of cerebrovascular disease

The signs and symptoms of cerebrovascular disease are listed in Box 18-4. The most common causes of cerebrovascular disease include hypertension and atherosclerosis. Cerebrovascular disease is generally divided into transient ischemic attack and cerebrovascular accident (CVA).

Transient Ischemic Attacks

Transient ischemic attacks are sometimes referred to as "mini-strokes." Neurologic deficits may result from embolism rather than ischemia, and they typically last for fewer than 24 hours. Secondary prevention with aspirin, ticlopidine, clopidrogel, or warfarin is warranted after an initial event, as is reduction in risk factors.

Cerebrovascular Accidents

The three major causes of **cerebrovascular accidents** are hemorrhagic, cardiogenic, and ischemic. On initial presentation to an emergency room, hemorrhagic events are ruled out with computed tomography or magnetic resonance imaging before initiation of therapy. Supportive therapy is the main option that is available for patients with hemorrhagic CVAs. Patients with cardiac disease (e.g., atrial fibrillation, valve replacement, and congestive heart failure) are at increased risk for developing a CVA, and primary prevention with warfarin or aspirin is indicated. Should a cardiogenic CVA occur in these patients, anticoagulation treatment, followed by secondary prevention, is generally effective. Ischemic events are the most common causes of CVAs. If a patient presents within 3 hours of the onset of symptoms, tissue plasminogen-activating factor can improve outcomes; after 3 hours from onset, it can cause an increase in intracranial hemorrhage and should be avoided. After completion of an ischemic stroke, secondary prevention with aspirin, ticlopidine, clopidrogel, or warfarin is warranted, as is management of preexisting risk factors.

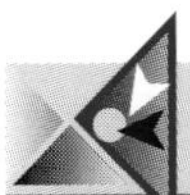

Box 18-4

SIGNS AND SYMPTOMS OF CEREBROVASCULAR DISEASE

SIGNS

- Infarct or hemorrhage on computed tomography scan
- Vital sign changes
- Pupil changes

SYMPTOMS

- Weakness
- Paralysis
- Numbness
- Aphasia
- Visual changes
- Dizziness
- Sudden, severe, and unexplained headache
- Slurred speech
- Paralysis

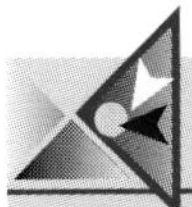

Box 18-5

SIGNS AND SYMPTOMS OF PERIPHERAL NEUROPATHY

SIGNS

- Decreased vibratory sensation
- Decreased temperature and touch sensation

SYMPTOMS

- Weakness
- Numbness
- Tingling
- Glove or stocking sensation
- Constipation
- Diarrhea

Peripheral Neuropathy

Neuropathy, or disease of the peripheral nerves, results from to destruction or dysfunction of the nerve cell body, the axon, or from demyelination. Peripheral neuropathies can be divided into motor, sensory, and autonomic neuropathies. Causes of peripheral neuropathies are numerous, including autoimmune processes, tumors (e.g., lung cancer, multiple myeloma, and chronic lymphocytic leukemia), radiation therapy, infections (e.g., human immunodeficiency virus), vitamin deficiencies, trauma or compression, and medications. The leading cause of peripheral neuropathies that a pharmacist will see is secondary to diabetes. Approximately half of all patients with diabetes develop some degree of peripheral neuropathy throughout their disease. Signs and symptoms of peripheral neuropathies are listed in Box 18-5 and are dependent on the nerves that are affected. Treatment is aimed at controlling symptoms but is generally unsatisfactory and includes medications such as tricyclic antidepressants, NSAIDs, narcotics, anticonvulsants, and capsaicin.

SYSTEM ASSESSMENT

Subjective Information

When assessing the nervous system, subjective patient information can provide valuable data; therefore, it is important for the pharmacist to ask the patient appropriate questions.

Headache

? INTERVIEW Do you ever experience headaches? If so, when does the pain start? How long does it last? Have you had this type of headache before? How often do you experience headaches? Can you tell that it is coming on?

ABNORMALITIES Approximately one-quarter of patients with migraine experience an aura before their headache. Patients with cluster headaches may be woken up from sleep, and the headache may last for only 30 to 90 minutes.

? INTERVIEW Describe the pain. Is it pulsating or throbbing? Is it a pressure or squeezing type of pain? A stabbing pain?

ABNORMALITIES Migraine headaches are generally described as a pulsating or throbbing pain, tension headaches as a pressure or squeezing pain, and cluster headaches as a sharp, stabbing pain.

? INTERVIEW Where is the pain? Is it on one side of the head or on both? Is it across the forehead? Behind one eye?

ABNORMALITIES Migraine and cluster headaches are more often unilateral, occurring on one side of the head. Tension headaches are generally bilateral.

? INTERVIEW What makes the headache better or go away? What makes it worse?

ABNORMALITIES Migraine headaches are worsened with activity; tension headaches are generally not affected by activity. A dark, quiet room or sleep will help to relieve migraine headaches.

? INTERVIEW Do you notice any other symptoms with your headache? Nausea or vomiting? Sensitivity to light or sound? Watery eyes or runny nose?

ABNORMALITIES During cluster headaches, patients can experience watery eyes and rhinorrhea, especially on the side affected by the pain. Nausea, vomiting, photophobia, and phonophobia classically occur with migraine headaches.

Seizures

? INTERVIEW Have you ever experienced any seizures? If so,

Onset and duration: When did your last seizure occur? How often do they occur? How long do they last?

Location: Where do the seizures begin? Do they travel through the body? They occur on one or both sides?

Symptoms: Describe the seizure.

ABNORMALITIES See Table 18-3 for the differences between seizure types.

? INTERVIEW

Causes: What can cause you to have a seizure?

Relief: Has anything helped you to have fewer seizures? Are you currently on, or have you ever been on, any medications for seizures?

Symptoms: Do you experience any other symptoms with your seizures? Do you ever know when you are going to have a seizure? After a seizure, are you told that you spend time sleeping or have any confusion, weakness, headaches, or muscle aches?

ABNORMALITIES Patients who experience an aura before a generalized seizure are actually having a partial seizure that secondarily generalizes. Patients with a tonic-clonic seizure disorder have a postictal phase, during which they may be tired, confused, weak, and complain of muscle pain.

Paresthesia

? INTERVIEW Do you ever have numbness or tingling in your hands or feet? If so, how long has the numbness and tingling been going on? How frequently does this occur?

ABNORMALITIES Peripheral neuropathies tend to be a chronic numbness and tingling, in which temporary nerve compression can also occur and cause similar symptoms, that resolves in a short period of time.

? INTERVIEW

Location: Where are the numbness and tingling occurring?

Symptoms: Describe the numbness and tingling. Do you have any other symptoms associated with the numbness and tingling? What makes it worse?

Relief: Does anything make it better or go away?

Past history: Do you have any past history of neurologic problems? Headaches? Epilepsy? Stroke? High cholesterol? Diabetes? Irregular heartbeat? Any cardiovascular problems? Parkinson's disease?

Family history: Have any immediate family members had neurologic disease? Seizures? Headaches? Stroke?

Medication history: What prescription and nonprescription medications are you currently taking? Do you currently, or have you ever taken in the past, any medications for seizures? For headaches? Stroke prevention? Mental illness?

Social history: Do you smoke or chew tobacco? If so, how much each day? For how many years? Do you drink caffeine? If so, how much each day? Has your intake changed? Do you drink alcohol? If so, how much each day or week? For how many years?

ABNORMALITIES The location of the numbness and tingling can guide the examiner in the physical examination to determine the placement of a nerve injury. Symmetrical distal sensory loss suggests a polyneuropathy. If bilateral, it suggests a "glove and stocking" sensory loss such as that seen with diabetes or alcoholism. Medication history can help rule out a drug-related cause of the paresthesia.

Objective Information

Objective information pertaining to the nervous system primarily includes the physical assessment and diagnostic tests.

Physical Assessment

Physical assessment of the nervous system is complex, and for efficiency, certain portions should be integrated with other parts of the patient's examination (e.g., cranial nerves can be observed during examination of the head and neck). A neurologic examination should be organized into five sections: (1) mental status (see Chapter 19), (2) cranial nerves, (3) the motor or musculoskeletal system (see Chapter 17), (4) the sensory system, and (5) reflexes.

Cranial Nerve I: Olfactory

Ordinarily, taste and smell are not evaluated unless a problem is suspected. Quite often, patients do not recognize that they have lost sensory activity. Therefore, when a sensory loss is suspected, test the relevant cranial nerve.

TECHNIQUE

STEP 1

Test for Sense of Smell

- Use the least irritating odor (e.g., peppermint, vanilla, or toothpaste).
- Ask the patient to close both eyes and to occlude one nostril.
- Place the substance beneath the patient's nose.
- Ask the patient to sniff and then identify the smell.

ABNORMALITIES Normally, smell decreases as patients age; however, any asymmetry is important. Upper respiratory tract infections, tobacco or cocaine use, a frontal lobe lesion, or a fracture in the nasal area can all cause an abnormal sense of smell.

Cranial Nerve II: Optic

The optic nerve is generally tested during the eye examination, which includes visual acuity, visual fields, light reflex, and direct inspection. (For the assessment of cranial nerve II, see Chapter 9.)

Cranial Nerves III, IV, and VI: Oculomotor, Trochlear, and Abducens

Movement of the eyes through the six cardinal points of gaze; pupil size, shape, response to light, and accommodation; and opening of upper eyelids are described in Chapter 9. Although the assessment technique is not described here, the pharmacist should be aware of potential abnormalities with cranial nerves III, IV, and VI that may relate to use of medication. Nystagmus is the constant, involuntary movement of the eye in a cyclical pattern and is a classic adverse effect associated with antiseizure medications, particularly in cases of toxicity or overdose.

Cranial Nerve V: Trigeminal

Assessment of cranial nerve V is illustrated in Figure 18-8.

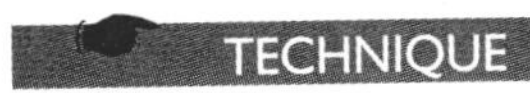

STEP 1

Inspect and Palpate the Face

- Observe the face for muscle atrophy or deviation of the jaw to one side.
- While palpating the masseter and temporal muscles, have the patient clench the teeth. Note the strength of the muscle contraction.

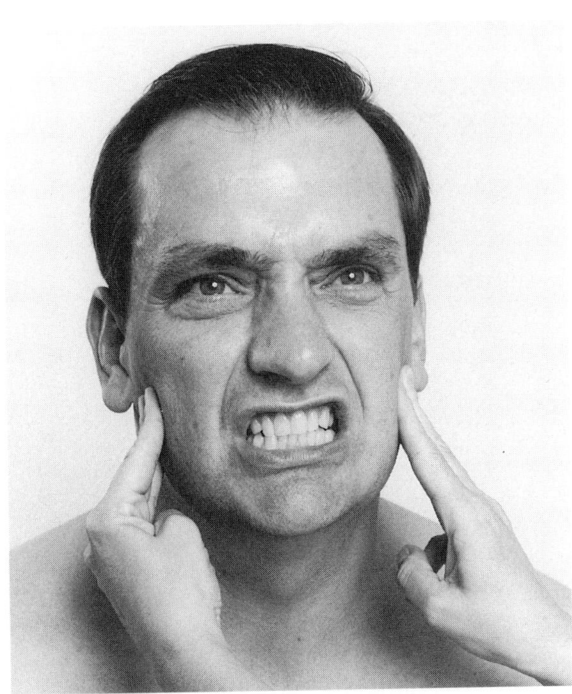

FIGURE 18-8 ■ Assessment of cranial nerve V.

ABNORMALITIES A unilateral weakness occurs with a cranial nerve V lesion. A bilateral weakness can occur with either peripheral nervous system or CNS involvement.

CAUTION Cranial nerve V may be difficult to assess in patients without teeth.

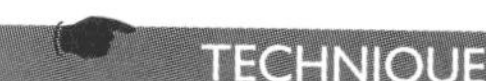

STEP 2

Evaluate Superficial Touch Sensations

- Have the patient close his or her eyes.
- Touch each side of the face at the scalp, cheek, and chin areas. Alternate using the sharp and smooth edge of a paper clip or a broken tongue blade.

CAUTION Do not use a predictable pattern. Do not scratch the patient.

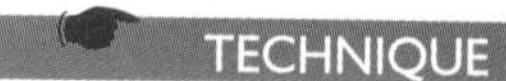

STEP 2 (Continued)

- Ask the patient to report the sensation of dull or sharp.
- Repeat with a cotton wisp or brush, and ask when the stimulus is felt.

ABNORMALITIES Absent touch and pain or paresthesias can be caused by tumor, trauma, trigeminal neuralgia, or sequelae of alcohol ingestion.

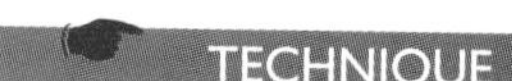

STEP 3

Test for the Corneal Reflex

Assessment of the corneal reflex is illustrated in Figure 18-9.

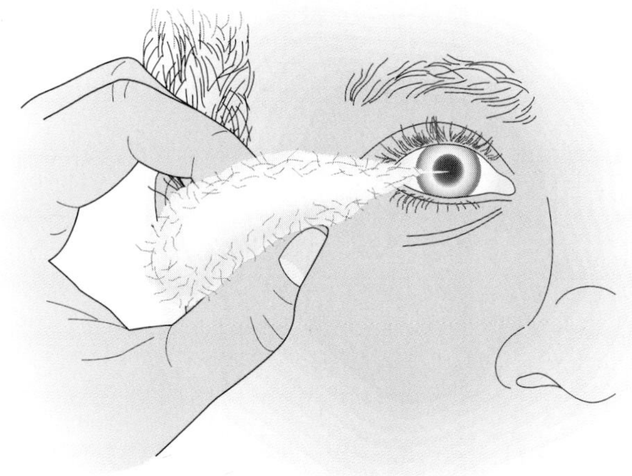

FIGURE 18-9 ■ Assessment of the corneal reflex.

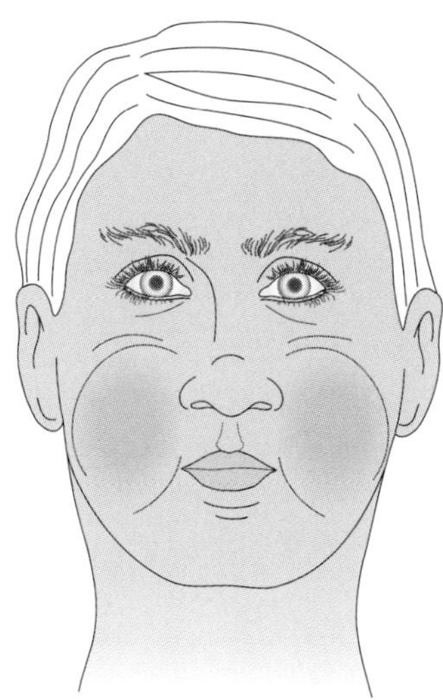

FIGURE 18-10 ■ Assessment of cranial nerve VII.

- Ask the patient look up and away from you, and approach from the other side.
- Lightly touch the cornea of one eye with a cotton wisp.
- Repeat with the other side.
- A symmetric blink reflex should occur.

CAUTION Contact lenses, if worn, should be removed. Patients with contact lenses may have a decreased or absent corneal reflex.

Cranial Nerve VII: Facial

Assessment of cranial nerve VII is illustrated in Figure 18-10.

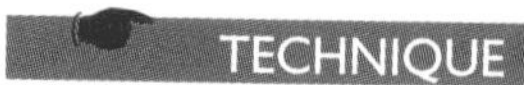

STEP 1

Observe Motor Function

- Have the patient perform the following expressions:
  Raise the eyebrows.
  Squeeze the eyes shut against force.
  Wrinkle the forehead.
  Frown.
  Smile.
  Show the teeth.
  Purse the lips to whistle.
  Puff out the cheeks.
- Observe for unusual facial movements, tics, and asymmetry of expression.

ABNORMALITIES A peripheral injury affects both the upper and lower face; a central lesion affects the lower face. In unilateral facial paralysis, the mouth droops on the affected side when the patient smiles or grimaces.

Cranial Nerve VIII: Acoustic

Hearing is evaluated using an audiometer or the simple screening tests described in Chapter 9. The Romberg test can be used to test vestibular function; however, because it is more commonly used to assess gait and balance, it is outlined later in this chapter.

Cranial Nerves IX and X: Glossopharyngeal and Vagus

The glossopharyngeal nerve is tested simultaneously with the vagus nerve for gag reflex and motor function of swallowing (see Chapter 10).

Cranial Nerve XI: Spinal Accessory

Assessment of cranial nerve X is illustrated in Figure 18-11.

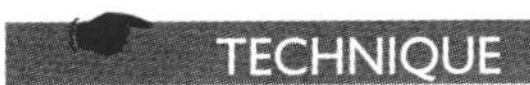
TECHNIQUE

STEP 1

Observe Motor Function

- Inspect for atrophy or abnormalities from behind the patient.
- Ask the patient to shrug both shoulders upward against your hands while applying a light pressure.
- Ask the patient to turn his or her head to each side against your hand.
- Observe the contraction of the sternocleidomastoid muscle, and note the force against your hand.

ABNORMALITIES Weakness with atrophy and fasciculation indicates a peripheral nerve disorder. When the trapezius muscle is paralyzed, the shoulder droops, and the scapula is displaced downward and laterally.

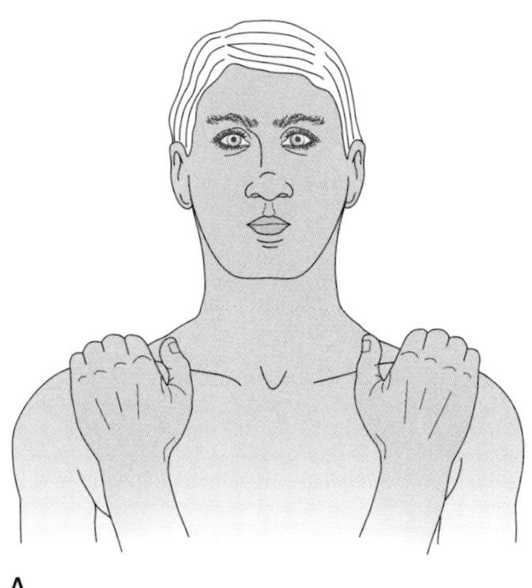

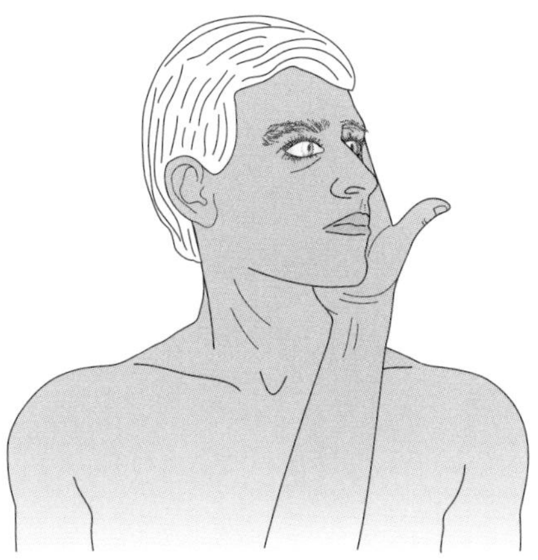

FIGURE 18-11 ■ Assessment of cranial nerve XI. **(A)** Shrugging shoulders against pressure. **(B)** Turning head against pressure.

Cranial Nerve XII: Hypoglossal

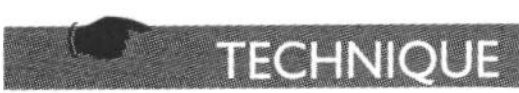
TECHNIQUE

STEP 1

Inspect the Tongue

- Inspect the tongue as it lies on the floor of the mouth. Look for any atrophy or fasciculations.
- Ask the patient to protrude his or her tongue. Look for any deviations, atrophy, or asymmetry.

ABNORMALITIES Atrophy and fasciculations suggest peripheral nerve disease. When protruded, the tongue deviates to the side of the lesion.

Motor System

Abnormal positions of the body during movement and at rest can alert you to neurologic deficits such as paralysis. Inspect for atrophy of muscles, muscle tone, and strength. In addition to the physical examination techniques described in Chapter 17, gait, balance, and coordination should be examined.

Gait and Balance

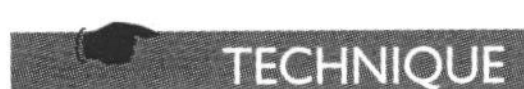
TECHNIQUE

STEP 1 Assess the Patient's Gait

Gait can be changed by both musculoskeletal and neurologic disorders. Chapter 17 details the technique to examine gait; however, alterations in gait that result from neurologic abnormalities are discussed here.

ABNORMALITIES Gait can be abnormal in many ways, including spastic hemiparesis, spastic diplegia (i.e., "scissoring"), steppage, cerebellar or sensory ataxia, and parkinsonian festinating (Fig. 18-12). Spastic hemiparesis typically occurs in patients with cerebrovascular accident. The paralyzed foot is fixed in a plantar flexion and is dragged in a semicircular fashion when walking. The paralyzed arm is fixed across the body and is flexed at the shoulder, elbow and wrist. Spastic diplegia often is associated with multiple sclerosis. In these cases, the knees cross or touch ("scissoring"), which requires short steps and great effort to walk effectively. Steppage typically occurs with lower motor nerve disease and may be associated with foot drop, diabetic neuropathy, or both. Patients who walk with a steppage gait lift their legs higher than normal, with knees bent and ankles flexed, as if walking up stairs. Cerebellar and sen-

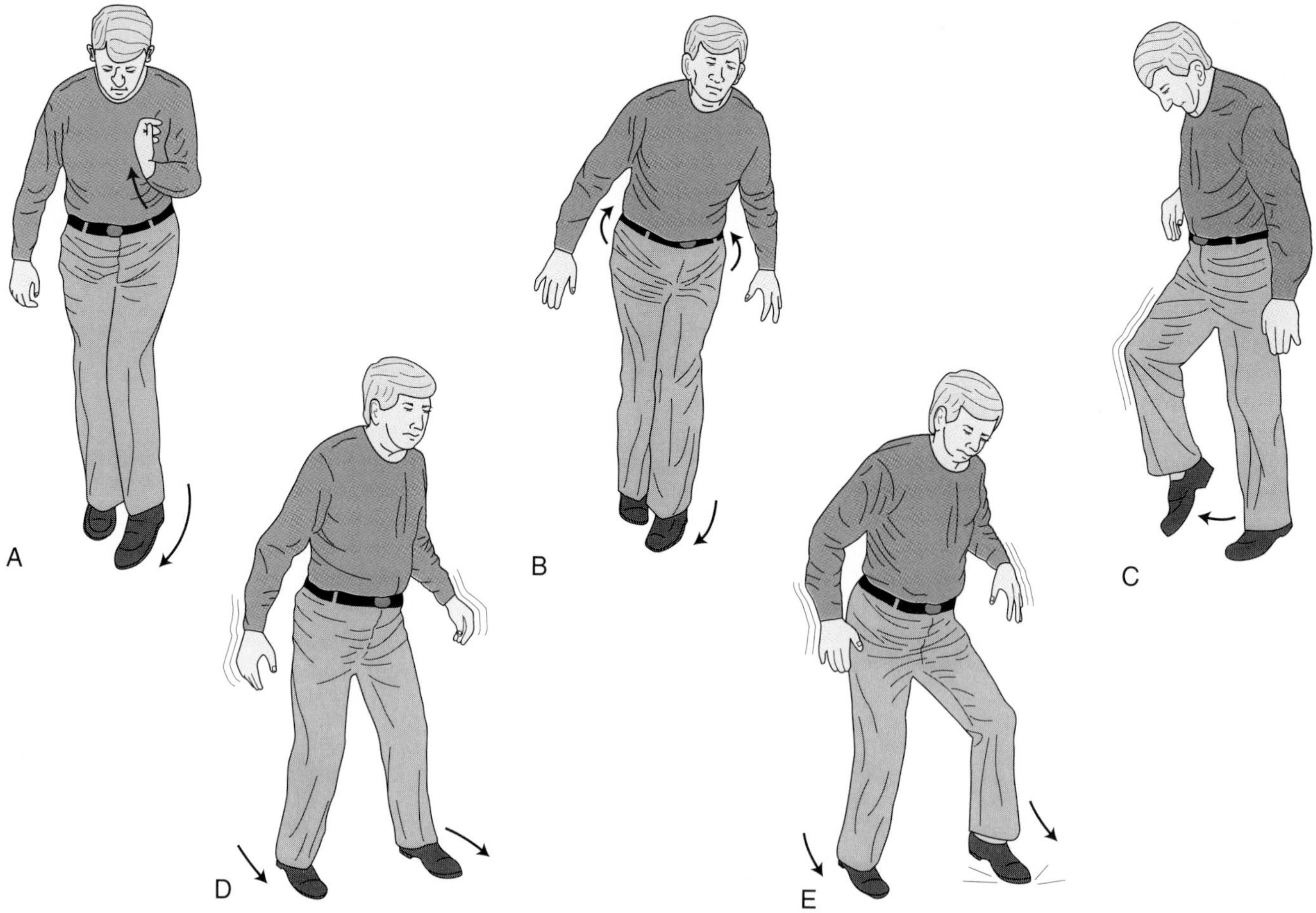

Figure 18-12 ■ Abnormalities of gait. **(A)** Spastic hemiparesis. **(B)** Spastic diplegia (scissoring). **(C)** Steppage gait. **(D)** Cerebellar ataxia. **(E)** Sensory ataxia.

sory ataxia are associated with a wide-based, staggering gait. Sensory ataxia is more commonly related to polyneuropathy; cerebellar ataxia is often a toxicity related to drugs. Alcohol, barbiturates, and phenytoin are associated with cerebellar ataxia. Festinating includes the stooped posture and classic shuffling (i.e., short, hurried steps) associated with Parkinson's disease.

TECHNIQUE

STEP 2

Perform the Romberg test

The Romberg test is illustrated in Figure 18-13.

- Ask the patient to stand up, with his or her feet together and arms to the side.
- Once the patient is in a stable position, ask the patient to close his or her eyes and then hold that position.
- Wait 20 to 30 seconds.
- A person should be able to maintain posture and balance even without visual orientation.

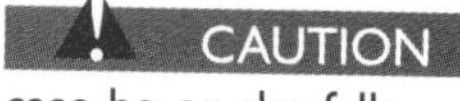

Stand close to catch the person in case he or she falls.

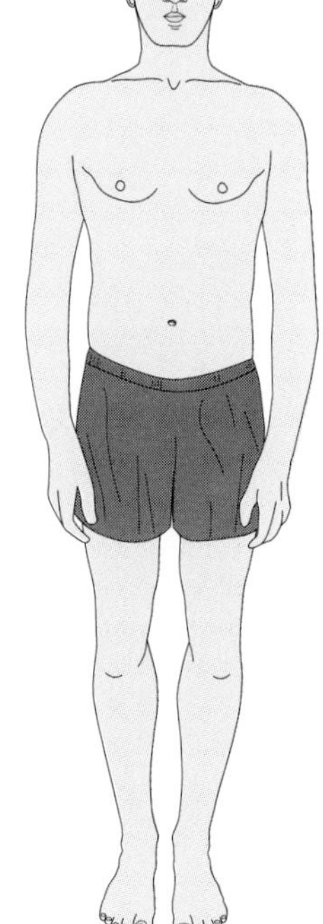

Figure 18-13 ■ Evaluation of balance with the Romberg test.

ABNORMALITIES A positive Romberg sign (i.e., swaying, falling, or widening the base of the feet to avoid falling) occurs in cerebellar ataxia, multiple sclerosis, alcohol intoxication, and vestibular dysfunction.

TECHNIQUE

STEP 3

Assess the Patient's Balance

- Have the patient stand in front of you.
- Pull backward on the patient's shoulders.

CAUTION Stand close enough to catch the patient in case he or she falls.

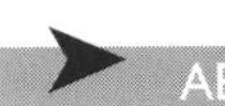

ABNORMALITIES **Retropulsion,** or falling backward when you pull on the patient's shoulders, is a sign of Parkinson's disease.

Coordination

Coordination requires that four areas of the nervous system work in an integrated way. These areas include:

- The motor system
- The cerebellar system
- The vestibular system
- The sensory system

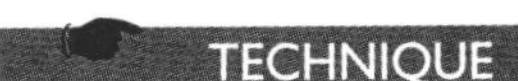

TECHNIQUE

STEP 1

Assess the Patient's Ability to Perform Rapid, Alternating Movements

- Ask the patient to pat his or her knees with both hands, lift the hands up, turn the hands over, and pat the knees with the back of the hands.
- Ask the patient to do this faster.
- Ask the person to tap the thumb to each finger on the same hand, starting with the index finger and then reversing directions.

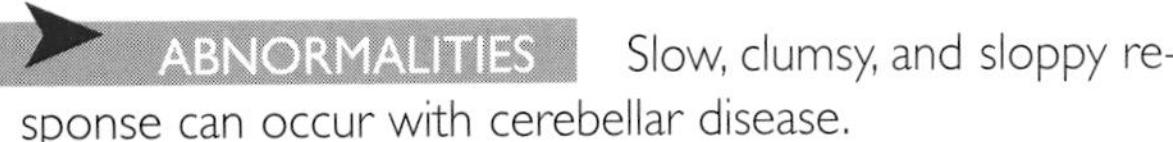

ABNORMALITIES Slow, clumsy, and sloppy response can occur with cerebellar disease.

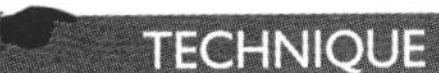

TECHNIQUE

STEP 2

Assess the Patient's Ability to Perform Point-to-Point Movements

- With the patient's eyes open, ask that he or she use the index finger to touch your finger and then his or her nose.
- After a few times, move your finger to a different spot.
- Ask the patient to place one heel on the opposite knee and then run it down the shin to the big toe.
- Repeat on each side, with and without the patient's eyes being open.

ABNORMALITIES With cerebellar disease, movements are uncoordinated, clumsy, and inappropriately varied in speed, force, and direction. The heel or finger may overshoot its mark, and performance with the eyes closed is generally poor.

Sensory Testing

To accurately assess the sensory system, patients must be calm, alert, and cooperative. If no abnormalities are suspected, then assessing light touch in the arms and legs or vibration and pain in the extremities is typically adequate. Adhere to the following guidelines when assessing sensory function:

- Assess body symmetry.
- When assessing position, perception, or vibration, examine the knuckles.
- When assessing touch, temperature, or pain, evaluate distal and proximal sensations in relation to each other.
- Avoid repetition to ensure true patient response.

ABNORMALITIES Unusual findings, including pain, weakness, or atrophy, require further investigation.

Evaluation of the primary sensory functions is illustrated in Figure 18-14.

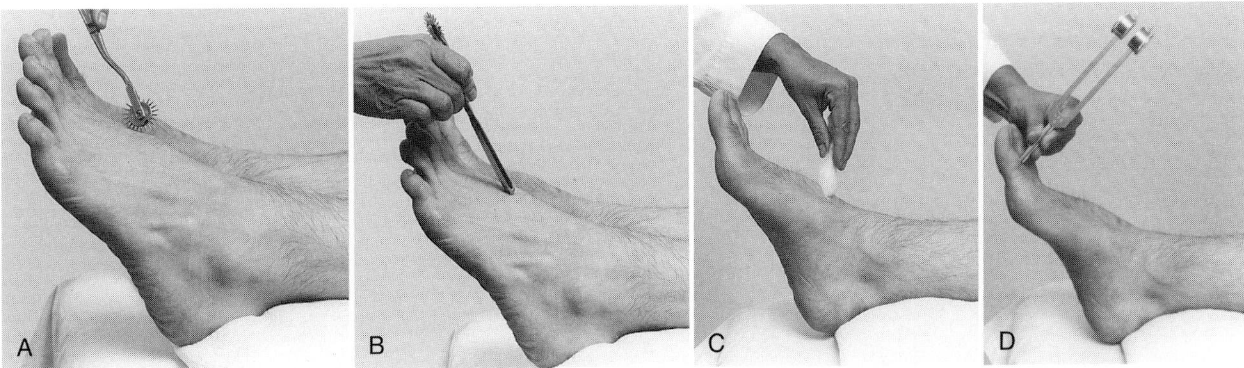

FIGURE 18-14 ■ Evaluation of primary sensory functions. **(A)** Sharp: touch various areas of the skin with a sharp object; alternate with a dull object. **(B)** Dull: touch various areas of the skin with a dull object; alternate with a sharp object. **(C)** Light touch: stroke a cotton wisp or brush lightly over the skin. **(D)** Vibration: place the stem of a vibrating tuning fork against bony prominences.

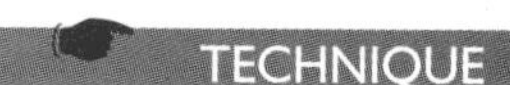

TECHNIQUE

STEP 1

Test the Response to Pain

- Using a safety pin or broken tongue blade, apply pressure of varying degrees with both the sharp and dull ends of the pin (Fig. 18-14*A*, *B*).
- Ask the patient, "Is this sharp or dull? Does this feel the same as this?"

CAUTION Use a light stimulus. Do not draw blood.

TECHNIQUE

STEP 2

Test the Ability to Sense Temperature, Light Touch, and Vibration

- Testing for temperature sensation is generally not done except when pain sensation is abnormal or in question. If necessary, distal and proximal sensations are tested using hot and cold water.
- Use a fine wisp of cotton to determine light touch (Fig. 18-14*C*).
- Brush cotton over the skin at varying areas and intervals.
- Ask the patient to identify when the touch is felt.
- To test vibration, tap on the heel of your hand with a low-pitched tuning fork, and place the tuning fork on the distal interphalangeal joint over a patient's finger and big toe (Fig. 18-14*D*).
- Ask the patient, "What do you feel?"
- If the patient is uncertain, ask "When does the vibration stop?"

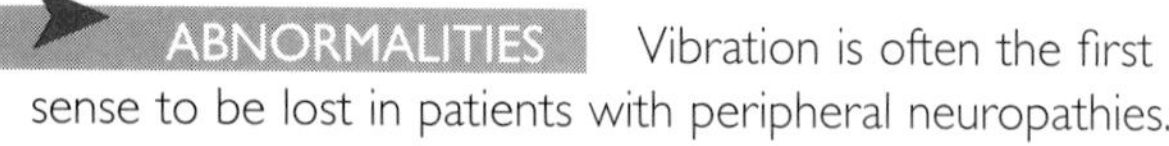

ABNORMALITIES Vibration is often the first sense to be lost in patients with peripheral neuropathies.

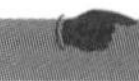

TECHNIQUE

STEP 3

Assess the Ability to Recognize Items by Touch and Manipulation

The ability to recognize items by touch and manipulation is termed **stereognosis.** Evaluation of stereognosis is illustrated in Figure 18-15.

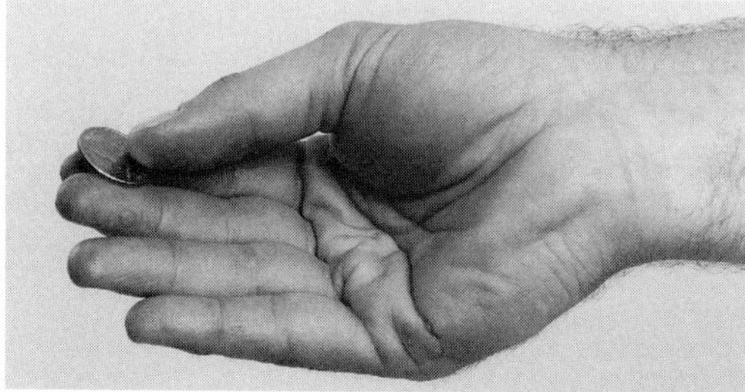

FIGURE 18-15 ■ Evaluation of stereognosis: patient identifies an object by touch.

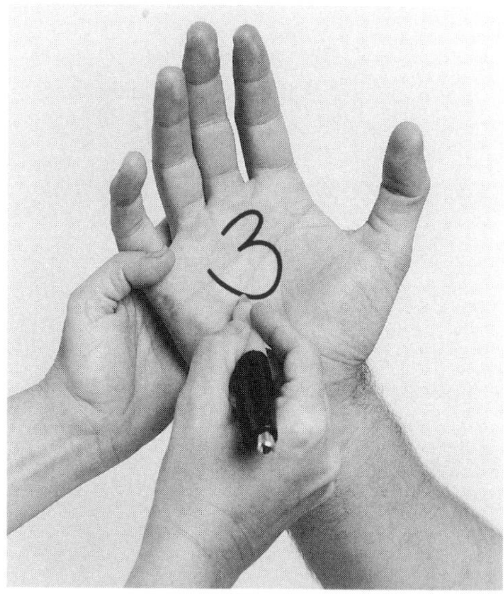

FIGURE 18-16 ■ Evaluation of graphesthesia: patient identifies a letter or number drawn on the body.

- Ask the patient to close his or her eyes.
- Hand the patient a familiar object (e.g., a key or paper clip), and ask the patient to identify the item by touch and manipulation.

ABNORMALITIES Inability to recognize objects by touch may indicate a parietal lobe or sensory cortex lesion.

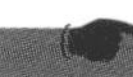

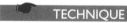

TECHNIQUE

STEP 4

Assess the Ability to Identify a Letter or Number Traced on the Skin

The ability to identify a letter or number traced on the skin is termed **graphesthesia.** Evaluation of graphesthesia is illustrated in Figure 18-16.

- Ask the patient to close his or her eyes.
- With a blunt object, trace a letter or number on the palm of the patient's hand, and ask the patient to identify it.

ABNORMALITIES Inability to identify the traced letter or number may indicate a sensory cortex lesion.

Reflexes

Reflex response partially depends on the force of the stimulus. Use only the force needed to elicit a definite response. It is easier to assess differences between sides than it is to assess symmetric changes in reflexes. Symmetrically diminished reflexes can be present in patients without pathology. Reflexes are usually graded on a 0 to 4+ scale:

- 4+: very brisk, hyperactive, with clonus.
- 3+: brisker than average; possibly, but not necessarily, indicative of disease.
- 2+: average, normal.
- 1+: somewhat diminished.
- 0: No response.

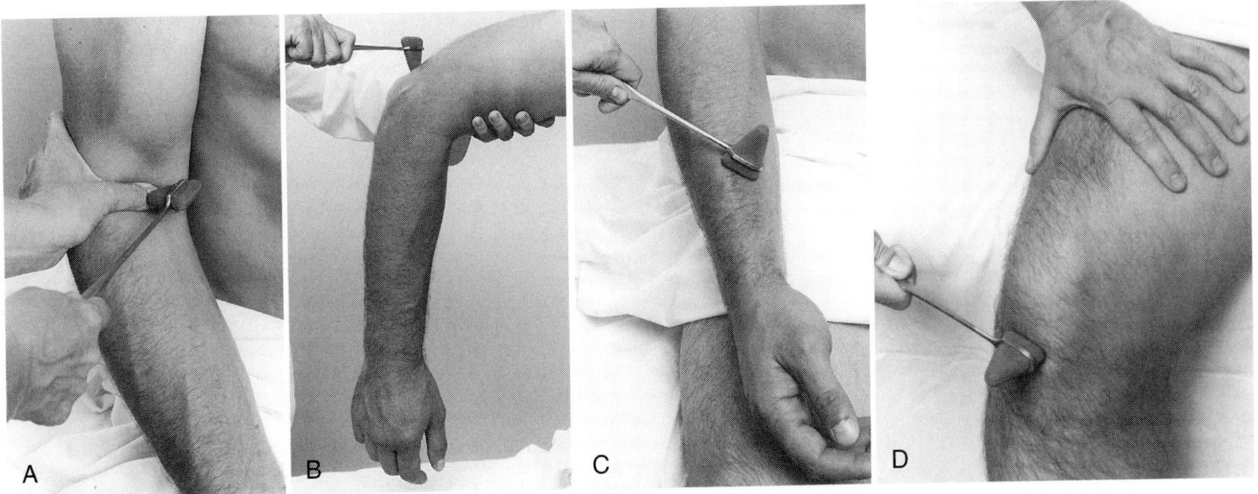

FIGURE 18-17 ■ Evaluation of deep tendon reflexes. **(A)** Biceps. **(B)** Triceps. **(C)** Brachioradialis. **(D)** Patellar (quadriceps).

Deep tendon reflexes include the biceps, brachioradial, triceps, patellar, and Achilles reflexes.

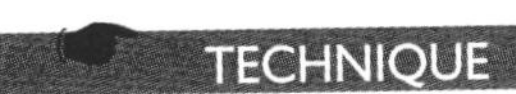

STEP 1

Assess for Deep Tendon Reflexes

Evaluation for deep tendon reflexes is illustrated in Figure 18-17.

- Persuade the patient to relax and to position properly and symmetrically, with the limbs relaxed and the muscles partially stretched.
- Swing the rubber hammer freely between your thumb and index finger, and strike the tendon briskly, using a rapid wrist movement. The strike should be quick and direct.

ABNORMALITIES Deep tendon reflexes can be diminished in patients with hypothyroidism and spinal cord injuries. **Hyperreflexia** (i.e., an exaggerated response) may be seen during a CVA.

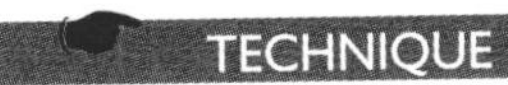

STEP 2

Evaluation of Plantar Reflex

Evaluation of the plantar reflex is illustrated in Figure 18-18.

- Have the patient sit or lie down, with the leg stretched out on the table in front.
- With an object such as a wooden end of an applicator stick, stroke the lateral aspect of the sole from the heel to the ball of the foot, curving medially across the ball.
- Note the movement of the toes (normally flexion).

ABNORMALITIES Dorsiflexion of the big toe, which is generally accompanied by fanning of the other toes, is a positive Babinski sign. It often indicates a CNS lesion, or it may occur in unconscious states resulting from drug and alcohol intoxication. This sign is normal in newborns and infants during the first year of life.

Laboratory and Diagnostic Tests

The following diagnostic tests may be useful when assessing the nervous system:

- A computed tomographic scan, with or without enhancement using contrast material, can be useful to identify areas of atrophy, trauma, hemorrhage, and tumors.
- An electroencephalogram is a graphic illustration of the brain's electrical impulses and can be useful in identifying seizure disorders and focal neurologic deficits.
- Magnetic resonance imaging is a noninvasive test that can be useful in depicting more defined areas of the brain and spinal cord to identify hemorrhage, ischemia, and other pathologies.
- A lumbar puncture is a procedure in which a needle is placed into the lumbar spine and CSF is withdrawn. It is commonly used in the diagnosis of meningitis and cancer.

Special Considerations

Pediatric Patients

Pediatric patients require additional questions to be asked of the parent or guardian.

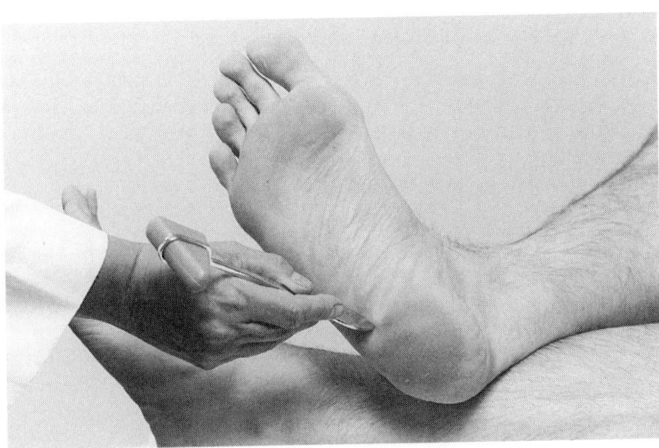

FIGURE 18-18 ■ Evaluation of plantar reflex.

? INTERVIEW Did the mother have any health problems during the pregnancy? Any illnesses, medications, hypertension, alcohol or drug use, diabetes, or seizures? Tell me about the baby's birth. Was the baby full-term or preterm? Any birth trauma or complications? Congenital defects? What have you noticed about the baby's behavior? Does the child seem to have any problems with balance? Did the child's motor or developmental milestones seem to come at the right age? How does the child compare to siblings or age-mates?

ABNORMALITIES Prenatal drug and alcohol use by the mother can result in deficiencies in the neurologic development of an infant (Fetal alcohol syndrome)

Developmental delays in motor skills may indicate a need to screen for muscular dystrophy or lead exposure.

The neurologic system shows dramatic growth and development during the first year of life. Assess an infant for milestones that you would normally expect to see achieved. After the newborn period, assess to determine whether the early, more primitive reflexes have disappeared. Generally, neurologic problems are suspected when the child is not doing something that most children of the same age can. A delay in motor activity can occur with brain damage, mental retardation, peripheral neuromuscular damage, prolonged illness, or parental neglect. In an older child, much of the motor assessment can be obtained from watching the child walk, dress, and manipulate buttons.

The patellar reflex is present at birth; however, the Achilles and brachioradial reflexes do not appear until 6 months of age. When testing reflexes in an infant, the examiner should tap with a finger instead of the reflex hammer. Deep tendon reflexes are rarely tested in children younger than 5 years, because they usually are unable to relax fully.

Sensory integrity is generally shown by withdrawal from painful stimuli. When assessing the cranial nerves, child-specific assessments may be required to accurately measure the response. When testing the olfactory nerve, children may recognize a certain smell, but they may not be able to connect it to a specific product. Instead, ask the child, "What does this smell like to you?" In examining the trigeminal nerve, observe the patient chewing to assess jaw strength. When examining the facial nerve, observe the child's facial expressions, including smiling, frowning, and crying. Ask the child to puff his or her cheeks or to show his teeth. The spinal accessory and hypoglossal nerves may be difficult to evaluate in young children; ask older children to shrug their shoulders or stick out their tongue.

Geriatric Patients

Geriatric patients also require additional questions to be asked of the patient or caregiver.

? INTERVIEW Do you take care of your medicine by yourself at home? Does anyone help you with your medicine? What do you do when you forget your medicine?

ABNORMALITIES Noncompliance with medications is a common problem in the elderly and could be related to forgetfulness or other neurologic deficits.

? INTERVIEW Any problem with dizziness? When you first stand up? When you move your head? When getting up during the night?

ABNORMALITIES Changes in vascular muscle tone can increase the incidence of dizziness in the elderly. Medications, such as β-blockers and other medication with anticholinergic side effects or used to treat hypertension, can cause orthostatic hypotension which may cause the elderly to experience dizziness with a change in body position.

The same examination is used with geriatric patients as with younger adults. Although nerves for taste and smell are not usually tested, they may have declined in function. Senile tremors, tremors on intention in the hands, head nodding, and tongue protrusion can occur. The gait may be slower and more deliberate than in younger adults and may deviate from midline. Loss of the sensation of vibration, especially in the ankle, is common once patients are older than 65 years. Deep tendon reflexes are less brisk.

Pregnant Patients

Pregnant patients also require additional questions to be asked.

? INTERVIEW Have you ever had a seizure in the past or during previous pregnancies? Hypertension during previous pregnancies? Headaches associated with previous pregnancies?

ABNORMALITIES Women with a history of seizures, diabetes, or hypertension are considered to have a high risk pregnancy and require closer monitoring for management of their chronic disease and minimalization of risk to the fetus from the disease itself (seizures), medications used to control the disease (diabetes), or complications from the disease (diabetes, hypertension). Migraines may worsen during pregnancy due to the hormone changes.

The neurologic physical examination is the same in pregnant women as in nonpregnant adults. Baseline deep tendon reflexes can be useful in monitoring symptoms of pregnancy-induced hypertension.

APPLICATION TO PATIENT SYMPTOMS

Because the pharmacist typically practices in a setting where the patient presents with a specific symptom, the pharmacist must be able to assess the patient's symptoms, to identify the probable cause, and to determine the most appropriate action. Common symptoms relating to the neurologic system include headache, seizure, and paresthesias.

TABLE 18-4 ➤ DIFFERENTIATING CHARACTERISTICS OF HEADACHE PAIN

CHARACTERISTICS	MIGRAINE	CLUSTER	TENSION	SINUS
Onset and duration	Morning hours most common, lasts 4–72 hours	Early morning hours, lasts 30–90 minutes	Later in the day, variable duration (hours to weeks)	Throughout the day, generally lasts for hours or until precipitating event is resolved.
Severity	Mild to severe	Excruciating	Mild to moderate	Mild to moderate
Type of pain	Throbbing, unilateral	Stabbing, unilateral	Pressure, bilateral	Pressure, primarily behind the eyes and forehead
Associated symptoms	Nausea, vomiting, photophobia, phonophobia	Tearing of the eye, rhinorrhea, drooping of the eye	Tiredness, irritability	Nasal stuffiness, rhinorrhea
Relieved by	Rest, quiet, dark space, medications	Short-acting medications (injectable or nasal spray)	Rest, exercise, analgesics	Hot showers, decongestants

Headache

Headaches are a common patient complaint and are routinely self-treated with both over-the-counter pharmacologic agents and nonpharmacologic therapies. Most headaches present with similar symptoms, but specific characteristics may differentiate the various classifications. Table 18-4 lists the differentiating characteristics of headache pain. Medications and other drugs that may cause headache pain are listed in Box 18-6.

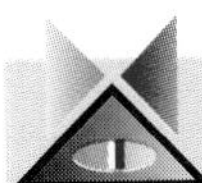

Box 18-6

MEDICATIONS THAT CAN CAUSE HEADACHES

- Alcohol
- Caffeine (and withdrawal)
- Cocaine
- Corticosteroids (and withdrawal)
- Ergotamine (and withdrawal)
- Estrogens and oral contraceptives
- Fluoxetine
- Nonsteroidal anti-inflammatory drugs
- Sympathomimetics
- Vasodilators

CASE STUDY

PM is a 39-year-old white woman who comes into the pharmacy to refill her medications for her headaches. She has a long history of headaches, dating back to when she was a teenager. She states that the medication does not seem to be working all that well anymore.

ASSESSMENT OF THE PATIENT

Subjective Information

39-year-old white woman complaining of headaches

WHERE IS THE PAIN? It normally occurs on the left side of my head.

COULD YOU DESCRIBE THE PAIN? It hurts tremendously, and my head feels like someone is hitting it. It throbs.

HOW LONG DOES IT LAST? Normally for a day, maybe two at the most, but it is pretty constant for the most part during that time.

HOW OFTEN DO THE HEADACHES OCCUR? About two or three times a month.

HAS THAT CHANGED? Yes, I used to only get them about once every couple of months, but over the last six months, it has become more consistent.

DO YOU EVER KNOW WHEN YOU ARE GOING TO GET A HEADACHE? Not really.

DO YOU EVER NOTICE ANYTHING ELSE WITH YOUR HEADACHES OTHER THAN THE PAIN? I get very nauseated and vomit. Bright lights and loud sounds really bother me.

IS THERE ANYTHING THAT CAUSES YOUR HEADACHES? I get one after I eat Chinese food, but that hasn't really changed.

DOES ANYTHING MAKE THE PAIN WORSE? It worsens the more I do.

DOES ANYTHING MAKE THE PAIN BETTER? If I can lie down and go to sleep in a quiet, dark room it seems to help, and the Imitrex.

DOES ANYONE ELSE IN YOUR FAMILY HAVE THE SAME KIND OF HEADACHES? No.

Continued

What medications do you take, both over-the-counter and prescription? I am taking Ortho-Novum 1/35, Imitrex, and verapamil.

Any vitamins or herbal products? I take a multivitamin every day, but that is all.

How often do you forget your medicines? I only take the Imitrex when I need it, but I don't miss my birth control, multivitamin, or verapamil.

How much caffeine do you have every day? I generally have two diet sodas a day.

Objective Information:

Computerized medication profile:

- Imitrex: 25 mg tablets, one at onset, may repeat in 2 hours; No. 9; Refills: 11; Patient obtains refills every 30 to 60 days.
- Ortho-Novum 1/35: 28-day pack, one tablet daily; No. 84; Refills: 2; Patient obtains refills every 84 days, started 6 months ago.
- Verapamil SR: 180 mg, one tablet daily; No. 30; Refills: 11; Patient obtains refills every 30 days.

Patient in no acute distress
Gait normal
Oriented to person, place, and time
Neurologic examination negative
Cranial nerves II–XII intact
Heart rate: 80 bpm
Blood pressure: 124/78 mm Hg
Respiratory rate: 18 rpm

DISCUSSION

The concern centers on the occurrence of PM's headaches. PM states that the quality and severity of her headaches have not changed, but that they have become more frequent during the past 6 months. The pharmacist first must try to determine why the headaches are changing in frequency. PM recently started on Ortho-Novum 1/35, which could exacerbate her migraine headaches. Her caffeine intake, although not identified as a trigger by PM, may aggravate her migraine headaches as well and should be avoided. PM states compliance with her medications, and this is supported by her refill history.

After evaluating and synthesizing all the patient's subjective and objective information, the pharmacist concludes that PM's increase in headache frequency is most likely caused by initiation of the oral contraceptive and may be further aggravated by her caffeine intake. The steps involved in this assessment process are illustrated in the accompanying decision tree (Fig. 18-19). Because PM is not currently having a headache or decreasing neurologic signs, the pharmacist calls the physician and discusses the probable exacerbation of the migraine headaches by the oral contraceptive. The pharmacist recommends either discontinuation of the oral contraceptive or switching to a lower estrogen-containing product. The physician decides to discontinue the oral contraceptive. The pharmacist educates PM about exacerbation of the migraine headaches by the oral contraceptives and caffeine and about tapering off of the caffeine and discontinuing the oral contraceptive. The pharmacist also schedules a follow-up in 1 month to assess changes in the frequency and severity of PM's migraine headaches. In addition, the pharmacist discusses alternative contraceptive options with the patient.

Pharmaceutical Care Plan

Patient Name: PM

Date: 5/19/02

Medical Problems:
Migraine headaches

Current Medications:
Verapamil SR, 180 mg, one tablet daily
Imitrex, 25 mg, one tablet at onset of headache, may repeat in 2 hours if needed
Ortho-Novum 1/35, one tablet daily
Multivitamin, one tablet daily

S: 39-year-old white woman complaining of increasing number of headaches. Unilateral throbbing headaches associated with nausea, vomiting, photophobia, and phonophobia. Previously occurred once every couple of months; however, patient states that during the last 6 months, their frequency has been increasing. No change in quality or severity. States compliance with all medications. Six months earlier, initiated on Ortho-Novum 1/35. Drinks two caffeinated beverages per day.

O: Patient in no acute distress.
Heart rate: 80 bpm
Blood pressure: 124/78 mm Hg
Respiratory rate: 18 rpm

A: Migraine headache exacerbation, possibly secondary to initiation of oral contraceptive and caffeine intake.

P:
1. Call physician, and recommend discontinuation of oral contraceptive.
2. Educate PM about triggers of migraine headaches, discontinuation of oral contraceptive, and slow tapering off of caffeine intake.
3. Discuss alternative contraceptive options with patient.
4. Schedule follow-up phone call with patient in 1 month to evaluate frequency and severity of migraine headaches.

Pharmacist: *John Doe, Pharm.D.*

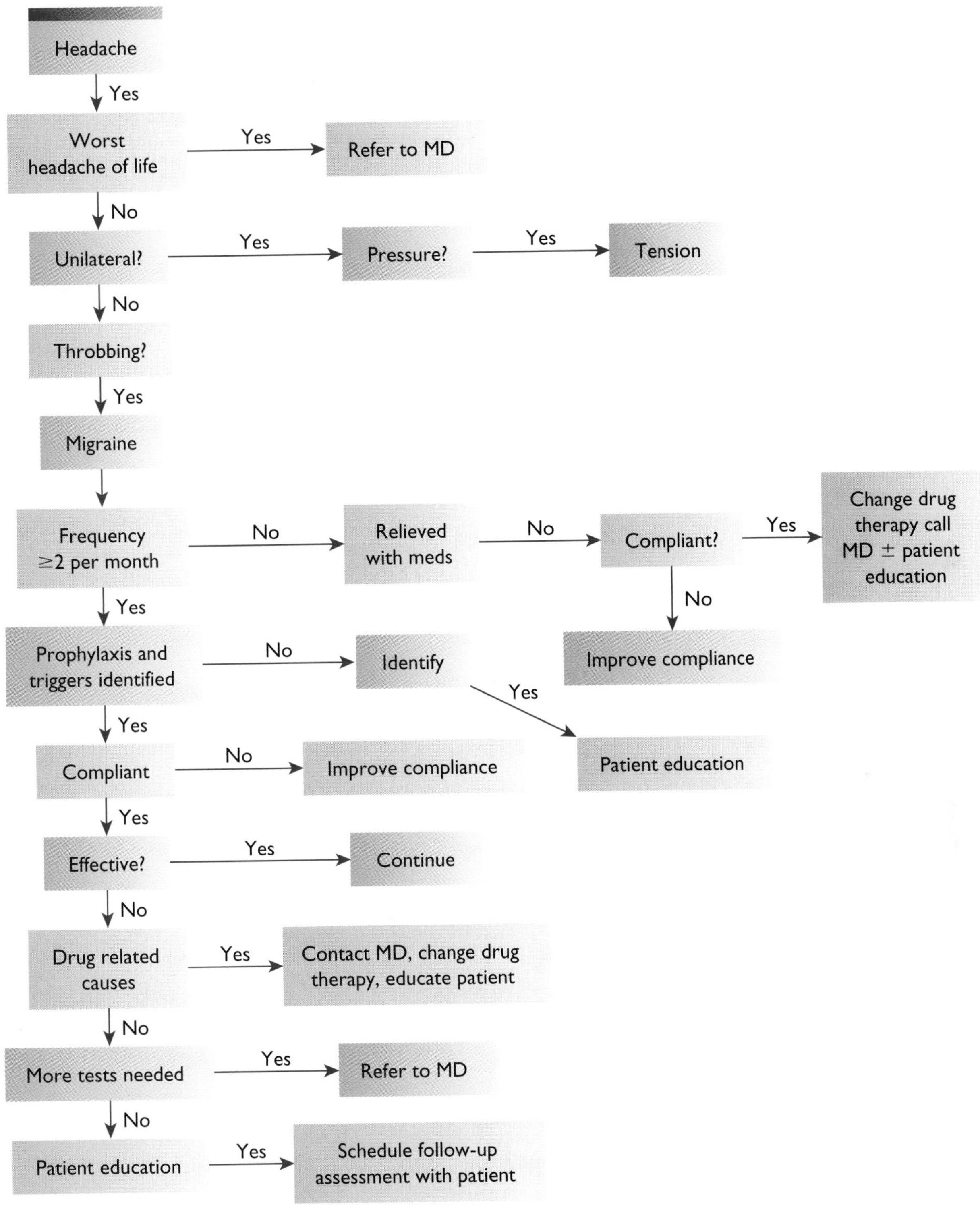

FIGURE 18-19 ■ Decision tree for headaches.

Self-Assessment Questions

1. How do you differentiate between the different types of headache pain?
2. What factors can precipitate headaches?
3. Which patients presenting with a headache should be immediately referred to medical care?

Critical Thinking Questions

1. In the case of PM, how would the pharmacist's assessment and plan change if the headaches were changing in quality and severity as well as in frequency?
2. What various physiologic changes occur during a migraine headache, and how would these affect drug therapy?

Seizures

Various causes of seizures include infection, trauma, metabolic disturbances, tumors, anoxia, and medications (Box 18-7). As discussed, seizures can have varying presentations and degrees of severity. Patients may present with a range of symptoms or a history of symptoms. Table 18-3 lists the criteria for differentiation between seizure types.

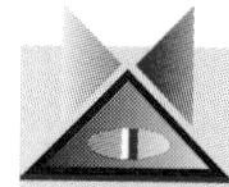

Box 18-7

MEDICATIONS THAT CAN CAUSE SEIZURES

- Alcohol
- Antidepressants
- Antipsychotics
- Antiepileptics
- β-Lactam antibiotics
- Drugs of abuse
- Lithium
- Quinolones
- Sedative-hypnotics
- Theophylline

CASE STUDY

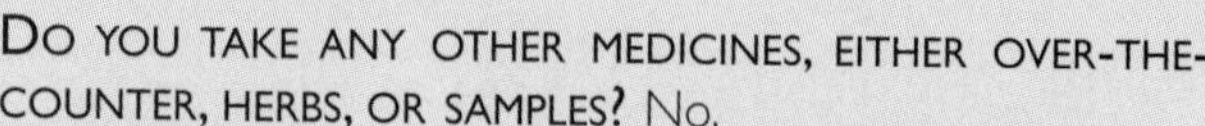

SE is a 15-year-old boy who comes into the pharmacy with his mother to pick up his prescriptions. He complains that he does not like to take his medication and wonders how much longer he will have to take them. The pharmacist knows that SE has been on numerous medications in the past for his seizure disorder, which is described as complex partial with secondary generalization.

ASSESSMENT OF THE PATIENT

Subjective Information

15-year-old boy with a history of complex partial seizures with secondary generalization

WHEN WAS YOUR LAST SEIZURE? A couple of months ago.

HOW OFTEN DO YOU HAVE A SEIZURE? I have a seizure every 2 to 4 months.

HOW LONG HAVE YOU HAD SEIZURES? Off and on since age 3, when I had meningitis.

DO YOU KNOW WHEN YOU ARE GOING TO HAVE A SEIZURE? I don't, but people say I start acting weird before I have a seizure. It's really embarrassing.

IS THERE ANYTHING THAT SEEMS TO MAKE THE SEIZURES COME ON? No.

WHAT HELPS TO PREVENT THE SEIZURES? I guess they are a little bit better on this medicine, but nothing really. I still get them.

WHAT MEDICATIONS DO YOU TAKE FOR YOUR SEIZURES? Just the ones that we're getting today.

DO YOU TAKE ANY OTHER MEDICINES, EITHER OVER-THE-COUNTER, HERBS, OR SAMPLES? No.

HOW OFTEN DO YOU FORGET TO TAKE YOUR MEDICINES? I sometimes forget to take them during the day at school. I have to go all the way to the nurse's station to get them. I don't like them anyway.

WHAT PROBLEMS ARE YOU HAVING WITH THE MEDICINES THAT CAUSE YOU NOT TO LIKE THEM? I feel slowed down and fuzzy after I take them. It makes it real hard to concentrate at school.

WHAT GRADE ARE YOU IN? HOW IS SCHOOL GOING? I'm in ninth grade, and I guess okay. I am passing with C's.

Objective Information

Computerized medication profile:

- Phenobarbital: 60 mg, one tablet twice daily; No. 60; Refills: 3; Patient obtains refills every 30 to 40 days, started 1 year ago.
- Carbamazepine, 200 mg, one tablet four times daily; No. 120; Refills: 6; Patient obtains refills every 30 to 40 days, started 6 months ago.

Patient in no acute distress
Slightly obese
Patient oriented to time, place, and person
Blood pressure: 110/70 mm Hg
Respiratory rate: 12 rpm
Heart rate: 64 bpm
Cranial nerves II–XII intact
Reflexes normal
Gait normal

Continued

CASE STUDY—continued

DISCUSSION

SE is concerned with his seizure control. He continues to have a seizure every couple of months and is worried about getting his driver's license when he turns 16. Because that time is coming closer, SE is becoming more concerned with his lack of seizure control. States vary on the requirements to obtain a driver's license after a seizure; however, most states require a seizure-free period ranging from 6 months to 1 year.

The pharmacist must decide the cause of SE's lack of seizure control, which includes several possibilities: physiologic worsening of the seizure disorder, improper medication selection, subtherapeutic drug dosing; patient noncompliance with medication, and drug interactions. No evidence suggests that SE is having physiologic worsening of his seizures. Their frequency has not increased; however, further evaluation may be warranted. Both phenobarbital and carbamazepine are indicated in complex partial seizures with secondary generalization. All antiepileptic medications have significant drug interactions. Both carbamazepine and phenobarbital are potent enzyme inducers and may decrease levels of the concomitant drug. Serum levels would be appropriate to obtain in SE. His lack of seizure control could be secondary to low levels resulting from drug interactions between carbamazepine and phenobarbital. SE states, however, that he doesn't like to go to the nurse's office to get his medication and that he misses taking his medication on occasion.

Side effects from antiepileptic medications can be quite bothersome and decrease cognitive functioning. SE complains of feeling tired and foggy when he takes his medication. The combination of not wanting to go to the nurse's office and of wanting to avoid these side effects indicates that SE's seizures are most likely not controlled because of noncompliance with his medication. The pharmacist therefore recommends to the physician that the carbamazepine be changed to an extended-release formulation to decrease the number of doses per day and, possibly, that the phenobarbital be changed to a less-sedating antiepileptic (e.g., valproic acid). The physician has the patient come into the office that afternoon for carbamazepine and phenobarbital levels and changes the carbamazepine to an extended-release formulation. Over the next month or two, the physician states that she will begin tapering the phenobarbital and, possibly, add the valproic acid at a later date. The pharmacist arranges the appointment, fills the new prescription, counsels the patient regarding the medication change, and schedules a follow-up assessment with SE in 3 weeks to evaluate his seizure control, to assess his medication's side effects, and to begin tapering off of the phenobarbital.

Pharmaceutical Care Plan

Patient Name: SE

Date: 9/4/02

Medical Problems:
Complex partial seizures with secondary generalization

Current Medications:
Carbamazepine, 200 mg, one tablet QID
Phenobarbital, 60 mg, one tablet BID

S: 15-year-old boy having a history of complex partial seizures with secondary generalization. Continues to have a seizure every 2 to 4 months. Complains of feeling slowed down and fuzzy after taking medication. Regularly misses midday doses of carbamazepine.

O: Slightly obese male in no apparent distress. Oriented to time, place, and person.

Blood pressure: 110/70 mm Hg

Respiratory rate: 12 rpm

Heart rate: 64 bpm

Neurologic: Cranial nerves II–XII intact.

Reflexes: Normal.

Gait: Normal.

A:
1. Uncontrolled seizure disorder, possibly caused by noncompliance with medications.
2. Adverse drug reaction of decreased cognitive function secondary to antiepileptic medications.

P:
1. Call physician to discuss patient's condition and to recommend change to extended-release carbamazepine.
2. Change carbamazepine, 200 mg QID, to extended-release carbamazepine, 400 mg BID.
3. Schedule appointment with physician today to check carbamazepine and phenobarbital levels.
4. Educate patient about proper use of extended-release carbamazepine.
5. Schedule a follow-up assessment in 3 weeks to assess SE's seizure control and side effects of medication and to begin tapering off of phenobarbital in conjunction with the physician.

Pharmacist: *Sally Smith, Pharm.D.*

Self-Assessment Questions

1. How do you differentiate between the different types of seizure disorders?
2. What medications may induce a seizure?
3. Describe an electroencephalogram and its use in evaluating seizures.

Critical Thinking Questions

1. A 72-year-old woman on phenytoin is experiencing ataxia, mental status changes, seizures, and decreasing levels of consciousness. She has a phenytoin level of 7.2 mg/dL and an albumin level of 2.5 g/dL. What would your assessment and plan be?
2. How do the different anticonvulsant medications differ in respect to side-effect profiles, and how would you assess the differences?

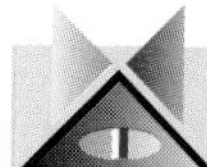

Box 18-8

MEDICATIONS THAT CAN CAUSE PERIPHERAL NEUROPATHY

- Antiretrovirals
- Chemotherapeutic agents
- Folic acid antagonists
- Alcohol
- Nitrofurantoin
- Amiodarone
- Dapsone
- High-dose vitamins

Paresthesia

Paresthesia, which is a spontaneously occurring, abnormal tingling sensation, is sometimes referred to as "pins and needles." Paresthesias are a very common complaint. Approximately 50% of patients with diabetes will experience paresthesias, a sign of peripheral neuropathy, during their lifetime. Paresthesias result from, among other reasons, damage to the peripheral nerve either by compression, trauma, infection, and autoimmune processes. Medications that can cause paresthesias are listed in Box 18-8.

CASE STUDY

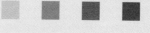

GL is a 59-year-old man with a history of type 2 diabetes mellitus and hypertension. He comes into the pharmacy complaining that his feet feel like they have tight socks on them all the time.

ASSESSMENT OF THE PATIENT

Subjective Information

59-year-old man with a history of type 2 diabetes mellitus and hypertension complaining of a constant tight feeling about his feet

HOW LONG HAS THIS BEEN GOING ON? Off and on for a couple of years, but it has been more consistent over the past 4 months.

DESCRIBE THE DISCOMFORT FOR ME. It feels like I have socks on my feet all the time. They feel kind of numb, and it feels like pins and needles when I walk.

DO YOU NOTICE THIS IN YOUR HANDS AS WELL? Not really.

DO YOU EVER NOTICE SHARP PAINS SHOOTING DOWN YOUR LEG? No.

WHAT MEDICAL CONDITIONS DO YOU CURRENTLY SEE YOUR DOCTOR FOR? I have diabetes, high blood pressure, and high cholesterol.

WHAT MEDICATIONS ARE YOU CURRENTLY TAKING? I take glyburide in the morning and at night, benazepril in the morning, and Lipitor at night.

HOW OFTEN DO YOU FORGET TO TAKE YOUR MEDICINES? I generally don't. Every once in a great while, I guess.

WHAT DO YOUR BLOOD SUGARS GENERALLY RUN? They run between 180 and 200 most of the time.

DO YOU HAVE ANY PROBLEMS WITH YOUR STOMACH? ANY CONSTIPATION OR DIARRHEA? I get heartburn if I'm not careful of what I eat. But I take a couple of Tums, and it generally goes away.

WHAT OTHER OVER-THE-COUNTER MEDICATIONS DO YOU TAKE? Just some ibuprofen every now and then for aches and pains, but that isn't very often.

HOW OFTEN DO YOU DRINK ALCOHOL? Two or three times a week, I'll have a couple of beers. I've done that for the last 20 to 30 years.

Objective Information

Computerized medication profile:

- Glyburide: 5 mg, two tablets twice daily; No. 120; Refills: 2; Patient obtains refills every 25 to 35 days.
- Lotensin: 10 mg, one tablet daily; No. 30; Refills: 2; Patient obtains refills every 25 to 35 days.
- Lipitor: 20 mg, one tablet at bedtime; No. 30; Refills: 2; Patient obtains refills every 25 to 35 days.

Patient in no apparent distress
Patient oriented to person, place, and time

Continued

CASE STUDY—continued

Blood pressure: 144/90 mm Hg
Respirations: 18 rpm
Heart rate: 78 bpm
Cranial nerves II–XII intact
Gait coordinated and even
Romberg sign negative
Deep tendon reflexes 2+ bilaterally
Decreased superficial touch, pain, and vibratory sensations bilaterally in feet and hands
No clonus

DISCUSSION

When a patient complains of paresthesias, the pharmacist needs to clarify the patient's symptoms and determine the most likely cause. GL's symptoms have developed during the last 2 years and have increased during the past 4 months. It is important, especially on the initial complaint, that the acuteness of the symptoms be ascertained. Paresthesias of acute onset may relate to Guillain-Barré syndrome, stroke, tumors, or medications, and they should be referred to a physician immediately, especially if they recur. GL is not experiencing shooting pains down his lower extremities, so sciatica is unlikely to be playing a role in his paresthesias. GL, however, does have poorly controlled diabetes and regularly consumes alcohol, both of which can cause or exacerbate peripheral neuropathies. GL is experiencing decreased sensation in his feet and hands as well as other symptoms associated with peripheral neuropathy. One of the concerns in patients with diabetes and peripheral neuropathy is the possibility of injury to the lower extremities without realization, along with complications of infection, possibly leading to amputation.

After evaluating GL's symptoms, the pharmacist concludes that GL's paresthesias probably result from peripheral neuropathies secondary to diabetes and, possibly, alcohol intake. To illustrate the steps involved with the assessment process, see the accompanying decision tree (Fig. 18-20). GL is supposed to return to his physician in 1 week for his 6-month visit. The pharmacist decides that the physician should be notified of GL's condition and writes a letter detailing GL's signs and symptoms. The pharmacist also counsels GL on improving his diet and diabetic control and decreasing his alcohol intake. The pharmacist also recommends an over-the-counter capsaicin product for topical use to decrease the paresthesias. A follow-up appointment is scheduled in 2 weeks to assess GL's signs, symptoms, and diabetic control.

PHARMACEUTICAL CARE PLAN

Patient Name: GL

Date: 10/25/01

Medical Problems:
Type 2 diabetes mellitus
Hypertension
Hyperlipidemia

Current Medications:
Glyburide, 5 mg, two tablets twice daily
Lotensin, 10 mg, one tablet daily
Lipitor, 20 mg, one tablet at bedtime

S: A 59-year-old man complaining of feeling as if he has tight socks on his feet all the time, with tingling and numbness in his feet. Has occurred during the last 2 years but has become more consistent during the last 4 months. No shooting pains or changes in mental status. Drinks two beers two to three times weekly for the past 20 to 30 years. Compliant with medications. States home blood sugars are from 180 to 200 mg/dL.

O: Patient in no apparent distress. Oriented to person, place, and time.

Blood pressure: 144/90 mm Hg

Respirations: 18 rpm

Heart rate: 78 bpm

Neurologic: Cranial nerves II–XII intact. Gait coordinated and even. Romberg sign negative. Deep tendon reflexes 2+ bilaterally. Decreased superficial touch, pain, and vibratory sensations bilaterally in feet and hands. No clonus.

A:
1. Paresthesias, probably caused by peripheral neuropathy secondary to diabetes and chronic alcohol intake.
2. Type 2 diabetes mellitus, poorly controlled.

P:
1. Educate patient to improve control of diet and diabetes, proper foot care, and decreasing alcohol intake.
2. Recommend capsaicin topical cream, four times daily.
3. Keep appointment with physician next week.
4. Follow-up assessment in 2 weeks to monitor signs and symptoms of peripheral neuropathy and diabetes control.

Pharmacist: *Ann Jones, Pharm.D.*

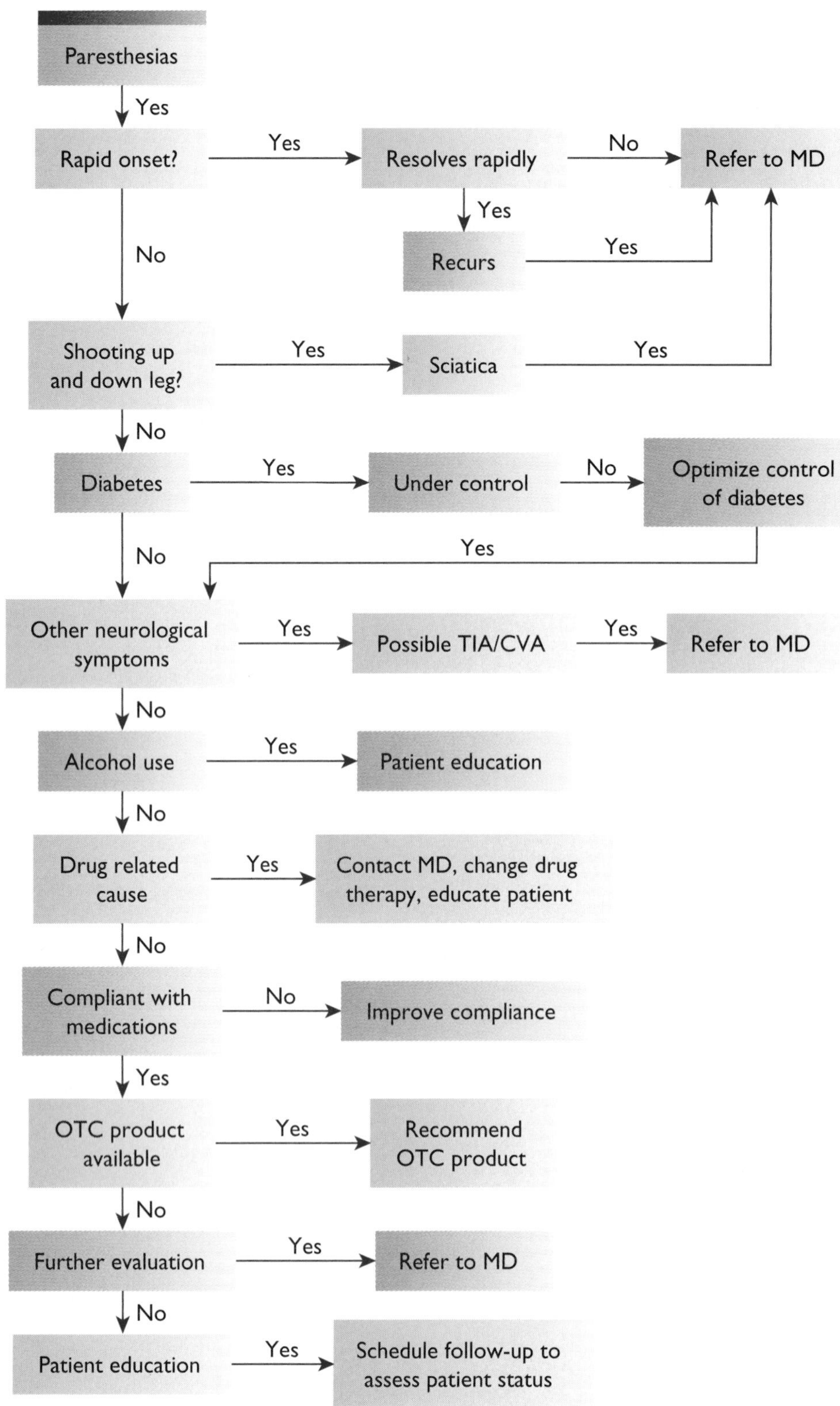

FIGURE 18-20 ■ Decision tree for paresthesias. *CVA,* cerebrovascular accident; *OTC,* over-the-counter; *TIA,* transient ischemic attack.

Self-Assessment Questions

1. What common signs and symptoms are associated with peripheral neuropathy?
2. What medications may induce or exacerbate peripheral neuropathies?
3. Which patients presenting with paresthesias should be referred for immediate medical attention?

Critical Thinking Questions

1. What measures can be instituted in a patient on antiretroviral therapy for human immunodeficiency infection to prevent peripheral neuropathies?
2. How would the pharmacist's assessment and plan change if GL was just experiencing gastrointestinal-related symptoms?

Bibliography

Bantam medical dictionary. New York: Bantam Books, 1990.

Bates B. A guide to physical examination and history taking. 7th ed. Philadelphia: JB Lippincott, 1999.

Dipiro JT, Talbert RL, Yee GC, Matske GR, Wells BG, Posey LM. Pharmacotherapy: a pathophysiologic approach. 4th ed. Stamford, CT: Appleton & Lange, 1999.

Goodman Gilman A, Hardman JG, Limbird LE. Goodman and Gilman's the pharmacological basis of therapeutics. 10th ed. New York: McGraw-Hill Medical Publishing, 2001.

Hauser R, Zesiewicz TA. Parkinson's disease: questions and answers. 2nd ed. Coral Springs, FL: Merit Publishing International, 1997.

Hawkes CH. Diagnosis of functional neurological disease. Br J Hosp Med 1997;57:373–377.

Herfindal ET, Gourley DR. Textbook of therapeutics: drug and disease management. 6th ed. Baltimore: Williams & Wilkins, 1996.

Jarvis C. Physical examination and health assessment. 3rd ed. Philadelphia: WB Saunders, 2000.

Kent TH, Hart MN. Introduction to human disease. 4th ed. Stamford, CT: Appleton & Lange, 1998.

LoVecchio F, Jacobson S. Approach to generalized weakness and peripheral neuromuscular disease. Emerg Med Clin North Am 1997;15:605–622.

Martini FH, Timmon MJ. Human anatomy. 2nd ed. Upper Saddle River, NJ: Prentice-Hall, 1997.

McGee JO, Isaacson PG, Wright NA. Oxford textbook of pathology. Volume 2b. Oxford, UK: Oxford University Press, 1992.

Novak G, Maytal J, Alshansky A, Ascher C. Risk factors for status epilepticus in children with symptomatic epilepsy. Neurology 1997;49:533–537.

Pagana KD, Pagana TJ. Mosby's diagnostic and laboratory test reference. 2nd ed. St Louis: Mosby–Yearbook, 1995.

Pinnell NL. Nursing pharmacology. Philadelphia: WB Saunders, 1996.

Seidel HM, Ball JW, Dains JE, Benedict GW. Mosby's guide to physical examination. 4th ed. St Louis: Mosby–Yearbook, 1999.

Sturmann K. The neurologic examination. Emerg Med Clin North Am 1997;15:491–506.

Tortora GJ, Grabowski SR. Principles of anatomy and physiology. 9th ed. New York: John Wiley and Sons, 2000.

Welty T. Managing the patient with epilepsy. Clinical Pharmacy Newswatch 1997;4:1–6.

Young LY, Koda-Kimble MA. Applied therapeutics: the clinical use of drugs. 6th ed. Philadelphia: Lippincott Williams & Wilkins, 2001.

CHAPTER

19

Mental Status

Karen M. Theesen and Sarah Shoemaker

GLOSSARY TERMS

- Adjustment disorder with anxiety
- Adjustment disorder with depressed mood
- Agnosia
- Alogia
- Anhedonia
- Anxiety disorder
- Apraxia
- Autism
- Avolition
- Bipolar disorder
- Circumstantiality
- Cognitive disorders
- Compulsion
- Confabulation
- Delirium
- Delusions
- Dementia
- Depressive disorders
- Dysthymic disorder
- Echolalia
- Flight of ideas
- Generalized anxiety disorder
- Hallucination
- Illusions
- Loosening of associations
- Major depressive disorder
- Mental disorder
- Mood disorders
- Neologism
- Obsessions
- Obsessive-compulsive disorder
- Panic attack
- Perseveration
- Posttraumatic stress disorder
- Psychotic disorders
- Schizophrenia
- Social phobia
- Specific phobia
- Substance abuse
- Substance dependence
- Tangentiality
- Thought blocking
- Word salad

ANATOMY AND PHYSIOLOGY OVERVIEW

Optimal functioning in a person is reflected by life satisfaction in work, in personal relationships, and within the self. There are numerous reasons why a person may not be functioning optimally, many of which are short term and will resolve with time. In other cases, people may not be optimally functioning because they are suffering from a change in mental status that suggests a more serious illness, which will not resolve on its own.

The Nervous System

The human nervous system is divided into three functional levels: (1) the spinal cord, (2) the lower brain, and (3) the higher brain. The spinal cord is responsible for motor activity. Its responses are automatic and occur almost instantaneously. The lower brain consists of the medulla, pons, mesencephalon, hypothalamus, thalamus, cerebellum, and basal ganglia. Most of the subconscious activities of the body (e.g., respiration, equilibrium) are controlled at the lower-brain level. Certain emotional responses (e.g., anger, excitement, reaction to pain) are also derived from lower-brain activity. The higher brain consists of the cerebral cortex and the limbic system. Together, these areas control our "mental state" (i.e., our higher functions and emotions). Higher functions of the human nervous system include thinking, learning and memory, language and communication, attention, sexual arousal, stages of sleep, and levels of consciousness. Emotions are complex feeling states with psychic, somatic, and behavioral components that relate to affect and mood. Examples include joy, anger, and fear.

Specifically, the cerebral cortex functions as a vast information-storage area. It is divided into four lobes: (1) frontal, (2) parietal, (3) occipital, and (4) temporal. Functions of the frontal lobe include complex motor movements, speech, and intellectual functioning (e.g., judgment, reasoning, abstract thinking). Functions of the parietal lobe include processing and perception of somatosensory information (e.g., touch or position sensations) and integration of visual and auditory stimuli. The occipital lobe receives and interprets visual stimuli. The temporal lobe's functions are varied and complex; they include receiving and interpreting auditory, gustatory, and olfactory impulses as well as language, emotional behavior, learning, memory, and sexual function.

In contrast, the limbic system is often referred to as the emotional circuit of the brain. The limbic system consists of the amygdala, hippocampus, hypothalamus, anterior thalamus, cingulate gyrus, basal ganglia, and septal nuclei. Although behavioral and emotional expressions are a function of the entire nervous system, a person's emotional status, subconscious motor and sensory drives, and intrinsic feelings of pain and pleasure are derived from activity in the limbic system.

On the cellular level, the brain is composed of billions of nerve cells, called neurons, that carry out the functions of the nervous system. Neurons are the information-processing elements that communicate chemically by releasing and responding to a wide range of chemical substances, called neurotransmitters. Neurotransmitters are classified as amino acid transmitters (e.g., glutamate, aspartate, gamma aminobutyrate, glycine), aminergic transmitters, and neuropeptides. The aminergic transmitters include acetylcholine, epinephrine, norepinephrine, dopamine, serotonin, and histamine. Examples of neuropeptides are substance P, opioid peptides, and somatostatin. There is a vast array of neurotransmitters, many of which have not been identified.

Special Considerations

Pediatric Patients

In a normal infant, the spinal cord and lower brain are fully functioning at birth. Higher-brain functioning (e.g. consciousness) is rudimentary at birth but continues to develop through adolescence. At 1 year of age, children typically begin to use one word at a time, followed by multiword sentences around the age of 2. Children begin to fully use language to communicate at 4 to 5 years. At age 7, children develop reasoning skills and begin to understand the moral concepts of right and wrong. In early adolescence, the development of abstract reasoning begins, which continues into late adolescence. The development of neuronal tracks and the functioning of neurotransmitters continue from birth through early adolescence.

Geriatric Patients

During the aging process, the brain decreases in weight and volume; however, there is no significant loss of higher cortical functioning. Elderly patients may have a slower response time to questions, and new learning is slower. Recent memory may be decreased, but long-term memory is not affected. Age-related changes in sensory perception (e.g., hearing loss) can affect the results of the mental status examination, and the elderly person may appear to be confused. The elderly person has more potential for loss of loved ones, job status, prestige, income, and physical health. Coping with both current and potential losses puts added stress on the elderly person.

Pregnant Patients

Pregnancy produces marked biologic, physiologic, and psychologic changes in the woman. There is no consensus on whether the incidence of psychiatric disorders during pregnancy is different from that of the general population. Factors that may alter the incidence of psychiatric disorders during pregnancy include predisposition to psychiatric disorders, past psychiatric history, physical health, and desirability of the pregnancy. The postpartum period is associated with an increased incidence of feelings of sadness, frequent tearfulness, and clinging dependency. The rapid changes in hormonal levels, stress of childbirth, and awareness of the increased responsibility of motherhood may contribute to these feelings. In rare cases, the mother develops postpartum psychosis, which is characterized by hallucinations or delusions. A history of development of a psychiatric disorder during a previous pregnancy is the strongest predictor of a psychiatric disorder during a subsequent pregnancy.

PATHOLOGY OVERVIEW

A **mental disorder** is defined by the American Psychiatric Association (APA) as a clinically significant behavioral or psychologic syndrome or pattern that occurs in an individual. Mental disorders are associated with distress or impairment in one or more areas of functioning or with a significantly increased risk of death, pain, disability, or an important loss of freedom. Often, the cause of mental disorders is not well understood. They may—or may not—be associated with observable stress. Patients without mental disorders who are under significant stress may function less than optimally until the stress is reduced.

The APA publishes the *Diagnostic and Statistical Manual of Mental Disorders* (DSM), which describes the official classification system of American psychiatry and reflects the consensus of current formulations for a psychiatric diagnosis. The purpose of the DSM is to provide a clear description of diagnostic categories to enable practitioners to diagnose, communicate about, study, and treat various mental disorders. The most recent edition of the DSM was published in 1994 and is the fourth edition (DSM-IV).

Anxiety Disorders

Anxiety disorders are frequently encountered in the general patient population. Approximately one-quarter of the general population will experience at least one anxiety disorder in their lifetime.

Anxiety disorders, according to the DSM-IV, include:

- Adjustment disorder with anxiety
- Generalized anxiety disorder
- Panic attacks, agoraphobia
- Specific phobias
- Social phobias
- Obsessive-compulsive disorder
- Posttraumatic stress disorder

Anxiety is also associated with many other disorders, thus, it is necessary to carefully question the patient to determine if he or she has an anxiety or a different mental disorder. Anxiety is also associated with physical illness and can be a drug side effect (e.g., from excessive intake of caffeine). Patients with anxiety disorders have a high utilization rate of health care services for a variety of specific or vague physical complaints, such as palpitations, tachycardia, chest pain or tightness, shortness of breath, and hyperventilation. The patient may develop significant disability if the symptoms of anxiety are unrecognized or misdiagnosed as a physical disorder.

Adjustment Disorder with Anxiety

Patients having an **adjustment disorder with anxiety** are experiencing a maladaptive reaction of nervousness, worry, or jitteriness to an identifiable environmental or psychosocial stressor that interferes with their functioning. In these cases, the degree of anxiety-related stress can be disabling, but the patient's anxiety is expected to resolve or an adaptation to be made within 6 months of the stressor. Potential stressors include physical illness, divorce, natural disasters, loss of a job, death of a loved one, and so on. Adjustment disorder with anxiety is usually treated with psychotherapy and/or short-term, low-dose benzodiazepines.

Generalized Anxiety Disorder

Generalized anxiety disorder (GAD) is characterized by excessive and uncontrollable worry that is out of proportion to the likelihood or impact of the feared events. The anxiety is focused on many life circumstances, is not associated with an obvious stressor, and is associated with at least three of the following symptoms: restlessness or feeling keyed up or on edge, being easily fatigued, difficulty concentrating or mind going blank, irritability, muscle tension, and difficulty falling or staying asleep or restless, unsatisfying sleep. The symptoms of GAD must be apparent for at least 6 months and cause significant impairment in occupational or social functioning. It may be treated with psychotherapy, benzodiazepines, buspirone, or low doses of antidepressants.

Phobias

Phobias are often frequently encountered in the general population. A patient with **social phobia** has a persistent and exaggerated fear of humiliation or embarrassment in social situations that results in distress and possible avoidance of social situations. Examples of such phobias include fear of choking on food when eating in front of others or fear of urinating in a public lavatory. The fear or avoidance must have a significant effect on the person's ability to function for it to be considered a phobia. Drug therapies for social phobias include routine antidepressants, benzodiazepines, or β-blocker before the social situation. In addition, behavioral therapies using increased exposure to the phobia or psychotherapy may be used.

A **specific phobia** is described as a marked and persistent fear that is excessive or unreasonable to the specific situation or object. Examples of specific phobias include fear of heights, dogs, tunnels, or flying. Patients with a specific phobia recognize that the fear is unreasonable, but they are still disabled by the fear. Some typical fears would not fulfill the criteria for a specific phobia. For example, a person who is afraid of snakes but is rarely, if ever, in contact with them and is not distressed about this fear would not have a diagnosis of specific phobia.

Posttraumatic Stress Disorder

Posttraumatic stress disorder (PTSD) can be an immediate or delayed response to a catastrophic life event. It was originally described as a post-war phenomenon, but currently, the term is applied when a person develops characteristic symptoms after experiencing a serious, life-threatening event, either to themselves or to others. Examples of a traumatic event include sexual assault, physical/sexual abuse, serious accidents, witnessing the death of another person, or being affected by a natural disaster. The characteristic symptoms of PTSD include persistently re-experiencing (in dreams or recollections) the traumatic event, persistently avoiding the stimuli associated with the trauma, numbing of general responsiveness, and persistent symptoms of increased arousal (e.g., difficulty falling asleep, irritability, difficulty concentrating, exaggerated startle response). The characteristic symptoms of PTSD must be present for 1 month, and the patient must experience significant occupational or social impairment to fulfill the DSM-IV criteria. Depending on the prominent symptoms in the patient, PTSD is treated with psychotherapy and a variety of psychotropic agents.

Panic Attacks

A **panic attack** is characterized by a discrete attack of intense fear or anxiety that is accompanied by several physical symptoms (Box 19-1). The symptoms of a panic attack reach peak intensity within 10 minutes. The patient describes the sensation as a fear of dying, of losing control, or of going crazy. Patients fre-

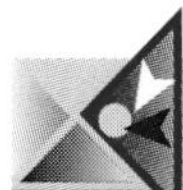

Box 19-1

SYMPTOMS OF A PANIC ATTACK

A discrete period of intense fear or discomfort in which four (or more) of the following symptoms developed abruptly and reached a peak within 10 minutes:

- Palpitations, pounding heart, or accelerated heart rate
- Sweating
- Trembling or shaking
- Sensations of shortness of breath or smothering
- Feeling of choking
- Chest pain or discomfort
- Nausea or abdominal distress
- Feeling dizzy, unsteady, light-headed, or faint
- Derealization (feelings of unreality) or depersonalization (being detached from oneself)
- Fear of losing control or going crazy
- Fear of dying
- Paresthesias (numbness or tingling sensations)
- Chills or hot flushes

Adapted from the DSM-IV (APA, 1994).

quently seek extensive medical treatment for the cardiovascular (heart attack) or endocrine (diabetes) symptoms, with negative results. The patient with panic attacks frequently develops symptoms of agoraphobia, an excessive fear and avoidance of situations in which they could not escape or in which help is not readily available. Patients with agoraphobia avoid driving, airplanes, crowded places, stores, elevators, or being alone. Agoraphobia usually develops from a fear of having another panic attack. The drug treatment of panic attacks and agoraphobia consists of antidepressants or benzodiazepines. Behavioral treatments focusing on gradual exposure may be used for agoraphobia.

Obsessive-Compulsive Disorder

Patients with **obsessive-compulsive disorder** (OCD) experience a recurrence of obsessions or compulsions that are frequent enough to interfere with normal daily activities. The patient feels compelled to perform the compulsion to avoid or reduce anxiety. Patients avoid revealing their symptoms because of embarrassment, and they often find ways to accommodate the disorder in their daily lives. OCD is a not a disorder of memory; rather, patients cannot be "certain" that they have completed a task. Physical symptoms may result from these compulsions (e.g. dermatitis caused by excessive handwashing). The primary drug therapy for OCD is antidepressants that increase the activity of serotonin. Behavioral treatments and psychotherapy are used as adjunct therapy with the antidepressants.

Mood Disorders

The term *mood* describes the long-term (i.e., sustained) emotional state, whereas the term *affect* describes a short-term emotional state. Mood is often compared to the climate of a geographical location and affect to the current weather. Terms that describe mood include *euthymic, depression, dysthymia,* and *euphoria.* Terms that describe different affects are numerous and include *sad, gloomy, happy, labile, worried, annoyed, impatient, furious, blunted, flat, inappropriate,* and *labile.* Mood disorders include several that are differentiated by the severity of the mood alteration and the duration of the symptoms. The DSM-IV divides the **mood disorders** into **depressive disorders,** including adjustment disorder with depressed mood, dysthymic disorder, and major depressive disorder, and bipolar disorders. Comorbid mood disorders are frequently found in patients with general conditions (e.g., cardiovascular disorders, cancer) or as a result of drug toxicity or withdrawal.

Adjustment Disorder with Depressed Mood

Patients having **adjustment disorder with depressed mood** have an identifiable environmental or psychosocial stressor that has resulted in sadness, social isolation, difficulty concentrating, and preoccupation with the stressful events in addition to changes in sleep and appetite. The potential stressors are similar to those for any adjustment disorder, including physical illness, divorce, job loss, or natural disaster. Adjustment disorder with depressed mood is considered to be a transient disorder and usually responds to supportive psychotherapy. People with poor coping skills and inadequate social support systems may be more likely to suffer from an adjustment disorder. Patients with more severe symptoms may have developed major depression.

Dysthymic Disorder

Dysthymic disorder is characterized by a chronically depressed mood for more days than not during the course of at least 2 years. The depressed mood is accompanied by changes in appetite and sleep as well as symptoms of low self-esteem, feelings of inadequacy, pessimism, decreased productivity, and low energy. The diagnosis of dysthymia is not made if the severity of the depressed mood fulfills the criteria for major depression. Patients with dysthymia may respond to antidepressant therapy in conjunction with psychotherapy.

Major Depressive Disorder

The criteria for a **major depressive disorder** is a period of at least 2 weeks during which there is either depressed mood or **anhedonia,** the loss of interest or pleasure in nearly all activities. The mood disturbance causes marked distress and results in significant impairment in activities of daily living and occupational functioning. In children, the mood may be irritable instead of sad. In addition, the patient must have at least five of the symptoms listed in Box 19-2. Patients describe the depressed mood as a feeling of sadness, hopelessness, or discouragement, although

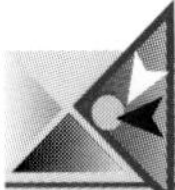

Box 19-2

SYMPTOMS ASSOCIATED WITH A MAJOR DEPRESSIVE EPISODE

At least five of the following symptoms must be present during a 2-week period:

- Depressed mood for most of the day[a]
- Markedly diminished interest or pleasure in all or almost all activities[a]
- Appetite disturbance with a 5% increase or decrease in weight within 1 month
- Sleep disturbance
- Psychomotor agitation or retardation that is observable by others
- Fatigue or loss of energy
- Feelings of worthlessness or excessive or inappropriate guilt
- Diminished ability to concentrate or indecisiveness
- Recurrent thoughts of death or suicidal thoughts, suicide attempt, or plan

Adapted from the DSM-IV (APA, 1994).
[a]The five symptoms must include at least one of these.

some individuals emphasize somatic complaints of body aches or pain. Patients may attribute the symptoms to another cause, such as stress or personal failure. Patients with anhedonia may describe a loss of interest in hobbies and/or sexual activity that is accompanied by a sense of not caring anymore. Frequently, the patient will report increased irritability, angry outbursts, or blaming others. The patient may describe a sense of worthlessness or guilty feelings about events that are out of proportion to those events. Patients may also describe difficulty concentrating and complain of memory problems.

The biologic signs associated with a major depressive disorder help to differentiate it from an adjustment disorder or a grief reaction. In a major depressive disorder, the appetite may be reduced or increased and is associated with the resultant change in body weight. The most common sleep disturbance is insomnia, although some patients describe hypersomnia instead. Psychomotor changes include agitation (e.g., inability to sit still, pulling or rubbing of the skin, clothing) or retardation (e.g., slow body movements, slow speech, long pauses before answering questions). The patient may also report feeling tired without physical exertion and state that daily activities take twice as long as usual.

Ideas of harming oneself, including suicidal plans or attempts, are associated with a major depressive disorder. Patients may describe the need to end their emotional suffering and that they perceive the obstacles in their life to be insurmountable. Patients who describe thoughts of suicide require immediate referral and, most likely, hospitalization. Patients suffering from major depression with features of psychosis have additional symptoms of delusions and/or hallucinations. Patients that have had a previous manic episode need to be identified and are diagnosed as bipolar, depressed phase.

Bipolar Disorder

Bipolar disorder describes the patient who experiences both episodes of depression and mania. The DSM-IV criteria for the diagnosis of bipolar disorder require at least one manic episode, which is a distinct period during which there is an abnormally and persistently elevated, expansive or irritable mood for a duration of at least 1 week. The manic episode causes marked distress, results in significant impairment in activities of daily living and occupational functioning, and usually requires hospitalization.

The elevated mood of mania may be described as euphoric and is recognized as being excessive for that person. The expansive quality of mood is characterized by the unceasing and indiscriminate need for interpersonal, sexual, or occupational interactions. Irritability is also associated with mania, especially if the person does not receive what he or she wants. The hallmark of a manic episode is the decreased need for sleep. Patients report that they sleep 3 to 4 hours per night and, at least for the first several nights, awaken energized. Grandiosity is a sense of inflated self-esteem that may be demonstrated by a patient claiming to be the superintendent of the hospital, to have discovered the cure for cancer, to be very rich, or to have a special relationship with God. As the mania progresses, the grandiosity may turn into a sense of persecution (i.e., paranoia). For example, if patients believe they have the cure for cancer, then they may fear that someone will try to harm them to learn about it.

Patients with mania may have pressured, loud, and rapid speech. In addition, the patient's thoughts may race, and the patient may jump from topic to topic (i.e., **flight of ideas**). Patients have difficulty screening out irrelevant stimuli and are easily distracted. They may also have an increase in goal-directed activity and will start—but not finish—multiple projects. Patients with mania report excessive involvement in pleasurable activities, such as shopping, indiscriminate sexual activity, and foolish business adventures. The impairment in judgment associated with mania usually requires hospitalization to protect the individual from the negative consequences of their behavior. As mania continues, patients may develop psychotic symptoms, such as delusions or hallucinations, and may appear to have paranoid schizophrenia.

Bipolar disorder is treated with lithium, carbamazepine, or valproic acid. If a patient develops the depressed phase of bipolar disorder, an antidepressant is used in conjunction with the bipolar agent. Symptoms of mania can be induced by antidepressant medications, which must be discontinued if symptoms of mania develop. During the manic phase, antipsychotic medications are used to treat the delusions and hallucinations.

Psychotic Disorders

Psychotic symptoms are the hallmark of disorders in this category and include delusions, hallucinations, and disorganized behavior, language, or thinking. Although a wide variety of psychiatric conditions may result in the manifestation of psychotic symptoms, the DSM-IV divides **psychotic disorders** into schizophrenia and other psychotic disorders, which includes schizoaffective disorder, psychotic disorder caused by medical conditions, and substance-induced psychotic disorder, to name a few. For the purposes of this book, the following discussion focuses on schizophrenia.

Schizophrenia

Schizophrenia is a complex syndrome that is associated with markedly impaired occupational or social functioning. The onset of schizophrenia typically occurs between the late teens and the mid-30s; it rarely occurs in childhood. To fulfill the DSM-IV criteria for schizophrenia, the signs and symptoms must be present for at least 1 month, with some signs of the disorder persisting for at least 6 months. Schizophrenia has been observed in all cultures and socioeconomic classes.

No one symptom is pathognomonic for schizophrenia; every sign and symptom observed in schizophrenia can be seen in other disorders. The symptoms of schizophrenia are divided into those that are added to the premorbid state (i.e., positive symptoms) and those that indicate a lack of function (i.e., negative symptoms). The positive symptoms of schizophrenia include hallucinations, delusions, disorganized speech, and bizarre behavior. The negative symptoms include emotional blunting, poverty of speech, avolition, anhedonia, and social isolation. It is important to note that patients with schizophrenia, even during the active phases, have a clear sensorium and are oriented.

During an acute psychotic episode of schizophrenia, the patient loses touch with reality and experiences a variety of positive symptoms. A **hallucination** is a sensory experience of something that does not exist outside the mind. The types of hallucinations vary but can occur in any sensory modality (e.g., auditory, visual, olfactory, gustatory, tactile). Auditory hallucinations, usually experienced as voices, are the most common and characteristic of schizophrenia. The patient can differentiate auditory hallucinations from the patient's own inner thoughts. The content of the auditory hallucination varies greatly but may include command hallucinations, in which the patient hears a voice that tells him or her to do something (e.g., "You need to kill yourself.").

Delusions are fixed, false beliefs that have a variety of themes (e.g., persecutory, religious, somatic, or grandiose). Delusions are fixed because the patient cannot be talked out of the delusions—even if evidence to the contrary is presented. Delusions are false because the delusion is not in keeping with reality and is a belief of the patient. For patients with schizophrenia, persecutory delusions are the most common (e.g., "The FBI is spying on me."). Bizarre delusions are especially suggestive of schizophrenia. For example, a patient who states that a sibling has wired the patient's brain to a computer and is reading the patient's thoughts is experiencing a bizarre delusion.

Patients with schizophrenia experience abnormalities in the form of thought that is observed through the individual's speech. Patients may not be able to carry on a logical conversation and may exhibit signs of loose associations, tangentiality, and incoherence, all of which are ineffective forms of communication. Incoherence is a condition in which each sentence is very difficult or impossible to understand. Infrequently, patients with schizophrenia use a neologism or a combination word in an attempt to communicate.

Bizarre or socially unacceptable behaviors may be observed in the patient with schizophrenia. Patients may wear a wool coat in the summer or hit themselves. Frequently, the seemingly bizarre behavior is a component of another symptom. For example, patients who are hitting themselves may be experiencing visual hallucinations of being on fire and, in their minds, are hitting the flames to put them out.

The negative symptoms of schizophrenia include affective flattening, poverty of speech, avolition, and social isolation (i.e., **autism**). Affective flattening is descriptive of when a patient has very little or a restricted range of emotional expression or affect. The examiner can observe that the patient's face is without expression or response, eye contact is poor, and body language is reduced. If the affect of the patient is not appropriate to the situation (e.g., the patient is laughing while describing a funeral), then the patient has an inappropriate affect. Poverty of speech (i.e., **alogia**) is manifested by brief replies to questions with little spontaneous speech and may result in mutism. Patients with **avolition** do not initiate or persist in goal-directed activities. The patient may be observed to sit for a long period of time and not show interest in activities. Autistic behavior is descriptive of when a patient appears withdrawn and inwardly directed.

The negative symptoms of schizophrenia are nonspecific and may be a consequence of the adverse effects of antipsychotic medications (e.g., sedation, pseudo-Parkinson's) or comorbid depression. In addition, the negative symptoms may result from the positive symptoms of schizophrenia. For example, patients with a delusional belief that they are at risk of being harmed may not talk and will remain isolated to protect themselves. A careful assessment is required to differentiate negative symptoms from the compounding factors.

Treatment of schizophrenia consists primarily of antipsychotic medications, which are most effective for the positive symptoms of schizophrenia. The negative symptoms of schizophrenia are more difficult to treat, with resultant continued disability. Patients that develop depression may also receive antidepressant medication in addition to the antipsychotic.

Cognitive Disorders

Cognitive function refers to an individual's ability to know or perceive. Therefore, patients with cognitive disorders present with deficiencies in cognitive function (e.g., attention, language, memory, construction) and higher functions (e.g., intellect, abstraction, judgment). The DSM-IV divides the **cognitive disorders** into three major categories: (1) delirium, (2) dementia, and (3) amnestic disorders. This section focuses on delirium and dementia as two common psychiatric disorders that pharmacists encounter.

Delirium

Delirium is characterized by alterations in consciousness and change in cognition that develops over a short period of time (Box 19-3). Patients with delirium may have fluctuating symptoms and appear to be normal in the morning, but during the

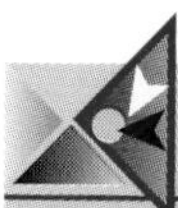

Box 19-3

SYMPTOMS OF DELIRIUM

- Disorientation
- Confusion
- Reduced attention, concentration, and memory
- Rambling speech
- Hallucinations
- Delusions
- Behavioral disinhibition
- Emotional lability
- Irritability
- Fragmented sleep/wake cycle (increased symptoms at night)
- Tremors and abnormal reflexes

Adapted from the DSM-IV (APA, 1994).

evening, they may become threatening, scream, curse, and attempt to pull out intravenous lines or other medical equipment. Patients with delirium are usually disoriented to time and/or place and are easily distracted, with a decreased ability to focus their attention. It is very difficult to conduct an interview with a patient suffering from delirium. The patient's speech may be rambling and irrelevant. The patient may also experience illusions and/or hallucinations and sleep disturbances. Neurologic findings include tremors and abnormal reflexes.

Patients with general medical conditions (e.g., congestive heart failure, pneumonia, urinary tract infections, electrolyte disturbances, cancer), especially those patients who are elderly, are at the greatest risk to develop delirium. Contributing factors include the toxicity from numerous medications, especially those with anticholinergic, analgesic, or sedative effects. In addition, the withdrawal of sedative hypnotics, including alcohol, may result in delirium. Determining and addressing the causative factor of delirium is the first step in treatment. Nondrug therapy, such as having a staff member or relative provide orientation for the patient, use of a clock or calendar, and sensory stimulation with lights or a television, may help to calm the patient. If delirium continues, short-term use of high-potency, low-anticholinergic, antipsychotic medications or short-acting benzodiazepines may be indicated.

Dementia

Dementia is characterized by a decline in social and/or occupational functioning and cognitive deficits that include impairment of memory. The onset of dementia depends on the cause, but it usually occurs later in life. Children 4 years and older may develop dementia because of a medical condition or head trauma. There are numerous causes of dementia, many of which are reversible after identification and treatment. These include hyponatremia, hypoglycemia, urinary tract infection, and especially, depression. In addition, signs and symptoms of dementia are frequently drug-induced (Box 19-4). The irreversible dementias include dementia of the Alzheimer's type, vascular dementia, dementia resulting from acquired immunodeficiency syndrome, head trauma, and Huntington's disease (Box 19-5).

Memory impairment is the hallmark of dementia. Patients with memory impairment have difficulty in recalling previously learned material or in learning new material. Patients misplace valuables (e.g., purse, eyeglasses), forget appointments, or get lost in familiar neighborhoods. The cognitive deficits of dementia include aphasia, apraxia, agnosia, or disturbance in executive functioning. Patients with aphasia have difficulty with spoken or written language. **Apraxia** describes the patient's impaired ability to perform motor activities, despite intact motor abilities, sensory function, and comprehension of the task. **Agnosia** is the inability to recognize or identify objects or people. The disturbance in executive functioning is a common finding in dementia. Patients describe a loss in the ability to perform higher-level cognitive functioning (e.g., abstract thinking, planning, completion of a complex task). Dementia is usually not associated with a disturbance of consciousness or perception.

The most important step in the assessment of a patient with delirium or dementia is to identify the disorder (Table 19-1) and then treat all reversible causes. For patients with irreversible dementia, treatment consists of assistance with daily activities and monitoring for additional complicating factors. For patients in the early phases of dementia of the Alzheimer's type, medication therapy with acetylcholinesterase inhibitors may be minimally effective in delaying progression of the illness.

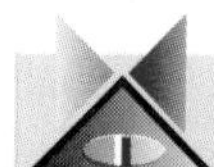

Box 19-4

MEDICATION-RELATED CAUSES OF DEMENTIA-LIKE SYMPTOMS

- Antiarrhythmics
- Antibiotics
- Anticholinergics
- Antidepressants
- Anticonvulsants
- Antiemetics
- Antihypertensives
- Antineoplastics
- Antiparkinsonian agents
- Antihistamine/decongestants
- Cardiac agents (e.g., digoxin)
- Corticosteroids
- Histamine-receptor antagonists
- Immunosuppressive agents
- Narcotic analgesics
- Muscle relaxants
- Nonsteroidal anti-inflammatory agents
- Sedative-hypnotic agents

Box 19-5

PHYSICAL CAUSES OF DEMENTIA-LIKE SYMPTOMS

IRREVERSIBLE

- Primary degenerative dementia of the Alzheimer's type
- Creutzfeldt-Jakob syndrome
- Multi-infarct dementia
- Head trauma

REVERSIBLE[a]

- Intracranial tumors or trauma
- Organ failure or insufficiency
- Metabolic/endocrine (e.g., anemia, electrolyte abnormalities, Wilson's disease, Addison's disease, hypothyroidism/hyperthyroidism, hypoparathyroidism/hyperparathyroidism)
- Heavy metal poisoning
- Infections
- Arteriosclerotic disease
- Vitamin-deficiency states
- Psychiatric disorders (e.g., depression, schizophrenic decompensation)
- Visual and hearing disorders

[a]Depending on recognition and treatment.

Substance Use Disorders

Substance use disorders present as a complication from the use of a substance and/or as the compounding factor of another psychiatric illness. **Substance dependence** is a behavioral pattern of compulsive drug use that results in tolerance and/or withdrawal despite significant substance-related problems. **Substance abuse** is a pattern of substance use that results in repeated and harmful consequences and does not include tolerance or withdrawal (DSM-IV). Because of the high incidence of people with substance abuse disorders, it is imperative that pharmacists understand the assessment of these disorders and the complications of drug abuse.

Patients who are intoxicated with a substance exhibit signs and symptoms according to the substance that was used. There are three primary difficulties in assessing a patient who is intoxicated: (1) Patients may not reveal—or may underreveal—all the substances that they have ingested, 2) the true contents of illegal substances may not be known, and (3) patients may have a variety of responses to substances, depending on their personality characteristics, compounding physical or mental illnesses, frequency of use, consumption, and environment. A wide variety of substances can be abused, but the most common are alcohol, sedative-hypnotics, marijuana, opioids, and stimulants.

Alcohol

Because of its availability, alcohol is the most commonly abused substance. Alcohol dependence is typified by the repetitive intake of alcoholic beverages to the degree that the patient is harmed physically, socially, or economically. In addition, the patient is not able to control the frequency or amount of ingestion. There are numerous risk factors for alcohol dependence, including occupation, religion, race, and socioeconomic status. Patients with anxiety or depression are frequently alcohol dependent; however, the use and withdrawal of alcohol contributes to these symptoms, resulting in a vicious cycle. Patients with alcohol dependency can have an extensive number of physical findings, including gastritis, diarrhea, liver damage, peripheral neuropathy, and cardiomyopathy. The signs and symptoms of alcohol intoxication and withdrawal are listed in Box 19-6.

Patients who are withdrawing from alcohol are generally treated with tapering doses of benzodiazepines and supportive care. In addition, patients must receive large doses of the B vitamins, particularly thiamine, to prevent peripheral neuropathy

TABLE 19-1 ➤ DIFFERENTIATING SIGNS AND SYMPTOMS OF DELIRIUM, DEMENTIA, AND DEPRESSION

CHARACTERISTICS	DELIRIUM	DEMENTIA	DEPRESSION
Onset	Rapid, acute	Usually insidious	Usually insidious
Precipitating factors	Present	Usually none	Possibly
Duration	<1 month	>1 month	>2 weeks
Course	Fluctuating	Steady	Steady
Sleep-wake cycle	Always disrupted	Normal	Usually disrupted
Memory	Recent impaired	Recent and remote impaired	Recent impaired
Thinking processes	Disorganized	Impoverished	Slower
Attention	Disturbed, fluctuating	May be intact	Slightly decreased
Awareness	Reduced	Intact	Normal
Alertness	Increased or decreased	Normal or decreased	Normal, increased, or decreased
Perception	Misperceptions often present	Misperceptions often present	Normal

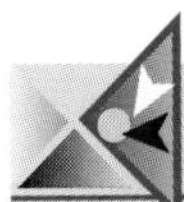

Box 19-6

SIGNS AND SYMPTOMS OF ALCOHOL INTOXICATION AND WITHDRAWAL

INTOXICATION

- Slurred speech
- Incoordination
- Unsteady gait
- Nystagmus
- Flushed face
- Disinhibition of sexual or aggressive impulses
- Mood lability
- Impaired judgment
- Impaired social or occupational functioning
- Impaired attention
- Sedation

WITHDRAWAL

- Nausea or vomiting
- Malaise or weakness
- Tremor
- Anxiety
- Depressed mood or irritability
- Autonomic hyperactivity (tachycardia, sweating, increased blood pressure)
- Headache
- Insomnia
- Hyperthermia
- Transient hallucinations or illusions
- Delirium
- Seizures

and Wernicke-Korsakoff syndrome. After withdrawal symptoms subside, treatment focuses on maintaining sobriety and addressing the concurrent psychiatric conditions. To maintain sobriety, participation in Alcoholics Anonymous is beneficial, and deterrents to the use of alcohol (e.g., disulfiram) may be helpful.

Sedative-Hypnotics

Abuse of sedative-hypnotics, including the benzodiazepines and barbiturates, is often attributed to overprescribing. Use of the barbiturates has dramatically decreased because of the availability of benzodiazepines. The pharmacist's role is to differentiate appropriate versus inappropriate use of sedative-hypnotics. Indications of inappropriate use would include multiple prescribers, multiple sedative-hypnotics, or excessive doses.

The signs and symptoms of intoxication from sedative-hypnotics are similar to those of intoxication from alcohol. The intoxicated patient exhibits unsteady gait, lack of coordination, slurred speech, inattention, impaired memory, impaired judgment, lethargy, and disinhibition. Signs and symptoms of withdrawal are dependent on the daily dose and duration of administration. The larger the dose and the longer the duration of treatment, the more severe the withdrawal process. The signs and symptoms of abrupt withdrawal include anxiety, irritability, nausea, vomiting, tachycardia, sweating, tremor, insomnia, and the possibility of tonic-clonic seizures. Patients are withdrawn from the sedative-hypnotics by gradually decreasing the dose. Abrupt withdrawal of any sedative-hypnotic (including alcohol) can be fatal.

Marijuana

Marijuana has sedative-hypnotic properties; however, it is also known to induce hallucinations and paranoia and is associated with all the risks of tobacco smoking. The active component of marijuana is γ-9-tetrahydrocannabinol (THC). The signs and symptoms of intoxication with marijuana include tachycardia, conjunctival congestion, increased appetite, dry mouth, euphoria, sensory intensification, and apathy. Chronic use of marijuana is associated with amenorrhea, decreased testosterone production, and inhibition of spermatogenesis. In addition, chronic use may cause an amotivational syndrome that is characterized by signs and symptoms of apathy, dullness, impaired judgment,

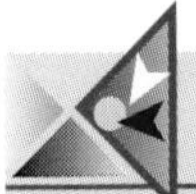

Box 19-7

SIGNS AND SYMPTOMS OF OPIOID INTOXICATION AND WITHDRAWAL

INTOXICATION

- Fluctuating mood (euphoria, dysphoria, apathy)
- Psychomotor retardation
- Impaired judgment
- Impaired attention and memory
- Pupillary constriction
- Drowsiness
- Slurred speech
- Impaired social and occupational functioning

WITHDRAWAL

- Lacrimation
- Rhinorrhea
- Mydriasis
- Piloerection
- Sweating
- Fever
- Nausea and vomiting
- Hypertension (tachycardia)
- Abdominal cramping
- Anxiety
- Craving for opioids
- Insomnia
- Anorexia
- Agitation

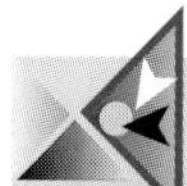

Box 19-8

SIGNS AND SYMPTOMS OF STIMULANT INTOXICATION AND WITHDRAWAL

INTOXICATION

- Tachycardia
- Pupillary dilation
- Hypertension
- Sweating or chills
- Nausea and vomiting
- Motor agitation
- Euphoria
- Grandiosity
- Increased talking
- Impaired in social and occupational functioning

WITHDRAWAL

- Fatigue
- Insomnia or hypersomnia
- Depression
- Irritability
- Anxiety

decreased concentration, decreased memory, decreased personal hygiene, and lack of goal-directed behavior. Treatment of the abuse of marijuana focuses on abstinence and the possibility of an underlying psychiatric disorder.

Opioids

The abused opioids include street drugs (e.g., heroin) and the prescription opioids. Patients may become dependent on opioids either through illicit use or during proper medical treatment. The signs and symptoms of opioid intoxication and withdrawal are listed in Box 19-7. Treatment of intoxication is the careful use of opioid antagonists and supportive care. Treatment of opioid withdrawal includes substitution with the long-acting opioid methadone and subsequent tapering. Alternatively, use of tapering doses of a central a_2-agonist, such as clonidine, to attenuate the noradrenergic hyperactivity of opiate withdrawal may alleviate the symptoms of withdrawal.

Stimulants

Stimulants include the amphetamines and their derivatives, cocaine, phenylpropanolamine, ephedrine, and caffeine. The effects of stimulants include reduced fatigue, increased alertness, and decreased appetite. The signs and symptoms of stimulant intoxication and withdrawal are listed in Box 19-8. Treatment of intoxication may involve antipsychotic or benzodiazepine antianxiety drugs. Treatment of stimulant abuse is focused on abstinence and treatment of any underlying psychiatric disorder.

SYSTEM ASSESSMENT

Subjective Information

The physical status of a patient can dramatically influence the mental status examination (MSE). Brain functioning can be modified by disease states, trauma, lack of sleep, changes in electrolyte levels, reduced energy sources, increased levels of perceived stress, and medications. For example, a patient with a fever or a metabolic process may not be able to abstract or make new memories until the physical illness is resolved. An increase in the level of stress that a patient experiences may result in transient dysfunction in mental capacity. Common stressful events would include the death of a close relative or the loss of a job.

The MSE assesses a patient's higher cortical functioning and emotional state. The MSE is not measured like a blood pressure, however. Rather, it is inferred through observation of the patient's behavior and a series of questions. Factors that affect the mental status include age, physical changes in health (e.g., lack of sleep, alcoholism, chronic renal disease), drugs of all kinds (e.g., illicit, alcohol, over-the-counter [OTC], prescription), stress (e.g., job, family, school, life events), level of education, and mental disorders. The definitive diagnosis of a psychiatric disorder includes the MSE, psychiatric history, medical history, physical examination, and appropriate laboratory test results.

Integrating parts of the MSE into the health history according to the patient's presentation is adequate for most people; however, it is necessary to perform a full MSE if the patient shows any abnormality in affect or behavior. The MSE does not have to be a separate part of the patient evaluation, but it should be based on the observation of the patient throughout the history and physical examination. Information that is acquired during the MSE may influence the physical examination, and vice versa.

The MSE should be conducted in a private, quiet, and comfortable area. If possible, both the examiner and the patient should be sitting. Patients usually have less anxiety if the examiner is at the same eye level. Because of possible fluctuations in mental status, the interviewer should note the specific time of the interview. Specific documentation of the results of the MSE allows subsequent assessment for deterioration or improvement over time.

The interviewer should cover most areas of the MSE, but not necessarily in the exact order described below. Flexibility in interviewing skills, however, requires practice. More difficult screening questions can be asked initially to determine the person's level of functioning in a specified area. A correct answer to a difficult question indicates an adequate level of functioning in that area, so further testing of that area is probably unnecessary. Throughout the interview, the examiner should also consider the patient's intellectual level, geographic region, and cultural background.

The four main areas of assessment for the MSE are (1) general appearance and attitude, (2) behavior, (3) cognitive functioning, and (4) thought processes, content, and perceptions. In practice, inspection of general appearance, attitude, and behavior are completed concurrently with the subjective evaluation of cognitive functioning and thought processes. As a student, you will notice that inspection is an "objective" physical examination skill and is usually covered in the "objective" section of each chapter. To accurately represent what is done in practice, however, inspection of general appearance, attitude, and behavior are addressed in the "subjective" section of this chapter. To maintain consistency, this chapter uses the "objective" format for those sections involving inspection or observation.

General Appearance and Attitude

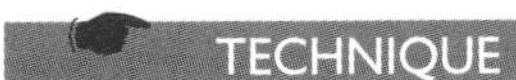

STEP 1

Observe the Patient's Appearance and Attitude

- Have the patient sit or stand in a relaxed position.
- Observe and document the patient's posture, body movements, grooming, hygiene, and clothing. (The documentation should be complete enough that another practitioner could recognize the patient from the description.)

ABNORMALITIES Body movements should be voluntary, deliberate, coordinated, and at the appropriate rate. The person should be clean and well groomed. Clothing should be appropriate for setting, season, age, gender, and social group; it should also fit and be put on appropriately. Sitting on the edge of the chair, restless pacing, frowning, scanning the environment, and tense muscles may indicate anxiety, whereas sitting slumped in a chair or slow gait are associated with depression. Poor hygiene or a lack of concern about appearance is associated with depression and Alzheimer's disease. Excessive grooming is associated with OCD. Patients with mental disorders are frequently observed to dress inappropriately. Patients with Alzheimer's disease may wear their pajamas over their daytime clothing. Patients with schizophrenia may wear a coat as a protective covering at all times, regardless of the environmental temperature, and patients in the manic phase of bipolar disorder may dress in a provocative manner.

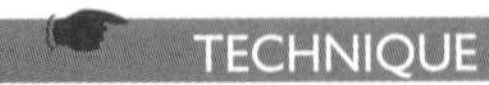

STEP 1 (Continued)

- Note the patient's attitude towards the examiner.

ABNORMALITIES The patient should be receptive and cooperative with your questions. Patients who are evasive, apathetic, hostile, or paranoid require further questioning to determine the cause.

Behavior

STEP 1

Assess the Patient's Level of Consciousness

- Observe and document the patient's level of consciousness.

ABNORMALITIES Consciousness is the most basic of the mental status functions and represents the person being aware of one's own existence, feelings, thoughts, and environment. The patient should be awake, alert, and appropriately responding to internal and external stimuli. Patients whose consciousness is found to be lethargic (hypersomnia), obtunded, stuporous, semicomatose (the patient requires vigorous and repeated stimulation for a response), and comatose (unarousable, unresponsive to noxious stimuli) require further evaluation to determine the cause.

 TECHNIQUE

STEP 2

Assess the Patient's Facial Expression and Reaction to Stimuli or Questioning

- Observe and document the patient's facial expressions and reaction to stimuli or questioning.

ABNORMALITIES The person should exhibit an appropriate facial expression, which should change appropriately with the situation. There should be an appropriate amount of eye contact within cultural norms. The person should share the conversation appropriately, at a moderate pace, and be able to clearly articulate. A flat or mask-like expression is associated with schizophrenia or parkinsonism. Dysarthria should be noted if the person exhibits distorted speech sounds and cannot articulate. Pace of the conversation can be increased by anxiety and reduced in patients with parkinsonism or depression.

 TECHNIQUE

STEP 3

Assess the Patient's Speech and Language Comprehension

- Observe and document the patient's speech and language comprehension.
- To test for aphasia, show the patient an item (e.g., watch, pen), and ask the person to name it.

ABNORMALITIES The patient should speak smoothly, use the correct words, and be able to name common objects. Patients with aphasia have difficulty with language comprehension and production related to certain types of brain damage. Patients with an inability to name an item respond with answers such as, "A thing you write with," or "A thing you tell time with."

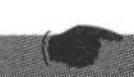 TECHNIQUE

STEP 4

Assess the Patient's Emotional State

- Assess and document the patient's mood and affect.

☛ Observe the range, intensity, lability and the appropriateness of the affect in relationship to the patient's content of thought.

ABNORMALITIES The patient should have an appropriate range and intensity of emotions according to the topic of conversation or the patient's situation. A labile or inappropriate affect may indicate a mood disorder or psychosis. An inappropriate affect is noted when a person is laughing but topic of conversation or the situation (e.g., a funeral) is appropriately serious or sad. A depressed mood is noted when the patient describes feelings of being low, down, or depressed. A patient with a euphoric mood describes feelings of elation and of being on top of the world.

Cognitive Functioning

Assessment of the patient's cognitive functioning can be completed by asking a variety of questions from various perspectives. Because the basis of this assessment is the interview, the common "subjective" format found in previous chapters is used here. The examples provided illustrate only one way of how this questioning might be completed. Interview questions are grouped in major sections according to the area of cognitive functioning being assessed.

Orientation to Time, Place, and Person

INTERVIEW What is today's date? What is the day of the week? What season are we in? Where are you? What time is it? What town are we in? What state are we in? Please state your name. What is my name? What is my occupation?

CAUTION When testing for a person's orientation to time, the examiner should ask the patient to tell the examiner the approximate time of day, day of week, date, year, and season. Asking the patient to state the year is very important in some cases, because the patient may be able to state the other time descriptors but not know the year or state a previous year.

ABNORMALITIES Time changes more frequently than place; therefore, orientation is lost first to time and then to place. Rarely does a person lose orientation to himself or herself, but this may be found in cases of amnesia. If the patient states that he or she is in a hospital but cannot state the exact name, this may be acceptable. However, patients in a hospital who state that they are in a hotel are obviously not oriented to place. Orientation may be altered by a variety of physical (e.g., electrolyte disturbances, pain) and mental (e.g., delirium, dementia) conditions. In addition, the side effects of a variety of drugs are some of the most frequent causes of disorientation.

Concentration and Attention Span

There are a variety of tests to assess the patient's concentration and attention span. The examiner can use simple mathematic calculations, spelling a five-letter word backward (e.g., *world*), digit-sequence recall that is presented at the rate of one digit per second, and serial 3's or 7's. For the serial 3's or 7's test, ask the patient to start with 100, subtract either 3 or 7 from it, and then continue from there. The patient should be able to do simple mathematic calculations or spelling tasks correctly and at a normal pace.

INTERVIEW Please spell the word *world* backward. Start at 100 and subtract 7 to get an answer, then continue subtracting 7 and stating the answer until I tell you to stop.

ABNORMALITIES Patients who cannot complete the simple tests of attention span and concentration may have a physical disorder, anxiety, drug use, or a variety of mental disorders.

Immediate, Recent, and Long-Term Memory

Recent memory of events that have happened within the last few days may be assessed with the following questions.

INTERVIEW Tell me what you have eaten in the last 24 hours. I am going to state four words; after I have said them all, please repeat them back to me: *ball, chair, clown, plant.*

In the latter question, the patient must repeat the four words back, or the test is invalid. The examiner then continues with typical interview questions that serve as a distracter for the patient. After approximately 5 minutes, the examiner asks the patient to recall the four words. The examiner should select four words from different categories (e.g., a specific animal, color, object).

Immediate memory is the ability to recall information, such as the seven-digit sequence recall. To have a valid test of immediate memory, the patient must have the ability to pay attention.

INTERVIEW Please repeat the following sequence of numbers back to me. 8, 1, 3, 6, 10, 15, 21.

For long-term memory, the examiner can ask verifiable chronologic events in the patient's life history concerning past health, first job, birthday, anniversary dates, and other relevant dates. Questions about past presidents, dates of wars, and other significant events are easier to use, because the information is more readily available to everyone. In contrast to recent or immediate memory, long-term memory is usually retained in most patients.

INTERVIEW What is your birthday? Who was the first president of the United States? On what date did the invasion of Pearl Harbor occur?

CAUTION Certain memories will be influenced by the patient's country of origin.

ABNORMALITIES A patient should be able to describe their diet and remember four out of four words after 5 minutes. A patient should be able to perform the seven digit-immediate recall with minimal effort. A patient should be able to recall events that happened years ago. Memory can be affected by a variety of causes, including Alzheimer's dementia, inattention, distractibility, amnesia, depression (i.e., lack of effort), and anxiety. A person who confabulates, especially to impress the interviewer, may be suffering from memory loss.

Abstract Reasoning

Abstract reasoning is a higher cortical function that is demonstrated by an ability to think beyond the concrete and literal. Ask the patient to state the similarities and differences of two items, such as an apple and an orange. Ask the patient to interpret a proverb, such "People who live in glass houses should not throw stones." The patient should be able to give examples of how an apple and an orange are similar (e.g., both grow on trees, both are fruit) and different (e.g., one is red, one is orange). The answers to the proverbs should demonstrate the ability to abstract a personal or reflective meaning (e.g. certain things happen in life, and it is best to carry on and not be stuck in the past).

INTERVIEW How are a cat and a mouse alike? What do people mean when they say "There is no use crying over spilled milk"? "Don't judge a book by its cover?"

ABNORMALITIES Concrete and literal interpretations of these proverbs may include answers such as, respectively, "The milk is dirty," or "The book may have dirty pictures in it." The inability to abstract may reflect a thought disorder but can also reflect cultural influences, educational level, and socioeconomic status.

Insight and Judgment

Ask the patient to explain their disorder to you. A patient with good insight should be able to recognize that the symptoms of the illness are abnormal and understand the origin and development of the symptoms. Also, ask the patient to describe their future plans or use a scenario such as, 'What would you do if you smelled smoke in a crowded movie theater?" Good judgment is demonstrated by acting responsibly and responding in an appropriate manner.

INTERVIEW What seems to be the trouble? What do you think is wrong? How are you going to manage if you lose your job?

ABNORMALITIES Lack of insight may be found in patients who deny that they are ill or in those with a formal thought disorder. Patients who would yell "Fire!" in a crowded movie theater would not be demonstrating good judgment. A lack of insight and poor judgment suggest that a patient may not be able—or may not be willing—to participate in their own health care.

Ability to Perform Complex Acts

Ask the patient to use a comb, drink from a glass, draw a house, copy geometric forms, or button their shirt. A patient should be able to perform any of these tasks with minimal effort and time.

INTERVIEW Can you draw me a picture of a house? Please draw a clock face with the numbers and the hands.

ABNORMALITIES Apraxia is the inability to perform these types of tasks and is associated with patients with cognitive decline because of Alzheimer's disease or other types of dementia.

Level of Ambivalence

Ambivalence is the coexistence of opposite thoughts, feelings, and will (e.g., wanting to eat but also not wanting to eat).

INTERVIEW Describe your plans for the next few days.

ABNORMALITIES A patient should be able to have a direction or goal and be able to make a decision requiring higher cortical functioning. A certain level of ambivalence is normal, however, and reflects the need for time to make a decision or to decide on a goal or direction.

INTERVIEW What is one thing that you would like to get done this week? What will do you to make this happen?

ABNORMALITIES A high level of ambivalence is disabling and associated with mental disorders, such as schizophrenia, bipolar disorder, and OCD.

Thought Process, Content, and Perceptions

Logic, Relevance, Organization, and Coherence of Thought Processes

The majority of this assessment is completed by listening to the words and speech of the patient throughout the interview. The interviewer should follow appropriate leads for further clarification. A normal patient will have a logical train of thought with an appropriate, timely response to a question.

A patient's thought process is the way a person thinks, and it is assessed by listening to the patient's speech or communication pattern. Several descriptors are used to describe a person's communication pattern. **Circumstantiality** describes when a patient includes peripheral details or minutiae that are assumed to be implicit to the conversation. **Tangentiality** is when the patient wanders to a distant point in the conversation and is unable to return spontaneously to the original point. Patients with flight of ideas change from topic to topic with more or less of an apparent connection between the topics. **Loosening of associations** is when an examiner cannot follow the patient's conversation because the patient combines unrelated topics or words. At the end of the patient's paragraph, it is difficult—and sometimes impossible—to interpret the meaning of the statements. **Word salad** is a rare form of communication in which the patient uses only jumbled words and not sentences. **Perseveration** is when patients repeat the same words over and over, and **echolalia** is when patients repeats the words the examiner stated. A **neologism** is a nonexistent word or a combination of words that the patient invents. Only the patient knows the meaning of the neologism. Patients who suddenly stop speaking in midsentence may be noted to have **thought blocking. Confabulation** is when a patient in clear consciousness fabricates a memory. The fabricated memory may be described in great detail and is not judged to be morally wrong. The patient is merely replacing lost memory with fantasy. Patients may confabulate to avoid embarrassment at the loss of true memory.

A certain amount of circumstantiality and tangentiality occurs in normal conversation, but it becomes problematic with extensive use. Flight of ideas is most frequently found in patients during the acute phases of mania. Loosening of associations is most commonly found in patients with schizophrenia or during the severe stages of mania. Word salad, perseveration, and echolalia are found in acute stages of schizophrenia or dementia. Neologisms are used by patients with schizophrenia. Thought blocking may be found in patients with schizophrenia and as an adverse drug effect. Confabulation may commonly be found in patients with dementia.

Thought Content

Thought content is used to describe what a person thinks, their specific ideas or beliefs, and it is assessed by listening to the patient's answers to questions. A patient with appropriate thought content will have ideas or beliefs that are within the normal range. In addition, a normal patient will not have excessive obsessions, compulsions, or phobias.

? INTERVIEW Describe any repetitive thoughts, ideas, impulses, or phobias that you regard as senseless. Can you tell me more about that? What do you think about at times like these?

➤ ABNORMALITIES Patients with abnormal thought content will have delusions, obsessions, and phobias. A delusion is a fixed, false belief that can have a variety of themes (e.g., persecutory, religious, somatic, or grandiose). Delusions are fixed because the patient cannot be talked out of the delusions—even if evidence to the contrary is presented. Delusions are false because the delusion is not in keeping with reality and, finally, is a belief of the patient. **Obsessions** are repetitive thoughts, ideas, or impulses that are recognized by the patient as senseless. A **compulsion** is a repetitive behavior (e.g., checking, handwashing) or a mental act (e.g., counting, repeating words silently) that the patient feels forced to complete. Obsessions or compulsions are considered to be normal if they do not substantially interfere with thinking or activities of daily living. Phobias are irrational fears that are associated with severe anxiety; people will avoid the object or situation to avoid embarrassment and the accompanying fear.

Risk for Suicide

Assessment for suicidal ideations requires a sense of trust and empathy from the practitioner. Often, it is more difficult for the practitioner to ask these types of questions than it is for the patient to answer. To assess the patient, begin with general questions, and if the answers suggest suicidal tendencies, ask more detailed questions.

These questions are very important, and contrary to popular belief, asking about suicide does not promote the idea of suicide. Patients will often report a sense of relief that someone has initiated the discussion. A patient who is not at risk of harming themselves or suicidal will answer these questions in a straightforward manner. In addition, the patient will indicate plans for the future.

? INTERVIEW Do you have any ideas or thought of harming yourself? Do you have any thoughts, ideas, or plans to commit suicide?

➤ ABNORMALITIES Patients will admit that they have had thoughts of harming themselves or of suicide. Indicators of suicidal intent are previous suicide attempts; symptoms of major depression or schizophrenia; verbal or written expressions relating to death, failure, or worthlessness; and giving away of personal possessions. A specific plan of suicide or an actual attempt requires immediate referral to a psychiatrist and almost always hospitalization. In some instances, it may be necessary to arrange for transportation to the hospital.

Altered Perceptions of the Senses

A perception is the awareness of stimuli through any of the five senses. A normal patient should not have any alterations to their five senses and should be able to describe normal perceptions.

? INTERVIEW Describe any changes in your senses. Are you hearing things that are not there? Do you see things that other people do not? Are you experiencing any unusual smells, tastes, or touches to your skin?

➤ ABNORMALITIES Illusions are when a person misperceives visual stimuli (e.g., a mirage in the desert). Hallucinations have no obvious stimuli and can occur in any of the five sensory modalities (i.e., auditory, visual, olfactory, gustatory, tactile). Hallucinations are associated with a variety of mental illnesses, adverse effects of medications, substances of abuse, and temporal lobe epilepsy. Hypnopompic hallucinations are noted when a person has a hallucination on arising from sleep. Hypnagogic hallucinations occur when a person is falling to sleep. Both phenomena should be differentiated from other types of hallucinations.

Objective Information

Physical Assessment

Normally, physical examination techniques are presented at this point in each chapter. As explained previously, however, completion of a MSE is unique. Therefore, to maintain an accurate representation of practice, all areas of a MSE have been presented in the subjective information section.

Laboratory and Diagnostic Tests

All patients with suspected changes in mental status should receive a complete physical examination by a primary care provider that includes a urinalysis and blood tests for electrolytes, glucose, complete blood cell count, as well as laboratory tests to establish renal, hepatic, and thyroid functioning. The patient will continue to display alterations in mental status until appropriate treatment for the underlying physical or laboratory abnormality is received.

Mini-Mental Status Examination

The Mini-Mental Status Examination (Fig. 19-1) is a formalized screening tool for cognitive functions. It requires only 5 to 10 minutes to administer, and it can be administered for both initial and serial measurement of worsening or improvement of cognition over time. The tool concentrates only on cognitive function, not on mood or thought processes; therefore, it is a

Patient ______________

Examiner ______________

Date ______________

"Mini-Mental State"

Maximum Score	Score	
		Orientation
5	( )	What is the (year) (season) (date) (day) (month)?
5	( )	Where are we: (State) (country) (town) (hospital) (floor).
		Registration
3	( )	Name 3 objects: give 1 second to say each. Then ask the patient all 3 after you have said them. Give 1 point for each correct answer. Then repeat them until he learns all 3. Count trials and record.
		Attention and calculation
5	( )	Serial 7's. 1 point for each correct. Stop after 5 answers. Alternatively spell "world" backwards.
		Recall
3	( )	Ask for the 3 objects repeated above. Give 1 point for each correct.
		Language
9	( )	Name a pencil, and watch (2 points) Repeat the following "No ifs, and or buts" (1 point) Follow a 3-stage command: "Take a paper in your right hand, fold in half and put it on the floor" (3 points) Read and obey the following: CLOSE YOUR EYES (1 point) Write a sentence (1 point) Copy a design (1 point)

______________ Total score

Assess level of consciousness along a continuum ______________

Alert   Drowsy   Stupor   Coma

FIGURE 19-1 ■ Mini-Mental Status Examination.

Instructions for administration of
Mini-mental state examination

Orientation

(1) Ask for the date. Then ask specifically for parts omitted, e.g., "Can you also tell me what season it is?" One point for each correct.

(2) Ask in turn "Can you tell me the name of this hospital?" (town, country, etc.) One point for each correct.

Registration

Ask the patient if you may test his memory. Then say the names of 3 unrelated objects, clearly and slowly, about one second for each. After you have said all 3, ask him to repeat them. This first repetition determines his score (0-3) but keep saying them until he can repeat all 3, up to 6 trials. If he does not eventually learn all 3, recall cannot be meaningfully tested.

Attention and calculation

Ask the patient to begin with 100 and count backwards by 7. Stop after 5 subtractions (93, 86, 79, 72, 65). Score the total number of correct answers.

If the patient cannot or will not perform this task, ask him to spell the word "world" backwards. The score is the number of letters in correct order. E.g. dlrow = 5, dlorw = 3.

Recall

Ask the patient if he can recall the 3 words you previously asked him to remember. Score 0-3

Language

Naming: Show the patient a wrist watch and ask him what it is. Repeat for pencil. Score 0-2.

Repetition: Ask the patient to repeat the sentence after you. Allow only one trial. Score 0 or 1.

3-Stage command: Give the patient a piece of plain blank paper and repeat the command. Score 1 point for each part correctly executed.

Reading: On a blank piece of paper print the sentence "Close your eyes," in letters large enough for the patient to see clearly. Ask him to read it and do what it says. Score 1 point only if he actually closes his eyes.

Writing: Give the patient a blank piece of paper and ask him to write a sentence for you. Do not dictate a sentence, it is to be written spontaneously. It must contain a subject and verb and be sensible. Correct grammar and punctuation are not necessary.

Copying: On a clean piece of paper, draw intersecting pentagons, each side about 1 in., and ask him to copy it exactly as it is. All 10 angles must be present and 2 must intersect to score 1 point. Tremor and rotation are ignored.

Estimate the patient's level of sensorium along a continuum, from alert on the left to coma on the right.

Reference:
Folstein MF, Folstein SE, McHugh PR. "Mini-Mental State": A practical method for grading the cognitive state of patients for the clinician. J Psychiat Res 1975, Volume 12, pp. 189-198.

FIGURE 19-1 ■ Continued

good screening tool to detect dementia or delirium. The maximum score is 30, and normal people average a score of 27.

Special Considerations

Pediatric Patients

Assessment of the pediatric patient is performed according to the developmental stage of the child. Adolescents can be assessed in a similar fashion as adults. Additional questions for the pediatric patient's parent or guardian include:

? INTERVIEW Has there been any change in the child's personality and/or behavior? Have you noticed any physical changes in your child? How has the child been performing in school? Have there been any changes in the child's school performance? Describe the child's peer relationships. How about the relationships between the child and the family? Mother? Father? Siblings? Has the child reached the developmentally appropriate milestones, such as toilet training?

ABNORMALITIES Developmental milestones are important in monitoring the mental as well as physical development of a child. Attention deficient hyperactivity disorder is often diagnosed when a child enters school, where either inattention or hyperactive-impulsive behavior becomes more noticeable and problematic. Inattention may be demonstrated by failure to pay close attention to details, trouble sustaining attention during tasks, easy distractibility, forgetfulness, and avoidance of schoolwork or homework. Hyperactivity-impulsivity can manifest as fidgeting, talking excessively, interrupting others, difficulty waiting their turn, difficulty playing quietly, running or climbing inappropriately, and leaving their seat in the classroom when seating is expected.

Although attention deficit hyperactivity disorder can be diagnosed for the first time in adolescence or adulthood, the answers to the previous questions in the teen years are often tools to determine whether an adolescent is struggling with depression or substance abuse. Signs and symptoms of depression are similar regardless of age. Puberty, however, can make it difficult to determine if common symptoms such as forgetfulness, negative attitude, and labile emotions are a normal part of development or a sign of more serious problems. To make it more difficult, some symptoms of depression, such as a change in eating or sleeping habits, may also be symptoms of a substance abuse problem. Symptoms that persist for more than a couple of weeks should raise concern and prompt referral to a mental health professional.

Substance abuse, as described earlier, can result in personality, behavioral, and physical changes in an adolescent as well as an adult. Drug-related personality changes are often obvious and noticeable and will worsen over time. Drug-related changes occur faster than personality changes because of normal development, and they often appear to have no obvious cause. These changes may include a sudden shift in a teen's interests or hobbies, irritability, withdrawal from family and friends, sudden mood swings, nervousness, lack of initiative, and defensiveness. Behavioral changes may include new friends, unwillingness to introduce friends to parents, lying, stealing, abusive behavior, unexplained phone calls, risky behavior, being late to events, and increased conflict with siblings. In school, grades may drop, discipline problems may develop, and the teen may skip classes and drop out of afterschool activities. Personal habits may also change, such as an increase or decrease in appetite, erratic sleep habits, excessive protection of the bedroom and personal space, and an excessively messy, cold, or frequently aired-out bedroom. Physical changes may include silliness, paranoia, weight loss, chronic cough, slurred speech, frequent colds or flu, and rapid muscle growth.

Geriatric Patients

Additional questions for the geriatric patient and/or caregiver include:

INTERVIEW Can you tell me what medications you are taking? For what conditions are you taking these medications? Are you having any side effects from these medications? Do you forget to take your medications? If so, how often? What do you do to help yourself remember?

ABNORMALITIES For the geriatric patient, start the assessment by checking for sensory changes in hearing and vision. Loss of hearing and vision is common in older adults, can make the elderly person look confused, and can produce social isolation, frustration, and possibly, suspicion. In general, there is no loss of general knowledge and little to no loss in vocabulary. In addition, during retirement, many elderly people do not know the exact date and time, but this is considered to be normal.

Pregnant Patients

Additional questions for the pregnant patient include:

INTERVIEW During your previous pregnancy, did you experience any changes in your mood? Did you become sad or depressed during your previous pregnancy? After the birth of the baby?

ABNORMALITIES Depression is twice as common in women as in men, and it reaches its peak incidence between 25 and 45 years, the primary reproductive age of a woman. It is becoming more recognized that childbirth is a major risk factor in development of mental illness. It is currently estimated that 40% of the 4 million births occurring every year in the United States are complicated by some form of postpartum mood disorder. Forty percent to eighty-five percent of women who deliver a baby experience a mild form of depression 3 to 5 days after delivery. Symptoms of this "normal" phenomenon are irritability, anxiety, confusion, crying spells, mood lability, and disturbances in sleep and appetite. These symptoms spontaneously resolve within 24 to 72 hours. Postpartum depression complicates 10% to 15% of all deliveries and is even more common following deliveries by adolescent women (26%–32%). The majority of patients have an onset of symptoms within 6 weeks of delivery and usually suffer from this illness for more than 6 months. Symptoms include dysphoric mood, loss of interest in usually pleasurable activities, difficulty concentrating or making decisions, psychomotor agitation or retardation, fatigue, changes in appetite or sleep, recurrent thoughts of death/suicide, feelings of worthlessness or guilt (especially failure at motherhood), and excessive anxiety over the child's health. Women who experience postpartum depression are at higher risk of recurrence following subsequent pregnancies.

APPLICATION TO PATIENT SYMPTOMS

The pharmacist needs to work to develop a therapeutic relationship with the patient for that patient to feel comfortable revealing their symptoms completely and accurately. If patients don't feel that they can trust the pharmacist, they may describe themselves in a positive way or simply describe vague symptoms that require further assessment. It is important that the pharmacist be able to recognize the signs and symptoms of a potential mental illness, assess the patient's presenting symptoms, make recommendations, and refer the patient to a mental health care practitioner, if necessary.

Memory Problems

Memory problems are associated with several mental illnesses and physical disorders. It is important that the patient receive a thorough medical assessment to eliminate any physical causes of dementia (see Box 19-5). A thorough assessment of the patient and their medications should be done to identify possible drug-therapy problems and, specifically, any medication-related causes (see Box 19-4).

CASE STUDY

WP is a 65-year-old man who comes into the pharmacy and states that he has been feeling rather strange lately. He explains that he has become more forgetful and that his wife has noticed he appears to be "spacey." He is worried that he is becoming senile. His past medical history includes hypertension, insomnia, and heartburn.

ASSESSMENT OF THE PATIENT

Subjective Information

65-year-old man complaining of forgetfulness

WHEN DID THESE SYMPTOMS START? Over the last couple of weeks.

COULD YOU PLEASE DESCRIBE HOW YOU HAVE BEEN FEELING? I feel like my head is not clear and that I cannot think as clearly.

HOW HAS YOUR MEMORY BEEN AFFECTED? I have forgotten where I have placed items, like my car keys. It is taking me more time to complete simple tasks.

IS THERE A TIME OF DAY OR NIGHT WHEN THE PROBLEM IS WORSE? No, I have not noticed any difference. The problem just comes and goes.

ARE YOU HAVING TROUBLE WITH TIME AND DATES? Sometimes I forget the day of the week.

CAN YOU TELL ME TODAY'S DATE AND APPROXIMATE TIME? Today is Sunday, October 31, 1999, about three in the afternoon.

I ASSUME THAT YOU KNOW WHERE YOU ARE. AM I CORRECT? Yes, I am at the pharmacy.

ARE YOU CURRENTLY HAVING ANY PHYSICAL PROBLEMS? No, not that I know of.

ARE YOU TAKING ANY MEDICATIONS? I have been taking enalapril for my blood pressure.

HOW LONG HAVE YOU BEEN TAKING ENALAPRIL? For over a year.

HOW IS YOUR BLOOD PRESSURE? Good, it was 140/85 last time I was at the doctor's office.

HAVE YOU HAD ANY SIDE EFFECTS FROM THE ENALAPRIL? No, not that I have noticed.

DO YOU HAVE TROUBLE REMEMBERING TO TAKE THE ENALAPRIL? No, I take it every morning when I brush my teeth.

ARE YOU TAKING ANY OTHER MEDICATIONS? No.

ARE YOU TAKING ANY OVER-THE-COUNTER OR HERBAL MEDICATIONS? No herbals, but I take Benadryl and cimetidine.

WHY ARE YOU TAKING THE BENADRYL? To help me sleep.

HOW LONG HAVE YOU BEEN HAVING TROUBLE SLEEPING? I have had trouble sleeping on and off, but over the last month, I have had more trouble getting to sleep.

IS THERE ANYTHING UNUSUAL THAT HAS BEEN HAPPENING OVER THE LAST MONTH? HAS THERE BEEN A CHANGE IN YOUR DAILY LIFE? Well, I am retiring in 2 weeks, but nothing else.

DO YOU HAVE PLANS FOR YOUR RETIREMENT? Some, but now I don't know. I can't do much, if I'm becoming senile.

HOW MUCH OF THE BENADRYL ARE YOU TAKING? I have been taking a couple of the Benadryl.

HOW MANY IS A "COUPLE?" I take two 25-mg capsules.

OVER THE LAST MONTH, HOW MANY TIMES HAVE YOU TAKEN THE BENADRYL? About three or four times per week.

EARLIER, YOU SAID YOU WERE TAKING CIMETIDINE AS WELL AS THE BENADRYL. CAN YOU TELL ME MORE ABOUT YOUR CIMETIDINE USE? Yes, I am taking cimetidine at night for heartburn.

HOW MUCH CIMETIDINE ARE YOU TAKING? I take 800 mg (four 200-mg over-the-counter pills), because that is what I took 10 years ago to treat my ulcer.

HOW LONG HAVE YOU BEEN TAKING THE CIMETIDINE? For the last couple of weeks.

HAS IT RELIEVED YOUR HEARTBURN? Yes, I'd say so.

Objective Information:

Computerized medication profile:

- Enalapril (Vasotec): 10 mg, one tablet a day; No. 30; Refills: 1.

Healthy male appearing his stated age and in no acute distress

Blood pressure: 140/85 mm Hg

Respiratory rate: 12 rpm

Heart rate: 60 bpm

Continued

CASE STUDY—continued

DISCUSSION

WP is concerned that he is developing dementia. He is retiring from his job in 2 weeks. Retirement is considered to be a major change in lifestyle and may be perceived as positive or negative. It is possible that WP perceives a great amount of stress because of the upcoming transition to retirement. WP is self-treating with OTC medications for insomnia and heartburn.

The pharmacist needs to determine the cause of WP's forgetfulness, which includes several possibilities to be ruled out:

- *Dementia of the Alzheimer's type (DAT):* This is a diagnosis of exclusion. All other possible causes of dementia must be ruled out before the assumption can be made that the patient has DAT. The definitive diagnosis of DAT is made at autopsy. Therefore, to rule out DAT, the patient would need an extensive physical assessment.
- *Vascular dementia:* To rule-out vascular dementia would also require an extensive assessment. Although early vascular dementia is a possibility, the patient's blood pressure is within the acceptable range.
- *Patient noncompliance with medication:* WP stated that he has no problems taking his enalapril, and it is unlikely that he is developing a new adverse reaction.
- *Perceived stress because of retirement:* WP may not be able to verbalize the stress that he perceives because of his pending retirement.
- *Anxiety/depression:* It is possible that WP is developing anxiety or depression and is treating the somatic symptoms with OTC medications.
- *Adverse or toxic effects of medications:* When assessing the course of events, the OTC medications are the most likely cause of WP's forgetfulness and confusion. Diphenhydramine's anticholinergic and antihistaminic effects have significant effects on immediate and recent memory. In addition, both diphenhydramine and cimetidine are associated with confusional states, especially in the elderly population. In addition to the pharmacodynamic effects of the medications, WP may have been experiencing toxicity because of the large doses of cimetidine and diphenhydramine that he was taking.

Based on the current status of this patient, the pharmacist has two options (Fig. 19-2). First, the pharmacist can immediately refer WP to his physician for further assessment. Second, the pharmacist can explain to WP the adverse effects of diphenhydramine and cimetidine and then suggest that WP discontinue the use of both diphenhydramine and the cimetidine and determine whether the change in memory and the confusional state remit within the next week. If the symptoms do not remit, WP will need further assessment by his physician to determine the cause of the memory problems and confusion. In addition, WP may need alternative medications for his insomnia and stomach upset. The pharmacist schedules a note to make a follow-up phone call to WP in 1 week to assess his status.

PHARMACEUTICAL CARE PLAN

Patient Name: WP

Date: 11/5/01

Medical Problems:
Hypertension
Insomnia
Heartburn

Current Medications:
Prescription:
Vasotec (enalapril), 10 mg, one table daily, No. 30, Refills: 1
OTC:
Diphenhydramine, 25 mg, two tablets at bedtime for insomnia
Cimetidine, 200 mg, four tablets at bedtime for heartburn

S: WP is a 65-year-old, 5'10" Caucasian man, retiring in 2 weeks, who is concerned about memory problems and confusional state. Patient states that he can't think as clearly. He has forgotten where he has placed items, like his car keys, and it takes more time to do simple tasks. These symptoms began over the last couple of weeks.

O: Healthy male appearing his stated age and in no acute distress.

Respiratory rate: 12 rpm

Heart rate: 60 bpm

Blood pressure: 140/85 mm Hg

Drug allergies: none known

A: 1. Dosage too high: wrong dose (cimetidine). Being an elderly patient and using high doses of cimetidine are most likely contributing to the patient's presenting symptoms.
2. Adverse drug reaction: undesirable effect (diphenhydramine). The antihistaminic and anticholinergic effects of diphenhydramine can certainly cause the patient's forgetfulness.

Continued

CASE STUDY—continued

■ Pharmaceutical Care Plan ■

3. Hypertension stable.

P: 1. Recommend that WP discontinue OTC medications, Benadryl, and cimetidine.
2. Educate WP about the adverse effects of diphenhydramine.
3. Recommend other OTC medications for sleep as well as healthy sleeping behavior: avoiding caffeine, not exercising at night, and trying to avoid or decrease stress.
4. Educate WP about the adverse effects of cimetidine, particularly when using a large dose.
5. Recommend using lower doses of other OTC heartburn medications.
6. Call 1 week after discontinuing OTC medications to evaluate for improvements in forgetfulness; if none, refer WP to physician for further assessment.

Pharmacist: *Boris Shintanko, Pharm.D.*

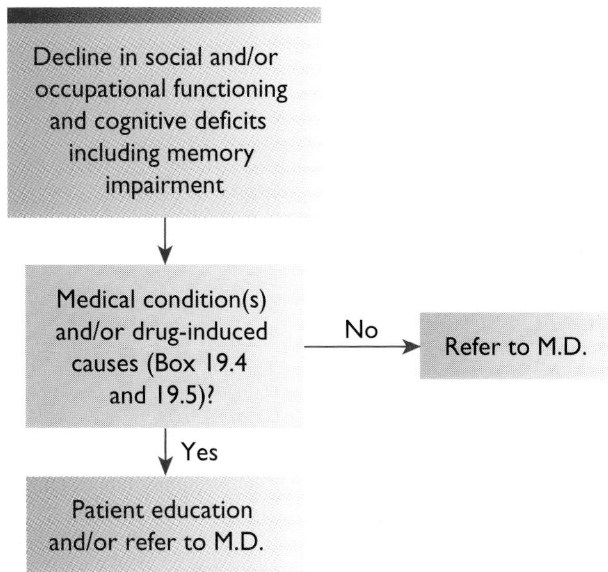

Figure 19-2 ■ Decision tree for memory impairment.

Self-Assessment Questions

1. How can you differentiate between dementia, delirium, and depression?
2. What physical causes of dementia must be ruled out before the presumptive diagnosis of DAT can be made?
3. What common symptoms are associated with dementia?

Critical Thinking Questions

1. In the case of WP, what would your assessment and plan be if his blood pressure was 140/110 mm Hg?
2. What is the relationship between DAT and the use of anticholinergic agents?

Depression

Major depression is a frequent finding in the general population and requires a thorough assessment. Patients with major depression may not complain of a depressed mood as the most prominent symptom. When assessing a patient's mental status, it is important to use open-ended questions and allow the patient to elaborate on their perception of the problem. A thorough assessment of patients and their medications should be done to identify possible drug therapy problems and, specifically, medication-related causes (Box 19-9).

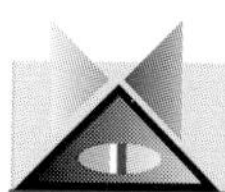

Box 19-9

MEDICATION-RELATED CAUSES OF DEPRESSION

- Antihypertensive agents (e.g., clonidine, methyldopa, reserpine)
- Antiparkinsonian agents
- Antipsychotic agents
- Corticosteroids
- Neoplastic agents
- Nonsteroidal anti-inflammatory agents
- Opioids
- Sedative-hypnotic agents
- Stimulant withdrawal

CASE STUDY

PL is a 55-year-old Hispanic man who comes into the pharmacy and states that he needs a medication for various aches and pains and some vitamins to boost his energy. Past medical history includes hypertension.

ASSESSMENT OF THE PATIENT

Subjective Information

55-year-old man complaining of aches, pains, and lack of energy

Hi, how are you today? Oh, not so good.

What's going on that you're "not so good?" I'm in pain.

When did your pain start? I don't know. It seems like it has been a long time.

Where are you experiencing the pain? In my back, and sometimes my head hurts.

Have you injured your back? No, not that I know of.

Can you describe the pain for me? It's just a dull ache.

About how many hours out of a day do you have pain? I don't know. It comes and goes.

Are there certain times of day that the pain is different? No, I don't think so.

Do certain activities or environmental factors affect the pain? Nothing in particular.

Is there anything that makes it better or worse? Nothing I have noticed.

Do you experience any other accompanying symptoms other than headache? No.

Do you take anything for the pain? Yes, I take some Tylenol.

What is the strength of the Tylenol, 325 or 500 mg? The 500-mg strength.

How many do you take a day? Usually about two.

Does the Tylenol help? Sometimes, but I want something better.

Have you tried any other medication for the pain? No, not yet.

Does the pain interfere with your sleep? No, not really, but I can't sleep anyway.

How has your sleep pattern changed? I wake up early in the morning, around four, and I cannot get back to sleep. I am tired the rest of the day.

Have you tried anything to help you sleep? Nope.

Do you drink coffee or other beverages with caffeine? I drink some coffee in the morning, and that's all.

How much alcohol do you drink per week? I have a couple of mixed drinks on the weekend.

How many is a "couple?" Two or three.

Have you changed your eating habits? No.

In the past, have you felt that you didn't need to sleep or that you felt extremely high, capable of doing anything, as if you were on top of the world? No, not that I remember.

What other medical problems do you have? High blood pressure.

Are you taking any prescription medications for your blood pressure? Yes, I take a water pill, hydrochlorothiazide.

What strength do you take and how often? I take 50 mg daily in the morning.

How long have you been taking the water pill? For a couple of years.

Continued

CASE STUDY—continued

HOW IS YOU BLOOD PRESSURE? Pretty good, it was 130/80 two weeks ago.

HAVE YOU NOTICED ANY PROBLEMS FROM TAKING THE WATER PILL? No, I don't think so.

ARE YOU TAKING ANY OTHER OVER-THE-COUNTER MEDICATIONS, ALTERNATIVES/HERBALS, OR VITAMINS? No.

ANYTHING TO HELP YOU TO SLEEP? Nope.

Objective Information

Computerized medication profile:

- Hydrochlorothiazide: 50 mg, one tablet daily.

Moderately overweight, irritable man appearing his stated age and in mild distress
Blood pressure: 132/75 mm Hg
Respiratory rate: 20 rpm
Heart rate: 65 bpm

DISCUSSION

PL is describing vague physical complaints and is not verbalizing complaints of depression. Patients often verbalize gastrointestinal complaints, neurologic complaints (e.g., dizziness, numbness), generalized fatigue, lack of energy, and pain. It is often difficult to ask questions more related to mental illness when the patient is focused on the somatic complaints. PL is typical, in that he is looking for a quick resolution to his problem.

The pharmacist must decide the cause of PL's symptoms, which may include the following possibilities:

- A physical condition
- Anxiety
- Depression
- Adverse effect from the hydrochlorothiazide (unlikely, but assessment for hypokalemia and hyponatremia is necessary)

Considering the vague physical complaints, the patient should be referred for a laboratory and physical assessment to rule out any nonpsychiatric cause of the symptoms.

PHARMACEUTICAL CARE PLAN

Patient Name: PL

Date: 11/7/01

Medical Problems:
Hypertension

Current Medications:
Prescription:
Hydrochlorothiazide, 50 mg, one tablet daily in the morning
OTC:
Acetaminophen, 500 mg, one tablet twice daily as needed

S: A 55-year-old man appearing his stated age and moderately overweight. He also appears to be irritable and in mild distress. Patient has a history of vague complaints of pain and lack of energy. Patient states that the pain is in his back and that sometimes his head hurts. The pain is more of a dull ache that comes and goes. The pain has no characteristic timing of symptoms or factors that improve or worsen it. Patient cannot pinpoint when these symptoms started. The patient is also overeating despite a lack of appetite and has used Tylenol, 500 mg, with minimal relief. Patient has a history of high blood pressure that is well maintained with hydrochlorothiazide, 50 mg once daily, and no reports of problems. His last blood pressure was 130/80 mm Hg. Patient has also had difficulty sleeping, waking up in the middle of the night, and being unable to return to sleep. He also feels tired throughout the day.

O: Moderately overweight, irritable man appearing his stated age and in mild distress.

Blood pressure: 132/75 mm Hg
Respiratory rate: 20 rpm
Heart rate: 65 bpm
Drug allergies: none known

A:
1. Wrong drug: not indicated for the condition (Tylenol). The patient isn't receiving relief with Tylenol use and there may be an underlying cause of the pain. The problem is that the pain may be a symptom of an underlying medical disorder, depression, or anxiety.
2. Stable condition: hypertension. Need for ongoing monitoring.
3. Untreated condition: insomnia.

P:
1. Explain to PL that the symptoms (e.g., aches, pains, lack of energy, insomnia) may indicate an underlying medical problem or that he may be developing depression.
2. Refer PL to his primary care physician for further assessment to determine if the symptoms are a result of a medical problem (e.g., metabolic disorders, anemia, cardiovascular disease) or possible depression.
3. Refer PL to laboratory for electrolyte blood work to ensure he is not hyponatremic or hypokalemic.
4. Schedule a follow-up call for a few days after PL sees his physician for further assessment. Follow up again in 1 month to see if blood pressure control is maintained.

Pharmacist: *Tanya Troublino, Pharm.D.*

Self-Assessment Questions

1. What are the signs and symptoms of depression?
2. Should a practitioner assess a patient's likelihood of self-harm?
3. Does the use of alcohol contribute to the signs and symptoms of depression?

Critical Thinking Questions

1. How would the treatment of PL differ if he had had a previous manic episode?
2. How does culture influence the diagnosis and treatment of depression?

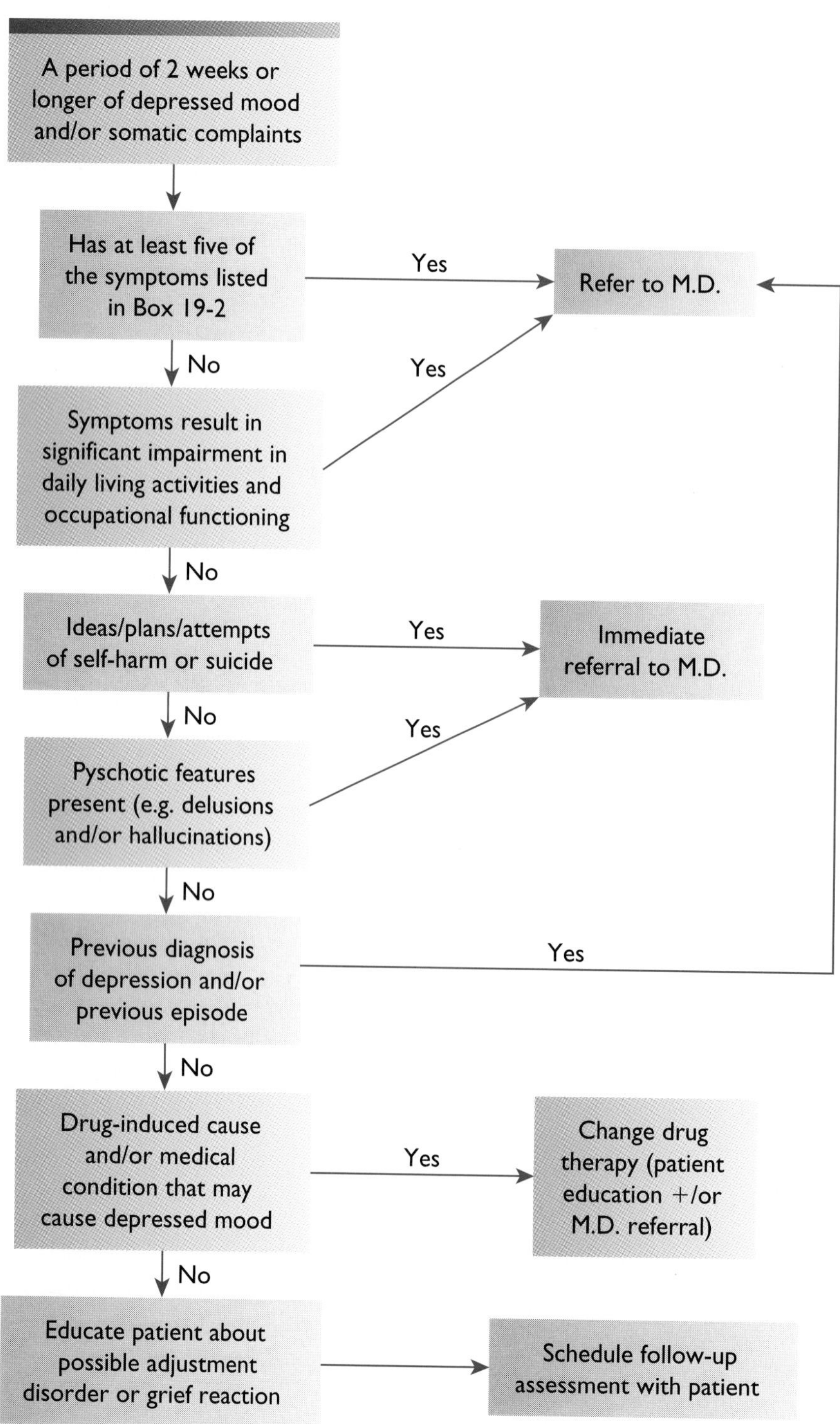

FIGURE 19-3 ■ Decision tree for depression.

Anxiety

Anxiety is a frequent finding in the general population and is associated with a variety of physical conditions. In addition, signs and symptoms of anxiety are associated with the use and withdrawal of various drugs (Box 19-10). When assessing a patient's mental status, it is important to determine contributing factors (e.g., stress) and to distinguish between normal and disabling levels of anxiety. Normal anxiety can be treated with reassurance and, possibly, brief psychotherapy. More severe anxiety requires further assessment and treatment.

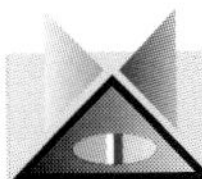

Box 19-10

MEDICATION-RELATED CAUSES OF ANXIETY

USE OF THE MEDICATION

- Antiasthma agents (e.g., albuterol, theophylline)
- Anticholinergics
- Digoxin
- Stimulants (e.g., amphetamines and related derivatives, caffeine, ephedrine, phenylpropanolamine, pseudoephedrine)

WITHDRAWAL OF THE MEDICATION

- Alcohol
- Antianxiety agents
- Opioids
- Sedative-hypnotics

CASE STUDY

SS is a 21-year-old, Asian-American man who comes into the pharmacy and begins to walk up and down the aisle looking for something. He picks up a package of an acetaminophen-and-diphenhydramine combination product and walks toward the pharmacy. His facial muscles look tense. He is shifting his weight from one leg to the other, and he looks apprehensive. He asks if the product will help him get some sleep.

ASSESSING THE PATIENT

Subjective Information

21-year-old, Asian-American man who appears tense and apprehensive and desires a sleep aid

HI, HOW ARE YOU? Just fine, but I need to get some sleep. Will this stuff work?

ARE YOU HAVING TROUBLE SLEEPING? Yes, so what do you think?

WELL, DO YOU HAVE TROUBLE FALLING ASLEEP OR STAYING ASLEEP? Both.

OKAY. HOW LONG HAVE YOU HAD TROUBLE WITH SLEEP? Just the last few nights.

HOW MANY HOURS ARE YOU SLEEPING PER NIGHT? Depends. Sometimes four, sometimes eight.

WHEN YOU TRY TO GO TO SLEEP, WHAT HAPPENS? I just lay there.

ARE YOU THINKING ABOUT THINGS IN YOUR LIFE? Yes, my mind is racing.

ARE YOU THINKING ABOUT SOMETHING IN PARTICULAR? Yes, I am freaking out about exams!

SO YOU ARE A STUDENT? Yes.

HAVE YOU BEEN ABLE TO STUDY DURING THE DAY? Yes.

OKAY, WELL SOMETIMES IT IS BEST TO NOT USE A DRUG AND TRY OTHER METHODS. Like what?

WELL, IT IS BEST TO PREPARE YOURSELF FOR SLEEP BY FOLLOWING A ROUTINE SCHEDULE OF GOING TO SLEEP AND WAKING UP. Well, I have early classes and late. Besides, I need to study.

I THINK A ROUTINE SCHEDULE MAY HELP. ARE YOU DRINKING A LOT OF COFFEE OR SODA POP THAT HAS CAFFEINE? Well, I try to drink caffeine only in the morning, but sometimes, I drink coffee all day long to stay up and study.

YOU KNOW THAT ALCOHOL CAN AFFECT SLEEP, TOO. HOW MUCH ALCOHOL ARE YOU DRINKING? Not that much.

WELL, HOW MUCH DID YOU DRINK THIS WEEK? A couple of nights, I went out with friends, and I probably had four or five beers each night.

ANY WINE OR OTHER LIQUOR? No.

OKAY. IS THERE ANYTHING ELSE THAT HAS BEEN HAPPENING OVER THE LAST FEW WEEKS? No, not that I know of.

DO YOU HAVE ANY MEDICAL PROBLEMS, LIKE ASTHMA, DIABETES, OR HIGH BLOOD PRESSURE? No.

ARE YOU TAKING ANY OTHER MEDICATIONS OR HERBAL PRODUCTS? No.

Continued

CASE STUDY—continued

Objective Information:

Asian American male appearing his stated age and anxious
Facial muscles look tense
Shifting weight from one leg to the other
Looks apprehensive

DISCUSSION

SS is suffering from insomnia. He is studying for examinations and is consuming a high amount of caffeine and alcohol. He wants to treat his insomnia with an acetaminophen-and-diphenhydramine combination product. The pharmacist must assess the cause of SS's insomnia, which includes several possibilities:

- Caffeine-induced insomnia.
- Insomnia caused by alcohol withdrawal.
- Perceived stress caused by examinations.
- Anxiety (if GAD is suspected, further assessment after completion of examinations is required).
- Manic phase of bipolar disorder, which would need to be ruled out with further assessment. (SS states that he's able to study during the day, however, so this is unlikely.)

SS's insomnia is of less than 3 weeks in duration. This is typical of individuals without a history of sleep problems, and it appears to be a result of a combination of factors: use of caffeine, alcohol, and high stress from examinations. If SS's insomnia was long term in duration (>3 weeks), a referral would be necessary, because this may be the result of a medical or a psychiatric disorder (e.g., GAD, depression). Refer to Figure 19-4 to aid in determining the need for a referral.

PHARMACEUTICAL CARE PLAN

Patient Name: SS

Date: 12/19/01

Medical Conditions:
None

Current Medications:
None

S: A 21-year-old, Asian-American man currently completing final examinations. Has had insomnia the last couple of nights and is under stress because of his finals. Using caffeine excessively and has been drinking alcohol during the last week. Has trouble falling and staying asleep.

O: 21-year-old, Asian American man appearing his stated age and anxious. Presents to the pharmacy a package of an acetaminophen-and-diphenhydramine combination product. His facial muscles look tense. He is shifting his weight from one leg to the other and looks apprehensive.

Drug allergies: none known

A: Untreated medical condition: insomnia.

P:
1. Explain the effects of caffeine and alcohol on sleep, and suggest a decrease in use of both drugs.
2. Recommend that SS not use diphenhydramine because of its anticholinergic and antihistaminic effects on immediate and recent memory, which could affect his ability to study for and take his examinations.
3. Suggest the use of nondrug methods for insomnia, such as a regular time to wake up and go to sleep; sleeping only until rested; going to bed only when sleepy; avoiding trying to force sleep; avoiding daytime naps; scheduling worry time during the day; exercising routinely but not close to bedtime; creating a comfortable sleep environment; discontinue use of alcohol, caffeine, and nicotine; avoiding excessive fullness or hunger at bedtime; avoiding drinking large quantities of fluids in the evening; and do something relaxing and enjoyable before bedtime.
4. If the symptoms do not remit, complete further assessment to determine the cause of the insomnia.
5. Schedule a follow-up in a few days (after examinations) to see if symptoms are improving.

Pharmacist: *Mohannad Said, Pharm.D.*

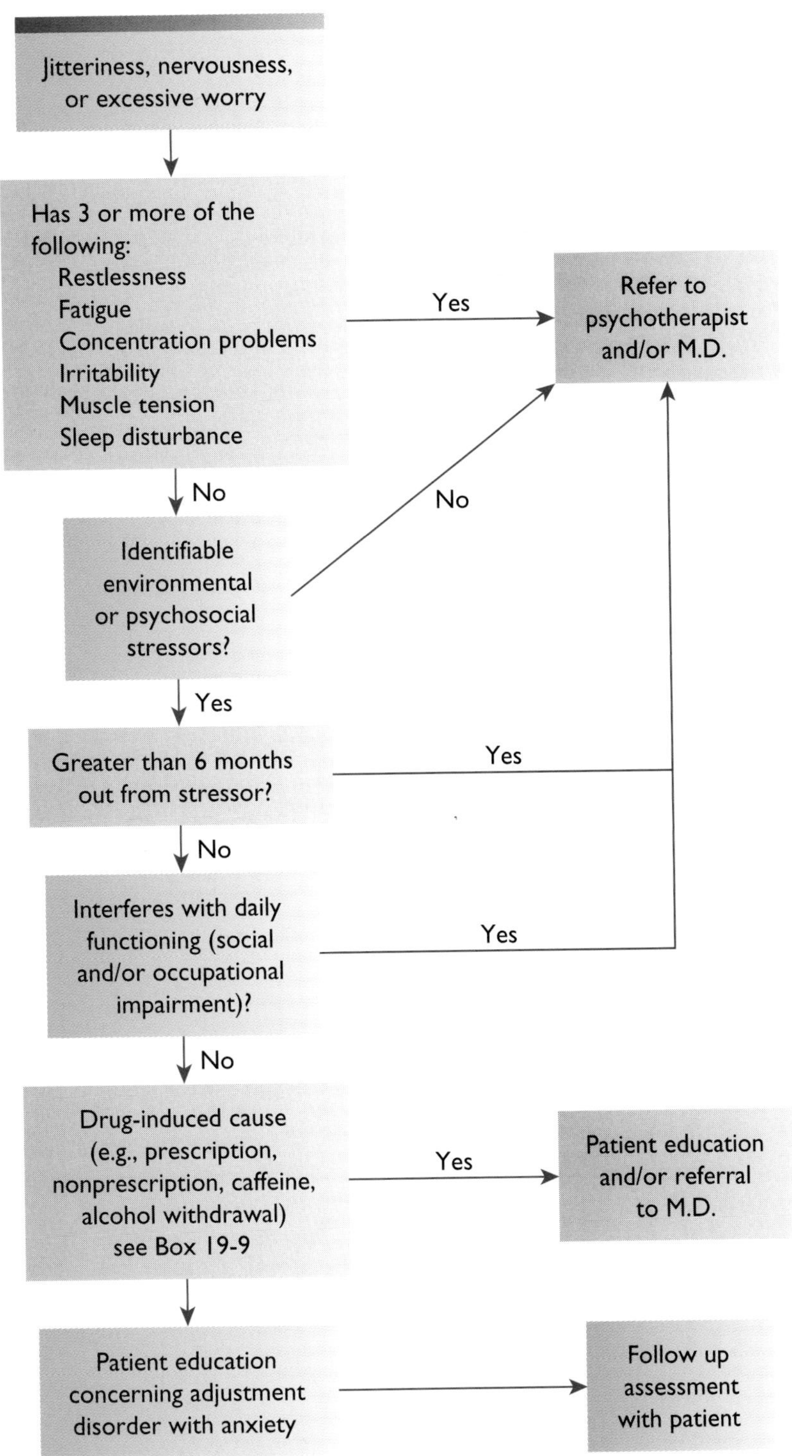

FIGURE 19-4 ■ Decision tree for anxiety.

Self-Assessment Questions

1. How can you differentiate the insomnia associated with anxiety versus that associated with depression?
2. What nondrug methods and sleep habits are helpful for treating insomnia?
3. How prevalent is anxiety in the general population, and what are the signs and symptoms?

Critical Thinking Questions

1. If SS had been experiencing mania, what other symptoms would have been present?
2. What other OTC medications are available for the treatment of insomnia? How effective are they? What are their side effects, if any?

Bibliography

American Psychiatric Association. Diagnostic and statistical manual of mental disorders. 4th ed., rev. Washington, DC: American Psychiatric Association, 1994.

Berne RM, Levy MN. Physiology. 4th ed. St. Louis: Mosby, 1998.

Bickley LS. Bates' guide to physical examination and history taking. 7th ed. Philadelphia: JB Lippincott, 1999.

Bloom FE, Kupfer DJ. Psychopharmacology: the fourth generation of progress. New York: Raven Press, 1995.

Cipolle RJ, Strand LM, Morley PC. Pharmaceutical care practice. New York: McGraw-Hill, 1998.

Davies DM. Textbook of adverse drug reactions. New York: Oxford University Press, 1991.

Dukes MG. Meyler's side effects of drugs. 13th ed. New York: Elsevier, 1996.

Folstein MF, Folstein SE, McHugh PR. "Mini-Mental State": a practical method for grading the cognitive state of patients for the clinician. J Psychiatr Res 1975;12(3):189–198.

Kaplan HI, Sadock BJ. Comprehensive textbook of psychiatry/VI. 6th ed. Baltimore: Williams & Wilkins, 1995.

Leopold KA, Zoschnick LB. Postpartum depression. Women's primary health grand rounds at the University of Michigan. In: Johnson TRB, Apgar B, eds. OBGYN.net: the female patient. Retrieved January 7, 2001, from http://www.obgyn.net/femalepatient/default.asp?page=leopold

Lowinson JH, Ruiz P, Millman RB, Langrod JG. Substance abuse: a comprehensive textbook. 3rd ed. Baltimore: Williams & Wilkins, 1997.

Chapter 20

Endocrine System

Maryann Skrabal

Glossary Terms

- Diabetes mellitus
- Diabetic ketoacidosis
- Exophthalmos
- Graves' disease
- Graves' ophthalmopathy
- Hashimoto's disease
- Hyperosmolar hyperglycemic nonketotic coma
- Hyperthyroidism
- Hypothyroidism
- Onycholysis
- Pretibial myxedema
- Retinopathy
- Syndrome X
- Thyroid storm

ANATOMY AND PHYSIOLOGY OVERVIEW

The endocrine system differs from other systems in that it is not localized. It is a complex regulatory system that releases chemical messengers, known as hormones, into the bloodstream. These hormones regulate the metabolic effects of all the body's cells. Glands and organs that comprise the endocrine system are located throughout the body and are shown in Figure 20-1.

The amount of a given hormone that is released by the endocrine glands and tissues is determined by the body's need for that hormone. The hormone itself, nerve impulses, and regulating factors control the levels of circulating hormone through negative feedback. Endocrine disorders often reflect overactive or underactive glands, and they are usually discovered because of a distant metabolic effect. They include pituitary, adrenal, and thyroid function problems in addition to disorders of carbohydrate metabolism. This chapter discusses the most common endocrine functions and their associated disorders, which include carbohydrate metabolism and thyroid function.

Carbohydrate Metabolism

The pancreas, an endocrine and exocrine gland, is located posteriorly and slightly inferior to the stomach. It has a head, a body, and a tail. Histologically, it consists of islets of Langerhans and acini. The islets are infiltrated by blood capillaries and cells that form the exocrine part of the gland. The islets include three types of cells: (1) alpha cells, (2) beta cells, and (3) delta cells. Alpha cells secrete the hormone glucagon in response to low blood glucose levels, and beta cells secrete the hormone insulin in response to high blood glucose levels. These cells perform the endocrine function of the pancreas.

Normal carbohydrate metabolism occurs in the body to keep blood glucose concentrations within certain narrow limits to ensure that an adequate supply of glucose reaches the central nervous system. Insulin works to decrease blood glucose levels by inhibiting glycogenolysis (i.e., the conversion of glycogen to glucose), stimulating lipogenesis (i.e., facilitating glucose transport into fat and muscle cells), and glycogenesis (i.e., the storage of glucose as glycogen). Insulin is released continuously at a basal rate of approximately 1 unit per hour and 5 to 10 unit bo-

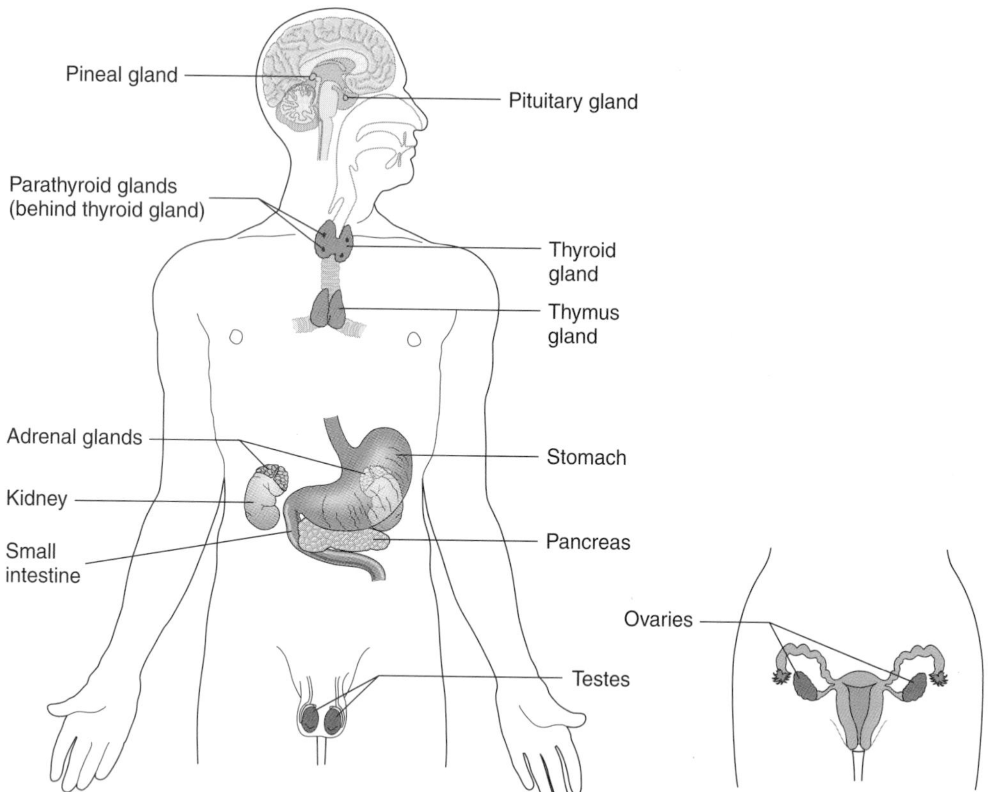

FIGURE 20-1 Glands and organs of the endocrine system.

luses for glucose loads, approximating 40 units per day. Its release is triggered by blood glucose levels of 100 mg/dL or greater. When blood glucose levels are low, the alpha cells stimulate the release of glucagon and other counterregulatory hormones (i.e., cortisol, epinephrine, growth hormone), which increase blood glucose levels by stimulating glycogenolysis and gluconeogenesis (i.e., the conversion of amino acids, glycerol, and lactic acid to glucose) followed by lipolysis (i.e., the breakdown of lipids into fatty acids). This is depicted in Figure 20-2.

Thyroid Function

Weighing approximately 25 g, the thyroid gland is the largest endocrine gland in the body. This highly vascular gland is the only one that is accessible to direct physical examination. Knowledge regarding the anatomy of the neck is important to understand the position of the gland (Fig. 20-3). It is made up of two lobes, known as the right lobe and left lobe, which appear in a butterfly-shape. The lobes are connected by an isthmus, which lies across the trachea below the cricoid cartilage of the larynx. The lobes are mostly covered by the sternocleidomastoid muscles. One-third of the population has a pyramidal lobe that extends upward from the isthmus slightly left of the tracheal midline.

The thyroid gland releases thyroid hormone in accordance with the body's metabolic needs. Decreased levels of thyroid hormone stimulate the hypothalamus to release thyrotropin-releasing factor, which in turn triggers the release of thyroid-stimulating hormone (TSH) from the pituitary. TSH causes the thyroid to release the two biologically active thyroid hormones into the blood: thyroxine (T_4), and triiodothyronine (T_3) (Fig. 20-4). These hormones are synthesized from iodine and tyrosine within thyroglobulin, and they are carried in the blood with plasma proteins, mostly thyroxine-binding globulin. The functions of the thyroid hormones are regulation of the metabolic rate, growth and development of children, and reactivity of the nervous system.

In comparison to T_4, T_3 is four times more potent but is present at a lower concentration and has a shorter half-life (T_3, half-life of 1.5 days; T_4, half-life of 7 days). In fact, T_4 serves as a precursor to T_3. Their binding to thyroxine-binding globulin prevents their metabolism and excretion. Iodide is necessary for thyroid hormone production and should be present in the diet as iodine at 100 μg/day, which is equivalent to what is found in 1 g of iodized salt.

Special Considerations

Pediatric Patients

Abnormalities in carbohydrate metabolism in pediatric patients most commonly present as type 1 diabetes. There is a peak in incidence around the onset of puberty, at the age of 11 to 14 years, that may relate to the hormonal changes occurring at that time. A rare type of type 2 diabetes, known as maturity-onset diabetes of youth, also occurs in this population. When diabetes occurs at a young age it is usually rapid in onset and quite severe. Patients presenting with type 1 diabetes may present with diabetic ketoacidosis (described later) as their first sign of disease. In those with the onset of diabetes before age 5, there may be an

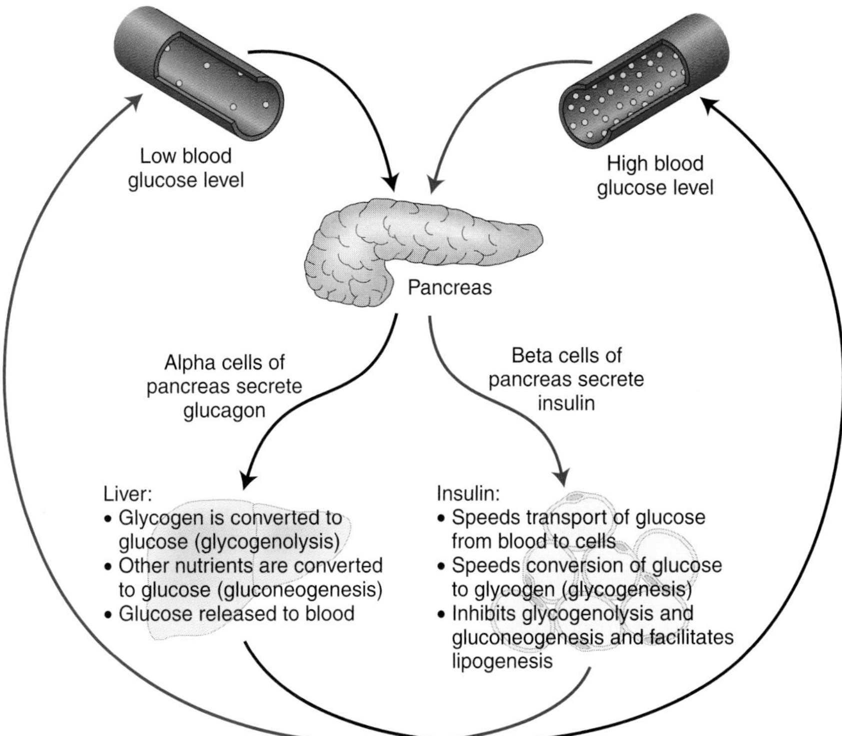

FIGURE 20-2 Regulation of glucagon and insulin secretion.

increased risk for problems with intellectual development because of the metabolic changes that occur during this crucial period of growth. Studies investigating this were completed before the widespread use of blood glucose monitoring, however, so their application is controversial. A "honeymoon" remission period may occur in children with diabetes where control of their condition improves. This gives both the patient and the family the false sense that they are cured. Patients should continue taking their insulin during this period, even if a only very small dose, because the period will end (usually predicated by some illness, infection, or the onset of puberty).

Thyroid hormone is important for normal growth and development during embryonic life and childhood. A deficiency of thyroid hormone during the early years of life results in fewer and smaller neurons, defective myelination of axons, and mental retardation. These effects can begin as early as fetal and

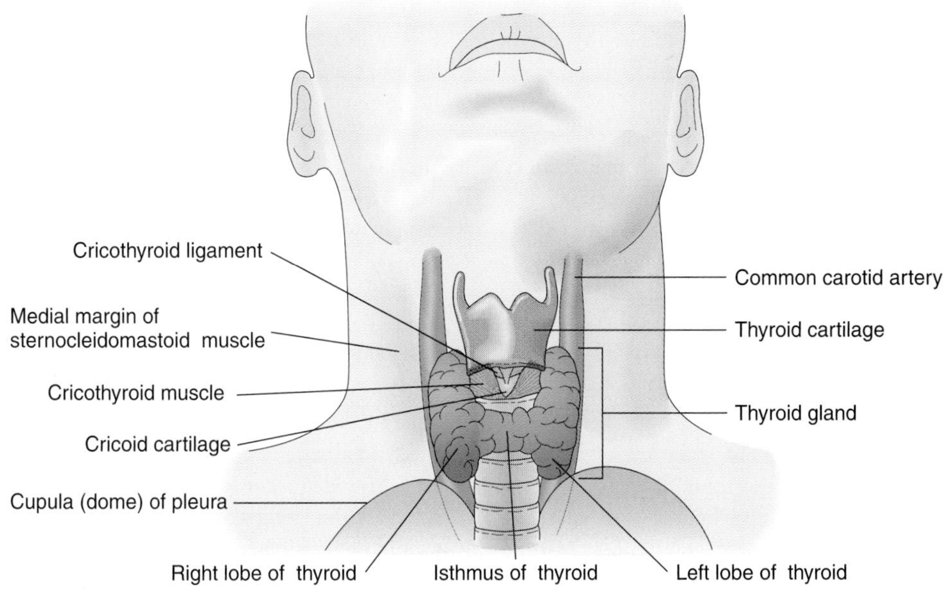

FIGURE 20-3 Thyroid gland.

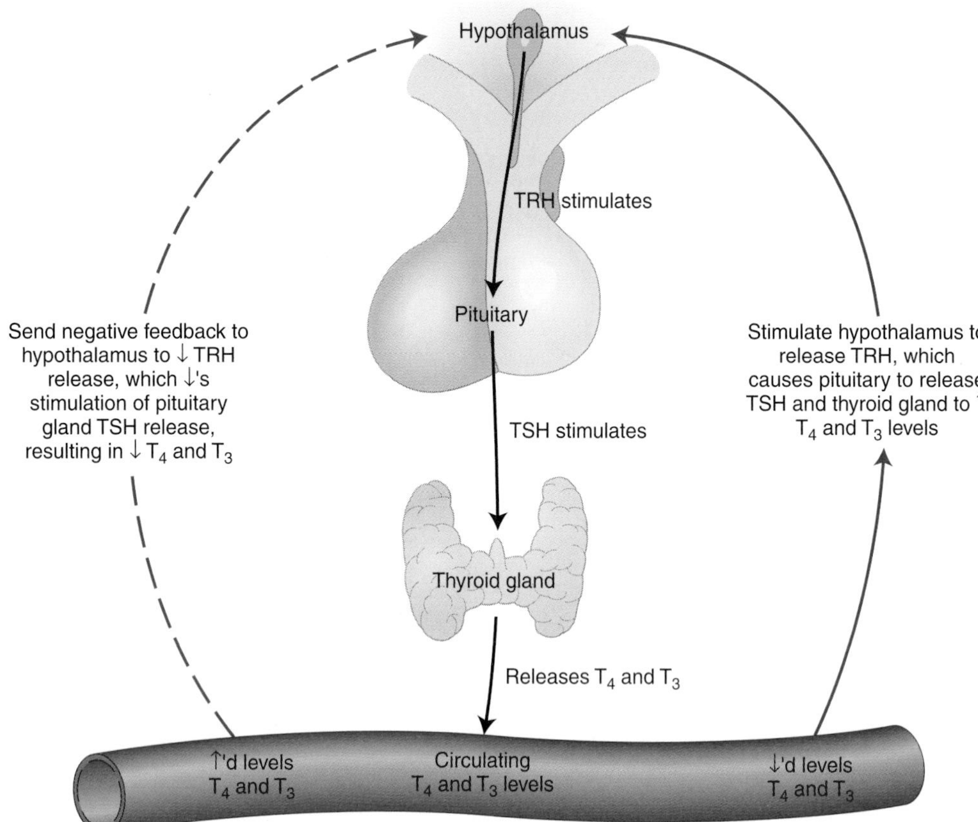

FIGURE 20-4 Thyroid hormone regulation. ↑, Increase; ↓, decrease.

neonatal development. The severity of retardation depends on the severity and duration of the condition. Profound retardation is known as cretinism. If uncorrected, cretinism may result in the child having smaller stature and poor development of certain organs. Cretinism most often occurs in areas where iodide is decreased in the diet or when thyroid dysfunction is congenital.

If maternal TSH antibody titers are high during pregnancy, transfer across the placenta may cause infants to have hyperthyroidism. This usually appears 8 to 10 days after the child is born, and the child may need to be treated for as long as 8 to 12 weeks (until the antibody is cleared). Hyperthyroidism in children is rare, and rapid gain in height not associated with puberty may be the only sign.

Geriatric Patients

Aging slows the activities of most glands. Thus, decreased activity of the endocrine system may not indicate an abnormality; instead, it may be occurring as a normal manifestation of aging itself. Glucose intolerance tends to increase with age and is responsible for a fasting blood glucose elevation of approximately 1 to 2 mg/dL and a 2-hour postprandial glucose elevation of approximately 8 to 20 mg/dL per decade of life after the age of 30 to 40 years. Secretion of insulin may decline, but the main effect is believed to be a decrease in insulin-mediated peripheral glucose metabolism. Insulin responsiveness also declines, but the number of insulin receptors does not. Elderly patients tend to have decreased lean body mass and increased adipose tissue, and they are less active, which also contributes to the development of glucose intolerance. Many of the organs that diabetes affects with long-term complications are identical to those that are also affected by aging. In older patients, there is a 25-fold increase in the incidence of renal disease and blindness, a 20-fold increase in gangrene and vascular insufficiency, a 3-fold increase in hypertension, a 1.5-fold increase in myocardial infarction, and a 2-fold increase in stroke.

As a person ages, the thyroid gland becomes more fibrotic and may feel more irregular and nodular on palpation. Thyroid hormone secretion decreases, the rate of T_4 production decreases, and the level of TSH tends to increase in elderly patients. The basal metabolic rate decreases with age and is related to the decrease in muscle mass that also occurs. The diagnosis of thyroid disorders may be more difficult in aging patients, because they may only exhibit symptomatology involving a single system (as opposed to symptomatology involving multiple systems in the younger population). This is caused by changes in the sympathetic nervous system in elderly patients.

Myxedema coma occurs most often in elderly patients and results from long-standing, uncorrected hypothyroidism. It should be considered a medical emergency when it occurs. The hallmark of this disorder is edema that causes facial tissues to swell and look puffy.

Pregnant Patients

The combined effects of placental hormones and fetal nutrient use alter carbohydrate metabolism during pregnancy. Human placental lactogen, progesterone, cortisol, and prolactin may impair glucose uptake by insulin target cells, and this impairment progresses as these hormones continue to increase during pregnancy. Fetal nutrient use increases as fetal mass increases, which may counteract some of the insulin resistance that occurs toward the end of the pregnancy. Gestational diabetes mellitus (GDM) is the term used to describe diabetes that occurs during pregnancy.

Preconception care is important in women with diabetes who plan to get pregnant, because good metabolic control is crucial during the earliest stages of pregnancy, when organogenesis occurs. The incidence of congenital malformations appears to be proportional to the level of maternal metabolic control and are two- to threefold more common in women with diabetes than in women among the general population.

Maternal thyroid function during pregnancy is modulated by three independent but interrelated factors: (1) an increase in chorionic gonadotropin concentrations that stimulate the thyroid gland, (2) a significant increase in urinary iodide excretion that results in a fall in plasma iodine concentrations, and (3) an increase in thyroxine-binding globulin during the first trimester. The effects of these factors on maternal thyroid function are most apparent when other conditions, such as iodine deficiency or autoimmune thyroid disease, are present.

Approximately 0.2% of pregnancies are affected by hyperthyroidism, most commonly Graves' disease. If left untreated, fetal loss could occur by spontaneous abortions or premature delivery. Thyroid-stimulating antibodies may cross the placenta and cause fetal and neonatal hyperthyroidism.

Hypothyroidism in pregnancy is uncommon, but when it occurs, it is thought to relate to a pharmacokinetic alteration. Thyroid hormone is necessary for proper fetal growth. If left untreated, hypothyroidism may lead to an increased risk of stillbirth and lower psychologic scores in infants.

PATHOLOGY OVERVIEW

Disorders of the endocrine system have significant effects on health and function. The pharmacist is in a perfect position to recognize potential disorders from a collection of presenting symptoms, and he or she should be able to evaluate patients and refer them to their primary care provider for diagnosis. More commonly, the pharmacist plays an active role in monitoring the efficacy of and side effects from treatment of the most common endocrine disorders: diabetes mellitus, and thyroid disorders (hyperthyroidism and hypothyroidism).

Diabetes Mellitus

Diabetes mellitus is a chronic, heterogeneous disorder that is characterized by increased fasting blood glucose levels. It is associated with abnormalities in carbohydrate, fat, and protein metabolism and, if not aggressively treated, quite often leads to renal, ocular, neurologic, and cardiovascular diseases.

There are two major types of diabetes mellitus: type 1, and type 2. Historically, type 1 has been referred to as juvenile-onset or insulin-dependent diabetes mellitus, whereas type 2 has been known as adult-onset or noninsulin-dependent diabetes mellitus. These latter terms have been dropped, however, and changed to identifications that more accurately describe the diagnosis of the condition as opposed to the treatment or the population type. This is because diabetes of either type may occur at any age, and both types may be dependent on insulin. Other types of diabetes include GDM and impaired glucose metabolism, which includes impaired fasting glucose and impaired glucose tolerance.

The main difference between the two major types of diabetes is the cause of the fasting hyperglycemia that occurs. In type 1, the primary defect is inadequate secretion of insulin by the pancreas caused by pancreatic islet beta-cell destruction, which is classified as immune-mediated or idiopathic. Patients at risk for developing type 1 diabetes show serologic evidence of an autoimmune pathologic process occurring or a genetic predisposition. Despite the possible involvement of genetics, however, environmental variables, such as viral illnesses and pancreatic toxins, may initiate the occurrence of the autoimmune process.

Type 2 diabetes exhibits impaired release of insulin by the pancreas and decreased peripheral tissue sensitivity to insulin (i.e., insulin resistance). Type 2 has a stronger connection to genetics than type 1, but environmental factors, such as obesity and age, also influence a person's chance of developing type 2 diabetes. Current guidelines recommend that screening should be considered in all individuals 45 years and older; if normal, screening should be repeated in 3 years. Testing should be considered at an earlier age in patients who are at risk. The risk factors for development of type 2 diabetes mellitus include:

- Family history of type 2 diabetes mellitus (first-degree relative)
- Increased age (>45 years)
- Obesity (≥120% desirable body weight, or body mass index ≥27)
- Physical inactivity
- History of gestational diabetes mellitus or delivering a baby weighing > 9 pounds
- Impaired glucose tolerance on previous testing
- Member of a high-risk ethnic population (African American, Hispanic, or Native American)
- Hypertension (≥140/90 mm Hg)
- High-density lipoprotein cholesterol ≤35 mg/dL and/or triglyceride ≥250 mg/dL

Syndrome X describes patients who are typically obese and have subsequently developed insulin resistance and hyperinsulinemia. This combination of increased insulin and increased glucose then causes atherosclerosis, hypertension, and hyperlipidemia. This syndrome has also been appropriately termed *CHAOS* because of the presence of cardiovascular disease, hypertension/hyperlipidemia, adult-onset diabetes, obesity, and stroke.

Many drugs cause glucose intolerance because of effects on insulin release, tissue responsiveness to insulin, or direct pancreatic effects. Drugs that have been associated with hyperglycemia are listed in Box 20-1.The signs and symptoms of type 1 and type 2 diabetes are related to hyperglycemia and quite often distinguish one type from the other (Box 20-2).Type 1 commonly presents with the "classic" symptoms, such as polydipsia, polyphagia, and polyuria. Weight loss tends to occur, and the onset of symptoms is more rapid and severe. The presentation of type 2 is more insidious because of slow development of symptoms and lesser severity resulting from the presence of some insulin activity. Fatigue, blurred vision, pruritis, polyuria, and recurrent vaginal infections occur more often in type 2 diabetes.

Short-term complications of diabetes mellitus include **diabetic ketoacidosis** in type 1 diabetes and **hyperosmolar hyperglycemic nonketotic coma** in type 2 diabetes. These result from excessively high blood glucose concentrations and occur most commonly when patients are sick and dehydrated. Both should be considered medical emergencies. Risk factors for hyperosmolar hyperglycemic nonketotic coma include acute illness, decreased thirst perception, noncompliance, dementia, limited fluid access, and new-onset diabetes.

The consequences of long-term hyperglycemia on the various tissues in the body include damage to various organs, especially the eyes, kidneys, nerves, heart, and blood vessels. Long-term complications include retinopathy with possible blindness, nephropathy with possible renal failure, peripheral neuropathy with risk of foot ulcers and amputation, sexual dysfunction, and autonomic neuropathy causing pupillary, gastrointestinal, genitourinary, and cardiovascular symptoms. Patients with diabetes are also at risk for atherosclerotic cardiovascular, peripheral, and cerebrovascular disease. Prevention of these complications is the goal of therapy for patients with diabetes.

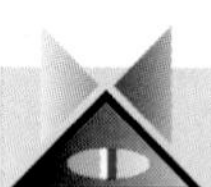

Box 20-1

MEDICATIONS THAT MAY CAUSE HYPERGLYCEMIA

- β-Blockers
- Calcium-channel blockers
- Diazoxide
- Diuretics (thiazides)
- Glucocorticoids
- L-asparaginase
- Niacin
- Estrogens
- Oral contraceptives
- Lithium
- Pentamidine
- Phenytoin
- Growth hormone
- Phenothiazines
- Isoniazid
- Sugar-containing medications
- Sympathomimetics

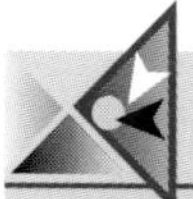

Box 20-2

SIGN AND SYMPTOMS OF HYPERGLYCEMIA (DIABETES MELLITUS)

SIGNS

- Blood glucose elevation (fasting level >126 mg/dL)
- Urine ketones
- Urine glucose

SYMPTOMS

- Polydipsia
- Polyuria
- Polyphagia
- Weight changes
- Blurred vision
- Fatigue
- Dry/itchy skin
- Recurrent/nonhealing infections
- Impotence/decreased libido
- Numbness of extremities
- Bloated feeling

Common drug treatment for type 1 diabetes involves the use of insulin. Insulin varies by species, type, time-course, purity, and concentration. Drug therapy for type 2 diabetes includes the second-generation sulfonylureas, metformin, acarbose, thiazoladinediones, repaglinide, and insulin. Because the mechanism of these therapies acts to decrease blood glucose levels, hypoglycemia (i.e., low blood glucose) may result. The level at which hypoglycemia occurs varies with each patient, but it generally occurs at approximately 50 to 70 mg/dL. Early signs and symptoms may include diaphoresis, pallor, tachycardia, palpitations, paresthesias, hunger, shakiness, and irritability. As the hypoglycemia progresses, neurologic evidence may include inability to concentrate, somnolence, confusion, slurred speech, irrational behavior, and blurred vision. The last stage also may include disoriented behavior, loss of consciousness, seizures, and even death. Pharmacists should be aware of these signs and symptoms and reinforce the importance of early recognition and treatment to prevent serious consequences. Treatment includes approximately 15 g of carbohydrates (e.g., half-cup of fruit juice, two tablespoons of raisins, five or six hard candies, glucose tablets or gel) for mild to moderate cases and glucagon or dextrose injections for the most severe cases.

Nonpharmacologic therapy is the cornerstone for treatment of diabetes. It includes a total lifestyle change that involves both diet therapy and exercise. An emphasis on weight loss is often needed in type 2 diabetes if the patient is overweight. Diet therapy may include food-exchange lists, preplanned daily menus, and counting-and-point systems. Exercise is recommended, because it helps to achieve weight loss and to improve glycemic control, lipid concentrations, and blood pressure. It also helps to decrease hyperinsulinemia, insulin resistance, and obesity. Aerobic exercise is recommended at 65% to 80% of maximal heart rate for 20 to 45 minutes most days each week. The pharmacist should have literature available with nutritional and exercise recommendations for patients with diabetes as well as the names of certified diabetes educators, clinical nutrition specialists, and physical therapists in the area.

Thyroid Disorders

Thyroid disorders are more common in those between the ages of 20 and 40 years. They are also more common in women than in men. Hyperthyroidism and hypothyroidism are thyroid disorders that pharmacists should be aware of for disease screening and treatment monitoring.

Hyperthyroidism is characterized by elevated levels of thyroid hormones in the blood. **Graves' disease** (i.e., toxic diffuse goiter), the most common cause, is an autoimmune disorder in which thyroid-stimulating immunoglobulins are present that stimulate the TSH receptor to cause overproduction of thyroid hormones. It affects multiple systems and most commonly is seen in women during the third or fourth decade of life. Other causes include iatrogenic reasons (e.g., excess thyroid replacement, amiodarone), excess iodine (i.e., nodular goiter), toxic multinodular goiter, tumors, and toxic uninodular goiter (i.e., Plummer's disease).

The signs and symptoms of hyperthyroidism include those related to adrenergic stimulation and are listed in Box 20-3.

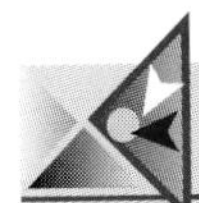

Box 20-3

SIGNS AND SYMPTOMS OF HYPERTHYROIDISM

SIGNS

- Tachycardia, atrial fibrillation
- Increased diastolic and decreased systolic blood pressures
- Eye signs such as stare, lid lag, and proptosis/exophthalmos[a]
- Pretibial myxedema
- Onycholysis
- Acropachy
- Silky, fine textured hair
- Flush, warm, smooth, and moist skin
- Fine tremor, proximal muscle weakness

SYMPTOMS

- Inappropriate weight loss (increased appetite)
- Increased sweating, heat intolerance
- Increased bowel habits
- Palpitations
- Increased agitation, irritability
- Rapid speech
- Amenorrhea

[a]With Graves' disease.

Graves' ophthalmopathy is the hallmark of Graves' disease and includes several characteristic features seen in the eyes, such as exophthalmos, proptosis, excess retro-orbital tissue, and blurred/double vision. Most cases are self-limited and require only local measures for symptomatic relief.

Thyroid storm is a life-threatening condition that includes exaggerated signs and symptoms of hyperthyroidism as well as altered mental status and fever. It warrants immediate control within 48 to 72 hours to avoid a 50% mortality rate. It is usually precipitated by injury but can occur after radioactive iodine therapy and sudden withdrawal of antithyroid medications.

The most common drug therapy for hyperthyroidism involves antithyroid medications, known as thioamides, which include propylthiouracil and methimazole. Because these drugs have a slow onset of action, adjunct agents are often needed initially for symptomatic relief until the antithyroid medications take effect; such agents include iodides and adrenergic blockers. Agranulocytosis may occur with antithyroid medications, so patients need to be educated to watch for signs of illness (e.g., fever, chills, sore throat, hoarseness) and, if they occur, to report immediately to their physician for a complete blood count workup.

Most common nonpharmacologic therapy for hyperthyroidism includes the use of radioactive iodine to destroy the thyroid gland or surgery (i.e., subtotal thyroidectomy). Surgery is indicated for rapid correction in patients who decline radioactive iodine or who may have contraindications to antithyroid medications.

Hypothyroidism occurs when there is a decrease in thyroid hormones. Primary hypothyroidism occurs when there is failure of the thyroid gland. Secondary hypothyroidism, which is less common, occurs when there is failure of the pituitary or hypothalamus. **Hashimoto's disease** (i.e., chronic autoimmune thyroiditis) is the most common cause of primary hypothyroidism. It is a chronic autoimmune disorder that occurs most often in children and in women between the ages of 30 and 50 years. Other causes of primary hypothyroidism include iatrogenic reasons (e.g., drugs, radiation, surgery), iodine deficiency (i.e., endemic goiter), enzyme defects, congenital defects (e.g., atresia, inborn errors of thyroxine metabolism), or ingestion of goitrogens (e.g., rutabagas, turnips, cabbage).

Drugs that inhibit thyroid hormone synthesis and secretion include agents that block iodide transport into the thyroid (e.g., fluorine, lithium), agents that impair organification and coupling of thyroid hormones (i.e., sulfonylureas), and agents that inhibit thyroid hormone secretion (e.g., large doses of iodide, lithium). The signs and symptoms of hypothyroidism include those that would be expected from inadequate adrenergic stimulation and are listed in Box 20-4.

Myxedema coma is a rare, life-threatening coma that can occur in persons with long-standing, uncontrolled hypothyroidism. It is most common in elderly patients, is often precipitated by illness, and may include hypothermia, bradycardia, respiratory failure, and cardiovascular collapse. It should be considered a medical emergency.

The most common drug therapy for hypothyroidism is the administration of thyroid-replacement therapy. Thyroid replacement is available as T_4 or T_3 (T_4 is preferred). Synthetic forms are recommended over natural forms (e.g., desiccated

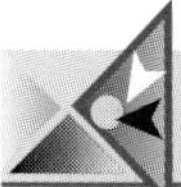

Box 20-4

SIGNS AND SYMPTOMS OF HYPOTHYROIDISM

SIGNS

- Bradycardia, S_3, S_4, or gallop rhythm
- Decreased systolic and increased diastolic blood pressures
- Decreased deep tendon reflexes
- Dry, coarse, and cold skin
- Brittle nails
- Periorbital and facial puffiness
- Carpal tunnel syndrome
- Coarse, thinning hair and hair loss
- Lateral eyebrow hair loss

SYMPTOMS

- Fatigue, lethargy
- Inappropriate weight gain (decreased appetite)
- Hoarse voice
- Decreased sweating, cold intolerance
- Decreased hearing
- Depression
- Constipation
- Decreased libido
- Menorrhagia

thyroid from hog, beef, sheep thyroid glands) because of antigenicity of the natural products. Bioequivalence is important, because in the past, some variation was found among brands. Recently, however, this situation has improved, and generics are now available that meet bioequivalence criteria. Blood levels should be monitored for success of therapy as well as for signs and symptoms of under- or overreplacement. Blood levels should also be monitored when switching from one brand of thyroid medication to another.

Nonpharmacologic therapy may include ensuring adequate iodine in the diet if a deficiency is expected. The approximate daily iodine requirement is 100 µg, which is the amount found in 1 g of iodized salt. Dietary sources of iodine include seafood, kelp, dairy products, eggs, and "conditioned" bread.

SYSTEM ASSESSMENT

Endocrine dysfunction produces many different systemic consequences depending on the disorder. Pharmacists need to evaluate each patient for a collection of signs and symptoms that may indicate inadequate control of a particular endocrine disorder. Recognition of signs and symptoms, however, as well as common physical presentation of these disorders, may help pharmacists to identify individuals who should be referred to their primary care provider for further evaluation.

Subjective Information

Polyuria

? INTERVIEW Do you ever experience increased urination, feeling like you have to go to the bathroom constantly? If yes,

Onset and duration: How often are you having to urinate? What times of the day or night is it occurring most frequently?

Appearance: Is the urine an unusual color? Does it have an odor?

Cause: Has your fluid intake increased? How many fluids or beverages containing caffeine are you drinking throughout the day? What problems have you noticed regarding your urine? Does it have an odor to it? Do you feel burning when urinating? Do you have difficulty starting a stream when going to the restroom? What other medications are you currently taking? If taking a diuretic, what time are you currently taking it?

ABNORMALITIES Polyuria occurs when a patient has an increased number of urinations and may present as nocturia or urinary incontinence when it occurs at night. Besides diabetes, an increase in urination may be caused by increased fluid intake, increased caffeine intake, urinary tract infections, prostate problems, or medication use (i.e., diuretics).

? INTERVIEW

Relief: Are there ever times that it seems to improve?

Symptoms: Do you experience any other symptoms? Increased thirst? Increased appetite? Weight loss or gain? Blurred vision? Dry, itchy skin? Increased or repeated infections? Sexual difficulties? Tingling in your fingers or toes? Bloated after eating?

ABNORMALITIES Hyperglycemia that occurs with diabetes may present with many different signs and symptoms, including polydipsia, polyphagia, weight changes, blurred vision, dry/pruritic skin, increased infections, impotence, paresthesias, and diabetic gastroparesis.

? INTERVIEW

Monitoring: When was the last time your eyes were examined?

ABNORMALITIES A dilated-eye examination by an ophthalmologist should be performed initially within 3 to 5 years of a diagnosis of type I diabetes in those patients 10 years or older to determine if retinopathy has occurred. Patients with type 2 diabetes should have an initial examination as soon as possible after diagnosis. Thereafter, eye examinations should be repeated at least annually. Microvascular disease with a thickening of the capillary membrane initially occurs and can lead to nonproliferative or proliferative retinopathy. The most serious case, with the worst prognosis, is proliferative diabetic **retinopathy,** the development of new vessels, and is caused by anoxic stimulation. The new vessels lack the supporting structure of normal vessels and are more likely to hemorrhage. Diabetes is the most common cause of legal blindness in the United States. After 20 years of diabetes, most patients with type I and more than 60% of patients with type 2 have some degree of retinopathy.

? INTERVIEW

Monitoring: When was the last time you had a dental examination?

ABNORMALITIES A dental examination should be performed twice annually by a dentist. Tooth and gum problems are common in patients with hyperglycemia.

Fatigue

? INTERVIEW Do you ever experience fatigue or extreme tiredness? If yes,

Onset and duration: How long have you been feeling tired and worn out?

Cause: Explain your sleep patterns lately. Have they been normal? What types of additional stress have you been experiencing lately? Any major lifestyle changes? What new prescription or over-the-counter medications have you been taking for allergies, cold, or other symptoms lately? What other medications are you currently taking? What dosage changes have occurred with your medications? What medical problems do you currently have or have you had in the past?

ABNORMALITIES Changes in sleep patterns, stress, lifestyle changes, medications, and certain diseases such as hypothyroidism and diabetes may all be associated with fatigue.

? INTERVIEW

Past history: Do you have any past history of thyroid problems? Have you ever had surgery on your thyroid? If taking thyroid medications, how many times do you think you missed your thyroid medicine in the last two weeks? Have any of your medications changed lately?

ABNORMALITIES History of thyroid surgery or thyroid problems and the use of thyroid medication may warrant a thyroid evaluation to determine if it is the cause of fatigue.

? INTERVIEW

Relief: What makes the tiredness go away?

Symptoms: Do you experience any other symptoms? Weight gain? Hoarseness in your voice? Difficulty hearing? Dry skin? Constipation? Hair loss? Inability to keep warm? Menstrual problems? Increased urination, thirst, hunger? Frequent infections?

ABNORMALITIES Hypothyroidism often presents with signs and symptoms that include inappropriate weight gain, hoarse voice, decreased hearing, dry skin, constipation, alopecia, cold intolerance, and menorrhagia. Diabetes often presents with polyuria, polydipsia, polyphagia, and frequent infections (see the diabetes section).

Objective Information

Objective patient information pertaining to the endocrine system includes the physical assessment and the results of laboratory and diagnostic tests.

Physical Assessment

The physical assessment is important if the patient has been diagnosed with an endocrine disorder or if one is suspected based on the subjective information collected. In patients suspected of having diabetes mellitus or a thyroid disorder, referral to a primary care provider for further evaluation is appropriate. In patients whose diabetes or thyroid disorders are being monitored by their pharmacists, however, more detailed understanding of and ability to perform the physical examination are needed to evaluate the heart, eyes, feet, nails, skin, hair, weight, height, and any signs of infection to determine the efficacy of treatment or the presence of complications. Lifestyle factors such as eating, drinking coffee, smoking, and exercise as well as medication intake and upright posture can affect the examination results in patients suffering from diabetic autonomic neuropathy.

Vital Signs

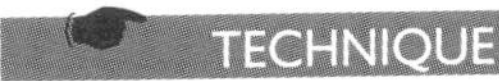

STEP 1

Assess the Vital Signs

See Chapter 5 for detailed instructions.

- Auscultate blood pressure and palpate the heart rate and rhythm with the patient both sitting and standing.

ABNORMALITIES Hypertension is usually defined by a blood pressure greater than 140/90 mm Hg, but blood pressures greater than 130/80 mm Hg in patients with diabetes should be treated aggressively to prevent complications. A resting heart rate greater than 100 bpm, orthostasis (fall in systolic blood pressure of >20 mm Hg on standing), edema, decreased ejection fraction, or decreased exercise tolerance may indicate autonomic neuropathy. Increased systolic and decreased diastolic blood pressures, tachycardia, atrial fibrillation, and hyperdynamic cardiac pulsations with an accentuated S_1 occur in hyperthyroidism. Decreased systolic and increased diastolic blood pressures, bradycardia, and decreased intensity of heart sounds occur in hypothyroidism.

Extremities (Feet and Hands)

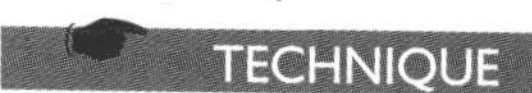

TECHNIQUE

STEP 1

Inspection of the Feet

- Ask patient to remove the shoes and socks from his or her feet.
- Put on gloves.
- Inspect the feet for changes, such as signs of an ulcer or history of an ulcer, toenails that are ingrown or too long, corns, calluses, pressure points, redness, swelling, warmth, dryness, maceration, or any obvious deformities.
- Record findings on a Diabetic Foot Assessment form (Fig. 20-5).
- Note any changes from previous evaluations, if appropriate.

ABNORMALITIES Treat calluses and corns carefully and without use of harsh over-the-counter (OTC) products. Bathroom surgery is not recommended. Nail grooming needs to be performed carefully (e.g., nails should be trimmed straight across). Referral to a podiatrist for nail care may be necessary in some cases. Ulcers and obvious deformities should be referred to the patient's physician.

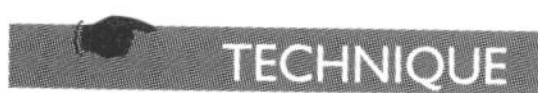

TECHNIQUE

STEP 2

Perform Monofilament Test and Palpate the Pedal Pulses

The monofilament (Fig. 20-6)test is a method of evaluating peripheral neuropathy by testing for touch sensation. Follow instructions similar to those above when inspecting the foot (e.g., have the patient remove shoes and socks, put on gloves).

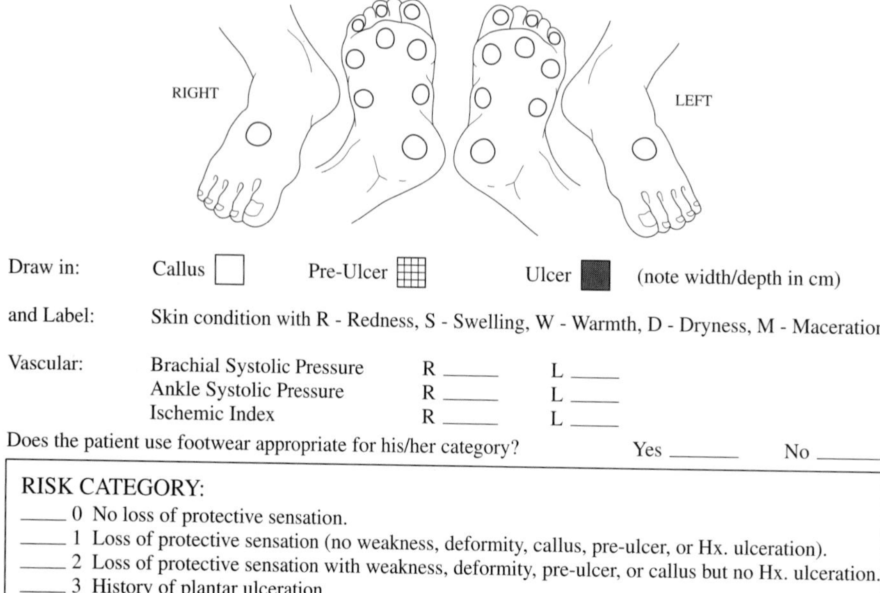

DIABETIC FOOT SCREEN	Date:
Patient's Name (Last, First, Middle) ________________	ID No.:

Fill in the following blanks with an "R", "L", or "B" to indicate positive findings on the right, left or both feet.

Has there been a change in the foot since last evaluation?	Yes ____	No ____
Is there a foot ulcer now or history of foot ulcer?	Yes ____	No ____
Does the foot have an abnormal shape?	Yes ____	No ____
Is there weakness in the ankle or foot?	Yes ____	No ____
Are the nails thick, too long, or ingrown?	Yes ____	No ____

Label: Sensory Level with a "+" in the circled areas of the foot if the patient can feel the 10 gram (5.07 Semmes-Weinstein) nylon filament and "–" if he/she cannot feel the 10 gram filament.

RIGHT LEFT

Draw in: Callus ☐ Pre-Ulcer ▦ Ulcer ■ (note width/depth in cm)

and Label: Skin condition with R - Redness, S - Swelling, W - Warmth, D - Dryness, M - Maceration

Vascular:			
	Brachial Systolic Pressure	R ____	L ____
	Ankle Systolic Pressure	R ____	L ____
	Ischemic Index	R ____	L ____

Does the patient use footwear appropriate for his/her category? Yes ____ No ____

RISK CATEGORY:
____ 0 No loss of protective sensation.
____ 1 Loss of protective sensation (no weakness, deformity, callus, pre-ulcer, or Hx. ulceration).
____ 2 Loss of protective sensation with weakness, deformity, pre-ulcer, or callus but no Hx. ulceration.
____ 3 History of plantar ulceration.

This diabetic foot screen may be reproduced and used without permission.

FIGURE 20-5 Diabetes foot assessment. *Hx*, history.

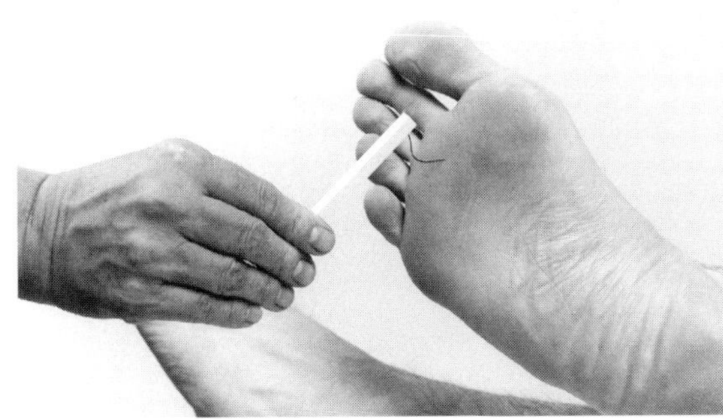

FIGURE 20-6 Monofilament.

- Ask the patient to place his or her foot on your lap or a chair.
- Ask the patient to close his or her eyes.
- Touch various areas of the patient's foot (see Fig. 20-5 for specific areas) with the 10-g monofilament. The monofilament should be applied perpendicularly and pushed until it is slightly bent in each area indicated (Fig. 20-6).
- Ask the patient to tell you each time a touch on his or her feet is felt. Place a plus (+) in the areas where the patient can feel the monofilament and a minus (−) in the areas where the patient doesn't respond.
- Palpate for the dorsalis pedal pulse (see Chapter 13 for details).
- Record the findings on the Diabetic Foot Assessment form.
- Repeat with the other foot.
- Assign a risk category dependent on the findings of the inspection and sensory testing.
- Refer patients with "risk" to their physician or a podiatrist, depending on the severity.

ABNORMALITIES Inability to detect sensation using a 10-g filament indicates the loss of protective sensation; refer such patients to their health care provider if loss has occurred. Signs and symptoms of peripheral arterial disease include intermittent claudication, cold feet, decreased or absent pulses, atrophy of subcutaneous tissues, and hair loss.

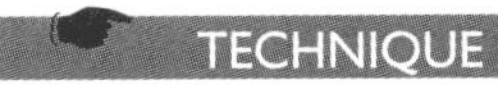

TECHNIQUE

STEP 3

Evaluate the Deep Tendon Reflexes

See Chapter 17 for detailed instructions.

ABNORMALITIES Patients with hypothyroidism may display decreased deep tendon reflexes.

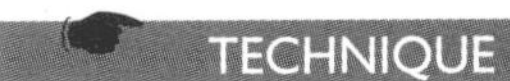

TECHNIQUE

STEP 4

Inspect the Fingers

- Ask the patient to sit comfortably with his or her palms on each leg.
- Inspect the back of the hands and fingers for color, lesions, and tremors.
- Ask the patient to turn his or her hands over (i.e., palms upward).
- Inspect the fingertips and palms for color, lesions, and tremors.

ABNORMALITIES Some patients have small bumps where their fingers are pricked. If no fingersticks are evident, ask the patient to demonstrate the technique for home monitoring of blood glucose to help assess his or her compliance and comfort with the procedure. A fine tremor may indicate hyperthyroidism.

Thyroid Gland

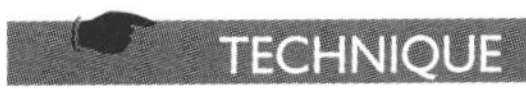

TECHNIQUE

STEP 1

Inspect the Neck for the Thyroid Gland

- Ask the patient to tip his or her head back slightly.
- Shine a light across the neck, pointing the light downward from the tip of the patient's chin.
- Inspect the area below the cricoid cartilage for the gland.
- Ask the patient to sip some water, tip the head back, and swallow.
- Note the upward movement of the thyroid gland, its contour, and its symmetry.

CAUTION The lower border of the thyroid gland rises when swallowing and may look less symmetric.

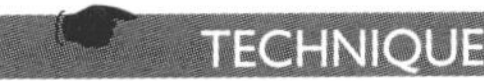

TECHNIQUE

STEP 2

Palpate the Thyroid Gland

- Stand behind the patient.
- Place the fingers of both hands on the patient's cricoid cartilage.
- Slowly move the fingers laterally, so that they rest on each side of the cricoid cartilage (Fig. 20-7).
- Ask the patient to tip his or her head back slightly.

CAUTION Overextension of the neck causes the neck muscles to tighten and obscures the ability to palpate the thyroid.

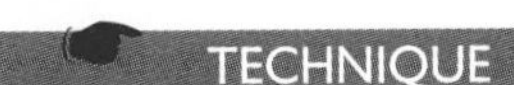

TECHNIQUE

STEP 2 (Continued)

- Ask the patient to sip some water, tip the head back, and swallow.
- Feel for the thyroid rising under your fingers.

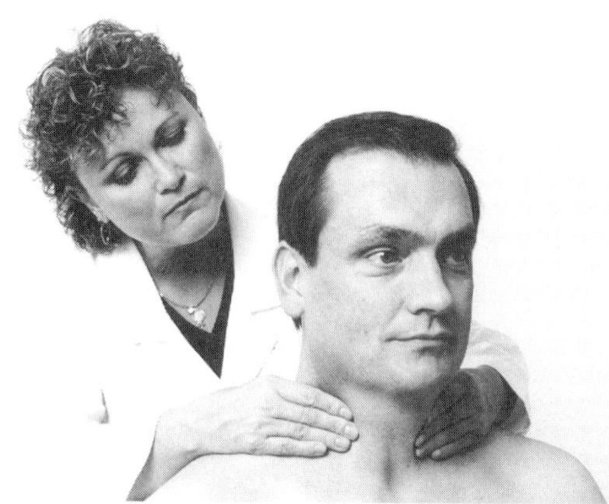

FIGURE 20-7 Palpation of the thyroid gland.

- Note the size, shape, and consistency of the thyroid.
- Document any nodules or tenderness.

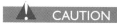

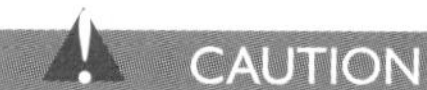
CAUTION The thyroid is not always palpable.

Eyes

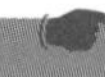
TECHNIQUE

STEP 1

Inspect the Eyes and Eyelids

See Chapter 9 for detailed instructions.

- Examine the eye for evidence of hyperthyroidism (Graves' ophthalmopathy) or other ophthalmic effects of thyroid dysfunction.

ABNORMALITIES Hyperthyroidism (Graves' ophthalmopathy) includes **exophthalmos** (i.e., protrusion of the eyeball), which may result from an increased volume of orbital content. It may appear unilateral or bilateral. Notice that the sclera is easily seen from above and below the limbus of the cornea. Scleral redness may indicate that the eyelids cannot close completely to keep the cornea and sclera moist. Exophthalmos commonly does not disappear after the thyroid dysfunction is corrected (Fig. 20-8). Fasciculations or tremors of eyelids may occur while examining lightly closed eyes. Myxedema of the eyelids (i.e., a dry, waxy swelling of abnormal deposits of mucin) may occur in hypothyroidism.

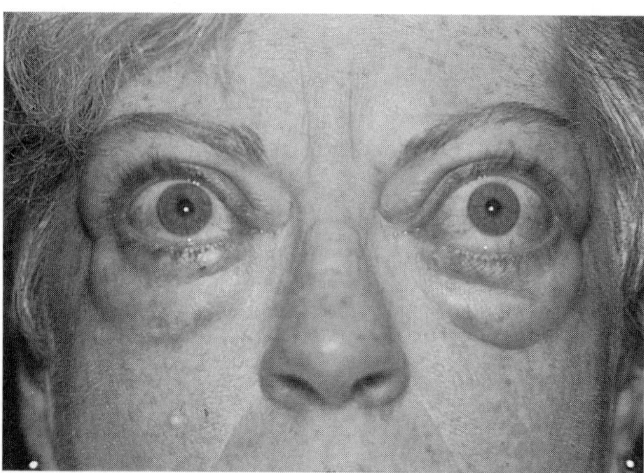

FIGURE 20-8 Exophthalmos of Graves' disease.

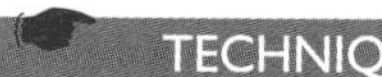
TECHNIQUE

STEP 2

Inspect the Pupils

See Chapter 9 for detailed instructions.

- Examine the pupils for effects of autonomic neuropathy from diabetes.

ABNORMALITIES Failure of the pupil to contract in light or to dilate in darkness may indicate pupillary autonomic neuropathy.

Skin

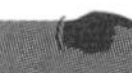
TECHNIQUE

STEP 1

Inspect the Skin

See Chapter 8 for detailed instructions.

- Inspect and palpate the skin.
- Note its appearance, temperature, and texture.

ABNORMALITIES Soft, smooth, and warm skin is consistent with hyperthyroidism. Rough, dry, and cold skin is consistent with hypothyroidism. **Pretibial myxedema** is a dry, firm, waxy swelling of the skin in the pretibial area and is characteristic of hypothyroidism. Periorbital and face puffiness may also be present in hypothyroidism. Frequent or slow-healing infections may be a sign of diabetes or lack of glucose control.

Hair

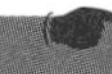
TECHNIQUE

STEP 1

Inspect the Hair

See Chapter 8 for detailed instructions.

- Inspect the hair.
- Note its texture, color, and distribution.

ABNORMALITIES Hair should be smooth, symmetrically distributed, and have no splitting or cracked ends. Coarse/dry/brittle hair, alopecia (i.e., hair loss), and lateral loss of eyebrow hair may occur in hypothyroidism.

Fine/silky hair may occur in hyperthyroidism. Itchy skin should be differentiated from dry skin, aging, drug reactions, allergies, obstructive jaundice, uremia, and lice.

Nails

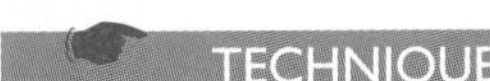

TECHNIQUE

STEP 1

Inspect the Nails

See Chapter 8 for detailed instructions.

ABNORMALITIES **Onycholysis** (i.e., separation of the nail bed from the plate) may occur in hyperthyroidism or hypothyroidism. Clubbing (i.e., a thickening of the tissues at the bases of the fingernails and toenails) may also occur in hypothyroidism and cause the normal angle between the nail and digit to be filled in. Most commonly, however, it is found in disorders of the lung and infective endocarditis.

Laboratory and Diagnostic Tests

The following laboratory and diagnostic tests may be useful in assessing for diabetes mellitus and thyroid disorders:

- *Blood glucose* should be tested to evaluate the level of diabetes or diabetes control. Normal fasting blood glucose levels are between 80 and 120 mg/dL. The diagnosis of diabetes mellitus is based on the presence of one of the following criteria using plasma blood glucose levels:
  1. Symptoms of diabetes plus casual plasma glucose ≥200 mg/dL. "Casual" is defined as any time of the day without regards to meals. Classic symptoms of diabetes include polyuria, polydipsia, and unexplained weight loss.
  2. Fasting blood glucose ≥126 mg/dL. Fasting is defined as no caloric intake for at least 8 hours.
  3. A 2-hour post glucose ≥200 mg/dL during an oral glucose tolerance test.

  If the blood glucose level meets one of the above criteria, it should be confirmed on a subsequent day. The treatment goal for patients with diabetes mellitus is a fasting blood glucose <120 mg/dL. Whole-blood glucose concentrations are 15% lower than plasma glucose concentrations, because the glucose is not distributed in the red blood cells. This should be noted, because it accounts for the differences between the results of hospital laboratories and some home blood glucose monitors.
- *Glycosylated hemoglobin* (HbA_{1c}) is used to determine achievement of treatment goals. Normal values are 4% to 6% and show an average blood glucose level over a period of 2 to 3 months. The level of glucose in the blood irreversibly glycosylates a proportional amount of the red blood cells, and because the average life span of a red blood cell is 120 days, this is a good determinant of average blood glucose concentrations. An HbA_{1c} of 7% and 9% correlates with a blood glucose value of 150 and 210 mg/dL, respectively. Values are falsely low in conditions with decreased red-blood-cell life span and in anemias. The treatment goal for patients with diabetes mellitus is HbA_{1c} <7%.
- *Urinalysis with microscopic examination* evaluates for the presence of urine protein to detect any early occurrence of renal dysfunction. Routine urinalysis should be performed annually in adults, and if positive for protein (proteinuria), a quantitative measure is helpful. Proteinuria usually indicates overt nephropathy. Initially, for type 2 diabetes, tests should be performed at diagnosis; for type 1 diabetes, tests should be tested at puberty or after 5 years of having the disease. If negative for protein, a test for microalbuminuria is necessary. This may be determined by three different methods of collection: (1) the random spot collection (i.e., albumin:creatinine ratio), (2) the 24-hour collection with creatinine (also allowing simultaneous creatinine clearance), and (3) timed collection (4 hour or overnight). Microalbuminuria is the appearance of low but abnormal levels of albumin in the urine (>30 mg/day or 20 μg/min), and if positive, it should be confirmed at two subsequent tests within a 3-month period. If at least two of the three tests are positive, the patient should begin treatment. These patients are referred to as having incipient nephropathy. If the test for microalbuminuria is negative, it should be repeated yearly.

  The presence of urine glucose was traditionally a common monitoring parameter in diabetes. It has fallen out of favor, however, because it only appears after blood glucose levels reach the renal threshold level of >180 mg/dL. Also, with this method, it is difficult to determine the actual blood glucose level. It may be an alternative for patients unable to use a home blood glucose monitor. Urine ketones should be checked in patients with type 1 diabetes who have blood glucose values >250 mg/dL. This occurs most frequently during sick days and when patients are noncompliant with insulin, and its presence warrants immediate evaluation and treatment.
- *Transient elevations in urinary albumin* excretion can occur with short-term hyperglycemia, exercise, urinary tract infections, marked hypertension, heart failure, and acute febrile illness. Two (of three) positive tests are needed to establish the diagnosis.
- *The presence of white blood cells, blood, or mucus* may indicate urinary tract or vaginal infection, which are common in patients with diabetes.
- *Serum creatinine* is measured in patients with diabetes to determine creatinine clearance and evaluate renal status.
- *Gastric emptying tests,* such as a barium swallow or manometric studies, are used to evaluate gastrointestinal function. Reduced or absent peristalsis, delayed emptying, or reduced lower esophageal sphincter tone may indicate gastrointestinal autonomic neuropathy.

- *Radiologic and urodynamic studies* are used to test for dysfunction of the genitourinary system. Genitourinary autonomic neuropathy may be suspected in patients with increased bladder capacity or postvoid residual volume, decreased bladder contractility, or impaired urine flow.
- *Angiography/Doppler ultrasound or nocturnal penile tumescence tests* are used to test for impotence, which can be related to genitourinary autonomic neuropathy.
- *Thyroid function tests* are used to diagnose and monitor patients with thyroid disorders. Clinical need determines which of the many available tests is indicated in each particular case. Many can be performed depending on the clinical situation, but only the most common tests are discussed here:
  - *Free T_4* is a measure of free thyroxine. It is the most sensitive test and is usually elevated (along with a suppressed TSH) in overt hyperthyroidism and suppressed (along with an elevated TSH) in overt hypothyroidism. Serum T_4 (total T_4) concentrations are also available, include both free and bound hormone, and may be abnormal because of changes in thyroxine-binding globulin.
  - *Thyroid-stimulating hormone (TSH)* is also known as thyrotropin. It should be checked on diagnosis and at 6 to 8 weeks for evaluation. Because the level takes 6 to 8 weeks to reach steady state because of the delayed pituitary effects, therapy should not be evaluated any sooner than this time. It is usually suppressed (along with an elevated free T_4) in overt hyperthyroidism and elevated (along with a suppressed free T_4) in overt hypothyroidism. Levels of >20 mU/L are considered to be diagnostic of hypothyroidism.

ABNORMALITIES TSH is increased with lithium and antithyroid medications and decreased by dopamine agonists, salicylic acid, steroids, and thyroid hormone replacement. If free T_4 is elevated and TSH is not suppressed, this may indicate that the hyperthyroidism is caused by a TSH-producing pituitary adenoma. If T_4 is normal and TSH is increased with few symptoms of hypothyroidism, this could indicate subclinical hypothyroidism. These patients have an increased chance of developing hyperlipidemia and progression to overt disease. The incidence is 4% to 17% and increases with age. If T_4 is normal and TSH is decreased, this may indicate subclinical hyperthyroidism. These patients have an increased chance of developing atrial fibrillation, osteoporosis, and progression to overt disease. Presently, the decision to treat or merely follow subclinical disease more closely to prevent complications is controversial. Evaluate each case individually to determine the benefits and risks of therapy. Conditions that increase the body's need for energy trigger the feedback system to increase thyroid hormone secretion. These include cold environment, high altitude, and pregnancy. Large amounts of sex hormones (e.g., androgens, estrogens) cause both TSH and secretion of thyroid hormone to decrease.

- *Thyroid scans* are used to determine the size, shape, and activity of the gland. Either I^{123} or Tc^{99m} are administered. The test is useful in patients with nodular disease to detect "hot" and "cold" spots, but it is usually avoided because of its cost.
- *Electrocardiograms* are useful to determine any cardiac involvement such as atrial fibrillation.
- *Cholesterol profiles* are used in patients with diabetes or hypothyroidism. Goal low-density lipoprotein cholesterol for patients with diabetes is <100 mg/dL. In patients with hypothyroidism, an elevated cholesterol is consistent with the diagnosis of hypothyroidism.

Special Considerations

Pediatric Patients

Additional questions for the pediatric patient's parent or guardian include:

? INTERVIEW

Diabetes: What symptoms is the child having? Excessive thirst? Bedwetting or frequent urination? Weight loss? Does the child have a family history of diabetes? What other medication is the child currently taking? What other health problems does the child have? Does the child have a history of thyroid problems?

ABNORMALITIES Tremendous thirst and frequent urination are quite common in affected children. Bedwetting may recur. Children with diabetes also seem to have a good appetite, to be eating a lot, and yet to be losing weight. An active and robust child may suddenly appear weak, be irritable, and have little energy. Family history and use of medications is important in establishing the diagnosis. The occurrence of more than one autoimmune disease, such as diabetes mellitus and hypothyroidism, is common.

? INTERVIEW

Thyroid: Does the child have a family history of thyroid disease? What other medication is the child taking? Did the biological mother have thyroid problems during pregnancy that were detected?

ABNORMALITIES Family history is important, as are any medications that the child could be taking that might be causing problems with the thyroid. If the biologic mother experienced thyroid problems during pregnancy, the newborn child may also exhibit effects.

Because retinopathy is rare before age 10 in children with diabetes, a dilated eye examination is not necessary until the patient reaches this age. In children 10 years or older who have type 1 diabetes, an eye examination should be performed within 3 to 5 years of the onset of disease. Microalbuminuria is rare and of short duration in type 1 diabetes and before puberty; therefore, screening is recommended to begin at puberty and after 5 years of diagnosis.

The thyroid gland is very difficult to palpate in infants because of their short, thick necks. If enlarged, it may be palpable. Goiter in infants may result from deprivation of thyroid hormone in utero. The thyroid of young children may normally be palpable because of their slender necks; therefore, the ability to palpate alone does not indicate the presence of a thyroid disorder in these patients. During adolescence, a noticeable enlargement of thyroid cartilage occurs. In boys, deepening of the voice occurs because of the effects of the enlarged cartilage on the larynx. In the United States, all newborns are screened for T_4 and TRH, and if low levels are discovered, thyroid supplements are given to prevent neurologic systemic effects.

In children, excessive sweating could accompany hypoglycemia, heart disease, or hyperthyroidism.

Geriatric Patients

Additional questions for the geriatric patient or caregiver include:

? INTERVIEW

Diabetes: When did the increased urination start? Do you have any problems with your prostate, bladder control, or urinary tract infections? What other medications are you currently taking?

ABNORMALITIES Elderly patients tend to take more medications than younger patients, and many medications can affect blood glucose. Elderly patients tend to present with more subtle signs and symptoms that have gradually worsened over time. These symptoms are often overlooked and unreported, because the patients think they are a normal part of aging. Thirst perception declines, masking polydipsia and often leading to dehydration, which is often the cause for the increase in emergency hyperosmolar states in elderly patients.

If treating elderly patients with diabetes, recognize that they are more prone to hypoglycemic episodes than younger patients. This is because hypoglycemic symptoms are normally both adrenergic and neuroglycopenic. As a person ages, the adrenergic symptoms (e.g., tachycardia, shakiness) decrease because of the loss of autonomic nerve function. Consequently, an elderly patient may only be able to detect low blood sugars from symptomatology relating to neuroglycopenic symptoms. This is serious, because neurologic symptoms occur as the hypoglycemia progresses and, quite often, are mistaken for confusion, dementia, and other psychologic changes normally associated with aging.

? INTERVIEW

Thyroid: Do you have any problems with your heart, such as atrial fibrillation or heart failure? Is your heart rate unusually fast or slow? What other medications are you currently taking?

ABNORMALITIES Diagnosing thyroid disorders is more difficult in elderly patients, because their symptomatology may involve only a single system (as opposed to multiple systems in younger patients). The only symptoms seen may include weight loss, a cardiac abnormality, atrial fibrillation, or heart failure. This is because of the changes in the sympathetic nervous system in the elderly.

Proteinuria in elderly patients may occur even in the absence of diabetes. Age specific norms are currently under development for microalbuminuria to aid in the diagnosis and management of nephropathy.

The thyroid gland becomes more fibrotic as a person ages, and it may feel more irregular and nodular upon palpation. With age, there is a modest decrease in T_4, a slight increase in TSH, and no change in T_3. The aging process also involves a slow atrophy of skin structures and a decrease in the number and function of sweat and sebaceous glands, leading to dry skin. Hair distribution changes as well, often becoming thin. The basal metabolic rate declines, which is related to a decrease in muscle mass. It is often more difficult to detect hyperthyroidism in elderly patients, because they often elicit few symptoms (except for those from single systems; e.g., weight loss, cardiac abnormalities). The cardiac abnormalities observed most frequently in elderly patients with hyperthyroidism include atrial fibrillation and congestive heart failure. Other subtle symptoms that may exist include hoarseness, deafness, confusion, dementia, ataxia, depression, dry skin, or hair loss.

As people age, they tend to sweat less, tolerate cold less well, and prefer warmer climates. Pruritis/itching is common in aging skin and needs to be distinguished from other systemic disorders, such as liver disease, diabetes mellitus, kidney disease, and thyroid disorders. Elderly patients with other autoimmune diseases or unexplained depression, cognitive dysfunction, or hypercholesterolemia should be screened with a TSH test.

Toxic nodular goiter or Plummer's disease is more common than Graves' disease in elderly patients. Ophthalmopathy is not present in toxic nodular goiter and, therefore, is not common in elderly patients.

Pregnant Patients

Additional questions for pregnant patients include:

? INTERVIEW

Diabetes: When did the first signs and symptoms appear? Were you diagnosed with diabetes before the pregnancy, or did it begin during the pregnancy? Did you have problems with diabetes during previous pregnancies?

Thyroid: When did the first signs appear? Were you diagnosed with thyroid problems before the pregnancy, or did they begin during the pregnancy? Did you have problems with your thyroid in previous pregnancies?

When planning pregnancy, women with preexisting diabetes should have a comprehensive eye examination and receive counseling on the risk of development and/or progression of diabetic retinopathy during pregnancy. If a woman with diabetes becomes pregnant, she should have an eye examination during the first trimester and close follow-up throughout the pregnancy. Those with GDM are not at increased risk of diabetic retinopathy, thus negating the need for intensive monitoring during pregnancy.

Screening for GDM should occur between 24 and 28 weeks of pregnancy in women with one or more of the following:

- Age ≥25 years
- Age <25 years and obese (≥120% of desired body weight, or body mass index ≥27 kg/m^2)
- Family history of diabetes in a first-degree relative
- Membership in an ethnic/racial group with a high prevalence rate of diabetes (e.g., Hispanic American, Native American, Asian American, African American, or Pacific Islander)

Pregnant women not meeting these criteria are considered at low risk, and it is often considered to be cost-ineffective to screen them. GDM is diagnosed if, during screening, the patient has a fasting plasma glucose of 105 mg/dL or greater; a 1-hour, post–100 g load of 190 mg/dL or greater; a 2-hour, post–100 g load of 165 mg/dL or greater; and a 3-hour, post–100 g load of 145 mg/dL or greater. If GDM occurs, the patient needs treatment accordingly and repeat testing for diabetes at 6-weeks postpartum. If at 6-weeks postpartum glucose levels are still diagnostic of diabetes mellitus, the patient should be reclassified. Because of the increased risk of diabetes in this population after pregnancy, educate the patient about the signs and symptoms of diabetes, modification of other risk factors for diabetes, and the need for more frequent monitoring for the disease.

Pregnant women with diabetes should check their urine for ketones daily. They also may need to perform more frequent blood glucose monitoring to ensure good metabolic control.

The thyroid gland increases in size because of hyperplasia of the glandular tissue and increased vascularity during pregnancy. It may become palpable during pregnancy because of this enlargement. During pregnancy, the body's metabolic rate increases, which causes increased sweating in an attempt to dissipate the additional heat that is produced. For women with hyperthyroidism who become pregnant, evaluate the TSH level more often (at least every trimester) to predict the chances of neonatal hyperthyroidism, and adjust therapy as indicated. For women with hyperthyroidism during pregnancy, check thyroid function tests at 6- to 8-weeks postpartum to assess for worsening of the disease, because exacerbations occur most frequently at this time.

APPLICATION TO PATIENT SYMPTOMS

Because pharmacists are readily accessible to patients who inquire about OTC remedies or regularly refill prescription medications and supplies for their endocrine disorders, they are in the optimal position to assist these patients. Pharmacists may evaluate a patient's symptomatology and either recommend therapy for relief of minor symptoms or refer appropriately to the patient's physician for further evaluation. Polyuria and fatigue are examples of two common symptoms that patients may present with to their pharmacist. These symptoms are discussed in further detail as they relate to the monitoring of patients with endocrine disorders.

Polyuria

Polyuria is the excessive secretion and discharge of urine, and it is one of the "classic" symptoms of patients who present with hyperglycemia of diabetes mellitus. Evaluation should include other causes of polyuria besides diabetes mellitus, which may include excessive fluid intake, diabetes insipidus, chronic nephritis, nephrosclerosis, diuretic use, prostate problems, and urinary tract infections. If these are ruled out, then the presence of other signs and symptoms associated with diabetes should be evaluated (Box 20-2). These include fatigue, polydipsia, weight loss, polyphagia, and blurred vision. The symptoms of type 2 diabetes are more nonspecific and gradual at onset. They may go unnoticed for many years before the diagnosis is established, which is why the pharmacist needs to be aware of the condition and to refer patients with suspected diabetes as soon as possible for appropriate evaluation and diagnosis. Quite often, by the time that diabetes is discovered, the onset of complications has already begun.

CASE STUDY

BS is a 67-year-old man who presents to the pharmacy counter complaining that lately he has been having to go to the bathroom so frequently that it keeps him up at night. It is frustrating him, because he has been much more tired and unproductive during the day. He asks for some more of the sleep medicine that he had taken previously when he was having trouble sleeping.

ASSESSMENT OF THE PATIENT

Subjective Information

67-year-old man complaining of polyuria and insomnia

HOW OFTEN ARE YOU HAVING TO URINATE? HOW MANY TIMES ARE YOU GETTING UP AT NIGHT? At least every hour during the day, and three times during the night.

Continued

CASE STUDY—continued

HOW MANY FLUIDS OR BEVERAGES CONTAINING CAFFEINE ARE YOU DRINKING THROUGHOUT THE DAY? HAS THIS INCREASED? No, although I have felt more thirsty lately, I'm still not drinking much more than usual. And I avoid caffeine-containing products because of my high blood pressure.

WHAT PROBLEMS HAVE YOU NOTICED REGARDING YOUR URINE? None that I know of.

DOES IT HAVE AN ODOR TO IT? DO YOU FEEL BURNING WHEN URINATING? No, it doesn't appear to have any smell to it, and it doesn't burn, either.

DO YOU HAVE DIFFICULTY WITH STARTING A STREAM WHEN GOING TO THE RESTROOM? No, I go very easily.

WHAT OTHER MEDICATIONS ARE YOU CURRENTLY TAKING? I'm taking a new water pill for my blood pressure and want something to help me sleep. I haven't been taking any other medications.

WHAT TIME ARE YOU TAKING YOUR WATER PILL? First thing in the morning when I get up.

HOW OFTEN DO YOU FORGET TO TAKE YOUR BLOOD PRESSURE MEDICATION? I never forget it. I always remember.

YOU MENTIONED FEELING A LITTLE MORE THIRSTY LATELY. IS THIS TRUE? Yes, I usually don't get thirsty in between breaks at work, but lately, it seems like my thirst is not quenched as easily as before.

WHAT CHANGES IN APPETITE HAVE YOU EXPERIENCED? Actually, I'm much more hungry lately. I just can't seem to satisfy my hunger like I used to.

WHAT WEIGHT CHANGES HAVE OCCURRED? It actually surprised me to step on the scale today and see that my weight was lower than before, when I'm eating quite a bit more.

WHAT PROBLEMS WITH YOUR VISION HAVE YOU BEEN EXPERIENCING? My eyes have been a little blurry lately, but my eyeglasses prescription is probably getting old.

IS YOUR SKIN DRY AND ITCHY? Not any more than usual.

WHAT TYPES OF INFECTIONS HAVE YOU EXPERIENCED LATELY? None that I know of. I haven't been really sick for a couple years.

WHAT DIFFICULTIES HAVE YOU HAD SEXUALLY? Uh [seems a little embarrassed], none, I'm just fine in that category.

ARE YOU EXPERIENCING ANY TINGLING IN YOUR FINGERS OR TOES? No.

DO YOU FEEL FULL AND LIKE YOUR FOOD ISN'T BEING DIGESTED VERY QUICKLY? No.

WHICH RELATIVES OF YOURS HAVE BEEN DIAGNOSED WITH HAVING HIGH BLOOD SUGAR OR DIABETES IN THE PAST? I'm not sure. None that I know of. Grandpa died of kidney failure, but I don't know why.

HAVE YOU EVER BEEN SCREENED FOR DIABETES WITH A BLOOD SUGAR TEST? Not that I know of.

WHEN WAS THE LAST TIME YOU ATE? Last night at supper. I got up too late today to get anything, because I was hoping to catch some extra rest.

Objective Information

Computerized medication profile:

- Hydrochlorothiazide (HCTZ): 50 mg, one tablet every morning; No. 30; Refills: 11; Patient obtains refills every 25–30 days.
- Nytol: As needed for sleep (OTC agent, last purchased 10/10/97)

Blood pressure: 150/94 mm Hg
Heart rate: 62 bpm
Glucose: 180 mg/dL

DISCUSSION

Before offering the patient a sleep-aid recommendation, the pharmacist should evaluate for other possible causes of polyuria, such as increased fluids, urinary tract infections, kidney problems, prostate problems, and medication (i.e., diuretic) use. Thus, while asking the appropriate questions to evaluate for secondary causes of polyuria, it is discovered that BS is taking a diuretic. BS is asked about the timing of the medication to determine if this alone may be contributing to his nocturia. BS indicates that he takes it first thing in the morning and never forgets. If he would have been taking it at bedtime, then simply changing his medication to the morning might have helped him make it through the night without having to get up to urinate.

During questioning about other symptoms BS may be experiencing, the pharmacist discovers that he has been thirstier (polydipsia), he has been hungrier (polyphagia), and his vision has been blurry lately, which are all symptoms of hyperglycemia. BS denies experiencing any tingling extremities (peripheral neuropathy), increased infections, or abdominal bloating (gastroparesis) that may indicate additional complications of hyperglycemia. BS also denies any family history of diabetes, but he does mention that his grandfather died of kidney disease, which is a common complication of diabetes.

Because this patient also indicates that he does not think he has ever been tested for blood sugar before, the pharmacist decides to check his blood glucose. (The patient said he hadn't had time to eat breakfast that morning, so he has fasted for 8 hours.) The blood glucose value is found to be 180 mg/dL, which is higher than the desired 126 mg/dL for fasting levels (the monitor used displayed the reading as a plasma level). Based on recommended guidelines, this blood glucose is too high, but the pharmacist notes this may be a result of the effects of HCTZ on blood glucose (especially at

Continued

CASE STUDY—continued

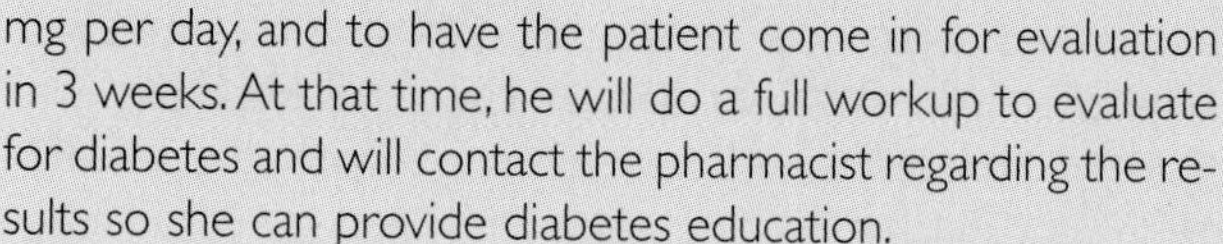

doses of >25 mg). The pharmacist calls the patient's physician, discusses this problem, and recommends that the physician either decrease the HCTZ to 25 mg or consider changing it to another blood pressure medication to see if changing the thiazide diuretic alone might improve BS' levels. The physician agreed to change from HCTZ to lisinopril, 10 mg per day, and to have the patient come in for evaluation in 3 weeks. At that time, he will do a full workup to evaluate for diabetes and will contact the pharmacist regarding the results so she can provide diabetes education.

Figure 20-9 shows the decision tree concerning how to evaluate patients with complaints of polyuria.

PHARMACEUTICAL CARE PLAN

Patient Name: BS

Date: 05/09/02

Medical Problems:
Hypertension

Current Medications:
HCTZ, 50 mg, one tablet every morning
Nytol, as needed for sleep (OTC agent, last purchased 10/10/97)

S: 67-year-old man complaining of increased urination in the day and at night, which appears to be causing insomnia. Also complains of polydipsia, polyphagia, and blurred vision. Denies any increase in fluids/beverages or caffeine use, foul-smelling urine, burning on urination, difficulty starting stream, dry/itchy skin, infections, tingling of extremities, sexual problems, or abdominal bloating. Compliant with HCTZ and requesting sleep-aid.

O: Fasting blood glucose of 180 mg/dL. No other labs available.

Blood pressure: 150/94 mm Hg

Heart rate: 62 bpm

A:
1. Polyuria, possibly caused by hyperglycemia.
2. HCTZ, 50 mg, may cause polyuria and hyperglycemia.
3. Possible diabetes mellitus caused by HCTZ; needs further evaluation for diagnosis.
4. Hypertension, uncontrolled.

P:
1. Call patient's physician to explain the problem and recommend a decrease in HCTZ to 25 mg per day or a switch to another antihypertensive, such as an angiotensin-converting enzyme inhibitor like lisinopril.
2. Educate BS about the importance of following up of the problems discovered today.
3. Explain the importance of adequate control of blood pressure and blood sugars.
4. Schedule phone follow-up appointment for 1 week with patient to assess symptomatology and tolerance of new blood pressure medication.
5. Schedule a visit (after appointment with physician; >3 weeks) to appropriately follow up and educate as needed at that time.
6. Blood pressure goal is <130/85 mm Hg, unless diagnosed with diabetes (then <130/80 mm Hg), and HbA_{1c} goal is <7 %.

Pharmacist: *Kathryn Klein, Pharm.D.*

Self-Assessment Questions

1. What are the signs and symptoms of hyperglycemia? (Differentiate between type 1 and type 2 symptomatology.)
2. What are the signs and symptoms of hypoglycemia?
3. What medications affect blood glucose levels?

Critical Thinking Questions

1. LS comes into the pharmacy with a recent urinalysis. The urinalysis showed that her protein was negative but that she had microalbuminuria. Her physician has prescribed lisinopril. LS heard that this medication was for high blood pressure, however, and the last time she checked, her blood pressure was controlled. Explain the reason for the prescription to LS, and differentiate between urine protein and microalbuminuria.
2. PT comes into your pharmacy and says his home blood glucose monitor isn't working. He explains that the reading his physician gave him from the clinic's lab was 124 mg/dL, but that he checked his blood glucose right before that with his home monitor, which gave a reading of 108 mg/dL. You check PT's monitor with the control solutions, and it appears to be working correctly. What do you think is the reason for the discrepancy?

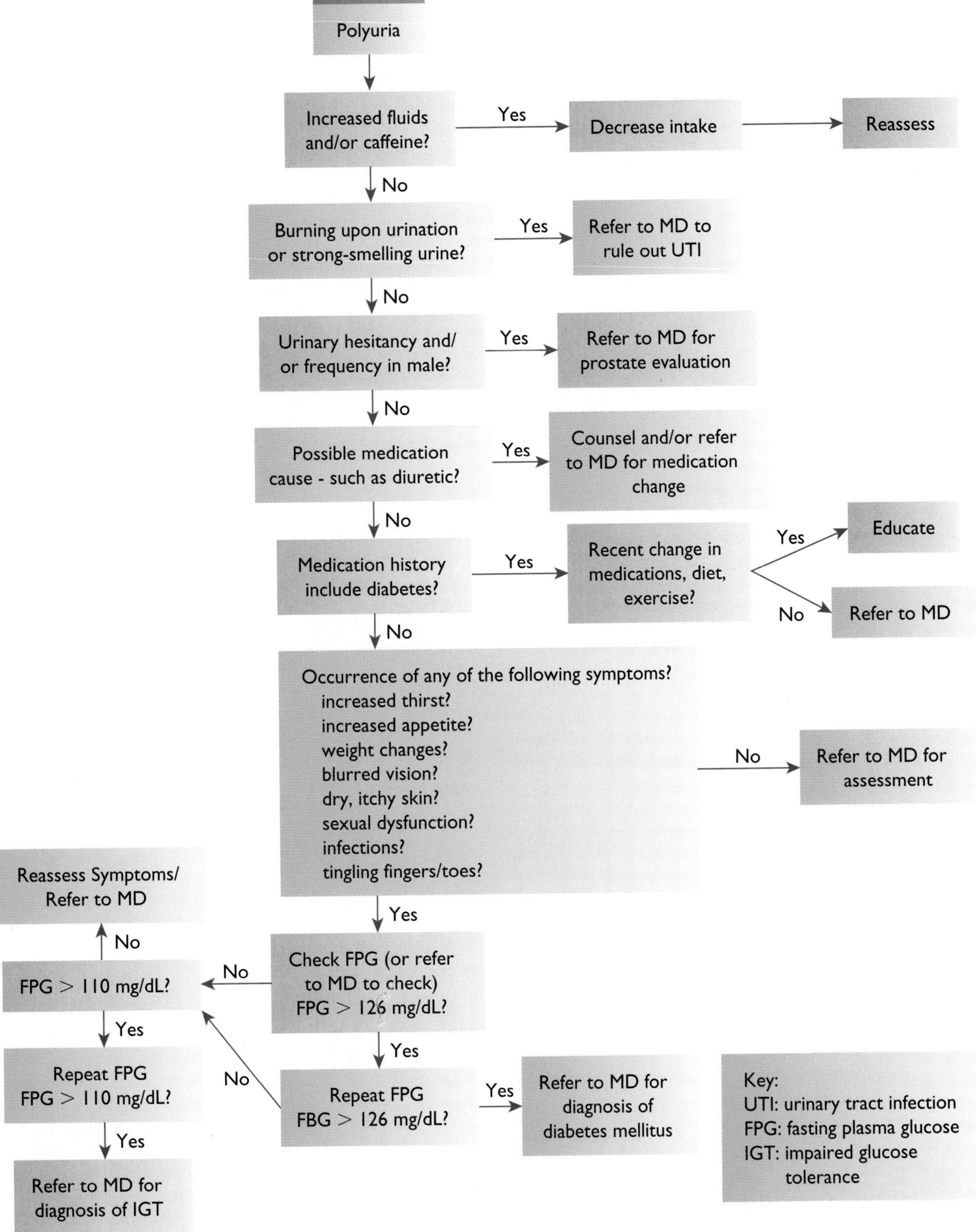

FIGURE 20-9 Decision tree for polyuria.

Fatigue

Fatigue is a feeling of tiredness or weariness, usually resulting from continued activity and inadequate rest. Causes of fatigue include the presence of or inadequate treatment of malnutrition, heart disease, anemia, respiratory disturbances, infectious diseases, endocrine disorders (e.g., diabetes, hypothyroidism), psychogenic factors (e.g., anxiety, frustration, boredom), medications (e.g., β-blockers, sedatives, anxiolytics), and environment. Patients with hypothyroidism that is inadequately treated or with hyperthyroidism that is overtreated may also experience fatigue. Causes of inadequate response or the appearance of undertreatment for hypothyroidism include poor compliance, inadequate dosage, decreased bioavailability, and drug interactions with thyroid medications. Medications causing hypothyroidism include lithium, antithyroid medications, and amiodarone (amiodarone may cause hypo- or hyperthyroidism). Inadequate iodine in the diet can also cause hypothyroidism. Medications known to interact with the absorption of thyroid medications include cholestyramine, colestipol, and ferrous sulfate; administration of such medications should be separated by at least 6 hours.

CASE STUDY

ML is a 45-year-old woman who appears at the pharmacy counter with a refill request of her cholesterol medication. She also says that she has been experiencing a tired, run-down feeling for the last few weeks and is requesting a medication to help increase her energy level throughout the day. She is wearing a wool sweater, which seems unusual for the summer months, during which temperatures are approximately 100°F outside. Her voice also sounds a little hoarse.

ASSESSMENT OF THE PATIENT

Subjective Information

45-year-old woman complaining of a tired, run-down feeling and wearing a wool sweater in 100°F weather.

HOW LONG HAVE YOU BEEN FEELING TIRED AND WORN OUT? The last month or so, maybe a little longer.

EXPLAIN YOUR SLEEP PATTERNS LATELY. HAVE THEY BEEN NORMAL? I've been sleeping normal amounts at the normal times, but possibly an extra hour each night because I feel so worn down.

WHAT TYPES OF ADDITIONAL STRESS HAVE YOU BEEN EXPERIENCING LATELY? ANY MAJOR LIFESTYLE CHANGES? None. Things have been going great for me at work and at home, and nothing has changed. I don't feel any pressures right now.

WHAT NEW PRESCRIPTION OR OVER-THE-COUNTER MEDICATIONS HAVE YOU BEEN TAKING FOR ALLERGIES, COLD, OR OTHER REASONS LATELY? I have been taking a stool softener for constipation lately, which troubles me because I am normally very regular.

WHAT OTHER MEDICATIONS ARE YOU CURRENTLY TAKING? The stool softener, cholesterol medicine for the last couple months, and my thyroid medicine. I don't remember the names; you'll have to look at my list in your computer.

WHAT DOSAGE CHANGES HAVE OCCURRED WITH YOUR MEDICATIONS? None for years. I just started my cholesterol medicine about 2 months ago, and the dose hasn't changed yet.

WHAT MEDICAL PROBLEMS DO YOU CURRENTLY HAVE OR HAVE YOU HAD IN THE PAST? High cholesterol right now, I guess.

HAVE YOU EVER HAD A HISTORY OF TROUBLE WITH YOUR THYROID? Oh, yeah, I used to have trouble, but then I had surgery on it a few years ago and I don't have a problem anymore.

SO, YOU HAD SURGERY ON YOUR THYROID? Yes. It was about 3 years ago. They started me on my thyroid medicine after that.

HOW MANY TIMES DO YOU THINK YOU MISSED YOUR THYROID MEDICINE IN THE LAST TWO WEEKS? Oh, I never miss it. I always take it in the morning at the same time as my other medicine before breakfast.

HAVE YOU EXPERIENCED ANY WEIGHT GAIN? Yes, I was surprised and disturbed by that, because I'm actually eating much less than normal this summer because we're going on a cruise and I want to fit into my bikini.

ANY HOARSENESS IN YOUR VOICE? Maybe a little.

ANY DIFFICULTY HEARING? Oh, I don't think so.

IS YOUR SKIN DRY? Yes, a little more than usual. Normally, the humidity in the summer keeps my skin moist, but this year, it seems drier and cracks easily.

ANY CONSTIPATION? Yes, like I said, I've been taking a stool softener for it.

ANY HAIR LOSS? Not that I've noticed.

DO YOU HAVE TROUBLE KEEPING WARM? Yes, I had to pull out my wool sweater to wear this morning. I can't seem to keep warm enough.

Objective Information

Computerized medication profile:

- Questran (cholestyramine): one packet two times daily with breakfast and supper; No. 60; Refills: 9; Patient obtained first refill in 25 days.
- Synthroid (levothyroxine): 0.125 mg, one tablet daily every morning; No. 30; Refills: 5; Patient obtains refills every 25-30 days.
- Docusate sodium: 100 mg as needed for constipation; No. 100. (OTC, filled 3 weeks ago.)

Continued

CASE STUDY—continued

Thyroid labs:

- On request today (7/25/02) from physician's clinic:
  - Free T_4: 0.1 (0.6–2.1 ng/dL).
  - TSH: 20 (0.5-5.5 μU/mL).
- From 03/08/02:
  - Free T_4: 0.9 (0.6–2.1 ng/dL)
  - TSH: 3 (0.5-5.5 μU/mL).

Blood pressure: 104/90 mm Hg
Heart rate: 48 bpm
Deep tendon reflexes: delayed relaxation phase
Hoarse voice
Cool, dry skin
Goiter +

DISCUSSION:

ML presents to the pharmacy complaining of extreme fatigue and requesting a stimulant to energize her. Before finding her a stimulant, the pharmacist needs to assess ML for secondary causes of fatigue, which may include insomnia, lifestyle changes, and medication changes (Fig. 20-10).

ML denies any changes in her sleep patterns or major lifestyle changes or stressors. She indicates that she has actually been sleeping a little more lately, because she feels so worn down, and that the only changes in her medicines are the addition of a cholesterol medication a couple of months ago and a stool softener for constipation approximately 3 weeks ago. Reviewing her information, it is found that she has a history of hypothyroidism that was last evaluated in March 2002 and considered to be normal at that time. She swears compliance with her thyroid medication, and judging from the computer profile's refill history, the pharmacist agrees.

While questioning ML and examining her profile, it became obvious that she started taking cholestyramine for elevated cholesterol a couple months ago and that her symptomatology began soon afterward. ML also indicates that she has been taking all her medications at the same time (before breakfast) each day. She is wearing a sweater in the middle of July, and she appears to be experiencing cold intolerance lately, which is another symptom of hypothyroidism. Signs that also indicate hypothyroidism include bradycardia, decreased systolic and increased diastolic blood pressure, and vocal hoarseness. These problems are noted, and permission is obtained from ML to contact her physician. Her physician agrees to have thyroid function tests performed today and wants ML to come to the clinic this afternoon for evaluation.

The pharmacist contacts the physician again after receiving laboratory values that indicate hypothyroidism and recommends separating the cholestyramine and levothyroxine dosage to eliminate the drug interaction and rechecking for effectiveness or switching to a new cholesterol medication that causes less gastrointestinal effects (e.g., constipation) and avoids the interaction with levothyroxine. The physician decides to give the cholestyramine another chance and asks the pharmacist to educate the patient appropriately about the timing of the medications. Part of the rationale for this decision is to avoid the more expensive cholesterol therapy, because the patient's insurance plan covers very little drug costs. In response, the pharmacist notes that the patient is taking a brand-name product of levothyroxine, which is more expensive than the generics that are currently available. The pharmacist recommends using the generic product of levothyroxine. The physician expresses concern but is reassured to learn that there are now agents that meet bioequivalence standards and that, as long as a TSH is evaluated in 6 to 8 weeks, conversion is usually successful.

■ PHARMACEUTICAL CARE PLAN ■

Patient Name: ML

Date: 07/25/02

Medical Problems:
Hypothyroidism (subtotal thyroidectomy on 08/7/95)
Hyperlipidemia

Current Medications:
Questran (cholestyramine), one packet two times daily with breakfast and supper
Synthroid (levothyroxine), 0.125 mg, one tablet daily every morning
Docusate sodium, 100 mg as needed for constipation (OTC agent, last purchased 3 weeks ago).

S: 45-year-old woman feeling tired and run-down for last few weeks. Presents wearing wool sweater in middle of 100°F summer weather. Denies stressors or lifestyle changes. Experiencing constipation, inappropriate weight gain, dry skin, some voice hoarseness, and cold intolerance. Denies difficulty hearing (although you had to repeat several questions), and hair loss. Compliant with medications. Takes cholestyramine, levothyroxine, and docusate in the morning before breakfast and cholestyramine again at supper. Docusate may be repeated one other time throughout the day if she doesn't have a bowel movement. Docusate added 3 weeks ago. Cholestyramine added 2 months ago. Denies dosage change/noncompliance with levothyroxine.

Continued

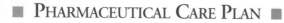

CASE STUDY—continued

PHARMACEUTICAL CARE PLAN

O: Hoarse voice. Cool, dry skin. Goiter +.

Thyroid labs: On request today (7/25/02) from physician's clinic: free T_4, 0.1 (0.6–2.1 ng/dL); TSH, 20 (0.5–5.5 μU/mL). 03/08/02: free T_4, 0.9 (0.6–2.1 ng/dL); TSH, 3 (0.5-5.5 μU/mL).
Blood pressure: 104/90 mm Hg
Heart rate: 48 bpm
Deep tendon reflexes: delayed relaxation phase

A:
1. Hypothyroidism secondary to drug interaction between cholestyramine and levothyroxine decreasing absorption of levothyroxine.
2. Constipation secondary to hypothyroidism and/or cholestyramine.
3. Therapy not the most cost-effective for patient's insurance coverage; taking brand name where generic levothyroxine available.

P:
1. Call the patient's physician to discuss problems with him.
2. Educate the patient to take cholestyramine and levothyroxine at least 6 hours apart, if possible.
3. Reinforce education concerning diet and exercise therapy to improve cholesterol, and educate patient about increasing fluid and fiber intake to help prevent further bouts of constipation. Explain that her constipation will most likely improve with thyroid control, but that her cholesterol medication may contribute, so any changes the patient can make to prevent it would be helpful.
4. Recheck free T_4 and TSH in 6–8 weeks

Pharmacist: *John Schultis, Pharm.D.*

Self-Assessment Questions

1. List the medications that interact with levothyroxine. What do you recommend when a patient is taking these medications concurrently?
2. What are the signs and symptoms of hyperthyroidism?
3. What are the signs and symptoms of hypothyroidism?

Critical Thinking Questions

1. A patient comes into the pharmacy complaining of a sore throat, hoarseness, chills, and other symptoms of illness. You notice that he has a history of hyperthyroidism and is taking antithyroid medication. What do you suspect the problem could be? (SOAP this patient.)
2. Explain the association between hypothyroidism and hyperlipidemia.

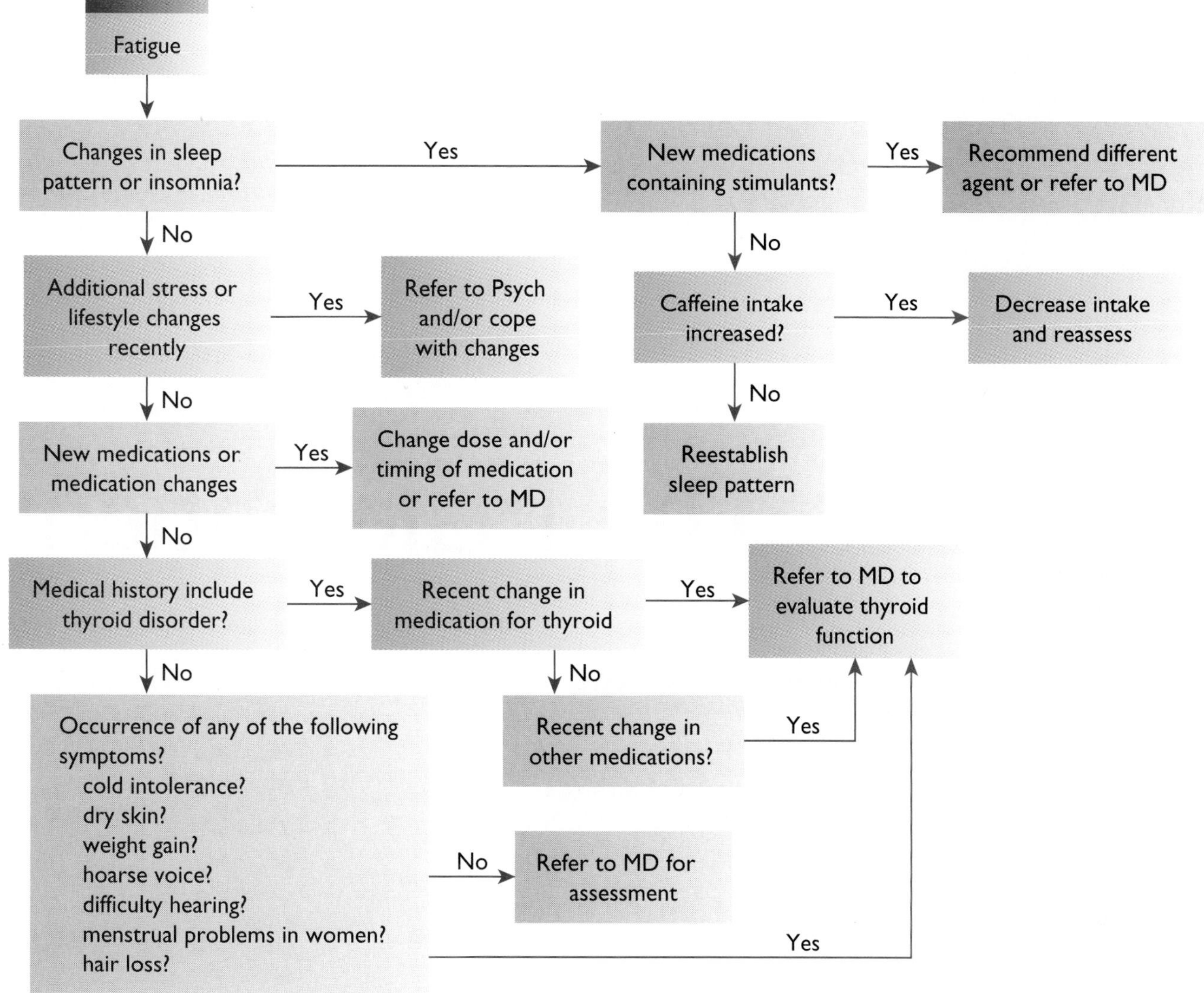

FIGURE 20-10 Decision tree for fatigue.

Bibliography

American Diabetes Association. Clinical practice recommendations 2002. American Diabetes Association. Volume 25, Supplement 1, January 2002.

Burch HB, Wartofsky L. Graves' ophthalmopathy: current concepts regarding pathogenesis and management. Endocr Rev 1993;14:747–793.

Burrow GN, Ferris TF. Medical complications during pregnancy. 4th ed. Philadelphia: WB Saunders, 1995.

DiPiro JT, Talbert RL, Yee GC, et al. Pharmacotherapy: a pathophysiologic approach. 4th ed. Stamford, CT: Appleton & Lange, 1999.

Expert Committee on the Diagnosis and Classification of Diabetes Mellitus. Diabetes Care 1997;20:1183–1197.

Klein I, Becker DV, Levey GS. Treatment of hyperthyroid disease. Ann Intern Med 1994;121:281–288.

Franklyn JA. The management of hyperthyroidism. N Engl J Med 1994;330:1731–1738.

Koda-Kimble, Young LY. Applied therapeutics: the clinical use of drugs. Baltimore: Lippincott Williams & Wilkins, 2001.

Mandel SJ, Brent GA, Larsen PR. Levothyroxine therapy in patients with thyroid disease. Ann Intern Med 1993;119:492–502.

Siminoski K. Does this patient have a goiter? JAMA 1995;273:813–817.

Singer PA, Cooper DS, Levy EG, et al. Treatment guidelines for patients with hyperthyroidism and hypothyroidism. JAMA 1995;273:808–812.

Surks MI, Sievert R. Drugs and thyroid function. N Engl J Med 1995;333:1688–1694.

CHAPTER

21

The Male Patient

Julie A. Hixson-Wallace and Raylene M. Rospond

GLOSSARY TERMS

- Benign prostatic hyperplasia
- Cryptorchidism
- Epidermoid cysts
- Erectile dysfunction
- Gynecomastia
- Hernia
- Hydrocele
- Incarcerated hernia
- Lipomastia
- Paraneoplastic syndrome
- Strangulated hernia
- Tinea capitis
- Tinea cruris
- Tinea pedis
- Tinea unguium
- Varicocele

ANATOMY AND PHYSIOLOGY OVERVIEW

Breasts

The breasts, or mammary glands, are present in both sexes. The male breast contains ducts that elongate and branch during childhood. The development of the breast in males is similar to that in females until puberty, when male breast development stops. A normal adult male breast resembles an immature female breast, consisting of a nipple and areola. The nipple is made of fibrous tissue interspersed with smooth muscle cells. The smooth muscle cells cause the nipple to be an erectile structure. Various stimuli, such as touch and temperature, can lead to puckering of the areola and a firmer, smaller, and more erect nipple. The breast tissue itself is often not distinguishable from other surrounding tissues.

External Genitalia

The external genitalia of the male are the penis and the scrotum (Fig. 21-1). Externally, the penis has four distinctive but continuous regions. The shaft is the main body of the penis. The corona is the expanded base of the cone-shaped glans. The urethral meatus is located at the distal end of the glans. The prepuce, commonly called the foreskin, covers the glans.

The penis is innervated by sympathetic, parasympathetic, and somatic fibers that interact with the vascular system in the erectile tissue. The erectile tissue is comprised of cavernous sinuses that normally are empty but dilate from arterial blood flow during erection. Specifically, the penis contains the corpora cavernosa, which are two cavities extending down either side of the penis, and the corpus spongiosum, which is a single cavity surrounding the urethra (Fig. 21-2). Somatic fibers relay sensations from the penile skin; parasympathetic impulses cause the arteries in the penis to dilate, leading to high pressure within the erectile tissue. Venous outflow is partially occluded, further contributing to the expansion of the sinusoidal spaces. Sympathetic innervation controls emission from the epididymis, vas deferens, seminal vesicles, and prostate as well as ejaculation. Various stimuli, including visual, auditory, olfactory, and imaginative, can elicit erectile responses through the hypothalamic area in the brain, mediated by the spinal reflex pathways.

The scrotum is a loose, bag-like structure that houses the testes. An increase in temperature can prevent spermatogenesis from occurring in the testes; therefore, the testes must be housed

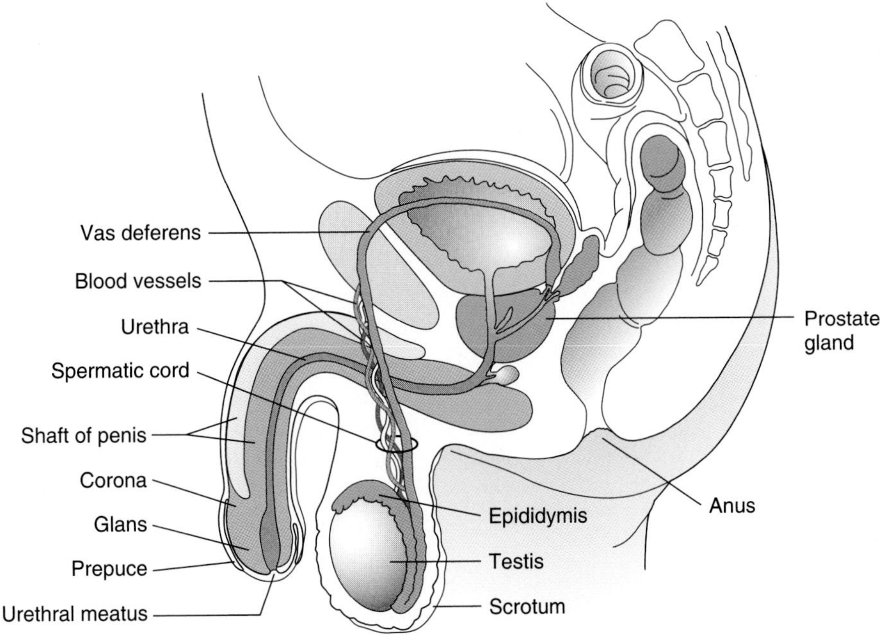

FIGURE 21-1 ■ Male genitalia (external and internal).

outside the abdominal cavity to maintain a lower temperature. Scrotal reflexes lead to contraction of the scrotum, so that the testicles hang close to the body, during cold situations and relaxation of the scrotum, so the testicles hang far from the body, in warm situations. The scrotum also contains many sweat glands to further aid in keeping the testes cool. The scrotum is generally wrinkled and covered with hair.

Internal Genitalia

The internal genitalia of the male include the vas deferens, the seminal vesicles, the testes, the epididymis, the spermatic cord, and the prostate gland (Fig. 21-1). The testes are two rubbery, ovoid structures that are responsible for spermatogenesis and steroid hormone production. It is normal for one testicle to be larger than the other. Each testis is made of approximately 900 seminiferous tubules, which are the sites of spermatogenesis. Sperm produced in the seminiferous tubules are nonmotile, but they mature and become motile during their 18-hour to 10-day journey from the seminiferous tubules through the epididymis. Clusters of Leydig cells within the testes convert cholesterol to testosterone, which is then either stored in the testes or secreted into the plasma. In the peripheral tissues, testosterone is further metabolized into dihydrotestosterone and estradiol.

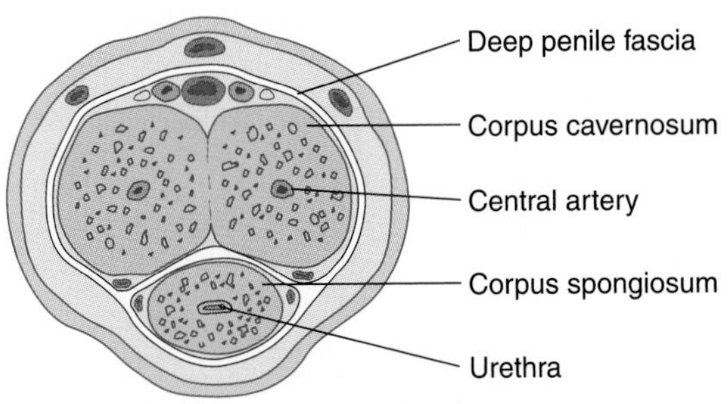

FIGURE 21-2 ■ Erectile tissues of the penis.

Some sperm are stored in the epididymis, but most are stored in the vas deferens, which connects the epididymis to the prostate gland. Adjacent to the vas deferens are the seminal vesicles, which secrete nutrient substances for the sperm as well as prostaglandins and fibrinogen. Both the vas deferens and the seminal vesicles empty into the prostate gland and provide a substantial portion of the semen.

The prostate gland surrounds the urethra, and its growth is regulated by dihydrotestosterone. The fluids of the vas deferens (and of the vagina) are acidic and can inhibit sperm function. The function, therefore, of the prostate gland is to contribute alkaline fluids to the semen to maintain healthy sperm that can fertilize an ovum. The semen is ejaculated via the ejaculatory duct through the penis during the male sexual act.

The musculature and supporting structures of the pelvis include the rectus abdominus muscle, the inguinal ligament, the inguinal canal, the femoral canal, the femoral ring, and the internal and external inguinal rings (Fig. 21-3). The area between the inferior epigastric artery, the edge of the rectus abdominus muscle, and the inguinal ligament is known as Hesselbach's triangle, and this is the location for development of direct inguinal hernias. Hernias can also develop through the femoral ring as well as through the processus vaginalis, a peritoneal-lined tract from the peritoneal cavity into the scrotum.

Special Considerations

Pediatric Patients

Newborns (of either sex) may have enlarged breast tissue caused by maternal estrogen that crosses the placenta. The nipples may also secrete a clear or white fluid that is not significant and

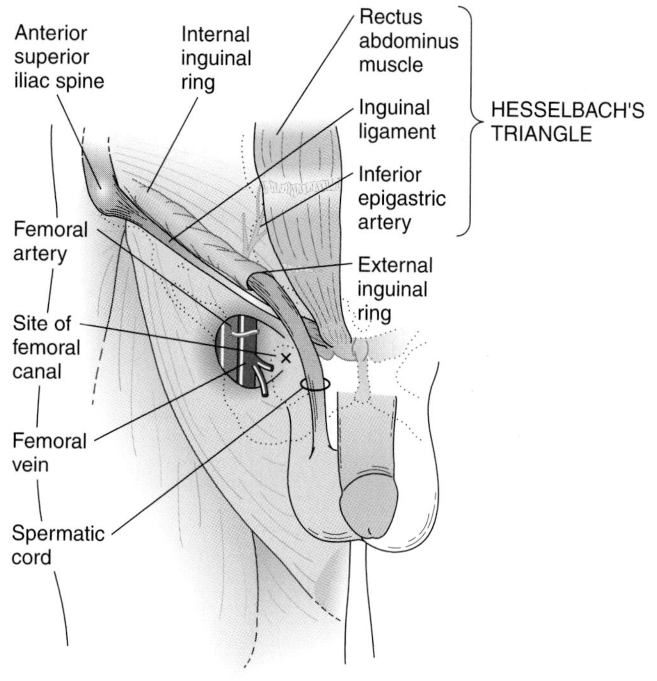

FIGURE 21-3 ■ Pelvic structures.

should stop within the first few weeks of life. At birth, the glans is covered by the foreskin, and the urethral orifice should be located at the end of the penis. The testes should be palpable in the scrotum; however, one or both testes may still be in the abdomen at birth. Undescended testes generally resolve by 1 year of age. The scrotum may be edematous for the first several days of life because of maternal estrogen. The penis may vary in size during early childhood until puberty, but unless it is unusually large, this is not significant.

During adolescence, testosterone stimulates the penis, the scrotum, and the testes to enlarge by approximately eightfold compared to their prepubescent sizes. This enlargement ends by the age of 20 years. The prostate gland also grows during puberty, because of the influence of testosterone, and reaches its adult weight of 20 g. Secondary sexual characteristics develop through the influence of testosterone as well; these characteristics include growth of body hair over the pubis, up the abdomen to the umbilicus, on the face, and on the chest. The Tanner staging scale (Table 21-1) can be used to assess sexual maturity. In addition, the voice becomes deeper in pitch and the skin thicker, a spurt in height occurs, and overall musculature increases. Starting around age 12, boys may experience nocturnal ejaculation.

TABLE 21-1 ➤ SEXUAL MATURITY RATING SCALE (TANNER SCALE)

STAGE	ILLUSTRATION	PUBIC HAIR	PENIS	TESTES AND SCROTUM
1–Preadolescent		No pubic hair	Same size as in childhood	Same size as in childhood
2		Long downy hair, straight or slightly curled, base of penis, sparse of growth	Slight or no enlargement	Testes and scrotum larger, somewhat reddened, texture altered
3		Coarse, curlier hair; darker; beginning to spread over pubic symphysis	Larger, especially in length	Further enlarged
4		Coarse, curly hair similar to that seen in an adult; covers greater area but not as fully as in an adult	Longer and thicker, with development of the glans	Further enlarged, with darkening of scrotal skin
5		Adult in quality, quantity; distribution incomplete to abdomen	Adult in size and shape	Adult in size and shape

Adapted from Bickley LS. Bates' Guide to Physical Examination and History Taking. 7th Edition. Philadelphia, PA: Lippincott Williams & Wilkins, 1999.

Geriatric Patients

In older men, the pubic hair may become gray and more sparse in distribution. Penile size decreases, and the testicles hang lower in the scrotum. The testes themselves do not change in size as a result of aging, but they may decrease in size after chronic illness. The prostate gland undergoes changes beginning around the age of 50. These changes can result in either atrophy or nodular hyperplasia. Often, both atrophy and hyperplasia may be present in the prostate glands of older men. Although testosterone secretion begins to decrease around the age of 25, sexual function generally remains unchanged until around the age of 50. At this time, the decrease in testosterone secretion becomes more pronounced, and sexual drive decreases.

PATHOLOGY OVERVIEW

Dysfunction of various parts of the male reproductive system is a common cause of medical problems in men. Common male reproductive pathologies include gynecomastia, testicular abnormalities, hernia, tinea infection, erectile dysfunction, and benign prostatic hyperplasia.

Gynecomastia

Gynecomastia is an abnormal hypertrophy of the male breasts (Fig. 21-4). If this enlargement occurs during or before puberty, it is referred to as neonatal, pubertal, or juvenile hypertrophy of the breasts. In adult males, however, it is always referred to as gynecomastia. Histologically, growth occurs in the branching ducts in the breasts, resembling normal adolescent breast tissue. This growth may be idiopathic or result from abnormally increased estrogens or a hormonal disturbance associated with a malignant neoplasm (**paraneoplastic syndrome**). Some risk factors for development of gynecomastia include:

- Liver disease in which estrogens are not metabolized normally
- Paraneoplastic syndrome associated with lung cancer
- Drug therapy (Box 21-1)
- Klinefelter's syndrome (a genetic disorder in which the male has an extra X chromosome)
- Rare, feminizing testicular tumors

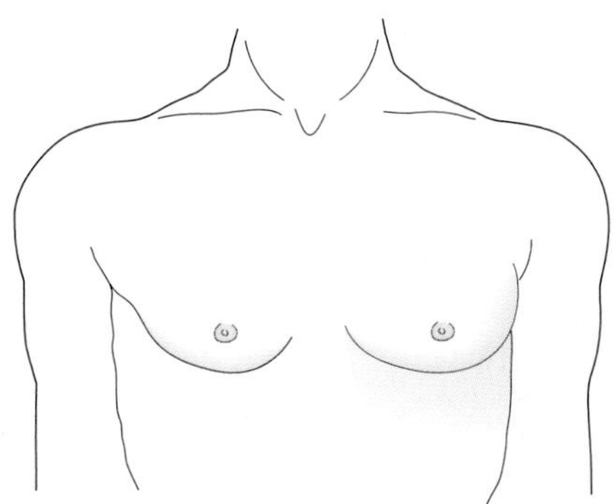

FIGURE 21-4 ■ Gynecomastia.

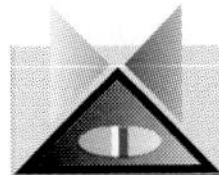

Box 21-1

DRUGS THAT CAN CAUSE GYNECOMASTIA

EXOGENOUS ESTROGEN

- Diethylstilbestrol
- Birth control pills
- Digitalis
- Estrogen-containing cosmetics
- Estrogen-contaminated foods
- Phytoestrogens

ENHANCEMENT OF ENDOGENOUS ESTROGEN SECRETION

- Gonadotropins
- Clomiphene

INHIBITORS OF TESTOSTERONE SYNTHESIS OR ACTION

- Spironolactone
- Cimetidine
- Flutamide
- Etomidate
- Alkylating agents
- Cisplatin
- Metronidazole
- Ketoconazole

UNKNOWN

- Busulfan
- Isoniazid
- Methyldopa
- Tricyclic antidepressants
- Penicillamine
- Diazepam
- Omeprazole
- Calcium-channel blockers
- Angiotensin-converting enzyme inhibitors
- Marijuana
- Heroin
- Finasteride

A false gynecomastia (**lipomastia**) can occur in older men in whom a natural decrease in chest muscle tissue is replaced by adipose tissue. The most common symptoms of gynecomastia are tender, bilaterally enlarged, subareolar areas of both breasts. Treatment of gynecomastia includes discontinuation of any causative drugs (if appropriate), resolution of the underlying endocrine cause, or surgical excision of the breast tissue.

In contrast to gynecomastia, breast cancer generally presents as a single, nontender mass in one breast. Pain accompanying breast cancer, though uncommon, is described as vague, pulling, or burning in nature. Discharge from the nipples and skin changes on the breast are more suggestive of breast cancer. Treatment of breast cancer may include surgery, radiation, chemotherapy, hormonal therapy, or some combination thereof.

Lesions Palpable in the Scrotum

Testicular tumors account for only 1% of all cancers in men but are of special interest. These tumors are frequent in young men, have a high degree of malignancy, and present in a variety of histopathologic patterns. Germ cell tumors account for more than 95% of testicular neoplasms. High rates of testicular germ cell tumors are found in the United States, as compared to low rates in Japan. The incidence rates are much higher in whites than in blacks in all geographic areas. Testicular cancer is the most common cancer in young men between the ages of 15 and 35. Most testicular tumors occur in only one of the two testes. Risk factors for testicular cancer include:

- **Cryptorchidism** (failure of the testes to descend into the scrotum)
- Previous testicular cancer in the contralateral testis
- Mumps orchitis (inflammation of the testes from mumps)
- Inguinal hernia
- **Hydrocele** (a collection of serous fluid in the scrotal sac)

Other conditions also may present with testicular abnormalities (Fig. 21-5). Mumps orchitis occurs in approximately 25% of men with mumps infection. It generally follows the traditional parotitis (i.e., inflammation of the parotid gland) of mumps, but it can also precede it. Mumps orchitis is bilateral in approximately 33% of cases and unilateral in the rest. The testes may return to normal size or atrophy following mumps orchitis. The testicles are generally painful and tender in acute orchitis.

Torsion or twisting of the testicle can produce a tender, swollen testicle that is retracted upward in the scrotum. Testicular torsion usually presents soon after vigorous physical exercise, but it can also occur at rest. Torsion is considered to be a surgical emergency that must be repaired quickly to limit obstruction of the circulation and subsequent necrosis of the area.

Acute epididymitis can present as a painful testicle, because the epididymis is often difficult to distinguish from the testicle. Epididymitis often occurs concurrently with urinary tract infections and prostatitis.

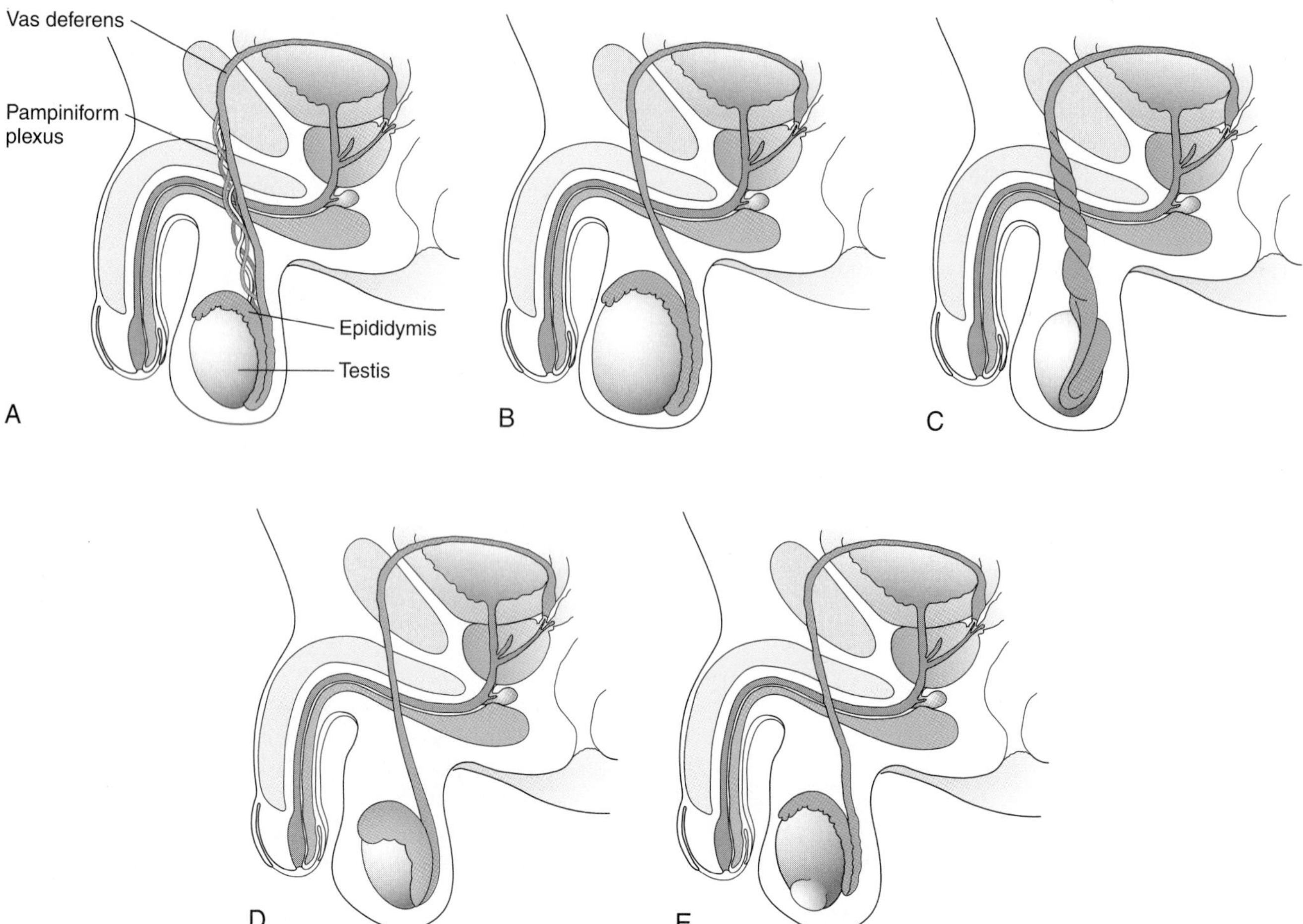

FIGURE 21-5 ■ Testicular abnormalities. **(A)** Normal. **(B)** Acute orchitis. Note the testicular enlargement. **(C)** Testicular torsion. Note the twisting of the spermatic cord. **(D)** Epididymitis. Note the enlarged epididymis. **(E)** Testicular tumor. Note the growth on the testicle.

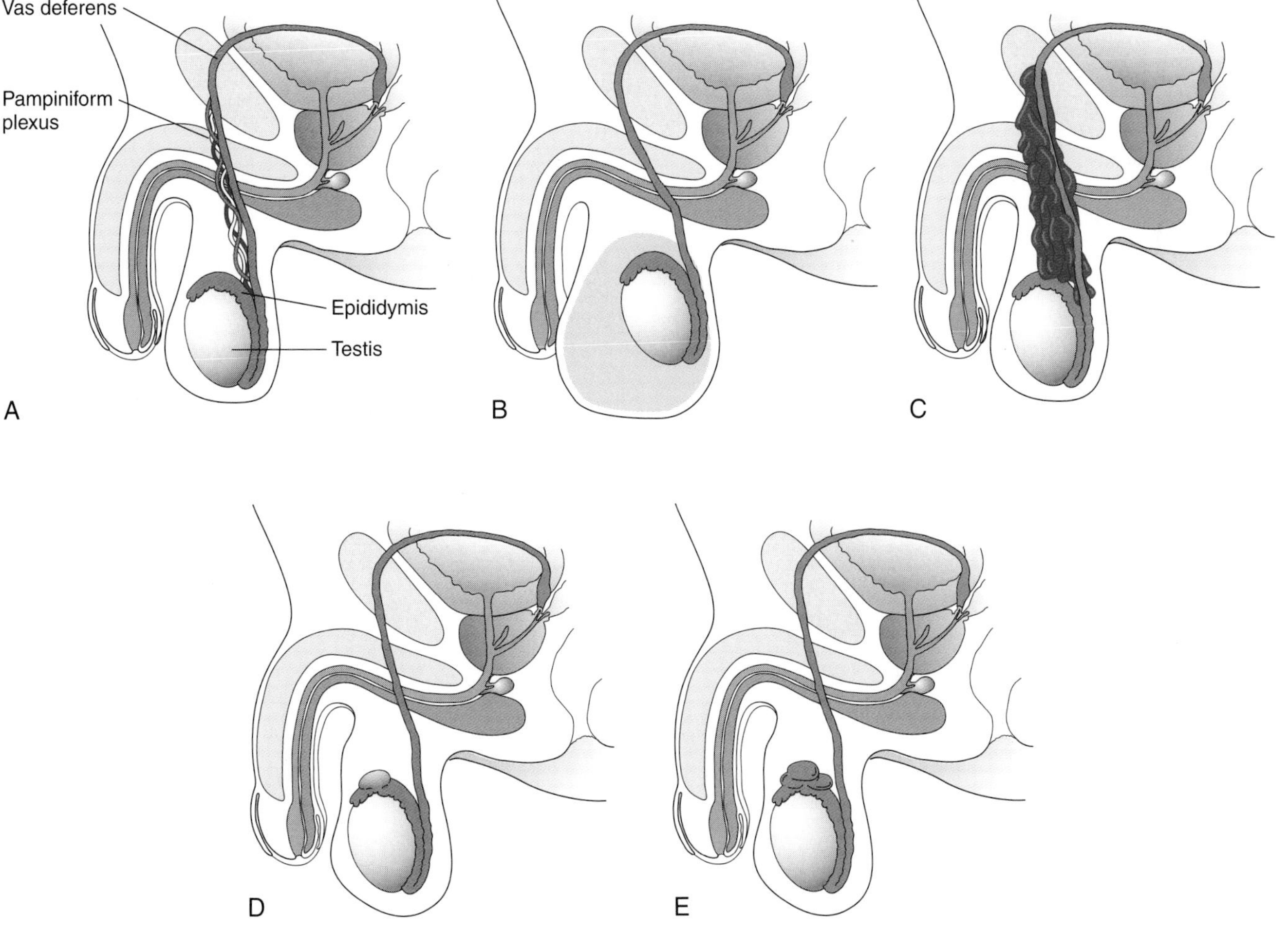

FIGURE 21-6 ■ Causes of scrotal swelling. **(A)** Normal. **(B)** Hydrocele. Note the collection of fluid in the scrotum. **(C)** Varicocele. Note the dilated spermatic veins. **(D)** Spermatocele. Note the outpouching of epididymis. **(E)** Epididymal cysts. Note the growth on the epididymis.

Sickle cell anemia can also lead to painless testicular atrophy in one-third of men with this condition.

Scrotal swelling may be confused with testicular abnormalities (Fig. 21-6). A hydrocele is the most common cause of scrotal swelling and results from a collection of serous fluid in the scrotal sac. Hydroceles can be complicated by infection or hemorrhage, are generally not painful, and can be transilluminated. A **varicocele** occurs in 10% to 15% of men and results from a retrograde flow of blood into the internal spermatic vein (i.e., varicose veins of the spermatic cord). Eventually, dilation of veins around the testes may become palpable. Eighty-five percent of varicoceles occur on the left side. Varicocele can lead to infertility, but it is generally painless and said to feel like "a soft bag of worms." A mass that is painless, movable, and located just above the testicle suggests a spermatocele or an epididymal cyst. Both spermatoceles and epididymal cysts will transilluminate. Scrotal edema in the absence of pain or erythema accompanied by taut scrotal skin is often associated with generalized edema, such as that in patients with heart failure or nephrotic syndrome.

Testicular tumors may present as testicular swelling or pain, but early symptoms are often not seen. A nontender testicular nodule is considered to be pathognomonic for testicular cancer. In some cases, the first symptoms arise from a metastatic site of tumor growth. Symptoms can include a change in the feel of the testicle, a feeling of fullness in the scrotum, an ache in the lower abdomen or scrotum, or an accumulation of blood or fluid in the scrotum. Rarely, men may experience breast tenderness as a sign of testicular cancer because of an increase in human chorionic gonadotropin. Treatment of testicular cancer includes orchiectomy; chemotherapy with agents such as etoposide, cisplatin, and bleomycin; and radiation therapy. If discovered early, the success rate for treating testicular cancer is 90%. Therefore, for men between the ages of 15 and 35, monthly testicular self-examination (TSE) is an important health promotion activity (Box 21-2).

Hernia

A hernia is caused by the protrusion of part of the intestine through a tear or weakened area in the abdominal muscles. In men, hernias often occur in the inguinal and femoral areas (Fig. 21-7). The intestine may be forced through the pelvic structures by any of the conditions listed below. The loop of intestine may slip back into the abdominal cavity or become lodged. Some risk factors for an inguinal or femoral hernia include:

- Obesity
- Heavy lifting
- Straining during defecation

Box 21-2

TESTICULAR SELF-EXAMINATION

- Examine your testicles on the first day of each month after a warm bath or shower. The warmth and moisture will cause the scrotal skin to relax and make any lumps easier to feel.
- Rolling each testicle between your thumb and finger (as illustrated), feel for hard lumps or bumps.
- One of your testicles may be larger than the other. This is normal and is not a cause for concern.
- Testicular lumps are generally about the size of a pea and may be on the front or side of the testicle.
- Lumps are generally not painful.
- If you feel a lump, schedule an appointment with your physician as soon as possible.

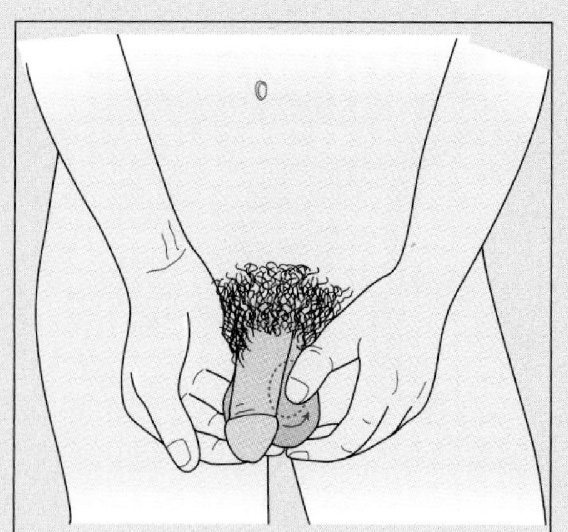

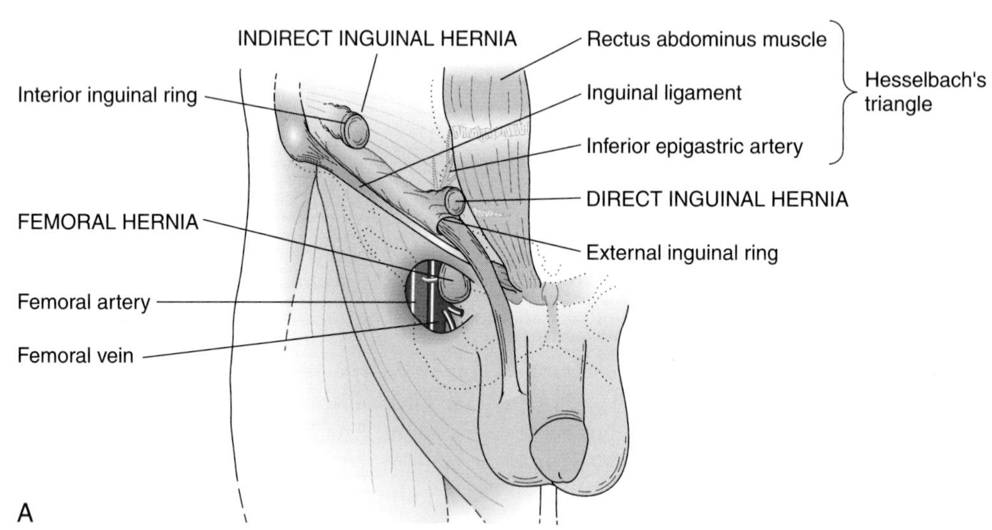

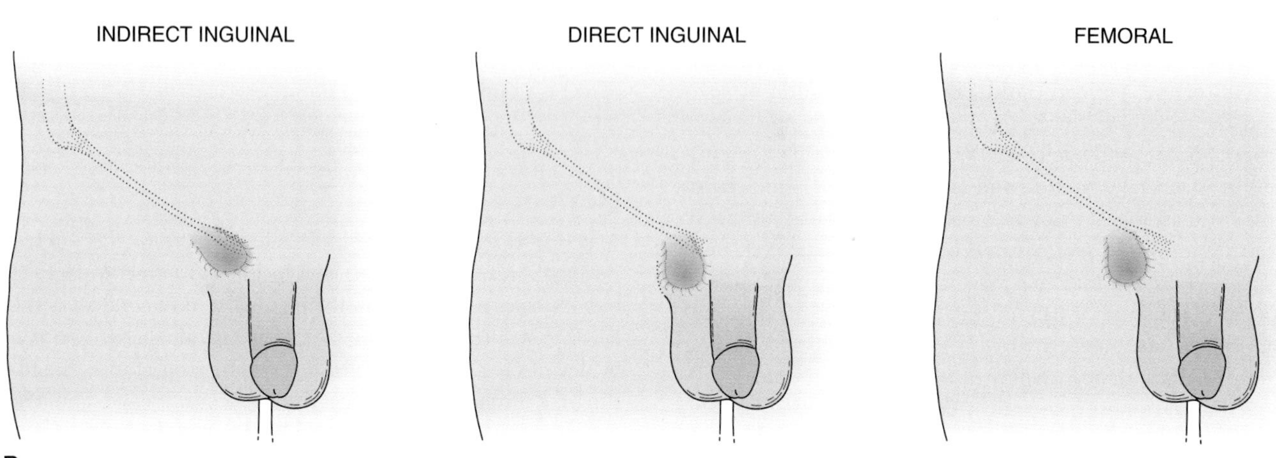

FIGURE 21-7 ■ Hernia locations and presentations. **(A)** Anatomy of hernia locations. **(B)** Appearance and location of groin bulges (shaded area) produced by various hernias.

Indirect inguinal hernias are the most common type, originate above the inguinal ligament, and often extend into the scrotum. Direct inguinal hernias are less common and originate above the inguinal ligament but close to the external inguinal ring. Direct inguinal hernias rarely extend into the scrotum and bulge anteriorly to push the examining finger forward from the inguinal canal during straining. Femoral hernias are the least common and present more often in women than in men. Femoral hernias originate below the inguinal ligament, and they never extend into the scrotum. The inguinal canal is empty on examination during straining. Femoral hernias appear more laterally in the groin.

Some of the symptoms of a hernia include a lump or bulge in the groin, a dull ache in the groin, a sensation of dragging during walking, or an obstruction of the intestine. Any bulge that appears when a person is asked to bear down is suggestive of a hernia.

Treatment of inguinal hernias generally consists of surgical repair. A truss can be used, but this often leads to enlargement of the hernia and complications when surgical repair is finally attempted. Femoral hernias also generally require surgical repair.

Tinea Infection

Fungi can infect the skin, hair, and nails and are most often of the genera *Trichophyton, Microsporum,* and *Epidermophyton.* Fungal growth is encouraged by a damp, alkaline environment. Infection can occur on the foot (**tinea pedis**), the nails (**tinea unguium**), the scalp (**tinea capitis**), or the groin (**tinea cruris**). Males are affected with tinea cruris much more often than females. Risk factors for tinea infection include:

- Damp environment
- Alkaline environment
- Excessive diaphoresis
- Obesity
- Warm weather
- Exposure to areas in which tinea infection is present (e.g., infected towels, hot tubs, swimming pools, and common showers)

Tinea cruris presents as a scaling, erythematous eruption that generally does not occur on the scrotum. The incidence may increase during periods of humid weather or participation in sports activities. Symptoms include chafed, itchy skin in the groin, inner thighs, and pubic or perianal areas. The fungal infection can be transmitted from the feet to the groin area, so it may occur in those with concurrent tinea pedis. Tinea infections can generally be treated with topical imidazoles, such as clotrimazole or ketoconazole, along with keeping the area as clean and dry as possible. Treatment may require several weeks of therapy to eradicate the fungus.

Erectile Dysfunction

Erectile dysfunction can be very troubling to a man. Pharmacists need to maintain open communication with patients so that discussion of such a personal issue is possible. Conversation is often the pharmacist's only tool for assessment of the male reproductive system. Therefore, an environment that encourages open discussion is vital.

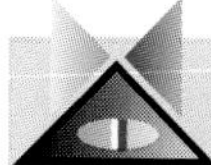

Box 21-3

DRUGS THAT CAN CAUSE ERECTILE DYSFUNCTION

- Antiandrogens:
  - Histamine (H_2) blockers
  - Spironolactone
  - Ketoconazole
  - Finasteride
- Antihypertensives:
  - Central-acting sympatholytics
  - Peripheral-acting sympatholytics
  - β-Blockers
  - Thiazide diuretics
- Anticholinergics
- Antidepressants:
  - Monoamine oxidase inhibitors
  - Tricyclic antidepressants
- Antipsychotics
- Central nervous system depressants:
  - Sedatives
  - Antianxiety drugs
- Drugs of habituation or addiction:
  - Alcohol
  - Methadone
  - Heroin
  - Tobacco

Erectile dysfunction can include loss of desire or libido, inability to initiate or to maintain an erection, failure to ejaculate, premature ejaculation, inability to achieve an orgasm, or some combination thereof. Causes of erectile dysfunction include systemic disease, drug therapy (Box 21-3), urogenital disorders, endocrine disorders, and psychologic disturbances. Risk factors for development of erectile dysfunction include:

- Diabetes mellitus
- Aortic occlusion
- Pelvic irradiation
- Prostate surgery

Some commonly used drug therapies for the treatment of erectile dysfunction include alprostadil urethral suppositories and intracavernosal injections, papaverine intracavernosal injections, and oral sildenafil. Other options include psychotherapy, vacuum devices, and surgically implanted penile prostheses.

Benign Prostatic Hyperplasia

Benign prostatic hyperplasia (BPH), a noncancerous enlargement in the prostate, occurs in almost all aging men. The prostate remains a constant size between the ages of 20 and 50,

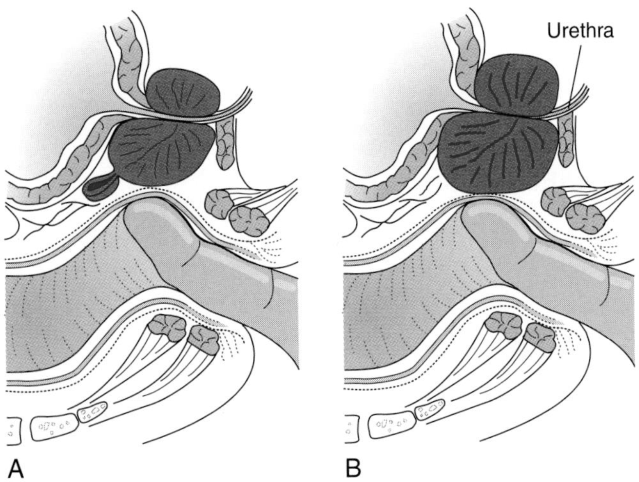

FIGURE 21-8 ■ Benign prostatic hyperplasia. **(A)** Normal prostate gland. **(B)** Benign prostatic hyperplasia.

but it undergoes a growth spurt during the sixth decade of life in most men. By the age of 80, more than 90% of men are affected by BPH. In normal development of the prostate gland during puberty, the entire gland grows. During the development of hyperplasia, however, the periurethral region of the prostate gland preferentially grows. The hyperplastic gland then compresses the urethra, obstructing the flow of urine (Fig. 21-8). The rectum can also be compressed by the hyperplastic gland, leading to constipation. The cause of BPH is not completely understood, but it seems to relate to a relative increase in estrogen in the aging man. This increase in estrogen acts synergistically with dihydrotestosterone to cause the proliferation of prostate tissue. Whether development of BPH is in any way related to the risk for prostate cancer remains unclear. The incidence of BPH is highest in Western Europe and least in Asian countries. In the United States, the incidence of BPH is between that of the two areas just mentioned. In addition, BPH is more common among African Americans than among European Americans.

Medically, BPH can be treated with α-adrenergic antagonists (e.g., terazosin or doxazosin) and with 5α-reductase inhibitors (e.g., finasteride). Surgical options include transurethral resection of the prostate, open prostatectomy, transurethral incision of the prostate, laser prostatectomy, balloon dilation of the urethra, urethral stents, and transrectal or transurethral microwave hyperthermia.

SYSTEM ASSESSMENT

Subjective Information

Obtaining subjective information regarding the male reproductive system requires pharmacists to maximally use their communication skills to put patients at ease. The goal is to obtain thorough and complete information without undue embarrassment on the part of the patient or the pharmacist. Enlarged breasts, lumps in the scrotum, bulges in the groin, genital itching, and urinary retention are all common symptoms for which a patient might ask the advice of a pharmacist.

Enlarged Breasts

? INTERVIEW Describe the pain or tenderness in your breasts. Does it seem localized to one spot, or is the whole breast tender? Do you feel a burning or a pulling sensation? Is the pain brought on by strenuous activity, especially involving one arm; a change in activity; manipulation during sex; or exercise? When did you first notice the enlargement? Are both your breasts enlarged, or is only one?

➤ ABNORMALITIES Breast pain is common in conjunction with gynecomastia but does not occur in most men with breast cancer. When pain accompanies breast cancer, it is described as vague, pulling, or burning in nature.

? INTERVIEW When did you first notice the enlargement? Are the breasts still continuing to enlarge? What medications do you take? Did you notice the breast enlargement before or after you started taking these medications? Do you use any illicit drugs?

➤ ABNORMALITIES Many medications and illicit drugs can cause gynecomastia (Box 21-1). A careful medication history may to help determine temporal relationships between medication or illicit drug use and the occurrence of gynecomastia.

? INTERVIEW Have you had any discharge from your nipples? If so, when did you notice it? What color is the discharge? Is it runny or thick? Is there an odor? Have you noticed any physical changes in the nipple?

➤ ABNORMALITIES Certain medications may cause a clear nipple discharge (Box 21-4), but this is less common in men than in women. Bloody or blood-tinged discharge is always significant. Any discharge in the presence of a lump is significant and needs further assessment.

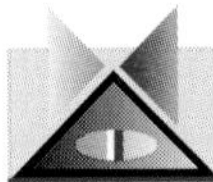

Box 21-4

MEDICATIONS THAT MAY CAUSE A CLEAR NIPPLE DISCHARGE

- Typical antipsychotics
- Oral contraceptives
- Phenothiazines
- Diuretics
- Digitalis
- Corticosteroids
- Tricyclic antidepressants
- Reserpine
- Methyldopa

Asymmetry in the nipples or change in nipple direction may indicate cancer.

? INTERVIEW Have you noticed any change in the skin of your breast? Any redness, warmth, dimpling, or swelling?

➤ ABNORMALITIES Breast cancer, especially in men, can lead to changes in the skin on the breast. The tumors can pull on the surrounding tissues and cause dimpling or other skin changes.

? INTERVIEW Have you had any trauma or injury to the breasts? If so, did it result in swelling, a lump, or a break in the skin?

➤ ABNORMALITIES A lump from injury is caused by local hematoma or edema and should resolve in a short period of time.

Lump in the Scrotum

? INTERVIEW Have you noticed a change in size of either testicle? If so, when did this change occur? Did you have any other symptoms, such as fever or swelling in the jaw or neck? Is the testicle tender to the touch? Have you injured the testicles or scrotum?

➤ ABNORMALITIES Testicular pain may be caused by mumps orchitis, testicular torsion, or epididymitis.

? INTERVIEW Is your scrotum red or inflamed? If so, how long has it been this way? Is the redness or inflammation associated with swelling?

➤ ABNORMALITIES Many acute processes, including acute orchitis, acute epididymitis, and torsion of the spermatic cord, can cause erythema of the scrotum along with edema.

? INTERVIEW Do you have any lumps or masses on your testicles? If so, how large is the lump? When did you first notice it? On which side is the lump? Is the lump painful to the touch?

➤ ABNORMALITIES Testicular cancer is associated with a unilateral lump on the top or side of the testicle and is generally not painful. As the tumor grows, the testicle may feel heavier than normal or the scrotum full.

? INTERVIEW Do you have any masses in your scrotum? Have you noticed any enlargement or swelling of your scrotum? Have you had any pain in your scrotum?

➤ ABNORMALITIES Many conditions can lead to scrotal swelling, including hydrocele, varicocele, scrotal hernia, spermatocele, epididymal cyst, heart failure, or nephrotic syndrome.

? INTERVIEW Have you ever been taught testicular self-examination? If so, how often do you perform it? What helps you remember to perform it?

➤ ABNORMALITIES Many testicular cancers are found during TSE. Early detection is the key to successful treatment. Monthly TSE is recommended for men between 15 and 35 years of age (Box 21-2).

Bulge in the Groin

? INTERVIEW Have you noticed any pain in the groin? If so, how long has the pain been present? What makes the pain better or worse?

➤ ABNORMALITIES Hernias can cause pain in the groin. Straining will generally cause the pain to become worse as the intestine slides through the weak musculature during the application of pressure.

? INTERVIEW Have you noticed any bulges in the groin? If so, where is the bulge?

➤ ABNORMALITIES Bulges in the groin can be caused by indirect inguinal hernias, direct inguinal hernias, and femoral hernias.

? INTERVIEW Can you push the bulge back into your abdomen? Have you had any other symptoms, such as tenderness, nausea, or vomiting?

➤ ABNORMALITIES A reducible hernia can be pushed back into the abdominal cavity. An **incarcerated hernia** cannot be pushed back into the abdominal cavity but still has blood flow to the intestine. A **strangulated hernia** occurs when the intestine is trapped to the extent that its blood supply is compressed. Strangulated hernias are often accompanied by tenderness, nausea, and vomiting, and they may need prompt surgical intervention.

Genital Itching

? INTERVIEW Can you tell me more about your itching? Is the itching accompanied by any skin changes? Where is the itching located? Where are the skin changes located? Do you have similar skin changes or itching anywhere else?

ABNORMALITIES Tinea cruris presents with inflammatory or noninflammatory, annular scaly plaques that occur throughout the groin area but spare the scrotum. Tinea pedis can be transferred to the groin area on damp towels, so concurrent infection may occur.

INTERVIEW Have you noticed any sores on your penis? Where are the sores located? Are the sores painful? Have you had any other symptoms, such as fever, headache, muscle pain, or penile discharge?

ABNORMALITIES Lesions can be caused by herpes simplex virus, syphilis, chancroid infection, or other infectious diseases. Herpes simplex and chancroid lesions are painful; syphilis lesions are painless and nontender. Herpes lesions are vesicular in nature, as compared to the larger ulcerations of syphilis and chancroid. Syphilis, chancroid, and herpes may present with enlarged inguinal lymph nodes. Patients in early stages of syphilis and chancroid are usually otherwise asymptomatic, as compared to the general feelings of fever, headache, malaise, myalgias, dysuria, and urethral discharge in patients seen with herpes simplex infection.

Urinary Retention

INTERVIEW Describe your urinary stream. Do you find that you stop and start several times during urination? Do you have a sensation of not completely emptying your bladder after finishing urination? Do you have to push or strain to begin urination? Do you have to stand closer to the toilet?

ABNORMALITIES BPH compresses the urethral lumen and leads to numerous urinary symptoms, including decreased force of stream, intermittency, incomplete bladder emptying, and straining on urination. Other conditions that can cause urethral obstruction include prostate cancer, urethral stricture, and neurologic deficits leading to improper sphincter relaxation (e.g., paraplegia and diabetic neuropathy). Medications can also cause urinary retention (Box 21-5).

INTERVIEW How often do you urinate in a 24-hour period? Do you find it difficult to postpone urination? How many times do you get up during the night to urinate?

ABNORMALITIES The urethral obstruction caused by BPH leads to bladder smooth muscle cell hypertrophy. In turn, this leads to decreased elasticity of the bladder and decreased bladder capacity. Storage symptoms, such as increased frequency of urination, increased urgency of urination, and nocturia, can result from this decrease in bladder capacity. Storage symptoms can also be caused by some neurologic conditions, such as stroke, multiple sclerosis, and Parkinson's disease.

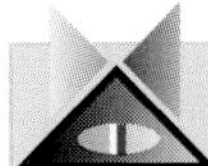

Box 21-5

DRUGS THAT CAN CAUSE URINARY RETENTION

- Bethanecol
- Typical antipsychotic agents
- Anticholinergic agents
- Calcium-channel blockers
- Prostaglandin inhibitors
- Tricyclic antidepressants
- β-Adrenergic blockers
- Sympathomimetic agents
- Antiparkinsonian drugs
- Estrogens

INTERVIEW Have you noticed any burning during urination? Have you had a fever? Do you have any tenderness in your lower back?

ABNORMALITIES BPH can lead to other complications, such as prostatitis or urinary tract infections. General symptoms of infection, such as fever, malaise, perineal pain, dysuria (i.e., painful urination), and costovertebral angle tenderness, may be present in these cases.

Impotence

INTERVIEW Tell me more about the problems you are having. How has this changed compared to your abilities to function in the past? Over what period of time has this occurred? How is your libido or sex drive? What medications are you taking? Did you notice your problems starting after you began any new medications? Do you have any new stressors in your life? At home? At work?

ABNORMALITIES Erectile dysfunction can result from psychologic or physiologic conditions or be a side effect of medications (Box 21-3).

Objective Information

Objective information regarding the male reproductive system primarily includes physical examination of the reproductive organs. Diagnostic tests may be used for screening or diagnosis of potential pathologic conditions. In all likelihood, a pharmacist will not examine the patient's reproductive system. Pharmacists, however, still need to understand these techniques to assess information provided by the patient or primary care provider or ascertained from the medical chart.

Physical Assessment

Physical assessment of the male reproductive system involves inspection and palpation of the penis, the scrotum, and the femoral and inguinal areas as well as palpation of the prostate gland.

Penis and Scrotum

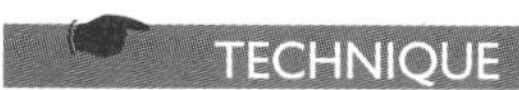

STEP 1

Inspect the Penis

- Ask the patient to stand in front of you, disrobed from the waist down, while you sit on a stool.
- Inspect the penis. Note the size, shape, and location of any lesions on the skin.
- If the prepuce is present, retract it, or ask the patient to do so. Note any lesions beneath the prepuce.
- Inspect the glans, looking for any ulcers, scars, nodules, or signs of inflammation.
- Inspect the base of the penis for inflammation or lesions. Check the pubic hair for nits or lice.
- Find the urethral meatus, and note its location. Gently compress the glans to open the urethral meatus to inspect for discharge (Fig. 21-9).

ABNORMALITIES Some abnormalities of the penis include hypospadias, syphilitic chancre, genital herpes, genital warts, penile cancer, and Peyronie's disease. In hypospadias, the urethral meatus is displaced to the posterior surface of the penis.

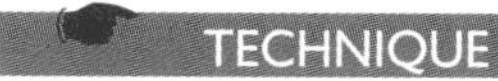

STEP 2

Inspect the scrotum

- Inspect the skin of the scrotum. Lift the scrotum to examine the posterior surface.
- Observe the contour of the scrotum. Note any edema, lumps, or vasculature.

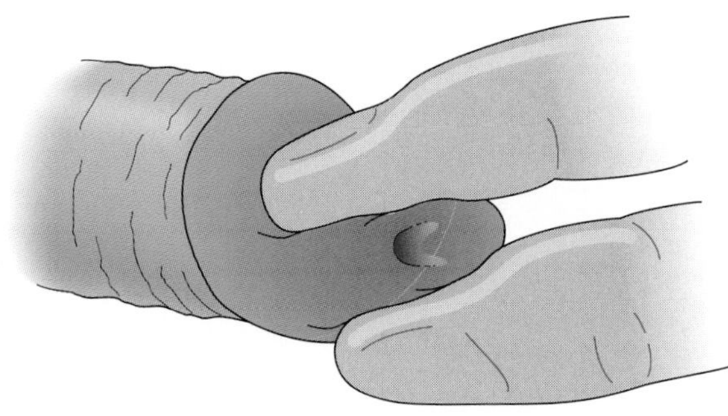

FIGURE 21-9 ■ Compression of the glans.

ABNORMALITIES Rashes on the scrotum are usually caused by heat in the moist environment of the groin. **Epidermoid cysts** are commonly present on the scrotum as firm, yellowish, nontender nodules approximately 1 cm in diameter. A very small scrotum indicates cryptorchidism, in which one of the testes is not palpable in the scrotal sac but, rather, may lie in the abdomen or inguinal canal.

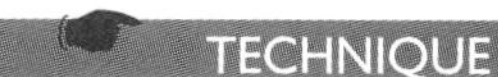

STEP 3

Palpate the Penis

- Using the thumb and first two fingers, palpate the penis. Note any tenderness or induration.

ABNORMALITIES Urethral stricture or penile cancer could produce indurations along the posterior surface of the penis. Areas of tenderness may suggest periurethral inflammation secondary to urethral stricture.

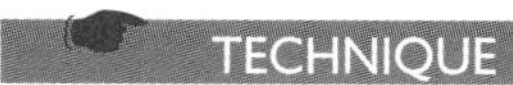

STEP 4

Palpate the scrotum

- Using the thumb and first two fingers, palpate each testicle and the epididymis. Note any tenderness as well as the size, shape, and consistency of the testes.
- Palpate both spermatic cords, following them from the epididymis to the superficial inguinal ring. Note any tenderness, nodules, or swelling.

ABNORMALITIES Painless nodules on the testicles suggest cancer. Palpable varicose veins, especially along the left spermatic cord, indicate a varicocele. Chronic infection of the vas deferens leads to a thickened or beaded feeling. Palpation of a cyst in the spermatic cord suggests a hydrocele of the cord. A scrotal mass that disappears when the patient lies down is most likely a scrotal hernia, which would also be suspected if bowel sounds are auscultated over the scrotal mass.

Femoral and Inguinal Areas

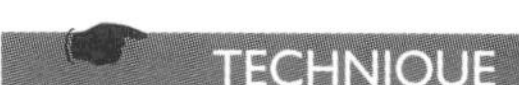

STEP 1

Inspect the Femoral and Inguinal Areas for Bulges

- Perform your inspection both while the patient is in a relaxed position and while the patient is straining. Ask the patient to bear down or cough.
- Palpate for an inguinal hernia, using your right hand for the patient's right side and your left hand for the patient's left side. Push some lose scrotal skin up into the inguinal canal using your index finger (Fig. 21-10).

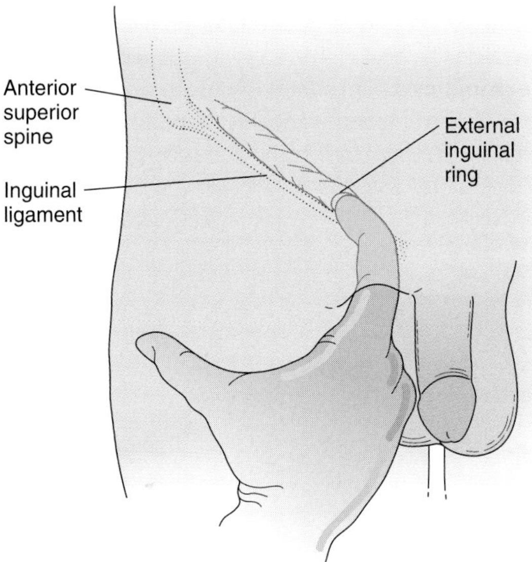

FIGURE 21-10 ■ Palpation for a hernia.

- Once your finger is positioned at the beginning of or within the canal, ask the patient to bear down or cough. Feel for any masses or bulges pressing against your finger.
- Place your fingers on the front of the thigh in the area of the femoral canal to palpate for a femoral hernia. Again, ask the patient to bear down or cough while feeling for any masses or bulges.

ABNORMALITIES Any mass or bulge noted in the inguinal canal or femoral area when a patient bears down or coughs suggests a hernia. Inguinal hernias can be palpated through the inguinal canal during straining. Direct inguinal hernias rarely extend into the scrotum and bulge anteriorly to push the examining finger forward from the inguinal canal during straining.

Prostate

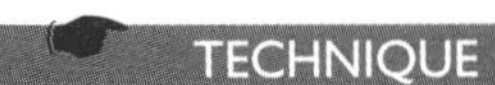

STEP 1

Palpate the Prostate

- Ask the patient to lean over the examining table.
- Spread the patient's buttocks apart to visualize the anus.
- Place your lubricated, gloved index finger against the anus, and ask the patient to bear down. As the patient bears down, slip your finger through the anus into the rectum.
- Insert your finger as far as possible into the rectum, and rotate your hand to palpate as much of the rectal surface as possible.
- To palpate the prostate gland, the finger must be turned counterclockwise. This may be easier if you also turn your body away from the patient. The prostate can be felt with your finger flexing toward the scrotum (Fig. 21-11).
- A normal prostate gland feels rubbery and is not tender.

ABNORMALITIES Palpable induration can indicate inflammation, scarring, or malignancy. Prostate cancer feels like a hard area in the prostate gland. Prostatic stones and chronic inflammation can also cause areas of hardness in the prostate gland. BPH leads to a symmetrically enlarged, smooth, firm, and elastic-feeling prostate gland. Acute prostatitis causes the gland to be extremely tender as well as swollen, firm, and warm. Chronic prostatitis does not result in any consistent physical findings.

Laboratory and Diagnostic Tests

The following laboratory and diagnostic tests may also be used for evaluation of the male reproductive system:

- *Prostate-specific antigen (PSA):* The PSA test can be used for early detection of prostate cancer, to measure the effectiveness of therapy for prostate cancer, and to detect recurrence of prostate cancer. Measurement of PSA requires a 5-mL venous blood sample. PSA is found in both normal prostate cells and prostate cancer cells. Levels of PSA increase with age because of enlargement of the prostate, an overall increase in prostate inflammation, microscopic prostate cancers that are not clinically significant, and PSA leakage into the serum. The level of PSA increases transiently following prostate palpation and digital rectal examination (DRE). The level can also be elevated in men with BPH and in a small percentage of men with no prostate abnormalities. Therefore, PSA is not considered to be a definitive marker for prostate cancer but, rather, a screening tool in addition to DRE. Table 21-2 lists normal, age-specific values for PSA reference ranges.
- *Potassium hydroxide test:* A potassium hydroxide preparation can be performed on skin scrapings from genital, pubic, perineal, or perianal areas to test for the presence of fungus. This is appropriate when yeast infections or tinea cruris is suspected.
- *Transrectal ultrasound (TRUS):* TRUS of the prostate can be performed to determine the gland's size and to delineate abnormal areas. A hypoechoic prostate gener-

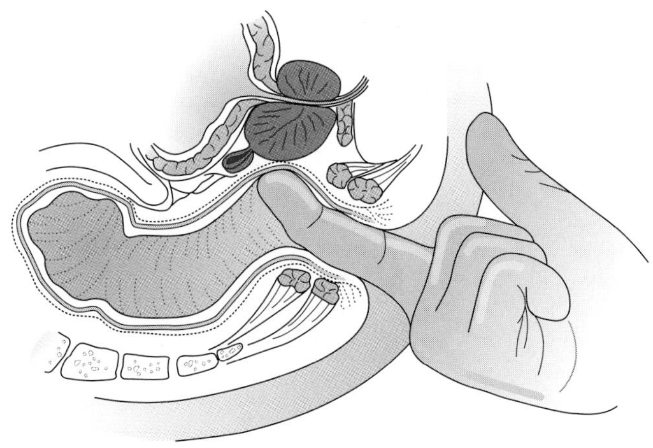

FIGURE 21-11 ■ Palpation of the prostate.

TABLE 21-2 ➤ AGE-SPECIFIC REFERENCE RANGES FOR PROSTATE-SPECIFIC ANTIGEN LEVELS

AGE (YEARS)	REFERENCE RANGE (ng/mL)
40–49	0.0–2.5
50–59	0.0–3.5
60–69	0.0–4.5
70–79	0.0–6.5

From Oesterling JE, Jacobsen SJ, Chute CG, et al. Serum prostate-specific antigen in a community-based population of healthy men: establishment of age-specific reference ranges. JAMA 1993;270:860–864.

ally indicates prostate cancer. TRUS can also be used to stage prostate cancer and to help in performing prostate biopsies.

- *Ultrasonography of the lower abdomen:* Ultrasonography of the abdomen may be used to measure the residual volume of urine left in the bladder after urination, which is helpful in evaluation of possible urinary retention. A more invasive means to obtain this measurement is by catheterization of the urinary bladder after urination, but ultrasonography has mostly replaced catheterization in this setting.
- *Gram stain and culture:* Urine and expressed prostatic secretions can be tested by Gram stain and culture to detect and to identify infecting organisms.
- *Ultrasonography of the testicles:* Testicular ultrasonography is indicated in any case of a painless testicular mass or persistent, painful testicular swelling. Ultrasound of intratesticular masses can be used to diagnose testicular cancer.

Special Considerations

Pediatric Patients

Pediatric patients require additional questions to be asked of the parent or guardian.

? INTERVIEW Does the child have any history of reproductive organ problems? Does the child have any trouble urinating? Has the child started puberty yet? Does the child wet the bed?

➤ ABNORMALITIES A history of undescended testes is associated with a higher incidence of testicular cancer. Onset of sexual maturity before 9 years of age is considered to be precocious puberty. Delayed puberty could relate to chronic illness, hypothalamic problems, abnormal anterior pituitary gland function, or testicular dysfunction. Bed wetting, or enuresis, is involuntary voiding of urine, which is not usually caused by any physical condition; rarely, enuresis may result from diabetes, seizure disorders, or urinary tract infections. A child at least 5 years of age and with voiding of urine at least twice per week for at least 3 months or with clinically significant distress or impairment in social, academic, or other important areas of functioning can be diagnosed with enuresis. Behavioral and conditioning methods are the primary mode of treatment, although drug therapy with tricyclic antidepressants or desmopressin may be required if other measures fail.

Examination of the reproductive organs in the pediatric male patient is generally limited to inspection and palpation of the external genitalia. Testicular descension is the main concern in children older than 1 year. The rectal examination is generally deferred.

Geriatric Patients

Geriatric patients also require additional questions to be asked of the patient or caregiver.

? INTERVIEW Do you have any problems with urinary incontinence? Do you have a history of prostate problems? Do you consume caffeinated beverages such as coffee? Do you take diuretics?

➤ ABNORMALITIES Any number of urinary symptoms are more common in elderly men because of BPH and prostate cancer. Consumption of caffeine and other diuretics can also contribute to urinary symptoms.

The DRE is the center of the evaluation of the elderly male reproductive organs. Men older than 50 years should undergo annual DRE and PSA as a screening tool for prostate cancer. The International Prostate Symptom Score can be used to assess lower urinary tract symptoms in aging males. Table 21-3 indicates the questions that are asked in the American Urological Association symptom index and the scoring system for them. The results from this symptom index yield the International Prostate Symptom Score.

APPLICATION TO PATIENT SYMPTOMS

Because the pharmacist typically practices in a setting where extensive patient examination is not practical, open discussion with the patient is all the more important. Many reproductive problems and concerns can be identified and addressed through careful interviewing and listening by the pharmacist. Although reproductive issues can be an uncomfortable subject, patients appreciate the concern and assistance that a pharmacist can offer. Common symptoms relating to the male reproductive system include enlarged breasts, testicular lumps, bulges in the groin, genital itching, urinary retention, and impotence.

Enlarged Breasts

True enlargement of the male breast tissue is termed gynecomastia. Enlargement of the breast area caused by an increase in fat deposits is termed pseudogynecomastia or lipomastia. Gynecomastia most commonly is caused by a build-up of estrogens, a paraneoplastic syndrome, or drugs (Box 21-1).

TABLE 21-3 ➤ INTERNATIONAL PROSTATE SYMPTOM SCORE (I-PSS)

	Not at All	Less Than 1 Time in 5	Less Than Half the Time	About Half the Time	More Than Half the Time	Almost Always	Your Score
1. **Incomplete emptying** Over the past month, how often have you had a sensation of not emptying your bladder completely after you finished urinating?	0	1	2	3	4	5	
2. **Frequency** Over the past month, how often have you had to urinate again less than 2 hours after you finished urinating?	0	1	2	3	4	5	
3. **Intermittency** Over the past month, how often have you found you stopped and started again several times when you urinated?	0	1	2	3	4	5	
4. **Urgency** Over the past month, how often have you found it difficult to postpone urination?	0	1	2	3	4	5	
5. **Weak stream** Over the past month, how often have you had a weak urinary stream?	0	1	2	3	4	5	
6. **Straining** Over the past month, how often have you had to push or strain to begin urination?	0	1	2	3	4	5	
	None	1 time	2 times	3 times	4 times	5 or more times	
7. **Nocturia** Over the past month, how many times did you most typically get up to urinate from the time you went to bed at night until the time you got up in the morning?	0	1	2	3	4	5	
					Total I-PSS Score =		

QUALITY OF LIFE DUE TO URINARY SYMPTOMS

	Delighted	Pleased	Mostly Satisfied	Mixed (About Equally Satisfied and Dissatisfied)	Mostly Dissatisfied	Unhappy	Terrible
If you were to spend the rest of your life with your urinary condition just the way it is now, how would you feel about that?	0	1	2	3	4	5	6

From International Consensus Committee under patronage of the World Health Organization (R. 20). Handy cards containing this information are currently available at no cost from Merck and Co., Inc. (215)652-7300.

CASE STUDY

RW is a 67-year-old man with a history of hepatic cirrhosis and hypertension. He returns to the pharmacy today requesting a refill of his spironolactone. The pharmacist notices that RW appears to be larger than she recalled from his last visit. When counseling RW, the pharmacist asks how he's been feeling, and RW states that he has been feeling bloated and that his breasts have seemed larger and are tender.

ASSESSMENT OF THE PATIENT

Subjective Information

67-year-old man complaining of bloating and breast enlargement/tenderness

WHERE IS THE BLOATING? In my stomach.

HAVE YOU NOTICED ANY CHANGE IN YOUR WAIST SIZE? Some days I can't button my pants, and I have had to let my belt out a notch or two.

HOW LONG HAVE YOUR BREASTS BEEN ENLARGED? About 1 month.

HOW LONG HAVE YOUR BREASTS BEEN TENDER? The same amount of time.

IN WHAT SPECIFIC AREA ARE YOUR BREASTS ENLARGED? Mainly right around the nipple.

IS ONLY ONE OR ARE BOTH BREASTS ENLARGED? Both breasts.

HAVE YOU NOTICED ANY CHANGES IN THE SKIN ON YOUR BREASTS? No.

HAVE YOU NOTICED ANY DISCHARGE FROM YOUR NIPPLES? No.

WHAT OTHER PRESCRIPTION MEDICATIONS DO YOU TAKE? Zestril.

HOW OFTEN DO YOU FORGET TO TAKE YOUR MEDICATIONS? Only about once a week.

HAS YOUR PHYSICIAN PRESCRIBED ANY NEW MEDICATIONS? No.

HAVE YOU BEEN TAKING ANY NONPRESCRIPTION MEDICATIONS? Just some Tylenol occasionally for headaches.

HAVE YOU CHANGED YOUR DIET OR ALCOHOL CONSUMPTION RECENTLY? No, I'm eating pretty much the same things. I stopped drinking 3 years ago. I'm still going to AA meetings.

HAVE YOU NOTICED ANY CHANGE IN YOUR WEIGHT? I've gained about 5 or 10 pounds in the last month.

Objective Information

Computerized medication profile:

- Aldactone (spironolactone): 100 mg, one tablet daily; No. 60; Refills: 6; Patient obtains refills every 25 to 35 days.
- Zestril (lisinopril): 20 mg, one tablet daily; No. 30; Refills: 6; Patient obtains refills every 25 to 35 days.

Patient in no acute distress
Heart rate: 88 bpm
Blood pressure: 148/88 mm Hg
Respiratory rate: 16 rpm
Extremities: 1+ pitting edema

DISCUSSION

The concern in this case centers around RW's bloating and gynecomastia. The pharmacist needs to determine whether the gynecomastia is caused by medications or by RW's cirrhosis. RW describes his bloating as being in his stomach. He describes his breast enlargement as being bilateral in the areolar area, accompanied by tenderness, but without skin changes or nipple discharge. RW is generally compliant with his medications and only takes occasional over-the-counter (OTC) Tylenol for headaches. On inspection, the pharmacist notices that RW appears to have gained weight, to be at rest, and to be in no distress currently. His vital signs reveal an elevated blood pressure but are otherwise normal. His extremities are somewhat edematous, with 1+ pitting edema.

After evaluating and synthesizing all the patient's subjective and objective information, the pharmacist concludes that RW's gynecomastia is most likely caused by a combination of chronic spironolactone therapy and a build-up of estrogens because of liver disease (Fig. 21-12). His stomach bloating and weight gain accompanied by a change in waist size indicate ascites, a common finding in patients with cirrhosis.

Because RW is not in any current distress and his blood pressure elevation is not critical, the pharmacist calls RW's physician and discusses his complaints and elevated blood pressure. The pharmacist suggests increasing the spironolactone to 100 mg taken twice a day to relieve RW's ascites and, possibly, decrease his blood pressure. The spironolactone may be contributing to RW's gynecomastia, but it is the drug of choice for cirrhotic ascites. If RW does not find the gynecomastia too distressing, he should continue the spironolactone therapy. Because of his chronic liver disease, RW's gynecomastia most likely would not resolve even with discontinuation of the spironolactone. The physician agrees with the increase in spironolactone dose, and the pharmacist fills the new prescription and explains the change in dose to RW. The pharmacist also explains the causes of gynecomastia to RW and reassures him that it is not a dangerous condition. In addition, the pharmacist makes arrangements to have RW come back in 1 week for a blood pressure check and follow-up on whether his ascites is resolving.

CASE STUDY

PHARMACEUTICAL CARE PLAN

Patient Name: RW

Date: 11/11/01

Medical Problems:
- Hepatic cirrhosis
- Hypertension

Current Medications:
- Aldactone (spironolactone), 100 mg, one tablet daily
- Zestril (lisinopril), 20 mg, one tablet daily

S: 67-year-old man complaining of bloating and breast enlargement/tenderness. Patient denies changes in skin of breast. No nipple discharge. Patient states that breast enlargement is bilateral and confined to areolar areas. Patient states bloating is located "in my stomach." Patient appears to have gained weight and reports a 5- to 10-pound increase in the last month. Forgets to take prescribed doses about once a week.

OTC medications: Takes Tylenol occasionally for headaches.

O: Patient in no acute distress.

Heart rate: 88 bpm

Blood pressure: 148/88 mm Hg

Respiratory rate: 16 rpm

A:
1. Cirrhotic ascites, possibly caused by inadequate spironolactone therapy.
2. Gynecomastia, possibly caused by cirrhosis and spironolactone therapy.
3. Elevated blood pressure, possibly caused by ascites.

P:
1. Call physician, and recommend increasing spironolactone dose.
2. New prescription: Aldactone, 100 mg BID
3. Educate RW about new Aldactone dose, causes of gynecomastia, and what gynecomastia is.
4. Follow up with RW in 1 week to recheck blood pressure and ascites.

Pharmacist: *Whitney Farris, Pharm.D.*

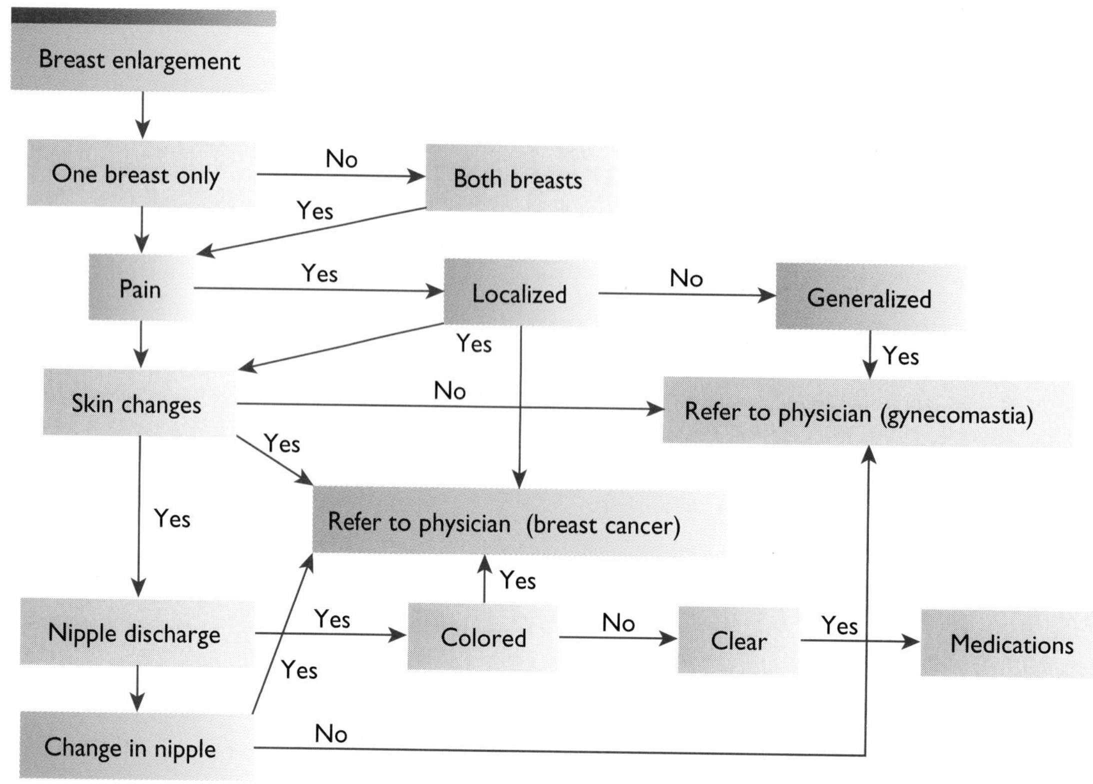

FIGURE 21-12 ■ Decision tree for breast enlargement.

Self-Assessment Questions

1. Compare and contrast the presentation of breast cancer versus gynecomastia.
2. What drugs can cause gynecomastia?
3. Compare and contrast the various interview questions that are useful in differentiating breast cancer and gynecomastia.
4. Explain lipomastia and how it would be differentiated from gynecomastia.

Critical Thinking Questions

1. In the case of RW, how would the pharmacist's assessment and plan change if RW had a single, nontender breast nodule?
2. A 54-year-old man complains of an increase in breast size during the past 5 to 10 years accompanied by a weight gain of 75 pounds during the same period. His breasts are not tender. What is your assessment and plan for this patient?

Testicular Lump

Any abnormal mass or swelling in the scrotum may be subjectively perceived by a man as a "lump in the testicle." The mass or swelling may not actually be located on the testicle but, rather, on the epididymis, on the spermatic cord, or within the scrotum itself. True testicular lumps are generally not painful; other masses on scrotal structures often are.

Patients with a true testicular lump caused by testicular cancer may have no other symptoms besides a feeling of fullness in the scrotum or an ache in the lower abdomen or scrotum. In addition to testicular cancer, other causes of scrotal or testicular abnormalities include:

- Epididymitis or epididymal cyst
- Testicular torsion
- Hydrocele
- Varicocele
- Scrotal hernia
- Spermatocele
- Generalized scrotal edema

CASE STUDY

MH is a 23-year-old man who comes to the pharmacy and asks to speak with the pharmacist. He seems rather embarrassed and uncomfortable but says he wants to ask a question. MH takes no routine medications besides occasional OTC pain relievers for muscle aches associated with weight-lifting exercises. MH tells the pharmacist that a few days ago in the shower, he noticed a lump on his right testicle. He also says that he has felt some fullness in his scrotum during the past month or so but that he "didn't think much of it." Now, since finding the lump, he is concerned that he may have a more serious problem and wants the pharmacist's opinion. Because the pharmacist is concerned that a mass could be either a serious condition such as cancer or a simple condition such as epididymitis, he asks MH to step into the patient consultation room to discuss his symptoms further.

ASSESSMENT OF THE PATIENT

Subjective Information

23-year-old man with a lump on his testicle

IS THERE ACTUALLY A LUMP ON THE TESTICLE, OR IS THE WHOLE TESTICLE ENLARGED? There is just a lump on the side of the right testicle.

DOES THE LEFT TESTICLE FEEL NORMAL? Yes.

IS THE LUMP PAINFUL TO THE TOUCH? No.

HAVE YOU NOTICED ANY SWELLING IN THE SCROTUM? No.

HAVE YOU HAD A FEVER RECENTLY? No.

DO YOU HAVE ANY BULGES IN YOUR GROIN AREA OR PAIN WHEN YOU STRAIN? No.

ARE YOU SEXUALLY ACTIVE? Yes.

HAVE YOU NOTICED ANY PROBLEMS IN YOUR SEXUAL PERFORMANCE? No.

DO YOU USE CONDOMS WHEN YOU HAVE SEX? My wife takes birth control pills, so I don't use condoms.

Objective Information

Computerized medication profile:

- No medications on record.

Patient in no acute distress
Vital signs not measured

DISCUSSION

Because a nontender lump on the testicle in a young man can indicate cancer, MH needs to see a physician for further evaluation. The lack of swelling, pain, fever, hernia, or other symptoms helps to rule out many causes besides testicular cancer (Fig. 21-13). MH seems to be in a committed relationship, so sexually transmitted diseases should also not be a concern. MH's complaint of a feeling of fullness in the scrotum for the past month also suggests testicular cancer, which often has very few symptoms until the disease is very advanced.

CASE STUDY

Pharmaceutical Care Plan

Patient Name: MH

Date: 11/15/01

Medical Problems:

No significant past medical history

Current Medications:

Occasional use of OTC pain relievers

S: 23-year-old man with a testicular lump discovered a few days ago and a feeling of fullness in the scrotum for the past month. Denies scrotal pain/swelling, fever, and groin bulges. In a committed relationship. No sexual performance difficulties.

OTC medications: Occasional pain relievers for muscle aches after weight lifting/exercise.

O: Patient in no acute distress. Vital signs not measured.

A: Symptoms suggestive of testicular cancer.

P: 1. Refer patient to physician for examination of testicular lump.
2. Educate patient about importance of follow-up with physician.
3. Reassure patient about the possible outcome of his follow-up examination and importance of TSE.

Pharmacist: Bill Jones, Pharm.D.

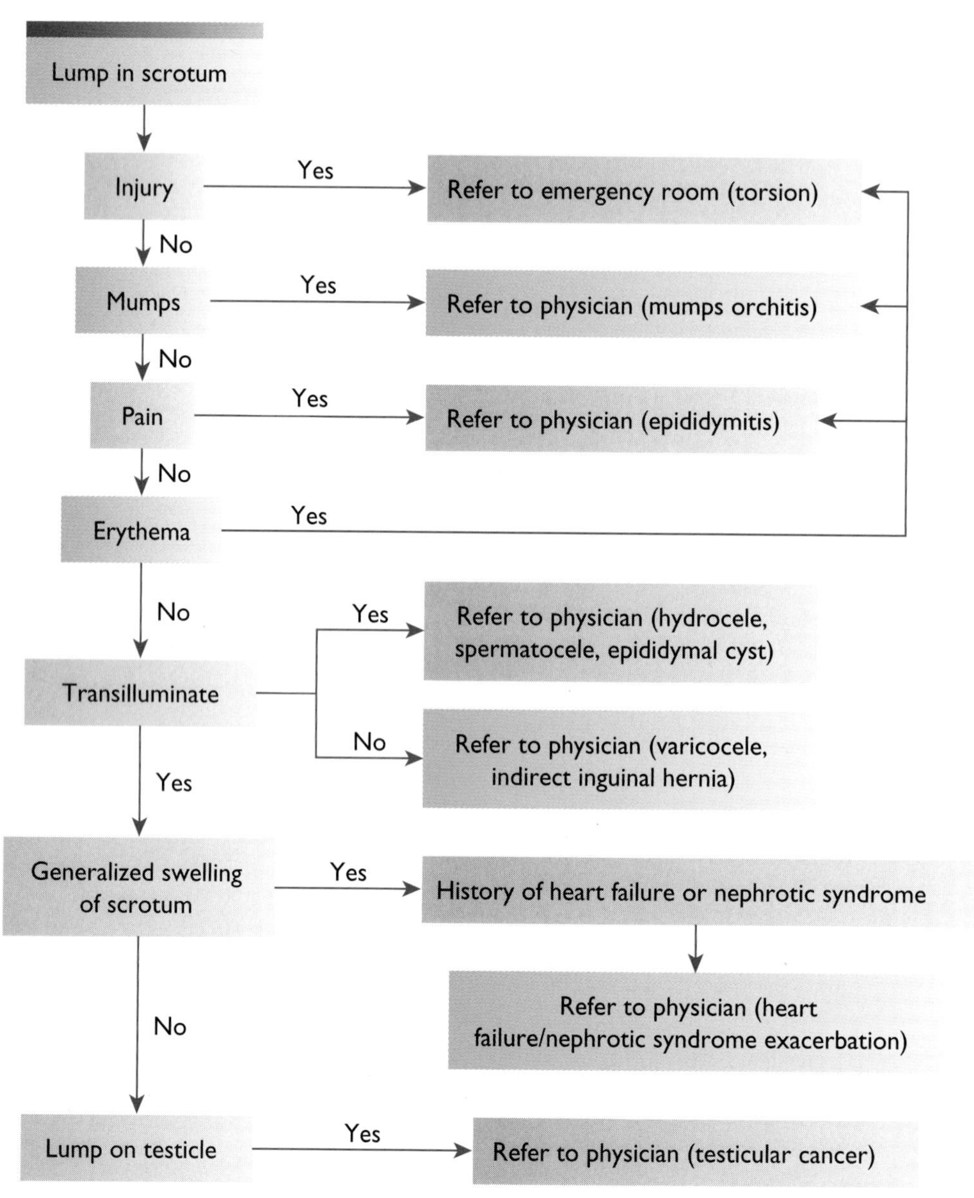

Figure 21-13 ■ Decision tree for lump in scrotum.

Self-Assessment Questions

1. What common signs and symptoms are associated with testicular cancer?
2. What other conditions can lead to testicular or scrotal lumps or swellings?
3. Differentiate the symptoms of testicular cancer from those of other testicular or scrotal abnormalities.
4. Outline how to complete a TSE.
5. Which testicular condition is considered to be an emergency, and why?
6. Which testicular condition is of concern in pediatric patients, and why?

Critical Thinking Questions

1. MH comes back to the pharmacy 3 weeks later and says that he did not keep the appointment with his physician to evaluate the testicular lump. He says that he is scared of what the outcome may be. How should the pharmacist handle this situation?
2. What physical examination procedures would be useful to further evaluate MH? What information would these procedures provide?

Bulge in the Groin

A bulge in the groin is generally caused by some type of hernia. A hernia occurs when a loop of the intestine protrudes through a weak area in the muscles of the abdomen. Various types of hernia include:

- Inguinal hernias
- Direct
- Indirect
- Femoral hernias

Patients with hernias often describe an area on the abdominal wall that bulges outward when they strain, bear down, or cough. In men, hernias can extend down into the scrotum. Hernias may be present for many years without the need for any type of treatment. If hernias become incarcerated or strangulated, however, treatment is often necessary.

CASE STUDY

DH is a 63-year-old man who presents to the pharmacy for a refill of his antihypertensive medications. While discussing his medications with the pharmacist, DH asks if any of these medicines can cause "lumps in the groin." Because the pharmacist is concerned that a mass could be either a serious condition such as cancer or a simple condition such as a hernia, he asks DH to step into the patient consultation room to discuss his symptoms further.

ASSESSMENT OF THE PATIENT

Subjective Information

63-year-old man who complains of "lumps in the groin"

HOW MANY LUMPS DO YOU HAVE IN YOUR GROIN? Just one, and it's kind of on the lower right side above my thigh.

IS THE LUMP PAINFUL? Yes. It's especially painful if I'm lifting something heavy.

HOW LONG HAVE YOU HAD THE LUMP? For about a year now.

IS THE LUMP ALWAYS PRESENT? No. It kind of comes and goes. When I'm bearing down for a bowel movement or lifting something heavy, it bulges out more.

HAVE YOU HAD ANY NAUSEA OR VOMITING? No.

HAVE YOU HAD ANY DIARRHEA? No. I have regular bowel movements every morning.

WHAT PRESCRIPTION MEDICATIONS ARE YOU TAKING? Vasotec and Lasix every morning.

HOW OFTEN DO YOU FORGET TO TAKE YOUR MEDICATIONS? Not very often. I don't think I've forgotten at all in the last month.

WHAT NONPRESCRIPTION MEDICATIONS ARE YOU TAKING? I'm taking saw palmetto. I heard it's good for the prostate. I also take vitamin E and vitamin C.

WHAT DO YOU DO FOR A LIVING? I'm a truck driver. I mainly deliver construction supplies like sheet rock and plywood. I transport the materials and help unload them at the worksites. I've been doing this for 20 years.

HAVE YOU EVER WORN A TRUSS? Yes, and it does seem to help, but it's uncomfortable, especially during the summer.

Objective Information

Computerized medication profile:

- Vasotec (enalapril): 10 mg, one tablet every day; No. 30; Refills: 6; Patient obtains refills every 25 to 35 days.
- Lasix (furosemide): 20 mg, one tablet every day; No. 30; Refills: 6; Patient obtains refills every 25 to 35 days.

Patient in no acute distress
Patient denies nausea and vomiting
Heart rate: 80 bpm
Blood pressure: 126/78 mm Hg
Respiratory rate: 14 rpm

DISCUSSION

When a patient complains of a "lump" in the groin, it is important to differentiate a discrete abdominal mass from a

Continued

CASE STUDY—continued

protrusion produced by a hernia. In the case of DH, the lump is in a single area, is intermittent, is not associated with any symptoms (e.g., nausea or vomiting), and occurs in predictable situations. DH's lump does produce some pain. DH's only medical problem is hypertension, which is being treated with Vasotec and Lasix. His blood pressure is well controlled. He is also using some OTC herbs and vitamins. Hernias are generally caused by mechanical changes to the normal abdominal anatomy and are not related to any specific disease states or medications. DH has found relief from the pain of the groin lump by using a truss. He is not currently using one, however, because it is summertime and the truss is particularly uncomfortable in hot weather.

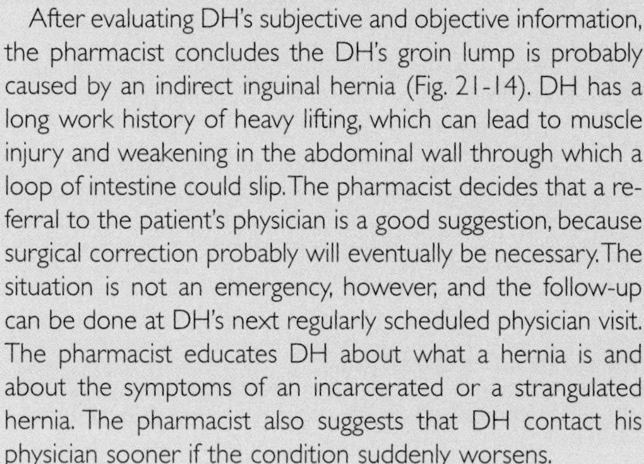

After evaluating DH's subjective and objective information, the pharmacist concludes the DH's groin lump is probably caused by an indirect inguinal hernia (Fig. 21-14). DH has a long work history of heavy lifting, which can lead to muscle injury and weakening in the abdominal wall through which a loop of intestine could slip. The pharmacist decides that a referral to the patient's physician is a good suggestion, because surgical correction probably will eventually be necessary. The situation is not an emergency, however, and the follow-up can be done at DH's next regularly scheduled physician visit. The pharmacist educates DH about what a hernia is and about the symptoms of an incarcerated or a strangulated hernia. The pharmacist also suggests that DH contact his physician sooner if the condition suddenly worsens.

Pharmaceutical Care Plan

Patient Name: DH

Date: 7/12/02

Medical Problems: Hypertension

Current Medications:

Vasotec (enalapril), 10 mg, one tablet every day
Lasix (furosemide), 20 mg, one tablet every day

S: 63-year-old man complaining of "lumps in my groin" for about 1 year. There is only a single lump in the right lower quadrant above the thigh. The lump is a bulge that occurs during straining and heavy lifting. The bulge is painful, especially during straining and heavy lifting. Denies any nausea, vomiting, or diarrhea. Compliant with Vasotec and Lasix therapy.

OTC medications: Takes saw palmetto (for prostate), vitamin E, and vitamin C.

O: Patient in no acute distress.

Heart rate: 80 bpm

Blood pressure: 126/78 mm Hg

Respiratory rate: 14 rpm

A: 1. Bulge in groin, most likely caused by an indirect inguinal hernia.

2. Hypertension: controlled.

P: 1. Educate DH about what a hernia is and about the signs and symptoms of a strangulated or incarcerated hernia.

2. Schedule follow-up assessment of blood pressure in 1 month. Also screen for changes in hernia at that time.

3. Advise patient to ask physician for a hernia assessment at his next scheduled visit.

Pharmacist: *Richard Silverstein, Pharm.D.*

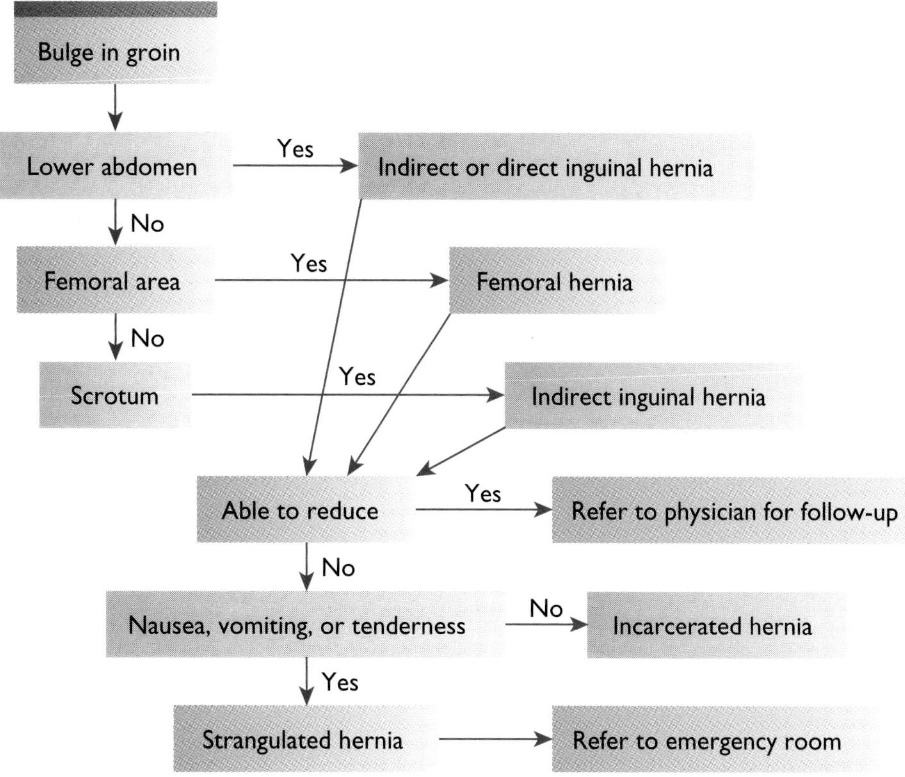

FIGURE 21-14 ■ Decision tree for bulge in groin.

Self-Assessment Questions

1. What signs and symptoms are associated with a hernia?
2. Differentiate between the various types of hernias.
3. Describe the signs and symptoms of a strangulated and an incarcerated hernia.
4. What factors predispose a patient to development of hernias?

Critical Thinking Questions

1. How would the pharmacist's assessment and plan change if DH had complained of nausea and vomiting?
2. A 69-year-old man states he has a lump in his lower abdomen that is always present and is hard and nonmobile. What would be your assessment and plan for this patient?

Genital Itching

Genital itching can be a common complaint among men. Some of the possible causes of genital itching include:

- Herpes simplex virus
- Heat rash
- Tinea cruris

Patients complaining of genital itching caused by tinea infection generally say they have scaly, erythematous plaques on the groin, inner thighs, and the pubic and perianal areas, but not on the scrotum. These symptoms are more likely to occur during periods of humid weather. Patients who are particularly hirsute will also have more problems with heat rash during periods of humid weather. Because tinea infection can be transferred from one part of the body to another, tinea pedis may spread to tinea cruris in the same person or between persons via shared, wet towels.

CASE STUDY

GS is a 37-year-old man who comes into the pharmacy and proceeds to the topical medications section. After GS has studied the "jock itch" section for several minutes, the pharmacist approaches to offer assistance in selecting a product. GS and the pharmacist step into the consultation room to discuss the patient's symptoms.

ASSESSMENT OF THE PATIENT

Subjective Information

37-year-old man seeking an OTC remedy for jock itch

WHAT TYPE OF SYMPTOMS ARE YOU HAVING? Genital itching.

WHERE IS THE ITCHING LOCATED? It is mainly on my inner thighs and in the pubic hair.

IS THERE ANY REDNESS OR SKIN CHANGE? The areas are very red and kind of scaly.

DO YOU HAVE ANY OPEN SORES OR BLISTERS? No.

HAVE YOU HAD ATHLETE'S FOOT RECENTLY? No, but my 15-year-old son did.

DO YOU EVER TOUCH YOUR SON'S TOWELS? He often leaves them on the floor in the bathroom, and I put them back on the rack beside mine.

HAVE YOU HAD ANY OTHER SYMPTOMS, LIKE FEVER, HEADACHES, OR MUSCLE PAIN? No.

WHAT PRESCRIPTION MEDICATIONS DO YOU TAKE? I don't take any prescriptions.

DO YOU USE ANY NONPRESCRIPTION MEDICATIONS? I use Rogaine to help stop my hair from thinning.

HOW LONG HAVE YOU BEEN HAVING THE ITCHING? For about a week now.

Objective Information

Computerized medication profile:

- No medications on record.

Patient in no acute distress
Vital signs not measured

DISCUSSION

Because genital itching can have various causes, it is important to gather information to help rule out specific causes (Fig. 21-15). Constitutional symptoms, such as fever, headache, and myalgia, are more common with outbreaks of herpes simplex virus. Herpes is also generally accompanied by small clusters of vesicles on the external genitalia. Because GS has none of these symptoms, herpes is not a likely cause. A heat rash could also lead to genital itching; however, it doesn't generally present as any lasting lesions but, rather, as transient erythema that resolves with cooling and drying of the area. GS' itching has been continuous for a week and accompanied by scaly patches that spare the scrotum. This sounds most consistent with tinea cruris. The temporal relationship to the tinea pedis of GS' son and GS' contact with his son's towels also suggests tinea cruris.

Appropriate treatment for tinea cruris consists of topical imidazole antifungal agents, such as clotrimazole or ketoconazole. The OTC antifungals are as effective as prescription products and significantly less expensive. Either clotrimazole or ketoconazole should be applied twice a day for 1 to 4 weeks, depending on response. A preparation such as a cream or ointment would be appropriate in the treatment of GS' tinea cruris.

PHARMACEUTICAL CARE PLAN

Patient Name: GS

Date: 8/13/02

Medical Problems:
No significant past medical history

Current Medications:
No medications on record

S: 37-year-old man with "jock itch." Has erythematous, scaly patches on inner thighs and in pubic area. Condition has been present for approximately 1 week. His son recently had a tinea pedis infection, and patient has been in contact with possibly infected towels. Takes no prescription medications.

OTC medications: Rogaine 2% solution to scalp daily.

O: Patient in no acute distress. Vital signs not measured.

A: Tinea cruris infection, possibly cross-infection from contact with tinea pedis.

P:
1. Recommend OTC treatment with Lotrimin AF 1% cream; apply to affected areas twice a day for 1 to 4 weeks, depending on response.
2. Educate patient to apply a thin layer and try to keep the area as dry as possible (use a hairdryer to dry the area after showering).
3. Ask patient to follow up with a physician if the condition does not improve within 1 month or if the scaly areas become worse.

Pharmacist: *James Lopez, Pharm.D.*

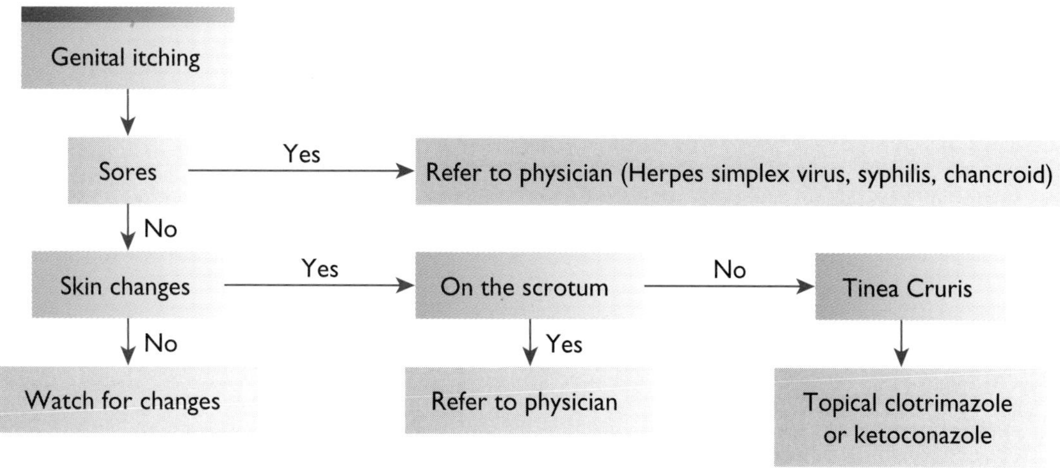

FIGURE 21-15 ■ Decision tree for genital itching.

Self-Assessment Questions

1. What common signs and symptoms are associated with tinea cruris?
2. What are risk factors for tinea cruris?
3. What questions would be useful in distinguishing tinea cruris from herpes simplex virus infection?

Critical Thinking Questions

1. GS comes back to the pharmacy in 2 weeks and still has red scaly patches on his groin. What questions should the pharmacist ask at this point?
2. GS comes back to the pharmacy and says that his son has "athlete's foot" again. GS wonders why this condition has returned. What explanations could the pharmacist offer GS?

Urinary Retention

Urinary retention is characterized by an uncomfortable feeling of a full bladder even after urination. Other symptoms that patients with urinary retention may experience include decreased force of the urinary stream, intermittency in the urinary stream, and straining during urination. The root of all these symptoms is compression of the urethral lumen by enlargement of the prostate. This enlargement most commonly occurs because of BPH as men age, but it can also result from prostate cancer. Decrease in the size of the urethral lumen can be caused by urethral strictures or neurologic deficits from spinal cord injury or diabetic neuropathy. Drugs that may induce urinary retention are listed in Box 21-5.

CASE STUDY

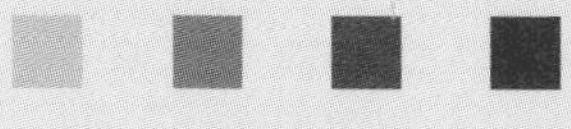

AC is a 72-year-old man who presents to the pharmacy for refills of his medications. He has recently moved to the area and has had prescriptions filled at the pharmacy before, but he is still getting to know the pharmacist and his new physician. The pharmacist asks AC to step into the patient consultation room so that she can interview AC and get to know him better. During this process, AC reveals that his new physician has changed the dose of his "prostate medicine." AC also complains of recent episodes of light-headedness and dizziness since the change in medication.

ASSESSMENT OF THE PATIENT

Subjective Information

72-year-old man complaining of light-headedness and dizziness since a change in dose of his "prostate medicine"

WHAT MEDICATION AND WHAT DOSE WERE YOU PREVIOUSLY TAKING FOR YOUR PROSTATE? I was taking Cardura, 2 mg at bedtime.

HOW LONG HAD YOU BEEN TAKING THAT MEDICATION? For 2 years.

HOW LONG HAD YOU BEEN TAKING THE 2-MG DOSE? For almost the same amount of time. I think I started out with 1 mg for about 2 weeks, then started the 2-mg dose and have been taking that ever since.

WHAT MEDICATION AND WHAT DOSE ARE YOU TAKING NOW FOR YOUR PROSTATE? My new doctor put me on Hytrin, 5 mg at bedtime.

DO YOU HAVE ANY OTHER MEDICAL CONDITIONS? I also have high blood pressure and diabetes. The high blood pressure was found about 10 years ago, and the diabetes was found around the same time.

Continued

CASE STUDY—continued

DO YOU TAKE MEDICATIONS FOR THESE CONDITIONS AS WELL? Yes. I take a water pill and glyburide.

DID YOUR NEW PHYSICIAN CHANGE THESE MEDICATIONS, TOO? No. Those are still the same and at the same doses.

DO YOU CHECK YOUR BLOOD PRESSURE AND BLOOD SUGAR REGULARLY? Yes. I have a blood pressure and blood glucose machine at home. My blood pressure is normally in the 130s, and my blood sugar runs around the 130s, too, as long as I don't cheat too much!

HAVE YOU NOTICED THAT YOUR BLOOD PRESSURE HAS BEEN LOWER ON THE HYTRIN? Actually, I haven't unpacked my blood pressure machine yet, so I haven't checked it in a couple of months. I am checking my blood sugar, though.

DO YOU TAKE ANY NONPRESCRIPTION MEDICATIONS? I do take a "baby aspirin" every morning and a multivitamin—whatever the generic "old folks" vitamin is at the pharmacy I'm going to.

HOW LONG HAVE YOU HAD THE LIGHT-HEADEDNESS AND DIZZINESS? I noticed it about 1 month after I moved here. I thought I had just been doing too much unpacking around the house.

HOW DID THE LIGHT-HEADEDNESS AND DIZZINESS RELATE TO WHEN YOU STARTED THE HYTRIN? Now that you mention it, I saw my new doctor the week after I moved here and started the new prescription after my old pills of the Cardura were gone. I guess that was a few days before I started getting dizzy.

DID YOU EVER ACTUALLY FAINT OR FALL WHEN YOU FELT DIZZY OR LIGHT-HEADED? No. I felt like I might, but I sat down quickly and never passed out.

HOW OFTEN DO YOU HAVE THESE EPISODES OF LIGHT-HEADEDNESS OR DIZZINESS? Once or twice a week, and mainly in the morning, right after I get up.

ARE YOU HAVING ANY LIGHT-HEADEDNESS OR DIZZINESS RIGHT NOW? No. I feel pretty good.

HAVE YOU NOTICED ANY CHANGE IN YOUR PROSTATE PROBLEMS SINCE YOU STARTED THE HYTRIN? No. It's the same as it was when I was on the Cardura. My prostate hasn't given me much trouble at all since I started taking the Cardura. Before that, I was having a hard time with my stream and feeling like I had to urinate all the time, but that's not a problem any more.

DO YOU SMOKE? No. I was lucky to have never started.

DO YOU CONSUME ALCOHOLIC BEVERAGES? Only very rarely. I haven't had any since my birthday 3 months ago.

HAS YOUR BLOOD SUGAR EVER BEEN LOW DURING YOUR DIZZY SPELLS? No. I did think to check that, and my blood sugar was always fine.

HOW OFTEN DO YOU FORGET TO TAKE YOUR MEDICATIONS? I am very careful about that, so I haven't forgotten at all that I know of. I made sure I had plenty of overlap before I moved and got to the doctor right quick after I moved here.

Objective Information

Computerized medication profile:

- DiaBeta (glyburide): 5 mg, one tablet in the morning and one tablet in the evening; No. 60; Refills: 3; Patient obtains refills every 20 to 25 days.
- Hydrochlorothiazide: 25 mg, one tablet daily; No. 30; Refills: 3; Patient obtains refills every 20 to 25 days.
- Hytrin: 5 mg, one tablet at bedtime; No. 30; Refills: 3; Patient obtains refills every 20 to 25 days.

Patient in no acute distress
No light-headedness or dizziness at this time
Heart rate: 110 bpm (regular rhythm)
Blood pressure: 124/70 mm Hg sitting, 100/62 mm Hg standing
Respiratory rate: 18 rpm
Blood sugar: 136 mg/dL (patient ate lunch 2 hours ago)
Extremities: no edema present

DISCUSSION

In this case, the pharmacist needs to determine if AC is experiencing dizziness as a side effect of his medications or as a result of his other medical conditions (Fig. 21-16). AC seems to relate the symptoms to the change in his medication for BPH from Cardura to Hytrin. Although AC was not having any worsening symptoms of BPH, the dose of his medication was drastically increased. This probably resulted from miscommunication between AC and his new physician when reviewing his previous medication therapy or from a misunderstanding of dose equivalency between Cardura and Hytrin by the physician. Hypoglycemia could also cause AC's symptoms, but AC says he has normal blood sugar during the episodes.

A possible side effect of α_1-blocker therapy for BPH is postural or orthostatic hypotension. The pharmacist evaluated AC for this side effect by measuring his blood pressure in both the sitting and the standing position. A fall in blood pressure of 20 mm Hg or more when the patient changes from a lying or sitting position to a standing position, especially if accompanied by symptoms of dizziness or light-headedness, would indicate orthostasis. It seems that AC's blood pressure is running lower than the values in the "130s" reported by AC, and that it falls even farther when AC assumes a standing position. These effects are probably greatest during the night or early morning, when the Hytrin's effects are at their greatest after bedtime administration. This time coincides with when AC has noticed his symptoms. AC

Continued

CASE STUDY—continued

is also experiencing tachycardia, which could be a side effect of α_1-blocker therapy as well. He is not experiencing peripheral edema, however.

Because AC was not experiencing any symptoms of BPH before the change from Cardura to Hytrin, it is unlikely that he needed a change in dose. The pharmacist contacts AC's physician and explains the situation to him while recommending either a change back to Cardura, 2 mg at bedtime, or to Hytrin, 2 mg at bedtime. The physician agrees with the change in therapy and gives an oral prescription for Hytrin, 2 mg at bedtime. The pharmacist explains the change to AC and what has most likely been causing his light-headedness and dizziness. She further educates AC that, when rising from a lying or a sitting position, he should move slowly to avoid the dizziness. The pharmacist arranges for AC to return in 1 week for follow-up blood pressure and heart rate measurements and encourages AC to unpack his home blood pressure monitoring system.

■ PHARMACEUTICAL CARE PLAN ■

Patient Name: AC

Date: 11/18/01

Medical Problems:

Hypertension
Diabetes mellitus, type 2
BPH

Current Medications:

DiaBeta (glyburide), 5 mg, one tablet in the morning and one tablet in the evening
Hydrochlorothiazide, 25 mg, one tablet daily
Hytrin, 5 mg, one tablet at bedtime

S: 72-year-old man complaining of light-headedness and dizziness for the past couple of months. Occurs about once or twice a week in the morning hours just after he arises. Denies any loss of consciousness or falls. Denies urinary symptoms or prostate complaints. "Prostate medicine" was switched by new physician and coincided with onset of symptoms. Compliant with Hytrin, hydrochlorothiazide, and DiaBeta. Does not smoke. Alcohol intake is rare. Measures blood pressure and blood glucose at home.

OTC medications: Takes a low-dose aspirin every morning and a geriatric multivitamin preparation.

O: Patient in no acute distress. No light-headedness or dizziness.

Heart rate: 110 bpm (regular rhythm)

Blood pressure: 124/70 mm Hg sitting, 100/62 mm Hg standing

Respiratory rate: 18 rpm

Blood sugar: 136 mg/dL (patient ate lunch 2 hours ago)

Extremities: No edema present.

A:
1. Light-headedness, dizziness, and tachycardia, most likely secondary to increased Hytrin dose.
2. Blood sugar well controlled on current medication.
3. Blood pressure at target for patient with diabetes mellitus; however, orthostasis is present.
4. Patient well educated regarding measurement of blood pressure and blood glucose at home.
5. BPH well controlled.

P:
1. Call physician, and recommend changing Hytrin, 5 mg QHS, to either Cardura, 2 mg QHS, or Hytrin, 2 mg QHS.
2. New prescription: Hytrin, 2 mg QHS.
3. Educate AC about change in medication, importance of rising slowly from a lying or sitting position to standing, and home measurement of blood pressure.
4. Schedule follow-up blood pressure and heart rate measurement at pharmacy in 1 week to assess effect of change in medication.

Pharmacist: *Josey Wells, Pharm.D.*

Self-Assessment Questions

1. What symptoms can occur as a result of BPH?
2. Compare and contrast the symptoms of BPH with those of acute prostatitis.
3. What drugs can cause urinary retention?
4. Compare and contrast the objective findings on palpation of the prostate in BPH, acute prostatitis, and prostate cancer.
5. What screening tests for prostate cancer are recommended in men older than 50 years of age?

Critical Thinking Questions

1. How will the pharmacist's assessment and plan change if AC's symptoms of BPH are not relieved?
2. A 68-year-old man complains of increased frequency of urination, nocturia, fever, and burning on urination. What is your assessment and plan for this patient?

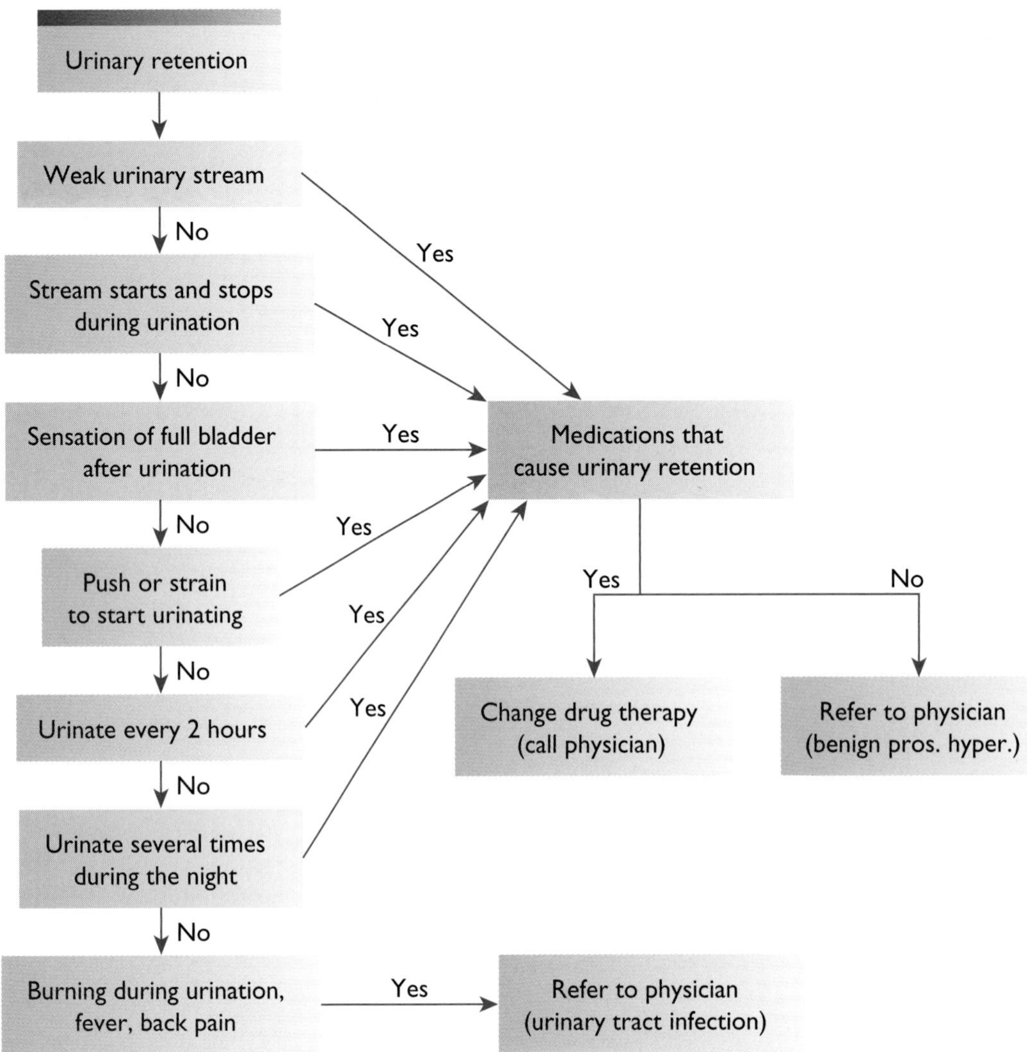

FIGURE 21-16 ■ Decision tree for urinary retention.

Bibliography

Barker LR, Burton JR, Zieve PD. Principles of ambulatory medicine. 4th ed. Baltimore: Williams & Wilkins, 1995.

Braunwald E, Fauci AS, Kasper DL, et al. Harrison's principles of internal medicine. 15th ed. New York: McGraw-Hill Health Professions Division, 2001.

DeSimone EM, Maag P. Common superficial fungal infections. Available at http://www.medscape.com/jobson/USPharmacist/1999/v24.n04/usp2404.desi/usp2404.desi-01.html

Fischbach F. A manual of laboratory and diagnostic tests. 6th ed. Baltimore: Lippincott Williams & Wilkins, 2000.

Henkel J. Testicular cancer: survival high with early treatment. Available at http://www.fda.gov/fdac/features/196_test.html

Kelley WN, DuPont HL, Glick JH, et al. Textbook of internal medicine. 3rd ed. Philadelphia: Lippincott-Raven, 1997.

Martini FH, Timmons MJ. Human anatomy. 2nd ed. Upper Saddle River, NJ: Prentice-Hall, 1997.

Nickel JC, Roehrborn CG. New dimensions in the pharmacologic treatment of benign prostatic hyperplasia. Available at http://www.medscape.com/CMECircle/Urology/2000/CME01/public/toc-CME01.html

Oesterling JE, Jacobsen SJ, Chute CG, et al. Serum prostate-specific antigen in a community-based population of healthy men: establishment of age-specific reference ranges. JAMA 1993;270:860–864.

Pharmacist's drug handbook. Bethesda, MD: Springhouse Corporation and American Society of Health-System Pharmacists, 2001.

Stedman's medical dictionary. 27th ed. Baltimore: Lippincott Williams & Wilkins, 2000.

CHAPTER

22

The Female Patient

Julie A. Hixson-Wallace and Raylene M. Rospond

GLOSSARY TERMS

- Acanthosis nigricans
- Cystocele
- Duct ectasia
- Dysmenhorrhea
- Dyspareunia
- Leukorrhea
- Peau d'orange
- Precocious puberty
- Premenstrual dysphoric disorder
- Rectocele
- Striae
- Vulvovaginitis

ANATOMY AND PHYSIOLOGY OVERVIEW

The primary components of the female reproductive system are the breasts, external genitalia, vagina, cervix, uterus, fallopian tubes, and ovaries.

Breasts and Axillae

The breasts, or mammary glands, are present in both sexes. The female breasts are accessory reproductive organs that function to produce milk with which to nourish the newborn infant.

Surface Anatomy

The female breast lies between the second and sixth ribs, between the sternal edge and the midaxillary line and anterior to the pectoralis major and serratus anterior muscles (Fig. 22-1). The nipple (Fig. 22-2) lies just lateral to the midline of the breast and is surrounded by the areola, which is comprised of small elevated sebaceous glands, called Montgomery's glands, that secrete a protective material during lactation. Smooth muscle fibers in the nipple and areola allow the areola to pucker and the nipple to become erect on tactile stimulation. The nipple and areola are more deeply pigmented than the rest of the breast surface; the color varies from pink to brown, depending on the person's skin color and parity (i.e., the condition of having given birth to an infant).

Internal Anatomy

The breast is composed of three types of tissue: (1) glandular, (2) fibrous, and (3) adipose. The proportion of these components varies with age, nutritional status, pregnancy, and lactation. The glandular tissue (Fig. 22-3) produces milk after childbirth and is organized into between 15 and 20 lobes radiating out from the nipple. Each lobe is composed of a number of lobules. Milk is produced by alveoli within the lobules and then travels through lactiferous ducts to lactiferous sinuses behind the nipple for storage. Cooper's ligaments are fibrous bands that extend vertically from the breast surface and attach to the muscles of the chest wall. These suspensory ligaments support the breast tissue. The lobes of the breast are surrounded by adipose tissue, which provides the bulk of the breast (Fig. 22-4). Breast tissue changes with the flow of hormones during the monthly menstrual cycle. Nodularity increases from midcycle to menstruation; during the 3 to 4 days before menstruation, the breast feels full, tight, heavy, and occasionally, sore.

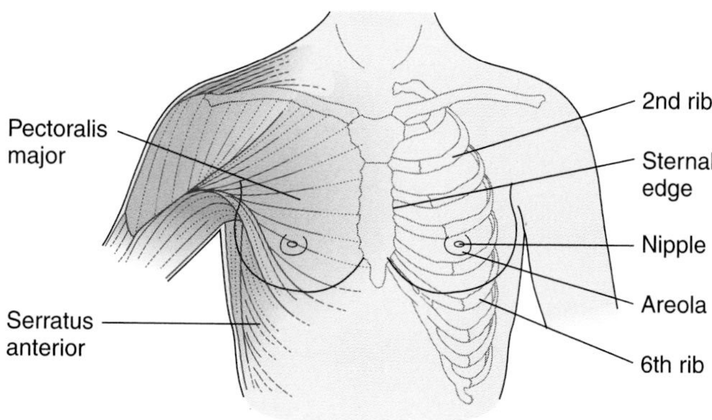

FIGURE 22-1 ■ Relationship of the breast to the chest muscles.

The superior lateral corner of the breast tissue, the axillary tail of Spence, projects up and laterally into the axilla. The breast has extensive lymphatic drainage, with 75% draining into the ipsilateral axillary nodes. The axillary lymph nodes (Fig. 22-5) are divided into four groups: (1) central, (2) pectoral (anterior), (3) subscapular (posterior), and (4) lateral.

External Genitalia

The external genitalia of the female is called the vulva (Fig. 22-6) and is comprised of the labia majora, labia minora, clitoris, and vestibule. The mons pubis is the round, firm fat pad overlying the symphysis pubis that is covered with hair after puberty. The labia majora are rounded folds of adipose tissue extending from the mons pubis down and about the area between the vulva and the anus (i.e., the perineum). The outer surface of the labia majora is also covered with pubic hair in adolescents and adults. The labia minora lie inside the labia majora and are thinner, darker, hairless folds that form the prepuce anteriorly and the frenulum posteriorly. The clitoris is a small, pea-shaped, erectile body (analagous to the male penis) that lies underneath

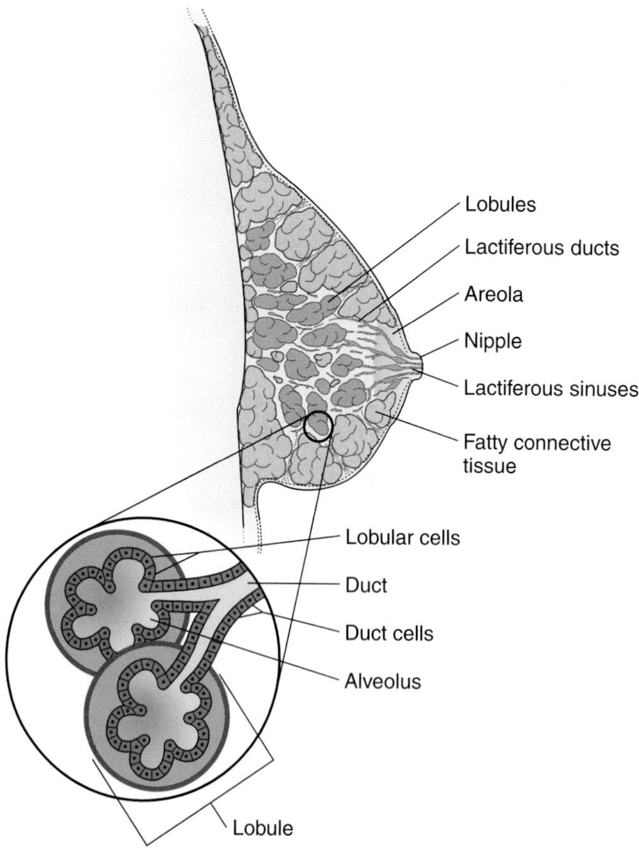

FIGURE 22-3 ■ Anatomy of the glandular breast tissue.

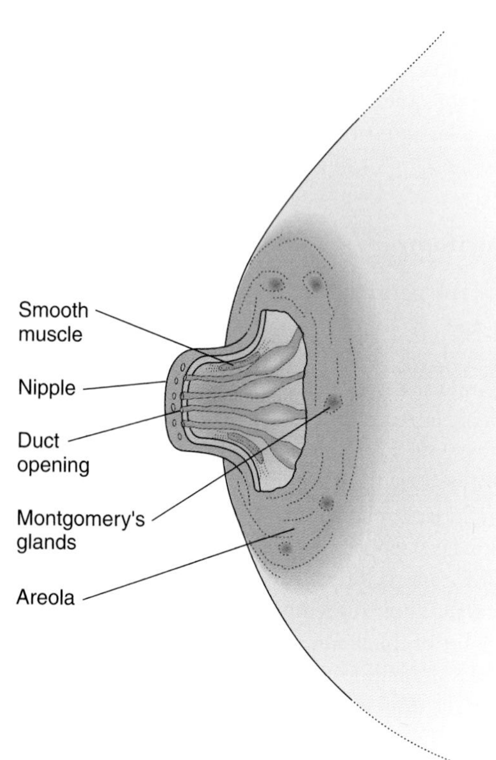

FIGURE 22-2 ■ Anatomy of the nipple.

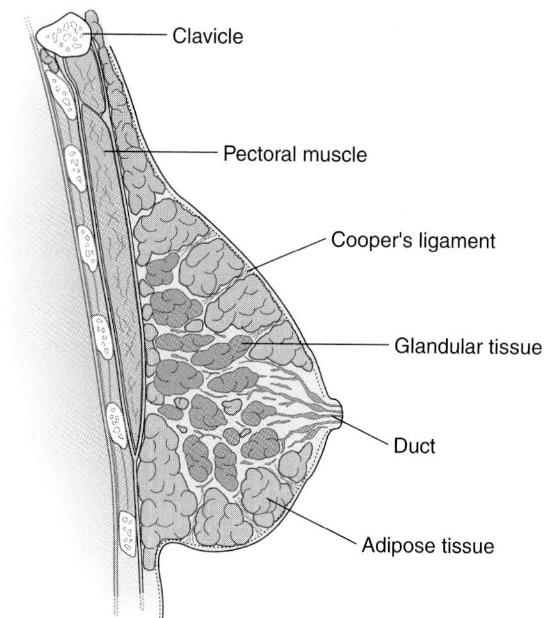

FIGURE 22-4 ■ Anatomy of the breast.

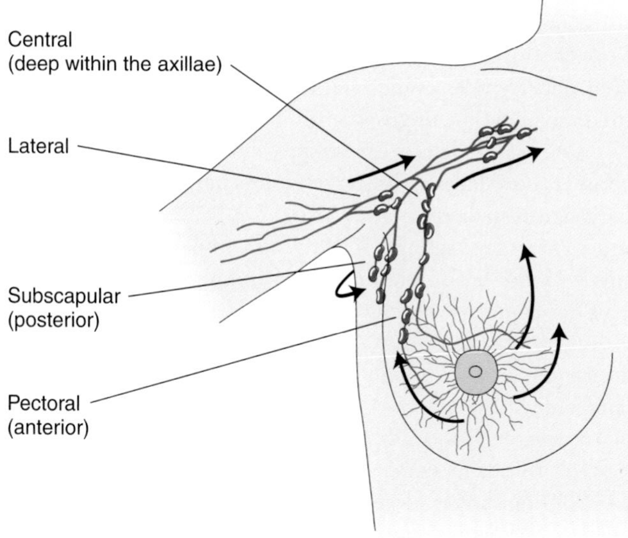

FIGURE 22-5 ■ Axillary lymph nodes. Arrows indicate the direction of lymph flow.

the prepuce. The labial structures encircle the vestibule, within which lie the urethral meatus, vaginal orifice, and Bartholin's glands. These glands secrete a clear mucus that provides lubrication during sexual intercourse.

Internal Genitalia

Anatomy

The internal genitalia of the female include the vagina, uterine cervix, uterus, fallopian tubes, and ovaries (Fig. 22-7). The vagina is a hollow tube that extends upward and posteriorly between the urethra and rectum. The mucosa is comprised of rugae, which are thick, transverse folds that can dilate during childbirth. The vagina sits at approximately a right angle to the uterus.

The uterus is a pear-shaped, thick-walled, muscular organ that is comprised of two parts, the corpus (body) and the cervix,

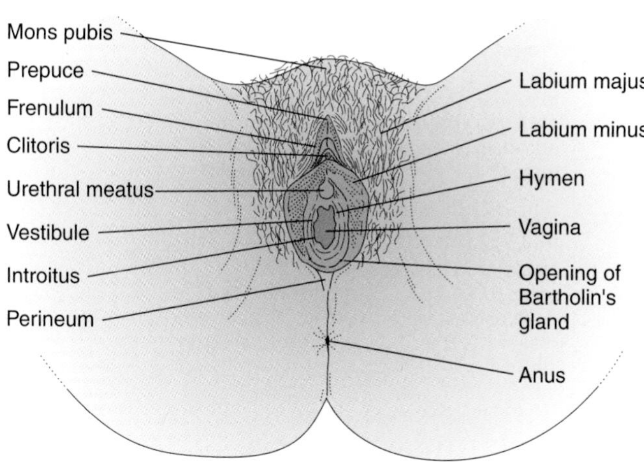

FIGURE 22-6 ■ Female external genitalia.

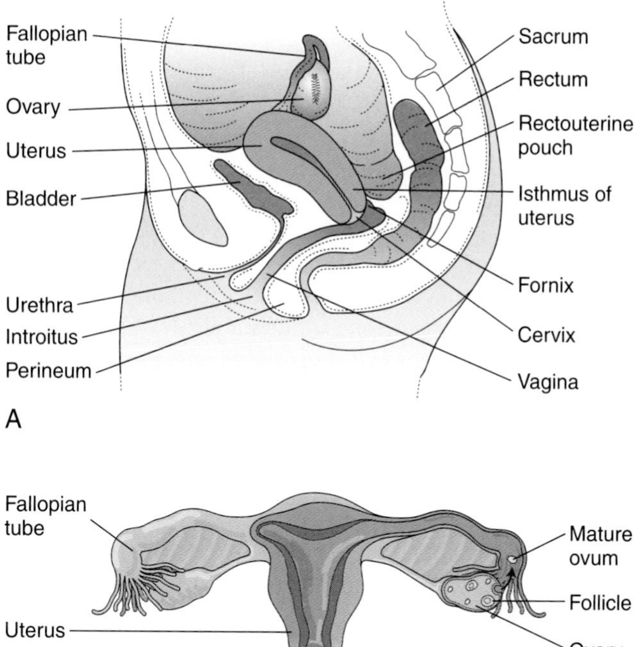

FIGURE 22-7 ■ Female internal reproductive organs. **(A)** Cross-section, side view. **(B)** Anterior view.

which are joined together by the isthmus. The uterine cervix projects into the vagina. The fallopian tubes extend from each side of the uterus toward the ovaries. The inner surface of the uterus is known as the endometrium, and it functions as the location for implantation of a fertilized ovum or egg.

The ovaries are located on each side of the uterus. Each is oval-shaped and approximately 3 cm in length, 2 cm in width, and 1 cm in thickness. The ovaries function in developing ova and female hormones and are regulated by follicle-stimulating hormone and luteinizing hormone (LH), both of which are produced in the pituitary gland. Production of ova begins in the female fetus, with 400,000 germ cells still present at menarche. These germ cells, or oogonia, are arrested in the midst of meiosis and remain in this state until the onset of puberty. With puberty, LH secretion increases during the nighttime hours, and ovarian estrogen secretion increases. This combination of LH and estrogen secretion eventually leads to ovulation and menarche. In the mature ovary, several follicles begin to mature each month, culminating in the production of a mature ovum (Fig. 22.7); the other follicles degenerate. The other function of the ovaries is the production of estrogens, progesterone, and androgens.

The fallopian tubes, ovaries, and supporting structures are often referred to as the adnexa.

Menstrual Cycle

The menstrual cycle is the monthly occurrence of endometrial proliferation, secretion, and desquamation. During the first 11 days of the cycle, the endometrium proliferates rapidly in response to the release of estrogen by the ovaries. By the time that ovulation begins, the endometrium is 3 to 4 mm in thickness and is secreting thin, stringy mucus. This mucus enters the cervix to guide sperm into the uterus. During the next 12 days of the cycle, the endometrium secretes nutrients, which are sometimes called "uterine milk," that are appropriate for the implantation of a fertilized ovum. This secretory phase results from the influence of progesterone on the endometrium. The endometrium is 5 to 6 mm in thickness by the end of the secretory phase. The last 5 days of the cycle are characterized by shedding of the endometrium from the uterine cavity. Both the levels of estrogen and of progesterone fall drastically during the end of the cycle, reversing the earlier expansion and secretion within the endometrium. During menstruation, approximately 35 mL of blood and 35 mL of serous fluid are lost along with the necrotic endometrial cells. If implantation of a fertilized ovum occurs in the uterus, progesterone secretion continues, and menstruation does not occur.

Special Considerations

Pediatric Patients

Newborns of either sex may have enlarged breast tissue because of maternal estrogen that crosses the placenta. The nipples may also secrete a clear or white fluid that is not significant and should stop within the first few weeks of life. At birth, the external genitalia are engorged because of the presence of maternal estrogen; this recedes after a few weeks and remains at a low level until puberty. The ovaries are located in the abdomen during childhood, and the uterus is small in size.

During adolescence, estrogen hormones stimulate the breast tissue to enlarge. Breast development (i.e., thelarche) is an early sign of puberty in girls, occurring between the ages of 8 and 13 years (average age, 10–11 years). Initial development begins with the breast and nipple protruding as a small mound. This development continues for an average of 3 years, until the breast reaches the mature stage (Table 22-1). The breasts may display tenderness during this time of development. Within the same individual, breasts may develop at different rates, resulting in asymmetry; if she is concerned, the girl should be reassured that this is usually temporary.

During breast development, pubic hair also develops (Table 22-1), with axillary hair following approximately 2 years later. The beginning of breast development precedes menarche (i.e., the beginning of menstruation) by approximately 2 years. African-American girls often develop secondary sex characteristics at an earlier age than European-American girls; axillary hair may also develop sooner, even before the appearance of pubic hair. Asian-American girls often display very fine, sparse pubic

TABLE 22-1 ➤ SEXUAL MATURING RATING SCALE

Stage	Breast	Pubic hair	Breast development	Pubic Hair
1 (Preadolescent)			Elevation of nipple	None
2			Elevation of breast and nipple as a small mound; enlargement of areolar diameter	Sparse growth, long, slightly pigmented, and downy hair, straight or slightly curled, mainly along the labia
3			Further enlargement of elevation of breast and areola, but no separation of contours	Darker, coarser, and curlier hair, spreading over the symphysis pubis sparsely
4			Projection of areola and nipple to form a secondary mound above level of the breast	Coarse and curly hair as in adults with area covered greater than in stage 3 but not as full as in an adult
5			Projection of nipple only; areola receded to general contour of breast; mature stage	Hair adult in quality and quantity; spread onto thighs but not on the abdomen

Adapted from Bickley LS. Bates' Guide to Physical Examination and History Taking. 7th Edition. Philadelphia, PA: Lippincott Williams & Wilkins, 1999.

hair. Menarche tends to occur between 9 and 16 years of age. Irregular menstrual cycles are common during adolescence. With the onset of menarche, the uterus increases in size, and the ovaries lie within the pelvic cavity.

Geriatric Patients

After menopause, the glandular and adipose tissue in the breast atrophies. The accompanying decrease in breast size and elasticity results in the breasts appearing flat, flabby, or droopy. Breast shrinkage and fibrosis may cause nipple retraction. Axillary hair diminishes. Ovarian function begins to diminish during a woman's forties, and on average, menopause occurs between the ages of 45 and 55 years. Pubic hair becomes sparse as well as gray. The labia and clitoris become smaller, the vagina narrows and shortens, vaginal mucosa thins and dries, and the uterus and ovaries diminish in size. A number of these changes result from the decline in estrogen levels in the body.

Pregnant Patients

Pregnancy stimulates expansion of the ductal system of the breast, supporting fatty tissues and secretory alveoli. These changes result in the breast enlarging and feeling more nodular. The nipples become larger, darker, and more erectile. The areolae also become larger, and they grow a darker brown as the pregnancy progresses. A venous pattern is prominent over the skin surface. Colostrum (i.e., the precursor of milk) may sometimes be expressed after the fourth or fifth month of pregnancy; this thick, yellow fluid contains protein and lactose but no fat. Lactation usually begins 1 to 3 days postpartum. During this time, the breast may become engorged; appear enlarged, reddened, and shiny; and feel both warm and hard. Frequent nursing will help to drain the ducts and sinuses as well as stimulate milk production. Nipple soreness is normal but usually lasts only 24 to 48 hours. The nipples may look red and irritated, and they may even crack. They will heal rapidly, however, if kept dry and exposed to the air.

With pregnancy, several changes occur in the female genitalia. By 4 to 6 weeks of pregnancy, the cervix softens, and the vaginal mucus and cervix appear cyanotic at 8 to 12 weeks. The uterus increases in capacity by 500- to 1,000-fold compared to its nonpregnant state and also becomes globular in shape. As the uterus increases in size, it presses on the bladder and rises outside the pelvis, displacing the intestines. Cervical and vaginal secretions increase in pregnancy and become thick, white, and more acidic.

Many drugs can be transferred in breast milk. The most important factor determining the transfer of a drug into breast milk is the maternal serum drug concentration. Physical and chemical properties of the drug also come into play. Molecules with molecular weights less than 200 daltons can pass through pores in the membranes of the mammary epithelium. Highly lipid-soluble drugs pass more readily into breast milk than do more water-soluble agents. Drugs must be in a free, unbound state to pass. Drugs with a higher pH will be trapped in breast milk as well.

PATHOLOGY OVERVIEW

Dysfunction of the female reproductive system is a common cause of morbidity. Common abnormalities of the female reproductive system include fibrocystic changes of the breast, breast cancer, vulvovaginal candidiasis, and premenstrual syndrome.

Fibrocystic Changes of the Breast

Fibrocystic changes of the breast occur in as many as 90% of women, making this condition one of normal variation rather than of actual disease. Fibrocystic changes often lead to patient complaints of dull, aching breast pain, most often during the premenstrual period. The pain generally is located in areas of the breast with more pronounced nodularity. The nodularity can be palpated as a "lumpy" character to the breast and is usually bilateral. Diffuse, easily movable, and poorly defined masses that are tender will be present in the fibrocystic breast. The upper outer quadrant of the breasts is most affected. The cysts are often difficult to distinguish from cancer, so many patients undergo at least one biopsy for differentiation of the lesion. Most biopsies show normal breast tissue, although approximately one-quarter show epithelial hyperplasia. Neither histopathologic finding increases an individual's risk of breast cancer. A biopsy showing hyperplasia with atypia, however, does warrant an increase in vigilance of follow up, because these patients have a higher risk of breast cancer. **Duct ectasia,** or dilation of the duct, can be associated with fibrocystic breast changes and results in a thick, gray-green nipple discharge. Such a discharge in the absence of palpable fibrocystic changes should prompt mammography and possible biopsy.

Fibrocystic breast changes generally resolve between the menstrual periods as the female hormones return to baseline. Most cysts or lumps that appear and resolve spontaneously are caused by fibrocystic changes in the breast. Monthly breast self-examination (BSE) will help a woman to become familiar with the normal condition of her breasts as well as with their cyclic changes (Box 22-1). Any lumps that persist or feel hard should be followed up by a physician.

Because many women are afraid that the nodularity in their breasts may indicate breast cancer, the pain caused by the condition is heightened. Once the condition has been shown to be fibrocystic changes with no adverse histopathologic findings, this fear can be allayed—and the pain often decreases as well. For patients who continue to experience pain, wearing a brassiere at night as well as during the day and avoiding caffeine may help to alleviate the pain. If pain relief from these nonpharmacologic measures is inadequate, danazol may be helpful in decreasing the growth and nodularity of breast tissue. Tamoxifen has also been used.

Breast Cancer

Breast cancer is the number one form of cancer and the second-leading cause of cancer deaths in women. Breast cancer can also occur in men, but this is extremely rare. Several different types of abnormal breast tumors, some of which are benign, occur.

Box 22-1

BREAST SELF-EXAMINATION

The breast self-examination (BSE) should be performed in both lying and standing positions.

- First, lie down with a pillow under your right shoulder and your right hand behind your head.
- Using the finger pads of the three middle fingers of your left hand, feel for lumps in your right breast.
- Press firmly enough to know how your breast feels.
- Move around your breast in a set way, such as those shown below. Remember how your breast feels from month to month.
- Repeat the examination on your left breast.
- Stand up, and place one arm behind your head. Check the part of the breasts toward your armpit using the same method described earlier.
- This process may be easier if done in the shower with soapy hands.
- Also, check your breasts by standing in front of a mirror with your hands on your hips. Look for any changes in the skin or changes in the nipples.
- If you find any changes, see your physician as soon as possible.

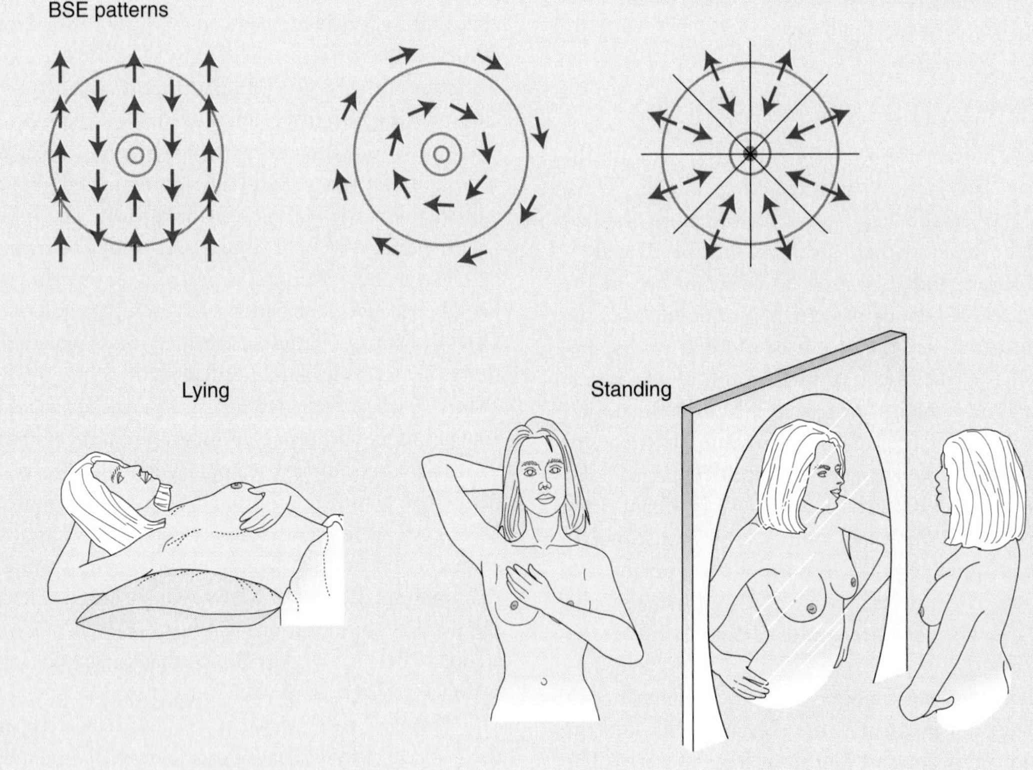

Fibroadenomas and papillomas are abnormal growths within the breast but are considered to be benign, because they cannot spread outside the breast tissue. Malignant tumors of the breast arise almost exclusively from the glandular tissues of the breast and, thus, fall into the general category of cancers known as adenocarcinoma. Ductal and lobular carcinomas account for most cases of breast cancer, with ductal carcinomas being the most common. Some less common types of breast cancer include inflammatory breast cancer, medullary carcinoma, mucinous carcinoma, phyllodes tumor, and tubular carcinoma. Paget's disease of the breast is also a type of cancer that starts in the ducts and then spreads to the skin of the nipple and areola.

The cause of breast cancer remains for the most part unknown. Ultimately, the interplay of many different factors in any given person resulting in DNA mutations leads to the development of breast cancer. Some of the known and probable risk factors include:

- Female gender
- Increasing age
- Mutations in the *BRCA1* and *BRCA2* genes
- Family history of breast cancer
- Personal history of breast cancer
- Caucasian race
- History of proliferative breast disease either without atypia, with usual hyperplasia, or with atypical hyperplasia
- Chest-area radiation therapy
- Menstruation before the age of 12 years

- Menopause after the age of 50 years
- Women without children or whose first child was born after the age of 30 years
- Long-term hormone replacement therapy
- Alcohol consumption
- Obesity

Early detection and risk factor modification are the best strategies for achieving good outcomes with breast cancer. Monthly BSE, clinician breast examination, and regular mammography are the best way to find breast cancer early and, thus, to decrease the mortality of this disease. Mammography is recommended by the American Cancer Society every 1 to 2 years for all women older than 40 years; more frequent examination may be warranted in those with a significant family history of breast cancer or with certain histopathologic changes in fibrocystic breast disease. Modifying risk factors may also reduce a woman's likelihood of developing breast cancer, although many women who develop breast cancer do not have identifiable risk factors. To reduce the risk of breast cancer in high-risk women, drug therapy with tamoxifen or raloxifene may be considered, or prophylactic mastectomy may be elected.

The signs and symptoms of breast cancer can be found in Box 22-2. Once breast cancer has been diagnosed, treatment is based on the stage and type of cancer identified. Treatment may be local, such as radiation or surgery (e.g., lumpectomy or mastectomy), or systemic, such as chemotherapy, hormonal therapy, or immunotherapy. Commonly used chemotherapeutic agents for breast cancer include cyclophosphamide, methotrexate, fluorouracil, doxorubicin, paclitaxel, epirubicin, docetaxel, venorelbine, gemcitabine, and capecitabine. Hormone therapy includes tamoxifen, raloxifene, toremifene, anastrozole, megestrol acetate, progestins, and androgens. Immunotherapy with trastuzumab is generally started after standard hormonal or chemotherapy is no longer effective.

Vulvovaginal Candidiasis

Vulvovaginitis is an inflammation of the vulva and vagina. The inflammation can result from various causes, including infection and local irritation. Among women with vulvovaginitis, approximately 40% are infected with *Candida albicans*. Colonization with *C. albicans* occurs in as many as 16% of nonpregnant, reproductive-aged women, however, so its presence does not establish the diagnosis.

Vulvovaginal candidiasis occurs when the balance of normal microbial flora is upset in the vagina. Some factors that can predispose one to infection with *C. albicans* include:

- Pregnancy
- Diabetes mellitus
- Immunosuppression
- Therapy with antibiotics or corticosteroids
- Iron-deficiency anemia
- Vaginal surgery
- Oral contraceptives
- Infection with the human immunodeficiency virus (HIV)
- Synthetic, occlusive items of clothing

Candida organisms thrive in conditions of persistent moisture, with resultant softening of the surrounding tissues. Increases in estrogen as well as vaginal pH also encourage *C. albicans* to proliferate. Candidal infections can become chronic or recurrent. Chronic infections result from inadequate treatment. Recurrent infections occur from reintroduction of the organism, which can occur through colonization of a sexual partner, improper perineal hygiene, or coitus. Some recurrences consistently occur during menstrual cycles.

Common symptoms caused by vulvovaginal candidiasis include vulvar itching and burning as well as vaginal discharge. Normal vaginal discharge has no odor and is floccular in consistency. In a candidal infection, vaginal discharge has a yeast-like odor and is thick and curd-like. Bacterial vaginosis causes a fishy- or musty-smelling vaginal discharge that is thin and creamy in consistency and is often most noticeable after coitus. A copius, frothy vaginal discharge occurs with trichomonal infection, as does dyspareunia (i.e., painful coitus). Atrophic vaginitis is a common disorder among postmenopausal women in which vaginal secretions become blood-tinged and the patient complains of vaginal and vulvar dryness. The diagnosis of vulvovaginal candidiasis can be confirmed by placing a few drops of 20% potassium hydroxide on a few drops of vaginal secretions on a glass slide to reveal budding filaments, pseudohyphae, and spores present from the fungus.

Vulvovaginal candidiasis can be treated with either topical or oral therapies. Some commonly used topical therapies include terconazole, butoconazole, miconazole, and clotrimazole. Orally, fluconazole can be given as a single dose. A topical steroid cream may also be used on the external structures to decrease burning, pain, and itching.

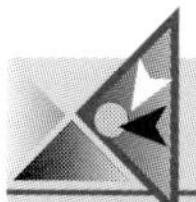

Box 22-2

SIGNS AND SYMPTOMS OF BREAST CANCER

- New lump or mass
- Painless lump
- Hard lump
- Lump with irregular edges
- Generalized swelling of part of the breast
- Skin irritation or dimpling
- Nipple pain or retraction
- Redness or scaliness of the skin of the breast or nipple
- Nipple discharge other than breast milk
- Enlarged axillary lymph nodes

Premenstrual Syndrome

During the period surrounding the menstrual cycle, many normal, ovulatory women experience various somatic symptoms, including edema, breast engorgement, abdominal bloating, abdominal cramping, irritability, depression, cravings for sweet or salty foods, tearfulness, headaches, mood swings, and lethargy.

This complex of symptoms is often referred to as premenstrual syndrome (PMS). There is no known cause of PMS; however, the mood and anxiety disturbances may relate to the effect of ovarian steroid hormones on serotonin and norepinephrine.

Abdominal cramping is often associated with menstruation and is termed **dysmenorrhea.** The pain may begin a few days before the onset of menses, is often most severe during the first several hours of the menstrual flow, and then abates over the next couple of days. Abdominal cramping can also occur in conjunction with ovulation. Primary dysmenorrhea occurs within the first couple of years after menarche. This type of dysmenorrhea is very common and is not considered to be a serious condition. It may continue throughout the menstrual life of the woman, or it may subside within a few years or with the use of oral contraceptives. Secondary dysmenorrhea occurs when menstrual pain or cramping begins or worsens in a more mature woman. Secondary dysmenorrhea often results from some type of gynecologic pathology, such as fibroids, endometriosis, or pelvic inflammatory disease, and should be investigated further.

Approximately 5% of women experiencing PMS find the condition to severely limit their activities of daily living. In such cases, the diagnosis of **premenstrual dysphoric disorder** is made, which includes the criteria for a major depressive episode. There is no specific treatment for PMS. Symptomatic therapies, such as pain relievers for the abdominal cramping and headaches, pyridoxine for the mood disorders, and diuretics for the bloating, have been used, but none has completely alleviated the syndrome in all women. In severe cases, patients should be referred to an endocrinologist or psychiatrist for trials of medications that alter ovarian function and mood. Fluoxetine has been approved for the treatment of premenstrual dysphoric disorder.

SYSTEM ASSESSMENT

Subjective Information

When assessing the female reproductive system, subjective patient information can be very valuable. It is important for the pharmacist to ask the patient appropriate questions to elicit the necessary information. Conversation is often the pharmacist's most valuable tool in performing the patient assessment.

Breast Lump

? INTERVIEW Do you have any pain or tenderness in your breasts? If so, when did you first notice it? Where is the pain? Does it seem to be localized or all over? Is the painful spot sore to touch? Do you feel a burning or pulling sensation? Is the pain cyclic? What relation does the pain have to your menstrual cycle? Is the pain brought on by strenuous activity, especially involving one arm? By a change in activity? Manipulation during sex? Part of an underwire bra? Exercise?

➤ ABNORMALITIES Breast pain does not occur in the majority of women with breast cancer. When pain has been documented, however, it has been described as vague, pulling, or burning in nature. Cyclic pain is common with normal breasts, use of oral contraceptives, and fibrocystic changes.

? INTERVIEW When did you first notice the lump in your breast? Where is it in the breast? Has it changed at all since then? Does the lump have any relation to your menstrual period? What changes have you noticed in the skin of your breast? Any redness, warmth, dimpling, or swelling?

➤ ABNORMALITIES Any lump in the breast should be thoroughly evaluated. Nodularity from fibrocystic changes often waxes and wanes in response to the menstrual cycle. Redness, warmth, and swelling may occur in disorders associated with lactation (e.g., plugged duct, mastitis, or breast abscess). Dimpling of the skin and edema resulting in an orange peel appearance (i.e., **peau d'orange**) of the skin are often associated with cancer.

? INTERVIEW Do you have any discharge from the nipple? If so, when did you notice it? What color is the discharge? Is it runny or thick? Is there an odor? Have you noticed any physical changes in the nipple?

➤ ABNORMALITIES Certain medications may cause a clear nipple discharge (Box 22-3). Bloody or blood-tinged discharge is always significant, as is any discharge in the presence of a lump. Asymmetry in the nipples or change in direction of the nipple may indicate cancer.

? INTERVIEW Have you noted any rash on the breast? If so, when did you first notice this? Where did it start? On the nipple, areola, or surrounding skin?

➤ ABNORMALITIES Paget's disease may start with a small crust on the nipple apex and then spread to the areola. Eczema or other dermatitis usually starts on the areola or surrounding skin.

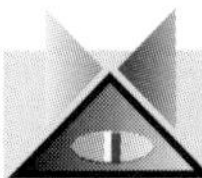

Box 22-3

MEDICATIONS THAT MAY CAUSE A CLEAR NIPPLE DISCHARGE

- Oral contraceptives
- Typical antipsychotics
- Diuretics
- Digitalis
- Corticosteroids
- Tricyclic antidepressants
- Reserpine
- Methyldopa

? INTERVIEW Have you noted any swelling in the breasts? If so, is this in one spot or all over? Does the swelling seem to be related to your menstrual period, pregnancy, or breast-feeding? Have you noticed any change in bra size?

ABNORMALITIES Swelling and tenderness of the breast are normal in relationship to the menstrual cycle. A sudden increase in the size of one breast may indicate an inflammatory process or new growth.

? INTERVIEW Have you had any trauma or injury to the breasts? If so, did it result in swelling, a lump, or any break in the skin?

ABNORMALITIES A lump from injury is caused by local hematoma or edema and should resolve in a short period of time.

? INTERVIEW Do you have any history of breast disease? If so, of what type? How was it diagnosed? When did this occur? How is it being treated? Has anyone in your family had breast cancer? If so, at what age did this relative have breast cancer?

ABNORMALITIES A history of breast cancer increases the risk of recurrent cancer. Fibrocystic changes may make it harder to examine the breasts, because the general lumpiness of the breast may conceal a new lump. A family history of breast cancer, especially in first-degree relatives, increases the risk for breast cancer.

? INTERVIEW Have you ever had surgery on your breasts? If so, was this a biopsy? Mastectomy? Mammoplasty? Augmentation or reduction?

ABNORMALITIES Augmentation or reconstruction of the breast using implants may make examination of the breasts more difficult.

? INTERVIEW Have you ever been taught breast self-examination? If so, how often do you perform it? What helps you to remember? Have you ever undergone mammography? If so, when was the last mammogram obtained?

ABNORMALITIES Most breast lumps are found through BSE.

? INTERVIEW Have you noticed any tenderness or a lump in the underarm area? If so, where? When did you first notice this?

ABNORMALITIES Enlarged axillary lymph nodes are usually associated with infection of the hand or arm or with recent immunizations or skin tests. Breast tissue extends into the axilla, however, and more than 50% of breast cancers occur in the upper outer quadrant of the breast. The axillae also contain numerous lymph nodes, which may enlarge as a first sign of breast cancer.

? INTERVIEW Do you have a rash in your underarm area? If so, please describe it. Does it seem to be a reaction to deodorant?

ABNORMALITIES Fragrances used in deodorants may cause allergic dermatitis.

Vaginal Discharge

? INTERVIEW Do you have any unusual vaginal discharge? Is there an increased amount? What is the color of the discharge? White? Yellow-green? Gray? What is the consistency of the discharge? Curd-like and thin? Does the discharge have an odor? When did it begin? Is the discharge associated with vaginal itching, rash, or pain with intercourse?

ABNORMALITIES Vaginal discharge varies in its characteristics depending on the causative factor. **Dyspareunia** (i.e., painful coitus) can occur with either trichomonal infection or atrophic vaginitis.

? INTERVIEW What medications are you currently taking?

ABNORMALITIES Some medications (e.g., antibiotics and corticosteroids) can predispose to candidal infections. Phenazopyridine may color all body secretions, including vaginal mucus, either red or orange.

? INTERVIEW Do you have a family history of diabetes? Have you ever been tested for diabetes?

ABNORMALITIES Recurrent vulvovaginal candidiasis can be a presenting symptom of the onset of diabetes mellitus in women.

? INTERVIEW What risk factors for infection with HIV, such as unprotected sex or intravenous drug use, do you have?

ABNORMALITIES Recurrent vulvovaginal candidiasis can be a presenting symptom of HIV infection in women.

Abdominal Cramping

INTERVIEW When does the cramping occur? Is there any relationship to your menstrual cycle? Do you have any other symptoms, such as nausea, vomiting, or fever?

ABNORMALITIES Dysmenorrhea is a common occurrence. Abdominal cramping unrelated to the menstrual cycle may result from other causes, such as gastrointestinal infection or upset as well as appendicitis. Nausea, vomiting, fever, and extreme abdominal pain often accompany the latter.

INTERVIEW Have you had a history of cramping since you began menstruating?

ABNORMALITIES Such a history would be consistent with primary dysmenorrhea as compared to secondary dysmenorrhea, which begins or worsens later during life.

INTERVIEW Do you have any other symptoms that you associate with your menstrual flow, such as headaches, bloating, irritability, or mood swings?

ABNORMALITIES All these symptoms are consistent with PMS.

Objective Information

Objective information pertaining to the female reproductive system primarily includes the results of physical examination of the breast and reproductive organs. Diagnostic tests may be used for screening or diagnosis of potential pathologic conditions. In all likelihood, a pharmacist will not be involved with completing the physical assessment; however, it is important to understand the techniques used when evaluating such information provided by the patient, primary care provider, or the medical chart. It is also vital that the pharmacist use conversation and appropriate questioning of the patient to obtain as many details as possible. The pharmacist should always remember that information retrieved by a thorough patient history might be more important than the physical findings in the process of patient assessment.

Physical Assessment

Physical assessment of the female reproductive system involves inspection and palpation of the breasts and reproductive organs.

Breasts and Axillae

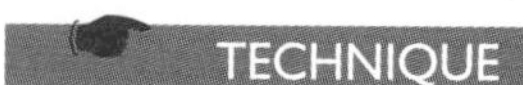

STEP 1

Inspect the Breasts

- Ask the patient sit on the examination table, disrobed to the waist and with arms at her side.
- Inspect the breasts. Note the color of the skin, size, symmetry, and contour.
- Inspect the nipples. Note the size, shape, and direction as well as any rash, ulcerations, or discharge.
- Ask the patient to raise her arms over her head. Observe for any dimpling or retraction on the breasts.
- Ask the patient to press her hands against her hips. Observe for any dimpling or retraction on the breasts.

ABNORMALITIES Redness of the breast may result from local infection or inflammatory carcinoma. Flattening of the breast, thickened and prominent pores, nipple retraction, nipple asymmetry, and dimpling or retraction of the tissue are suggestive of an underlying cancer. Pale, linear **striae,** or stretch marks, often follow pregnancy. Although nipples usually protrude, they may also be flat or inverted. Normal nipple inversion may be unilateral or bilateral, and it usually can be pulled out. Supernumerary nipples are normally present in 1% of men and women; these nipples are usually 5 to 6 cm below the breast, near the midline, and have no glandular tissues. Supernumerary nipples look like a mole, but close inspection reveals a tiny nipple and areola. These are not clinically significant.

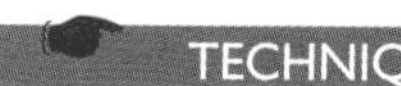

STEP 2

Inspect the Axillae

- Ask the patient to raise both arms.
- Inspect the axillae. Note any rash, infection, swelling, or unusual pigmentation.

ABNORMALITIES Rashes of the axillae are usually contact dermatitis from deodorants or other causes. Deeply pigmented velvety axillary skin may be **acanthosis nigricans,** which can be associated with internal malignancy.

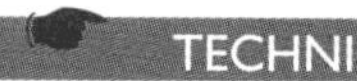

STEP 3

Palpate the Breasts

- Ask the patient to lie down.
- Place a pillow under the shoulder on the side you are examining.
- Ask the patient to rest her arm over her head.
- Place your fingers flat on the breast.
- Compress the tissues gently, in a rotary motion, against the chest wall and moving systematically from periphery to tail to areola. Press firmly to reach the deeper tissues.
- Palpate the entire breast from clavicle to inframammary fold and from midsternal line to posterior axillary line. Use a pattern of concentric circles, parallel lines, or consecutive clock times (Box 22-1). Note consistency of the tissues as well as any areas of tenderness or nodules.

TABLE 22-2 ➤ PHYSICAL EXAMINATION AND DOCUMENTATION OF BREAST MASSES

CHARACTERISTIC	NOTATION
Location	Several methods may be best. Note the quadrant, clock-face (e.g., 3-o'clock position), and distance (in cm) from the nipple. A diagram of the breast may also be used to mark the location of the nodule.
Size	Note in centimeters and in three dimensions (width × length × thickness).
Shape	Oval, round, lobulated, disk-like, regular, or irregular.
Consistency	Soft, hard, or firm.
Delimitation	Well-circumscribed or not; margins of lump distinct or not.
Mobility	Freely mobile or fixed. Note the relationship to the skin, pectoral fascia, and chest wall.
Distinctness	Solitary or multiple.
Nipple	Displaced or retracted.
Skin	Erythematous, dimpled, or retracted.
Tenderness	Tender to palpation?
Lymphadenopathy	Any regional lymph nodes palpable?

- If a nodule is found, note its location, size, shape, consistency, delimitation, and mobility (Table 22-2). Location is usually noted by referring to the quadrant of the breast (Fig. 22-8).
- Palpate each nipple. Note its elasticity, and watch for discharge. If discharge is observed, note its color, consistency, quantity, and location of appearance.

ABNORMALITIES Heat, redness, and swelling not associated with pregnancy and lactation may indicate inflammation. Hard, irregular, and poorly circumscribed nodules fixed to the skin or underlying tissue suggest a cancerous lesion. A mobile mass that becomes fixed when the patient presses her hand against her hip indicates that the mass is attached to the pectoral fascia. If the nodule is immobile when the patient is relaxed, it is attached to the ribs and intercostal muscles. Areas that may be tender include cysts, inflammation, and sometimes, cancerous lesions. If the nipple is thickened and has lost its elasticity, an underlying cancer should be suspected. A milky discharge in the absence of pregnancy and lactation usually relates to hormones or medication. Local breast disease should be suspected in the presence of a nonmilky, unilateral discharge.

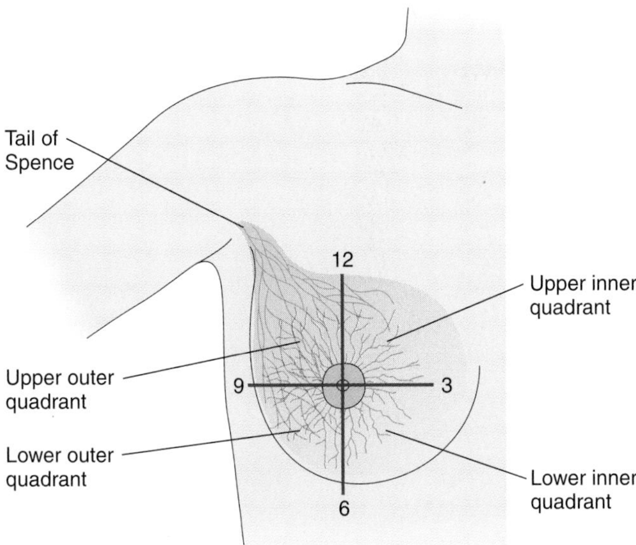

FIGURE 22-8 ■ Quadrants of the breast.

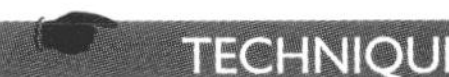

TECHNIQUE

STEP 4

Palpate the Axillae

- Have the patient sit relaxed, with her arms at the side.
- Lift the left arm.
- Support the left wrist or hand with your left hand.
- Cup together the fingers of your right hand.
- Reach as high as you can toward the apex of the axilla.
- Move your fingers firmly down in four directions: down the chest wall in a line from the middle of the axilla, the anterior border of the axilla, the posterior border, and along the inner aspect of the upper arm.

ABNORMALITIES Enlarged axillary nodes most commonly result from infection. Nodes that are large (≥1 cm), firm, matted, or fixed to the skin or the underlying tissues are suggestive of malignancy.

External Genitalia and Internal Organs

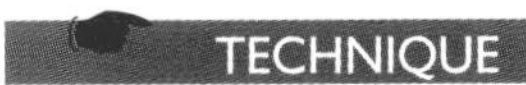

TECHNIQUE

STEP 1

Inspect the External Genitalia

- Drape the patient, and have her lie in a lithotomy position (i.e., on her back with thighs flexed on the abdomen and legs on the thighs, which are abducted) with her feet in the stirrups.
- Inspect the mons pubis, labia, and perineum.
- Look for nits or lice in the pubic hair as well as for any erythema or lesions.
- Separate the labia, and inspect the labia minora, clitoris, urethral meatus, and vaginal opening.
- Note any inflammation, discharge, lesions, swelling, or nodules.

ABNORMALITIES The clitoris may be enlarged in masculinizing conditions. Bartholin's gland may become infected, either acutely or chronically, which would lead to swelling of the area.

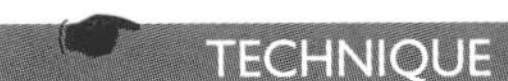

STEP 2

Palpate the Internal Organs

- Warn the patient that you will be touching her genitalia, and touch her thigh first before proceeding with the internal examination.
- Insert your index finger into the vagina, and feel for the round, firm surface of the cervix. During this examination, you can estimate the size of the vaginal canal to guide your choice of speculum.
- Feel the vaginal walls while having the patient bear down.
- Select a speculum of appropriate size, and lubricate it with warm water.
- Insert two fingers into the lower end of the vagina, and press down to enlarge the opening and help introduce the speculum.
- Insert the closed speculum over your two fingers at a downward angle and slightly to the left.

CAUTION **Do not pull the pubic hair or pinch the labia with the speculum.**

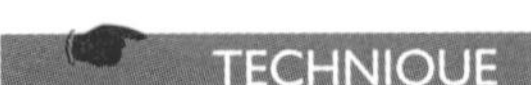

STEP 2 (Continued)

- When the speculum has entered the vagina, remove your fingers and rotate the speculum to the horizontal position. Once it is horizontal, advance the speculum to its full length (Fig. 22-9).
- Open the speculum, and adjust it to cup the cervix into full view. Lock the speculum into position. Be sure you have a well-positioned light.
- Inspect the cervix and the os. Note its color, position, any lesions on the surface, bleeding, discharge, or masses (Fig. 22-10).

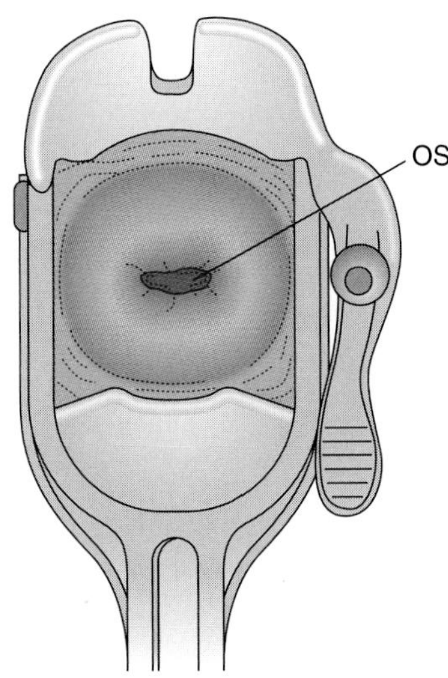

FIGURE 22-10 ■ View of the cervix through the speculum.

- An endocervical swab should be taken by inserting a cotton swab into the cervical os and rolling it clockwise and counterclockwise. Smear the swab onto a glass slide, and fix it promptly with ether alcohol or a fixative spray.
- A scraper or cervical broom can be used to obtain a sample of epithelial cells from the cervical os. Either instrument should be rotated in the cervical os. The sample should be placed on a glass slide and fixed as described previously.
- Unlock and withdraw the speculum slowly while observing the vagina. Close the speculum as it emerges from the vagina.
- Insert your lubricated index and middle fingers into the vagina, and palpate its walls.
- Palpate the cervix, and note its position, shape, consistency, mobility, and tenderness.
- Palpate the uterus by placing your other hand on the abdomen midway between the umbilicus and the symphysis pubis. Press down with the outside hand and up with the

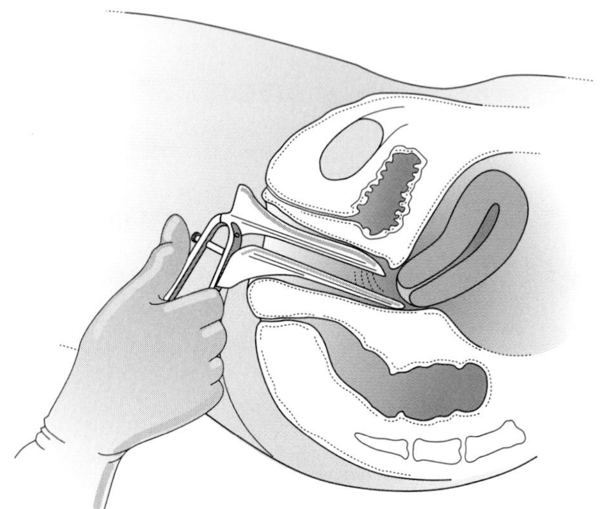

FIGURE 22-9 ■ Positioning the speculum.

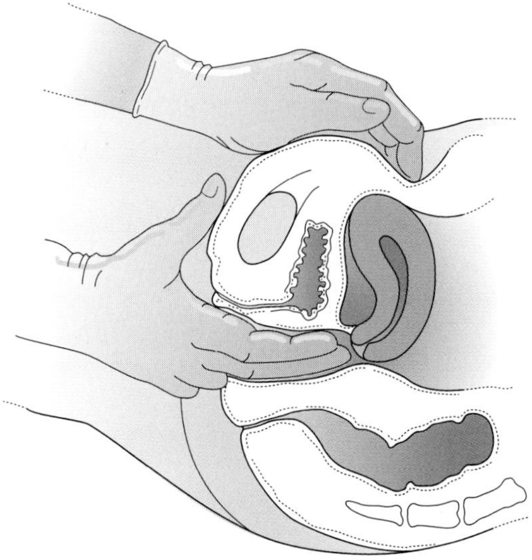

FIGURE 22-11 ■ Bimanual examination.

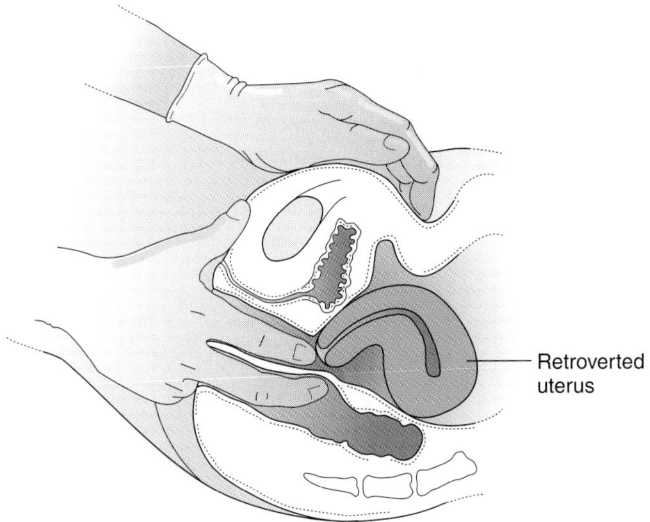

FIGURE 22-12 ■ Rectovaginal examination.

inside hand, trying to grasp the uterus between the two while assessing its size, shape, consistency, mobility, and any masses (Fig. 22-11).

☛ Palpate each ovary, again placing your outside hand on the abdomen in the right and left lower quadrants to feel the size, shape, consistency, mobility, and any masses in each.

☛ Withdraw your fingers, and then reinsert them with one in the vagina and one in the rectum. Repeat the maneuvers just described, trying to feel behind the cervix in the area you can only reach with the rectal finger (Fig. 22-12).

➤ ABNORMALITIES A bulge noted in the vagina may be either a **cystocele** or **rectocele.** A cystocele is a herniation of the bladder, usually into the vagina or introitus. A rectocele is a prolapse or herniation of the rectum. Both are more prominent during pregnancy. The uterus may be retroverted, leading to a difficult-to-view cervix; this is a normal variation in uterine location. The cervix may be round, oval, or slit-like. After vaginal deliveries, cervical lacerations may occur. A yellowish cervical discharge suggests infection with *Chlamydia trachomatis* or *Neisseria gonorrhoeae.* Normal ovaries may be slightly tender. Ovaries should not be palpable 3 to 5 years after menopause; if they are, this suggests an ovarian cyst or tumor. Movement of the cervix and adnexa should not cause pain; if the maneuver does, this suggests pelvic inflammatory disease. An enlarged uterus could be caused by pregnancy or malignancy.

Laboratory and Diagnostic Tests

Diagnostic tests that can be used in the evaluation of a patient with a breast lump include:

- *Mammography:* This radiologic examination of the breast identifies areas of calcification within breast masses and is used primarily in the diagnosis of cancer. Annual mammograms are recommended by the American Cancer Society for all women older than 40 years.
- *Ultrasound:* This imaging modality outlines the shape of breast masses. This is used in differentiating solid masses from cysts.
- *Biopsy:* This is excision of a small piece of tissue or an entire breast lump for microscopic examination.

Diagnostic tests that can be used in the evaluation of a patient with vaginal discharge include:

- *Papanicolaou (Pap) smear:* A Pap smear, which is used to detect cervical cancer, should be performed starting either at 18 years of age or with the onset of sexual activity. If the examination is normal for the first 3 years, then it should be repeated every 3 years, unless risk factors are present (Box 22-4).
- *Potassium hydroxide test:* This can be used to detect fungus in vaginal secretions.
- *Saline wet preparation:* This can be used to detect blood cells, fungus, and bacteria in vaginal secretions.
- *Ultrasound:* If an abnormal mass, size, or shape of the reproductive organs is palpated, ultrasonography can be used to further assess the condition.

Special Considerations

Pediatric Patients

Pediatric patients require additional questions to be asked of the parent or guardian.

? INTERVIEW Have you noticed any increase in vaginal secretions?

➤ ABNORMALITIES An increase in vaginal secretions is normal just before menarche. This increase in secretions is termed **leukorrhea** and is also associated with ovulation and with sexual excitement. Normal secretions should be distinguished from those caused by infection. Young girls will often insert foreign bodies into their vaginas, which can lead to infection and vaginal discharge.

Examination of the reproductive organs in the pediatric female patient is generally limited to the external genitalia. Sexual maturity can be rated using the Tanner staging scale for breast and

Box 22-4

RISK FACTORS REQUIRING MORE FREQUENT PAP SMEAR SCREENING

- Early onset of sexual activity
- Multiple sexual partners
- Infection with human papillomavirus
- Infection with human immunodeficiency virus

pubic hair development (Table 22-1). If pubic hair or breast enlargement occurs before the age of 8 years, **precocious puberty** is present and should be evaluated. A rectal examination is not part of a routine pediatric examination.

Geriatric Patients

Geriatric patients also require additional questions to be asked.

? INTERVIEW At what age did you experience menopause? Have you noticed any decrease in vaginal secretions? Do you experience pain during sexual intercourse because of vaginal dryness? Do you take calcium supplements? Do you take hormone replacement therapy?

ABNORMALITIES The vaginal mucosa normally thins after menopause; this is termed *atrophic vaginitis.* A decrease in estrogen can also result from oophorectomy and lead to the same symptoms. Topical estrogen and lubricating products can be used to ease the discomfort of atrophic vaginitis. Following menopause, it is also important that women investigate hormone replacement therapy with estrogen and progestin to prevent cardiovascular and bone-related complications. Calcium supplementation can also be beneficial in this group.

A full reproductive organ examination can be performed in elderly women, although it is not routinely necessary. The ovaries should not be palpable 3 to 5 years after menopause. If they remain palpable, a cyst or tumor should be suspected. Atrophic vaginitis is the main finding in geriatric female reproductive systems, and this may manifest as vaginal soreness, dryness, pruritis, and dyspareunia. The vaginal mucosa may be red, bleed easily, and have erosions.

Pregnant Patients

Many additional questions should be asked of the pregnant patient.

? INTERVIEW Have you noticed any breast tingling or tenderness?

ABNORMALITIES During pregnancy, hormones stimulate the breast tissue. This may lead to findings of tingling or tenderness in the breasts as they prepare for lactation. The increase in breast size may also lead to upper back pain.

? INTERVIEW Have you noticed any change in vaginal discharge?

ABNORMALITIES The hormones and resulting vasocongestion of the uterus and cervix during pregnancy can lead to an increase in vaginal secretions. These secretions will be seen as a milky white vaginal discharge. A vaginal discharge that contains blood, is malodorous, or is accompanied by symptoms of burning, itching, or pain needs further evaluation. Vaginal infections are more common during pregnancy.

Pregnant women may develop hemorrhoids, which can become larger, more painful, and bleed as pregnancy progresses. Bimanual examination of the reproductive organs is generally easier during pregnancy because of relaxation of the muscles. The examiner may feel that his or her fingers are immersed in a bowl of oatmeal, because the vaginal walls are softer and close around the fingers. The weeks of gestation can be estimated based on the size and position of the uterus. A rectovaginal examination may be performed if necessary to confirm uterine size, especially in the woman with a retroverted or retroflexed uterus.

APPLICATION TO PATIENT SYMPTOMS

Common symptoms relating to the female reproductive system include breast lump, vaginal discharge, and abdominal cramping.

Breast Lump

A breast lump can be a manifestation of breast cancer, fibrocystic breast changes, infection, or injury. The most common cause is fibrocystic breast changes, but any breast lump can be distressing to a patient. Breast lumps that are nontender, immobile, and hard are more suspicious of cancer, whereas lumps that are transient, mobile, and painful tend to be less of a cause for alarm. Nipple discharge, especially when associated with a breast lump, should also be investigated; nipple discharge can also be caused by various medications (Box 22-3).

CASE STUDY

MG is a 48-year-old woman going through menopause. She comes to the pharmacy for a refill on her Premarin, which she has been taking for 6 months now. The pharmacist often chats with MG about her children, but she seems distracted today. When the pharmacist asks MG if everything is all right, MG asks if she can speak to the pharmacist in private. The pharmacist invites MG into the patient consultation room.

ASSESSMENT OF THE PATIENT

Subjective Information

48-year-old woman who appears distracted and somewhat upset

DO YOU HAVE A SPECIFIC CONCERN TODAY? I noticed a lump in my breast when I got out of the shower this morning.

HAVE YOU EVER NOTICED THIS LUMP BEFORE? No. I do monthly breast self-examination, and this is the first time I've ever felt anything.

IS THE LUMP PAINFUL? No.

DOES THE LUMP MOVE AROUND UNDER THE SKIN? No. It is pretty much in one place.

HOW LARGE IS THE LUMP? About the size of a pea.

DO YOU HAVE ANY DISCHARGE FROM THE NIPPLE? There was a little bit of pinkish liquid that came out when I squeezed on it.

DO YOU HAVE YOUR MENSTRUAL PERIOD RIGHT NOW? I'm going through menopause and haven't really had a period in several months.

DO YOU HAVE A HISTORY OF FIBROCYSTIC BREAST CHANGES? No.

DO YOU HAVE A HISTORY OF BREAST CANCER IN YOUR FAMILY? No.

WHERE IN YOUR BREAST IS THE LUMP LOCATED? On the upper and outer portion of my right breast, near my armpit.

Objective Information

Computerized medication profile:

- Premarin (conjugated estrogens): 0.625 mg, one tablet daily; No. 30; Refills: 11; Patient obtains refills every 35 to 45 days.

Patient in no acute distress

Vital signs not measured

DISCUSSION

The concern in this case centers around the breast lump that MG has discovered. Because MG performs monthly BSE, she is familiar with her breast tissue and is confident that this lump is a change from the normal condition. MG is perimenopausal and has no history of fibrocystic breast changes, so the likelihood that this is a cyst associated with hormonal fluctuation is low. In addition, the lump is fixed and hard, neither of which are common characteristics of fibrocystic changes. The lump is not painful, which is also more typical of cancer. The presence of a nipple discharge, especially one that sounds like it may contain blood, is very suspicious. Although MG does not have a family history of breast cancer, most people who are diagnosed with breast cancer have no family history. (Risk does increase, however, for those who have first-degree relatives with breast cancer.)

After evaluating and synthesizing all the patient's subjective and objective information, the pharmacist concludes that MG's breast lump is highly suspicious for cancer. Because early treatment is more likely to lead to clinical cure and MG will feel more at ease once she knows what she's dealing with, the pharmacist advises MG to call a local mammography center that provides same-day appointments and evaluation for breast lumps. The pharmacist reassures MG that a thorough examination would be the most prudent course of action at this time.

Figure 22-13 may be useful in the assessment of patients complaining of a breast lump.

PHARMACEUTICAL CARE PLAN

Patient Name: MG

Date: 11/19/01

Medical Problems:
Menopause

Current Medications:
Premarin (conjugated estrogens), 0.625 mg, one tablet daily

S: 48-year-old woman complaining of a pea-sized lump in her breast that she discovered today. Patient appears to be distracted. The lump is nontender, immobile, and located in the upper outer quadrant of the right breast. Patient was able to express a "pinkish" liquid from the right nipple, has no history of fibrocystic breast changes, and is perimenopausal. Denies family history of breast cancer. Performs monthly BSE.

Compliance: Gets refills of monthly medication every 35 to 45 days.

O: Patient in no acute distress. Vital signs not measured.

A:
1. Breast lump suspicious for cancer by history.
2. Improper refill rate of Premarin prescription.

P:
1. Advise patient to call for same-day appointment at a local mammography center for evaluation of breast lump and appropriate referral.
2. Schedule follow-up phone call with the patient in 1 week to ascertain outcome of mammography.

Pharmacist: *Jill Delaney, Pharm.D.*

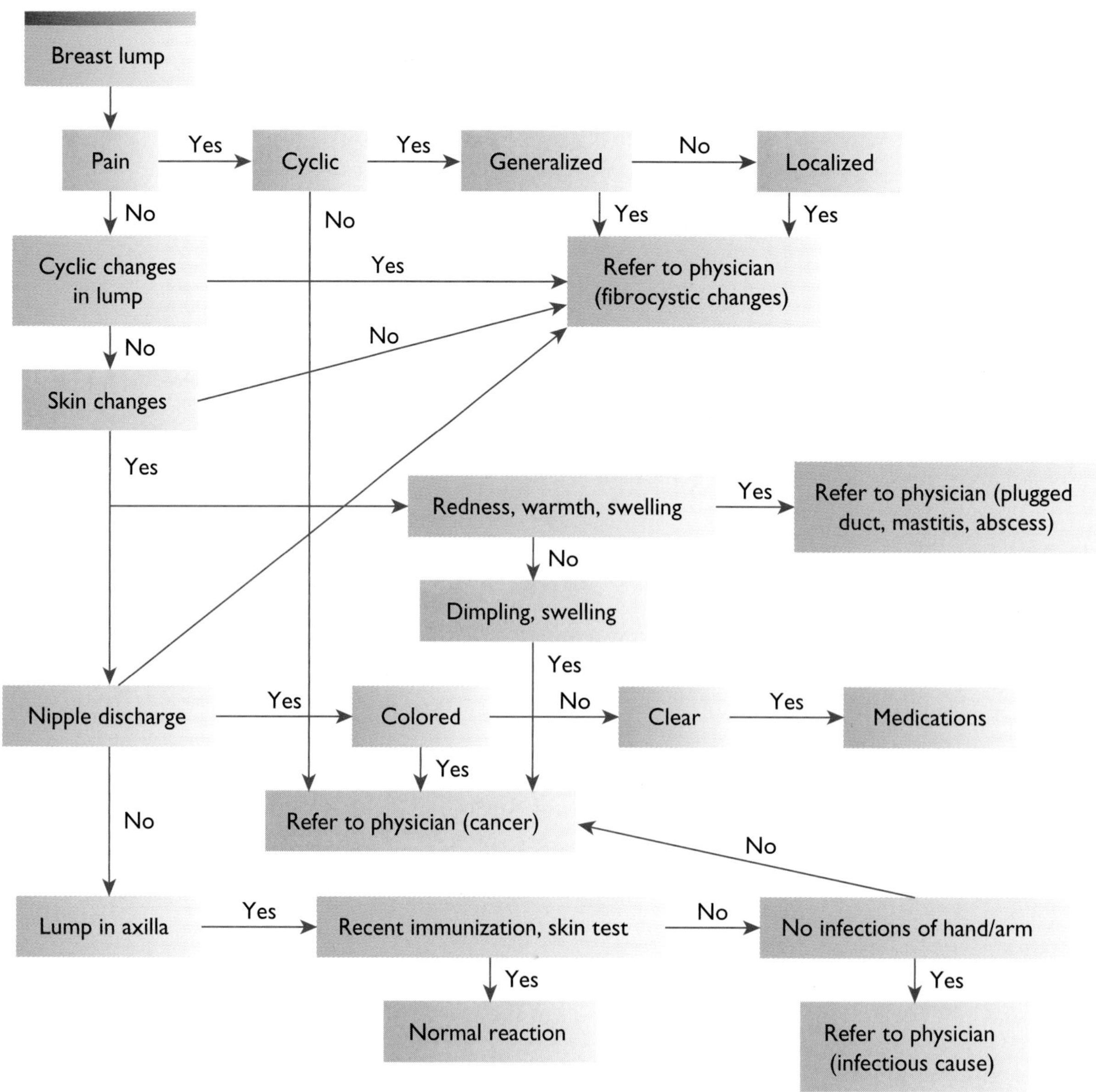

FIGURE 22-13 ■ Decision tree for breast lumps.

Self-Assessment Questions

1. Differentiate the varying characteristics of breast cancer versus fibrocystic breast changes.
2. What medications can cause a nipple discharge?
3. Compare and contrast the various interview questions that are useful in differentiating between breast cancer and fibrocystic breast changes.
4. Explain the procedure for completing a BSE.
5. List the known risk factors for breast cancer.

Critical Thinking Questions

1. How would the pharmacist's assessment and plan change if MG had painful nodules in both breasts similar to those she used to experience in conjunction with her menstrual cycle?
2. A 24-year-old woman complains of nodularity in her breasts that comes and goes in conjunction with her menstrual cycle. She currently drinks approximately six diet colas a day. What would be your assessment and plan for this patient?

Vaginal Discharge

Vaginal discharge can have many causes. Starting before puberty, leukorrhea occurs and will persist throughout adulthood and even past menopause. Abnormal vaginal discharge can be caused by various infections. Candidal infections can be effectively treated with over-the-counter (OTC) measures; all other infections require diagnosis by a physician and prescription therapy. Abnormal vaginal discharge is accompanied by other symptoms, such as vaginal itching, odor, burning, and dyspareunia.

CASE STUDY

SB is a 31-year-old woman who returns to the pharmacy 2 weeks after having a prescription filled for an upper respiratory tract infection. Before that, she had received a prescription allergy medication. She comes in today, says hi, and proceeds to the feminine products aisle. A few minutes later, she comes to the counter and asks what the difference is between two products for treatment of yeast infections. The pharmacist asks SB to step into the patient consultation room for further discussion.

ASSESSMENT OF THE PATIENT

Subjective Information

31-year-old woman with a yeast infection

HAVE YOU EVER HAD A YEAST INFECTION BEFORE? Yes, once a few years ago.

WHAT DID YOU USE TO TREAT THE PREVIOUS INFECTION? A cream my gynecologist prescribed.

WAS THE TREATMENT EFFECTIVE? Yes. The infection cleared up within a week or so.

WHAT SYMPTOMS DO YOU HAVE NOW THAT MAKE YOU THINK YOU HAVE A YEAST INFECTION? I'm having a lot of vaginal itching and burning, and I have a thick discharge that is kind of white and lumpy.

DOES THE DISCHARGE HAVE AN ODOR? Not really.

ARE YOU HAVING ANY BURNING WHEN YOU URINATE? Not that I've noticed. I mean, the whole area is kind of inflamed, but there is no particular burning there.

WHAT PRESCRIPTION MEDICATIONS ARE YOU TAKING? I take birth control pills, a prescription antihistamine, and I just finished up some antibiotics for a sinus infection.

DO YOU TAKE ANY NONPRESCRIPTION MEDICATIONS? I use naproxen for headaches about once a week, and I take calcium every day.

WHEN WAS YOUR LAST PAP SMEAR? I go to my OB/GYN every year. My last appointment was about 8 months ago.

WHEN WAS YOUR LAST MENSTRUAL PERIOD? Three weeks ago.

HAVE YOU BEEN USING AN ALTERNATE FORM OF BIRTH CONTROL SINCE YOU'VE BEEN TAKING ANTIBIOTICS? No. I didn't know I needed to.

Objective Information

Computerized medication profile:

- Triphasil (ethinyl estradiol/levonorgestrel): 28, one tablet daily; No. 1 pack; Refills: 3; Patient obtains refills every 25 to 30 days.
- Claritin (loratadine): 10 mg, one tablet daily; No. 30; Refills: 5; Patient obtains refills every 25 to 30 days.
- Zithromax (azithromycin): Dose Pak: as directed; No. 1 pack; Refills: 0.

Patient in no acute distress

Vital signs not measured

DISCUSSION

Because vaginal discharge can be physiologic or pathologic, the pharmacist must ask questions to elicit distinguishing symptoms (Fig. 22-14). In the case of SB, her symptoms are consistent with a candidal or yeast infection. Risk factors that SB has for vulvovaginal candidiasis include use of oral contraceptives and recent antibiotic therapy. Her infection does not appear to be either chronic or recurrent, because it has been years since her last episode. SB receives regular gynecologic care and is not in a high risk group requiring more frequent Pap smears.

The pharmacist feels that SB can be safely treated for her vulvovaginal candidiasis with an OTC preparation. Because creams can be messy and longer-term therapies harder to comply with, the pharmacist recommends a 3-day treatment with miconazole, 200-mg vaginal suppositories. The pharmacist also tells SB that a topical hydrocortisone cream applied to the vulva will help with the itching and burning and that she should wear natural-fiber, loose-fitting undergarments until the yeast infection resolves. In addition, the pharmacist advises SB to use an alternate form of birth control whenever she has to take antibiotics, which can cause failure of oral contraceptives.

■ PHARMACEUTICAL CARE PLAN ■

Patient Name: SB

Date: 10/29/02

Medical Problems:
Seasonal allergies
Resolving sinusitis

Current Medications:
Triphasil (ethinyl estradiol/levonorgestrel) 28: one tablet daily
Claritin (loratadine), 10 mg, one tablet daily
Zithromax (azithromycin), Dose Pak, as directed

Continued

CASE STUDY—continued

PHARMACEUTICAL CARE PLAN

S: 31-year-old woman complaining of a "yeast infection." Infection has occurred following a 5-day course of azithromycin for a sinus infection. Denies malodorous discharge. Describes discharge as "white and lumpy." Is also experiencing vaginal itching and burning. Compliant with medications.

OTC medications: Naproxen for headaches, approximately once a week. Calcium supplement daily.

O: Patient in no acute distress. Vital signs not measured.

A: Probable vulvovaginal candidiasis secondary to antibiotic therapy.

P:
1. Recommend OTC treatment with Monistat 3 suppositories and hydrocortisone cream.
2. Educate the patient regarding appropriate use of vaginal suppositories.
3. Educate the patient regarding need for alternative method of birth control during antibiotic therapy.
4. Instruct patient to see her physician if symptoms do not improve within 3 days.

Pharmacist: Donna Jiminez, Pharm.D.

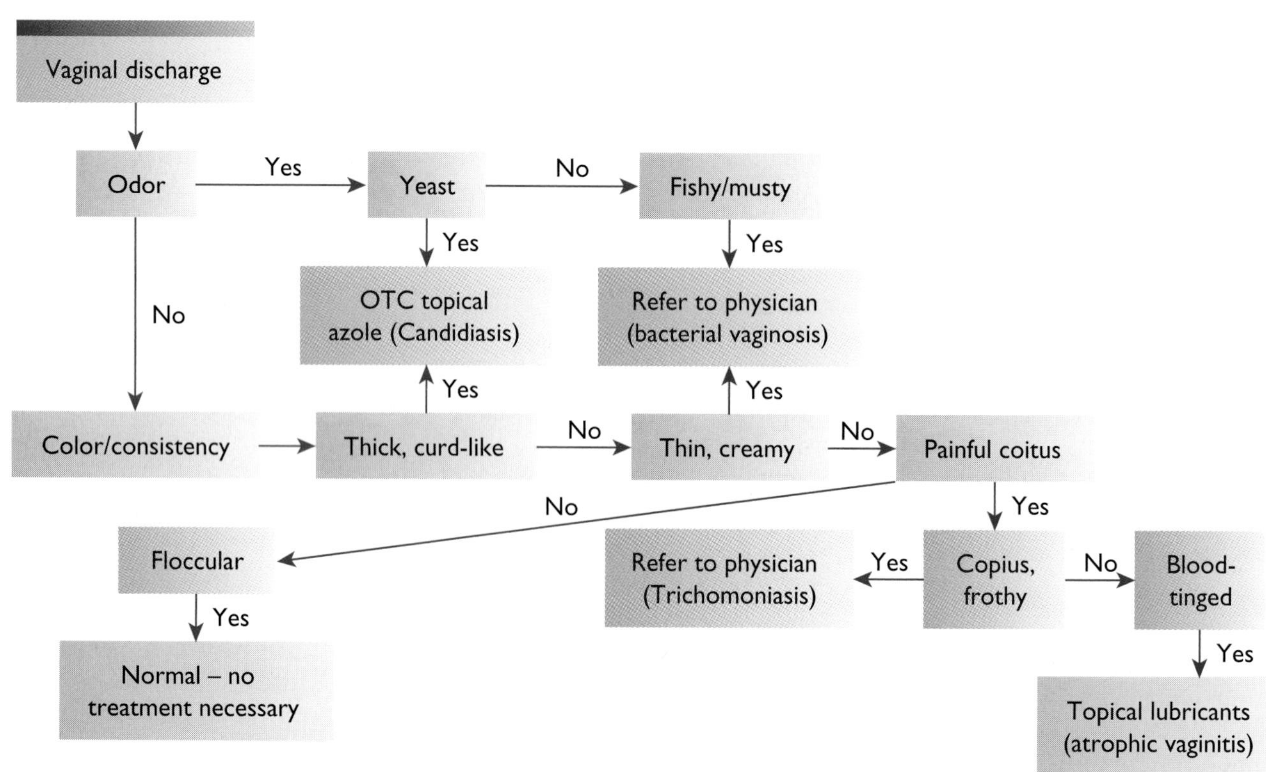

FIGURE 22-14 ■ Decision tree for vaginal discharge. *OTC*, over-the-counter.

Self-Assessment Questions

1. Compare and contrast the common signs and symptoms associated with vulvovaginal candidiasis and bacterial vaginal infections.
2. What are some risk factors for developing vulvovaginal candidiasis?
3. What is the usefulness of a potassium hydroxide test in evaluation of vulvovaginal candidiasis?
4. How would you differentiate a vaginal infection from atrophic vaginitis in an elderly woman?
5. What type of discharge normally occurs during pregnancy?

Critical Thinking Questions

1. SB comes back to the pharmacy in 3 weeks and says she's having the same symptoms again. What would the pharmacist's assessment and plan be now?
2. An 18-year-old female comes into the pharmacy seeking treatment for a yeast infection. This is the third time she has purchased such a product at the pharmacy, and she has never seen a gynecologist. What questions should the pharmacist ask to evaluate her situation?

Abdominal Cramping

Abdominal cramping associated with the menstrual period is termed *dysmenorrhea* and is very common. It may also be accompanied by other somatic symptoms, such as bloating, irritability, mood swings, and headaches. Most patients self-treat dysmenorrhea and other symptoms of PMS with OTC medications. Numerous products are available containing various ingredients such as pain relievers and diuretics. No product has been proven to be more effective than any other, so product selection is generally based on personal preference.

CASE STUDY

AH is a 26-year-old woman who comes to the pharmacy for her monthly refill of oral contraceptives. While checking out, she asks the pharmacist to recommend a "PMS remedy."

ASSESSMENT OF THE PATIENT

Subjective Information

26-year-old woman who complains of PMS

HOW LONG HAVE YOU HAD PMS? Pretty much ever since I started my period when I was 13.

WHAT MEDICATIONS HAVE YOU TRIED IN THE PAST? Aspirin, ibuprofen, Tylenol, and Midol.

DID YOU FIND MORE RELIEF FROM ONE PRODUCT THAN FROM ANOTHER? No. I guess I've just been searching for the "magic pill."

WHAT PMS SYMPTOMS DO YOU HAVE? I have cramps for the first couple of days of my period. I usually also have a dull headache.

DO YOU EXPERIENCE BLOATING? No.

WHEN DO YOU TAKE THE MEDICATIONS YOU'VE TRIED IN THE PAST? As soon as I have the first cramp or headache.

DO YOU HAVE PMS WITH EVERY PERIOD? I would say so.

ARE YOU ALLERGIC TO ANY MEDICATIONS? No.

DO YOU TAKE ANY PRESCRIPTION MEDICATIONS? Just the birth control pills.

DO YOU HAVE ANY MEDICAL CONDITIONS? No.

DO YOU TAKE ANY OTHER NONPRESCRIPTION MEDICATIONS? No.

DO YOU DRINK MUCH MILK OR EAT DAIRY PRODUCTS? I have a glass of milk about once a week.

Objective Information

Computerized medication profile:

- Ortho-Cyclen (ethinyl estradiol/norgestimate) 21: One tablet daily for 21 days of the month; No. 21; Refills: 10; Patient obtains refills every 20 to 30 days.

Patient in no acute distress
Vital signs not measured

DISCUSSION

When a woman complains of dysmenorrhea, any number of suggestions can be made for treatment options. As in AH's case, primary dysmenorrhea is not a cause for alarm. If an older patient presents for whom dysmenorrhea is a new or significantly worsened symptom, however, further investigation is warranted, because the cause could be a gynecologic pathology. In this case, AH only experiences abdominal cramping and headaches, so pain relief should be sufficient. The pharmacist recognizes that choosing a single-ingredient product, such as ibuprofen or acetaminophen, would avoid excessive exposure to unnecessary agents.

After evaluating AH's subjective and objective information, the pharmacist recommends that AH take ibuprofen, 400 mg three times a day, starting the day before she expects her pe-

Continued

CASE STUDY—continued

riod to begin. This will provide coverage before the onset of symptoms and may help to prevent the symptoms before they start. Given AH's age and lack of calcium intake in her diet, the pharmacist also recommends that AH take a calcium supplement daily to help maintain strong bones and prevent early bone loss. Some nonpharmacologic therapies that the pharmacist recommends for AH's dysmenorrhea include use of a heating pad or warm baths to help relieve the cramps.

Figure 22-15 may be useful in the assessment of patients complaining of abdominal cramping.

PHARMACEUTICAL CARE PLAN

Patient Name: AH

Date: 11/19/01

Medical Problems:

No significant medical history

Current Medications:

Ortho-Cyclen (ethinyl estradiol/norgestimate) 21, one tablet daily for 21 days of the month

S: 26-year-old female complaining of dysmenorrhea and PMS. Specific symptoms include abdominal cramping and headache during the first couple of days of her menstrual period. Denies other medical problems. Denies allergies to medications. Has tried aspirin, ibuprofen, Tylenol, and Midol, with no advantage of one over the others. Denies bloating. Has had PMS since thelarche at age 13. Compliant with Ortho-Cyclen. Uses no regular OTC medication.

O: Patient in no acute distress. Vital signs not measured.

A: PMS with primary dysmenorrhea.

P:
1. Recommend ibuprofen. 400 mg TID, beginning the day before the anticipated start of menstruation and to be taken with food or milk.
2. Recommend a daily calcium supplement.
3. Use heating pad or warm baths PRN for abdominal cramping.

Pharmacist: *Sue Ellen Hardy, Pharm.D.*

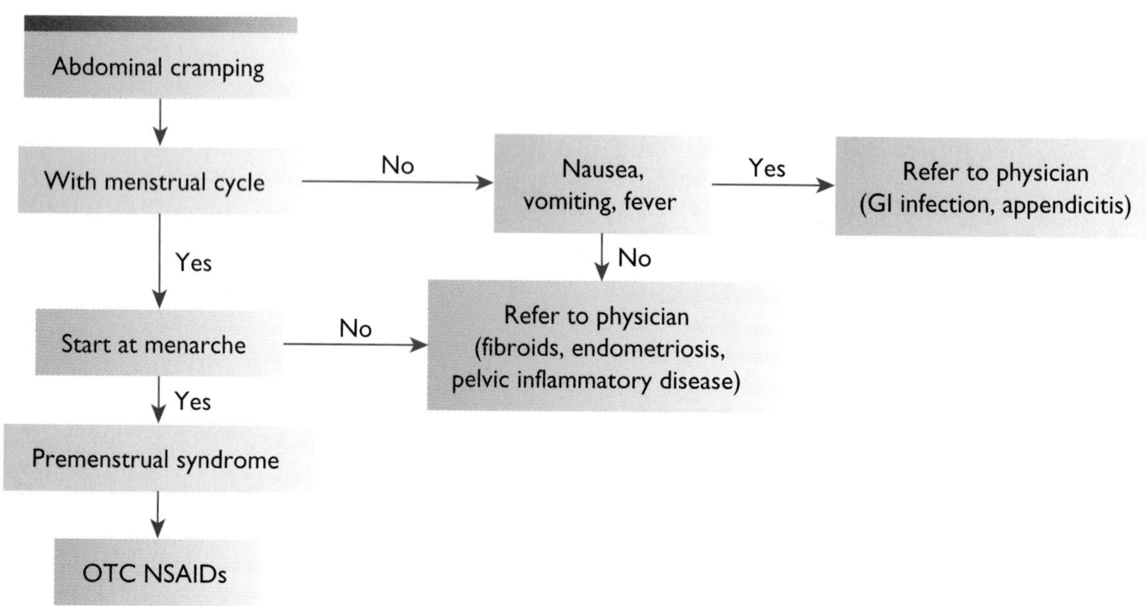

FIGURE 22-15 ■ Decision tree for abdominal cramping. *GI*, gastrointestinal; *NSAIDs*, nonsteroidal anti-inflammatory drugs; *OTC*, over-the-counter.

Self-Assessment Questions

1. What is the difference between primary and secondary dysmenorrhea?
2. What causes PMS?
3. What are the common signs and symptoms of PMS?
4. What medications may be useful in the treatment of PMS?
5. What signs and symptoms, if they present along with abdominal cramping, should result in a patient's referral to a physician?

Critical Thinking Questions

1. AH returns to the pharmacy a month later and says she is experiencing stomach upset. She also looks rather pale. She tells the pharmacist that she's been taking the ibuprofen and that her PMS is much improved. In fact, she has been taking the ibuprofen for about 2 weeks out of every month. What questions should the pharmacist ask to assess her symptoms?
2. A 42-year-old woman comes into the pharmacy looking for something to relieve abdominal cramps. She says that she hasn't had cramps like this in years. What would be your assessment and plan for this situation?

Bibliography

Allen KM, Phillips JM. Women's health across the lifespan: a comprehensive perspective. Philadelphia: Lippincott-Raven, 1997.

American Cancer Society. Breast cancer resource center. Available at http://www3.cancer.org/cancerinfo/load_cont.asp

Barker LR, Burton JR, Zieve PD. Principles of ambulatory medicine. 4th ed. Baltimore: Williams & Wilkins, 1995.

Dipiro JT, Talbert RL, Yee GC, et al. Pharmacotherapy: a pathophysiologic approach. 4th ed. Stamford, CT: Appleton & Lange, 1999.

Braunwald E, Fauci AS, Kasper DL, et al. Harrison's principles of internal medicine. 15th ed. New York: McGraw-Hill Health Professions Division, 2001.

Fischbach F. A manual of laboratory and diagnostic tests. 6th ed. Baltimore: Lippincott Williams & Wilkins, 2000.

Knoppert DC. Safety of drugs in pregnancy and lactation: pharmacotherapy self-assessment program. 3rd ed. Module 11: women's health. Kansas City, MO: American College of Clinical Pharmacy, 2000.

Martini FH, Timmons MJ. Human anatomy. 2nd ed. Upper Saddle River, NJ: Prentice-Hall, 1997.

Pharmacist's drug handbook. Bethesda, MD: Springhouse Corporation and American Society of Health-System Pharmacists, 2001.

Pray WS. Dysmenorrhea: how to relieve cramps. Available at http://www.medscape.com/jobson/USPharmacist/2000/v25.n09/usp2509.01.pray/usp2509.01.pray-01.html

Quan M. Vaginitis: meeting the clinical challenge. Clinical Cornerstone 2000;3(1):36-47, 2000.

Stedman's medical dictionary. 27th ed. Baltimore: Lippincott Williams & Wilkins, 2000.

Answers to Self-Assessment Questions

CHAPTER 1

1. Pharmaceutical care is a philosophy of caring about the patient's welfare through the responsible provision of drug therapy. The drug therapy should achieve definite health outcomes that improve a patient's quality of life.
2. Please refer to the discussion of the pharmacist's responsibilities within the pharmaceutical care process in the "Pharmaceutical Care" section.
3. The primary responsibility of a pharmacist who provides pharmaceutical care to patients is to identify, resolve, and prevent drug-related problems. For the pharmacist to adequately do this, he or she must continuously assess patient information, both subjective and objective. Thus, a pharmacist cannot provide pharmaceutical care without patient assessment.

CHAPTER 2

1. Culture is a complex pattern of shared meanings, beliefs, and behaviors that are learned and acquired by a group of people during the course of history. Culture reflects the whole of human behavior, including values, attitudes, and ways of relating to and communicating with each other.

   Ethnocentrism is the belief that one's own group or culture is superior while expressing disdain and contempt for other groups and cultures.

   Prejudice is the preconceived judgment or opinion of another person based on direct or indirect experiences.

   Stereotypes are fixed perceptions or images of a group while rejecting or ignoring the indivual existence within that group.
2. The three most common cultural variables that affect patient assessment include (1) health beliefs and practices, (2) family relationships, (3) communication.
3. Ways to enhance cultural sensitivity include: do a cultural self-assessment; get to know the patient and members of the patient's family if possible; listen actively and observe the patient's verbal and nonverbal cues; develop a genuine tolerance, acceptance, and respect for the patient's cultural values; ask questions about different features of your patient's culture; have a nonjudgmental approach with your patient; be empathetic; be willing to encounter new experiences; get to know others in various cultural groups.

CHAPTER 3

1. Comfortable room temperature, sufficient lighting, quiet surroundings, clean and organized setting, 4 to 5 feet of distance between the patient and the pharmacist, private area, and equal-status seating.
2. Open-ended questions are most useful in beginning a patient interaction, starting a new set of questions, or when the patient switches to a new topic. Closed-ended questions are most useful in obtaining detailed information. They also assist in speeding up the patient interaction.
3. Timing, location, quality or character, quantity or severity, setting, aggravating and relieving factors, and associated symptoms.
4. By asking open-ended questions (e.g., what medications do you take, and how often do you take them?), having the patient describe his or her daily routine for taking medications, asking the patient how often he or she needs to obtain a new supply of medication, and reviewing pharmacy refill records.

CHAPTER 4

1. Inspection, palpation, percussion, and auscultation. For a description of each, please review the "Methods of Assessment" section.
2. See Box 4-1.
3. See Box 4-3.
4. For key points in assessing elderly patients, review the "Geriatric Patients" section.

CHAPTER 5

1. BMI = (weight [lbs]/height [in]^2) × 703 = (225/69^2) × 703 = 33.2, which is classified as obese
2. See the "Vital Signs" section.
3. See the "Vital Signs" section.
4. Follow these guidelines:
   - Always check for appropriate cuff size.
   - Always make sure that the patient's arm is well supported and at heart level.
   - Allow the patient at least 5 minutes to rest and relax before obtaining a blood pressure reading.
   - If a measurement (systolic or diastolic) needs to be rechecked, the cuff should be completely deflated and a new reading obtained after waiting at least 1 to 2 minutes.
   - Always deflate the cuff at an appropriate speed (~2 mm Hg/sec).

CHAPTER 6

1. Calories or energy, protein, and fat.
2. 1750 kcal (25 kcal/kg), 70 g of protein (1.0 g/kg), and 2100 mL (30 mL/kg).
3. Electrolytes, vitamins, and trace minerals.
4. Marasmus, kwashiorkor, and mixed marasmus-kwashiorkor.

5. Marasmus, calorie deficiency; kwashiorkor, protein deficiency; mixed, both deficient.
6. Anorexia nervosa is a syndrome characterized by self-starvation, extreme weight loss, disturbance of body image, and intense fear of becoming obese.
7. Bulimia nervosa is characterized by binge eating that is usually followed by some form of purging, such as self-induced vomiting, laxative abuse, or associated behaviors (e.g., diuretic use, diet pill use, or compulsive exercising).
8. Adults: diabetes, anemia; pregnant women: preeclampsia, low-birth-weight infant; children: food allergies, failure to thrive; adolescents: pregnancy, eating disorder; elderly: medications, economic hardship.
9. Eating patterns, food allergies and intolerances, medications, gastrointestinal symptoms (e.g., vomiting, diarrhea, and constipation), and exercise patterns.
10. 24-hour recall or 3-day food record.
11. Semiquantitative food-frequency questionnaire or dietary history.
12. Weight
13. Body fat
14. Serum albumin concentration
15. Iron deficiency anemia, infection, inflammation, malignancy, and increased erythropoiesis.
16. Thin, shiny, scaly skin; decubitus ulcers; ecchymoses (bruising); easily plucked, lackluster hair; and thin, brittle nails.
17. Flushing of the skin, headache, dizziness, nausea, and anorexia.
18. Have the patient lie on one side with the uppermost arm fully extended and the palm of the hand resting on the thigh.

CHAPTER 7

1. Acute pain is related to an event, is linear in nature, has a beginning and an end, has a positive connotation, has a treatment goal of pain relief, and demonstrates physiologic manifestations of pain. Chronic pain is related to a situation, is circular in nature, has no definite beginning and no end in sight, has negative connotations, has a treatment goal of pain prevention, and often does not result in any physiologic changes.
2. Somatic pain is often characterized as throbbing, burning, or pricking. Visceral pain is usually described as deep, dull, aching, dragging, squeezing, or pressure-like.
3. Neuropathic pain is often described as burning, tingling, numbing, pressing, squeezing, itching, sharp, lacinating, electrical, shocking, searing, or jolting.
4. Self-report
5. *P,* palliative or precipitating factors associated with the pain; *Q,* quality of the pain; *R,* region where the pain is located, or radiation of the pain; *S,* subjective description of severity of the pain; *T,* temporal or time-related nature of the pain.
6. Visual analog scale, verbal numeric scale, and verbal rating scale.
7. Pain diaries, pain drawings, Wisconsin Brief Pain Questionnaire, and McGill Pain Questionnaire.
8. Faces pain scale, poker chip scale, and color scales.
9. Behavior and physiologic
10. In both children and the elderly, behavioral manifestations may include impaired or changed physical or social functioning, facial expressions, body movements, lack of usual movements, and vocalizations. For full list of behaviors in each of these categories, see Box 7-2.
11. Increased heart rate, increased respiratory rate, pallor, sweating, fatigue, swelling, and redness.

CHAPTER 8

Rash

1. The patient's history of poison ivy dermatitis is an excellent starting point. He presents with erythematous papules and vesicles. The fact that the rash is localized to the face and to the arms below the elbows indicates contact dermatitis. The fact that he worked in the garage several days before the eruption also indicates the possibility of touching something in the garage with the resin on it.
2. Poison ivy dermatitis can be contracted by touching an inanimate object that came in contact with the plant resin. Such objects can include tools, clothes, and shoes. It can also be contracted by touching an animal, such as a cat or dog, that has run through the poison ivy and gotten the resin on its skin.

Folliculitis

1. Folliculitis is inflammation of a hair follicle. His condition started out as a pimple (consistent with folliculitis), but it has progressed to form a painful erosion with a central necrotic plug. The spreading of folliculitis to surrounding tissue indicates development of furunculosis.
2. A small area of erythematous papules and pustules is not consistent with folliculitis. This would be suggestive of a new, developing rash.
3. The patient used the same antibiotic ointment a year ago. Before an allergic reaction takes place, a person must first be exposed to the antigen that triggers an immune response. The next time the person comes in contact with the allergen, a reaction will occur. Use of the antibiotic ointment with a known sensitizer indicates a possible allergic reaction.

Nail Infection

1. Dermatophytic infections produce drying of the nail, with thick patches under the nail between the nail and the nail bed. Candidal onychomycosis appears in the lateral nail folds and is painful to the touch. In addition, pus may be expressible from the nail folds.

CHAPTER 9

Red Eye

1. Viral conjunctivitis caused by adenovirus is the most common form of conjunctivitis.
2. Signs and symptoms of primary angle-closure glaucoma include blurred or hazy vision, halos around lights, headache (around the eye), ocular pain or discomfort, nausea, vomiting, diaphoresis, and abdominal pain.
3. The hallmark symptom of allergic conjunctivitis is itching.
4. A history of injury to the eye, loss of vision, or pain inside the eye are all indications of possible emergency situations, such as retinal detachment or iritis. In these situations, refer the patient to the nearest emergency room. Urgent referral to a physician should occur for symptoms of blurred vision or seeing halos around lights. These symptoms may be from glaucoma, which can cause permanent damage or blindness if the eye is untended. A fever in conjunction with a red eye that is swollen or tender to the touch may represent periorbital cellulitis. Refer these patients to their primary care provider immediately.
5. Inspection of the eye should include the following: position and alignment of the eyes in the face; quantity, distribution, and position of the eyebrows and eyelashes; ability of the eyelids to open and close completely; color and skin of the eyelids; conjunctiva and sclera for color, injection, drainage, swelling, and lesions; puncta of the lacrimal apparatus for swelling or excessive tearing or dryness; smoothness and clarity of the cornea and lens; color and markings on the iris; size, shape, and symmetry of the pupils.
6. *PERRLA,* pupils equal round reactive to light and accommodation; *EMOI,* extraocular muscles intact.

Ear Pain

1. Refer to Box 9-5 and Box 9-6.
2. As the pharmacist prepares to insert the otoscope, pull the auricle of the adult up and back. In infants and children younger than 3 years, pull the auricle back and down before inserting the otoscope. This helps to straighten the S-shape of the canal.
3. Portions of the malleus are visible through the translucent drum: the umbo, manubrium, and short process. In some cases, the incus may be visible as a whitish haze in the upper posterior area of the membrane. The cone-shaped light reflex is not an anatomic landmark but, rather, is a reflection of the otoscope light. During a normal examination, it should be visible at the 5-o'clock position on the right eardrum and the 7-o'clock position on the left eardrum.
4. Weber Test: Stand to the side of the patient. Instruct the patient to indicate if the tone sounds the same in both ears or better in one. Hold the tuning fork by the stem, and strike the tines softly on the back of your hand. Place the vibrating fork in the midline of the patient's skull. Normally, the sound is heard in the midline or equally loud in both ears. Rinne Test: Stand to the side and back of the patient. Instruct the patient to tell you when the sound can no longer be heard. Hold the tuning fork by the stem, and strike the tines softly on the back of your hand. Place the stem of the vibrating tuning fork on the patient's mastoid process. Once the patient indicates that the sound has gone away, quickly invert the fork so that the vibrating end is near the ear canal. Ask the patient if he or she can hear the sound. Instruct the patient to tell you when the sound can no longer be heard. Repeat with the opposite ear.
5. Lateralization of sound during the Weber test, or hearing the sound only on one side, is an abnormal result. During conductive hearing loss, sound lateralizes or is heard in the "bad" ear. The ear with conductive hearing loss has a better chance to hear bone-conducted sound, because it is not distracted by background noise. During sensorineural hearing loss, the sound lateralizes to the "good" or unaffected ear. The ear with nerve-based hearing loss is unable to perceive the sound.
6. Abnormal results of the Rinne test occur when AC is not greater than BC. When conductive hearing loss is present, the patient should have a negative Rinne test, which is air conduction being less than or equal to bone conduction ($AC = BC$, or $AC < BC$). A patient suffering from sensorineural hearing loss will hear poorly both ways, but the ratio of $AC > BC$ is maintained.

CHAPTER 10

Headache Pain

1. Band-like pain, usually diffuse and bilateral. May also describe the pain as tightness or pressure. Onset is usually acute in nature.
2. Stress, anxiety, muscle tension, and temporomandibular joint disease.

Facial Pain

1. Signs of sinusitis include mucopurulent nasal discharge, abnormal transillumination, poor response to decongestants, and headaches that respond poorly to analgesics. Symptoms of sinusitis include colored nasal discharge, nasal congestion, facial pain, maxillary toothache, fever, and cough.
2. Frontal sinus involvement often results in frontal headache. Maxillary sinus involvement can cause pain in the cheek area or teeth. Ethmoid sinus involvement can result in pain deep and medial to the eye.
3. Radiologic procedures currently are not warranted in the diagnosis of acute sinusitis.

Sore Throat

1. Viral pharyngitis predominates in children <4 years of age, recent history of cold or other viral infection, bacterial pharyngitis, especially streptococcal pharyngitis common between age 4–14 years, white exudates on throat, no history of cold or viral infection.

2. Abscesses, rheumatic fever, and streptococcal glomerulonephritis.
3. To provide rapid confirmation of group A. β-hemolytic streptococcus in the office environment. Because of lower rates of sensitivity, however, negative rapid "strep" tests must be verified by throat culture.

CHAPTER 11

Dyspnea

1. See Boxes 11-1, 11-2, and 11-6.
2. Pulmonary: chronic obstructive pulmonary disease, asthma, emphysema; cardiac: congestive heart failure, coronary artery disease; emotional: anxiety.
3. When do you become short of breath? What brings it on? Exertion? At rest? Lying down? What relieves it? Does it occur at any specific time of day? At night? If so, how many pillows do you need to use to sleep comfortably at night? Any other symptoms? Chest pain? Wheezing? Fever? Cough? Any bluish discoloration (cyanosis) around the lips, nose, fingers, or toes? Do you smoke? Have you smoked in the past?
4. See Table 11-7.
5. Typical signs and symptoms of respiratory distress include severe shortness of breath or tachypnea, use of accessory muscles, cyanosis of lips, nostrils, or wheezing.

Wheezing

1. See Box 11-1.
2. Exposure of sensitive patients to inhalant allergens (e.g., tobacco smoke, animal dander, dust mites, fungi/molds, pollen, exercise). See Box 11-7 for medications that may induce wheezing in sensitive patients.
3. Pulmonary functions tests (arterial blood gases, spirometry, oxygen saturation), peak expiratory flow rate, observation for shortness of breath or respiratory distress.
4. See Table 11-9.

Cough

1. How long have you had the cough? What time of the day does it usually occur? Early morning? Does it wake you up at night? Do you cough up any sputum, or is it a dry, hacking cough? What makes the cough worse? What relieves it? Do you have any other symptoms with it? Fever? Chest pain? Runny nose? Nasal congestion?
2. See Tables 11-5 and 11-6.
3. Bronchophony: an increase in loudness and clarity of vocal resonance as heard through the stethoscope when it is placed over the lungs. Egophony: a nasal or bleating quality of voice sounds as heard through the stethoscope when it is placed over the lungs; whispered pectoriloquy: an increase in the loudness and clarity of vocal resonance when the person whispers, as heard through the stethoscope when it is placed over the lungs.

CHAPTER 12

Chest Pain

1. See Table 12-1.
2. Factors that may precipitate angina include exercise or strenuous activity, activity that involves use of arms above the head, cold environment, emotional stress, extreme fear or anger, and coitus.
3. Do you ever have any chest pain or discomfort? If yes:

   Onset and duration: When did the pain start? How long did it last? Have you had this type of chest pain before? How often do you experience the chest pain?

   Characteristics: Describe the pain. Is it a severe crushing or pressure feeling or sharp/stabbing pain? Burning sensation?

   Location: Where is the pain? Does it radiate to any other areas?

   Cause: What brought on the pain? Physical exertion? Cold weather? Intercourse? Stressful situation?

   Relief: What relieves the pain? Rest or nitroglycerin?

   Symptoms: Do you experience any other symptoms? Nausea/vomiting? Sweating? Shortness of breath? Lightheadedness?

Dyspnea

1. Symptoms of congestive heart failure include shortness of breath, dyspnea on exertion, orthopnea, paroxysmal nocturnal dyspnea, peripheral edema, cough, weakness, and fatigue. Objective signs include tachycardia, S_3 gallop, left ventricular hypertrophy, rales, ejection fraction $< 40\%$, weight gain, increased blood urea nitrogen, jugular venous distension, hepatomegaly, and hepatojugular reflex.
2. Medications that may induce or worsen congestive heart failure include β-blockers, calcium-channel blockers, amphetamines, nonsteroidal anti-inflammatory drugs, corticosteroids, estrogens, hydralazine, methyldopa, prazosin, and minoxidil.
3. The S_3 heart sound is an abnormal heart sound that occurs immediately after the normally occurring first and second heart sounds. The third heart sound is a sign of volume overload in the ventricle and, thus, can occur with congestive heart failure.

Palpitations

1. Common symptoms of arrhythmias include palpitations, shortness of breath, dizziness/light-headedness, syncope, nervousness, and anxiety. Signs associated with arrhythmia include an irregular heart rhythm, normal heart rate, bradycardia, or tachycardia, and an abnormal electrocardiogram.
2. Medications that may induce palpitations are digoxin, sympathomimetic amines, antiarrhythmics, terfenadine (when used with erythromycin or ketoconazole), caffeine,

bronchodilators, decongestants, appetite suppressants, amphetamines, and antidepressants.

3. The electrocardiogram is a graphic illustration of the heart's electrical impulses that occur during the cardiac cycle. Since it provides an illustration of the heart's rhythm, it is useful in identifying an abnormal heart rhythm or, in other words, an arrhythmia.

Risk Factors for CHD

1. See Box 12-1, Risk factors for coronary heart disease.
2. Secondary prevention are those patients with CHD, including those with previous MI, cerebrovascular accident, transient ischemic attack, PVD, CABG, or angina. Primary prevention are those patients without CHD. For goals, see **Tables 12-3** and **12-4**
3. HDL is the "good cholesterol" that is responsible for removal of cholesterol from the arterial wall and peripheral tissues and carrying it back to the liver for disposal. LDL is considered the "bad cholesterol" and is the subfraction that lodges into the arterial wall, becomes oxidized, and stimulates the development of atherosclerotic plaque. Desirable levels of each are listed in **Tables 12-3** and **12-4** and include high HDL and low LDL cholesterol.

CHAPTER 13

1. ■ Age: males, >45 years; females, >55 years
   ■ Sex: women are at lower risk than men until after menopause
   ■ Familial predisposition
   ■ Hyperlipidemia (high LDL or low HDL cholesterol)
   ■ Hypertension
   ■ Diabetes
   ■ Cigarette smoking
2. See Box 13-1
3. **? INTERVIEW** Describe the type of pain that you are experiencing. Is it burning, aching, cramping? How long have you been experiencing it? Did it come on suddenly or gradually? What brings it on? What makes it better or go away? Does it come on with walking or activity? If yes, how many blocks can you walk before the pain begins? Have you recently started a new exercise?

   ➤ ABNORMALITIES Leg pain associated with peripheral vascular disease is usually an aching/cramping/weak type of pain that is brought on by walking or exertion and is relieved with rest. As the disease progresses, the shorter the distance the patient will be able to walk before experiencing leg pain. Keep in mind that leg cramping at night is common in elderly patients and may not be a sign of peripheral vascular disease.

   ? INTERVIEW Any history of smoking, high blood pressure, high cholesterol, diabetes, heart problems, recent trauma, bedrest, or surgery?

   ➤ ABNORMALITIES A history of these would put the client at increased risk for peripheral vascular disease or deep venous thrombosis.

CHAPTER 14

Abdominal Pain

1. See Box 14-1.
2. See Box 14-3.
3. **? INTERVIEW** How would you describe your pain? Can you point to where the pain is? What makes your pain better? What makes your pain worse? Do you have any other symptoms that occur when you are having your pain? Describe them for me.

   ➤ ABNORMALITIES Typically, epigastric pain is more common in PUD, whereas the pain in GERD is described more as "heartburn." In PUD, the pain is generally worse at night and relieved by food. In GERD, the pain is worse when lying down and may be aggravated by food. Patients with PUD more commonly have bloating or distention symptoms, whereas patients with GERD complain of regurgitation symptoms that may influence swallowing and breathing. In terms of signs, melena is more common with PUD.
4. Presence of severe unrelenting pain. Blood in vomitus or stool. Decreased nutritional intake. Weight loss. Pallor or fatigue. Previous history of PUD, GERD, or gastrointestinal bleeding. History of self-treatment that has been ineffective. If concomitant chronic diseases are flaring (e.g., increased shortness of breath from COPD or CHF, increased palpitations in heart patient).

Nausea and Vomiting

1. Ask all the regular questions, but add the following: Have you been experiencing any fecal incontinence ? How much water do you drink per day? How many meals do you eat per day? Do you eat fruit and vegetables? Describe your normal day to me. Are you able to complete all your normal activities? Cooking? Cleaning? Laundry? If not, how much can you do? Do you every feel confused?
2. Ask all the regular questions, but add the following: What does the child's typical diet include? Has the child been able to hold down fluids? Does the child cry if you press on his or her abdomen? Did the child sustain an injury to the head before the nausea and vomiting started? Has the child been near any toxic or poisonous materials such as household cleaners?

3. How are you or your child feeling? Are you having any other symptoms besides the vomiting and diarrhea? Can you describe them for me? Do you feel like you have to drink all the time? Have your bathroom habits changed? If so, how? Are you experiencing any dry mouth, dizziness, fatigue, or fever? Has your child's behavior changed? If so, how? Do your children have tears when they cry? Do they have the same number of wet diapers?
4. See Box 14-9.

Change in Bowel Habits

1. See Box 14-5.
2. Describe your diarrhea to me. How many bowel movements do you have per day? How has this changed over the last 4 weeks? Has the appearance/color of your bowel movements changed? Describe this change to me. Do you have any other symptoms along with your diarrhea? Any blood in your stool? Abdominal pain? Fatigue? Fever? Dizziness? Weakness? What makes it better? What makes it worse? What treatment have you tried? Does it help?
3. See Box 14-11.

CHAPTER 15

Abdominal Pain

1. Interview questions that may be useful in differentiating abdominal pain include:

   Onset and duration: When did the pain start? Did the pain start suddenly? How long does it last? How does it change through the day? Have you had this type of abdominal pain before? How often do you experience abdominal pain?

   Characteristics: Describe the pain. Is it severe and stabbing or dull and constant? Aching? Cramping? Burning? Gnawing? Have you ever had this type of pain before? Is it the same or different? How severe is it?

   Location: Where is the pain located? Does the pain radiate to any other areas? What brings on the pain? What makes it worse? Does it get worse with food intake? Does it get worse with change in position?

   Relief: What relieves the pain? Food? Lying down?

   Symptoms: Do you experience any other symptoms with it? Nausea? Vomiting? Diarrhea? Itching? Yellow skin?
2. Signs and symptoms of cholelithiasis or cholestasis include abdominal pain, nausea, vomiting, anorexia, fever, mildly elevated serum bilirubin, and mildly elevated serum alkaline phosphatase.
3. See Box 15-8.

Ascites

1. A fluid wave can sometimes be felt in people without ascites and, conversely, may not occur in patients with early ascites.
2. See Box 15-7.
3. First, percuss for areas of dullness and resonance on the abdomen with the patient supine. Mark the area. Then, have the patient lie on one side, and again percuss for tympany and dullness. Mark the area. The dullness will change positions in patients with ascites, because ascitic fluid characteristically sinks with gravity. Percussion gives a dull note in the dependent areas of the abdomen. The dullness will shift to the more dependent side, whereas the tympany will shift to the top.

Jaundice

1. See Table 15-2.
2. See Box 15-3.
3. HCV has a higher chronic carrier rate (80%) than HBV (20%). HCV evades the immune system more readily and mutates more rapidly than HBV. Subsequently, patients generally have less of an immune response to HCV than to HBV. The majority of patients with acute and chronic HCV infection are asymptomatic. The more of an immune response a patient has, the more severe the signs and symptoms that he or she will experience. Because the body is less able to rid itself of the initial infection, there is a high HCV chronic carrier rate.

CHAPTER 16

1. Renal system functions include:
   - Regulation of sodium, potassium, chloride, calcium, and other ion concentrations in the plasma.
   - Regulation of blood volume and blood pressure by controlling the volume of water excreted in the urine, releasing erythropoietin, and releasing renin.
   - Excretion of urea and uric acid, toxic substances, and drugs.
   - Stabilization of blood pH.
   - Synthesizing of calcitriol, a vitamin D_3 derivative that stimulates calcium ion absorption by the intestines.
2. See Box 16-2.
3. CrCl [mL/min] = $([140 - \text{age}]/\text{LBW}) \div (72 \times Cr_s)$

   The LBW is the person's lean body weight in kilograms, and the Cr_s is the serum creatinine concentration. Because females have a lower muscle mass than men, this equation must be multiplied by 0.85 for females:

   CrCl = $([140 = 82]/66) \div 72(1.4) = 38$ mL/min $\times$ 0.85 = 32 mL/min

CHAPTER 17

Musculoskeletal Pain

1. The pain of gout is typically sudden in onset with extreme tenderness. Usually, no history of recent injury will be recalled. Normally localized to a very specific area, the pain often has a "burning" quality. Many times, patients with gout also have associated risk factors that will lead to either increased production or decreased excretion of uric acid.

2. Questions pertaining to the diagnosis of gout should revolve around the onset and quality of pain, any recent injuries or trauma to the area, current medications, and concomitant disease states. Also important is social history, particularly recently, to determine if anything has "triggered" an attack. Answers that reflect chronic moderate pain or current injury would eliminate the diagnosis.
3. Because of the nature of the disease, nonpharmacologic therapies do not have a large role in the treatment of gout. Patients should be counseled to avoid any foods that may trigger an attack. Patients should also avoid alcohol, especially in excessive quantities. Cold applied directly to the area may be of some relief for the burning sensation associated with gout.

Musculoskeletal Swell or Edema

1. See Table 17-4.
2. The important symptoms to establish when differentiating between OA and RA include the presence of inflammation, distribution of the disease, whether symmetric involvement is present, and any pertinent laboratory results. The general condition of the patient should also be assessed through subjective questioning, because RA is often associated with a chronic illness state.
3. Nondrug therapy consisting of rest, exercise, and heat is also part of the regimen for treating RA. Both physical and occupational therapy, as well as ongoing emotional support, may be of benefit to the patient. In patients with disease that is difficult to manage, surgical removal of the synovium may be an option.

Stiffness and Decreased ROM

1. The fact that the patient has the disease appearing to be limited to one joint, is noninflamed, and has noted crepitus on examination and morning stiffness that is quickly resolved indicates that this condition is most likely OA. Also important is the history of possible trauma and the impact the patient experiences from running.
2. Chronic, high-dose acetaminophen therapy may be associated with hepatotoxicity, particularly in combination with alcohol use. Patients with any predisposing liver dysfunction should be carefully monitored if they are receiving chronic acetaminophen therapy.
3. NSAIDs are an option, assuming that the patient's peptic ulcer disease can be controlled. Nabumetone may also be an option; clinical literature suggests it may have a more favorable gastrointestinal side effect compared with other agents. Caution is warranted, however, with any of the "gastrointestinal-sparing" NSAIDs, because all drugs in this class have the potential to cause gastrointestinal bleeding. Injectable hyaluronic products have recently been introduced to the market and may be of benefit in some patients who have not responded to traditional therapies. Currently, these products are only approved for use in OA of the knee.

CHAPTER 18

Headache

1. See Table 18-4.
2. Factors that may precipitate headaches include medications, emotional stress, depression, tobacco smoke, sensory stimulation (e.g., light, sound, odors), diet, hormonal changes, changes in sleep or exercise patterns, hypoglycemia, medical conditions such as stroke, hypertension, tumors, infections, and pregnancy.
3. Patients with headaches described as the "worst headache" of their life; other neurologic signs and symptoms, such as weakness, paralysis, and changes in vision or ability to speak; and patients with chronic headaches unresponsive to over-the-counter medications should be immediately referred to medical care.

Seizures

1. See Table 18-2.
2. See Box 18-7.
3. The electroencephalogram is a graphic illustration of the brain's electrical activity. Because it illustrates the brain's activity, it is useful in identifying abnormal electrical activity as well as focal points for this seizure activity.

Paresthesia

1. Signs and symptoms of peripheral neuropathy depend on the nerves affected. Common signs and symptoms of peripheral neuropathy involving sensory nerves include tingling, numbness, weakness, a glove or stocking sensation, and decreased temperature, pain, and vibratory sensation. Signs and symptoms of autonomic peripheral neuropathy include heartburn, diarrhea, constipation, erectile dysfunction, and incontinence.
2. Medications that can cause peripheral neuropathies are listed in Box 18-8.
3. Patients should be referred immediately to medical care if they have recurrent paresthesias; concomitant neurologic symptoms such as mental status changes, paralysis, or weakness; pain shooting down a leg; or acute onset of severe symptoms.

CHAPTER 19

Memory Problems

1. See Table 19-1.
2. See Box 19-5.
3. Memory impairment is the hallmark of dementia. This impairment may manifest as difficulty in recalling previously learned material or in learning new material. Patients will misplace valuables (e.g., purse, eyeglasses), forget appointments, or get lost in a familiar neighborhood. The cognitive deficits of dementia include aphasia, apraxia, agnosia, or a disturbance in executive functioning.

Depression

1. See Box 19-2.
2. Yes.
3. Patients with anxiety or depression are frequently alcohol dependent; however, the use and withdrawal of alcohol contributes to these symptoms, resulting in a vicious cycle.

Nervousness

1. Insomnia of less than 3 weeks in duration is typical of individuals without a history of sleep problems and may result from transient anxiety-provoking events. Long-term or chronic insomnia (>3 weeks) may relate to medical or psychiatric disorders (e.g., depression).
2. Regular time to wake up and go to sleep; sleep only until rested; go to bed only when sleepy; avoid trying to force sleep; avoid daytime naps; schedule worry time during the day; exercise routinely but not close to bedtime; create a comfortable sleep environment; discontinue use of alcohol, caffeine, and nicotine; avoid excessive fullness or hunger at bedtime; avoid drinking large quantities of fluids in the evening; do something relaxing and enjoyable before bedtime.
3. Prevalence is frequent, with one-quarter of the general population experiencing at least one anxiety disorder in their lifetime. Signs and symptoms of anxiety include excessive and uncontrollable worry that is out of proportion to the likelihood or impact of the feared events, restlessness or feeling keyed up or on edge, being easily fatigued, difficulty concentrating or mind going blank, irritability, muscle tension, difficulty falling or staying asleep, restless and unsatisfying sleep, palpitations, tachycardia, chest pain or tightness, shortness of breath, and hyperventilation.

CHAPTER 20

Polyuria

1. See Box 20-2. Type 1 has a quick onset and presents with more severe symptoms, often including the "classic" symptoms, such as polydipsia, polyuria, and polyphagia, with weight loss also commonly occurring. At diagnosis, type 1 may present with diabetic ketoacidosis. Type 2 presents more slowly, with insidious onset and less severity because of residual insulin activity. Fatigue, blurred vision, pruritis, polyuria, and recurrent vaginal infections are more common in type 2.
2. Early signs and symptoms may include diaphoresis, pallor, tachycardia, palpitations, paresthesias, hunger, and shakiness. As it progresses, neurologic evidence may include inability to concentrate, somnolence, confusion, slurred speech, irrational behavior, and blurred vision. The last stage may include disoriented behavior, loss of consciousness, seizures, and even death.
3. β-Blockers, calcium-channel blockers, diazoxide, diuretics (thiazide), glucocorticoids, L-asparaginase, niacin, estrogens, oral contraceptives, lithium, pentamidine, phenytoin, growth hormone, phenothiazines, isoniazid, sugar-containing medications, and sympathomimetics.

Fatigue

1. Bile acid–binding resins (cholestyramine and colestipol) and ferrous sulfate interact with the absorption of levothyroxine. When used concurrently, they should be separated by 6 hours.
2. See Box 20-3.
3. See Box 20-4.

CHAPTER 21

Enlarged Breasts

1. Breast cancer is characterized by a unilateral, nontender, discrete, and immobile nodule that may be accompanied by nipple discharge. Gynecomastia is characterized by bilateral, tender, and generalized enlargement of the breast tissue surrounding the areolae.
2. See Box 21-1.
3. Is one or are both breasts involved? Is the lump tender? Is there a nipple discharge? What area of the breast is involved?
4. Lipomastia can occur in older men. This condition develops normally through aging and is characterized by the normal chest muscle tissue being replaced by adipose tissue.

Scrotum Lump

1. Testicular cancer often has no obvious signs until the disease has advanced to other structures in the scrotum or metastasized. Some symptoms that may be noticed are a nontender lump on the top or side of the testicle, a feeling of fullness in the abdomen or scrotum, or an ache in the lower abdomen or scrotum.
2. Epididymitis or epididymal cyst, testicular torsion, hydrocele, varicocele, scrotal hernia, spermatocele, or generalized scrotal edema.
3. Testicular cancer is characterized by the symptoms listed in answer 1, whereas other testicular or scrotal abnormalities are accompanied by pain, swelling, erythema, and fever.
4. Refer to Box 21-2.
5. Testicular torsion is considered a surgical emergency and must be repaired quickly to prevent loss of a testis as a result of the obstruction in blood flow and resulting necrosis that can occur.
6. The presence of an undescended testicle in a child older than 1 year is of concern, because this condition can increase the risk of testicular cancer.

Bulge in the Groin

1. The signs and symptoms associated with a hernia include a bulge in the groin area (especially on straining), a dull ache

or pain associated with the bulge, a feeling of pulling in the groin area, and intestinal obstruction.

2. An indirect inguinal hernia is above the inguinal ligament near the internal inguinal ring, often extends into the scrotum, and touches the examiner's fingertip in the inguinal canal. A direct inguinal hernia is above the inguinal ligament near the external inguinal ring, rarely extends into the scrotum, and pushes the side of the examiner's finger forward. A femoral hernia is below the inguinal ligament and never extends into the scrotum; the inguinal canal is empty on examination.
3. An incarcerated hernia cannot be reduced or pushed back into the abdomen. A strangulated hernia can lead to tenderness, nausea, and vomiting in addition to the nonreducible lesion.
4. Factors that can predispose an individual to development of inguinal or femoral hernias include obesity, heavy lifting, and straining during defecation.

Genital Itching

1. Tinea cruris leads to genital itching, erythema, and scaly patches in the groin but sparing the scrotum.
2. Risk factors for tinea cruris include damp environment, alkaline environment, excessive diaphoresis, obesity, warm weather, and exposure to areas where tinea infection is present (e.g., infected towels, hot tubs, swimming pools, common showers).
3. Do you have any blisters? Are there any lesions on your penis? Do you have a fever? Do you feel tired? Is the condition on your scrotum? Have you recently had athlete's foot or been around anyone who has?

Urinary Retention

1. BPH can lead to a feeling of fullness in the bladder after urination, difficulty in beginning a urine stream, nocturia, difficulty in maintaining a urine stream, frequent urination, and constipation.
2. BPH can lead to the symptoms listed in answer 1, whereas acute prostatitis would also be accompanied by fever, chills, low back pain, perineal pain, and burning on urination.
3. See Box 21-5.
4. A normal prostate feels rubbery or "boggey" on palpation. Prostate cancer presents as a hard nodule within the normal prostate; BPH presents as symmetric, enlarged, smooth, firm, and elastic on palpation. Acute prostatitis presents as swollen, firm, warm, and extremely tender on palpation.
5. An annual digital rectal examination and a prostate-specific antigen level are recommended as screening tests for prostate cancer in men older than 50 years.

CHAPTER 22

Breast Lump

1. Breast cancer is characterized by a single, hard, nontender, and immobile lump possibly accompanied by nipple discharge, displacement of the nipple, or changes in the skin of the breast. Fibrocystic breast changes are characterized by waxing and waning, multiple, bilateral breast nodules, and tenderness.
2. See Box 22-3.
3. Is one or are both breasts involved? Is the lump painful? Does the lump come and go? Is the lump associated with your menstrual cycle? Are there any changes in the skin of your breast? Are there any changes in your nipples?
4. See Box 22-1.
5. Known risk factors for breast cancer include female gender, increasing age (especially >60 years), mutations in the *BRCA1* and *BRCA2* genes, family history of breast cancer, personal history of breast cancer, Caucasian race, history of proliferative breast disease, chest area radiation therapy, menstruation before the age of 12 years, menopause after the age of 50 years, women without children or whose first child was born after the age of 30 years, long-term hormone replacement therapy, and alcohol consumption.

Vaginal Discharge

1. Vulvovaginal candidiasis causes a white, curd-like discharge that is not malodorous, vaginal itching and soreness, pain on urination, and inflammation of the vulva. Bacterial vaginosis causes a gray or white, thin discharge with a fishy or musty odor but without vaginal or vulvar irritation.
2. Pregnancy, diabetes mellitus, immunosuppression, therapy with antibiotics or corticosteroids, iron deficiency anemia, vaginal surgery, oral contraceptives, infection with the human immunodeficiency virus, and synthetic or occlusive items of clothing.
3. A potassium hydroxide test allows for visualization of the branching hyphae of *Candida* sp.
4. Atropic vaginitis can present with vaginal soreness and itching similar to vaginal infections, especially candidiasis. Vaginal dryness and dyspareunia are common with atrophic vaginitis. A vaginal discharge is usually not present in atropic vaginitis, although bleeding may occur. Age of the patient and menopausal status may often help in differentiating the two conditions.
5. A milky white discharge is normal during pregnancy. Hormone shifts result in vasocongestion of the uterus and cervix, leading to increased vaginal secretions.

Abdominal Cramping

1. Primary dysmenorrhea occurs early after menarche and is a common finding. Secondary dysmenorrhea occurs or worsens years after menstruation begins and can often be an indicator of gynecologic pathology.

2. There is no well-defined cause of PMS.
3. Somatic symptoms, including edema, breast engorgement, abdominal bloating, abdominal cramping, irritability, depression, cravings for sweet or salty foods, tearfulness, headaches, mood swings, and lethargy, are common with PMS.
4. Pain relievers, pyridoxine, and diuretics may be useful in treating PMS.
5. A patient suffering from abdominal cramping accompanied by nausea, vomiting, and fever should be referred to a physician for further evaluation.

Glossary

Absence seizures Generalized seizures that are most common in children and are sometimes confused with daydreaming; loss of consciousness and return to consciousness occur rapidly.

Acanthosis nigricans Deeply pigmented, velvety axillary skin; can be associated with internal malignancy.

Acne An inflammatory disease of the skin with follicular, papular, and pustular eruption involving the pilosebaceous apparatus.

Acromegaly Abnormal enlargement of the bones of both the face and the skull resulting from hyperactivity of the pituitary gland.

Acute pain Pain that arises from injury, trauma, spasm, or disease to the skin, muscles, somatic structures, or viscera of the body. The intensity of the pain is proportional to the degree of injury and decreases as the tissue damage heals.

Acute renal failure Decline in renal function that occurs rapidly and results in azotemia.

Acute sinusitis Inflammation of the sinuses that remains for 7 to 10 days or longer; associated with bacterial and viral infections of the upper respiratory tract.

Adjustment disorder with anxiety Maladaptive reaction of nervousness, worry, or jitteriness to an identifiable environmental or psychosocial stressor that interferes with a person's functioning.

Adjustment disorder with depressed mood Disorder with an identifiable environmental or psychosocial stressor that results in sadness, social isolation, difficulty concentrating, and preoccupation with the stressful events in addition to changes in sleep and appetite.

Adverse drug reaction An unwanted pharmacologic effect associated with a medication the patient is taking; commonly termed a *side effect.*

Afterload Vascular resistance against which the ventricle must contract.

Agnosia Inability to recognize or identify objects or people.

Allergic reaction Hypersensitivity to a particular antigen or allergen that provokes characteristic symptoms whenever it is encountered.

Alogia Poverty of speech.

Alopecia Baldness.

Angina pectoris Presence of intermittent chest pain caused by temporary oxygen insufficiency and myocardial ischemia.

Angioplasty Nonsurgical method of mechanically dilating a partially obstructed coronary artery.

Anhedonia Loss of interest or pleasure in nearly all activities.

Anorexia nervosa Syndrome characterized by self-starvation, extreme weight loss, body image disturbance, and an intense fear of becoming obese.

Antalgic gait A limping walk used to avoid pain.

Anuria Urine output of less than 50 mL/day.

Anxiety disorder Broad term encompassing a category of mental disorders; may include adjustment disorder with anxiety, generalized anxiety disorder, panic attacks, agoraphobia, specific phobias, social phobias, obsessive-compulsive disorder, and posttraumatic stress disorder.

Apraxia Impaired ability to perform motor activities despite intact motor abilities, sensory function, and comprehension of the task.

Arcus senilis Gray-white arc or circle around cornea.

Arrhythmia Irregular pulse rhythm or rate of cardiac contraction.

Arteriosclerosis Condition in which the blood vessels become more rigid, lose elasticity, and become thicker as the body ages; calcification of weakened vessel walls.

Ascites Effusion and collection of serous fluid in the abdominal cavity.

Asthma Chronic inflammatory disorder of the airways.

Ataxia Staggering, unsteady gait that can occur with excessive alcohol or drug ingestion (e.g., barbiturates, benzodiazepines, or central-nervous-system stimulants).

Atherosclerosis Condition in which atherosclerotic plaques are deposited in the vascular system as the body ages.

Atonic seizures Generalized seizures that are characterized by a sudden loss of postural muscle tone, usually lasting only 1 to 2 seconds.

Auscultation Listening to the sounds made by various body structures and functions as a diagnostic method, usually with a stethoscope.

Autism Condition of social isolation.

Avolition Lack of initiative or persistence in goal-directed activities.

Azotemia Accumulation in the blood of nitrogenous waste products (i.e., blood urea nitrogen and creatinine) that are normally excreted in the urine.

Ballottement Palpatory technique to examine for excess fluid on the patella.

Benign prostatic hyperplasia Noncancerous enlargement in the prostate.

Bipolar disorder Condition in which the patient experiences episodes of both depression and mania.

Blood pressure Force of blood as it pushes against the arterial walls; dependent on cardiac output, volume of blood ejected by the ventricles per minute, and peripheral vascular resistance.

Blood urea nitrogen Measurement of the amount of urea nitrogen in the blood.

Body mass index Concept used to determine the appropriateness of an individual's weight-to-height ratio.

Boutonniere deformities Deformities of the hand that are marked by proximal interphalangeal joint flexion and distal interphalangeal joint hyperextension.

Bradycardia Adult heart rate of less than 60 bpm.

Bradypnea Adult respiratory rate of less than 12 rpm.

Bronchitis Inflammation and edema of the bronchioles causing excessive mucus production and airway obstruction.

Bronchophony Condition in which the word "ninety-nine" spoken by the patient is heard clear and loud through a stethoscope placed over the lungs, possibly indicating consolidation or atelectasis. In a normal test, the word would sound muffled.

Bruit Blowing, murmur-like sound of vascular rather than cardiac origin.

Bulimia nervosa Syndrome characterized by binge eating that is usually followed by some form of purging, such as self-induced vomiting, laxative abuse, or associated behaviors (e.g., diuretic use, diet pill use, or compulsive exercising).

Bulge sign Test used to confirm the presence of small amounts of fluid (4–8 mL) in the suprapellar pouch.

Bursitis Inflammation of the bursa, which is a sac or cavity filled with synovial fluid and usually located near joints.

Cachectic Condition in which the patient looks emaciated or very thin, with sunken eyes and hollowed cheeks; associated with chronic wasting diseases such as cancer, starvation, and dehydration.

Candidiasis Fungal infections caused by *Candida albicans.*

Carbuncle Boil that forms from the coalescence of adjacent furuncles and that can penetrate beyond the dermis into the subcutaneous layer.

Cardiac output Volume of blood pumped from each ventricle in 1 minute; product of the heart rate and stroke volume.

Carpal tunnel syndrome Entrapment of the median nerve of the wrist.

Cataracts Complete or partial opacity of the ocular lens.

Cerebrovascular accidents Strokes; sudden neurologic afflictions usually related to cerebral blood supply; classified as hemorrhagic, cardiogenic, and ischemic.

Cerebrovascular disease Broad term encompassing diseases relating to the blood vessels of the central nervous system.

Chickenpox (varicella) Highly infectious childhood disease caused by the varicella-zoster virus.

Chief complaint Brief statement of why the patient is seeking care; typically includes one or two primary symptoms, along with their duration, and is recorded in the patient's own words.

Chloasma Hyperpigmentation of the face.

Cholecystitis Inflammation of the gallbladder.

Chronic obstructive pulmonary disease Disease characterized by airflow limitation (primarily expiratory flow) that is not fully reversible.

Chronic pain Pain that persists for a minimum of 6 months.

Chronic renal failure Diminished renal function that occurs for an extended amount of time and is unlikely to improve.

Chronic sinusitis Inflammation of the sinuses that is present for 8 weeks, occurs for periods of longer than 10 days on more than four occasions during a 1-year period, or is repeatedly unresponsive to medical therapy.

Circumstantiality Inclusion by a patient of peripheral details or minutiae that are assumed to be implicit to the conversation.

Circus senilis White circle around the cornea that results from deposits of fat.

Cirrhosis Chronic disease of the liver in which widespread hepatic cell destruction leads to the formation of connective tissue and nodular regeneration, with consequent disorganization of the normal architecture.

Closed-ended questions Questions that require the patient to respond with specific information and details; questions that elicits short, one- or two-word or yes/no answers; sometimes called *direct questions.*

Cluster headache Headache characterized by excruciating, stabbing pain that is unilateral and clusters over an eye.

Cognitive disorders Broad term encompassing a range of psychologic disorders that are divided into three major categories: delirium, dementia, and amnestic disorders.

Coma Condition in which the patient is completely unconscious and does not respond to any external stimuli or pain.

Compulsion Repetitive behavior (e.g., checking or handwashing) or mental act (e.g., counting or repeating words silently) that the patient feels forced to complete.

Confabulation Fabrication of a memory in clear consciousness.

Congestive heart failure Condition in which the heart cannot pump a sufficient amount of blood to meet the metabolic needs of the body.

Conjunctivitis Inflammation of the clear mucous membrane of the eye.

Constipation Sporadic or arduous passage of stool.

Contractility Ability of the cardiac muscle, when given a load, to shorten and contract.

Corneal arcus Lipid deposits in the periphery of eye that may be detected when light is directed to the iris.

Coronary heart disease Degenerative changes in coronary circulation that are caused by an imbalance between myocardial oxygen demand and blood supply; also termed *coronary artery disease* or *ischemic heart disease.*

Crackles Short, sharp, or rough sounds heard with a stethoscope over the chest. Most often heard in pleurisy with fibrinous exudate.

Creatinine clearance A measure of the glomerular filtration rate; an evaluative measure of renal function.

Crepitus Crackling sound heard during the movement of joints that is caused by irregularities in the articulating surfaces.

Crohn's disease Chronic inflammatory process involving any portion of the gastrointestinal tract from the mouth to the anus.

Cryptorchidism Failure of the testes to descend into the scrotum.

Cultural pluralism Diversity of culture (as opposed to a single, dominant culture).

Culture Complex pattern of shared meanings, beliefs, and behaviors that are learned and acquired by a group of people during the course of history.

Cushing's disease Excessive plasma cortisol resulting in a central obesity, abnormal rounding of the face, excess hair above the lip and on the chin. These individuals may also present with striae, myopathy, muscular weakness, hypertension, glucose intolerance, menstrual abnormalities, osteoporosis, and psychiatric changes.

Cyanosis Bluish discoloration of the skin caused by an inadequate amount of oxygen in the blood; can be associated with shortness of breath, lung disease, heart failure, or suffocation.

Cystocele Herniation of the bladder, usually into the vagina or introitus.

Deep venous thrombosis Presence of a thrombus (i.e., a blood clot) in a deep vein and an accompanying inflammatory process in the vessel wall; also known as *thrombophlebitis.*

Degenerative joint disease Disease characterized by deterioration of articular cartilage resulting in formation of new bone at the surfaces of the joint; also known as *osteoarthritis.*

Delirium Cognitive disorder characterized by alterations in consciousness and a change in cognition that develops over a short period of time.

Delusions Fixed false beliefs with a variety of themes.

Dementia Cognitive disorder characterized by a decline in social and/or occupational functioning and cognitive deficits that include impairment of memory.

Depressive disorders Subcategory of mood disorders that includes adjustment disorder with depressed mood, dysthymic disorder, and major depressive disorder.

Dermatomyositis Inflammatory disease of the connective tissue leading to muscle inflammation, edema, and dermatitis.

Dermis Second layer of the skin.

Diabetes mellitus Chronic heterogeneous disorder that is characterized by increased fasting blood glucose levels.

Diabetic ketoacidosis Acidosis, as in diabetes or starvation, caused by the enhanced production of ketone bodies.

Diaper rash Acute inflammatory condition in the area of the buttocks, genitalia, perineum, and abdomen.

Diarrhea Increase in the number and fluid content of bowel movements.

Diastole Phase of the cardiac cycle during which the ventricles relax, the atrioventricular valves open, and blood passively flows from the pressure-filled atria into the low-pressure ventricles.

Diastolic blood pressure Resting pressure that the blood exerts between each ventricular contraction.

Diplopia Double vision.

Dislocation Displacement of a bone from a joint, with subsequent tearing of ligaments, tendons, and articular capsules.

Drug therapy problem Any undesirable event experienced by the patient that involves drug therapy and that actually or potentially interferes with a desired outcome.

Duct ectasia Dilation of the lactiferous ducts in the breast.

Dysesthetic pain Neuropathic pain categorized by discomfort and altered sensations that are distinct from the usual sensation of pain.

Dysmenorrhea Abdominal cramping associated with menstruation.

Dyspareunia Female condition characterized by painful coitus.

Dyspnea Shortness of breath.

Dysthymic disorder Condition characterized by a chronically depressed mood for more days than not during a period of at least 2 years.

Echolalia Repetition by the patient of words that are stated by the examiner.

Eclampsia Occurrence of seizures that cannot be attributed to other causes in a woman with preeclampsia.

Ecthyma Ulcerative impetigo involving both the epidermis and the dermis.

Ectropion Turning outward of the lower lid of the eye.

Eczema Broad term used for a variety of inflammatory skin conditions.

Egophany Condition in which the sound "ee" spoken by the patient is heard as "ay" through a stethoscope placed over the lungs, possibly indicating consolidation. In a normal test, the "ee" sound would be heard.

Emphysema Respiratory disease characterized by an abnormal, permanent enlargement of airspaces distal to the bronchioles.

Enteral Oral route of nutritional intake.

Entropion Turning inward of the lower lid of the eye.

Epidermis Outer layer of the skin.

Epidermoid cysts Firm, yellowish, nontender nodules that are approximately 1 cm in diameter and are commonly present on the scrotum.

Epilepsy Condition defined as two or more unprovoked seizures without an identifiable cause.

Erectile dysfunction Male condition characterized by loss of desire or libido, inability to initiate or maintain an erection, failure to ejaculate, premature ejaculation, and/or inability to achieve an orgasm.

Ethnicity Unique set of characteristics shared by a socially, culturally, and politically defined group of people.

Ethnocentrism Belief in the superiority of one's own group or culture while expressing disdain and contempt for other groups or cultures.

Evoked pain Neuropathic pain accompanied by altered sensory thresholds and, possibly, by hyperalgesia, allodynia, hyperethesia, and hyperpathia.

Exophthalmos Protrusion of the eyeball as a result of an increased volume of orbital content; also known as *proptosis.*

Fibromyalgia Systemic condition resulting in chronic muscle and soft-tissue pain.

First heart sound (S_1) Heart sound that is produced by closure of the atrioventricular valves and that signals the beginning of systole; characterized as "lub" and usually loudest over the apex area of the heart.

Flight of ideas Condition in which thoughts may race and the patient may jump from topic to topic; often accompanies mania.

Folliculitis Inflammation of hair follicles.

Fracture A break in a bone.

Friction rub The sound, heard on auscultation, made by the rubbing of two opposed serious surfaces roughened by an inflammatory exudate, or, if chronic, by nonadhesive fibrosis.

Furuncle Deep-seated folliculitis caused by *Staphylococcus aureus.*

Gastroesophageal reflux disease Disorder in which gastric contents are refluxed into the esophagus.

Generalized anxiety disorder Excessive and uncontrollable worry that is out of proportion to the likelihood or impact of the feared events.

Generalized seizures Seizures in which the patient usually loses consciousness; classified as either tonic-clonic seizures, absence seizures, myoclonic seizures, or atonic seizures.

Gingivitis Inflammation of the gingivae; the most common and mildest form of periodontal disease.

Glaucoma Group of eye disorders involving optic neuropathy and characterized by changes in the optic disc and loss of visual sensitivity and field.

Goniometer A protractor with moveable arms that is used to measure the range of joint motion in degrees.

Gout Disorder of uric acid metabolism.

Graphesthesia Ability to identify a letter or number traced on the skin.

Graves' disease Autoimmune disorder in which thyroid-stimulating immunoglobulins stimulate the thyroid-stimulating hormone receptor to cause overproduction of thyroid hormones; characterized by thinning of the face and protruding or bulging eyes; also known as *toxic diffuse goiter.*

Graves' ophthalmopathy Hallmark of Graves' disease; includes several characteristic features that are seen in the eyes, such as exophthalmos, proptosis, excess retro-orbital tissue, and blurred/double vision.

Gynecomastia Abnormal hypertrophy of the male breasts.

Hallucination Sensory experience of something that does not exist outside the mind.

Hashimoto's disease Chronic autoimmune disorder most often seen in children and women between the ages of 30 and 50 years; the most common cause of primary hypothyroidism; also known as *chronic autoimmune thyroiditis.*

Health history Concise summary of the patient's current and past medical problems, medication history, family history, social history, and review of systems. The purpose of the health history is to obtain subjective patient information (i.e., what the patient says about his or her own health, medications, and so on).

Heberden's or Bouchard's nodules Hard, nontender nodules on the distal interphalangeal joints.

Hematuria Blood in the urine.

Hepatitis Inflammation of the liver.

Hepatojugular reflex Sustained elevated jugular venous pressure that occurs during abdominal compression; indicates that hepatic venous congestion is present.

Hernia Protrusion of part of the intestine through a tear or weakened area in the abdominal muscles.

History of present illness Thorough description and expansion of the patient's chief complaint. Specific characteristics should be obtained on all presenting symptoms and recorded in a precise and chronologic sequence.

Hydrocele Collection of serous fluid in the scrotal sac.

Hydrocephalus Excess fluid in the skull; seen as an enlargement of the head without a change in the face.

Hyperosmolar hyperglycemic nonketotic coma A complication seen in diabetes mellitus in which marked hyperglycemia occurs (such as levels over 800 mg/dL), causing osmotic shifts in water in brain cells and resulting in coma. It can be fatal or lead to permanent neurologic damage. Ketoacidosis does not occur.

Hyperpnea Fast, deep breathing that occurs normally with exercise or with forms of metabolic acidosis; also known as *Kussmaul respirations.*

Hyperreflexia Exaggerated reflex response.

Hyperresonance Abnormally long, low-pitched sound that is heard with emphysema or a pneumothorax in which a large amount of air is present.

Hypertension Elevated systolic blood pressure (>140 mm Hg) and/or diastolic blood pressure (>90 mm Hg) measured on at least two separate occasions; classified according to severity as stage 1, 2, or 3.

Hyperthyroidism Elevated levels of thyroid hormones in the blood.

Hypodermis Third layer of skin; also called the *subcutis.*

Hypothyroidism Decreased levels of thyroid hormones.

Hypoxemia Low oxygen concentration in the blood.

Hypoxia Lack of oxygen.

Illusions Misperceived visual stimuli (e.g., mirage in the desert).

Impetigo Cutaneous bacterial infection caused by *Staphylococcus aureus* and group A β-hemolytic *Streptococcus pyogenes.*

Incarcerated hernia Hernia that cannot be pushed back into the abdominal cavity but that still allows blood flow to the intestine.

Incontinence Inability to prevent the discharge of any of the excretions, especially of urine or feces.

Inspection Visual evaluation/assessment of the patient; first step in the physical examination process.

Ischemia Deficiency of blood in a part, usually due to functional constriction or actual obstruction of a blood vessel.

Isolated systolic hypertension Systolic blood pressure of 140 mm Hg or greater and diastolic blood pressure of 90 mm Hg or lower; should be staged appropriately (e.g., 170/82 mm Hg is stage 2 isolated systolic hypertension).

Jaundice Yellowing of the skin caused by an excessive amount of bilirubin (a bile pigment) in the blood; can be an indication of liver disease or obstruction of the bile ducts by gallstones.

Kwashiorkor Disease resulting from a deficiency of protein in infancy or early childhood.

Kyphosis Hunched back; commonly associated with osteoporosis (i.e., loss of bone density).

Lesion Area of tissue with impaired function resulting from disease or physical trauma.

Lethargy Condition in which the patient drifts off to sleep easily, looks drowsy, and responds to questions very slowly.

Leukorrhea Increase in vaginal secretions just before menarche.

Linea nigra Pregnancy-related, brownish-black line down the middle of the abdomen.

Lipomastia False gynecomastia; can occur in older men in whom a natural decrease in chest muscle tissue is replaced by adipose tissue.

Loosening of associations Inability of the examiner to follow a conversation because the patient combines unrelated topics or words.

Lordosis Inward curvature of the spine, typically located in the lower back; commonly associated with osteoporosis (i.e., loss of bone density).

Macroencephalopathy Disease of the brain resulting from an abnormally enlarged skull.

Macronutrients Nutrients required in the greatest amount (e.g., carbohydrates, protein, and fat).

Major depressive disorder Disorder characterized by a period of at least 2 weeks with either depressed mood or anhedonia.

Malignant pain Cancer pain; may arise at the primary site of the cancer as a result of tumor expansion, nerve compression or infiltration by the tumor, malignant obstruction, or infections in a malignant ulcer.

Marasmus Chronic condition resulting from a deficiency in total energy intake; severe cases result in impaired cell-mediated immunity and muscle function.

McMurray's test Rotation of the tibia on the femur to determine injury to meniscal structures.

Measles Highly infectious childhood viral disease; causative organism has been categorized as a paramyxovirus.

Mental disorder Clinically significant behavioral or psychologic syndrome or pattern that occurs in an individual.

Microencephalopathy Disease of the brain resulting from an abnormally small skull.

Micronutrients Nutrients required for the proper use of macronutrients and involved in a wide variety of physiologic functions (e.g., electrolytes, vitamins, and trace minerals).

Migraine headaches Headaches thought to result from a combination of vascular and neurohormonal mechanisms; symptoms may include aura or visual disturbances, unilateral pulsating pain, and nausea.

Miosos Contraction of the pupil.

Mood disorders Broad term encompassing a category of mental disorders involving the long-term state of an individual; may include depressive disorders and bipolar disorders.

Murmur Gentle, blowing, swishing sound heard on the chest wall.

Musculoskeletal pain Subcategory of nonmalignant pain; arises from muscles, bones, joints, or connective tissue.

Myasthenia gravis Autoimmune disease marked by skeletal muscle fatigue.

Mydriasis Long-continued or excessive dilatation of the pupil of the eye.

Myocardial infarction Occurrence of myocardial cell death and necrosis caused by local, severe, or prolonged ischemia.

Myoclonic seizures Generalized seizures characterized by sudden and brief muscle contraction in either a single part of the body or the entire body.

Myopathy Disease of the muscle.

Neologism Nonexistent word or a combination of words that the patient invents.

Neuropathic pain Subcategory of nonmalignant pain; can be idiopathic in nature or arise from discrete or generalized sites of nerve injury.

Neuropathy Disease of the peripheral nervous system.

Nonmalignant pain Noncancerous chronic pain.

Nutrition Cumulative processes involved during the taking in and utilization of food substances.

Nystagmus Involuntary oscillating eye movements.

Obesity Excessive accumulation of body fat.

Obsessions Repetitive thoughts, ideas, or impulses that are recognized by the patient as being senseless.

Obsessive-compulsive disorder Mental disorder characterized by a recurrence of obsessions or compulsions that are frequent enough to interfere with normal daily activities.

Oliguria Decrease in urine output.

Onycholysis Separation of the nail bed from the plate that may occur in hyperthyroidism or hypothyroidism.

Onychomycosis Infection of the nail caused by yeasts, molds, and/or fungi.

Open-ended questions Questions that require the patient to respond in a narrative or paragraph format rather than with a simple yes/no answer.

Orthopnea Shortness of breath that occurs while the patient is lying flat.

Osteoarthritis Disease characterized by deterioration of articular cartilage resulting in the formation of new bone at the surfaces of the joint; also known as *degenerative joint disease.*

Osteomyelitis Inflammation of the bone marrow and surrounding bone caused by an infecting organism.

Osteoporosis Disease characterized by low bone mass and microarchitectural deterioration of bone tissue leading to increased bone fragility and susceptibility to fracture.

Otalgia Ear pain.

Otitis externa Inflammation of the skin lining the external auditory canal.

Otitis media Inflammation of the middle ear.

Pallor Abnormal paleness of the skin resulting from reduced blood flow or decreased hemoglobin level; can be associated with a wide range of diseases (e.g., anemia, shock, and cancer).

Palpation Touching or feeling the patient with the hand to augment the data gathered through inspection; second step in the physical examination process.

Pancreatitis Inflammation of the pancreas.

Panic attack Discrete attack of intense fear or anxiety accompanied by physical symptoms such as palpitations, sweating, or trembling.

Paraneoplastic syndrome Clinical or biochemical (e.g., hormonal) disturbance associated with a malignant neoplasm but not directly related to invasion by the primary tumor or its metastases.

Parenteral Intravenous route of nutritional intake.

Paresthesia Spontaneously occurring, abnormal tingling sensations; sometimes referred to as *pins and needles.*

Parkinson's disease Chronic, progressive neurologic condition characterized by muscular tremors, rigid movement, postural instability, and mask-like face.

Paroxysmal nocturnal dyspnea Sudden gasping for air that occurs while sleeping at night.

Partial seizures Seizures that begin in an area of the brain limited to one hemisphere; often suggestive of an underlying focal brain lesion.

Past medical history Brief description of the patient's past medical problems that may or may not be related to the patient's current medical condition.

Patient assessment Evaluation of subjective/objective patient information to enable decisions regarding health status of the patient, drug therapy needs and problems, interventions to resolve identified drug problems and prevent future drug therapy problems, and follow-up to make sure that patient outcomes are met. The primary purpose of the patient assessment is to identify, resolve, and prevent drug therapy problems.

Peau d'orange Dimpling of the skin of the breast and edema resulting in an orange peel appearance; often associated with cancer.

Pediculosis Louse-borne infestations; typically involve the head (pediculosis capitis), body (pediculosis corporis), or pubic region (pediculosis pubis).

Peptic ulcer disease Heterogeneous group of disorders characterized by ulceration of the upper gastrointestinal tract.

Percussion Striking of the body surface lightly but sharply to determine the position, size, and density of underlying structures as well as to detect fluid or air in a cavity; third step in the physical examination process.

Periodontitis Inflammation of the tissue supporting the teeth.

Peristalsis Progressive, involuntary, wave-like movements of the alimentary canal.

Perseveration Continuous repetition of the same words by a patient.

Pharmaceutical care Provision of drug therapy to achieve definite outcomes that improve a patient's quality of life.

Pharyngitis Inflammation of the pharynx and surrounding lymphoid tissues; often caused by viruses or bacteria.

Phonophobia Sensitivity to sound; associated with migraine headaches.

Photophobia Sensitivity to light; associated with migraine headaches.

Pneumonia Inflammation of the lungs; most commonly caused by a community-acquired bacterial infection (*Streptococcus pneumoniae*).

Polymyositis Inflammatory disease of the skeletal muscle tissue characterized by symmetric weakness of proximal muscles of the limbs, neck, and pharynx.

Posttraumatic stress disorder Immediate or delayed response to a catastrophic life event characterized by persistent re-experience (in dreams or recollections) of the traumatic event, persistent avoidance of the stimuli associated with the trauma, numbing of general responsiveness, and persistent symptoms of increased arousal (e.g., difficulty falling asleep, irritability, difficulty concentrating, or exaggerated startle response).

"PQRST" mnemonic Mnemonic aid used by clinician to evaluate a patient's pain. P, palliative or precipitating factors associated with the pain; Q, quality of the pain; R, region in which the pain is located or radiation of the pain; S, subjective description of severity of the pain; and T, temporal or time-related nature of the pain.

Precocious puberty Appearance of pubic hair or breast enlargement before the age of 8 years.

Preeclampsia Pregnancy-specific syndrome of reduced organ perfusion secondary to vasospasm and activation of the coagulation cascade.

Prejudice Preconceived judgment or opinion of another person based on direct or indirect experiences.

Preload Passive stretching of the ventricular muscle as the volume of blood in the ventricle at the end of diastole increases

Premenstrual dysphoric disorder Severe form of premenstrual syndrome in which activities of daily living are limited and a major depressive episode is experienced.

Presbycussis Hearing loss that occurs with aging as the auditory nerve degenerates.

Presbyopia Far-sightedness.

Pretibial myxedema Dry, firm, waxy swelling of the skin in the pretibial area; characteristic of hypothyroidism.

Prinzmetal angina Angina that occurs at rest.

Proptosis Bulging eyes; also known as *exophthalmos.*

Proteinuria Protein in the urine.

Pseudoptosis Upper lid of the eye resting on the lashes.

Psychotic disorders Broad term encompassing a category of psychologic disorders that includes schizophrenia and other psychotic disorders such as schizoaffective disorder, psychotic disorder caused by medical conditions, and substance-induced psychotic disorder.

Pulmonary embolism Movement of a thrombus to the lung.

Pulse pressure Difference between the systolic and diastolic pressure; reflects stroke volume.

Purpura Hemorrhage into the skin with obvious discoloration.

Pyelonephritis Inflammation of the kidney caused by a severe bacterial infection.

Pyuria Presence of pus/white blood cells in the urine.

Race Groupings of people with the same biologic and familial heredity; typically reflected in physical characteristics (e.g., skin color) and continued through generations.

Rectocele Prolapse or herniation of the rectum.

Referred pain Localization of pain to superficial or deep tissues distant from the source of pathology.

Renal insufficiency Mild reduction in the glomerular filtration rate with no occurrence of signs or symptoms.

Resonance Long, low-pitched sound that can usually be heard over all the lung fields.

Retinopathy Development of new vessels in the eye caused by anoxic stimulation.

Retropulsion Condition in which the patient falls backward when pulled on the shoulders; sign of Parkinson's disease.

Review of systems General description of patient symptoms per each body system.

Rheumatoid arthritis Systemic musculoskeletal disease characterized by symmetric inflammation of synovial tissues.

Rhinitis Inflammation of the nasal mucous membrane.

Rhinorrhea Recurrent or chronic watery nasal discharge.

Rhonchi An added sound with a musical pitch occurring during inspiration or expiration, heard on auscultation of the chest, and caused by air passing through bronchi that are narrowed by inflammation, spasm of smooth muscle, or presence of mucus in the lumen.

Schizophrenia Complex psychologic syndrome associated with markedly impaired occupational or social functioning.

Sciatica Severe pain in the leg that is felt at the back of the thigh and running down along the sciatic nerve.

Scoliosis Abnormal lateral curvature of the vertebral column. Depending on the etiology, there may be one curve, or primary and secondary compensatory curves; scoliosis may be "fixed" as a result of muscle and/or bone deformity or "mobile" as a result of unequal muscle contraction.

Scotoma Blind spot in the visual field surrounded by an area of normal or decreased vision.

Second heart sound (S_2) Heart sound produced by closure of the semilunar valves; signals the ending of systole.

Seizure Focal and/or generalized disturbance of neuronal electrical activity; sometimes manifested by abnormal movements or sensations and a loss of reflexes, memory, or consciousness.

Sensitization Increased sensitivity of the receptors following repeated application of a noxious stimulus.

Serum creatinine Normal metabolic product of skeletal muscle breakdown in the body.

Social phobia Persistent and exaggerated fear of humiliation or embarrassment that results in distress and possible avoidance of social situations.

Somatic pain Pain that results from activation of nociceptors in cutaneous and deep tissues.

Specific phobia Marked and persistent fear that is excessive or unreasonable to a specific situation or object.

Sprain Trauma to a joint that includes damage to the ligaments.

Stable angina Angina that occurs most commonly when the workload of the heart increases through exertion or stress; usually associated with a significant amount of atherosclerotic narrowing of one or more coronary arteries.

Status epilepticus Repetitive seizure activity (with or without convulsions) without recovery of consciousness between attacks that can last 30 minutes or more.

Stereognosis Ability to recognize items by touch and manipulation.

Stereotype Fixed perception or image of a group that rejects the existence of individuality within that group.

Stevens-Johnson syndrome Serious, drug-related cutaneous diseases that are characterized by widespread lesions covering most of the body, including the mucous membranes.

Strabismus Deviation of one eye.

Strain Overstretching of a muscle.

Strangulated hernia Type of hernia in which the intestine is trapped, compressing the blood supply.

Stratum corneum Outermost layer of the epidermis; also called the *horny layer.*

Stratum germinativum Innermost layer of the epidermis; also called the *basal cell layer.*

Striae Pregnancy-related, silver to pink jagged lines on the skin; more commonly known as *stretch marks.*

Stroke volume Amount of blood ejected in one full heartbeat

Stupor Condition in which patient responds only to persistent and vigorous shaking and answers questions with only a mumble.

Styes Acute pustular infections of an eyelash follicle or sebaceous glands of the eye.

Subculture Separate groups within a larger cultural context.

Substance abuse Pattern of substance use that results in repeated and harmful consequences and that does not include tolerance or withdrawal.

Substance dependence Behavioral pattern of compulsive drug use that results in tolerance and/or withdrawal despite significant substance-related problems.

Swan-neck deformities Deformities of the hand marked by flexion of the distal interphalangeal joints and hyperextension of the proximal interphalangeal joints.

Syndrome X Term used to describe patients who are typically obese and have subsequently developed insulin resistance and hyperinsulinemia.

Systole Phase of the cardiac cycle during which pressure in the ventricles exceeds pressure in the aorta and pulmonary artery, the ventricles contract, the semilunar valves open, and blood is ejected into the pulmonary and systemic arteries.

Systolic blood pressure Maximum pressure felt on the arteries during left ventricular contraction (or systole); regulated by stroke volume (i.e., volume of blood ejected with each heartbeat).

Tachycardia Adult heart rate greater than 100 bpm.

Tachypnea Adult respiratory rate greater than 20 rpm.

Tactile fremitus Palpable vibrations that are transmitted through the bronchial tree to the chest wall when a patient speaks.

Tangentiality Situation in which the patient wanders to a distant point in the conversation and is unable to return spontaneously to the original point.

Temporomandibular joint syndrome Painful jaw movement characterized by dull pain and tenderness in the joint area.

Tendinitis Inflammation of the tendon (i.e., the connective tissue that attaches muscle to bone).

Tenosynovitis Inflammation of the tendon and the synovial membrane at the joint.

Tension headaches Most common type of headache; generally a pressing/tightening, nonpulsating, bilateral pain.

Thought blocking Condition in which a patient suddenly stops speaking in midsentence.

Thyroid storm Life-threatening condition that includes exaggerated signs and symptoms of hyperthyroidism as well as altered mental status and fever.

Tinea capitis A common form of fungus infection of the scalp caused by various species of Microsporum and Trichophyton on or within hair shafts, occurring almost exclusively in children and characterized by irregularly placed and variously sized patches of apparent baldness because of hairs breaking off at the surface of the scalp, scaling, black dots, and occasionally erythema and pyoderma.

Tinea cruris A form of tinea imbricata occurring in the genitocrural region, including the inner side of the thighs, the perineal region, and the groin.

Tinea pedis Dermatophytosis of the feet, especially of the skin between the toes, caused by one of the dermatophytes, usually species of Trichophyton or Epidermophyton; the disease consists of small vesicles, fissures, scaling, maceration, and eroded areas between the toes and on the plantar surface of the foot; other skin areas may be involved.

Tinea unguium Ringworm of the nails due to a dermatophyte.

Tonic-clonic seizures Generalized seizures characterized by a prolonged postseizure (or postictal) stage in which the patient can experience symptoms such as fatigue, muscle pain, and confusion.

Transient ischemic attacks Neurologic deficit possibly resulting from embolism rather than ischemia and typically lasting fewer than 24 hours; sometimes referred to as a *mini-stroke.*

Ulcerative colitis Chronic inflammatory process affecting the mucosa and submucosa of the colon only.

Unstable angina Angina characterized by an increased frequency of anginal pain; anginal attacks are usually precipitated by less exertion or may occur at rest, are more intense, and last longer than episodes of stable angina.

Uremia Accumulation of toxic urine-substances in the blood.

Urinalysis Dipstick examination of a urine specimen.

Varicocele Varicose veins of the spermatic cord; caused by a retrograde flow of blood into the internal spermatic vein.

Visceral pain Pain that occurs following injury to sympathetically innervated organs.

Vulvovaginitis Inflammation of the vulva and vagina.

Wheezes Whistling respiratory sounds caused by turbulent airflow through constricted bronchi.

Whispered pectoriloquy Condition in which the words "one-two-three" whispered by the patient are heard distinctively and clearly through a stethoscope placed over the lungs; possibly indicative of consolidation and pleural effusions. In a normal test, words would sound faint and muffled.

Word salad A rare form of communication in which only jumbled words and not sentences are used.

Xanthelasma Soft, raised, yellow plaques on lid at inner canthus.

Xanthomas Soft, yellowish, raised waxy lesions on or beneath the eyelid.

Xerosis Pathologic dryness of the skin (xeroderma), the conjunctive (xerophthalmia), or mucous membranes.

Index

Note: Page numbers followed by f *indicate figures; those followed by* t *indicate tables; and those followed by* b *indicate boxed material. Drugs are listed under the generic name.*

H

I

J

T